CURRENT THERAPY IN CARDIOTHORACIC SURGERY

Surgical Titles in the Current Therapy Series

Callaham:
Current Therapy in Emergency Medicine
Cameron:
Current Surgical Therapy
Charles, Glover:
Current Therapy in Obstetrics
Ernst, Stanley:
Current Therapy in Vascular Surgery
Fazio:
Current Therapy in Colon and Rectal Surgery
Foley, Payne:
Current Therapy of Pain
Garcia, Mastroianni, Amelar, Dubin:
Current Therapy of Infertility
Garcia, Mikuta, Rosenblum:
Current Therapy in Surgical Gynecology
Gates:
Current Therapy in Otolaryngology—Head and Neck Surgery
Grillo, Austen, Wilkins, Mathisen, Vlahakes:
Current Therapy in Cardiothoracic Surgery
Jay:
Current Therapy in Podiatric Surgery
Long:
Current Therapy in Neurological Surgery
Marsh:
Current Therapy in Plastic and Reconstructive Surgery
McGinty, Jackson:
Current Therapy in Orthopaedic Surgery
Parrillo:
Current Therapy in Critical Care Medicine
Resnick, Kursh:
Current Therapy in Genitourinary Surgery
Rogers:
Current Practice in Anesthesiology
Spaeth, Katz:
Current Therapy in Ophthalmic Surgery
Trunkey, Lewis:
Current Therapy of Trauma
Welsh, Torg, Shephard:
Current Therapy in Sports Medicine

CURRENT THERAPY IN CARDIOTHORACIC SURGERY

Editors

HERMES C. GRILLO, M.D.
Professor of Surgery
Harvard Medical School
Visiting Surgeon and
Chief of General Thoracic Surgery
Massachusetts General Hospital
Boston, Massachusetts

W. GERALD AUSTEN, M.D.
The Edward D. Churchill
Professor of Surgery
Harvard Medical School
Chief of Surgical Services
Massachusetts General Hospital
Boston, Massachusetts

EARLE W. WILKINS JR., M.D.
Clinical Professor of Surgery
Harvard Medical School
Visiting Surgeon
Massachusetts General Hospital
Boston, Massachusetts

DOUGLAS J. MATHISEN, M.D.
Assistant Professor of Surgery
Harvard Medical School
Assistant Surgeon
Massachusetts General Hospital
Boston, Massachusetts

GUS J. VLAHAKES, M.D.
Assistant Professor of Surgery
Harvard Medical School
Assistant Surgeon
Massachusetts General Hospital
Boston, Massachusetts

1989

B.C. Decker Inc • Toronto • Philadelphia

Publisher — **B.C. Decker Inc**
3228 South Service Road
Burlington, Ontario L7N 3H8

B.C. Decker Inc
320 Walnut Street
Suite 400
Philadelphia, Pennsylvania 19106

Sales and Distribution

United States and Possessions — **The C.V. Mosby Company**
11830 Westline Industrial Drive
Saint Louis, Missouri 63146

Canada — **The C.V. Mosby Company, Ltd.**
5240 Finch Avenue East, Unit No. 1
Scarborough, Ontario M1S 5P2

United Kingdom, Europe and the Middle East — **Blackwell Scientific Publications, Ltd.**
Osney Mead, Oxford OX2 OEL, England

Australia and New Zealand — **Harcourt Brace Jovanovich Group (Australia) Pty Limited**
30–52 Smidmore Street
Marrickville, N.S.W. 2204
Australia

Japan — **Igaku-Shoin Ltd.**
Tokyo International P.O. Box 5063
1–28–36 Hongo, Bunkyo-ku, Tokyo 113, Japan

Asia — **Info-Med Ltd.**
802–3 Ruttonjee House
11 Duddell Street
Central Hong Kong

South Africa — **Libriger Book Distributors**
Warehouse Number 8
"Die Ou Looiery"
Tannery Road
Hamilton, Bloemfontein 9300

South America — **Inter-Book Marketing Services**
Rua das Palmeriras, 32
Apto. 701
222–70 Rio de Janeiro
RJ, Brazil

NOTICE

The authors and publisher have made every effort to ensure that the patient care recommended herein, including choice of drugs and drug dosages, is in accord with the accepted standards and practice at the time of publication. However, since research and regulation constantly change clinical standards, the reader is urged to check the product information sheet included in the package of each drug, which includes recommended doses, warnings, and contra-indications. This is particularly important with new or infrequently used drugs.

Current Therapy in Cardiothoracic Surgery

ISBN 1–55664–001–1

Library of Congress catalog card number: 88–71655

10 9 8 7 6 5 4 3 2 1

CONTRIBUTORS

CARY W. AKINS, M.D.

Associate Clinical Professor of Surgery, Harvard Medical School; Staff Surgeon, Cardiovascular Surgical Unit, Massachusetts General Hospital, Boston, Massachusetts

Composite Aortic Valve and Aortic Root Replacement in Aneurysmal Disease
Coronary Surgery Without Cardioplegia

KATHRYN D. ANDERSON, M.D.

Professor of Surgery and Child Health, George Washington University School of Medicine and Health Sciences; Senior Attending Surgeon, Children's Hospital National Medical Center, Washington, D.C.

Congenital Tracheoesophageal Fistula

EDUARDO ARCINIEGAS, M.D.

Clinical Professor, Department of Surgery, Wayne State University School of Medicine; Chief, Department of Cardiovascular Surgery, Children's Hospital of Michigan, Detroit, Michigan

Pulmonary Atresia with Intact Ventricular Septum

PHILLIP G. ARNOLD, M.D.

Professor, Department of Plastic Surgery, Mayo Medical School; Consultant, Section of Plastic and Reconstructive Surgery, Mayo Clinic, Rochester, Minnesota

Muscle Flaps
Muscle Flap in Bronchopleural Fistula

CHRISTOS A. ATHANASOULIS, M.D.

Professor of Radiology, Harvard Medical School; Head, Section of Vascular Radiology, Massachusetts General Hospital, Boston, Massachusetts

Massive Hemoptysis: Control with Transcatheter Vessel Embolization

W. GERALD AUSTEN, M.D.

Edward D. Churchill Professor of Surgery, Harvard Medical School; Chief of Surgical Services and Visiting Surgeon, Massachusetts General Hospital, Boston, Massachusetts

Surgical Valvotomy and Percutaneous Balloon Valvotomy for Mitral Stenosis
Choosing a Heart Valve Substitute
Tricuspid Valve Replacement

JOHN C. BALDWIN, M.D.

Chief of Cardiothoracic Surgery, Yale University School of Medicine; Chief of Cardiothoracic Surgery, Yale-New Haven Medical Center, New Haven, Connecticut

Heart-Lung Transplantation

ARTHUR E. BAUE, M.D.

Professor of Surgery, Saint Louis University School of Medicine; Vice President, Saint Louis University Medical Center, Saint Louis, Missouri

Mallory-Weiss Syndrome

DOUGLAS M. BEHRENDT, M.D.

Professor of Surgery, University of Iowa College of Medicine; Chairman, Cardiothoracic Surgery, The University of Iowa Hospitals and Clinics, Iowa City, Iowa

Cardiac Transplantation in Children

PHILIP BELCHER, M.B., B.S., F.R.C.S.

Senior Registrar, National Heart and Chest Hospitals, London, England

Complications of Aortic Valve Endocarditis

JEAN-PAUL BELLER, M.D.

Practicing Hospitaler, Louis Pasteur University of Strasbourg; Anesthetist, University Hospital of Strasbourg, Strasbourg, France

Pulmonary Circulation: Pharmacologic Management

JOHN R. BENFIELD, M.D.

Professor and Chief, Division of Cardiothoracic Surgery, University of California at Davis, Sacramento, California

Benign and Low Grade Malignant Tumors
Anastomotic Leak

JEAN BERJAUD, M.D.

Chief of Clinic, University of Toulouse; Thoracic Surgeon, Purpan Hospital, Toulouse, France

Flail Chest and Pulmonary Contusion: Operative Management

PHILIP E. BERNATZ, M.D.

Professor, Mayo Medical School, Mayo Clinic, Rochester, Minnesota

Chest Wall Invasion in Non–Small-Cell Carcinoma

PETER C. BLOCK, M.D.

Associate Professor of Medicine, Harvard Medical School; Director, Cardiac Catheterization Laboratory and Physician, Massachusetts General Hospital, Boston, Massachusetts

Surgical Valvotomy and Percutaneous Balloon Valvotomy for Mitral Stenosis

DAVID F. BLYTH, F.R.C.S.(Edin)

Honorary Lecturer in Thoracic Surgery, University of Natal; Cardiothoracic Surgeon, Natal Provincial Administration, Natal, South Africa
Hydatid Disease

CHARLES A. BOUCHER, M.D.

Associate Professor of Medicine, Harvard Medical School; Associate Physician, Massachusetts General Hospital, Boston, Massachusetts
Noninvasive Evaluation of Patients with Cardiac Disease

FREDERICK O. BOWMAN Jr., M.D.

Professor of Clinical Surgery, Columbia University College of Physicians and Surgeons; Attending Surgeon, The Presbyterian Hospital at the Columbia-Presbyterian Medical Center, New York, New York
Constrictive Pericarditis

DAVID P. BOYD, M.D., F.R.C.S.(C)

Lecturer in Surgery, Harvard Medical School, Boston; Chairman Emeritus, Department of Thoracic and Cardiovascular Surgery, Lahey Clinic Medical Center, Burlington, Massachusetts
Bronchobiliary Fistula

JEROLD B. BRENOWITZ, M.D.

Associate, Milwaukee Heart Surgery Associates, S.C., Milwaukee, Wisconsin
Diffuse Coronary Artery Disease

MORTIMER J. BUCKLEY, M.D.

Professor of Surgery, Harvard Medical School; Chief, Cardiac Surgical Unit, Massachusetts General Hospital, Boston, Massachusetts
Intra-Aortic Balloon Circulatory Support

HEINRICH BÜLZEBRUCK, Ph.D.

Department of Medical Informatics and Biostatistics, Clinic for Thoracic Medicine, Heidelberg, Federal Republic of Germany
Sleeve Lobectomy

JEAN BUSSIÈRES, M.D., F.R.C.P.(C)

Associate Clinical Professor, Department of Anesthesiology, Laval University Faculty of Medicine; Anesthetist, Laval Hospital, Quebec, Quebec, Canada
Bronchial Rupture

CIRO CAMPANELLA, M.D.

Senior Lecturer in Cardiac Surgery, University of Edinburgh; Cardiac Surgeon, Royal Infirmary, Edinburgh, Scotland
Lung Amebiasis

DAVID B. CAMPBELL, M.D.

Associate Professor of Surgery, Pennsylvania State University College of Medicine, Milton S. Hershey Medical Center, Hershey, Pennsylvania
Coarctation of the Aorta

GERSON C. CARR, M.D., S.B.

Director of Research, The Heimlich Institute, Xavier University, Cincinnati, Ohio
Reversed Gastric Tube Graft

ALDO R. CASTAÑEDA, M.D., Ph.D.

William E. Ladd Professor of Surgery, Harvard Medical School; Surgeon in Chief and Chief of Cardiac Surgery, Children's Hospital, Boston, Massachusetts
Correction of Transposition: Arterial Switch Procedure

NOAH C. CHOI, M.D.

Assistant Professor, Department of Radiation Therapy, Harvard Medical School; Associate Radiation Oncologist, Department of Radiation Medicine, Massachusetts General Hospital, Boston, Massachusetts
Radiation Therapy
Radiation Therapy in Esophageal Neoplasia

DAVID R. CLARKE, M.D.

Associate Professor of Surgery, University of Colorado Health Sciences Center School of Medicine, Denver; Chief, Cardiothoracic Surgery, University Hospital and Children's Hospital, Denver, Colorado
Options in the Treatment of Aortic and Subaortic Stenosis in Children: Role of Aortoventriculoplasty

ADNAN COBANOGLU, M.D.

Associate Professor of Surgery and Assistant Chief of Cardiopulmonary Surgery, Oregon Health Sciences University School of Medicine; Attending Surgeon, University Hospital, Portland, Oregon
Mitral Valve Replacement

LAWRENCE H. COHN, M.D.

Professor of Surgery, Harvard Medical School; Chief, Division of Cardiac Surgery, Brigham and Women's Hospital, Boston, Massachusetts
Aortic Valve Replacement in the Adult with Small Aortic Annulus

EDWARD V. COLVIN, M.D.

Assistant Professor, Division of Pediatric Cardiology, University of Alabama School of Medicine; Staff Physician, Children's Hospital, Birmingham, Alabama
Cardiac Pacing in Children

STEPHEN B. COLVIN, M.D.

Associate Professor of Surgery, New York University School of Medicine; Chief of Cardiothoracic Surgery, Bellevue Hospital, New York, New York
Mitral Valve Reconstruction

DENTON A. COOLEY, M.D.

Clinical Professor of Surgery, University of Texas Medical School; Surgeon-in-Chief, Texas Heart Institute, Houston, Texas
Apicoaortic Conduits

JOEL D. COOPER, M.D., F.R.C.S., F.A.C.S.(C)

Professor of Surgery and Head, Section of Thoracic Surgery, Division of Cardiothoracic Surgery, Barnes Hospital, Saint Louis, Missouri
Cautery Excision
Lung Transplantation
Esophageal Dilation
Median Sternotomy

DELOS M. COSGROVE III, M.D.

Staff Surgeon, Department of Thoracic and Cardiovascular Surgery, The Cleveland Clinic Foundation, Cleveland, Ohio
Reoperation for Coronary Artery Disease

E. STANLEY CRAWFORD, M.D.

Professor of Surgery, Baylor College of Medicine; Senior Attending Surgeon, The Methodist Hospital, Houston, Texas
Replacement of the Thoracic Aorta
Acute and Chronic Aortic Dissection

WILLARD M. DAGGETT Jr., M.D.

Professor of Surgery, Harvard Medical School; Visiting Surgeon, Massachusetts General Hospital, Boston, Massachusetts
Myocardial Protection
Mediastinitis and Thoracic Space Infection
Postinfarction Ventricular Septal Rupture

MARCEL DAHAN, M.D.

Professor of Thoracic and Cardiovascular Surgery, University of Toulouse; Surgeon and Head of Thoracic Unit, Purpan Hospital, Toulouse, France
Flail Chest and Pulmonary Contusion: Operative Management

BENEDICT D. T. DALY, M.D.

Professor of Cardiothoracic Surgery, Tufts University School of Medicine; Senior Staff Surgeon, New England Medical Center and Chief of Cardiothoracic Surgery, Boston Veterans Administration Medical Center, Boston, Massachusetts
Open Lung Biopsy

MICHAEL N. D'AMBRA, M.D.

Assistant Professor, Harvard Medical School; Assistant Anesthetist, Cardiac Anesthesia Group, Massachusetts General Hospital, Boston, Massachusetts
Pulmonary Circulation: Pharmacologic Management

TIRONE E. DAVID, M.D., F.R.C.S.(C), F.A.C.S.

Associate Professor of Surgery, University of Toronto Faculty of Medicine; Head, Division of Cardiovascular Surgery, The Toronto General and Western Hospitals, Toronto, Ontario, Canada
Preservation of the Posterior Chordae Tendinae in Mitral Valve Replacement

G. MICHAEL DEEB, M.D.

Assistant Professor of Surgery, University of Michigan Medical School, Ann Arbor, Michigan
Cardiac Transplantation in Children

MARC R. DE LEVAL, M.D.

Consultant Cardiothoracic Surgeon, The Hospital for Sick Children, London, England
Palliation in Congenital Heart Disease

ALFRED A. DELORIMIER, M.D.

Professor of Surgery and Chief, Division of Pediatric Surgery, University of California School of Medicine, San Francisco, California
Tracheal Problems in Children
Vascular Rings

TOM R. DEMEESTER, M.D.

Professor and Chairman, Creighton University School of Medicine; Chief of Surgery, Department of Surgery, Creighton University School of Medicine, Omaha, Nebraska
Preoperative Evaluation of Gastroesophageal Reflux

JANETTE S. DENHAM, M.D.

Clinical Fellow, Department of Radiology—Vascular Section, Massachusetts General Hospital, Boston, Massachusetts
Massive Hemoptysis: Control with Transcatheter Vessel Embolization

JEAN DESLAURIERS, M.D., F.R.C.S.(C)

Professor, Department of Surgery, Laval University Faculty of Medicine; Chief, Department of Thoracic Surgery, Laval Pulmonary Disease Center, Ste-Foy, Quebec, Canada
Bronchial Rupture

JOHN DISIERE, M.D.

Thoracic and Cardiovascular Surgical Fellow, Baylor University Medical Center, Houston, Texas
Sternal Fractures and Myocardial Contusions
Eventration and Plication

DONALD B. DOTY, M.D.

Clinical Professor, Department of Surgery, University of Utah School of Medicine; Chairman, Division of Cardiovascular and Thoracic Surgery, Los Hospital, Salt Lake City, Utah
Spiral Vein Graft

CARLOS M. G. DURAN, M.D., Ph.D.

Professor, Cardiovascular Surgery and Chairman, Department of Cardiovascular Diseases, King Faisal Specialist Hospital and Research Center, Riyadh, Saudi Arabia
Tricuspid Valve Repair

ANDRÉ DURANCEAU, M.D., F.R.C.S., F.A.C.S.

Professor of Surgery, University of Montreal Faculty of Medicine; Division of Thoracic Surgery, Hôtel-Dieu, Montreal, Quebec, Canada
Cricopharyngeal Dysfunction and Myotomy

PAUL A. EBERT, M.D., F.A.C.S.

Director, American College of Surgeons, Chicago, Illinois
The Univentricular Heart: Role of Ventricular Septation

NABIL EL-BAZ, M.D.

Associate Professor, Rush Medical College of Rush University; Associate Attending, Rush-Presbyterian-St. Luke's Medical Center, Chicago, Illinois
Postoperative Pain Control

JOHN A. ELEFTERIADES, M.D.

Assistant Professor, Cardiothoracic Surgery, Yale University School of Medicine; Attending Physician, Yale-New Haven Hospital, New Haven, Connecticut
Diaphragm Pacing

F. HENRY ELLIS Jr., M.D., Ph.D.

Clinical Professor of Surgery, Harvard Medical School, Boston; Senior Consultant, Department of Thoracic and Cardiovascular Surgery, Lahey Clinic Medical Center, Burlington, and Chief, Division of Thoracic and Cardiovascular Surgery, New England Deaconess Hospital, Boston, Massachusetts
Upper Thoracic Esophageal Cancer
Nissen Fundoplication for Gastroesophageal Reflux
Achalasia

M. ARISAN ERGIN, M.D.

Associate Professor of Surgery, Division of Cardiothoracic Surgery, The Mount Sinai Hospital and Mount Sinai School of Medicine, City University of New York, New York, New York
Aortic Arch Replacement

HENRY ESCHAPASSE, M.D.

Honorary Professor of Thoracic Surgery, Paul Sabatier University; Past Chief of Thoracic Unit, Purpan Hospital, Toulouse, France
Prosthetic Substitutes of the Chest Wall

L. PENFIELD FABER, M.D.

Professor and Associate Dean of Surgery, Rush Medical College of Rush University; Senior Attending Surgeon, Rush-Presbyterian-St. Luke's Medical Center, Chicago, Illinois
Lung-Sparing Procedures: Segmental Resection
Broncholithiasis

MARK K. FERGUSON, M.D.

Associate Professor, Department of Surgery, University of Chicago Pritzker School of Medicine, Chicago, Illinois
Belsey Mark IV Hiatal Herniorrhaphy

THOMAS B. FERGUSON, M.D.

Professor of Clinical Surgery, Division of Cardiothoracic Surgery, Washington University School of Medicine; Attending Surgeon, Barnes Hospital, Saint Louis, Missouri
Sequestration

M. WAYNE FLYE, M.D., Ph.D.

Professor of Surgery and Immunology, Washington University School of Medicine; Director of Organ Transplantation, Washington University Medical Center, Saint Louis, Missouri
Malignant Pleural Effusion

KARL H. FUCHS, M.D.

Research Fellow, Department of Surgery, Creighton University School of Medicine, Omaha, Nebraska
Preoperative Evaluation of Gastroesophageal Reflux

JACQUES GAILLARD, M.D.

Professor of Thoracic and Cardiovascular Surgery, University of Toulouse; Surgeon and Chief of Thoracic Unit, Purpan Hospital, Toulouse, France
Flail Chest and Pulmonary Contusion: Operative Management
Prosthetic Substitutes of the Chest Wall

AUBREY C. GALLOWAY, M.D.

Assistant Professor of Surgery, New York University School of Medicine; Attending Surgeon and Director of Surgical Research, New York University Medical Center, New York, New York
Mitral Valve Reconstruction

ANTONIO A. GARZON, M.D.

Professor, SUNY Health Science Center, Brooklyn; Director of Surgery, St. Vincent's Medical Center of Richmond, Staten Island, New York
Massive Hemoptysis: Surgical and Tamponade Therapy

ROBERT J. GINSBERG, M.D., F.R.C.S.(C)

Professor of Surgery, University of Toronto Faculty of Medicine; Surgeon-in-Chief and Head, Division of Thoracic Surgery, Mount Sinai Hospital, Toronto, Ontario, Canada
Bronchogenic Cysts

WILLIAM W. L. GLENN, M.D.

Charles W. Ohse Professor Emeritus and Senior Research Scientist, Surgery, Yale University School of Medicine; Attending Surgeon, Yale-New Haven Hospital, New Haven, Connecticut
Diaphragm Pacing

MARSHALL D. GOLDIN, M.D.

Associate Professor of Surgery, Department of Cardiovascular-Thoracic Surgery, Rush Medical College of Rush University; Director, Surgical Intensive Care Unit and Senior Attending, Rush-Presbyterian-St. Luke's Medical Center, Chicago, Illinois
Acute and Chronic Mitral Regurgitation in the Ischemic Heart

RANDALL B. GRIEPP, M.D., Ph.D.

Professor of Surgery and Chief, Division of Cardiothoracic Surgery, The Mount Sinai Hospital and Mount Sinai School of Medicine, City University of New York, New York, New York
Aortic Arch Replacement

HERMES C. GRILLO, M.D.

Professor of Surgery, Harvard Medical School; Chief of General Thoracic Surgery, Massachusetts General Hospital, Boston, Massachusetts
Pneumomediastinum
Acquired Tracheoesophageal Fistula
Acquired Tracheal Stenosis
Mediastinal Exenteration
Substernal Goiter
Carinal Neoplasia
Carcinoma of the Cervical Esophagus
Spontaneous and Iatrogenic Esophageal Perforation

FREDERICK L. GROVER, M.D.

Professor of Surgery, Division of Cardiothoracic Surgery, University of Texas Health Science Center, San Antonio, Texas
Flail Chest and Pulmonary Contusion: Nonoperative Management

GERARD M. GUIRAUDON, M.D., F.R.C.S.(C), F.A.C.C.

Professor of Surgery, University of Western Ontario Faculty of Medicine; Consultant, University Hospital, London, Ontario, Canada
Wolff-Parkinson-White Syndrome

ROBERT A. GUSTAFSON, M.D.

Associate Professor of Surgery and Pediatrics, Section of Cardiovascular and Thoracic Surgery, West Virginia University School of Medicine, Morgantown, West Virginia
Esophageal Neoplasia: Benign Tumor

J. ALEX HALLER Jr., M.D.

Robert Garrett Professor of Pediatric Surgery, Professor of Pediatrics, and Professor of Emergency Medicine, The Johns Hopkins University School of Medicine; Children's Surgeon-in-Charge, The Johns Hopkins Hospital, Baltimore, Maryland
Caustic Burns of the Esophagus

GRADY L. HALLMAN, M.D.

Clinical Professor of Cardiac and Thoracic Surgery, University of Texas Medical School; Senior Consultant in Surgery, The Texas Heart Institute, Houston, Texas
Cardiac Tumors

ALDEN H. HARKEN, M.D.

Professor and Chairman, Department of Surgery, University of Colorado Health Sciences Center School of Medicine, Denver, Colorado
Recurrent Ventricular Tachycardia: Surgical Management

P. KENT HARMAN, M.D.

Assistant Professor of Surgery and Pediatrics, University of Texas Medical School, San Antonio, Texas
Flail Chest and Pulmonary Contusion: Nonoperative Management

MICHAEL R. HARRISON, M.D.

Associate Professor of Surgery, University of California School of Medicine, San Francisco, California
Tracheal Problems in Children

J. WARREN HARTHORNE, M.D.

Associate Professor, Harvard Medical School; Director, Pacemaker Lab and Physician, Massachusetts General Hospital, Boston, Massachusetts
Cardiac Pacing

HENRY J. HEIMLICH, M.D., D.Sc.(Hon), F.A.C.S., F.C.C.P.

President, The Heimlich Institute, Professor of Advanced Clinical Sciences, Xavier University, and Associate Clinical Professor of Surgery, University of Cincinnati College of Medicine; Attending Surgeon, Deaconess Hospital, Cincinnati, Ohio
Reversed Gastric Tube Graft

RICHARD F. HEITMILLER, M.D.

Assistant Professor, Department of Surgery and Thoracic Surgeon, The Johns Hopkins Hospital, Baltimore, Maryland
Esophagoscopy
French Incision

ROBERT D. HENDERSON, M.B., F.R.C.S.(C), F.A.C.S.

Professor of Surgery, University of Toronto Faculty of Medicine; Chief of Surgery, Women's College Hospital, Toronto, Ontario, Canada
Recurrent Hiatal Hernia
Scleroderma and Diffuse Spasm

W. HARDY HENDREN, M.D.

Robert E. Gross Professor of Surgery, Harvard Medical School; Chief of Surgery, The Children's Hospital and Visiting Surgeon, Massachusetts General Hospital, Boston, Massachusetts
Lobar Emphysema

ALAN D. HILGENBERG, M.D.

Assistant Professor of Surgery, Harvard Medical School; Associate Visiting Surgeon, Massachusetts General Hospital, Boston, Massachusetts
Esophageal Neoplasm: Palliation with Salivary Tubes
Cardiac and Thoracic Aortic Trauma

J. DONALD HILL, M.D.

Chairman, Department of Cardiovascular Surgery, Pacific Presbyterian Medical Center, San Francisco, California
The Artificial Heart: A Bridge to Cardiac Transplantation

LUCIUS D. HILL, M.D.

Clinical Professor of Surgery, University of Washington School of Medicine; General, Thoracoesophageal, and Vascular Surgeon, Virginia Mason and Swedish Medical Centers, Seattle, Washington
Hill Procedure for Gastroesophageal Reflux

RONALD C. HILL, M.D.

Assistant Professor of Surgery and Cardiothoracic Surgery, West Virginia University School of Medicine, Morgantown; Consultant, Veterans Administration Hospital, Clarksburg, West Virginia
Malignant Tracheoesophageal Fistula

E. CARMACK HOLMES, M.D.

Professor of Surgery, Divisions of Surgical Oncology and Cardiothoracic Surgery, University of California School of Medicine, Los Angeles, California
Chemotherapy for Non-Small-Cell Carcinoma

MARSHALL L. JACOBS, M.D.

Associate Professor of Surgery, George Washington University School of Medicine and Health Sciences; Attending Cardiovascular Surgeon, Children's Hospital National Medical Center, Washington, D.C.
Coronary Revascularization: Proximal Anastomoses Preceding Distal Anastomoses
Postinfarction Ventricular Septal Rupture
Correction of Tetralogy of Fallot

W. DUDLEY JOHNSON, M.D.

Associate Clinical Professor, Department of Thoracic-Cardiovascular Surgery, Medical College of Wisconsin; Medical Director, Cardiovascular Surgery, The Heart Institute of Milwaukee and Associate, Milwaukee Heart Surgery Associates, S.C., Milwaukee, Wisconsin
Diffuse Coronary Artery Disease

RICHARD A. JONAS, M.D.

Assistant Professor of Surgery, Harvard Medical School; Associate in Cardiac Surgery, The Children's Hospital, Boston, Massachusetts
Interrupted Aortic Arch

ELLIS L. JONES, M.D.

Professor, Cardiothoracic Surgery, Emory University School of Medicine, Atlanta, Georgia
Combined Carotid and Coronary Artery Disease

M. J. JURKIEWICZ, M.D., F.A.C.S.

Professor of Surgery, Emory University School of Medicine; Chief, Section of Plastic and Reconstructive Surgery, The Emory Clinic, Atlanta, Georgia
Free Jejunal Graft

JEAN S. KAN, M.D.

Associate Professor of Pediatrics, The Johns Hopkins University School of Medicine; Associate Professor of Pediatrics and Pediatric Cardiologist, Helen B. Taussig Children's Heart Center, The Johns Hopkins Hospital, Baltimore, Maryland
Percutaneous Intervention in Congenital Heart Disease

DAVID J. KANAREK, M.D.

Associate Clinical Professor of Medicine, Harvard Medical School; Associate Physician, Pulmonary Medicine, Massachusetts General Hospital, Boston, Massachusetts
Evaluation for Pulmonary Resection

ADOLF W. KARCHMER, M.D.

Associate Professor of Medicine, Harvard Medical School; Chief, Infectious Disease Section, New England Deaconess Hospital, Boston, Massachusetts
Prosthetic and Native Valve Endocarditis

MARK R. KATLIC, M.D.

Chief of Thoracic Surgery, Wilkes-Barre General Hospital, Wilkes-Barre, Pennsylvania
Substernal Goiter

KENNETH L. KAYSER, M.S.

Associate, Milwaukee Heart Surgery Associates, S.C., Milwaukee, Wisconsin
Diffuse Coronary Artery Disease

BLAIR A. KEAGY, M.D.

Associate Professor, Divisions of Cardiothoracic and Vascular Surgery, University of North Carolina School of Medicine, Chapel Hill, North Carolina
Spontaneous Pneumothorax

JAMES W. KILMAN, M.D.

Professor, Department of Surgery, Ohio State University College of Medicine and Professor, Department of Veterinary Clinical Sciences, Ohio State University School of Veterinary Sciences; Chief, Department of Thoracic Surgery, Columbus Children's Hospital and Attending Surgeon, Ohio State University Hospital, Columbus, Ohio
Congenital Mitral Stenosis and Atresia

THOMAS J. KIRBY, B.Sc., M.D., F.R.C.S.(C)

Lecturer, University of Toronto Faculty of Medicine; General Thoracic Surgeon, Toronto Western Hospital, Toronto, Ontario, Canada
Bronchogenic Cysts

JAMES K. KIRKLIN, M.D.

Professor of Surgery, Department of Surgery, University of Alabama School of Medicine, Birmingham, Alabama
Ebstein's Anomaly

JOHN W. KIRKLIN, M.D.

Professor of Surgery, Department of Surgery, University of Alabama School of Medicine, Birmingham, Alabama
Ebstein's Anomaly

C. FREDERICK KITTLE, D.B., M.S., M.D.

Professor of Surgery, Rush Medical College of Rush University; Senior Attending and Director, Section of Thoracic Surgery, Rush-Presbyterian-St. Luke's Medical Center, Chicago, and Provisional Staff, MacNeal Hospital, Berwyn, Illinois
Pleural Mesothelioma

GEORGE J. KLEIN, M.D., F.R.C.P.(C), F.A.C.C.

Professor of Medicine, University of Western Ontario Faculty of Medicine; Consultant, University Hospital, London, Ontario, Canada
Wolff-Parkinson-White Syndrome

NICHOLAS T. KOUCHOUKOS, M.D.

John M. Shoenberg Professor of Cardiovascular Surgery, Washington University School of Medicine; Cardiovascular and Thoracic Surgeon-in-Chief, The Jewish Hospital of Saint Louis, Saint Louis, Missouri
Aortic Valve Replacement

R. CRAIG KUYKENDALL, M.D.

Resident in Cardiovascular Surgery, The Texas Heart Institute, Houston, Texas
Cardiac Tumors

G. HUGH LAWRENCE, M.D., F.A.C.S.

Professor and Chairman, Department of Surgery, King Saud College of Medicine, Abha, Saudi Arabia; Associate Clinical Professor of Surgery, University of Washington School of Medicine, Seattle, Washington
Empyema and Bronchopleural Fistula
The Clagett Procedure

RAYMOND LEE, M.D.

Department of Surgery, Massachusetts General Hospital, Boston, Massachusetts
Primum Atrial Septal Defects

BERNARD T. LE ROUX, Ch.M., F.R.C.S.(Edin)

Professor of Thoracic Surgery, University of Natal; Chief Thoracic Surgeon, Wentworth Hospital and Natal Provincial Administration, Durban, Natal, South Africa
Bronchography
Hydatid Disease
Lung Amebiasis

RALPH J. LEWIS, M.D., F.A.C.S.

Clinical Professor of Surgery, University of Medicine and Dentistry of New Jersey, Robert Wood Johnson Medical School, New Brunswick, New Jersey
Thoracoscopy and the Chamberlain Procedure

CHRISTOPHER LINCOLN, F.R.C.S.

Senior Lecturer in Paediatrics, University of London; Consultant Cardiothoracic Surgeon, Brompton Hospital, London, England
Anomalous Pulmonary Venous Connection

ALEX G. LITTLE, M.D.

Associate Professor, University of Chicago Pritzker School of Medicine; Chief of Thoracic Surgery, University of Chicago Medical Center, Chicago, Illinois
Superior Vena Cava Syndrome

FLOYD D. LOOP, M.D.

Chairman, Department of Thoracic and Cardiovascular Surgery, Cleveland Clinic Foundation, Cleveland, Ohio
Coronary Revascularization: Distal Anastomoses Preceding Proximal Anastomoses

JACQUES G. LOSMAN, M.D., F.A.C.C.

Attending Cardiothoracic Surgeon, Newark Beth Israel Medical Center and St. Michael's Medical Center, Newark, New Jersey
Thrombolytic Therapy

JAMES E. LOWE, M.D.

Associate Professor of Surgery, Duke University School of Medicine; Director, Surgical Electrophysiology Service, Durham, North Carolina
Coronary Artery Anomalies

BRUCE W. LYTLE, M.D.

Staff Surgeon, Department of Thoracic and Cardiovascular Surgery, The Cleveland Clinic Foundation, Cleveland, Ohio
Conduit Options for Coronary Artery Bypass Surgery

WERNER MAASSEN, M.D.

Professor of Pneumonology and Thoracic Surgeon; Former Head of the Ruhrland Clinic, Essen, Federal Republic of Germany
Mediastinoscopy

JAMES W. MACKENZIE, M.D., F.A.C.S.

Professor and Chairman, Department of Surgery, University of Medicine and Dentistry of New Jersey, Robert Wood Johnson Medical School, New Brunswick, New Jersey
Thoracoscopy and the Chamberlain Procedure

JAMES A. MAGOVERN, M.D.

Instructor in Cardiothoracic Surgery, Pennsylvania State University College of Medicine, Milton S. Hershey Medical Center, Hershey, Pennsylvania
Support of the Failing Heart: Left Heart Assistance

WILLIAM G. MARSHALL Jr., M.D., F.A.C.C.

Assistant Professor of Surgery, Washington University School of Medicine; Staff Cardiovascular Surgeon, The Jewish Hospital of Saint Louis, Saint Louis, Missouri
Aortic Valve Replacement

NAEL MARTINI, M.D.

Professor of Surgery, Cornell University Medical College; Chief, Thoracic Surgery, Memorial Sloan-Kettering Cancer Center, New York, New York
Unresectable Neoplasms of the Lung

DOUGLAS J. MATHISEN, M.D.

Assistant Professor of Surgery, Harvard Medical School; Assistant Surgeon, Massachusetts General Hospital, Boston, Massachusetts
Bronchoscopy
Esophagoscopy
Penetrating Trauma: Hemothorax
Tracheostomy
Laryngotracheal Trauma
Acute Airway Obstruction
Pulmonary Arteriovenous Malformations
Short-Segment Colon Interposition
Barrett's Esophagus
French Incision
Mediastinitis and Thoracic Space Infection

HUGOE R. MATTHEWS, F.R.C.S.

Senior Clinical Lecturer, University of Birmingham; Consultant Thoracic Surgeon, Regional Department of Thoracic Surgery, East Birmingham Hospital, Birmingham, England
The Surgical Management of Giant Bullae

KENNETH L. MATTOX, M.D.

Professor of Surgery, Baylor College of Medicine; Deputy Surgeon-in-Chief and Director of Emergency Surgical Services, Ben Taub General Hospital, Houston, Texas
Penetrating Pulmonary and Esophageal Trauma

CONSTANTINE MAVROUDIS, M.D.

Associate Professor of Surgery, University of Louisville School of Medicine; Chief of Cardiothoracic Surgery, Kosair-Children's Hospital, Louisville, Kentucky
Patent Ductus Arteriosus

JOHN E. MAYER Jr., M.D.

Assistant Professor of Surgery, Harvard Medical School; Associate in Cardiovascular Surgery, Children's Hospital, Boston, Massachusetts
Ventricular Septal Defect

JOHN R. McCORMICK, M.D.

Clinical Associate Professor of Surgery, University of Pennsylvania School of Medicine; Attending Surgeon, Presbyterian-University of Pennsylvania Medical Center, Philadelphia, Pennsylvania
Coronary Artery Spasm

RICHARD B. McELVEIN, M.D.

Associate Professor of Surgery, University of Alabama School of Medicine, Birmingham, Alabama
Laser Techniques in Pulmonary Problems
Laser Techniques in Esophageal Problems

CHARLES L. McINTOSH, M.D., Ph.D.

Senior Attending Surgeon, Surgery Branch, National Heart, Lung, and Blood Institute, National Institutes of Health, Bethesda, Maryland
Idiopathic Hypertrophic Subaortic Stenosis

THERESA C. McLOUD, M.D.

Associate Professor of Radiology, Harvard Medical School; Chief of Thoracic Radiology, Massachusetts General Hospital, Boston, Massachusetts
Radiologic Assessment

WROTEN M. McQUIRTER Jr., M.D.

Thoracic and Cardiovascular Surgical Fellow, Baylor University Medical Center, Houston, Texas
Sternal Fractures and Myocardial Contusions
Eventration and Plication

GÜNTHER MEYER, M.D.

Surgical Department, Clinic for Thoracic Medicine, Heidelberg, Federal Republic of Germany
Sleeve Lobectomy

JOHN A. MEYER, M.D.

Professor of Surgery, SUNY Health Science Center; Attending Thoracic Surgeon, State University and Crouse-Irving Memorial Hospitals, Syracuse, New York
Small-Cell Carcinoma

NOEL L. MILLS, M.D.

Associate Clinical Professor in Surgery, Tulane University Medical Center, New Orleans; Surgical Director, Cardiology Center, Marrero, Louisiana
Intraoperative Coronary Angioplasty

ASHBY C. MONCURE, M.D.

Associate Clinical Professor of Surgery, Harvard Medical School; Visiting Surgeon, Massachusetts General Hospital, Boston, Massachusetts
Paraesophageal Hernia
Diaphragmatic Injury

JAMES L. MONRO, M.B., B.S., F.R.C.S.

Consultant Cardiac Surgeon, The General Hospital, Southampton, England
Homograft Material in Cardiac Surgery

JOHN M. MORAN, M.D.

Professor of Surgery, Brown University Program in Medicine; Surgeon-in-Charge, Division of Cardiothoracic Surgery, Rhode Island Hospital, Providence, Rhode Island
Cardiogenic Shock

ELDRED D. MUNDTH, M.D.

Professor of Surgery, Hahnemann University Hospital; Chief, Division of Cardiac Surgery and Senior Attending Surgeon, Bryn Mawr Hospital, Bryn Mawr, Pennsylvania
Ventricular Aneurysm

DOUGLAS A. MURPHY, M.D.

Assistant Professor, Department of Surgery, Emory University School of Medicine; Staff Surgeon, St. Joseph's Hospital, Atlanta, Georgia
Percutaneous Angioplasty: The Role of the Cardiac Surgeon

GORDON F. MURRAY, M.D.

Professor and Chairman of Surgery, West Virginia University School of Medicine, Morgantown, West Virginia
Malignant Tracheoesophageal Fistula
Esophageal Neoplasia: Benign Tumor

JOHN L. MYERS, M.D.

Assistant Professor of Cardiothoracic Surgery, Assistant Professor of Pediatric Cardiology, Pennsylvania State University College of Medicine, Milton S. Hershey Medical Center, Hershey, Pennsylvania
Coarctation of the Aorta

HASSAN NAJAFI, M.D.

Professor and Chairman, Department of Cardiovascular-Thoracic Surgery, Rush Medical College of Rush University; Senior Attending, Rush-Presbyterian-St. Luke's Medical Center, Chicago, Illinois
Acute and Chronic Mitral Regurgitation in the Ischemic Heart

KEITH S. NAUNHEIM, M.D.

Assistant Professor of Surgery, Saint Louis University School of Medicine, Saint Louis, Missouri
Mallory-Weiss Syndrome

WILLIAM I. NORWOOD, M.D., Ph.D.

Professor of Surgery, University of Pennsylvania School of Medicine; Chief of Cardiac Surgery, Children's Hospital of Philadelphia, Philadelphia, Pennsylvania
Hypoplastic Left-Sided Heart Syndrome

MARK B. ORRINGER, M.D.

Professor and Head, Section of Thoracic Surgery, University of Michigan Medical School, Ann Arbor, Michigan
Transhiatal Esophagectomy
Esophageal Infection: Moniliasis
Morgagni Hernia

ALBERT D. PACIFICO, M.D.

John W. Kirklin Professor of Cardiovascular Surgery, Department of Surgery and Director, Division of Cardiothoracic Surgery, University of Alabama School of Medicine, Birmingham, Alabama
Cardiopulmonary Bypass and Hypothermic Circulatory Arrest in Congenital Heart Surgery
Ebstein's Anomaly

PETER C. PAIROLERO, M.D.

Professor of Surgery, Mayo Medical School; Consultant, Section of Thoracic and Cardiovascular Surgery, Department of Surgery, Mayo Clinic and Mayo Foundation, Rochester, Minnesota
Chest Wall Neoplasia
Muscle Flaps
Muscle Flap in Bronchopleural Fistula
Occult Neoplasia
Cervical and Thoracic Esophageal Diverticulum

CHRISTIAN E. PALETTA, M.D.

Assistant Professor of Surgery, Division of Plastic Surgery, Saint Louis University School of Medicine; Division of Plastic Surgery, Saint Louis University Hospital and John Cochran Veterans Administration Medical Center and Director of Cleft Palate Clinic, Cardinal Glennon Children's Hospital, Saint Louis, Missouri
Free Jejunal Graft

DONALD L. PAULSON, M.D., Ph.D.

Clinical Professor, Thoracic and Cardiovascular Surgery, University of Texas Southwestern Medical Center, Dallas, Texas
Superior Sulcus Tumor

W. SPENCER PAYNE, M.D.

Professor of Surgery, Mayo Medical School; Consultant, Section of Thoracic and Cardiovascular Surgery, Mayo Clinic and Mayo Foundation, Rochester, Minnesota
Occult Neoplasia
Cervical and Thoracic Esophageal Diverticulum

F. GRIFFITH PEARSON, M.D., B.Sc.(Med), F.R.C.S.(C), F.A.C.S.

Professor, Department of Surgery, University of Toronto Faculty of Medicine; Surgeon-in-Chief, Toronto General Hospital, Toronto, Ontario, Canada
N_2 Disease in Non-Small-Cell Lung Cancer
Collis-Belsey Hiatal Herniorrhaphy
Management of Peptic Stricture of the Esophagus

MIKHAIL I. PERELMAN, M.D.

Professor of Surgery, Academician of the USSR Academy of Medical Science; Chair of Pulmonology, I Moscow Medical Institute, Department of Thoracic Surgery, Chief, All-Union Center of Surgery, and Consulting Surgeon, Moscow, USSR
Tracheal Tumor
Transsternal Technique for Bronchopleural Fistula

WILLIAM S. PIERCE, M.D.

Evan Pugh and Jane A. Fetter Professor of Surgery and Chief, Division of Artificial Organs, Department of Surgery, Pennsylvania State University College of Medicine, Hershey, Pennsylvania
Support of the Failing Heart: Left Heart Assistance

JOHN D. PIGOTT, M.D.

Assistant Professor of Surgery, University of Pennsylvania School of Medicine; Assistant Surgeon, Children's Hospital of Philadelphia, Philadelphia, Pennsylvania
Hypoplastic Left-Sided Heart Syndrome

HIRAM C. POLK Jr., M.D.

Professor and Chairman, Department of Surgery, University of Louisville, Louisville, Kentucky
Short Segment Jejunal Interposition

JUDSON RANDOLPH, M.D., F.A.C.S.

Professor of Surgery, George Washington University School of Medicine and Health Sciences; Surgeon-in-Chief, Children's Hospital National Medical Center, Washington, D.C.
Hiatal Hernia and Esophageal Reflux

BRUCE A. REITZ, M.D.

Professor of Surgery, The Johns Hopkins University School of Medicine; Cardiac Surgeon-in-Charge, The Johns Hopkins Hospital, Baltimore, Maryland
Cardiac Transplantation

JAMES M. RICHTER, M.D., M.A.

Assistant Professor of Medicine, Harvard Medical School; Assistant Physician, Massachusetts General Hospital, Boston, Massachusetts
Endoscopic Sclerotherapy in Esophageal Varices

ARTHUR J. ROBERTS, M.D.

Chief, Department of Cardiac Surgery, The Heart Institute, Wilkes-Barre General Hospital, Wilkes-Barre, Pennsylvania
Coronary Artery Spasm

FRANCIS ROBICSEK, M.D.

Clinical Professor of Surgery, University of North Carolina School of Medicine, Chapel Hill; Chairman, Department of Thoracic and Cardiovascular Surgery, Charlotte Memorial Hospital and Medical Center, Charlotte, North Carolina
Pectus Excavatum and Carinatum

DAVID A. ROCKE, M.R.C.P.(UK), F.F.A.S.A.

Professor of Anaesthetics, University of Natal; Chief Anaesthetist, King Edward VIII Hospital, Durban, Natal, South Africa
Bronchography

DAVID B. ROOS, M.D.

Professor of Surgery, University of Colorado Health Sciences Center; Teaching Staff, Presbyterian-Denver Hospital, Denver, Colorado
Operative Management of Thoracic Outlet Syndrome

DONALD ROSS, D.Sc., F.R.C.S.

Director of Surgery, National Heart Hospital and Consultant Cardiac Surgeon, London, England
Complications of Aortic Valve Endocarditis

THOMAS M. ROUSE, M.D.

Chief Resident in Surgery, Children's Hospital National Medical Center, Washington, D.C.
Hiatal Hernia and Esophageal Reflux

DANIEL P. RYAN, M.D.

Instructor in Surgery, Harvard Medical School; Assistant in Surgery, Massachusetts General Hospital, Boston, Massachusetts
Extracorporeal Membrane Oxygenation for Infants and Children

ROBERT M. SADE, M.D.

Professor of Cardiothoracic Surgery, Medical University of South Carolina College of Medicine; Attending Surgeon and Chief of Pediatric Cardiac Surgery, Medical University of South Carolina Medical Center, Charleston, South Carolina
Diaphragmatic Eventration—Diaphragmatic Plication
Tricuspid Atresia

SAED F. SAEDI, M.D.

Associate, Milwaukee Heart Surgery Associates, S.C., Milwaukee, Wisconsin
Diffuse Coronary Artery Disease

MARK E. SAND, M.D.

Clinical Assistant Professor of Surgery, F. Edward Hebert School of Medicine, Uniformed Services University of the Health Sciences, Bethesda, Maryland; Staff, Cardiothoracic Surgery, United States Air Force Medical Center, Keesler Air Force Base, Mississippi
Cardiac Pacing in Children

J. GORDON SCANNELL, M.D.

Clinical Professor of Surgery, Emeritus, Harvard Medical School; Senior Surgeon, Massachusetts General Hospital, Boston, Massachusetts
Tuberculosis
Lung Abscess
Malignant Pericardial Effusion

ROBERT H. SCHAPIRO, M.D.

Clinical Associate Professor of Medicine, Harvard Medical School; Physician, Massachusetts General Hospital, Boston, Massachusetts
Endoscopic Sclerotherapy in Esophageal Varices

ROBERT C. SCHNEIDER, M.D.

Assistant Professor, Harvard Medical School; Associate Anesthetist, Massachusetts General Hospital, Boston, Massachusetts
Anesthesia for Cardiac Surgery

SAMUEL R. SCHUSTER, M.D.

Associate Professor of Surgery, Harvard Medical School; Senior Associate in Surgery, The Children's Hospital, Boston, Massachusetts
Cystic Fibrosis

WILL C. SEALY, M.D.

Professor of Surgery, Mercer University School of Medicine, Macon, Georgia and Professor Emeritus, Thoracic Surgery, Duke University School of Medicine, Durham, North Carolina
Bronchiectasis

SAMUEL L. SELINGER, M.D.

Cardiovascular Surgeon, Sacred Heart and Deaconess Medical Centers, Spokane, Washington
Coronary Revascularization During Acute Myocardial Infarction

ÅKE SENNING, M.D.

Professor of Surgery, University of Zurich, Zurich, Switzerland
Correction of Transposition: The Senning Procedure

B. SETHIA, F.R.C.S.

Senior Surgical Registrar, The Hospital for Sick Children, London, England
The Double-Outlet Right Ventricle

DAVID M. SHAHIAN, M.D.

Assistant Clinical Professor of Surgery, Harvard Medical School, Boston; Chairman, Department of Thoracic and Cardiovascular Surgery, Lahey Clinic Medical Center, Burlington, Massachusetts
Upper Thoracic Esophageal Cancer

ARJUN D. SHARMA, M.D., F.R.C.P.(C), F.A.C.C.

Assistant Professor of Medicine, University of Western Ontario Faculty of Medicine; Consultant, University Hospital, London, Ontario, Canada
Wolff-Parkinson-White Syndrome

RICHARD B. SHEPARD, M.D.

Associate Professor of Surgery, Division of Cardiovascular and Thoracic Surgery, University of Alabama School of Medicine, Birmingham, Alabama
Cardiac Pacing in Children

DARRYL SHORE, F.R.C.S.

Consultant, Cardiac Surgeon, The Brompton Hospital, London, England
Selection and Postoperative Management of Prosthetic Valves in Children

ARUN K. SINGH, M.D., F.R.C.S.(C)

Assistant Clinical Professor of Surgery, Brown University Program in Medicine; Surgeon, Division of Cardiothoracic Surgery, Rhode Island Hospital, Providence, Rhode Island
Cardiogenic Shock

LELAND G. SIWEK, M.D.

Cardiovascular and Thoracic Surgeon, Spokane, Washington
Myocardial Protection

DAVID B. SKINNER, M.D.

Professor of Surgery, Cornell University Medical College; Attending Surgeon, President, and Chief Executive Officer, The New York Hospital, New York, New York
Belsey Mark IV Hiatal Herniorrhaphy

CHARLES D. SMITH, M.D.

Associate Professor of Surgery and Pediatrics, Medical University of South Carolina; Attending Surgeon, MUSC Medical Center, Charleston, South Carolina
Diaphragmatic Eventration—Diaphagmatic Plication

FRANK C. SPENCER, M.D.

George David Stewart Professor of Surgery, New York University School of Medicine; Chairman, Department of Surgery, New York University Medical Center, New York, New York
Mitral Valve Reconstruction

JAROSLAV F. STARK, M.D., F.R.C.S., F.A.C.S.

Consultant Cardiothoracic Surgeon, The Hospital for Sick Children, London, England
The Double-Outlet Right Ventricle

ALBERT STARR, M.D.

Professor of Surgery and Chief of Cardiopulmonary Surgery, Oregon Health Sciences University School of Medicine; Attending Surgeon, University Hospital, Portland, Oregon
Mitral Valve Replacement

FELICIEN M. STEICHEN, M.D.

Professor of Surgery, New York Medical College, Valhalla, New York
Staplers

ZWI STEIGER, M.D., F.A.C.S.

Professor of Surgery, Department of Surgery, Wayne State University School of Medicine; Chief, Division of Thoracic Surgery, Veterans Administration Medical Center, Allen Park and Attending Surgeon, Harper Hospital and Detroit Receiving Hospital, Detroit, Michigan
Chemotherapy, Radiation, and Surgery in Esophageal Neoplasia

SCOTT STEWART, M.D.

Professor, Department of Surgery, Division of Cardiothoracic Surgery, University of Rochester School of Medicine and Dentistry, Rochester, New York
Atrioventricular Canal Defect

EDWARD B. STINSON, M.D.

Professor of Cardiovascular Surgery, Stanford University School of Medicine, Stanford, California
Recurrent Ventricular Tachycardia and Fibrillation: The Automatic Internal Defibrillator

CHARLES D. SWERDLOW, M.D.

Assistant Professor of Medicine (Cardiology), Director, Cardiac Arrhythmia Study Unit, Stanford University School of Medicine, Stanford, California
Recurrent Ventricular Tachycardia and Fibrillation: The Automatic Internal Defibrillator

RAYMOND TAILLEFER, M.D.

Associate Professor of Radiology and Nuclear Medicine, University of Montreal; Department of Nuclear Medicine, Hôtel-Dieu, Montreal, Quebec, Canada
Cricopharyngeal Dysfunction and Myotomy

TIMOTHY TAKARO, M.D.

Consulting Professor of Surgery, Duke University School of Medicine, Durham; Chief of Staff, Veterans Administration Medical Center, Asheville, North Carolina
Fungal Infection

KJELL THOR, M.D.

Staff, Ersta Hospital, Stockholm, Sweden
Hill Procedure for Gastroesophageal Reflux

ROBERT L. THURER, M.D.

Assistant Professor of Surgery, Harvard Medical School; Associate Cardiothoracic Surgeon, Beth Israel Hospital, Boston, Massachusetts
Blood Conservation

THOMAS R. TODD, M.D., F.R.C.S.(C)

Associate Professor, University of Toronto Faculty of Medicine, Department of Surgery; Acting Head, Division of Thoracic Surgery, Toronto General Hospital, Toronto, Ontario, Canada
The Respiratory Intensive Care Unit

EDWARD R. TOWNSEND, M.B., B.S., F.R.C.S.

Consultant Thoracic Surgeon, Harefield Hospital, Harefield, Uxbridge, England
Space Problems During and After Lung Resection

VICTOR F. TRASTEK, M.D.

Associate Professor of Surgery, Mayo Medical School; Consultant, Section of Thoracic and Cardiovascular Surgery, Mayo Clinic and Mayo Foundation, Rochester, Minnesota
Occult Neoplasia
Cervical and Thoracic Esophageal Diverticulum

J. KENT TRINKLE, M.D.

Professor and Head, Division of Cardiothoracic Surgery, University of Texas Health Science Center, San Antonio, Texas
Flail Chest and Pulmonary Contusion: Nonoperative Management

GEORGE A. TRUSLER, M.D., B.Sc.(Med), M.S., F.R.C.S.(C), F.A.C.S.

Professor of Surgery, University of Toronto Faculty of Medicine; Head, Division of Cardiovascular Surgery, The Hospital for Sick Children, Toronto, Ontario, Canada

Congenital Aortic Stenosis

KEVIN TURLEY, M.D.

Associate Professor of Surgery, University of California School of Medicine; Attending Cardiac Surgeon and Acting Chief, Division of Cardiothoracic Surgery, University of California Medical Center, San Francisco, California

Truncus Arteriosus

HAROLD C. URSCHEL Jr., M.D., LL.D.(Hon), D.Sc.(Hon)

Professor of Thoracic and Cardiovascular Surgery, Baylor University Medical Center and University of Texas Southwestern Medical School; Senior Attending in Cardiovascular and Thoracic Surgery, Baylor University Medical Center, Dallas, Texas

Sternal Fractures and Myocardial Contusions
Eventration and Plication

JOE R. UTLEY, M.D.

Clinical Professor, University of South Carolina School of Medicine, Columbia and Medical University of South Carolina College of Medicine, Charleston; Chief of Cardiac Surgery, Spartanburg Regional Medical Center, Spartanburg, South Carolina

Cardiopulmonary Bypass in the Adult

JOSEPH P. VACANTI, M.D.

Assistant Professor of Surgery, Harvard Medical School; Assistant Surgeon, The Children's Hospital, Boston, Massachusetts

Congenital Diaphragmatic Hernia
Lobar Emphysema

PETER VAN TRIGT, M.D.

Assistant Professor of Surgery, Duke University School of Medicine, Durham, North Carolina

Pulmonary Embolism

EDWARD D. VERRIER, M.D.

Assistant Professor of Surgery, University of California School of Medicine; Attending Surgeon, H.C. Moffitt Hospital and Chief, Cardiothoracic Surgery, San Francisco Veterans Administration Hospital, San Francisco, California

Secundum Atrial Septal Defects

LAURI VIRKKULA, M.D.

Associate Professor of Surgery, University of Helsinki; Thoracic Surgeon, Department of Thoracic and Cardiovascular Surgery, University Central Hospital, Helsinki, Finland

Omentoplasty for Bronchopleural Fistula

GUS J. VLAHAKES, M.D.

Assistant Professor of Surgery, Harvard Medical School; Assistant Surgeon, Massachusetts General Hospital, Boston, Massachusetts

Mediastinitis and Thoracic Space Infection
Tricuspid Valve Replacement
Primum Atrial Septal Defects

INGOLF VOGT-MOYKOPF, M.D.

Professor of Thoracic Surgery, University of Heidelberg; Medical Director, Rohrbach Hospital and Chief of Surgical Department, Clinic for Thoracic Medicine, Heidelberg, Federal Republic of Germany

Sleeve Lobectomy

JOHN C. WAIN Jr., M.D.

Instructor in Surgery, Harvard Medical School; Assistant in Surgery, Massachusetts General Hospital, Boston, Massachusetts

Benign and Low Grade Malignant Tumors
Anastomotic Leak

JOHN A. WALDHAUSEN, M.D.

John W. Oswald Professor of Surgery and Chairman, Department of Surgery, Pennsylvania State University College of Medicine, The Milton S. Hershey Medical Center, Hershey, Pennsylvania

Coarctation of the Aorta

ALBERT L. WALDO, M.D.

Walter H. Pritchard Professor of Cardiology, Professor of Medicine, and Professor of Biomedical Engineering, Case Western Reserve University School of Medicine; Staff Physician and Director, Adult Cardiac Electrophysiology, Division of Cardiology, University Hospitals of Cleveland, Cleveland, Ohio

Arrhythmias Following Open Heart Surgery: Role of Cardiac Pacing and Recording

WILLIAM H. WARREN, M.D.

Assistant Professor, Department of Cardiovascular-Thoracic Surgery, Rush Medical College of Rush University; Assistant Attending, Department of Cardiovascular-Thoracic Surgery, Rush-Presbyterian-St. Luke's Medical Center, Chicago, Illinois

Lateral Thoracotomy: Technique, Indications, and Complications

RONALD M. WEINTRAUB, M.D.

Associate Professor of Surgery, Harvard Medical School; Head, Division of Cardiothoracic Surgery, Beth Israel Hospital, Boston, Massachusetts

Selection of Patients for Coronary Artery Surgery

STEPHEN WESTABY, B.S., M.S., F.R.C.S.

Consultant Cardiothoracic Surgeon, John Radcliffe Hospital, Oxford, England

Space Problems During and After Lung Resection

BENSON R. WILCOX, M.D.

Professor of Surgery and Chief, Division of Cardiothoracic Surgery, University of North Carolina School of Medicine, Chapel Hill, North Carolina
Spontaneous Pneumothorax

EARLE W. WILKINS Jr., M.D.

Clinical Professor of Surgery, Harvard Medical School; Visiting Surgeon, Massachusetts General Hospital, Boston, Massachusetts
Thymus: Myasthenia Gravis and Thymoma
Mediastinal Tumor
Solitary Pulmonary Nodule
Malignant Tumor of the Lower Third of the Esophagus
Esophageal Replacement

WILLIAM G. WILLIAMS, M.D., F.R.C.S.(C)

Associate Professor of Surgery, University of Toronto Faculty of Medicine; Staff Surgeon, Department of Cardiovascular Surgery, The Hospital for Sick Children and Toronto General Hospital, Toronto, Ontario, Canada
Congenital Aortic Stenosis

WILLIS H. WILLIAMS, M.D.

Professor of Cardiothoracic Surgery, Emory University School of Medicine; Chief of Cardiothoracic Surgery, Henrietta Egleston Hospital for Children, Inc., Atlanta, Georgia
Pulmonary Valvar and Infundibular Stenosis

ROGER S. WILSON, M.D.

Associate Professor of Anaesthesia, Harvard Medical School; Anesthetist, Department of Anesthesia, Massachusetts General Hospital, Boston, Massachusetts
General Principles of Anesthesia and High Frequency Ventilation

WALTER G. WOLFE, M.D.

Professor of Surgery, Duke University School of Medicine, Durham, North Carolina
Pulmonary Embolism

WARREN M. ZAPOL, M.D.

Professor of Anaesthesia, Harvard Medical School; Anesthetist, Massachusetts General Hospital, Department of Anesthesia, Boston, Massachusetts
Adult Respiratory Distress Syndrome
Extracorporeal Membrane Oxygenation

GEORGE L. ZORN Jr., M.D.

Associate Professor of Surgery, University of Alabama School of Medicine, Birmingham, Alabama
Laser Techniques in Pulmonary Problems
Laser Techniques in Esophageal Problems

PREFACE

Current Therapy in Cardiothoracic Surgery is intended to be just what the title says. We offer an up-to-date guide to the treatment of cardiac and general thoracic surgical problems. To that goal we invited, importuned, and cajoled a broad panel of experts to describe succinctly and personally their views on management of each condition. Many of the authors are prominent, and all are actively and expertly involved in the care which they describe. We do not present a compendium of opinions, but have preferred to offer you authoritative statements by surgeons respected for their work in particular fields.

Current Therapy is meant to be useful. Emphasis is on the practical and often the technical, with additional pointers on work-up, postoperative management, and avoidance of pitfalls. The book is organized in multiple small sections so that the surgeon may expeditiously find specific information about a specific problem. The book does not pretend to be a mini-textbook of cardiothoracic surgery. It does not at all replace the surgeon's readings in the literature. This is intended as an authoritative guide to dependable methods of treatment of each condition enumerated. A small number of selected readings are included in most chapters.

We requested the authors to address the practicing cardiothoracic surgeon, who may be assumed to possess basic information and more. For this reason the editors do not believe that the limited number of illustrations will detract from the value of the book.

As this book is *current* therapy, we look forward to future editions that will reflect changes and evolution in the fields of cardiac and thoracic surgery. The material presented in this volume is, therefore, the state of the art at the time of this publication, but it will certainly change in the future. We sincerely solicit our readers' opinions, both general and specific, in order to improve future editions.

The editors are grateful to the many busy surgeons who contributed. We appreciate the encouragement given by Mr. Brian Decker, the publisher who envisioned this series.

Hermes C. Grillo, M.D.
W. Gerald Austen, M.D.
Earle W. Wilkins Jr., M.D.
Douglas J. Mathisen, M.D.
Gus J. Vlahakes, M.D.

CONTENTS

CONGENITAL ANOMALIES

THORACIC SURGERY | PRE- AND POSTOPERATIVE CARE

EVALUATION FOR PULMONARY RESECTION

DAVID J. KANAREK, M.D.

Surgical treatment of lung cancer remains the most effective form of therapy in properly selected cases. However, lung cancer frequently occurs in the setting of compromised pulmonary function, generally due to the presence of severe obstructive lung disease, although pulmonary fibrosis may also be the culprit (as in asbestosis). With increasing frequency, in many of these cases there has been previous resection for lung cancer. In addition, lung cancer is much more likely to occur in older individuals in whom other diseases, principally heart disease, may also be present. The evaluation of the patient with lung cancer for surgery therefore consists of establishing (1) whether the tumor is capable of being removed by surgery with a reasonable chance of cure; (2) the degree of further impairment that may be expected as a result of lung surgery; and (3) the effect of other disease conditions on the perioperative and postoperative course.

Impaired pulmonary function leads to the development of postoperative complications. Certain clinical features are associated with the development of atelectasis and postoperative infection. These include:

1. A history of cigarette smoking,
2. Obesity,
3. Chronic cough and sputum production,
4. A history of wheezing,
5. Any neuromuscular condition leading to pulmonary restriction,
6. Clinical findings, particularly prolonged exhalation time or wheezing, that demonstrate the presence of obstructive lung disease, and
7. A history of cor pulmonale.

Obstructive lung disease diagnosed by pulmonary function studies also correlates with the development of postoperative complications. These postoperative complications do not necessarily occur in direct proportion to the severity of the disease.

In 1971 Stein showed that preoperative diagnosis was important because preoperative therapy of obstructive lung disease reduced the incidence of postoperative problems from 71 to 23 percent. In addition, he showed that the hospital stay for such patients was markedly reduced. That same study also indicated that high abdominal and thoracic surgery had the greatest propensity for producing certain postoperative complications.

The complications that can be avoided by the use of careful observation of preoperative warning signals are infection, postoperative atelectasis, and respiratory failure. Some complications, such as a pneumothorax or pulmonary embolism, are not predictable by such tests. The possibility of their occurrence may be predicted from the presence of risk factors such as previous deep venous thrombosis or emboli, or multiple bullae on the x-ray film. Hence, a full history and physical examination are as important as pulmonary function studies.

A wide range of pulmonary function studies is available. No single pulmonary function test provides an overall evaluation of pulmonary function or cardiopulmonary integration. Table 1 lists the common tests and the important information each provides. Therefore, the choice regarding appropriate testing is made with respect to the clinical assessment of the patient and the findings on the chest x-ray film.

TABLE 1 Common Tests and the Important Information Each Provides

Test	*Measurement*
FEV_1, $FEV_1\%$	Flow rate
Vital capacity, maximal breathing capacity	Mass air displacement
Total lung capacity	Gas exchange volume
Diffusing capacity	Alveolocapillary membrane surface
Pco_2	Global ventilation
Po_2, A-aDO_2, V_D/V_T	Overall ventilation: blood flow matching
Regional function	Radioisotope scans
Pulmonary vascular system	Examination, electrocardiogram, catheterization
Exercise	Cardiopulmonary integration during stress
Respiratory center control	Response to hypercarbia, hypoxia

Since obstructive lung disease is the commonest problem, the initial test is a flow volume loop from which the FEV_1 (forced expiratory volume in 1 second), the vital capacity, and the peak flow rate can be obtained. The FEV_1 is a measurement of flow, i.e., how fast air can be moved; the vital capacity is a measurement of the volume of air that can be moved. The peak flow rate is an assessment of the potential strength of cough. It should be at least 25 percent of that predicted, about 120 L per minute preoperatively, since it will certainly be reduced below that value postoperatively. The FEV_1 as a percent of that predicted and the FEV_1/FVC (forced vital capacity) ratio are the best measurements of obstructive lung disease. The latter value serves as a correction for a reduction in FEV_1 due to restrictive disease, since the FEV_1 may be lowered by a reduction in flow or available volume. Broadly, values below 75 percent are abnormal and those below 55 percent represent severe obstructive lung disease.

Although these tests provide an accurate estimate of the severity of the obstructive lung disease, interpretation must go beyond the value alone. For example, individuals with the same FEV_1 may have a different exercise capacity and different arterial blood gas measurements. Several reasons account for the variability. First, an FEV_1 of 0.8 L represents a marked difference as a percent of that predicted in, for example, a small elderly woman versus a large younger male. Second, the pathology of obstructive lung disease consists of various mixtures of emphysema and chronic bronchitis with divergent effects on blood gases, lung compliance, and pulmonary vascular resistance. Third, other factors, such as left ventricular function and general physical condition, intrude on overall exercise tolerance. Hence, although the FEV_1 is the most important measurement to be taken into account when assessing an individual's ability to tolerate lung resection, it must be tempered by an assessment of the entire clinical condition.

An FEV_1 of 0.8 L has come to be a generally accepted lower limit of postoperative function that should not be exceeded except under exceptional circumstances. There are no controlled trials that have shown this to be a critical level. Rather, the figure has been chosen because below an FEV_1 of 0.8 L (1) there is a tendency to develop an elevated PCO_2, and (2) exercise tolerance is almost always severely impaired. In brief, there is little reserve capacity.

The most common method of predicting the postoperative FEV_1 is from a radionuclide scan, either the ventilation or perfusion scan providing similar information. The simplest formula for prediction is:

$$\text{predicted postoperative } FEV_1 = \text{preoperative } FEV_1 \times \text{percent of lung remaining after resection}$$

In practical terms, a ventilation or perfusion scan is obtained from which the number of counts representing the region of lung that will remain is expressed as a percentage of the total counts and multiplied by the preoperative FEV_1. A typical example might be a man with a left upper lobe carcinoma and a preoperative FEV_1 of 1.2 L who has 30 percent of his function in the lobe to be removed. By calculation (70/100 × 1.2 L), 0.84 L will be the postoperative function, just within the acceptable level. Split function studies are indicated when the preoperative FEV_1 is less than 2 L, even in the case of an intended lobectomy, since one can never be certain that pulmonary function is evenly distributed between the lungs. Inspection of the washout phase of ventilation scans performed during tidal ventilation rather than the full inspiration used for standard ventilation scans provides further sophisticated evidence of the relative distribution of ventilation. In patients with obstructive lung disease it is very important that studies be carried out after a full therapeutic regimen has been instituted. Patients may be changed from a high to a much lower risk category when reversible airway disease has been diagnosed and treated.

Arterial blood gas values are very important in the evaluation. An elevated PCO_2, in conjunction with obstructive lung disease, is an absolute contraindication to further resection unless it can be shown to relate to other factors, such as central hypoventilation or metabolic alkalosis. In these instances, provided that the PCO_2 is less than 50 mm Hg, lobar resection may be attempted. A low PO_2 is rarely found in the absence of severe obstructive lung disease, and there is almost always other disease present to be taken into account.

The diffusing capacity is very useful as a measurement of the available pulmonary vascular bed. Destruction of the vascular bed, such as in emphysema or interstitial fibrosis, reduces the diffusing capacity and manifests as a fall in PO_2 during exercise but is unlikely to affect the PO_2 at rest. A normal or even elevated diffusing capacity is found in asthma and chronic bronchitis, even when the FEV_1 is reduced to the same degree as in severe emphysema, since the parenchyma of the lung remains functional. A diffusing capacity below 50 percent of that predicted represents a severe loss of reserve capacity and serves as a warning of significant postoperative problems, such as difficulty in ventilator weaning and prolonged air leaks because of the diffuse emphysema.

Stair climbing is helpful in the overall evaluation of a patient's reserve and should always be a part of the clinical evaluation. Patients who climb stairs easily in the face of obstructive lung disease generally do better than patients who have little reserve capacity. However, when obstructive lung disease is severe, considerable caution should be exercised against overemphasizing the value of exertional capacity. Patients may exercise with surprisingly little dyspnea because they hypoventilate and allow the PCO_2 to rise during exercise. Such patients do not tolerate the stress of resection well.

In addition, the lung to be resected may play an important role during exercise, resulting in an unexpected loss of function following the resection. Therefore when a patient is apparently able to climb stairs well in the face of severe obstructive lung disease, it is advisable to perform exercise studies with evaluation of blood gases and a regional functional study to guard against surprises. Measurements of pulmonary vascular resistance are hardly ever required when the previous steps have been carried out. An evaluation of the literature suggests that measurements of pulmonary vascular resistance would be difficult to use preoperatively, since many patients with relatively high vascular resistances have survived surgery well, whereas those with relatively low resistances appear to have done poorly. It is unlikely that measurements of pulmonary artery pressure and pulmonary vascular resistance add information that provides prognostic significance beyond that already obtained from flow volume loops, arterial blood gas measurements, split function studies, and, occasionally, exercise studies. These statements are necessarily based upon anecdotal and personal experience, since properly controlled studies have not been nor are they likely to be performed.

Preoperative therapy consists of (1) bronchodilators, including the institution of corticosteroids when necessary, (2) evaluation of sputum samples, and (3) chest physical therapy. Intravenous aminophylline is the commonest drug used in the perioperative period, together with inhaled bronchodilators such as metaproterenol or albuterol. Corticosteroids are useful when there is a history of response to corticosteroid therapy or an insufficient response to bronchodilators has been obtained. Although surgeons are rightly concerned about steroids retarding healing in addition to their other side effects, corticosteroids may also make the difference between a reasonable versus a highly risky operation. A dose of 40 mg of prednisone daily is sufficient. Reduction of the volume of sputum and clearing of infection are the most important factors in the preoperative management. All patients must stop smoking at least 2 weeks before surgery. A preoperative course of antibiotics is indicated when sputum examination suggests infection. Chest physical therapy may be helpful in the preoperative preparation and in teaching patients what to expect postoperatively. Sulfamethoxazole-trimethoprim or ampicillin is generally the drug of choice in treating exacerbations of chronic bronchitis. The reliability of the patient is crucial in deciding whether these measures are suitable for outpatient or inpatient therapy.

Lung cancer also occurs in the age group in which ischemic heart disease is common. The evaluation of patients who have lung cancer must include a careful search for coronary artery disease. A history of angina, exertional dyspnea (particularly if there is insufficient obstructive lung disease to explain the symptom), previous episodes of pulmonary edema or congestive heart failure, a coronary artery bypass graft, and an enumeration of any cardiac drugs are important clues to assessing the presence of ischemic heart disease. Mitral and aortic valvular heart disease are also important although less common problems than ischemic heart disease. The physical examination includes a search for the presence of arrhythmias, cardiomegaly, a cardiac murmur or gallop, congestive heart failure, and vascular disease in the carotid arteries or the peripheral circulation. The chest x-ray film may show cardiomegaly, individual chamber enlargement, congestive heart failure, or the redistribution of blood vessels. An electrocardiogram to look for evidence of ischemic heart disease, arrhythmia, or ventricular hypertrophy is mandatory. The presence of any of the risk factors listed above requires either an exercise thallium scan or, when exercise is not feasible, a Persantine thallium scan to assess myocardial ischemia and regional wall motion as well as overall function. In exceptional cases, cardiac catheterization may also be required. At our institution, a combined cardiopulmonary technique has been developed whereby the cardiac scans are obtained during an exercise study at the same time as maximum oxygen uptake, minute ventilation, an exercise electrocardiogram, and arterial blood gas determinations to obtain a comprehensive picture of the role of the pulmonary and cardiac systems in influencing exercise performance, symptoms, and reserve capacity.

The management of ischemic heart disease consists of the application of vasodilators such as nitrates, calcium-channel blockers, and beta-blockers in various combinations. Any evidence of congestive heart failure should be actively treated with diuretics and digoxin when indicated. A pulmonary artery catheter is inserted preoperatively to measure the capillary wedge pressure and assist in managing any left ventricular dysfunction.

Using these techniques of successive concentration on the history, physical examination, x-ray examination, and functional studies, the cardiopulmonary systems can be intensively evaluated and appropriate management instituted for any dysfunction. Mortality and morbidity can be lowered and the risks of pneumonia, pulmonary emboli, respiratory failure, myocardial infarction, and congestive heart failure can be considerably reduced.

SUGGESTED READING

Bria WF, Kanarek DJ, Kazemi H. Prediction of postoperative pulmonary function following thoracic operation. Value of ventilation-perfusion scanning. J Thorac Cardiovasc Surg 1983; 86:186–192.

Gass GD, Olsen GN. Preoperative pulmonary function testing to predict postoperative morbidity and mortality. Chest 1986; 89:127–135.

Stein M, Cassara EL. Preoperative pulmonary evaluation and therapy for surgery patients. JAMA 1970; 211:787–790.

Tisi GM. Preoperative evaluation of pulmonary function: validity, indications and benefits. Am Rev Respir Dis 1979; 119:293–310.

THE RESPIRATORY INTENSIVE CARE UNIT

THOMAS R. TODD, M.D., F.R.C.S.(C)

Respiratory intensive care for the postoperative thoracic surgical patient involves the management of several organ systems and a thorough understanding of their interrelationships. In particular, the thoracic surgeon must realize the unique interdependence of hemodynamic and ventilatory functions that exist in each individual patient.

VENTILATION

Indications

There are several reasons why ventilation may be required in the postoperative period. These are listed in Table 1. The most obvious situations in which benefit from elective postoperative ventilation can be obtained are those where potential space problems exist, and complete expansion of the lungs is desirable. We routinely provide ventilation for 24 hours following decortication, particularly if the compliance of the underlying lung is decreased. Such is often the case in tuberculosis or when decortication is performed after several years of pulmonary entrapment. In such cases, elective mechanical ventilatory support may ensure full lung expansion and obliteration of potential pleural air space, even though accompanying peripheral bronchopleural fistulas may be aggravated. Likewise, following bullectomy for major bullous disease, the assurance of adequate expansion may lead to the closure of potential air spaces and the early cessation of postoperative bronchopleural fistulas. Prolonged operative procedures resulting in large fluid losses and excessive narcotic administration may warrant elective ventilatory support. The provision of ventilatory support also allows safe and efficient management of gas exchange while hemodynamics, analgesia, and other postoperative difficulties are corrected. In that regard, it is our common practice to provide overnight ventilation following esophagectomy.

TABLE 1 Indications for Postoperative Ventilation

Elective:
Potential space problems—decortication, major bullectomy
Prolonged anesthesia
Large fluid requirements with associated pulmonary injury
Hemodynamic instability
Myocardial ischemia and/or recent infarction
Respiratory Failure

Ventilation for acute respiratory failure is much more straightforward, since the abnormalities are clearly recognized. Before extubation in the intensive care unit or recovery room, each patient should have a trial of spontaneous breathing with continuous positive airway pressure (CPAP). The ability to sustain spontaneous ventilation and satisfactory gas exchange can be further assessed by the measurement of vital capacity and negative inspiratory force. The vital capacity should be at least 10 ml per kilogram body weight and the negative inspiratory force greater than or equal to 25 cm of water before proceeding with extubation.

Type of Ventilatory Support

At present in our intensive care unit we employ only two types of ventilators—a standard volume cycled machine and high frequency jet ventilation. The former is the mode of ventilation employed in 90 percent of our patients, but the latter is specifically indicated in the management of (1) large bronchopleural fistulas, (2) post-tracheal resection, (3) high airway pressures following pulmonary resection, (4) high airway pressures that result in hemodynamic instability, and (5) high oxygen requirements.

Specifics of Ventilatory Support

There are two major objectives in ventilatory management. First, one must strive for the lowest possible fraction of inspired oxygen (F_{IO_2}). There have been several experimental studies as well as considerable clinical experience to suggest that levels of inspired oxygen above 50 percent are deleterious. There are several methods by which this might be achieved. Positive end-expiratory pressure (PEEP) is the obvious first choice. PEEP increases functional residual capacity and moves the lung up the limb of the pressure volume hysteresis curve. Ventilation-perfusion matching is maximized, and the F_{IO_2} frequently can be lowered. There are several methods for evaluating the appropriateness of a given level of PEEP. At low levels of PEEP (< 10 cm of water), the ability to improve oxygenation is probably sufficient. The measurement of static pulmonary compliance is more accurate. In the end, however, the desired outcome is the maximization of oxygen transport, which is calculated by the following formula:

$$O_2 \text{ Trans} = (\text{Hgb} \times 1.34 \times O_2 \text{ Sat}) + PaO_2 \times .031) \times CO^\circ$$

where Hgb = hemoglobin; O_2 Sat = oxygen saturation; PaO_2 = partial pressure of arterial oxygen; CO° = cardiac output. The formula illustrates the small contribution of Po_2 to transport and emphasizes why the simple measurement of Po_2 is an insufficient method of evaluating PEEP therapy.

PEEP usually improves oxygenation. However, in cases of unilateral lung disease, it may prove detrimental. The increase in alveolar pressure is conducted to the pulmonary capillary more readily in the compliant normal lung than in the contralateral noncompliant or diseased lung. Thus pulmonary arterial flow may shift from the normal to the diseased lung, with a resultant fall in PaO_2. This is not routine, but increments in PEEP should be assessed with caution in situations of unilateral pneumonitis.

Diuresis is another maneuver that frequently results in an improvement in oxygenation and hence a lower FIO_2. The principle applies even in the face of pulmonary pathology other than high pressure pulmonary edema. Most cases of acute or chronic respiratory failure are accompanied by an increase in the permeability characteristics of the pulmonary capillary. This is particularly true in the adult respiratory distress syndrome (ARDS) but applies to a lesser extent in pneumonia and pulmonary aspiration.

In the clinical setting, we are clearly unable to influence anything but hydrostatic capillary pressure and capillary osmotic pressure. The latter may be affected by transfusion of plasma protein. However, if permeability is altered, it is controversial whether or not the alteration in osmotic pressure is effective for long. Thus the clinician should attempt to manage the patient at the lowest possible pulmonary wedge pressure that is compatible with maintenance of systemic perfusion. In our intensive care unit, we often employ low doses of dopamine (< 5 μg per kilogram per minute) in order to achieve systemic perfusion and yet obtain a low wedge pressure.

Changes in posture can produce immediate changes in oxygenation. This simply makes practical use of gravity, in assuring that the majority of pulmonary arterial flow is directed to the areas of lung that are best ventilated. When patients are placed in one position for extended periods of time, progressive atelectasis occurs in the dependent areas. These are also the areas receiving the largest proportion of pulmonary blood flow. Thus it may be important in cases of severe hypoxemia and high FIO_2 to frequently change the patient's posture from side to side or even from prone to supine. The latter is easily accomplished with a circle electric bed or Strykers frame. Likewise, pulmonary pathology may be unilateral, suggesting that "the good side" should be most dependent.

An additional means of decreasing FIO_2 is high frequency jet ventilation. In our recent experience with 67 hypoxemic patients, high frequency jet ventilation was successful in lowering FIO_2 in 48 of the total.

Last, one can attempt to direct pulmonary artery flow away from the maximal disease to better areas of ventilation-perfusion matching. This can be achieved by the use of a pulmonary artery balloon catheter (Fig. 1). This should be reserved for the most severe cases of hypoxemic respiratory failure as a lifesaving measure.

The second major objective in ventilatory management is the achievement of the lowest possible peak airway pressure (Table 2). This is important in order to prevent barotrauma and also to minimize hemodynamic compromise. The former is particularly important in thoracic surgical patients, in whom suture line integrity must be maintained. The maneuvers to obtain this end are simple. A decrease in tidal volume always decreases peak airway pressure. In order to maintain the same PCO_2, the rate must be increased to provide the same minute ventilation. Thus one must simply calculate current minute ventilation (rate $\times$ tidal volume), pick the desired lower tidal volume, and calculate the new rate. Normal inspiratory to expiratory time ratios vary but are frequently less than unity. An increase in inspired time lowers peak airway pressure and yet tends to maintain the same mean airway pressure—the latter being the most important determinant of proper ventilation-perfusion matching. Aspiration of the pleural space is obvious to all thoracic surgeons. It becomes particularly important if airway pressures are high.

Bronchoscopy should be employed in every case of high peak airway pressure to ensure the patency of the endotracheal tube and the distal airway. The easy passage of a suction catheter is not an assurance of an open airway. The use of an oximeter provides constant monitoring of satisfactory oxygen saturation during bronchoscopy.

Just as diuresis may improve oxygenation, likewise the decrease in lung water improves compliance and airway pressure. The role of high frequency jet ventilation to lower airway pressure is particularly pertinent in situa-

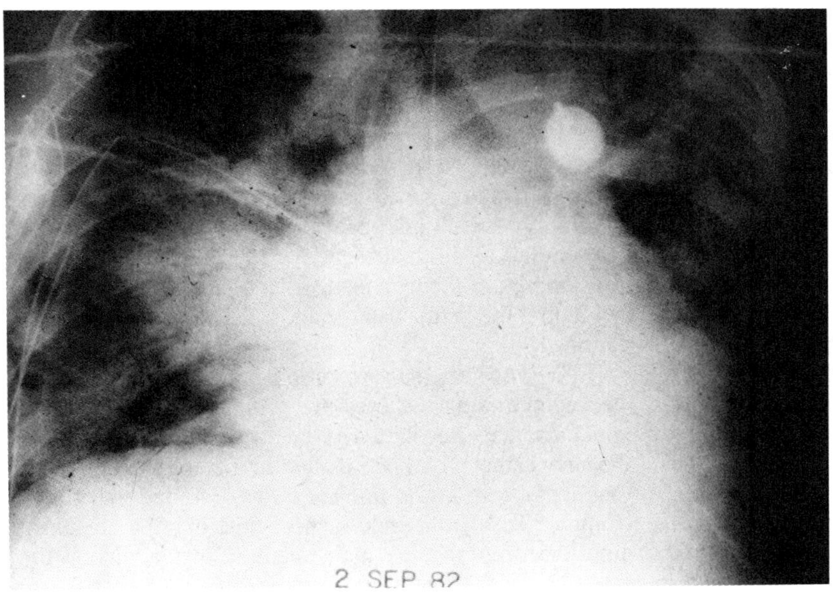

Figure 1 Chest x-ray with an indwelling pulmonary arterial line with a balloon inflated with contrast material. The balloon was inflated to divert blood from the left lung to the right.

TABLE 2 Achieving Lowest Peak Airway Pressure

1. Rate vs. volume
2. Alteration in inspiratory-expiratory ratio
3. Bronchoscopy
4. Diuresis
5. Evacuation of pleural space
6. High frequency ventilation

tions in which bronchial suture lines are at risk. We would not hesitate to employ jet ventilation in such cases when airway pressure exceeds 50 cm of water.

Weaning

There are basically two methods of weaning patients from mechanical ventilation: (1) CPAP or classic wean, and (2) IMV or intermittent mandatory ventilation.

Before weaning commences, it is important to recognize whether patients are actually ready for the weaning process. For the patient who has been electively ventilated, i.e., for less than 24 hours, the decision is straightforward. If the patient's vital capacity is greater than or equal to 10 ml per kilogram of body weight and the negative inspiratory force is greater than minus 25 cm of water, he or she can either be extubated immediately or, if there is still some concern about readiness, given a trial of CPAP for 1 or 2 hours.

The patient who has undergone prolonged ventilation for respiratory failure is somewhat different. Again, it is important to do an accurate assessment of the ventilatory function via a vital capacity and inspiratory force maneuver. However, one should also ensure that the FiO_2 is less than 50 percent, PEEP is less than or equal to 5 cm of water, and dead space to tidal volume ratio (V_D/V_T) is less than 0.65. The next decision to be made in this group of patients is whether to try a classic wean (CPAP) or an IMV wean. Proponents will be found for both types. My personal bias is to proceed initially with the classic wean in this group. It has been demonstrated that such patients frequently have discoordinate breathing patterns, which in our experience were overcome more readily during CPAP than IMV. In addition, CPAP weaning allows for rest periods with maximal work in-between. IMV places respiratory work on the patient constantly, and fatigue and subsequent failure may result. Nevertheless, there are patients who fail with CPAP and proceed nicely with IMV. The important point is that failure of one weaning system does not preclude an attempt at the other.

Two additional points should be made concerning classic weans. The first is that it is important to employ CPAP and not a T-piece. The absence of PEEP will be tolerated for short periods of time. However, with time, progressive atelectasis occurs, with accompanying increases in the alveoloarterial oxygen gradient and the work of breathing. Second, classic weans generally proceed slowly. Many patients fail to tolerate CPAP for 5 minutes but tolerate periods of 1 minute. Even when a 1-minute wean is poorly tolerated, it is important to persist, because it may take time for coordinate respiratory patterns to resume.

Extubation

At extubation, one must check to be certain that

1. The patient can protect his or her airway.
2. There is a leak around the endotracheal tube when the cuff is deflated.
3. The pharynx is aspirated of secretions.
4. The patient has a gag reflex and coughs on suctioning.

Failure to demonstrate a leak about the tube with the cuff deflated should alert the physician that significant upper airway obstruction exists. A useful method to be certain is to disconnect the patient from the ventilator, deflate the endotracheal tube cuff, and have him or her inspire maximally. At end-inspiration, occlude the tube with your thumb and instruct the patient to forcibly exhale. If exhalation takes place, then the tracheal lumen is adequate.

If there is no leak with the cuff deflated, we recommend transnasal bronchoscopy to assess the glottis and upper airway. Frequently the bronchoscope can be passed through the anterior commissure beside the endotracheal tube and down to the cuff. If that is possible, we proceed with extubation. If it is impossible, extubation should be withheld, and if no improvement is seen within 48 hours, a tracheostomy should be considered.

Postextubation stridor is not infrequent and can be handled with racemic epinephrine and heliox (30 percent oxygen, 70 percent helium) in the majority of cases. Immediate attempts at reintubation often make matters worse and should be withheld until a trial of epinephrine and heliox has been undertaken.

SPECIAL VENTILATORY CIRCUMSTANCES

Bronchopleural Fistula

There are several important points to note in the management of significant bronchopleural fistulas. In our institution, we do not hesitate to employ high frequency jet ventilation. In the absence of high frequency ventilation, there are other maneuvers available to the thoracic surgeon if the fistula is large and is interfering with ventilation.

First, one can place more saline in the drainage bottle, hence increasing the pressure against which the fistula must operate. Second, a bronchus blocker (Fig. 2) or Fogarty catheter can be inserted in the appropriate lobar segmental orifice and inflated to prevent the loss of tidal volume. Third, the endotracheal tube may be advanced into the contralateral main stem bronchus under the

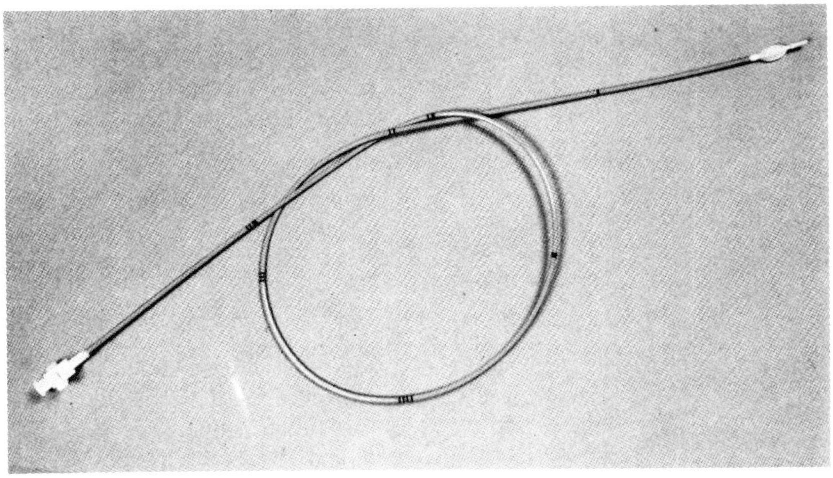

Figure 2 Bronchus blocker, which is inserted beside endotracheal tubes for the purposes of bronchial occlusion.

guidance of a flexible bronchoscope. Initially, one should place the bronchoscope as distally as possible to the desired side. The endotracheal tube is then advanced over the scope, the latter serving as a stent to guide the passage of the former. As the scope is withdrawn, the position of the tube is verified or adjusted. Last, in the case of postpneumonectomy fistulas, the pleural space can be opened and packed until jet ventilation becomes available.

Pain

Patients with thoracic incisions frequently have significant pain, which results in hypoventilation of the affected side and resultant ventilation-perfusion mismatching. Consequently, the liberal use of intravenous narcotic is recommended. If this is ineffective, consideration should be given to epidural morphine. There are specific opiate receptors on the dorsal columns that provide virtually complete analgesia if subjected to low doses of morphine in the epidural space. Constant nursing care is required to ensure that the narcotic does not rise to the brain stem and result in apnea. Bladder atony is common, but full skeletal muscle function persists and patients can be ambulatory. Intercostal blockade with Marcaine is occasionally feasible but requires the availability of physicians, and should not be employed in ventilated patients.

Pulmonary Sepsis

Postoperative pneumonitis is a significant complication for the thoracic patient. Sputum can be readily assessed, and antibiotics should be ordered based on the initial Gram's stain results. Subsequent alterations in antimicrobial therapy depend on the resultant culture and sensitivity findings. It is important to recognize that cultures of tracheal aspirates are frequently not representative of lower airway pathology. The availability of protected specimen brushes has overcome this difficulty. They are easy to use and provide accurate information about the offending organism. When employed quantitatively (which requires that the brush be immersed in a standard volume of sterile saline), they allow definite conclusions to be reached concerning the presence or absence of contamination from upper airway secretions.

The persistence of pulmonary infiltrates when protected specimen brushings are nondiagnostic warrants open lung biopsy. We do not favor transbronchial biopsy in ventilated patients due to the risk of pneumothorax and endobronchial hemorrhage.

One must be aware of the problems of prolonged antimicrobial therapy in intensive care unit patients, particularly the increasing incidence of fungemia. As a result, cultures should be reassessed frequently and consideration given to discontinuing all antibiotics after 2 weeks of therapy unless specific indications persist. One of the commonest errors of therapy seen in our institution is the continued use of antibiotics after the drainage of either intrathoracic or intra-abdominal abscesses. The latter group has the higher incidence of candidal sepsis.

When is Enough Enough?

Making the decision that recovery from respiratory failure is not possible is difficult. Following acute lung injury, our experience suggests that 12 weeks of relative stability are required before one can begin to seriously suggest that weaning cannot be successfully initiated. Although no measurements are absolute, several things should be considered before you conclude that you have failed.

A dead space to tidal volume ratio greater than 0.7 suggests an inability to wean. However, our experience has shown that the V_D/V_T may improve even after 12 weeks of relative stability. In addition, successful weaning with V_D/V_T ratios between 0.6 and 0.7 is possible.

A slow classic wean should have been attempted, as previously described. Once the patient has been successfully weaned during the day, cautious increases in spontaneous breathing should be made at either end of the nocturnal sleep time. In this regard, it is imperative to ensure that the patients sleep when not being weaned.

Occasionally the failure to wean is the result of hemodynamic derangements. Thus the wean should not be considered impossible until it has been attempted with a Swan-Ganz catheter in place. Only then are alterations in preload or afterload subsequent to the weaning process itself appreciated. Some are surprisingly found to have significant elevations of pulmonary artery pressure only during weaning. Pharmacologic decreases in pulmonary artery pressure with nitrates may result in a rapid and successful wean.

If respiratory failure persists in the face of diffuse pulmonary infiltrates that remain etiologically uncertain, a lung biopsy should be considered. This applies even if the original pathology was clearly pneumonitis, but adequate treatment has resulted in incomplete resolution. Surprising information is sometimes discovered.

Last, when all other efforts have failed, we try a course of corticosteroids in the hope that clinically inapparent small airway disease or early fibrosis may respond favorably. This is a completely unscientific approach, but in the patient with unisystem (i.e., pulmonary) failure it should be considered before concluding that the cessation of mechanical ventilatory support is impossible.

HEMODYNAMIC CONSIDERATIONS

Support of the circulation is paramount. Our maxim in the presence of respiratory failure is to keep preload as low as possible as long as the urine output is 50 ml per hour and inotropes are restricted to dopamine at 5 μg per kilogram per minute or less. As a result, careful hemodynamic monitoring is essential. The insertion of a Swan-Ganz catheter may greatly aid the decision-making as far as fluid requirements are concerned. Our indications for Swan-Ganz catheterization are listed in Table 3.

Swan-Ganz catheters are useful adjuncts in the evaluation of circulatory support but they are not innocuous. Arrhythmias are commonly encountered during insertion and usually consist of ventricular premature beats. The ectopics disappear once the catheter is withdrawn or advanced into the pulmonary artery. Their recurrence should be treated with 50 to 100 mg of intravenous lidocaine, following which a repeated attempt at insertion is permissible. The more worrisome arrhythmia is a bundle branch block. In our opinion a left bundle branch block is a relative contraindication to insertion of pulmonary artery lines. If it proves necessary to insert a Swan-Ganz catheter under such circumstances, a temporary pacemaker should be at the bedside.

TABLE 3 Indications for Swan-Ganz Catheterization

1. Pulmonary edema with normal central venous pressure
2. Hypotension with either normal or high central venous pressure
3. PEEP > 10 cm H_2O
4. Recent myocardial ischemia or infarction
5. Previous failed weaning attempt
6. Significant inotropic requirements

The surgeon is more familiar with pulmonary artery rupture from Swan-Ganz catheters. This usually occurs during insertion, generally in elderly patients or in those with pulmonary artery hypertension. The commonest site is the right middle lobe. The scenario is one of significant endobronchial hemorrhage upon inflation of the balloon. The bleeding usually stops, and morbidity and mortality are frequently related more to asphyxiation than to hemorrhage itself. Management consists of leaving the catheter in place, particularly if it has just been inserted and it is not known to which side it has migrated. Some have advocated reinflating the balloon to decrease hemorrhage. However, as noted, the bleeding almost always stops spontaneously, and uncontrolled reinflation of the balloon may extend the laceration in the pulmonary artery. The airway must be cleared, and this usually cannot be adequately performed with a flexible bronchoscope through the endotracheal tube; a rigid bronchoscope is required. Once airway patency is reestablished, the appropriate bronchus can be intubated with a bronchus blocker to protect the contralateral side in the event that hemorrhage recurs.

Since the bleeding usually stops spontaneously, the patient should survive as long as asphyxiation has been prevented. Thus a hiatus occurs when the surgeon must decide whether operative intervention is indicated. Our experience suggests that if there is no intraparenchymal hematoma and no hemothorax, conservative treatment will be uniformly successful. The presence of either of the above suggests that a thoracotomy should be undertaken.

Prevention of this complication demands that care be exercised on insertion of the catheter. It should not be advanced through the pulmonary valve, unless the balloon is inflated. Once the pulmonary artery has been entered, the catheter is advanced until the wedge position is reached. Upon deflation of the balloon, a pulmonary artery trace should return. The wedge pressure is checked a second time with reinflation, ensuring that at least 1 ml of air is required. If a wedge tracing is produced with less than 1 ml of air, the catheter should be withdrawn. This does not avoid all pulmonary artery ruptures, since catheter migration can occur even after satisfactory insertion.

The choice of fluid to be administered remains controversial in the surgical literature. It is apparent that colloid and crystalloid are equivalent as long as it is realized that approximately four to five times as much crystalloid as colloid must be given for the same hemodynamic benefit. Our preference, particularly in situations in which capillary permeability is likely to be altered, is to administer colloid. This results in less total administered volume and may result in preservation of intravascular fluid, although only transiently.

Following pneumonectomy or severe lung injury, significant increases in pulmonary artery pressure may ensue. Eventually they may result in hypotension due to right ventricular failure and consequent decreases in left ventricular loading. Although this is a difficult problem to manage, there are therapeutic alternatives. The use of sublingual (isosorbide dinitrate or Isordil) or intravenous nitrates may decrease pulmonary artery pressure sufficiently to improve left ventricular filling and cardiac output. If intravenous nitrates are to be used, one must be careful to ensure that preload is adequate in order to prevent systemic hypotension. A high left ventricular preload is usually required to overcome the deleterious hemodynamic effects of a high right ventricular afterload.

Patients with pre-existing coronary artery disease or those in whom myocardial ischemia develops postoperatively require careful monitoring. It is important to reduce the work of breathing and myocardial strain. As a result, weaning should be delayed until the patient is maximized and then should be undertaken with care, usually with a Swan-Ganz catheter in place.

NUTRITION

The provision of adequate nutritional support is an essential component of postoperative intensive care. Most patients can manage 48 hours without protein calorie supplementation, but it is imperative beyond that time. Fortunately, most thoracic patients can be managed with enteral feeding via nasogastric tubes or jejunostomy tubes inserted at the time of esophageal resection. Intravenous nutrition should be instituted immediately if enteral feeds either fail or are contraindicated.

It has been pointed out in the literature that caloric requirements are much less than suggested several years ago. We thus usually aim for approximately 2,000 to 2,400 calories per day in the noninfected patient, providing 1 g of protein per gram of nitrogen. Approximately 40 percent of calories are supplied with lipid. The septic patient usually receives 3,000 calories and 1.5 g of protein per gram of nitrogen. In the patient with respiratory and/or renal failure, fluid balance may be a problem during intravenous nutrition. Careful assessment of fluid gains and daily weights allows the addition of diuresis, dialysis, or ultrafiltration to properly balance the fluid requirements.

In the ventilated patient, it is important to remember that high glucose loads may sufficiently alter the respiratory quotient to the point that carbon dioxide production may exceed the ability of the patient to eliminate it without excessive respiratory work. Appropriate alternatives in the alimentation mixture are required.

SUGGESTED READING

Jackson RM. Pulmonary oxygen toxicity. Chest 1985; 88:900–905.

Morganroth ML, Morganroth JL, Nett LM, et al. Criteria for weaning from prolonged mechanical ventilation. Arch Int Med 1984; 144:1012–1016.

Shapiro BA, Cane RD, Harrison RA. Positive end-expiratory pressure therapy in adults with special reference to acute lung injury: a review of the literature and suggested clinical correlations. Crit Care Med 1984; 12:127–141.

Soutter I, Todd TR. Systemic candidiasis in a surgical intensive care unit. Can J Surg 1986; 29:197–199.

Stauffer JL, Olson DE, Petty TL. Complications and consequences of endotracheal intubation and tracheostomy. Am J Med 1981; 70:65–76.

Suter PM, Fairley B, Isenberg MD. Optimum end-expiratory airway pressure in patients with acute respiratory failure. N Engl J Med 1975; 292:284–289.

Vincent JL, Suter PM. Cardiopulmonary interactions in acute respiratory failure. In: Vincent JL, ed. Update in intensive care and emergency medicine. New York: Springer-Verlag, 1987.

POSTOPERATIVE PAIN CONTROL

NABIL EL-BAZ, M.D.

The recent advances and discoveries in pain research have led to the development and evaluation of new therapeutic modalities. Pain control after cardiothoracic surgery is achieved by blocking the transmission and processing of nociceptive impulses at the level of the brain, spinal cord, or peripheral nerves.

SYSTEMIC NARCOTICS

Narcotics bind to opiate receptors in the periaqueductal gray matter in brain stem, posterior thalamus, and amygdala, blocking central transmission and processing of pain. Intermittent injections of narcotics (intravenously, intramuscularly, and subcutaneously) remain the most widely used method for pain relief after cardiothoracic surgery. This method is easy to administer by nurses, has a high margin of safety, causes minimal cardiorespiratory impairment, and requires minimal monitoring and medical supervision. However, intermittent injections of narcotics are associated with inadequate pain relief in the majority of patients, fluctuation in serum narcotic levels, and alternating periods of analgesia and severe pain. Continuous intravenous infusion of narcotics and patient-controlled analgesia have been evaluated to improve postoperative analgesia and minimize serum narcotic fluctuations. These techniques require special delivery systems, intensive cardiorespiratory monitoring, and proper nursing and medical supervision for detection and treatment of central narcosis.

INTERCOSTAL NERVE BLOCK

Multiple intercostal nerve blocks with local anesthetics prevent the conduction of nociceptive impulses to the central nervous system and provide segmental postoperative analgesia. The intercostal nerve in the space used to enter the chest, the one above, the one below, and the one used for insertion of chest tubes should be blocked. These nerves, which lie in the subcostal groove of the rib of the same segment, should be injected under direct vision (transthoracic) before closing the chest. Bupivacaine (Marcaine) 0.5 percent with epinephrine 1:100,000 is injected near the nerve with a volume of 3 to 5 ml per nerve. This method provides short duration of analgesia, and repeated percutaneous injections are frequently required to provide continued pain relief. Repeated intercostal blocks are painful and increase the risk of infection, injury to the nerve and adjacent vessels, and pneumothorax, as well as the systemic toxicity of local anesthetics. Intercostal nerve block with neurolytic agents (phenol 6 percent, alcohol 100 percent) and cryocoagulation induce permanent or transient nerve degeneration and prolonged conduction anesthesia that is in excess of that needed for the postoperative period.

EPIDURAL SPINAL ANALGESIA

Epidural injection of local anesthetics in the thoracic region blocks the conduction of nociceptive impulses in the mixed spinal nerve and in the spinal cord. Intermittent epidural injection of 5 ml of bupivacaine (Marcaine) 0.5 percent, or continuous epidural infusion of 7 to 10 ml per hour, provides effective segmental analgesia after cardiothoracic surgery. However, this use of local anesthetics is associated with a high incidence of bradycardia and hypotension, numbness and weakness of the arms, and urinary retention. Epidural injection of morphine, 5 mg per 5 ml, provides segmental postoperative analgesia without alteration of neuronal conduction in mixed spinal nerves. Epidural morphine analgesia is the result of selective binding of morphine to opiate receptors in the substantia gelatinosa in posterior spinal gray matter, causing selective synaptic blockade of nociceptive impulses. Epidural injections of high doses of morphine, 2 to 10 mg, are associated with a high serum morphine level, causing a high incidence of nausea, vomiting, itching, urinary retention, central narcosis, and, occasionally, respiratory depression. The alternative use of continuous epidural infusion of a low dose of morphine, 0.1 mg per hour, achieves effective postoperative analgesia with minimal side effects. This low dose of morphine achieves effective blockade of opiate nociceptive receptors and is associated with undetectable morphine levels in blood and a low incidence of nausea, vomiting, and itching.

PREFERRED APPROACH

We routinely use a continuous epidural infusion of meperidine (Demerol), 2 mg in 2 ml of 2 percent lidocaine per hour, for pain relief after thoracic surgery. This technique is not used in patients with neurologic disorders, coagulation abnormalities, back infection, and tumors involving the vertebrae. We prefer to place the epidural catheter near spinal segment T5 preoperatively to allow for early institution of epidural infusion. The epidural solution is prepared in the operating room pharmacy by mixing 1 ml of meperidine 100 mg with 99 ml of lidocaine 2 percent (total 100 ml). Epidural infusion is used intraoperatively and postoperatively for 3 days at a fixed rate of 2 ml per hour through a volumetric infusion pump (IMED).

MECHANISM OF ACTION

Meperidine binds to opiate receptors in laminae I, II, III, and V of the posterior spinal gray matter. This presynaptic binding prevents the release of neurotransmitters, thus blocking the synaptic conduction of nociceptive stimuli. The other afferent nociceptive fibers that do not synapse in the posterior horn are blocked by lidocaine. The low dose and volume of lidocaine block neuronal conduction in the small nociceptive delta A and C fibers, potentiating the analgesia achieved with meperidine. Continuous infusion of small doses of meperidine and lidocaine avoids the problems associated with epidural injections of high doses of local anesthetics and narcotics.

CLINICAL EXPERIENCE

Continuous epidural infusion of meperidine-lidocaine achieves effective postoperative analgesia in 90 percent of our patients. Inadequate pain relief is probably the result of misplacement of the catheter or nociceptive transmission through alternative pathways. This method of analgesia is associated with a low incidence of nausea, vomiting, and itching but does cause urinary retention in all patients. This method of analgesia also requires occasional supplementation with intravenous narcotics, which are made available at the request of the patient. Thoracic epidurals are technically difficult to perform and should be done by an experienced anesthesiologist in order to minimize the risk of neurologic sequelae. This method of analgesia has proved safe, in our hands, and provides a specific approach to the problems of postoperative pain.

SUGGESTED READING

Bromage PR, Campores E, Chestnut D. Epidural narcotics for postoperative analgesia. Anesth Analg 1980; 59:473–480.

El-Baz N, Faber LP, Jensik RJ. Continuous epidural infusion of morphine for treatment of pain after thoracic surgery. Anesth Analg 1984; 63:757–764.

Rawal IV, Sjostrand UH, Dahlstrom B, et al. Epidural morphine for postoperative pain relief: a comparative study with intramuscular narcotic and intercostal nerve block. Anesth Analg 1982; 61:93–98.

Staren ED, Cullen ML. Epidural catheter analgesia for the management of postoperative pain. J Surg Gynecol Obstet 1986; 162:389–404.

Yaksh TL. Spinal opiate analgesia: characteristics and principles of action. Pain 1981; 11:293–346.

ADULT RESPIRATORY DISTRESS SYNDROME

WARREN M. ZAPOL, M.D.

DIAGNOSIS

Adult respiratory distress syndrome (ARDS) is a severe form of acute respiratory failure characterized by diffuse and bilateral pulmonary inflammation. The syndrome is easy to diagnose when it is acute and severe, with diffuse bilateral chest infiltrates seen radiologically and severe hypoxemia (PaO_2 less than 50 mm Hg at FIO_2 1.0) caused by a right-to-left intrapulmonary shunt. Other characteristics are reduced lung compliance and mild pulmonary arterial hypertension (mean pulmonary artery pressure [PAP] near 30 mm Hg) with a pulmonary capillary wedge pressure (PCWP) below 18 mm Hg.

A milder form of ARDS may develop in a large number of patients who have minor inflammatory lung lesions, fever, leukocytosis, and panlobar infiltrates that requires lower FIO_2 ventilation (0.5 to 0.8). Such patients should be observed closely, examined, and treated for possible causes of ARDS. A list of causes of ARDS appears in Table 1.

ARDS must be differentiated from congestive heart failure as well as from postoperative atelectasis; the latter is a different type of acute respiratory failure without pulmonary inflammation that responds readily to chest physiotherapy, postural drainage, suctioning, and, when necessary, mechanical ventilation with positive end-expiratory pressure (PEEP).

Sepsis

The physician must be vigilant whenever a potential cause of acute lung injury is present in the patient. The most common cause of ARDS after surgery is sepsis. Thus, any patient with culture-proven septicemia, a septic focus, or a septic syndrome is at high risk for developing diffuse inflammatory lung injury. A septic syndrome can occur with or without a proven septic focus (e.g., abscess, peritonitis, mediastinitis) and is diagnosed by the coexistence of several of the following systemic signs or symptoms: fever, leukocytosis or leukopenia, and the characteristic hemodynamic alterations of an increased cardiac output and a reduced systemic vascular resistance. These hemodynamic changes in themselves can provide sufficient reason to obtain all the appropriate cultures (blood, tracheal aspirate, urine, and wounds or drains) and to commence antibiotic therapy in patients with acute respiratory failure.

Once a presumptive diagnosis of acute respiratory failure caused by sepsis is made, the septic focus must be sought. Beginning with a thorough physical examination, the intensive care unit physician must examine and take x-ray films of the sinuses for evidence of sinusitis caused by nasotracheal intubation and search for a pharyngeal abscess or other complication of oral trauma. The abdo-

TABLE 1 Mechanisms of Postoperative Acute Lung Injury

Injury	*Mechanism*
Noninflammatory Acute Respiratory Failure	
Atelectasis	Airway occlusion, pulmonary compression, alveolar gas absorption and collapse
Inflammatory ARDS	
Lung Trauma	Direct injury to lung cells. Usually deceleration injury or crushing, intrapulmonary hemorrhage
Bacterial-viral pneumonia	Inflammatory edema due to direct alveolar and/or capillary cell injury
Endotoxemia-bacteremia	Increased capillary permeability, endothelial cell death, secondary mediator release by white cells, e.g., free radicals
Toxic oxygen breathing	Direct and indirect lung injury
Aspiration pneumonia	Acid burn of lung tissue, obstruction of airways by aspirated particles and bacteria
Fat embolism	Following skeletal trauma or orthopedic surgery, free fatty acids cause endothelial injury and pulmonary vascular occlusion
Massive transfusions	Leukocyte and platelet aggregates occlude vessels, probably prevented by fine pore filtration
Immunologic reactions	Drug hypersensitivity, anaphylaxis (e.g., heparin-protamine, antibiotics), an acute allergic vasculitis
Microembolization	Diffuse endothelial cell damage, occlusion of lung vessels, mediator release (serotonin, fibrin peptides)

men is a common locus of postoperative sepsis, but the drugs employed to allow mechanical ventilation (narcotics, sedatives, and neuromuscular blocking agents) often obscure physical findings. Occasionally the physician may need to withhold these drugs in order to thoroughly examine the abdomen. Either repeated portable ultrasonographic study or computed tomographic (CT) scanning may be required to diagnose abscesses, fluid accumulation, or acute acalculous cholecystitis. If sepsis is not discovered in this way, and all the other myriad causes have been ruled out (e.g., phlebitis, endocarditis), and if bacterial or viral pneumonia is not found to be the cause of acute lung disease, then the abdomen remains a likely source of sepsis, and an exploratory laparotomy must be considered. This decision is based upon the clinical dictum that an undrained source of sepsis can cause severe ARDS remediable only by removing the septic source. Few triumphs of surgical intensive care surpass that of draining a covert abdominal abscess and reversing severe ARDS. The physician is urged to find the septic source as quickly as possible, as systemic sepsis can also injure the kidneys, causing acute renal failure, and can damage other organs such as the liver. Indeed, it it not unusual for a patient to overcome septic ARDS once an abscess is drained and later succumb to multiple organ failure, often renal and hepatic.

Lung Contusion

Many trauma patients have acutely injured lungs, but few develop ARDS. Lung contusion usually produces local hemorrhage and pulmonary thrombosis. The majority of lung contusions improve rapidly after the tracheobronchial tree is cleared of blood and the patient is mechanically ventilated. Transpulmonary shunting is an uncommon problem if fat embolism does not occur.

Aspiration Pneumonia

Aspiration pneumonia is associated with high morbidity and mortality rates. It is a frequent diagnosis because some element of aspiration probably complicates most post-traumatic acute respiratory failure patients. Common after an alcoholic binge, a motor vehicle accident, head trauma with unconsciousness, and other orthopedic or abdominal trauma, aspiration also can occur accidentally during anesthetic induction or termination. Perhaps the most malignant aspiration syndromes are those associated with aspirating large quantities of highly acid gastric juice, causing rapid coagulative necrosis of lung tissue in almost any lung lobe, depending upon the patient's position. Immediate bronchoscopy is indicated to suction any food or other particles from large airways and to culture the aspirate. Although there is no proven value to administering antibiotic or corticosteroid therapy after a patient has aspirated acid gastric juice, strong evidence supports antibiotic therapy for aspiration of grossly infected matter (pus or feces) in order to prevent pneumonia. Following a major aspiration, the trachea should always be intubated and cleared, mechanical ventilation instituted, gas exchange measured, and chest films taken. If the radiologic findings clear rapidly and gas exchange is not impaired, tracheal extubation is imminent. If, however, there is progressive radiographic infiltration and deterioration of gas exchange, mechanical ventilation with PEEP will optimize gas exchange.

Nosocomial Pneumonia

Although it is beyond the scope of this chapter to deal in depth with the differential diagnosis and treatment of pneumonia, a few salient points require mention. All patients develop bacterial colonization of the upper respiratory tract after several days of tracheal intubation. The presence of these bacteria, usually gram-negative rods, often leads to pneumonia. Bacterial pneumonia occurs in 5 to 40 percent of postsurgical cases. The fatality rate varies with the pathogen and may be as high as 70 percent (as with *Pseudomonas aeruginosa*).

The intensive care unit physician must watch for large concentrations of microorganisms invading the distal lung and then must treat the responsible organism. This may not be easy; it is often difficult to diagnose a lower respiratory tract pneumonia in the presence of upper airway colonization, since fever and leukocytosis, both common signs of pneumonia, can follow surgery and atelectasis without pneumonia. One method to selectively sample bacteria from distal lung regions is to use a protected specimen brush culture, but the results of such cultures are often false and negative. Because of the treacherous nature of hospital-acquired pneumonia, the intensive care unit physician should first culture specimens from and then treat with specific antibiotics postsurgical patients who develop new chest infiltrates and whose Gram stain of tracheal aspirate shows a predominance of intra- and extracellular microorganisms and polymorphonuclear cells.

THERAPY OF ARDS

In brief, the therapy of ARDS requires the following:

Mechanical Ventilation with PEEP. This is done to increase the functional residual capacity, thereby recruiting collapsed lung and hopefully reducing the right-to-left shunt. Endotracheal intubation with a low pressure cuff is required. Sedation, muscle paralysis, and possibly hypothermia can be added in the severest cases. Increasing PEEP levels up to 20 to 30 cm H_2O may be necessary in severe hypoxemia.

Hemodynamic Monitoring. Usually, a Swan-Ganz catheter is placed in severe ARDS patients to measure the PCWP and PAP. Maintaining an adequate cardiac output at the lowest possible PCWP is the best strategy for minimizing the microvascular force that favors lung fluid filtration. If the PAP rises markedly because of an elevated pulmonary vascular resistance it is a poor sign, suggesting destruction of the pulmonary vasculature. Cardiac output must be measured frequently, and sufficient flow must be provided to the kidneys, liver, and brain; if necessary, cardiotonics should be infused. Renal function must be maintained. Death following ARDS most often results from multiple organ failure with kidney and hepatic failure, diffuse intravascular coagulation, and coma. Prevention is vital, because at this time it is not known how to effectively treat this syndrome of multi-organ failure.

Finding and Removing Any Source of Sepsis. If the cause of ARDS is septicemia, the septic source must be found and drained. Only then can the patient survive this syndrome. Appropriate antibiotics must then be delivered at correct dosages.

Effective General Support Measures. Chest physiotherapy and frequent suctioning are vital to prevent superinfection and atelectasis. Water balance must be maintained and, if necessary, excessive fluid removed with diuretics. Nutrition should be provided to allow immune systems to combat infection and to allow lung repair.

SUGGESTED READING

Higuchi JH, Johanson WG Jr. Colonization and bronchopulmonary infection. Clin Chest Med 1982; 3:133–142.

Hudson LD. Causes of the adult respiratory distress syndrome. Clinical recognition. Clin Chest Med 1982; 3:195–212.

Rajagopalan B, Lowenstein E, Zapol W. Cardiac function in the adult respiratory distress syndrome. In: Zapol W, Falke K, eds. Acute respiratory failure. New York: Marcel Dekker, 1985:555.

Rie MA, Wilson RS. Acute respiratory failure. In: Tinker J, Rapin M, eds. Care of the critically ill patient. New York: Springer-Verlag, 1983:311.

Zapol WM, Snider MT, Rie MA, Frikker M, Quinn DA. Pulmonary circulation during adult respiratory distress syndrome. In: Zapol W, Falke K, eds. Acute respiratory failure. New York: Dekker, 1985:241.

RADIOLOGIC ASSESSMENT

THERESA C. McLOUD, M.D.

Three common clinical problems in the thoracic patient require radiologic imaging: (1) mediastinal masses; (2) the staging of bronchogenic carcinoma; and (3) the solitary pulmonary nodule. With each situation, the choice and sequence of imaging studies, the value of such studies in diagnosis and preoperative management, and the use of radiologic interventional techniques, particularly percutaneous needle biopsy, will be discussed.

THE MEDIASTINUM

Computed tomography (CT) is the imaging method of choice in the evaluation of mediastinal lesions. The standard chest roentgenogram is relatively inexpensive and universally available and continues to serve as the initial radiologic examination in patients with suspected chest disease. Indeed, most mediastinal abnormalities are originally detected on the standard chest roentgenogram. CT is particularly useful as a supplemental technique that allows both accurate localization and characterization of pathologic processes within the mediastinum.

Generally, CT has supplanted other diagnostic imaging procedures previously used in the study of mediastinal lesions, including conventional tomography, radionuclide scans, and angiographic procedures such as cavography, pulmonary arteriography, and aortography. However, the barium-filled esophagus is still a good marker of disease in the mediastinum. A barium esophagogram should be obtained whenever a primary esophageal lesion is suspected.

CT of the mediastinum should be performed in suspended inspiration, that is, at total lung capacity. It is preferable to obtain 10-mm thick sections without any interval gaps. We recommend performing a standard CT without contrast as the initial step in the evaluation of the mediastinum. If a vascular lesion such as an aneurysm is suspected, then contrast should be administered in the bolus form in the amount of approximately 80 to 100 cc. Rapid dynamic scanning through the lesion should then be obtained. The contrast material is best delivered with a power injector at an injection rate of 2 cc per second. If this is not available, a forceful hand injection may be satisfactory.

In regard to characterizing mediastinal lesions, CT often permits a definitive noninvasive diagnosis by determination of relative attenuation values. CT numbers are precise enough to permit rapid identification of air, fat, serous fluid, and calcium within suspicious tissues. Lesions that contain homogeneous fatty tissue with attenuation values in the range of −80 to −160 Hounsfield units are invariably benign. They include such entities as lipomas, pericardial fat pads, and lipomatous herniations through the esophageal foramen or foramen of Morgagni or Bochdalek. In such instances, the CT diagnosis is usually conclusive, and surgery is not required. Although some other tumors in the mediastinum contain fat, such as liposarcomas, teratomas, and thymolipomas, they appear inhomogeneous on CT scanning. Some benign cysts in the mediastinum, such as pericardial cysts, can also be diagnosed confidently on CT scans. Most pericardial cysts are of near water equivalent density and have a Hounsfield number very close to zero. However, most bronchogenic cysts are filled with proteinaceous material and the attenuation value is higher, often close to that of solid tumors.

Other benign mediastinal masses that may be diagnosed confidently with CT scanning are mediastinal goiters. They are usually found in a paratracheal location, although occasionally they can be directly substernal or located posterior to the trachea. Because the thyroid gland concentrates iodine, such masses usually appear dense (higher than 80 Hounsfield units) on CT. They are almost always contiguous with the cervical thyroid gland and may demonstrate areas of calcification and of low attenuation that correspond to colloid cysts. Finally, they show evidence of marked and prolonged enhancement after intravenous administration of contrast material.

Most malignant mediastinal tumors are of soft tissue density. The CT findings are usually not diagnostic, but CT may be of value in determining the extent and origin of a mass and its relationship to other mediastinal structures. Invasion of surrounding mediastinal fat and of other structures in the mediastinum, the pleura, the pericardium, and the adjacent lung can be demonstrated.

Another common radiologic abnormality detected on the standard chest roentgenogram is a nonspecific widening of the mediastinum. This may be related to a normal variant, such as abundant fat deposition in an obese patient or possibly vascular tortuosity in the elderly patient. However, it may also be caused by vascular lesions, such as aneurysms, neoplasms, or diffuse adenopathy. CT can define the precise cause of such mediastinal widening, and the necessity for further invasive procedures, such as mediastinoscopy or aortography, may be avoided.

Aneurysms are easily diagnosable by CT, often without the need for angiography. The CT features of aneurysms include both a fine rim of calcification at the periphery of the lesion and a substantial increase in attenuation value following injection of a bolus of contrast material. Solid mediastinal lesions do not enhance to the same degree as aneurysms. If an aneurysm is almost entirely filled with thrombus, it may not enhance, although a small jet of contrast can usually be identified in the region of the neck of the aneurysm. If surgical resection of an aneurysm is necessary, then aortography may be required for preoperative planning. CT evaluation of aortic dissection should include dynamic scanning of at least three levels of the aorta, i.e., the ascending aorta, aortic arch, and descending aorta. CT can often identify both the true and false lumina as well as the intimal flap separating them. False-negative CT examinations sometimes occur when the false lumen is completely thrombosed. In such situations, a dissection cannot be distinguished from a fusiform aneurysm with extensive mural thrombus. If the dissection is of type B, that is, distal to the subclavian artery, CT may be the only procedure necessary for both diagnosis and follow-up. Type A dissections involving the entire aorta or the ascending aorta, aortic root, and aortic arch may require angiography prior to surgical management in order to assess involvement of branch vessels and the exact determination of the sites of intimal tear and re-entry.

STAGING OF BRONCHOGENIC CARCINOMA

Two major imaging studies are used in staging lung carcinoma, plain roentgenograms and CT. A bronchogenic carcinoma often is first suspected on standard chest roentgenograms. Occasionally the extent of tumor can be assessed accurately on standard roentgenograms, allowing invasive diagnostic or staging procedures such as bronchoscopy and mediastinoscopy to be performed without further radiologic studies. However, in most cases, an additional imaging procedure, namely, CT scanning, is required. CT is used for staging local disease, that is, determining the presence of mediastinal lymph node metastases, direct mediastinal invasion, and chest wall involvement. Radionuclide imaging can be helpful in detecting distant metastases to bone or liver, but such studies are not generally obtained unless symptoms or laboratory abnormalities suggest metastases. Some exceptions to this may be made, depending upon the histologic type of the tumor, its size, and whether it is located centrally or peripherally.

When CT is performed in the patient with lung cancer, the radiologist attempts not only to stage the tumor with reference to the TNM (tumor, nodes, and metastases) classification but also to determine its extent. The anatomic extent of the tumor can indicate whether or not the lesion is surgically resectable and to some degree what surgical procedure is required. This information is of importance in planning therapy.

Generally, tumors are considered unresectable if they are classified as T_3, N_2, or M_1. However, there are exceptions to this generalization. Tumors involving the chest wall that are classified as T_3 may successfully be resected if a lobectomy and chest wall resection are performed. In addition, selected tumors involving the carina may be successfully resected with new surgical techniques, provided there is no evidence of mediastinal metastases.

T_1 Lesions. T_1 lesions are peripheral lesions less than 3 cm in diameter that are limited to the lung. In such cases it is controversial whether radiologic staging should be performed. Often surgical staging, such as mediastinoscopy, is not required because of the low prevalence of mediastinal nodal metastases. The efficacy of CT scanning in such lesions for staging purposes remains an open question.

T_3 Lesions. A primary tumor is considered to be T_3 if it has invaded extrapulmonary structures such as the parietal pleura, chest wall, mediastinum and its contents, pericardium, or diaphragm, or if it results in a pleural effusion. Tumors involving a main bronchus less than 2 cm from the carina are also included in this category.

Direct Invasion of the Chest Wall. Occasionally chest wall invasion can be detected on standard chest roentgenograms when there is obvious rib destruction. The CT diagnosis of chest wall invasion is not very accurate, although its sensitivity is better than that of standard roentgenograms. Although radiologic signs of chest wall invasion on CT scanning have been described, such as the presence of obtuse angles between the mass and the pleura, increased density of extrapleural fat, and rib destruction, none of these findings has proved to be of great value. In one study, the overall accuracy of CT in regard to chest wall and parietal pleural involvement was only 39 percent. It appears that the presence of local chest pain is a much more sensitive and specific indicator of chest wall invasion. However, CT can be particularly useful in the evaluation of superior sulcus carcinomas. CT evidence of destruction of the vertebral bodies precludes surgical resection.

Mediastinal Invasion. The demonstration of tumor mass in contiguity with the mediastinal pleura or thickening of the mediastinal pleura on CT scanning does not necessarily indicate mediastinal invasion. However, direct interdigitations of tumor with mediastinal fat certainly suggest that mediastinal extension is present. In such patients, mediastinoscopy or mediastinal biopsy should be performed prior to an attempt at surgical cure. On standard x-ray films elevation of a hemidiaphragm may suggest phrenic nerve paralysis. This can be confirmed by fluoroscopy.

Pleural Effusion. Pleural effusions in patients with bronchogenic carcinoma can usually be diagnosed readily on standard roentgenograms. However, CT may show small effusions that are not readily apparent on standard films. Although all patients who have pleural effusions with bronchogenic carcinoma have a poor prognosis, only those patients in whom tumor cells can be demonstrated in the pleural fluid are considered to have unresectable disease.

Central Bronchial Lesions. Either plain roentgenograms or CT scans can be used to demonstrate the relationship of a proximal tumor mass to a main bronchus, carina, or trachea. However, we personally prefer the use of conventional tomography in both the anteroposterior and lateral planes to demonstrate such involvement. Because of the orientation of the tracheobronchial tree, imaging in the coronal or sagittal plane is preferable to the cross-sectional imaging of CT.

N_2 Lesions. Tumors that have spread to involve mediastinal lymph nodes are classified as N_2 and are generally considered unresectable. If enlarged mediastinal nodes are detectable on standard posteroanterior and lateral chest roentgenograms, a CT scan is usually not required. In such instances, surgical staging with mediastinoscopy should be performed to confirm the presence of mediastinal nodal metastases. However, plain x-ray films are relatively insensitive in the detection of mediastinal adenopathy. Most patients, therefore, require CT scanning. Lymph nodes larger than 1 cm are usually considered abnormal. However, large mediastinal nodes in patients with bronchogenic carcinoma are not always involved by tumor; reactive lymph node enlargement in the mediastinum is common. There are a number of studies evaluating the accuracy of CT in diagnosing mediastinal nodal metastases from bronchogenic carcinoma. These studies have varying results and cannot easily be compared because of different size criteria used to assess abnormal nodes, varying mediastinal mapping techniques, and different surgical methods for confirming or ruling out the presence of lymph node metastases (i.e., mediastinoscopy, palpation, total nodal dissection). Generally speaking, the larger the diameter used to distinguish malignant from benign nodes, the more specific but less sensitive CT becomes in detecting metastases. On the other hand, the use of a small node diameter increases sensitivity but at the expense of specificity. When the mediastinum is carefully explored surgically and all nodes are submitted for histologic study, the sensitivity of CT is lower than when the mediastinum is evaluated only by mediastinoscopy or palpation at surgery. Despite these problems, CT can be quite helpful in staging malignant disease in the mediastinum. Although it cannot be considered accurate enough to determine with certainty that mediastinal lymph nodes are or are not involved by tumor, it can provide information of value in guiding therapy and invasive diagnostic procedures. If the criterion of normal lymph node size is 1 cm or less, then metastases to mediastinal nodes larger than 1 cm can be diagnosed with an accuracy of 80 to 90 percent. Many authors suggest that mediastinoscopy is not necessary if the CT scan shows no evidence of adenopathy. Although some patients in this group will be found to have microscopic intranodal metastases at surgery, the vast majority of such tumors are resectable. Therefore, CT is useful in predicting surgical resectability. Nodes larger than 1 cm cannot be considered to contain metastatic disease in all instances. Many such nodes are hyperplastic and are seen in the setting of obstructive pneumonitis. In the presence of enlarged nodes, a surgical staging procedure, either mediastinoscopy or anterior mediastinotomy, is required.

A word should be said about alternatives to surgical staging of mediastinal lymph nodes. In addition to mediastinoscopy, such nodes can also be staged with other procedures that do not require general anesthesia. The advent of CT scanning has made it possible to approach many nodes by fine needle percutaneous biopsy. Clear visualization of mediastinal vessels allows for safe biopsy of these lesions. A diagnostic yield in the range of 85 to 95 percent can be obtained in those enlarged nodes that contain metastatic tumor. Biopsy of mediastinal nodes can also be achieved transtracheally or through the carina utilizing the Wang needle during bronchoscopy. CT scanning is recommended prior to Wang needle biopsy to define the exact site of enlarged nodes.

M_1 Lesions. Most radiologists include the adrenal glands as part of the routine CT scanning for staging bronchogenic carcinoma. The adrenal glands are common sites for extrathoracic metastases in patients with lung cancer. However, asymptomatic adrenal adenomas occur frequently in the general population, with a prevalence rate of approximately 5 percent. A recent report indicated that two-thirds of adrenal masses in patients with lung cancer were found to represent adrenal adenomas. Thus, biopsy of an enlarged adrenal gland is usually necessary to confirm metastatic disease.

Evaluation of the liver for metastases can also be carried out at the time of CT scanning of the chest. However, imaging procedures of other organs, such as CT of the brain or radionuclide bone scans, are not recommended unless there are specific symptoms or abnormal laboratory tests to suggest metastatic disease.

THE SOLITARY PULMONARY NODULE

Solitary pulmonary nodules are frequently identified on standard chest roentgenograms obtained because of pulmonary symptoms or for other reasons. In patients over the age of 40, approximately 50 percent of such nodules are malignant. The diagnosis of malignancy can usually be made easily with percutaneous biopsy. However, despite recent advances in the assessment of pulmonary nodules with conventional tomography, bronchoscopy, and percutaneous biopsy, surgical resection is still required in a number of patients with benign lesions to exclude the possibility of malignancy. Regarding radiologic assessment, there are only two criteria that support the benign nature of solitary pulmonary nodules: (1) no growth over at least a 2-year period, and (2) the presence of characteristic calcifications. The calcifications that are identified as signs that the nodule is benign include diffuse calcification, target or rim calcification, or calcification scattered throughout a nodule, i.e., the "popcorn" variety. If a solitary nodule is detected on standard posteroanterior and lateral chest roentgenograms, standard tomography may be the best initial screening procedure. Tomography done at low kilovoltage will detect most discrete calcifications, i.e., target, rim, or popcorn varieties. Unfortunately, lesions that are diffusely calcified may be difficult to evaluate. The presence of diffuse calcification often requires quantitative rather than qualitative assessment. If there is no evidence of calcification on standard tomography, a CT scan should then be performed. The advantage of CT is that attenuation coefficients can be measured directly. Such CT numbers correlate with the physical density of the lesion, permitting more accurate detection of calcification. The procedure should be done with thin sections to prevent partial volume averaging. Definite calcification can often be seen by simple inspection of the scans at narrow windows and measurement of the CT number using a cursor. However, in some cases, a reference "phantom" can be used as a comparison with the nodule. This phantom consists of two transaxial sections that simulate the anatomy of the thorax. Reference nodules composed of various sized cylinders made up of resins containing calcium carbonate can then be used to compare with the patient's nodule. Recent studies have shown that this method is highly accurate in determining the presence of calcification and also in establishing the benign nature of a lesion. However, CT is most effective in establishing the benign nature of nodules that are 3 cm or less in diameter and that have discrete or smooth margins. Occasionally calcification may occur in malignant lesions, but such nodules are usually larger than 3 cm in diameter and have irregular borders. In these larger lesions, biopsy or surgery is required.

NEEDLE ASPIRATION BIOPSY OF CHEST LESIONS

Percutaneous needle aspiration biopsy of lesions in the lung or mediastinum is a procedure frequently performed by radiologists. It is highly diagnostic and safe. Such procedures are done under fluoroscopic guidance, but they may also be done under CT guidance. A variety of needles of different gauges may be used, but the current approach is to use fine 20- or 22-gauge needles. Generally speaking, the material that is obtained is suitable for cytologic analysis. Occasionally small cores of tissue can also be retrieved for histologic processing. Lesions that are amenable to needle aspiration biopsy are lung nodules or masses that are peripheral in location, that is, beyond the central or segmental bronchi. The vast majority of patients referred for transthoracic needle aspiration biopsy have carcinoma of the lung. The decision to perform a needle aspiration biopsy in a patient with probable lung carcinoma is somewhat a matter of choice. Some surgeons may prefer to send such patients directly to surgery. However, the following are some suggested indications for needle aspiration biopsy: (1) an undiagnosed lung lesion occurring in a patient for whom the hazard of a thoracotomy is higher than normal; (2) undiagnosed lung lesions that have a low probability of requiring resection for treatment, i.e., stable lesions or lesions with atypical appearances for cancer; (3) patients with highly probable but confirmed inoperable primary or metastatic cancers in the lungs; (4) patients with multiple nodules with or without a past medical history of cancer; (5) two undiagnosed lesions in different lobes of the lungs; (6) undiagnosed lung cancers that require pneumonectomy for resection; (7) undiagnosed lung lesions in immunosuppressed patients; and (8) patients desiring a confirmed diagnosis prior to agreeing to a thoracotomy. Fine needle aspiration biopsy is highly accurate in the diagnosis of bronchogenic carcinoma. Most series indicate an 85 to 95 percent sensitivity. Results vary, depending upon the skill of the operator and also the availability and interest of the cytologist.

Ideally, patients who may benefit most from a needle aspiration biopsy of a solitary nodule are those in whom a definite benign diagnosis can be confirmed. Unfortunately, the results are not as good for specific diagnosis of benign legions, but approach the range of 30 to 60 percent. Specific benign diagnoses that can be confirmed by needle aspiration biopsy include hamartomas and granulomas. Active infections, such as tuberculosis, can easily be diagnosed, provided that material is obtained for smear and culture.

The most common complication of needle aspiration biopsy is pneumothorax; which occurs in 15 to 25 percent of cases. However, only approximately 5 to 10 percent of patients require chest tubes for treatment. Most radiologists manage such pneumothoraces by inserting small 9 F chest tubes that can be attached either to a Pleur-Evac or to a Heimlich valve. Such tubes are quite adequate to treat most postbiopsy pneumothoraces. Hemoptysis occurs in 2 to 3 percent of patients. In order to avoid any serious bleeding, a coagulation profile, including prothrombin time, partial thromboplastin time, and platelet count, should be obtained prior to the biopsy.

Fine needle aspiration biopsy can also be performed on mediastinal lesions. The yield for carcinoma in hilar or mediastinal lymph nodes is equally as high as it is in lung lesions. Most of these biopsies are done under CT guidance. However, the yield is considerably lower in diagnosing lesions of more complex histology, such as lymphomas and thymomas. Often sufficient tissue is not obtained for specific characterization.

SUGGESTED READING

Baron RL, Levitt RG, Sagel SS, et al. Computed tomography in the evaluation of mediastinal widening. Radiology 1981; 138:107–113.
Daly BDT, Faling LJ, Pugatch RD, et al. Computed tomography. An effective technique for mediastinal staging in lung cancer. J Thorac Cardiovasc Surg 1984; 88:486–494.
Sagel SS, Aronberg DJ. Thoracic anatomy and mediastinum. In: Lee JKT, Sagel SS, Stanley RJ, eds. Computed tomography. New York: Raven Press, 1983: 55–97.
Webb WR. Plain radiography and computed tomography in the staging of bronchogenic carcinoma: a practical approach. J Thorac Imaging 1987; 2:57–65.
Westcott JL. Direct percutaneous needle aspiration of localized pulmonary lesions: Results in 422 patients. Radiology 1980; 137:31–35.

BRONCHOGRAPHY

BERNARD T. LE ROUX, Ch.M., F.R.C.S.(Edin)
DAVID A. ROCKE, M.R.C.P.(UK), F.F.A.S.A.

Bronchography as an investigative procedure for respiratory disease has, at least in the Western world, fallen into disrepute. In the Third World, however, where those diseases for whose investigation bronchography was originally introduced are still common, this diagnostic technique is still widely used. Bronchography has a far wider application than mapping the precise distribution of bronchiectasis, for which computed tomography (CT) is not a substitute. Bronchial anatomy is so variable that segmentectomy for any purpose cannot be accurately planned without a bronchogram. Many plain film abnormalities that are difficult to interpret become crystal clear with the additional information obtained by bronchography. It is unwise, for example, to rely upon pulmonary angiography to determine operability of bullous emphysema, since this study does not reveal the intrinsic state of displaced bronchi, as does bronchography.

Many techniques of bronchography have been described, but none has been generally accepted. There have been many comprehensive reviews of the subject, and except in children, topical anesthesia in the conscious patient whose cooperation is required is the most widely used technique. For the conscious patient, bronchography is an uncomfortable experience; it has been described as an inelegant provocative test, the purpose of which is to ascertain the patient's ability to withstand drowning. Physicians responsible for the diagnosis of patients with respiratory disease have, over the last 20 or 30 years, become increasingly reluctant to recommend and radiologists to undertake bronchography, and they have tended to discount the value of bronchography because of the generally imperfect bronchograms achieved with topical anesthesia in the conscious patient. Localized bronchography with the fiberoptic bronchoscope deprives the interpretor of the subsequent x-ray films thus the opportunity of comparing bronchi with one another in a particular patient, an exercise that is an invaluable part of the interpretation of complete bilateral bronchograms because there are few absolute criteria of normality. Localized absence of bronchiolar filling, if there is uniformly good filling elsewhere in a bilateral bronchogram, is of profound significance, whereas if this is a feature of a limited bronchogram, it may be no more than evidence of technical failure.

TECHNIQUE

The technique of bronchography favored in children and adults is with general anesthesia, the use of a relaxant, and lung insufflation.

The patient is prepared for bronchography over a period of days by postural drainage and the administration of appropriate antibiotics. Premedication should be appropriate for the age and weight of the patient and should include atropine (0.01 mg per kilogram) as an antisialogogue. The patient's electrocardiogram is monitored, and electrodes must be so situated that they do not interfere radiologically. An intravenous line is established (a 20-gauge plastic cannula) in the dorsum of the hand. The anesthetic is given intravenously (thiopental 4 mg per kilogram) and includes the use of a short-acting relaxant (suxamethonium 1 mg per kilogram). A low dose of a nondepolarizing agent such as alcuronium, given before induction of anesthesia, reduces the incidence and severity of pain from suxamethonium. The lungs are inflated with oxygen delivered through a face mask, and when the patient is apneic and fully oxygenated, the bronchi are examined under direct vision with the rigid bronchoscope. Ventilation can be continued through the side arm of the bronchoscope using the Magill circuit (Mapleson A). Bronchoscopy is an essential preliminary to bronchography; it enables abnormalities to be detected in the proximal major bronchi and allows the air passages to be cleared of mucus by suction. The procedures of combined bronchoscopy and bronchography are primarily functions of surgeons and anesthetists.

On completion of bronchoscopy, the lungs are again inflated with oxygen, and a cuffed endotracheal tube is inserted into the trachea under direct vision. The cuff of the tube is inflated, and the endotracheal tube is connected to the anesthetic circuit. The endotracheal tube must be of an appropriate length to avoid endobronchial intubation. Intermittent ventilation is continued with oxygen or an oxygen and nitrous oxide mixture. The examination thus far is unlikely to have taken longer than 2 or 3 minutes.

The patient, who is lying on a mobile x-ray table top, is now turned onto the right side, and a film is positioned in the Potter-Bucky undercouch grid and the tube anode is positioned above.

The patient is momentarily detached from the

anesthetic circuit, most simply by detaching the catheter mount from the endotracheal tube, and a catheter of appropriate diameter, previously trimmed so that it is a centimeter longer than the endotracheal tube, is passed through the endotracheal tube. From a 20-ml syringe, the contrast medium, previously well agitated to ensure that it is thoroughly mixed, is injected rapidly into the trachea. The catheter mount is replaced to reestablish the anesthetic circuit and, using the reservoir bag on the Magill circuit, the lungs are inflated twice, firmly but not violently, to disperse the contrast agent. The contrast medium is insufflated into the dependent lung by pulmonary inflation. The radiologic plate for the right lateral bronchogram is then exposed; during the moments of radiographic exposure the anesthetist keeps the lungs inflated in order to depress the domes of the diaphragm—this constitutes a third inflation.

The patient is now turned to the right posterior oblique position, and a second cassette is exposed. Thereafter the patient is turned to the left posterior oblique position, and a further bolus of contrast material is rapidly injected into the trachea. The lungs are again inflated twice. A left posterior oblique exposure is then made with the lungs fully inflated, and the patient is turned to the supine position. An anteroposterior exposure is made to include the whole chest, again with the lungs fully inflated. All radiologic exposures are made with the lungs inflated and the diaphragmatic domes depressed.

Although an intravenous induction of anesthetic is preferred in all cases, in some small children venous access is difficult, and an inhalation induction with oxygen and halothane is used.

The entire procedure, including bronchoscopy, usually takes less than 7 minutes, and it is rarely necessary to inject a supplementary dose of relaxant. The anesthetist has full control of ventilation, even during bronchoscopy, if a Storz bronchoscope or similar equipment is used, with the eye piece in situ. Moreover, the technique of bronchography by insufflation, as opposed to a technique that demands many changes in posture and patient collaboration, is time-saving. Tracheobronchial toilet at the end of the procedure usually results in the elimination of most of the contrast medium by suction. The aspirate is sent for microbiologic examination, especially for a search for tubercle bacilli, since bronchography promotes their appearance in sputum, where they had not previously been found.

A feature of this technique of bronchography is that it has removed all elements of mystery from the investigation. For the uninitiated, the need for positioning the patient at a number of arbitrary angles for arbitrary periods of time lent a spurious air of profundity to the experienced bronchographer; there are no longer those moments of suspense while the films are being developed to ascertain how complete a bronchogram has been achieved or whether only the outline of the esophagus is visible.

CONTRAST MEDIUM AND DOSE

The contrast agent most readily available is propyliodone (oily Dionosil). This produces uniformly satisfactory bronchograms, as did Hytrast, made according to the original French formula. The dose of contrast used in adults is 15 to 18 ml per side depending on the patient's size. The quantity used in children is arbitrarily calculated as age in years plus 2 ml per side. In very young children, who tolerate bronchography as well as adults, bilateral filling with the first injection is so common that generally only one injection is given through the endotracheal tube, into the trachea, with the child supine, and then serially an anteroposterior, a right, and a left oblique view are done, without a right lateral view. It has only occasionally been thought appropriate to make unilateral bronchograms, with an interval between right and left, and only in patients with some other significant, usually cardiac, disorder. There is no evidence of detriment to properly selected patients from bilateral bronchograms. Pulmonary function capacity, in comparison with that before bronchography, is slightly reduced on the first day after bronchography and thereafter returns to normal. Only rarely are blood gas measurements modified by bronchography, and they return to prebronchographic levels by the second day after the test. It is sound practice to take a chest film on the second day after bronchography, by which time oily Dionosil or Hytrast has almost always disappeared from normal areas of lung; retention of contrast material is additional evidence of abnormality.

In order for bronchography with general anesthesia to be safe, quick, and effective, the collaboration of a large team is necessary. Required are an anesthetist and an aide; two radiology technicians and a darkroom attendant with no other responsibility during a bronchography session; and an expert bronchoscopist and an attendant operating room nurse. Rapid dry film development enables early scrutiny of the bronchogram, and there is time for rarely needed further contrast insufflation if bronchi are insufficiently outlined.

For the display of right bronchi, right lateral and right posterior oblique views are necessary. The somewhat jumbled right basal bronchi are well displayed in the oblique view, in which the right upper bronchi are jumbled and the middle bronchi obscured unless the right upper lobe is contracted upward, pulling the middle lobe with it. The right posterior oblique view is also advantageous when bilateral filling has occurred with the first insufflation of contrast agent and if there is a left-sided radiologic, usually pleural, abnormality. Left bronchial filling or a left radiologic opacity is rotated to the left side of the right posterior oblique film and is no longer superimposed on the right bronchi, as it is in a lateral view.

COMPLICATIONS

With the technique described, first in Edinburgh and more recently in Natal more than 10,000 bronchograms have been made and fewer than 2 percent have been found inadequate for a decision as to management of a patient. Needlessly forceful inflation of the lungs has resulted in the development of pneumothorax in five patients, quickly recognized in four without detriment to the patient, and unrecognized in one who subsequently died. In an inappropriately selected patient with a large pleural shadow that was not recognized as a florid empyema, bronchography by this technique resulted in endobronchial rupture of the empyema, and the patient drowned. Morbidity and mortality are never negligible, but this incidence of complication and death in over 10,000 bronchograms is small, a complication rate lower than from percutaneous fine needle aspiration of intrapulmonary lesions for cytologic purposes.

SUGGESTED READING

Flower CDR, Schneerson JM. Bronchography via the fibreoptic bronchoscope. Thorax 1984; 39:260–263.

Le Roux BT, Masson AHB. Bronchography under general anesthesia. Brit J Anaesth 1962; 34:200–202.

Le Roux BT, Mohlala ML, Odell JA, Whitton ID. Suppurative diseases of the lung and pleural space. Part 11:Bronchiectasis. Curr Probl Surg 1986; 22:111–117.

Love SHS, Morrow WFK. Anaesthesia for bronchography in children. Anaesthesia 1954; 9:74–76.

Olsen AM, O'Neil JJ. Bronchography: a report of the committee in bronchoesophyology. Dis Chest 1967; 51:663–668.

I ANESTHESIA

GENERAL PRINCIPLES OF ANESTHESIA AND HIGH FREQUENCY VENTILATION

ROGER S. WILSON, M.D.

This chapter focuses on the anesthetic management of the patient undergoing noncardiac thoracic surgery. It covers the salient features of the specific problems and anesthetic techniques used during the surgical resection of benign and malignant lesions of the lung, esophagus, and trachea.

PREOPERATIVE EVALUATION

The preoperative evaluation of the thoracic surgical patient is somewhat different from the approach used for most other surgical candidates. Several factors, including advanced age, generalized sequelae of preexisting neoplastic and/or infectious pulmonary pathology, and cardiovascular disease, can predispose this patient population to multiple organ system dysfunction during the intraoperative and immediate postoperative period. The patient with preexisting cardiopulmonary disease can be adversely affected by intraoperative events such as posture, e.g., the lateral decubitus position with head and feet in a dependent position, especially when combined with intraoperative compression of pulmonary and intrathoracic vascular structures.

Preexisting cardiac disease, including any history of atrial and ventricular arrhythmias, valvular pathology, and the existence of coronary artery disease (especially with evidence of ventricular dysfunction and congestive heart failure), requires special consideration in the thoracic surgical patient. Any significant intraoperative and/or postoperative alteration in gas exchange, with potential for hypercarbia and hypoxemia, creates a circumstance for acute deterioration of previously well-controlled cardiac disease and produces a need for emergent, specific, and often aggressive therapy.

PREMEDICATION

The standard approach to preoperative therapy using barbiturates, narcotics, tranquilizers, and antisialagogues frequently requires modification when used in thoracic surgical patients. Although the specific objectives of therapy differ little from those for other surgical patients, undesirable side effects, especially those involving postoperative pulmonary function, require special consideration in these patients. Special attention also must be given to patients with tracheal pathology in whom there is potential for exacerbation of airway obstruction with drugs that produce central respiratory depression or with the use of drying agents that result in production of inspissated secretions.

MONITORING

Although there are no universally recognized standards, a minimally acceptable approach probably would include an intermittent noninvasive measurement of blood pressure with continuous recording of electrocardiogram and body temperature. These techniques are frequently supplemented with the use of a precordial or esophageal stethoscope. Additional noninvasive techniques used to monitor the efficiency of gas exchange include the use of pulse oximetry and capnography. These latter techniques are of special value during the periods of prolonged airway manipulation that occur with laryngoscopy, bronchoscopy, and during intubation, especially with the placement of double-lumen endobronchial tubes. Peripheral arterial cannulation is generally dictated by the usual indications, including anticipation of any adverse hemodynamic effects of anesthesia and surgery and the specific need to obtain arterial blood gas readings to monitor respiratory gas exchange during the intraoperative and immediate postoperative periods. Invasive vascular monitoring for central venous and pulmonary artery pressures is dictated by criteria similar to those used for any patient with preexisting cardiopulmonary disease requiring anesthesia for a major surgical procedure. Of special consideration in certain thoracic surgical patients is the need for specific anatomic placement of the pulmonary artery catheter. When pulmonary resection is anticipated, it is advisable to place the catheter in the nonsurgical, dependent lung. This minimizes interference of measurement during the procedure and ensures that the catheter is not located in an area of the lung that will undergo resection.

Special consideration is necessary to minimize the potential occurrence of iatrogenic injury as a direct result of the surgical or anesthetic procedures or as a consequence of the unusual operative positioning required in this patient population. Of concern are accidental injuries to eyes, teeth, and soft tissue during airway manipulation procedures such as laryngoscopy, bronchoscopy, and placement of specialized endotracheal tubes. Various other injuries can result from placement of the patient in the lateral position, which is most frequently used for thoracotomy, including compression-related damage to one of several peripheral nerves, digits, and the dependent ear.

SELECTION OF ANESTHETIC

The choice of a specific anesthetic technique, including the use of local, regional, or general anesthesia, either individually or in combination, is dictated by several factors. These include the nature of the procedure itself and any specific objectives that need to be considered during the intraoperative and immediate postoperative periods.

Bronchoscopy

The choice of a regional, local, or general anesthetic is dictated in part by the bronchoscopic technique utilized, the extent of anticipated patient cooperation, and other associated conditions including the nature, location, and extent of the surgical lesion and the presence and severity of preexisting cardiopulmonary disease. The anesthetic objectives, regardless of the surgical technique utilized, include the need for analgesia; maintenance of gas exchange, including oxygenation and carbon dioxide elimination; and the ability to eliminate or to minimize reflex activity of the airways, including coughing, straining, and bucking. In certain patients it may be mandatory to prevent untoward side effects of surgical stimulation, including tachycardia, hypertension, and cardiac arrhythmias.

Flexible fiberoptic bronchoscopy is easily accomplished in cooperative patients using local anesthesia, frequently supplemented by intravenous narcotics and sedatives. Complete anesthesia of the posterior pharynx, larynx, and trachea can be produced using a variety of agents and techniques. General anesthesia is generally utilized when bronchoscopy is done in conjunction with mediastinoscopy, immediately prior to the thoracotomy or in the uncooperative or medically unfit patient. One prerequisite is the use of a sufficiently large size endotracheal tube (generally oral) to provide an adequate lumen for the endoscope and also sufficient for adequate gas exchange. The use of intravenously administered muscle relaxants with controlled positive pressure ventilation provides optimal surgical conditions by minimizing respiratory motion and eliminating the potential for coughing during critical periods of the procedure, such as during biopsy of airway or parenchymal tumors.

Rigid bronchoscopy is often the technique of choice in the evaluation of obstructing tracheal lesions and in patients with copious secretions or in the case of active hemoptysis. A general anesthetic is generally preferred. In most circumstances, one of the three major potent inhalation anesthetics is used, preceded by induction with an intravenous barbiturate. Use of a narcotic technique, generally supplemented with nitrous oxide, is suitable, provided that the technique is compatible with the ability to provide adequate gas exchange with anticipated respiratory depression and the reduced inspired oxygen concentration. Maintaining adequate ventilation necessary to provide for gas exchange and the administration of inhalation anesthetics is generally possible using a rigid bronchoscope adapted with a side arm and a glass window cap on the proximal end of the scope. Muscle relaxation is important to facilitate passage of the rigid bronchoscope through the oral pharynx, larynx, and trachea. Suitable techniques include use of intravenous succinylcholine, administered as a bolus or continuous infusion, or use of one of a number of nondepolarizing muscle relaxants.

Mediastinoscopy

Airway control utilizing endotracheal intubation obviates most problems concerned with ventilation and gas exchange. Specific complications relating to the procedure include the risk of uncontrolled hemorrhage within the confines of mediastinum, the compression of vascular structures such as the innominate artery (leading to temporary occlusion of flow and hence loss of measurable blood pressure in the right upper extremity), and reflex activity involving the cardiovascular and respiratory systems. The last is often induced by stimulation of the trachea and carina and other mediastinal structures during the digital exploration or during direct stimulation from the endoscope. The sequelae of such stimulation include tachycardia, bradycardia, and hypertension; in addition, it can produce adverse respiratory effects such as coughing and bucking. A variety of anesthetic techniques, including the use of potent inhalation agents or nitrous/narcotic anesthesia, are suitable and generally utilized. Muscle relaxation, although not necessary for the surgical procedure per se, may be advantageous in reducing activities such as coughing, straining, and bucking.

Thoracotomy

A unique consideration, common to the anesthetic management of all such noncardiac thoracic surgical procedures, is the need to consider use of one of several techniques for isolation of portions of the airway. Specific use of isolation techniques is indicated for a variety of reasons. Absolute indications for intraoperative isolation include (1) control of secretions, especially during surgery for pulmonary abscess or in the presence of bronchiectasis; (2) airway control, specifically in the presence of chronic or acute bronchopleural fistula or during sleeve resection; and (3) for improving operating conditions and surgical exposure. Other relative indications would include frequent use of the technique for the purpose of training and during thoracotomy in the presence of active hemoptysis.

Three techniques have been used to facilitate isolation during thoracic surgery. These include (1) endobronchial blockers, (2) single-lumen endobronchial tubes, and (3) double-lumen endobronchial tubes.

Endobronchial blockers, the oldest of the isolation techniques, have limited application in current practice. Indications for considering use of this technique include the need to isolate a peripheral airway rather than an entire lung in order to locate the lesion, or the necessity to utilize the maximum amount of pulmonary parenchyma for gas exchange because of extensive preexisting pulmonary disease. In addition, the presence of significant quantities of blood in the airway with potential for obstruction of "small lumen" single- and double-lumen endobronchial tubes creates a situation in which the use of endobronchial blockers may be advantageous. Finally, certain severe anatomic situations can be resolved using this technique, including the presence of an abnormally small oral pharynx, especially when associated with limitation of jaw motion. This situation can limit visualization with direct laryngoscopy and thus create a difficult circumstance for intubation with large endobronchial tubes. Also, prior surgery such as laryngectomy and unusual airway anomalies creates conditions in which the use of endobronchial tubes is difficult or impossible.

One approach to this technique of isolation is the use of a venous occlusion Fogarty catheter suitably positioned with the aid of a fiberoptic bronchoscope. A No. 8–14 Fogarty (10-cc volume balloon) provides a satisfactory and inexpensive technique for airway occlusion. Simultaneous placement of a conventional endotracheal tube and a Fogarty catheter into the trachea is accomplished using standard techniques of direct laryngoscopy. The Fogarty catheter is placed through the cords, external to and alongside the endotracheal tube. Localization and placement of the Fogarty catheter into the appropriate portion of the airway are accomplished with the flexible fiberoptic bronchoscope. Inflation of the cuff in the bronchus is confirmed to guarantee adequate inflation volume and to assure the position that will minimize proximal movement with coughing or interoperative surgical manipulation. Such movement, accompanied by dislodgement of the blocker into the trachea and the potential for total airway obstruction, must be constantly anticipated. Intraoperative bronchoscopic confirmation of catheter position and balloon inflation is frequently necessary when this technique is used. Several technical problems are associated with balloon occlusion. One problem is the inability to remove foreign material in the airways distal to the catheter tip. This creates the potential for major contamination when use of the catheter is terminated and undrained material is allowed to spill into the proximal airway. In addition, inability to allow for passive flow of gas from the operative lung into the proximal airway results in the slow collapse of lung distal to the catheter. Atelectasis results primarily from absorption of gas secondary to continued perfusion.

Two existing designs of single-lumen tubes are the Macintosh-Leatherdale (left endobronchial) and the Gordon-Green (right endobronchial). The design of these tubes is similar in that both are equipped with dual cuffs: an endobronchial cuff situated on the endobronchial portion of the tube and a tracheal cuff located in position to inflate in the distal trachea.

The Gordon-Green tube, designed for intubation of the right main stem bronchus, employs a carinal spur to maintain stability of the tube and a slit-like orifice in the distal underbronchial cuff for ventilation of the right upper lobe bronchus. This tube is designed with a lesser angulation (30 degrees) of the distal end of the tube from the midline when compared with the more acute (45 degrees) angulation of the left-sided Macintosh-Leatherdale tube. A disadvantage of all single-lumen endobronchial tubes is the inability to suction material from the operative lung and the potential limitation of ventilation to the nonintubated, surgical lung. The latter condition results from the fact that ventilation to the surgical lung must pass from the intubated bronchus and travel retrograde up around the endobronchial portion of the tube and ultimately over the carina into the nonintubated bronchus. Inadvertent positioning of the tube in a distal position in the bronchus can result in a seal without inflation of the endobronchial cuff. The small (20 × 5 mm) slit in the lateral wall of the endobronchial limb of the Gordon-Green tube poses potential problems with inadequacy of ventilation and drainage of secretions to the right upper lobe.

The double-lumen endobronchial tubes are the third and most popular technique used for isolation. Double-lumen endobronchial tubes, although used for bronchospirometry since 1949, were not utilized for thoracic surgery until 1951. Since that time a variety of tubes designed for placement into the right or left main stem bronchus have been clinically utilized. The Carlens tube (left) and the White tube (right), although once used exclusively for isolation techniques, have been discarded because of problems relating to the presence of the carinal hook and subsequent problems with intubation, cuff design with high pressure—low volume properties, and difficulties associated with ventilation of the right upper lobe when using the White tube. Current practice has shifted to use of the Robertshaw (nondisposable) right and left endobronchial tubes or one of a variety of polyvinylchloride (disposable) right and left endobronchial tubes.

The advantages of the Robertshaw double-lumen tube relate to the design characteristics, which include: (1) the wide lumen, allowing passage of large suction catheters and low resistance of gas flow; (2) the absence of a carinal hook, making intubation easier and not limiting surgical resection of a bronchial stump during pneumonectomy; (3) the simplified selection of appropriate size (although three sizes are available, the medium and large sizes are suited for female and male adult patients, respectively); (4) the right side endobronchial tube is designed to minimize occlusion of the right upper lobe bronchus, and (5) a preform bite block serves as a guide for adequate placement of the distal tip of the tube within the airway.

In more recent years, a variety of disposable polyvinylchloride tubes have received favorable attention in clinical use. Such tubes are available in right- and left-sided versions and are manufactured in French sizes 35, 37, 39, and 41. These tubes are designed for single use and have the advantage of improved characteristics of cuff design, including low pressure–high residual volume characteristics. In addition, advantages of the polyvinylchloride tubes are found in the improved cross-sectional diameter of the lumen compared with the external size of the tube as opposed to tubes of the Carlens, Gordon-Green, or Robertshaw design, and in the ability to conform the distal endobronchial portion of the tube to a stylet to facilitate intubation in patients in whom direct visualization of the airway is a problem.

Complications of use of isolation techniques primarily relate to three areas: (1) trauma, (2) malposition, and (3) hypoxemia during one-lung anesthesia. Trauma secondary to tube placement can be produced throughout the airway. This includes soft tissue injury to the oral and posterior pharynx, dislocation of the arytenoid, and similar injuries caused by the increased bulk of these tubes. True tracheobronchial rupture, a rare reported complication, has occurred with all types of double-lumen tubes. The location of the laceration is usually the membranous wall of the distal trachea or the proximal main stem bronchi. When reported, interoperative detection has been associated with development of a large air leak with positive pressure ventilation, visualization of air bubbles within the mediastinal structure, and/or direct visualization of the endobronchial cuff or tube tip within the surgical field. Surgical repair of the tracheal laceration is essential and, as reported, survival is the rule.

Malpositioning of double-lumen tubes within the airway is a second important complication to consider. A variety of malpositions generally can be classified under a number of circumstances, including position of the tube in a distal or too proximal position with the airway, malposition of the endobronchial cuff relative to the carina, and problems associated with the position of the slotted right endobronchial cuff adjacent to the right upper lobe bronchus. A potential cause for malposition would appear to be the selection of the tube that is inappropriate in size—generally one that is too small and thus does not advance far enough into the bronchus. Several factors necessitate selection of a small tube, including inability to pass the ideal size because of limitations in diameter of the upper airway at the laryngeal aperture or at the level of the cricoid and, in addition, inability to advance the distal tip of the appropriate sized tube into the bronchus because of bronchial narrowing, extrinsic compression, or endobronchial pathology. The result is that the endobronchial cuff does not advance far enough into the bronchus. Under such circumstances, it is common for the endobronchial cuff to be inflated in a position that is too proximal in the airway, thus producing partial or complete occlusion of gas flow from the tracheal port into the nonintubated (surgical) bronchus. This creates a situation in which it is possible to ventilate both lungs when the endobronchial cuff is deflated and only the nonsurgical lung when the cuff is in the inflated state. Abnormalities arising from such malpositioning should be detected if a carefully designed program for cuff inflation is carried out. A second complication relates to malposition of the tube secondary to advancement of the endobronchial limb too distally into the tracheobronchial tree. Owing to anatomic differences, the right upper lobe bronchus is subject to potential occlusion somewhat more frequently than would be anticipated for the left main stem bronchus. It appears that polyvinylchloride tubes, by virtue of their smaller cross-sectional configuration of the endobronchial lumen when combined with the more than adequate length of the tube itself, are somewhat easier to position too distally than the Robertshaw type tubes. A third specific form of malpositioning relates to inadequate positioning of the right endobronchial cuff and lateral slot adjacent to the right upper lobe bronchus. Previously mentioned characteristics of the polyvinylchloride tubes, when complicated by difficulties in design of an appropriate slotted cuff compared with older latex designs, create a situation in which right-sided tubes of this type are perhaps associated with a greater degree of malpositioning than are the nondisposable types.

Avoidance of malpositioning is based on a careful, meticulous approach to tube placement with use of visual inspection during subsequent isolation of both hemithoraces and confirmation with auscultation. Use of flexible fiberoptic bronchoscopy to determine absolute tube position, although it is almost never contraindicated, appears to be unnecessary with Robertshaw nondisposable types, optional with left-sided polyvinylchloride type, and desirable when right-sided polyvinylchloride tubes are utilized. Placement of a fiberopticscope into the tracheal lumen will confirm the position of the endobronchial cuff within the desired bronchus just distal to the carina. Inability to visualize the cuff necessitates withdrawal of the tube from the airway until appropriate cuff position can be determined. Optional inspection of the endobronchial lumen when right-sided tubes are used should be done to visualize adequacy of the slotted cuff in juxtaposition to the right upper lobe bronchus.

Hypoxemia during one-lung anesthesia is a well-recognized, well-documented problem associated with any and all isolation techniques. Numerous studies have confirmed that a significant percentage of patients undergoing thoracic surgical procedures for pulmonary and nonpulmonary resection, experience arterial hypoxemia in spite of administration of oxygen concentrations approximating 100 percent. In general, carbon dioxide elimination is not compromised provided that mechanical function and absence of airway obstruction during one-lung ventilation are not present and that the total minute volume used during two-lung ventilation is utilized during the one-lung procedure.

Arterial hypoxemia occurring during one-lung anesthesia is a result of many factors, including: (1) a fractional distribution of blood flow to the operative (nondependent) and nonoperative (dependent) lungs; (2) presence of alveolar collapse and/or vascular disease in the dependent lung; (3) inspired oxygen concentration, and (4) cardiac output. In general, optimal oxygenation is anticipated when minimal blood flow is distributed to the collapsed surgical lung and optimal alveolar expansion is produced in the nonoperative dependent lung. Extremes of cardiac output exist, including low output resulting in markedly reduced mixed venous saturation and oxygen tension and markedly elevated cardiac output with preferential distribution of blood flow due to increased hydrostatic pressure to the operative lung.

A variety of therapies have been advocated to minimize arterial hypoxemia during one-lung ventilation. These include use of positive end-expiratory pressure in the dependent lung, use of large (12 to 15 ml per kilogram body weight) tidal volumes in the dependent lung, continuous positive airway pressure and/or residual gas in the operative lung, and use of high frequency ventilation. Use of positive end-expiratory pressure in the dependent lung should be limited to relatively minimal levels approximating 5 cm of water. Levels in excess of this may increase pulmonary vascular resistance by virtue of overdistention of the dependent lung and redistribute blood flow to the collapsed operative lung, thus potentially increasing shunt. Use of continuous positive airway pressure to the nondependent lung provides oxygen for any blood continuing to flow through this lung but increases the complexity of equipment and, if carried to an extreme, obviates surgical exposure. Another option is to produce intermittent minimal inflation (approximately 200 ml of oxygen) periodically every 10 to 15 minutes with maintenance of the closed airway in the operative lung. This facilitates a partial supply of oxygen for any residual perfusion and does not interfere with surgical exposure.

Tracheal Resection and Reconstruction

It is essential for the anesthesiologist to have a complete understanding of the airway pathology and the plan for the surgical approach in order to structure optimal techniques for premedication, monitoring, induction, airway management, and postoperative care.

Premedication is selected using a conservative approach to minimize complications resulting from respiratory depression and airway obstruction and to prevent any residual postoperative effect.

Caution is exercised during induction of anesthesia, especially when there are critical limitations of airflow, to ensure continued spontaneous respiratory effort and minimal compromise to the upper airway resulting from soft tissue obstruction. Except in cases demonstrating little to no airway compromise, induction is accomplished with high inspired oxygen concentration, potent inhalation agents (halothane is optimal), and careful use of an intravenous barbiturate (only when dictated by need—generally during an exaggerated excitement phase). Bronchoscopy, generally the rigid technique, is accomplished with deep anesthesia, supplemented by topical anesthesia to the airway, with spontaneous, assisted ventilation. Following determination of the extent of the tracheal pathology and evaluation and estimation of the airway diameter at the level of the lesion, endotracheal intubation is performed. The type of tube is determined by the location of disease and the surgical approach. For the surgical approach to the upper one-half of the trachea, with cervical incision, an uncut, standard red rubber endotracheal tube is most suitable; size 26 or 28 F is optimal for gas exchange, suctioning of secretions, surgical exposure, and intraoperative manipulation. When the airway diameter is less than 5 to 6 cm, endoscopic dilation, if it can be accomplished with a degree of safety, is performed to allow the endotracheal tube to be passed distal to the lesion in order to maximize gas exchange and to ensure an unobstructed airway during initial surgical dissection. Pathology involving the distal trachea, carina, or bronchi, especially requiring a right thoracotomy, mandates special consideration and a variety of modified endotracheal tubes and is beyond the scope of this discussion. Anesthesia is maintained with an inhalation technique, usually with maximal inspired oxygen concentration.

Airway management during tracheal resection and suture placement for reconstruction is accomplished with a sterile, flexible, wire-reinforced endotracheal tube inserted into the distal tracheal lumen and connected to the anesthesia machine with sterile anesthesia tubes and a "Y" piece. Following the placement of all sutures, the trachea is approximated once the "field tube" is removed, and the translaryngeal endotracheal tube is advanced through the anastomosis.

In most uncomplicated cases, extubation is accomplished in the operating room. This is done at a deep level of anesthesia or once the patient is awake. The approach is determined by the anticipated need for immediate reintubation, usually optimal in anesthetized patients, and the achievement of minimal soft tissue obstruction to airflow and protection from aspiration in awake patients. The approach to optimal anesthetic management is designed to result in a comfortable, cooperative awake patient with adequate spontaneous respiration in the immediate postoperative period.

HIGH FREQUENCY VENTILATION

High frequency (small volume) ventilation (HFV) has been successfully utilized to effect adequate pulmonary gas exchange during a variety of laboratory and clinical conditions. Several techniques have been developed for use in patients with normal and abnormal lung function undergoing a wide range of thoracic surgical procedures. Such applications include use of HFV during (1) bronchoscopy or laryngoscopy, (2) pulmonary resection including lobectomy and sleeve pneumonectomy, and (3) during tracheal or carinal resection.

HFV is a generic term used to describe a variety of ventilatory techniques that provide partial or total respiratory gas exchange. HFV is frequently divided into three somewhat distinct methods: high frequency positive pressure ventilation, high frequency jet ventilation, and high frequency oscillation. The designated difference between these methods, although somewhat arbitrary and not consistent as described in the literature, are determined by several factors; including the respiratory frequency, size of the tidal volume, and the type of device used to produce the ventilatory pattern. Although HFV, which is similar to conventional positive pressure ventilation, depends in part on convective flow for gas transport, other mechanisms such as enhanced or augmented diffusion appear to be more prominent factors in effecting gas exchange with this method. Although gas exchange, including efficiency of oxygenation and carbon dioxide elimination, is similar to HFV when compared with conventional positive pressure methods, the mechanical and physical aspects of HFV are advantageous during certain surgical procedures. Any potential use of HFV during thoracic surgery must be considered in light of the availability and versatility of existing (although limited) technology, the advantages of this technology over standard techniques, and the potential for complications.

One important application is the use of HFV during thoracotomy under circumstances when one-lung ventilation techniques would be utilized for improved operating conditions. Advantages of HFV include the ability to provide for gas exchange in the operative lung while being able to minimize lung movement with use of the higher rate and smaller tidal volume (lower peak airway pressure) when compared with standard large volume and conventional rate positive pressure ventilation or one-lung isolation without gas exchange. High frequency jet ventilation has been used in patients during thoracotomy for pulmonary resection. Small tidal volumes, approximately 150 to 200 ml, at rates of 60 to 150 breaths per minute, provide adequate gas exchange when delivered into a standard endotracheal tube with the distal end located in the trachea. Another technique, isolated one-lung HFV, has been evaluated in patients during thoracotomy for pulmonary resection, including lobectomy, pneumonectomy, and esophagectomy. One-lung HVF is similar to standard one-lung isolation, using a single-lumen (but standard single cuff) tube with the distal portion of the tube located in the nonoperative bronchus. Again, small tidal volumes produced at a driving (inflation) pressure of 25 psi are delivered 150 times each minute. With this method, certain patients fail to achieve adequate levels of arterial oxygen tension generally considered to be less than 80 mm Hg. Modification of this technique is achieved using an uncuffed endobronchial tube. With the modified technique a small, uncontrolled fraction of ventilation escapes from the dependent lung in retrograde fashion to enter the nondependent, surgical lung. This, in most cases, would be expected to improve arterial oxygenation in a manner previously described with standard one-lung techniques.

A second clinical situation in which HFV could prove to be beneficial is in the setting of pulmonary resection with concomitant loss of large airway integrity such as occurs in sleeve lobectomy or pneumonectomy. In addition, the preoperative presence of acute or chronic bronchopleural fistula, especially when of a magnitude to limit gas exchange with conventional positive pressure ventilation, would warrant consideration for use of HFV. A potential approach in such cases is delivery of HFV into the distal trachea or a more distal airway using a small-bore catheter, e.g., 14 F advanced through a normal or small endotracheal tube. Improved gas exchange and operating conditions are possible when compared with conditions existing with standard intubation and ventilation. Also, this technique serves as an alternative method in cases in which bulkier single-lumen or double-lumen tubes could cause iatrogenic injury during placement or limit surgical technique.

Tracheal resection and reconstruction, especially when involving the carina, are surgical techniques most amenable to the use of HFV. Following airway transection, ventilation of distal lung can be achieved using a catheter passed into the distal airway via an endotracheal tube and thus spanning the gap between the tracheal ends or simply placed into the distal airway in the surgical field. Our experience with this approach, utilizing rates of 60 to 150 breaths per minute delivered via a suction-type catheter, has proved beneficial during surgery of the distal trachea and with carinal resection. During the former, use of standard cuffed endotracheal tubes with conventional ventilation following transection is often difficult because of a short length of trachea remaining proximal to the carina. When conditions necessitate two-lung ventilation during the "open-airway" interval of the procedure, use of a bifid or "Y"-shaped catheter with one limb advanced into each bronchus has provided a suitable means for gas exchange. Although this catheter is suitable for use during uncomplicated resection of the cervical trachea, the standard approach using an endotracheal tube (24 to 28 F) passed through the larynx for the initial and terminal periods of operation and a flexible (Tovell or Armored) tube introduced into the distal trachea via the surgical field is generally utilized. We favor this approach because it is functional, simple, and avoids exposure to the undesirable consequences of HFV, including: (1) the potential for hypoventilation with an open airway and trial-and-error method needed to determine appropriate pressure and rate settings, (2) noise and air-borne foreign material, including sputum and blood with retrograde flow of gas from the airway, (3) increased complexity of anesthetic management due to the need to convert from inhalation agents to intravenous drugs during HFV, thus potentially obviating the ability to awaken the patient for extubation in the operating room at the conclusion of the procedure, and (4) the potential for severe barotrauma with inadvertent slippage of the catheter tip into peripheral lung with high gas flow and pressure.

Finally, other examples of operative procedures in which use of HFV has been shown to be beneficial include bronchoscopy and laryngoscopy. During the latter, HFV is of significant benefit when visual or surgical exposure would be complicated by the use of standard large-size endotracheal tubes.

There are, undoubtedly, other potential applications for HFV techniques in conjunction with anesthesia for thoracic surgery. Current limitations of technology, especially limits of respiratory rate at 150 breaths with commercial devices, inadequate humidification, and lack of complete understanding concerning the basic principles that govern gas exchange, most notably with lung pathology, pose a natural restriction against more widespread use. At present, application of these methods should be limited to situations in which significant advantages exist when compared with more conventional, time proven approaches.

SUGGESTED READING

Capan LM, Turndorf H, Patel C, et al. Optimization of arterial oxygenation during one-lung anesthesia. Anesth Analg 1980; 59:847–851.

El-Baz NM, Kittle CF, Faber LP, et al. High-frequency ventilation with an uncuffed endobronchial tube. A new technique for one-lung anesthesia. J Thorac Cardiovasc Surg 1982; 84:823–828.

El-Baz N, Jensik R, Faber LP, et al. One-lung high-frequency ventilation for tracheoplasty and bronchoplasty: a new technique. Ann Thorac Surg 1982; 34:564–571.

Katz JA, Laverne RG, Fairley HB, et al. Pulmonary oxygen exchange during endobronchial anesthesia: effect of tidal volume and PEEP. Anesthesiology 1982; 56:164–171.

Seki S, Gotta K, Kondo T, et al. Gas exchange and facilitation of high-frequency ventilation in intrathoracic surgery. Ann Thorac Surg 1984; 37:491–496.

EXTRACORPOREAL MEMBRANE OXYGENATION

WARREN M. ZAPOL, M.D.

The membrane lung is an extracorporeal device for directly exchanging respiratory gases in blood. By preventing hypoxia and hyercapnia in some patients for days or weeks, the membrane lung can sustain life while otherwise intolerable pulmonary damage heals. Lung repair is made possible, since bypass with the artificial lung relieves the patient's lungs of their primary burden of respiratory gas exchange and avoids the handicaps of conventional ventilator therapy, high ventilator pressures, and inspired oxygen tensions. Temporary circulatory assistance can also be delivered to assist the heart. In newborns with congenital diaphragmatic hernia after surgical repair or meconium aspiration and an unstable pulmonary circulation (pulmonary vasoconstriction and ductal shunting), partial venoarterial perfusion appears to improve survival rates.

INDICATIONS

Adults

At present, treatment by extracorporeal membrane oxygenation (ECMO) patients is only useful for tiding patients over a week-long crisis of insufficient pulmonary gas exchange. The hope that large numbers of patients with respiratory failure due to septicemia or pneumonia would survive with ECMO support has proved fruitless, and ECMO should not be used to treat such patients. Indeed, the best use of ECMO is to tide patients over a brief crisis of insufficient gas exchange, especially when respiratory failure is provoked by reversible circulatory insufficiency. Acute pulmonary embolism is an excellent example of a major respiratory embarrassment with a reduced cardiac output, amenable to ECMO therapy if surgical embolectomy or thrombolytic therapy is undertaken. Another noninflammatory cause of respiratory failure, e.g., severe hypoxemic pulmonary alveolar proteinosis that cannot be lavaged with a double-lumen tube, has been successfully treated with 36 hours of ECMO to support bronchoalveolar lavage. Other transient and reversible causes of cardiorespiratory failure (e.g., iatrogenic venous gas embolism) can be successfully treated with ECMO and such illnesses are now the only appropriate ones for ECMO therapy.

Before ECMO is instituted for respiratory failure, an adequate duration trial of conservative therapy with conventional mechanical ventilation, suctioning, chest physiotherapy, muscle paralysis, positive end-expiratory pressure, cardiotonics, and diuretics must be carried out. However, an evaluation of the failure of conventional therapy and a decision to institute ECMO must be done early, before oxygen toxicity, barotrauma, and superinfection render attempts at ECMO futile. Most survivors of ECMO have been given this bypass early in the course of their disease, after receiving a single reversible pulmonary insult. Although determining the reversibility of any pulmonary insult is difficult, patients with several weeks of respiratory illlness, extensive pulmonary or multi-organ pathologic changes, or advanced age make survival after ECMO for respiratory failure unlikely.

Children

Success has been reported by Bartlett et al with ECMO venoarterial bypass therapy for neonatal respiratory failure in infants weighing more than 2 kg. These infants had persistent fetal circulation, meconium aspiration syndrome, and congenital diaphragmatic hernia (CDH). They were treated with ECMO after several different criteria were met for acute deterioration (PaO_2 less than 40 mm Hg or pH less than 7.15 for 2 hours), barotrauma, or CDH (PaO_2 less than 80 mm Hg at FIO_2 more than 0.8 after honeymoon period).

CONTRAINDICATIONS

ECMO causes thrombocytopenia and requires heparin therapy; bleeding is a common complication. Some patients with recent abdominal surgery (less than 24 hours) have been bypassed successfully, but patients with recent head trauma can develop intracerebral bleeding. There are reports of thoracic or abdominal surgery during ECMO, but hemostasis is difficult to achieve without reducing heparin anticoagulation and clotting the ECMO circuit. Patients often cure their respiratory failure on ECMO, but then after disconnection die of multiple organ failure. Thus patients with renal or hepatic failure are unsuitable for ECMO therapy. However, several adult respiratory distress syndrome (ARDS) patients have survived concomitant ECMO and hemodialysis or hemo-ultrafiltration. In neonates Bartlett considers as contraindications to the use of ECMO, an intracranial hemorrhage, age over 7 days, or a concomitant condition incompatible with a normal quality of life.

TYPES OF ECMO

Briefly, two types of ECMO are in common use: partial venovenous (VV) bypass and partial venoarterial (VA) bypass. Both perfusion routes have advantages and disadvantages that must be weighed in each patient. Both routes can be performed with a single blood pump and a simple extracorporeal circuit.

Venovenous bypass can be used in children and adults. Venovenous or prepulmonary bypass allows the arterial tree to distribute oxygenated blood in a uniform pattern through the left ventricle. Venous blood is drained from the inferior vena cava through the common femoral vein and oxygenated blood returned to the superior vena cava. A double-lumen catheter for both venous drainage and return of arterialized blood to the thoracic inferior vena cava is available and simplifies VV perfusion to use of only a single femoral vein cannulation. This simplified cannulation allows blood flows of 2 to 3 L per min. Venovenous perfusion can be used for infants to drain the right atrium via the internal jugular vein and return via the femoral vein, when possible below the sapheno femoral junction. Venovenous perfusion is believed best for adult perfusions for respiratory failure without cardiac failure, since VV bypass does not reduce the pulmonary blood flow.

Venoarterial bypass decreases pulmonary blood flow and requires large-bore cannulation of the arterial circulation. The major flaw of VA bypass is the inappropriate distribution of arterialized blood. Oxygenated blood returned to the distal aorta is distributed to the kidneys, mesenteric bed, and lower limbs. In severe ARDS we often see a combination of a large cardiac index, intrapulmonary shunt over 50 percent and a small A-VO_2 content difference. Venoarterial perfusion with distal aortic return is then ineffective to increase heart and brain PaO_2, and proximal aortic cannulation is required. Bartlett et al cannulate the internal carotid artery of neonates to improve cerebral oxygenation. Venoarterial bypass for ECMO in newborns has been extensively explored in recent times, and this route is recommended for this reason. Venoarterial bypass can support the heart by increasing the cardiac output and has been helpful in supporting adults with reversible right ventricular dysfunction or acute pulmonary embolism.

TABLE 1 Reported Bypass Survivors with Adult Respiratory Distress Syndrome* to 1986

Disease	*Survivors*
Shock, trauma, fat embolism	11
Bacterial pneumonia, septicemia	8
Viral pneumonia	5
Cardiac failure after cardiac surgery	4
Goodpasture's syndrome	3
Pulmonary embolism	2
Drowning, inhalation injury	2
Varicella pneumonia	2
Pneumocystis carinii pneumonia	2
Aspiration pneumonia	1
TOTAL	40

* Surviving patients over 10 years of age reported from approximately 250 to 300 adult bypass trials.

RESULTS OF BYPASS

About 40 adult patients have survived about 300 bypass procedures in my review of known cases (1986). The survivors are listed in Table 1. The shock and trauma group has provided the largest number of survivors. Although I cannot be certain that these patients would not have survived with conventional therapy, I am convinced by the outcome of a number of my own bypass and shock and trauma patients that hypoxemia and low cardiac output would have killed them unless sufficient time had been bought with an ECMO procedure. Clearly, membrane oxygenator perfusion can powerfully support gas exchange and cardiac output. However, each ECMO procedure must be accompanied by strenuous efforts to improve lung function and remove any reversible causes of respiratory or cardiac failure (e.g., clot, sepsis). Only by permanently reversing the natural lung or heart injury in adults or relieving the instability of the pulmonary circulation in neonates can extracorporeal perfusion with a membrane lung allow the natural organ to heal and the patient to survive.

SUGGESTED READING

Bartlett RH, Roloff DW, Cornell RG, et al. Extracorporeal circulation in neonatal respiratory failure: a prospective randomized study. Pediatrics 1985; 76:479-487.

Gattinoni L, Pesenti A, Mascheroni D, et al. Low- frequency positive-pressure ventilation with extracorporeal CO_2 removal in severe acute respiratory failure. JAMA 1986; 256:881-886.

Loyd JE, Newman JH, Brigham KL. Permeability pulmonary edema. Diagnosis and management. Arch Intern Med 1984; 144:143-147.

Rie MA, Wilson RS. Acute respiratory failure. In: Tinker J, Rapin M, eds. Care of the critically ill patient. New York: Springer-Verlag, 1983:311.

Rinaldo JE, Rogers RW. Adult respiratory distress syndrome: changing concepts of lung injury and repair. N Engl J Med 36:900–909.

Zapol WM, Qvist J, eds. Artifical lungs for acute respiratory failure: theory and practice. New York: Academic Press, 1976.

Zapol WM, Snider MT, Hill JR, et al. Extracorporeal membrane oxygenation in severe acute respiratory failure: a randomized prospective study. JAMA 1979; 242:2193–2196.

Zapol WM, Snider MT, Rie M, Frikker M, Quinn D. Pulmonary circulation during ARDS. In: Zapol WM, Falke K, eds. Acute respiratory failure. New York:Marcel Dekker 1985:241.

I ENDOSCOPY

BRONCHOSCOPY

DOUGLAS J. MATHISEN, M.D.

Introduction of the flexible bronchoscope has changed the practice of bronchoscopy dramatically. It has opened the field of bronchoscopy to the internist and, at the same time, diminished the experience with the rigid bronchoscope for the surgeon. However, specific situations continue to exist that demand only the use of the rigid bronchoscope.

RIGID BRONCHOSCOPY

Specific indications for rigid bronchoscopy include massive hemoptysis, aspirated foreign bodies, tracheal stenosis, and emergency control of the airway secondary to obstructing tumors of the trachea or main stem bronchi. The use of various telescopes and biopsy forceps allow the application of rigid bronchoscopy to virtually any situation requiring endoscopy of the tracheobronchial tree.

For the most part rigid bronchoscopy is perfomed under general anesthesia. Proper preparation of the patient while anesthesia is being induced includes positioning the head in the sniffing position, taping the eyelids, and protection of the teeth. A range of rigid bronchoscopes should be available, from pediatric sizes to the largest adult size.

Technique of Insertion

The patient's upper teeth should be grasped with the middle three fingers and the thumb used to lever the rigid bronchoscope off the teeth. The epiglottis is identified and then the bronchoscope rotated 90 degrees so that it is insinuated between the vocal cords at its narrowest diameter. Inspection then commences using 0-degree, 45-degree, and 90-degree telescopes for more direct visualization of each lobe and segment. Washings, brushings, and biopsies are then taken as necessary.

Brief mention should be made of those specific situations that require rigid bronchoscopy. Patients with tight tracheal stenosis should ideally be bronchoscoped with rigid instruments. This is best done after the patient is deeply anesthetized with halothane. Rigid bronchoscopes in a variety of sizes should be available to dilate tight strictures if necessary. This must be done very carefully in order to avoid perforation of the trachea. The proper measurements can then be taken as to the degree of involvement of the trachea and the amount of trachea remaining for reconstruction. Trying to examine a tracheal stenosis with a flexible bronchoscope in an awake patient may result in sudden airway obstruction, loss of the patient, or inadequate measurements. Aspirated foreign bodies are best managed with a rigid bronchoscope. The objects can be grasped and removed either through the bronchoscope or with the object held securely by the forceps as the bronchoscope is removed. Massive hemoptysis requires rigid bronchoscopy to allow adequate suctioning and to determine the origin of bleeding. The rigid bronchoscope can also be used to establish an airway by placing it into the unaffected lung. Bronchial blockers and packs can also be placed through a rigid bronchoscope, which might be much more difficult using flexible bronchoscopy. Patients who have airway obstruction secondary to malignant strictures can be managed by the use of rigid bronchoscopy, permitting removal of the tumor with biopsy forceps or actual coring out of the tumor with the tip of the bronchoscope. This can be done safely with little bleeding and with the expectation of a satisfactorily patent airway at completion.

FLEXIBLE BRONCHOSCOPY

Flexible bronchoscopy allows the quiet and easy visualization of the tracheobronchial tree in the awake patient. It can be performed safely at the bedside for purposes of inspecting the tracheobronchial tree or of aiding in clearing secretions in the patient with sputum retention.

Flexible bronchoscopy begins with proper premedication of the patient. Atropine 0.5 mg, diazepam 5 mg, and meperidine 50 mg, are given to the patient on call to the endoscopy suite. These doses are adjusted for age and size of the patient. Electrocardiographic electrodes and nasal prongs for oxygen administration are placed on the patient. Approximately 20 cc of 2 percent lidocaine are placed into a nebulizer and then sprayed into the pharynx to anesthetize the area. The patient is instructed to gargle and then expectorate the lidocaine. Use of a tongue blade is helpful for direct spraying of the most posterior aspect of the pharynx. Five cc of 2 percent lidocaine are then drawn into a syringe and connected to a 21-gauge butterfly needle. The cricothyroid membrane is palpated and the butterfly inserted in a caudad fashion at approximately 30 degrees to the patient's neck to avoid injecting into the larynx. The syringe is then aspirated to be certain that air returns, and the 5 cc of 2 percent lidocaine are slowly injected into the trachea. The patient should be instructed not to cough or swallow during this period. If the lidocaine is injected slowly enough, the patient will not cough.

Proper equipment needed to perform flexible bronchoscopy includes 10 cc of 2 percent lidocaine, a basin of sterile saline for irrigation, four cytology slides, a sputum trap, a small vial or piece of filter paper to collect biopsies, a brush, biopsy forceps, and a number 7.5 or 8 uncuffed endotracheal tube; epinephrine should be available in case of excessive bleeding. The uncuffed endotracheal tube is threaded over the flexible bronchoscope. When the flexible bronchoscope has been passed between the vocal cords and advanced into the trachea, the uncuffed endotracheal tube can easily be passed into the trachea. The tube is then secured by passing a gauze sponge around the base of it and having an assistant hold it. This allows for control of the airway and enables the examiner to go in and out of the tracheobronchial tree with ease when collecting multiple specimens. The flexible bronchoscope is passed by grasping the tongue and pulling it forward and using the oral route of intubation with the bronchoscope and endotracheal tube. If the examiner holds the tongue, the patient will not bite the bronchoscope. Additional lidocaine may be required in the area in which specimens and biopsies are taken. The judicious use of 2 percent lidocaine should prevent an overdose. A 1:10,000 concentration of epinephrine can be used to stop excessive bleeding by injecting 3- to 4-ml aliquots through the flexible bronchoscope directly into the bleeding area.

Transbronchial biopsy is best performed using the flexible bronchoscope. It must be carried out under fluoroscopic guidance and control. The use of a C-arm allows visualization of the area of interest and assures that the biopsy is taken in this area. If no specific target is to be biopsied, the biopsy forceps should be visualized near the periphery of the lung. It should then be withdrawn approximately 1 to 2 cm and the patient's jaws opened; the biopsy forceps is then advanced and a biopsy taken. Multiple biopsies should be taken to obtain representative samples. The management of complications from flexible bronchoscopy includes control of hemorrhage and the management of pneumothorax. Bleeding following transbronchial or other biopsy may be troublesome. The previously mentioned technique of using small aliquots of epinephrine in 1:10,000 concentration is effective for most cases. The affected area can also be lavaged with cold saline, although this has been reported to cause bronchospasm. Balloon catheters can be threaded through the flexible bronchoscope and placed in the affected area if massive bleeding continues. If bleeding continues to be a problem, rigid bronchoscopy may be required to isolate the area so as to permit control and tamponade of the bleeding.

SUGGESTED READING

Ikeda S. Atlas of flexible bronchoscopy. Tokyo: Igaku-Shoin, 1974.

ESOPHAGOSCOPY

RICHARD F. HEITMILLER, M.D.
DOUGLAS J. MATHISEN, M.D.

Esophagoscopy is an important procedure that should be considered in the evaluation of all esophageal disorders. There are few contraindications to its use, and it can be used in conjunction with other diagnostic procedures such as barium swallow and esophageal motility studies. Despite numerous developments in the field of esophagoscopy, which include improved anesthesia, superior optics, and the introduction of the flexible esophagoscope, it is still an artful procedure with serious potential complications.

ANATOMY

The esophagus is a musculomembranous tube about 25 cm in length that connects the pharynx and the stomach. It begins at the lower border of the cricoid cartilage opposite the sixth and seventh cervical vertebrae and ends below the diaphragm at the level of the tenth and eleventh thoracic vertebrae. The intra-abdominal portion of the esophagus is short, approximately 1.25 cm in length, and lies posterior to the left lobe of the liver. The esophagus is neither straight nor of constant luminal diameter. It has three important narrowings. The first and tightest of these narrowings is at its origin, where it has a luminal diameter of approximately 14 mm. The second is at the level of the aortic arch, where its lumen narrows to 15 to 17 mm, and the third area of narrowing is at the level of the diaphragmatic hiatus, where it again narrows down to a luminal size of 16 to 19 mm. The esophagus is broadest in the lower third of the thorax, where it reaches a luminal diameter of 22 mm. By convention endoscopic position is measured as distance from the incisor teeth. The origin of the esophagus, therefore, at the level of the cricopharyngeal sphincter is at 15 cm, the aortic arch is at 18 to 20 cm, and the diaphragmatic hiatus is at 40 cm.

INDICATIONS

Esophagoscopy is considered a complementary procedure to other diagnostic tests such as barium swallow, esophageal manometry, and pH testing. Esophagoscopy should be considered in the evaluation of all symptoms of esophageal disease. Visual inspection and biopsy allow for evaluation of esophageal masses, strictures, and mucosal abnormalities, such as esophagitis, Barrett's mucosa, and moniliasis. Therapeutic interventions include removal of foreign bodies, sclerosing varices, dilating esophageal strictures, and endoscopic positioning of intraluminal funnel tubes. Indications for use of the flexible esophagoscope versus the rigid esophagoscope are generally ones of personal preference. Flexible esophagoscopy can be done under local anesthesia, allows inspection of the stomach and duodenum, and because of the smaller size of the pediatric esophagoscope, may allow inspection beyond either a mass or stricture. The flexible esophagoscope is also generally safer in patients with severe kyphoscoliosis or cervical osteophytes. The rigid esophagoscope allows for larger biopsies, more aggressive suctioning in the face of massive bleeding, and easier removal of foreign bodies.

CONTRAINDICATIONS

There are few contraindications to the use of esophagoscopy. Relative contraindications include cervicothoracic spine problems such as degenerative disorders that would lead to cervical instability; kyphoscoliosis; cervical osteophytes that often protrude against the esophagus, increasing the risk of perforation; and cervical spine injuries that might jeopardize the spinal cord.

TECHNIQUE

Preparation of the patient includes removal of any dental prostheses and emptying of the esophagus. General anesthesia is used with rigid esophagoscopy and endoscopy in children, and a combination of sedation and topical anesthesia is generally used in adults. When utilizing topical anesthesia, the esophageal mucosa is insensitive, and therefore the posterior pharynx and the arytenoepiglottic folds need to be anesthetized. This can be accomplished with a 2 percent viscous lidocaine solution. Sedation is accomplished with a combination of benzodiazepam and narcotics, with the option of reversing the narcotics at the conclusion of the procedure.

For rigid esophagoscopy, the patient should be positioned in the supine position with the head and neck in the sniff position, as for a tracheal intubation. The patient should be positioned on a table such that the neck can be flexed and extended easily. Suction must be available. The first steps in performing esophagoscopy are identical to those for laryngeal intubation. The rigid endoscope is introduced at the base of the tongue and the epiglottis is visualized. Using the tip of the endoscope, the epiglottis is then picked up, and the scope is advanced slowly to the posterior pharynx. The cricopharyngeal sphincter is then identified as a horizontal groove approximately halfway between the posterior larynx and the posterior pharyngeal wall. If the sphincter is identified, the esophagus can be intubated under direct vision. A small Jackson's dilator can be used to locate the cricopharyngeal sphincter, and then the scope can be advanced over this dilator. This is the most dangerous part of the procedure, and it must be performed with care. Once the scope is inside the esophagus, the patient's neck is extended and then the endoscope is advanced only while visualizing the esophageal lumen. Throughout the procedure, the patient's upper teeth and lip are protected with a mouth guard or gauze sponge in addition to the endoscopist's left fingers and thumb.

For flexible endoscopy, the patient is positioned in the left lateral decubitus position. Two fingers are introduced into the mouth to lift the tongue, jaw, and epiglottis. The flexible esophagoscope is then introduced into the posterior pharynx, maintained in the midline, and guided between the two fingers. The cricopharyngeal sphincter is usually intubated "blindly," but it may be visually guided as well. This often involves an assistant. The endoscope is only advanced while visualizing the lumen. If the patient is intubated, entry into the esophagus often involves letting down the endotracheal tube cuff, visualizing the cricopharyngeal sphincter, and passing the scope under direct vision.

COMPLICATIONS

The most feared complication of endoscopy is esophageal perforation. The most common sites of perforation are the cricopharyngeal and cervical regions. The next most common areas are the points of relative narrowing of the esophagus or the level of any esophageal disease. Perforation can occur with both flexible and rigid endoscopy. Prevention by careful technique is far preferable to the management of esophageal perforation. Following completion of the procedure, each patient undergoing endoscopy should be checked for signs of perforation, such as severe localized pain, subcutaneous emphysema, pneumothorax, pleural effusion, and elevation in temperature. Suspicion of perforation should immediately be followed up by meglucamine diatrizoate (Gastrografin) barium swallow to identify the site of perforation. Treatment of esophageal perforation should be prompt and is discussed in the chapter *Spontaneous and Iatrogenic Esophageal Perforation.*

SUGGESTED READING

Jackson C, Jackson CL. Bronchoesophagology. Philadelphia: WB Saunders, 1950.

Palmer E, Wirts EW. Survey of gastroscopic and esophagoscopic accidents. JAMA 1957; 164:2012.

Postelthwait RW. Surgery of the esophagus. 2nd ed. Norwalk, CT: Appleton-Century Crofts, 1986.

Shalimier M, Schuman BM. Complication of fiberoptic endoscopy. Gastrointest Endosc 1980; 26:86.

Sweet RH, Terracol J. Diseases of the esophagus. Philadelphia: WB Saunders, 1958.

THORACOSCOPY AND THE CHAMBERLAIN PROCEDURE

JAMES W. MACKENZIE, M.D., F.A.C.S.
RALPH J. LEWIS, M.D., F.A.C.S.

THORACOSCOPY

Despite the numerous methods available to detect and confirm the presence of intrathoracic disease, on occasion a more direct look and biopsy may be necessary to establish a diagnosis. Exploratory thoracotomy, with its inherent morbidity, mortality, and prolonged hospitalization, often can be avoided by utilizing thoracoscopy.

Since 1970 we have performed 383 thoracoscopies without a death. The patients had a wide variety of intrathoracic disease, including mesothelioma, bronchogenic carcinoma, and carcinoma metastatic to the thorax, as well as chronic and acute inflammatory disease.

We have tried various instruments such as the flexible fiberoptic bronchoscope, rigid bronchoscope, peritoneoscope, and special thoracoscopes. However, we have found the standard Carlens mediastinoscope to be eminently satisfactory for use in adults. Although we have performed lung biopsy via the thoracoscope, we have usually confined thoracoscopy to patients with pleural disease.

The procedure is performed in the operating room with the use of endotracheal anesthesia; either side of the thorax can be readily approached. One-lung anesthesia simplifies the procedure. The patient is supine on the table which is in the reversed Trendelenberg position of about 20 degrees to prevent the abdominal viscera from elevating the diaphragm and thereby decreasing the intrathoracic volume. The side to be examined is elevated 30 degrees by means of folded sheets or a vacuum device. Slight flexion of the elbow at the side will permit more adequate exposure of the surface of the chest. The elbow is appropriately padded to avoid neural injury.

A transverse 2-inch incision is made in the midaxillary line at the level of the fifth or sixth interspace and carried through the skin, subcutaneous tissue, and extracostal muscles. Usually the muscle fibers can be separated and need not be divided, thus avoiding unnecessary bleeding. The intercostal muscles similarly are bluntly separated by the index finger, which enters the pleural cavity and can readily appreciate any adhesions between the visceral and parietal pleurae.

The parietal and visceral pleurae and lung in the immediate area can be palpated for consistency, nodules, and masses. Adhesions are gently divided by finger dissection when possible, and any fluid present is aspirated and collected for appropriate studies. The Carlens mediastinoscope is positioned between the ribs, and with appropriate manipulation in an organized and sequential manner the parietal and visceral pleurae, diaphragm, fissures, pericardium, hilum, and apex sulcus can be directly evaluated. At times, a sterile rigid bronchoscope is necessary to see the apex. Bleeding points may be controlled by pressure from the scope or by cauterization. Under direct vision, generous biopsy specimens can be safely obtained and then sent for frozen section to confirm the diagnosis. Deep parietal pleural biopsies should be avoided to prevent injury to the intercostal vessels. Visceral biopsies should not be attempted unless there is consolidation of the underlying lung, otherwise, bleeding and air leaks may occur. Pericardial biopsies should be approached with caution because of possible adherence between the visceral and parietal layers. Obviously, the phrenic nerve must be seen before any biopsy of the pericardium. Similarly, biopsy tissue from the diaphragm, if too generous, may produce defects in this muscle, causing herniation at a later time.

The biopsy areas are now inspected, and if hemostasis is satisfactory, the instrument is removed and a No. 28 chest tube is passed through the wound. The muscles are approximated with two or three sutures, the subcutaneous tissue with interrupted absorbable sutures, and the skin with an intradermal absorbable suture. The tube is sutured in place and connected to an underwater sealed bottle. The wound is dressed, and the patient is transferred to the recovery room where a chest radiograph is taken with a portable machine. When vital signs are stable, the patient is returned to the hospital floor. Fluids are permitted on the evening of operation and the patient rapidly progresses to a regular diet. Ambulation is begun on the evening of operation. A chest radiograph is taken the following day. The tube is usually removed within 48 hours. Antitubercular drugs are given on the day of operation if tuberculosis seems likely. On occasion, medication (bleomycin or tetracycline) is instilled into the intrathoracic tube to prevent the recurrence of pleural fluid. Depending upon the disease process, the patient may be discharged within 2 days of the operation.

Complications are rare and usually related to the general anesthesia. As with any intrathoracic procedure, bleeding may occur unless structures are carefully identified.

CHAMBERLAIN PROCEDURE

The theoretic drainage of lymphatics from the left upper lobe of the lung is to the subcarinal nodes and then to the ipsilateral peritracheal nodes. In practice, however, left upper-lobe lesions often drain to the right side as well. Therefore, because of its greater simplicity, we usually perform cervical mediastinoscopy first. In patients with lesions of the left upper lobe where the cervical mediastinoscopy is not diagnostic, and particularly if there is clinical suspicion of intrathoracic nodal metastases on which biopsy was not done, the Chamberlain procedure is employed.

As described by McNeill and Chamberlain, a 4-inch incision is made over the second costal cartilage. Guided by the radiologic findings, we may make the incision over the third cartilage or over the second interspace. The costal cartilage is totally excised subperichondrially, and the posterior periosteum is then incised. Alternatively, the intercostal muscles may be separated by a hemostat. The internal mammary artery vessels may be retracted laterally, but we often find it best to ligate them individually. With lateral mobilization of the pleura, it is possible to enter the mediastinum without entry into the pleural cavity. More commonly, however, the pleural space is entered either inadvertently or by design. In either case, a simple underwater seal apparatus is all that is needed.

Principally by blunt finger dissection, the region of the subaortic nodes is approached. The aorta should be identified, as should the main pulmonary artery. The mediastinoscope is inserted. Appropriate biopsies are taken. Through this incision, or with a slight lateral extension, biopsies of the lung itself may also be obtained. The use of a cautery and headlight significantly increases the ease of this procedure.

As stated above, we have usually preceded this procedure with cervical mediastinoscopy. In such cases the cervical wound is not closed prior to the mediastinotomy. Therefore, bimanual palpation of the subaortic area may be carried out.

Complications are remarkably infrequent. Obviously, bleeding may occur if care is not taken to securely ligate the mammary vessels or if care is not taken to differentiate lymph nodes (by aspiration if necessary) from major vascular structures. Again, we have found the standard mediastinoscope to be a most satisfactory instrument. Care should also be taken to avoid the vagus nerve and its recurrent branch as it lies just above the pulmonary artery on the left. An arteriovenous fistula is possible if the internal mammary artery and its vein are ligated together.

SUGGESTED READING

Jacobaeus H. The practical importance of thoracoscopy in surgery of the chest. Surg Gynecol Obstet 1922; 34:289–296.

Lewis RJ, Kunderman PJ, Sisler GE, Mackenzie JW. Direct diagnostic thoracoscopy. Ann Thorac Surg 1976; 21:536–539.

McNeill T, Chamberlain J. Diagnostic anterior mediastinotomy. Ann Thorac Surg 1966; 2:532–539.

Rodgers BM, Ryckman FC, Moazam F, Talbert JL. Thoracoscopy for intrathoracic tumors. Ann Thorac Surg 1981; 31:414–420.

Stemmer EA, Calvin JW, Chandor SB, Connolly JE. Mediastinal biopsy for indeterminate pulmonary and mediastinal lesions. J Thorac Cardiovasc Surg 1965; 49:405–411.

MEDIASTINOSCOPY

WERNER MAASSEN, M.D.

We have undertaken more than 11,500 mediastinoscopies in our clinic, with only five deaths. The immediate value of the examination is purely diagnostic. Its therapeutic use is seen in the results of the histologic examinations, which facilitate and ensure the differential diagnosis. In our experience mediastinoscopy has been effective in directing management in 82 percent of patients with changes of the mediastinum and/or pulmonary roots of uncertain origin and in 44 percent of those with ambiguous changes of the pulmonary parenchyma. The negative histologic results in the latter group are explainable in terms of nonspecific inflammatory pulmonary infections and benign tumors suspicious for bronchial carcinoma (BC). In both these groups, the examination initially often helps to plan internal medical or oncologic therapy. For thoracic surgeons, the results are mostly of interest (apart from a few cases of mediastinal tumors) for the preoperative staging of BC (36 percent of our patients undergoing mediastinoscopy have had results positive for BC).

INDICATIONS

In the two different patient groups mentioned above, mediastinoscopy is indicated when all less invasive methods have failed to establish a clear diagnosis. In cases of sarcoidosis, in particular, the results of bronchoscopy with mucosal biopsy, transbronchial pulmonary biopsy, and bronchoalveolar lavage must first be awaited. A mediastinoscopy is of no diagnostic assistance in cases of tumors in the anterior mediastinum in front of the heart and the great vessels (a parasternal mediastinotomy would be of more value because it is less dangerous than the retrosternal approach). When palpable supraclavicular lymph nodes are present, these should be examined first. In our clinic, in 575 patients examined simultaneously by mediastinoscopy and a classic Daniel's lymph node biopsy (in patients without palpable nodes), 54 percent had positive findings on the strength of the mediastinoscopy alone and 46 percent from the two procedures together. In patients with bronchial carcinoma, these percentages were 74 percent and 26 percent, respectively, and 57 percent and 43 percent for other malignant diseases. An inoperability rate of 30 percent must be expected in cases of BC with a negative supraclavicular lymph node biopsy, whereas this rate is only 5 percent to 8 percent after negative mediastinoscopy findings. In patients with cancer of the esophagus, mediastinal exploration provides information about metastasis in the upper mediastinum. When malignant or tuberculous changes of the pleura cannot be determined by puncture and thoracoscopy, mediastinoscopy can still lead to histologically useful results; the same is true in silicosis. In some patients with inflammatory suppuration (tuberculosis or mediastinal abscess) or mediastinal emphysema, the typical access path to the mediastinum can be used for drainage.

CONTRAINDICATIONS

Contraindications to mediastinoscopy are aortic aneurysm and extreme superior vena cava syndrome. If the latter is improved by a course of irradiation treatment, mediastinoscopy can be carried out without hesitation. Caution is advisable in cases in which extensive tumor growth necessitates high dose radiotherapy; in such instances, the histologic findings are usually no longer of interest anyway. There is no contraindication in patients without tracheostomies who have undergone laryngectomy. The examination is usually easier after thyroidectomy. We have performed repeat mediastinoscopies without incident in about 100 patients already examined in other hospitals. As a rule, in those who were not examined successfully, adhesions between the anterior surface of the trachea and the left brachiocephalic vein are found; when these are loosened, an almost normal procedure is possible. It has been proved histologically that mediastinoscopy does not lead to the formation of fibrosis of the mediastinum, and it does not cause any complications after a pneumonectomy.

TECHNIQUE

The patient lies in the supine position with the head extremely reclined, and endotracheal anesthesia is administered. A 3- to 4-cm skin incision is made in the jugulum, followed by separation of the platysma, incision of the superficial cervical fascia, blunt dissociation of the straight muscles, and exposure of the anterior surface of the trachea, as for an inferior tracheotomy. To perform this, only the assistant nurse's attendance is necessary. The pretracheal cervical fascia is lifted with a dissecting scissors and the layer between this and the trachea in front of it is opened at both sides. Then the inspection area is exposed by blunt finger preparation in a caudal direction; the finger should reach as far as the main bronchi, if possible. The mediastinoscope is then inserted, and further preparation is carried out by means of a suction rod. In cases of generalized disease, one or two tissue samples are usually sufficient, and this also applies for idiopathic tumors. In cases of suspected silicosis, tissue must be taken from the bifurcation lymph node, since it is most representative. Proof of silicates is not enough: a thickened silicotic transformation must also be present. In cases of BC, all lymph nodes in the upper mediastinum must be examined by means of biopsy—even apparently healthy ones—paratracheal on both sides, in both tracheobronchial and subcarinal angles. To sample the bifurcation lymph node, a bronchopericardial membrane must be perforated. When taking the sample, there is a risk of passing under the subcarinal nodes and injuring the esophagus.

Local or general antibiotic therapy is not necessary, except probably when lymph nodes involved by caseous tuberculosis are entered. When taking all samples, the trachea must be used as a guideline, and the exits of the two main bronchi must be established. On the right, it is possible for the partly exposed azygos vein to protrude and be mistaken for an anthracotic lymph node. This danger is limited if an exploratory puncture is undertaken using a fine needle, and every node is freed to the extent that it can almost be removed with large forceps. Bleeding during the procedure mostly arises from small vessels and stops by itself. More severe hemorrhages can normally be stopped by tamponade in 15 to 20 minutes. Injuries to a bronchial artery in the area of bifurcation usually have to be repaired by means of coagulation; a compact tamponade with resorbable gauze (Tabotamp) often suffices. Lymph nodes on the left paratracheal side cannot always be freed; no forced attempts should be made to do this because of the risk of damage of the recurrent nerve. Postoperative drainage is not necessary. The straight cervical muscles are joined by one suture, and three subcutaneous and three cutaneous sutures (perhaps intradermal) are sufficient. X-ray films of the thorax should be taken a few hours later to check for pneumothorax or pleural effusion.

COMPLICATIONS

Complications associated with this procedure are rare: the mortality rate according to collected statistics is 1.14 percent and in our clinic 0.04 percent. Paresis of the recurrent nerve can occur in 0.5 percent, even when the examiner is skilled, sometimes as a result of injury to the nerve caused by instrument pressure, but this resolves itself after 6 to 8 weeks. Occasional vascular injuries of the brachiocephalic trunk have been reported that were corrected by suturing or a prosthetic patch. In cases of esophageal lesions, including the mucosa, parenteral feeding is sufficient for healing as a rule. About 50 percent of the mediastinoscopies we undertake are performed on an ambulatory basis, either on patients from other hospitals or outpatients. Mediastinoscopy is mostly carried out in conjunction with bronchoscopy.

SPECIAL INDICATIONS FOR BRONCHIAL CARCINOMA

In our experience, there are varying prognostic assessments for the different lymph nodes within the N_2 classification, namely, for those nodes proved metastatic by mediastinoscopy and those found during thoracotomy (parabronchial, paraesophageal, and those in the pulmonary ligament). A surgeon who considers metastatic involvement of the upper mediastinal lymph nodes to be grounds for inoperability should routinely examine this area via a mediastinoscopy before surgery. The sensitivity of this procedure is 95 percent, depending on experience, its specificity 100 percent, and its accuracy 98 percent. The predictive value of a positive test is therefore 95 percent.

Contralateral dissemination in cases of middle lobe tumors and BC of the right lower lobe is relatively common in our experience, so mediastinoscopy is indicated in these patients too. Because of the frequent formation of contralateral metastases in cases of left-sided carcinoma and the difficulty of removing these during a left-sided thoracotomy, the right paratracheal and trachcobronchial area in left-sided BC should always be examined preoperatively.

When the mediastinum is shown to be free of growth on mediastinoscopy, lymph node dissection in the posterior

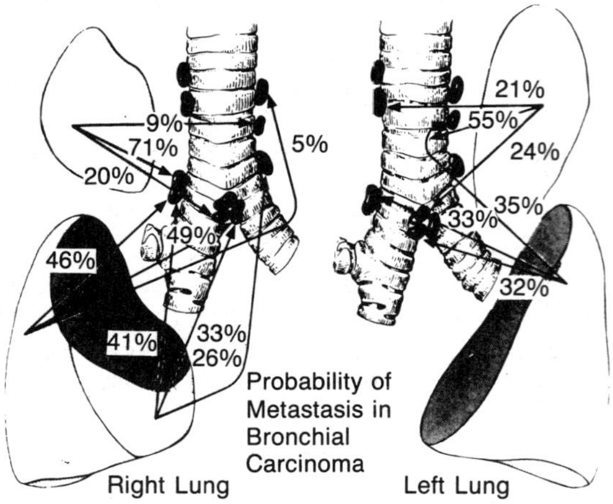

Figure 1 Incidence of lymph node metastases according to location of primary tumor.

mediastinum is unnecessary during thoracotomy and, thus, the operation time can be shortened and the extent of resection often limited. It is not possible to have the indication for mediastinoscopy depend on the size and localization of peripheral and highly differentiated BCs. Routine results in 400 patients with peripheral squamous cell BC were positive in 28 percent (33 percent right-sided, 22 percent left-sided; 18 percent in stage I, 33 percent in stage II, and 44 percent in stage III for the right lung and 18 percent, 29 percent; and 15 percent, respectively, for the left lung). The corresponding figures for 143 patients with peripheral adenocarcinomas were 33 percent positive (40 percent right-sided, 24 percent left-sided; with 26 percent, 45 percent, and 45 percent, respectively, in stages I, II, and III on the right and 16 percent, 25 percent, and 42 percent, respectively, for the same stages on the left).

Gallium scintigraphy and oblique hilar tomography seem ill-suited for a guided mediastinoscopy because of insufficient sensitivity and accuracy. Computed tomography of the mediastinum is suitable. According to a double-blind study carried out in our clinic, the critical size of the involved lymph node seems to be 1.5 cm. Metastases are rare in nodes any smaller than this, and preoperative mediastinoscopy is not useful unless several nodes of from 10.0 to 10.5 cm are present. The larger the lymph node is, the more likely proof of metastasis can be found. However, a clearly enlarged lymph node in the mediastinum with known histologic diagnosis of BC does not necessarily mean a metastasis, for no noninvasive procedure can differentiate between lymph nodes that are enlarged because of metastasis and reactive-hyperplastic ones.

SUGGESTED READING

Carlens E. Mediastinoscopy: a method for inspection and tissue biopsy in the superior mediastinum. Dis Chest 1959; 36:343–352.

Jepsen OH. Rahbek Sorensen: mediastinoscopy. Proceedings of an international symposium. Odense: Odense University Press, 1971.

Maassen W. Results and importance of mediastinoscopy and other thoracic bioptic investigations (in German). Berlin: Springer-Verlag, 1967.

Maassen W. Accuracy of mediastinoscopy. In: Delarue NC, Eschapasse H, eds. International trends in general thoracic surgery. Vol I. Lung cancer. Philadelphia: WB Saunders, 1985:42.

Nohl-Oser HC. The long-term survival of patients with lung cancer after selection by mediastinoscopy. Thorac Cardiovasc Surg 1980; 28:158–161.

Pearson FG, Delarue NC, Ilves R, Todd TRJ, Cooper JD. Significance of positive superior mediastinal nodes identified at mediastinoscopy in patients with resectable cancer of the lung. J Thorac Cardiovasc Surg 1982; 83:1–11.

I TRAUMA

PNEUMOMEDIASTINUM

HERMES C. GRILLO, M.D.

Pneumomediastinum means air in the mediastinum outside of its usual containers, the trachea and the esophagus. The causes of pneumomediastinum are (1) spontaneous, or, more correctly, effort, (2) trauma, (3) inflammatory, (4) neoplastic diseases of the thorax, and (5) abdominal processes with dissection into the mediastinum. There are some additional miscellaneous causes.

SPONTANEOUS OR EFFORT PNEUMOMEDIASTINUM

The amount of effort needed to produce pneumomediastinum may be minimal. Less often, the pneumomediastinum actually seems to be spontaneous. Causes of such effort leakage of air are (1) respiratory distress in infants (2) asthma, especially in children, (3) inspired foreign bodies, usually accompanied by significant cough, (4) strenuous or moderate effort in work or at play, and (5) labor. Lifting heavy objects, bouts of coughing, excessive phonation, pulmonary function tests, stress, mountain climbing, and a variety of other associated causes have been noted. History is usually obtained of a preceding event of the types noted. The principal symptoms are dyspnea with pain, especially on deep inspiration. The pain is centrally located in the chest. It is retrosternal, sometimes radiates to the neck and shoulders and down the arms, and sometimes penetrates to the back. The patient may describe a sense of chest tightness, and there may also be some dysphagia. Dyspnea may be minimal or severe. Hamman's sign—mediastinal crunch—which accompanies heartbeat and respiration may be noted. This may also be seen, however, in simple pneumothorax.

The mechanism of spontaneous or effort pneumomediastinum is related to alveolar rupture, which occurs in marginally situated alveoli with forced hyperexpansion. There may be coexisting bronchiolar obstruction, which serves as a check valve. Rupture tends to occur in the more central alveoli, which have fixed bases. The air dissects along the blood vessels, impelled by respiratory movement. Air thus tracks through the interstitial spaces to the hilus and thence to the mediastinum. If the amount of air continues to build up, rupture of the pleura may occur, with secondary pneumothorax. Subpleural dissection may then occur into the chest wall and also beneath the diaphragmatic pleura. The air may break through the fascial planes of the mediastinum and dissect up into the neck to create subcutaneous emphysema. In infants, the air may more frequently dissect through the interface of pericardial attachments in the mediastinum and present as pneumopericardium. It is thought that this may occur also along the vessels as they exit from the pericardium. Both clinically and experimentally, air from pneumomediastinum has been shown to dissect into the retroperitoneal plane and in some cases to break into the free peritoneal cavity, producing pneumoperitoneum. In most cases spontaneous or effort pneumomediastinum does not produce significant physiologic consequences. However, in infants it is possible for the pneumomediastinum and its associated pneumothoraces and pneumopericardium and even pneumoperitoneum to produce physiologic consequences that can become life-threatening. Hypotension and bradycardia are seen in these infants.

Radiologic findings show streak-like shadows of air dissecting interstitially toward and appearing in the mediastinum. The mediastinal pleura is displaced laterally, as seen on the posteroanterior chest x-ray film, and linear shadows are produced parallel to the heart border. The pleura is separated from the heart by gas, especially on the left side and also along the ascending and descending aorta. Lateral views show retrosternal air and clear-cut outlines of the aortic shadow. In the adult, air dissects up into the neck and out over the thoracic wall. In children, the thymus may be elevated by the air and produce a "sail sign." Air may also be seen between the parietal pleura and the diaphragm. In children it has been found that air leak syndromes are produced in 45 percent of cases in children with asthma and in 22 percent following pneumonia. In reverse, 2 percent of children admitted to a hospital with acute asthma may have pneumomediastinum. Treatment is rarely indicated for these cases produced by effort. Observation and rest are all that is needed. In a few infants, however, pneumothoraces or pneumopericardium may require tube drainage.

Effort perforation of the esophagus, the Boerhaave syndrome, initially produces mediastinal emphysema with the early "V" sign of air at the junction of the mediastinum and the diaphragm.

TRAUMA

Traumatic pneumomediastinum may be produced by either external injury or internal instrument perforation. *External injuries* may include thoracic contusion with or without rib fracture. When pneumomediastinum is seen following blunt chest trauma, there must also be suspicion of injury to major bronchi or the trachea or even rarely to the esophagus. Presentation with bronchial injury may range from tension pneumothorax to complete pneumothorax that fails to respond to suction, or pneumothorax that does respond to suction, or the complete absence of pneumothorax. The last circumstance is seen when there has been pleural obliteration or when the peribronchial connective tissue provides a seal despite total severance of the bronchus. In this case, the air dissection is confined to the mediastinum. Rupture of the trachea in the neck by direct contusion leads to escape of air into the cervical mediastinal tissue planes. There is usually a major dissection of air in the neck in these cases. Perforation of the esophagus by *instrumentation* may also produce mediastinal air, with dissection into the neck seen especially in upper esophageal perforations. Postsurgical mediastinal air is also seen after tracheostomy with dissection from the neck, and as a complication of bronchial and esophageal surgery with leakage.

Barotrauma is another type of injury that can lead to pneumomediastinum. Although this can occur with rapid ascent either in air or water owing to sudden drops in atmospheric pressure with expansion and rupture of alveoli (seen in pilots and scuba divers and also with the excessive airway pressure used during anesthesia or with the Venturi apparatus for bronchoscopic anesthesia), it is most commonly seen with the use of pressure ventilators. Neonates are particularly susceptible to this type of trauma. In adults, the syndrome is seen in patients who require high ventilatory pressures and particularly in those who have destructive lung disease. Thus, mediastinal air was frequently seen in patients requiring continuous positive airway pressure. Peak airway pressures greater than 25 cm of water may produce extra-alveolar air, and pressures greater than 80 cm are extremely hazardous in this respect. Interstitial emphysema usually precedes the pneumomediastinum.

INFLAMMATORY, NEOPLASTIC, AND OTHER CAUSES

On rare occasions pneumomediastinum may result from inflammatory diseases such as viral disease or tuberculosis, diphtheria, influenza, and pneumonia. It has also been described with neoplasms involving the airways, presumably resulting from cough. Abdominal processes such as duodenal perforation, perforation of the colon, and rectal surgery have preceded pneumomediastinum. Miscellaneous causes include therapeutic and diagnostic pneumoperitoneum with upward dissection, facial fractures, dental drilling and tonsillectomy.

In summary, pneumomediastinum can often be a distressing finding. Usually, especially in the adult, it does not require active treatment. It should be observed carefully in the infant so that the occasional case with cardiovascular effects or respiratory compromise can be treated promptly by catheter suction.

SUGGESTED READING

Grillo HC. Air in the mediastinum. The Fifth Coventry Conference. In: Doyle JA, Smith RE, eds. The present state of thoracic surgery. London: Pitman, 1981:49.

FLAIL CHEST AND PULMONARY CONTUSION: NONOPERATIVE MANAGEMENT

P. KENT HARMAN, M.D.
J. KENT TRINKLE, M.D.
FREDERICK L. GROVER, M.D.

Pulmonary contusion may result from blunt external chest trauma, penetrating high-velocity gunshot wounds, or shotgun blasts. Severe chest trauma may produce multiple rib fractures and flail segments. Common associated injuries include myocardial contusion, aortic transection, vertebral disruption, and solid viscus fracture.

The classic therapeutic approach to chest trauma had been external stabilization of the chest wall using tethering towel clips or sandbags. Subsequently, internal pneumatic chest wall support using endotracheal intubation and positive-pressure ventilation became common. Considerable evidence indicates that external modes of stabilization promote atelectasis and subsequent pneumonitis. Endotracheal intubation and positive end expiratory pressure preserve functional residual capacity, but the immediate gains produced by a closed positive-pressure breathing circuit are often negated by the propensity for bacterial colonization and barotrauma.

The primary respiratory pathophysiology of major chest trauma is not the obvious dramatic disruption of rib segments but the extent of the underlying pulmonary contusion. A conservative approach to pulmonary contusion is preferred for all patients who do not require emergent operative therapy for associated injuries. The emphasis is directed toward the reduction of edema and hemorrhage in the area of pulmonary trauma. Accumulated blood and serum in the pleural space are meticulously drained. Most bleeding from fractured ribs and pulmonary wounds is self-limited.

A single 34 or 36 F chest tube usually sufficiently evacuates a hemothorax. Thoracostomy tubes are placed away from obvious fracture sites and open wounds. Tubes inserted in the fifth or sixth intercostal space, midaxillary line, are usually adequate. The tip of the chest tube should be directed superiorly and posteriorly to facilitate pleural drainage in the supine patient.

Emergent thoracotomy is performed only when blood drainage from the ipsilateral hemithorax exceeds 300 ml per hour during the first 1 to 4 hours. Exceptions are rare and include massive initial hemothorax greater than 1,500 ml or suspected cardiac-great vessel injury.

Occasionally clotted blood does not undergo complete spontaneous lysis and a thick pleural peel forms. Lung "trapped" by a chronic hemothorax becomes atelectatic, and vital capacity is reduced. Undrained blood in the pleural space may progress to an empyema. Chronic hemothorax may be prevented by the early placement of multiple chest drainage tubes. If a chronic sanguineous peel develops, it should be removed by open thoracotomy 1 to 3 weeks after the injury.

Significant chest wall fractures are palliated with intramuscular and regional analgesics. The "pulmonary contusion regimen" is instituted in all patients arriving at our emergency department with severe blunt chest trauma: (1) Crystalloid resuscitation is restricted to less than 1,000 ml during the immediate period of stabilization and less than 50 ml per hour as an intravenous maintenance dose. (2) The hematocrit is maintained over 30 ml per deciliter using packed red blood cells. (3) Furosemide, 20 mg, is injected intravenously twice each day. (4) Methylprednisolone, 5 mg per kilogram, is administered intravenously every 6 hours for the first 72 hours. (5) Fresh frozen plasma or synthetic fractional protein is infused at 50 ml per hour to maintain a normal serum oncotic pressure. (6) Intercostal nerve blocks are used frequently for the control of rib pain. Bupivicaine (Marcaine), 0.25 percent, provides reliable pain relief for 8 to 12 hours. Three to five milliliters are injected around involved intercostal nerves. Lidocaine 1 percent in similar quantities is effective for 4 to 6 hours. The injection site is 8 to 10 cm lateral to the midline of the spine. The intercostal nerve is immediately beneath the rib. The intercostal artery and vein are avoided. Intravascular injection of lidocaine is relatively benign, but bupivicaine may produce serious systemic hypotension. The intercostal nerve to all fractured ribs and one intercostal nerve above and below the area of injury are injected. (7) Postural drainage, external vibratory pulmonary thoracic massage, extensive use of incentive inspiratory bottles, and, when necessary, liberal use of endotracheal suctioning are used. (8) Early ambulation is required of all patients, including those with thoracostomy tubes.

Endotracheal intubation can almost always be avoided, even in elderly patients. If an operative procedure is required for a concurrent injury, extubation is expedited soon after the general anesthetic. Upper airway control can be more difficult in patients with moderate to severe head injuries, and for this particular subset, endotracheal intubation, for airway control, is used more liberally. Although we make every attempt to avoid endotracheal intubation, we feel that subsequent airway strictures can usually be avoided by the use of high-volume, low-pressure endotracheal cuffs. We prefer nasotracheal or endotracheal intubation to cricothyroidotomy or tracheostomy, even for periods up to 10 to 14 days.

Prophylactic antibiotics are not used. Daily sputum cultures are obtained, and antibiotic therapy is instituted if the clinical appearance and cultures indicate a bacterial pneumonia.

The previously accepted theory of Pendelluft has been largely discarded. We ignore traumatic chest wall paradoxical motion, and mechanical ventilation is instituted largely using blood gas criteria. These criteria include an arterial PaO_2 of less than 60 mm Hg using supplemental oxygen, a P_{CO_2} greater than 48 mm Hg, acidosis, or obvious respiratory distress that predicts imminent respiratory failure. We have come to the realization that paradoxical motion of the chest wall is a relatively minor factor in the total respiratory injury and that the major problem is the underlying pulmonary contusion.

The avoidance of fluid overloading is paramount. The efficacy of free water depletion can be monitored accurately by serum sodium determinations obtained at 6-hour intervals for the first 72 hours. In the absence of obvious renal injury, a serum sodium level of greater than 140 mEq per liter is optimal. Additional 10 to 20 mg intravenous doses of furosemide are useful for purposes of free water diuresis. This facilitates desiccation of the traumatized lung.

This approach is based on extensive experimental and clinical prospective trials from our own institution and includes treatment of over 1,100 penetrating wounds and a similar number of blunt chest injuries during the past 12 years.

SUGGESTED READING

Avery EE, Morsch ET, Benson DW. Critically crushed chests: a new method of treatment with continuous mechanical hyperventilation to produce alkalotic apnea and internal pneumatic stabilization. J Thorac Surg 1956; 32:291–311.

Cullen P, Modell JH, Kirby RR, et al. Treatment of flail chest: use of intermittent mandatory ventilation and positive end-expiratory pressure. Arch Surg 1975; 110:1099–1103.

Trinkle JK. Flail chest and pulmonary contusion. In: Trinkle JK, Grover FL, eds. Management of thoracic trauma victims. Philadelphia: JB Lippincott, 1980:39.

Trinkle JK, Furman RW, Hinshaw MA, et al. Pulmonary contusion—pathogenesis and effect of various resuscitative measures. Ann Thorac Surg 1973; 16:568–573.

Trinkle JK, Richardson JD, Franz JL, et al. Management of flail chest without mechanical ventilation. Ann Thorac Surg 1975; 19:355–363.

FLAIL CHEST AND PULMONARY CONTUSION: OPERATIVE MANAGEMENT

MARCEL DAHAN, M.D.
JEAN BERJAUD, M.D.
JACQUES GAILLARD, M.D.

Unstable flail chest combines four respiratory deficiency factors: (1) pain of multiple rib fractures, which reduces respiratory motion and cough, (2) pleural effusion, which decreases respiratory capacity, reduces the shock of cough, and aggravates hypoxia because of anemia, (3) pulmonary contusion, which is maximal in 48 hours, increased by perfusion, and maintained by chest mobility, and (4) alveolar hypoventilation (paradoxical respiration), which is below the site of this abnormal mobility.

Indications for treatment by osteosynthesis are presented in Figure 1. The purpose of osteosynthesis is to transform a "soft and complicated thorax" into "simple thorax" of thoracotomy by repairing rib fractures, cleaning and good drainage of the pleural cavity, and permitting the checking and treatment of possible endothoracic injuries.

This technique reduces the risks of flail chest, the duration of hospitalization, and minimizes respiratory sequelae.

OPERATIVE TECHNIQUE

Anesthesia

Surgery is performed with the patient under general anesthesia and intubated. The patient must be resuscitated prior to the start of anesthesia. Pain and respiratory distress are important factors in assessing the degree of cardiovascular disorder. Analgesia and ventilation are sometimes effective in controlling these factors.

After surgery, mechanical ventilation is recommended for 12 to 24 hours and sometimes longer. It permits optimal ventilation and clearing of the tracheobronchial tree until the patient is completely awake.

Surgical Technique

Approach. The usual approach is a posterolateral thoracotomy incision in the middle of the flail chest. The patient is placed in the lateral position. If the high ribs are broken, the parietal incision can be lengthened upward toward the spine of the scapula. Better rib cage exposure can be obtained if a thoracoplasty valve is attached to the

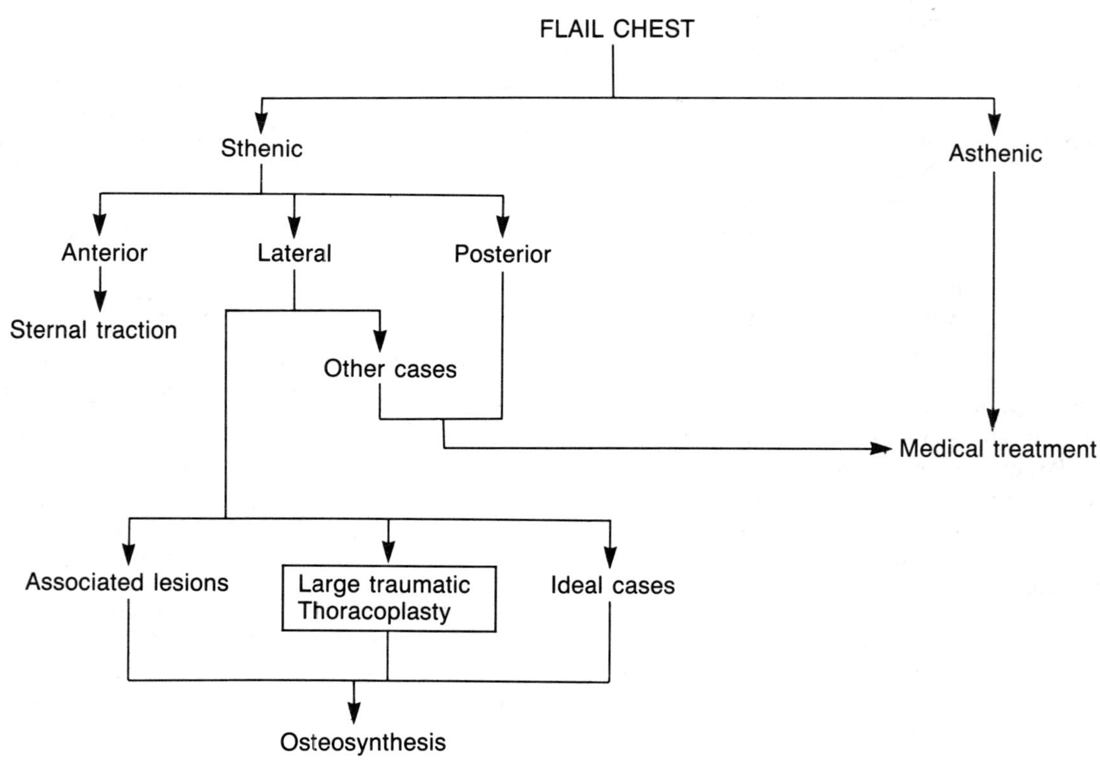

Figure 1 Therapeutic indications for flail chest.

frame of the table. In the case of an associated abdominal lesion, we prefer to start the operation with a separate laparotomy.

Visceral Exploration. Visceral exploration must be quick, systematic, and conservative. Double pleural drainage is used before beginning chest wall fixation. Pleural toilet is carried out at the end of the repair, before closure of the thoracotomy.

Rib Fixation. The spreader is removed, and the surgeon inserts his hand into the pleural cavity to examine the topography and mobility of the fractures. Every mobile fracture must be successively reduced and fixed. We start the fixation farthest from the thoracotomy incision. It is indispensible to have a set of Judet's struts of various sizes (from 14 to 20) with Nos. 8 and 12 staples and two pliers, one straight and one bent at a right angle.

The strut is chosen in proportion to the size of the fracture (No. 8 staples for simple, No. 12 staples for oblique or comminuted fractures). It is curved according to the curvature of the rib. The edges of the rib are cleaned with an electrical scalpel. The fracture is reduced, and the strut is maintained in strong contact with the reduced rib.

The strut must be placed so that the inferior edge of the rib fits the acute angle of the strut. Then it is necessary to clip on the superior part to fix it. The best sized strut is one that stabilizes rib without any tightening. The strut is tightened with pliers, made tighter for a young patient and looser for an older one.

If the strut is too large, it will deform while being tightened and will not hold the rib. If it is too small, it may not enclose the rib. Excessive tightening is to be avoided particularly if the bone is porotic (Fig. 2).

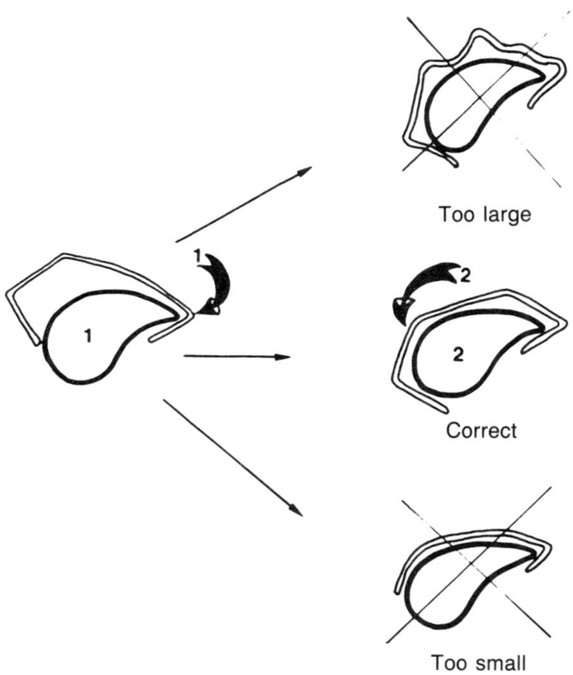

Figure 2 Judet's strut technique.

The posterior arch of the rib has a circular section and is curved sharply. The strut chosen must be larger, formed with care, and tightened with caution.

When there is shattered rib with substantial loss of bone, it is possible to join the two parts of the rib by using three struts, the middle one of which is fixed on the other two (Fig.3).

After cleaning of the pleura, the closure of muscles and skin is done in a standard manner, followed by insertion of the peridural analgesia catheter.

Placement of strong, elastic, semicircular bandage will avoid parietal expansion when the patient coughs.

POSTOPERATIVE CARE

Usually postoperative care is very simple and routine. The analysis of our results shows that patient mortality rate is directly related to the number of extrathoracic injuries sustained. Head injury is the first cause of mortality, followed by advanced age of the patient. Bronchopulmonary infection caused by prolonged mechanical ventilation preceding the operation creates the third highest risk of mortality. As we acquired experience, we modified our indications for surgery and reduced the incidence of the complications.

Osteosynthesis can result in two types of complications: parietal infections, which is exceptional, and pain or strut mobility, which is also unusual. These two complications require removal of the strut under general anesthesia.

There is no easy way to appreciate true respiratory sequelae, since it is difficult to evaluate the consequences of preoperative ventilation. A few problems related to previous chronic bronchitis have been noted. Subjective complaints are frequent, and we think that the same subjective syndrome exists in severe flail chest as in head injury.

INDICATIONS

The indications for management of flail chest with Judet's struts are determined on the basis of topography of flail chest, initial state of the patient, respiratory state of the patient, period of time elapsed since the injury, and associated injuries.

Topography. The center of paradoxical motion defines the topography of the flail chest. In our experience,

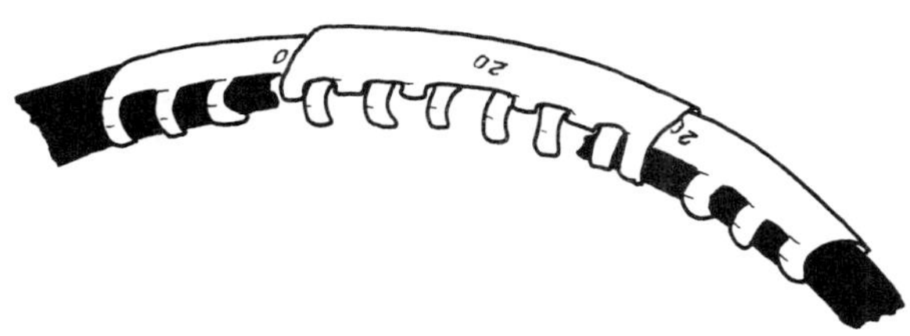

Figure 3 Technique of the "strut bridge".

anterior flail chest involves sternocostal disruption. In this circumstance, we use sternal traction by means of a retrosternal thread. Posterior flail chest is not very mobile. However, secondary displacement downward into the chest may be an indication for fixation. In lateral flail chest, paradoxical motion is often great and respiratory function is significantly impaired; this is the best indication for fixation with Judet's struts.

Initial State of the Patient. Sthenic patients are able to participate in the postoperative physiotherapy program. They constitute the ideal candidates for surgical fixation. Asthenic patients are debilitated by previous disease or associated trauma (head or spinal cord injury). They must receive assisted ventilation and cannot be operated on, and they would be unable to participate in the recovery program.

Respiratory State of the Patient. If the patient has respiratory distress, intensive care preparation is needed prior to surgery. However, early secondary surgical fixation can be considered.

Delay Between Injury and Operation. After 72 hours, surgical fixation is rarely useful. It is reserved for extensive traumatic thoracoplasty, because bronchopulmonary infection is often present. This is an indication for secondary osteosynthesis.

Associated Injuries. When such injuries are associated lesions (endothoracic, abdominal, skeletal), we extend the indications for surgical fixation because the same anesthesia permits repair of these other injuries. Secondary motion can occur when the patient awakens and he or she can ambulate more easily; this is an indication for opportunistic osteosynthesis.

Operative stabilization appears to be indicated in the following conditions: If the patient is conscious, before any signs of pulmonary infection, and if mechanical ventilation would be unavoidable without this procedure. The therapeutic choice must be made in the first 24 hours. This ideal osteosynthesis is performed on the first day on sthenic patients who have large, mobile, lateral flail chest.

In our experience, surgical stabilization of flail chest with Judet's struts is the main treatment for severe lateral flail chest.

SUGGESTED READING

Besson A, Saegesser F. Color atlas of chest trauma and associated injuries. Vol. 1 and 2. Oradell, NJ: Medical Economics, 1982.

Dahan M, Vanche J, Chauveau N. Etude expérimentale de la respiration paradoxale. Rev Med Toul 1982; 33:32.

Eschapasse H, Gaillard J. Volets thoraciques, principes du traitement. Ann Chir Thorac Cardio-Vasc 1973; 12:14.

Glintz W. Chest trauma: diagnosis and management. New York: Springer Verlag, 1981.

Richardson JD. Chest wall fractures. In: Trinkle JK, ed. Management of thoracic trauma victims. Philadelphia: JB Lippincott, 1980:31.

STERNAL FRACTURES AND MYOCARDIAL CONTUSIONS

HAROLD C. URSCHEL Jr., M.D., LL.D.(Hon), D.Sc.(Hon)
WROTEN McQUIRTER Jr., M.D.
JOHN DISIERE, M.D.

STERNAL FRACTURES

Sternal fractures are uncommon and usually secondary to steering wheel injuries during automobile accidents. Although they are generally indicative of a severe degree of trauma, only 25 percent of sternal fractures are related to cardiac contusion. Simple sternal fractures are often unrecognized and usually are treated conservatively. A displaced or overlapping sternal fracture is often painful, and if left untreated it usually results in a pseudarthrosis. The most common location of displaced sternal fractures is the sternal manubrial joint. Open reduction and wiring are indicated for those in severe pain and should be performed prior to 2 weeks after the fracture because of the rapid callus formation, assuming that the other injuries are not prohibitive for the procedure.

MYOCARDIAL CONTUSION

Myocardial contusion represents a pathologic spectrum that can involve subepicardial, subendocardial, and/or intramyocardial hemorrhage with various degrees of muscle fragmentation. This lesion was initially described in 1676 via Borch. The primary etiologic agent is blunt trauma, usually occurring in motor vehicle accidents with steering wheel trauma. The work of Kissane and Osborn on unselected motor vehicle accident victim autopsies cites an incidence of 15 to 17 percent.

Pathology

The heart is a pendular muscle between two bony structures, the thoracic spine and the sternum. This predisposes it to acceleration and deceleration injuries. A variety of lesions, from mild to extensive myocardial contusion, may be encountered, depending on the extent of muscle damage. If the injury is extensive with significant myocardial fragmentation, it results in myocardial rupture or ventricular aneurysm. Depending on the intravascular and intrathoracic pressures, this would present as an acute or delayed rupture secondary to myocardial necrosis.

However, in minor muscle fragmentation there may be no clinically significant manifestations. Enzyme level

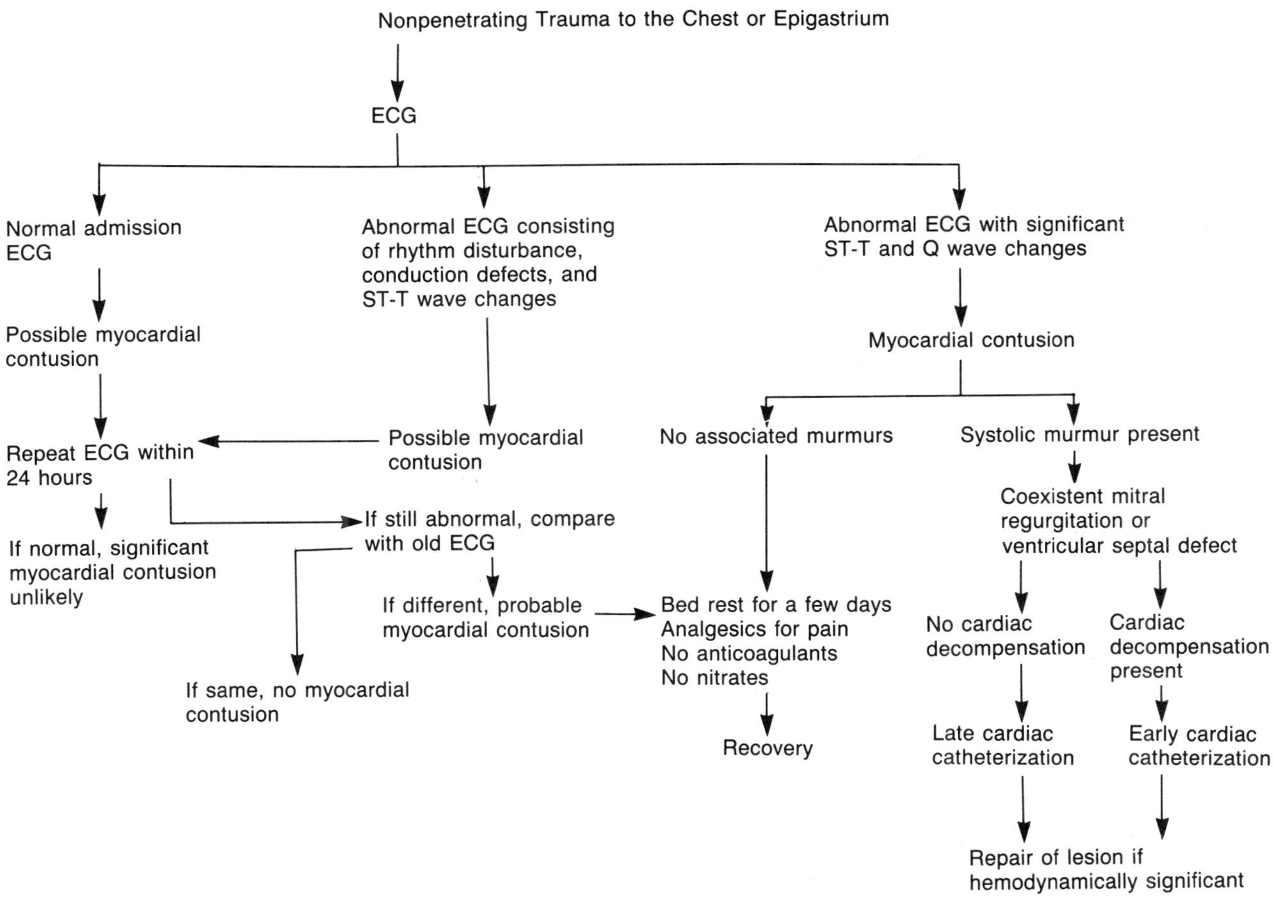

Figure 1 Algorithm for diagnosis and management of cardiac contusion. (From Symbas PN. Trauma to the heart and great vessels. New York: Grune & Stratton, 1978:39.)

elevations or cardiac arrhythmias may or may not be associated. The subepicardial hemorrhages are usually located near large coronary arteries on the anterior surface of the heart. Most lesions from low-level injuries heal without scarring or functional alterations.

Clinical Manifestation

The clinical manifestation of these lesions is complex and varies, depending on the pathologic nature of the injury and coexisting cardiac injuries.

Most cardiac contusions are mild and the patient is free of any cardiac symptoms or at most has only transient complaints. The most common complaint is pain with similar referred patterns as angina pectoris. However, the pain of cardiac contusion does not respond to nitroglycerin.

Cardiac failure may accompany cardiac contusion and is often associated with concomitant cardiac injuries such as ventricular septum or valve ruptures. Auscultation demonstrates hemodynamically significant murmurs. Myocardial contusions associated with hemopericardium, rupture, or exudation of fluid through the epicardium can produce cardiac tamponade.

Cardiac dysrhythmias are the most frequent significant sequelae of myocardial contusions and can be fatal. These include atrial or ventricular irregularities. Other symptoms may be dysrhythmia, hypotention, or symptoms related to ventricular septal defect or mitral regurgitation. Physical findings include pericardial friction rub secondary to pericarditis, heart murmurs resulting from rupture of the ventricular septum or cardiac valves, and tachycardia. Thus adequate clinical suspicion, prompt diagnosis, and appropriate treatment may be lifesaving.

Diagnosis

Cardiac contusion must always be considered in the differential diagnosis of each significant trauma case. When the physician is suspicious of the lesion, the most reliable diagnostic tool is the serial 12-lead electrocardiogram, which at best is nonspecific. Electrocardiographic variability depends on the extent of the injury; the abnormalities range from transient to long-lasting disturbances of rhythm, evidence of pericarditis, focal muscle damage, or change suggestive of typical myocardial infarction. One must keep in mind that the pathologic nature of the injury is not vascular insufficiency and that subsequently the healing is much faster in myocardial contusions. When cardiac contusion is suspected, serial electrocardiograms should be performed for at least 3 days after the trauma.

These changes are usually seen soon after injury but may not occur for 24 to 48 hours. Other helpful tests are serial serum cardiac enzyme profiles with myocardial enzyme fractions, radioisotope scanning, and two-dimensional echocardiograms. Chest ultrasonography is helpful in the diagnosis of cardiac tamponade.

Treatment

Treatment, as with diagnosis, varies from simple clinical observation of the mild syndrome to arrhythmia management or surgical repair, depending on the extent of the lesion (Fig. 1). The treatment of myocardial contusion is similar to that of myocardial infarction and in addition to the control of arrhythmias includes bed rest, oxygen therapy, and treatment of pain with narcotics. Anticoagulants are contraindicated. Congestive heart failure is managed with diuretic fluid restrictions and other conservative measures. If ventricular septal defect or mitral regurgitation is suspected, cardiac catheterization should be performed early. Surgical repair is indicated at the proper time. Myocardial rupture either early or late requires emergency repair, often with cardiopulmonary bypass.

Cardiac tamponade is treated by pericardiocentesis and surgery if serious bleeding is confirmed.

The prognosis for patients with cardiac contusion is generally good. Most patients revert to relatively normal electrocardiogram findings after 1 month.

SUGGESTED READING

Flancbaum L, Wright J, Siegel JH. Emergency surgery in patients with post-traumatic myocardial contusion. J Trauma 1986; 26:795–803.

Hamilton JR, Dearden C, Rutherford WH. Myocardial contusion associated with fractures of the sternum: important features of the seatbelt syndrome. Injury 1984; 16:155–156.

Harley DP, Mena I. Cardiac and vascular sequelae of sternal fractures. J Trauma 1986; 26:553–555.

Kumar S, Puri V, Mittal V, Cortez J. Myocardial contusion following nonfatal blunt chest trauma. J Trauma 1983; 23:327–331.

Moore EE, Eiseman B, Van Way CW III. Chest wall injuries and flail chest. In: Critical decision in trauma. St. Louis: CV Mosby, 1984:147.

Oreskovich M, Larrico J. Trauma: management of the acutely injured patient. In: Sabiston D, ed. Textbook of surgery. Philadelphia: WB Saunders, 1986:294.

Tenzer ML. The spectrum of myocardial contusion: a review. J Trauma 1985; 25:620–627.

BRONCHIAL RUPTURE

JEAN DESLAURIERS, M.D., F.R.C.S.(C)
JEAN BUSSIÈRES, M.D., F.R.C.P.(C)

Most bronchial tears are associated with crushing injuries suffered in high-speed motor vehicle accidents. Forceful compression of the chest produces lateral widening with distracting forces acting mostly at the carina (80 percent of all tears involve the main brochi within 2.5 cm of the carina). When trauma occurs on a closed glottis, resulting in high intraluminal pressure, this substantially increases the potential for rupture.

The nature of the lesion varies from a small tear to extensive linear laceration and from partial to complete separation. Concurrent esophageal injuries with resultant bronchoesophageal fistula are exceedingly rare. Failure to perform early repair of a bronchial injury ultimately results in stricture formation with secondary atelectasis and/or bronchiectasis of the distal lung.

The true incidence of bronchial trauma is unknown because patients often die (from the disruption or from associated injuries) before getting to the hospital. The overall mortality is estimated at 30 percent, but 90 percent of patients reaching the hospital alive can expect full recovery. Early diagnosis and treatment greatly reduce morbidity and increase the chances of restoring normal pulmonary function.

MANAGEMENT OF A PATIENT SUSPECTED OF HAVING A BRONCHIAL INJURY

Successful management of a trauma patient suspected of having a bronchial injury must be considered from several viewpoints: (1) a high index of suspicion about a possible bronchial tear, (2) prompt cardiopulmonary resuscitation with skillful management of airway obstruction, tension pneumothorax, and/or associated injuries, (3) confirmation of the nature, site, and extent of the lesion, and (4) definitive repair without undue delays.

Prompt Recognition of the Injury

The possibility of bronchial injury should be entertained in every patient with blunt chest trauma (Table 1). The clinical presentation depends not only on the nature, site, and extent of injury, but also on the degree of communication between the disrupted bronchus and the pleural space. With a free communication, the patient is in respiratory distress (loss of functioning lung and loss of inspired air), with hemoptysis and rapidly progressive surgical emphysema. Tension pneumothorax, persistent lung collapse, and large inexhaustible air leak are major diagnostic clues. Increased respiratory distress on high tube suction is virtually diagnostic of a large bronchial defect.

If there is no pleural communication, the symptoms are more subtle, since bronchial continuity is often maintained by opposition of peribronchial soft tissues, and the tear is sealed by fibrin or blood clot deposits. Pneumo-

TABLE 1 Conditions in Which a Bronchial Rupture Must be Suspected

Upper thoracic crushing injury
Fracture of upper ribs (ribs one to three)
Respiratory distress, subcutaneous emphysema, hemoptysis
Pneumothorax (tension or bilateral), pneumomediastinum
Persistent collapse despite adequate pleural drainage
Large air leak
Increased respiratory distress when high suction is applied to the chest tube
Radiologic obstruction in the course of an air-filled bronchus

thorax may or may not be present but in most cases, the lung expands readily with tube drainage.

Resuscitation and Early Management

Immediate consideration should be given to ensure a free airway with adequate ventilation. Contrary to what one might expect, the airway is seldom obstructed, and it is possible to manage most of these patients without ventilatory support until such time as bronchoscopy and surgical repair are carried out.

If intubation is deemed necessary, blind insertion of an endotracheal tube can be extremely hazardous and should probably be avoided if one is not ready to proceed immediately with bronchoscopy or thoracotomy. The endotracheal tube may extend an unknown tracheal laceration or even be advanced through it in the mediastinum. The use of muscle relaxants and/or deep sedation (often necessary to intubate these restless and anoxic patients) eliminates any respiratory drive that may still be present and that is in fact keeping the patient alive. Emergency tracheotomy is therefore preferable to blind intubation. The most significant advantage of a tracheotomy is the easy access given to the airway (for aspiration of blood or retained secretions) if the patient requires transportation from a peripheral medical center to a major trauma unit. Tracheotomy also provides an opening by which trapped mediastinal air can be released, and it considerably reduces intratracheal pressure by eliminating glottic closure.

Thoracostomy tubes should be inserted bilaterally because a tension pneumothorax is often present or can rapidly develop. If there is a large air leak, the chest tube should be connected to an underwater seal without suction.

Assessment of the Lesion

Bronchoscopy is the most useful procedure to confirm the diagnosis of bronchial injury, determine its location and extent, and plan the operative repair. It should be done under operating room conditions in the event that the injury is aggravated by endobronchial manipulations and immediate thoracotomy is needed. Although there is often abundance of blood in the tracheobronchial tree, we prefer the use of flexible bronchoscopy (following local topical anesthesia and light sedation) over rigid bronchoscopy. Further, an endotracheal tube can sometimes be placed over the flexible bronchoscope. Flexible bronchoscopy is always indicated when associated injuries of the head or cervical spine are suspected.

Most ruptures can be clearly seen, although the full extent of injury may not be apparent. If the site of rupture is not seen, indirect endoscopic signs such as local bleeding, air bubbling, or local edema should be looked for and may suggest the diagnosis. When the tear cannot be identified, bronchoscopy should be repeated as often as necessary if clinical or radiologic findings remain consistent with the diagnosis. Bronchography is almost never needed during the acute phase, but may be useful to assess the distal lung in the face of a chronic bronchial stricture.

DEFINITIVE MANAGEMENT OF SMALL BRONCHIAL TEARS

Most minor tears can be managed conservatively if the patient has few symptoms and the lung has fully expanded on x-ray examination. These lesions usually consist of a linear tear on the membranous portion of the bronchial wall or a local separation between membrane and cartilage. The use of tracheotomy has been advocated (to decrease intraluminal pressure), but for most cases it is unnecessary. All patients should be bronchoscoped at regular intervals until the laceration has healed perfectly.

DEFINITIVE MANAGEMENT OF MAJOR BRONCHIAL TEARS DIAGNOSED AT AN EARLY STAGE

All major bronchial disruptions require immediate operative repair, and the procedure should be carefully planned at the time of endoscopy.

Anesthesia

Four important rules must be observed by the anesthetist inducing a patient with bronchial rupture:

1. The patient should be intubated while breathing spontaneously. This can be done under topical anesthesia (with the patient fully awake) or under general anesthesia with halogenated (not curarized) anesthetics.
2. The surgeon and operating room personnel must be ready to perform immediate thoracotomy if needed.
3. Thoracostomy tubes must remain connected to an underwater seal until the chest is opened.
4. The ultimate and only goal of all anesthetic maneuvers is to gain control of the normally functioning lung.

There are two currently acceptable methods for intubation of a patient with proven bronchial rupture. An extra long straight cuffed endotracheal tube can be advanced under direct vision (by passage over a flexible fiberoptic bronchoscope) into the bronchus of the normal lung (or beyond the injury site if at the carinal level). Single-lung ventilation is then provided until such time as the surgeon gains full control of the airway. The greatest disadvantage of this technique is the possibility of tube displacement during positioning of the patient for thoracotomy or during opening of the hemithorax.

Although it is more dangerous (because of the possibility of extending the injury), we prefer intubation with a double-lumen catheter that can be more firmly anchored at the tracheobronchial bifurcation. For some of these tubes, proper positioning can be checked by flexible bronchoscopy (small diameter tracheoscope inserted into the tube lumen).*

Operation

The main goal of surgery is primary repair of the bronchial tear without unnecessary sacrifice of functional parenchyma. Thoracotomy must be done on the side of injury because the trauma is often more extensive than previously assessed and may have to be dealt with by complex reconstruction or by pulmonary resection. Bilateral main brochus tears (an uncommon injury) are repaired through a right posterolateral thoracotomy.

The surgical principles involved in the repair of a torn bronchus are the same as in any other tracheobronchial reconstruction and are as follows:

1. Thorough exploration of the pulmonary and mediastinal structures with particular attention to unrecognized tears of the distal bronchial tree, pulmonary artery, or esophagus.
2. Proper exposure of the site of injury (division of the azygos vein and tape passed around the lower trachea may be useful).
3. Full assessment of the extent of damage by mobilization of the lower trachea, carina, and lobar bronchi if necessary.
4. Excision of all devitalized and necrotic tissues, mostly at the bronchial edges (necrotic cartilage) and in the soft tissues surrounding the site of rupture.
5. Primary repair by end-to-end approximation (mucosa-to-mucosa and cartilage-to-cartilage) using interrupted absorbable sutures. Our preference goes to Vicryl 3–0 for the anastomosis of bronchial cartilage and 4–0 for the membrane.
6. Use of pedicled flaps (intercostal muscle, pleura, pericardium, pericardial fat) to protect the reconstruction and increase local vascular supply.
7. At completion of the reconstruction, air tightness should be carefully checked and the endotracheal tube pulled back to a sufficient distance above the suture line. In order to aspirate blood, remove necrotic debris, and check the reconstruction, fiberoptic bronchoscopy must be performed before the patient leaves the operating room.

In the event of difficulties with ventilation, the surgeon must be ready to manipulate the endotracheal tube into proper position or even intubate the opposite lung across the operating field (by means of an armored tube with sterile connecting tubing passed to the anesthetist). This latter maneuver is seldom necessary with simple ruptures but may be needed in complex disruptions involving the main carina.

Fortunately, pulmonary resection is needed infrequently to treat a rupture of a main bronchus. In our experience, it is more often required in lobar or segmental tears because reconstruction of small airways may prove difficult or because parenchymal damage is more severe.

Postoperative Care and Results

Complications are unusual, and the advent of epidural morphine analgesia has considerably lowered the immediate postoperative morbidity. Routine bronchoscopy is performed before hospital discharge, and excellent functional results can be expected in nearly 100 percent of patients.

DEFINITIVE MANAGEMENT OF MAJOR BRONCHIAL TEARS DIAGNOSED AT A LATE STAGE

The management of late sequelae of undiagnosed or untreated injuries of the bronchial tree is more challenging, but unless there is distal suppuration, preservation of lung function should be attempted with local resection of the stricture and reanastomosis of the bronchi.

If the rupture was only partial, a bronchial stenosis develops at the site of disruption and leads within 4 to 6 weeks to saccular bronchiectasis and irreversible lung damage. In this event, pulmonary resection (lobectomy or pneumonectomy) is the only therapeutic alternative.

If the rupture was initially complete, each of the two stumps heals separately by granulation, the lung becomes atelectatic, and the distal tree fills with noninfected mucus. These patients can be asymptomatic for a long period of time or present with signs of arterial desaturation due to physiologic intrapulmonary shunting. In this situation, every effort should be made to preserve the distal lung, and bronchoplastic reconstruction should be attempted no matter how long it has been since the initial injury. The surgical principles involved in the repair of a late stricture are similar to those in the acute phase, but specific aspects of this type of surgery should be emphasized:

1. Proper exposure of the site of injury is difficult, especially on the left side where the aortic arch may have to be mobilized in order to gain access to the main carina.
2. Primary suture is more difficult because of dense

* Editor's note: We would concur with the concern expressed regarding double-lumen tubes. We prefer advancement of single-lumen tubes with bronchoscopic control or the use of bronchial blockers placed with the aid of a flexible bronchoscope.

peribronchial scarred tissues and because the anastomosis has to be done very proximally on the main bronchus.
3. There may be a pathologic process (fibrosis and loss of elasticity) in the lung that prevents expansion despite adequate reconstruction. In this event, pneumonectomy may be necessary.

Excellent functional results are obtained in most patients treated by surgical intervention within 6 months of the injury. With longer delays between trauma and repair, some return of pulmonary function can be expected, but usually not to a normal level.

SUGGESTED READING

Grover FL, Ellestad C, Arom KU, et al. Diagnosis and management of major tracheobronchial injuries. Ann Thorac Surg 1979; 28:384–391.
Kirsh MM, Orringer MB, Benrendt DM, Sloan H. Management of tracheobronchial disruption secondary to nonpenetrating trauma. Ann Thorac Surg 1976; 22:93–101.
Mills SA, Johnston FR, Hudspeth AS, et al. Clinical spectrum of blunt tracheobronchial disruption illustrated by seven cases. J Thorac Cardiovasc Surg 1982; 84:59–58.
Urschel HC, Razzuk MA. Management of acute traumatic injuries of tracheobronchial tree. Surg Gynecol Obstet 1973; 136:113–117.

PENETRATING TRAUMA: HEMOTHORAX

DOUGLAS J. MATHISEN, M.D.

Hemothorax refers to blood in the pleural cavity. The most common cause in contemporary practice is related to trauma, either blunt or penetrating. Iatrogenic causes occur secondary to subclavian vein cannulation and insertion of chest tubes and as a result of percutaneous needle biopsy. There are many other uncommon causes too numerous to mention that also might lead to hemothorax. The source of bleeding can be from many different sites: from the pulmonary vasculature secondary to penetrating trauma, the intercostals, the heart, the great vessels, or the abdominal viscera if the diaphragm is ruptured. The diagnosis is usually made by physical examination, chest x-ray, and thoracentesis.

When evaluating a patient with hemothorax, one must consider associated injuries that frequently occur; especially when trauma has been involved. Pneumothorax, cardiac tamponade, cardiac contusion, diaphragmatic rupture, transection of the thoracic aorta, and abdominal injuries are only a few of the associated problems that must be carefully considered in any patient with a traumatic hemothorax. The presence of these injuries may obviously dictate the course of management, not only of these problems but of the hemothorax as well.

Hemothorax can be arbitrarily divided into minimal (0 to 500 ml of blood), moderate (500 to 1,500 ml of blood), and massive (more than 1,500 ml of blood). One must consider the source of the bleeding, i.e., whether it is dark blood suggestive of pulmonary artery hemorrhage, which usually stops because of the low pressure system from which it comes, or bright red arterial bleeding from the intercostals or great vessel injury, which is unlikely to stop. The initial management of any significant amount of blood in the pleural space is by tube thoracostomy. This is generally placed in the midaxillary line and directed posteriorly. It is best done with a large chest tube size No. 28 F or larger to avoid possible clotting and plugging of the catheter. The first consideration after placement of a tube thoracostomy is whether or not surgical intervention will be needed. Guidelines must be established as to when surgical exploration should be undertaken. Depending on the circumstances and if the patient's condition permits, angiography might be considered prior to surgical intervention. If a large hemothorax is suspected, preparation should be made for autotransfusion to avoid delay for crossmatching blood. My guidelines for exploration are as follows: (1) immediate removal of more than 1,500 ml of blood and continued bleeding is indication for surgical intervention, (2) removal of 500 ml of blood an hour for 3 consecutive hours warrants surgical intervention, and (3) removal of 200 to 300 ml of blood for 5 or 6 consecutive hours warrants surgical intervention. These are rules of thumb and need to be evaluated in the context of each clinical situation.

The next goal in management of hemothorax is the removal of all blood and reexpansion of the underlying lung. This again is best accomplished by tube thoracostomy. A second chest tube is sometimes necessary, especially for loculated collections. Early surgical intervention is rarely indicated for a hemothorax. The one exception may be in patients with a large clotted hemothorax causing significant restriction of their breathing capacity. One concern of any hemothorax is the development of a fibrous peel leading to restrictive lung function. Any patient who is discharged from the hospital with a significant hemothorax should be followed carefully for the development of this problem. If the hemothorax has not been absorbed after a month, a diminished vital capacity of 75 percent predicted warrants consideration of decortication. Historically this has been performed between 3 and 5 weeks after the occurrence of the hemothorax, when the clot has had a chance to organize and therefore is easily peeled off the underlying lung. This again should only be necessary in a small percentage of patients (5 percent).

The next major concern is the development of empyema. Blood is obviously an ideal culture medium. Factors that predispose to subsequent empyema are the initial presentation of shock, gross contamination of the pleural space, the development of subsequent pneumonia, and prolonged catheter drainage. Gross contamination of the pleural cavity may dictate early surgical intervention; however, again this would be unusual. Early management in this setting should consist of total evacuation of the hemothorax with complete reexpansion of the underlying lung. Patients who have had a hemothorax regardless of whether or not it has been completely evacuated should be followed in the early postdischarge period for the development of empyema (5 percent). The management of empyema is dealt with in the chapter *Empyema and Bronchopleural Fistula*. One additional precautionary note should be raised about early intervention and decortication. One should always consider the status of the underlying lung. If the underlying lung has been severely damaged from contusion or infection, early exploration and decortication are not warranted. They must be delayed until the status of that lung has been clarified so that if decortication is performed, the underlying lung can reexpand to fill the thoracic cavity. Failure to heed this advice may lead to more significant problems.

Fibrinolytic agents have been recommended by some to help liquefy the hemothorax and aid in evaluation. I have never found this effective and do not recommend them.

SUGGESTED READING

Chetty KG, Davidson PT. A guide to management of hemothorax. Hosp Med 1975; June, 25–29.

Wilson JM, Boren CH, Peterson SR, Thomas AN. Traumatic hemothorax: is decortication necessary? J Thorac Cardiovasc Surg 1979; 77:489–494.

PENETRATING PULMONARY AND ESOPHAGEAL TRAUMA

KENNETH L. MATTOX, M.D.

Every 24-hour period approximately 12 patients per one million population will sustain a thoracic injury. Four of these patients will require hospitalization, and one patient every 48 hours will have a severe thoracic injury. These wounds may be produced by firearms or knives, or may be the result of blunt trauma. Iatrogenic injury during thoracentesis, lung biopsy, tube thoracostomy, or esophageal endoscopy is perhaps almost as common as injury resulting from social violence or automobile accidents. Except for minor injuries to the chest wall, penetrating lung injuries are probably the most common thoracic visceral injuries, whereas penetrating esophageal wounds are among the rarest injuries of intrathoracic organs.

PULMONARY INJURY

The *therapeutic alternatives* include observation only, tube thoracostomy in conjunction with observation, and/or operation. Flexible or rigid bronchoscopy may be required in instances of aspiration or to remove intrabronchial blood. Bronchoscopy is also an aid in the removal of mucous plugs in atelectasis.

Conservative (non-surgical) therapy is indicated in over 85 percent of patients with isolated penetrating wounds of the lung. Early tube thoracostomy or thoracentesis to achieve lung reexpansion and removal of blood and air from the pleural space aids not only in stabilizing respiratory dynamics but also in restoring lung parenchymal hemostasis.

Surgery

Indications

The three indications for operation in acute pulmonary injury are (1) bleeding, (2) air leak, and (3) air embolism. The average amount of blood in the pleural space following penetrating lung injury is usually between 500 and 1,000 ml. If blood loss exceeds 1,000 ml and bleeding continues at a constant rate, immediate thoracotomy should be performed. Even if the rate of bleeding slows, the loss of an additional 1,000 ml during the 3 hours following chest tube insertion is an indication for thoracotomy.

The patient with a massive air leak has major disruption to pulmonary parenchyma or to major tracheobronchial structures. With high pressure aspiration on the chest tube, the entire tidal volume can be evacuated through the chest tube. In such instances, the chest tube should be placed only to the underwater seal with no negative pressure on the chest drainage apparatus, and the patient should be taken immediately to the operating room for closure or repair or both of the air leak.

Systemic air embolism can occur with penetrating injuries to the lung and intrabronchial pressures in excess of 60 torr. This may occur either during a forced Valsalva maneuver or during positive-pressure ventilation, and it results in a bronchiolar-pulmonary vein fistula. Many such cases occur shortly after an endotracheal tube has been inserted and the patient is receiving assisted ventilation via a ventilating bag. The air embolism is manifested by cardiac arrhythmias, cerebral insufficiency, lateralizing neurologic signs, seizure activity and/or cardiac arrest. Immediate thoracotomy, cross-clamping of the pulmonary hilus, evacuation of all air from the aorta and cardiac chambers, cardiac resuscitation, and lobectomy of the injured lung should be performed.

One additional indication for thoracotomy is a penetrating injury to the lung parenchyma caused by a high-velocity gunshot or an industrial petroleum product. These two types of wounds are not commonly seen in civilian practice.

Contraindications to Surgery

The mere presence of a bullet in the lung parenchyma with a suspicion of significant injury is not an indication for performing thoracotomy. Neither is the presence of a pulmonary hematoma or pulmonary contusion, because both will resolve in the majority of instances. With both blunt and penetrating trauma, air sacs are virtually always seen on a routine computed tomographic scan of the chest. These are not seen on routine and lateral chest x-ray films. They virtually always clear, and their exact pathophysiologic significance has not been determined.

Incisions

For penetrating injuries of the lung, a standard fourth or fifth interspace anterolateral or posterolateral incision is the incision of choice. The anterolateral incision is chosen if multiple concomitant injuries exist that might require cardiorrhaphy or transsternal extension into a bilateral anterolateral thoracotomy. If concomitant esophageal or descending aortic injury exists, a posterolateral incision is preferred.

Techniques of Repair

Penetrating pulmonary injuries are basically approached using one of three techniques: pneumonorrhaphy, tractotomy, or resection. Resection is accomplished by lobectomy or pneumonectomy.

Over 75 percent of surgically treated penetrating pulmonary injuries can be managed by simple pneumonorrhaphy. Pneumonorrhaphy is assisted at times when the lung is decompressed via anesthesia of one lung (Carlens' tube or Robertshaw's tube). Pneumonorrhaphy can be accomplished using a variety of sutures, including absorbable, polypropylene, and staples. Its purpose is to control air leaks and hemorrhage, and it is best applied to more peripheral lesions.

With large through-and-through holes in the center of a lobe without obvious injury to a major pulmonary artery or vein, tractotomy may be indicated. With such injuries, hemoptysis or systemic air embolism may occur if simple pneumonorrhaphy at the entrance and exit sites is performed. Tractotomy is performed by placing a large instrument completely through the wound, from entrance to exit, and dividing all lung tissue between the tract and the closest surface of the lung. Digital compression limits the amount of blood loss during this maneuver. By using staples or precise running polypropylene suture and by specifically ligating bleeding points and subsequently closing the visceral pleura over the open iatrogenically created laceration of the lung, both air leaks and blood loss may be controlled. Recent experience of 12 such repairs during the last 6 months has been extremely satisfactory.

Formal resection is employed only for hilar injuries or in instances of uncontrollable bleeding into the substance of the lung. Resection may also be required for high-velocity injuries and systemic air emboli. Although formal resection with ligation of specific lobar arteries and veins and subsequent division of the bronchus might be accomplished, more often cross-clamping of the hilus with lobar debridement followed by specific suture ligation of lobar arteries, veins, and bronchus is necessary. Such resections are for control of hemorrhage and air leak rather than for resection of a pulmonary cancer. During such procedures, the use of one-lung anesthesia and autotransfusion is extremely helpful.

Outcome

Survival

In the absence of associated disease, death from simple lung injury is extremely uncommon. When simple pneumonorrhaphy is possible, the mortality is less than 1 percent. No deaths have occurred in our recent experience with pulmonary tractotomy. When major resection is required, the mortality rate may exceed 25 percent because of the high incidence of associated injuries. In patients with systemic air embolism secondary to penetrating pulmonary injury, the mortality rate exceeds 90 percent.

Complications

The major complications following penetrating lung injury include unevacuated hemothorax, pulmonary hematoma and contusion, and pneumonia. With atelectasis or pneumonia, early bronchoscopy for bronchial toilet is indicated. If there is an unevacuated hemothorax, early evacuation lessens the chances of empyema, shortens the hospitalization, and precludes the development of a fibrothorax in most instances. Most interparenchymal hematomas and contusions clear between 5 days and 2 weeks after injury.

Special Problems

Air embolism is avoided by preventing intrabronchial pressures in excess of 60 torr for the patient in whom the potential for bronchopulmonary vein fistula exists. With penetrating lung injuries, especially at the hilus, the normal anatomy may be grossly distorted because of the hematoma and blood staining of the tissues. If lobectomy is performed, special care is required not to injure the vasculature of the remaining lung. If time permits, the use of a double-lumen endotracheal tube to allow for one-lung anesthesia is extremely helpful in managing pulmonary injury. The high rate of associated injury demands a thorough search and evaluation of other intrathoracic and intra-abdominal organs.

ESOPHAGEAL TRAUMA

Blunt and/or penetrating injuries of the thoracic esophagus are extremely rare. In the reports in the literature from busy trauma centers, only one or two penetrating esophageal injuries are seen each year. No diagnostic maneuver is absolutely certain. Esophageal injury may be discovered while performing surgery for associated injuries through an anterolateral incision with the patient in the supine position, making repair difficult or impossible during this procedure.

Therapeutic Alternatives

The injured esophagus may be repaired directly with or without supportive viable muscle flaps. It may be diverted or even resected, with later esophageal reconstruction or conduit replacement. Although some gastroenterologists treat small iatrogenic perforations with antibiotics only, trauma to the esophagus virtually always requires surgical intervention.

Preferred Approach

For most simple penetrating esophageal wounds, direct lateral esophagorrhaphy is the preferred method of repair. Diversionary procedures, including creation of a deliberate fistula over a large T-tube, are reserved for extensive injuries or those that are discovered late and in which considerable mediastinal contamination is present.

Surgery

Indications

Endoscopic or radiologic evidence of esophageal trauma or findings of esophageal injury at the time of thoracotomy are indications for surgery on the esophagus. Even in the patient who is extremely septic from mediastinitis and empyema secondary to esophageal injury, surgical treatment by mediastinal and thoracic drainage and cervical esophagostomy diversion is indicated. Once an injury is recognized, there are no contraindications to surgically treating the injured esophagus.

Incisions

For an injured esophagus, a posterolateral incision is indicated. For upper esophageal injuries, a fourth *right* interspace incision is preferable, and for lower esophageal injuries a *left* sixth or seventh interspace incision is preferred.

If an esophageal injury is discovered at the time of thoracotomy for associated injury through a median sternotomy or anterolateral or bilateral anterolateral thoracotomies, the anterior injury and incision should be repaired, the patient put into the lateral recumbent position, and an appropriate posterolateral incision made specifically for treatment of the esophageal injury. Esophageal repairs through an anterior incision have a 50 percent incidence of breakdown.

Techniques of Esophageal Repair

The mediastinal pleura over the hematoma around the esophagus is divided, the esophagus is encircled using the nasogastric tube within it as a guide, and the entrance and exit wounds are identified. Two-layer closure is accomplished. An intercostal muscle flap based posteriorly is used to reinforce the entire suture line.

With extensive injuries, such as those encountered with large-caliber or high-velocity missiles, deliberate fistula formation or diversion is indicated. This may be accomplished by placing a large T-tube (preferably made from a soft Silastic type material) through the injury, with loose approximation at the tissue over the arms of the T-tube. This procedure is done in conjunction with a cervical lateral esophagostomy. Alternately, the distal esophagus may be encircled with either umbilical tape or heavy absorbable suture, taking care not to encircle the vagus nerves. This maneuver is accompanied by a mediastinal drainage and cervical esophagostomy, either lateral or end, depending on how complete a diversion is desired. Subsequent reconstruction may be accomplished when healing has occurred and the patient is in a good nutritional state. A tube gastrostomy or jejunostomy or both are performed at the time of the diversion. Esophageal diversion should not be performed without considerable forethought. Patients undergoing diversion incur a considerable longer hospitalization than those who have simple repair. Such patients also must face at least one or more secondary procedures, some of which are extremely extensive.

Recognition of Complications

A major complication of a missed esophageal lesion or a breakdown of an esophageal repair is infection, manifested by mediastinitis, empyema, leukocytosis, and fever. An additional complication of stricture at the site of distal occlusion of the esophagus may require secondary surgical operations. In a patient who has had a simple repair that breaks down, diversion or T-tube placement with deliberate fistula formation at the time of mediastinal and pleural drainage should be given strong consideration.

Special Problems

A missed esophageal injury carries a 50 percent mortality rate, which underscores the need for early diagnosis. When the surgeon is confronted with combined injuries to the esophagus, trachea, and vasculature at the thoracic outlet, difficult management decisions must be made. Following the repair, all tubular structures should be separated with a muscle flap, and deliberate lateral exteriorization of the esophageal injury should be considered. Closure of the esophageal stoma at a later operation is a simple procedure.

Outcome

Patients with isolated esophageal injuries that are successfully repaired or diverted have a mortality rate of less than 10 percent and a relatively low morbidity. When an esophageal injury is missed or breakdown of a thoracic esophageal repair occurs, the mortality rate approaches 50 percent. The complication rate increases in proportion to both extent of injury and number of associated organs injured.

SUGGESTED READING

Coselli JS, Mattox KL, Beall AC. Re-evaluation of early evacuation of clotted hemothorax. Am J Surg 1984; 148:785–787.
Defore WW, Mattox KL, Hansen HA, et al. Surgical management of penetrating injuries of the esophagus. Am J Surg 1977; 134:734–738.
Glatterer MS Jr, Toon RS, Ellestad D, et al. Management of blunt and penetrating external trauma. J Trauma 1985; 25:784–792.
Graham JM, Mattox KL, Beall AC. Penetrating trauma of the lung. J Trauma 1979; 19:665–669.

THE TRACHEA

TRACHEOSTOMY

DOUGLAS J. MATHISEN, M.D.

Tracheostomy is a simple surgical procedure. Although it has been in use for centuries, many variations in technique still exist.

Prolonged mechanical ventilation and pulmonary toilet are the major indications for tracheostomy. Tracheostomy should be considered after 7 to 10 days of mechanical ventilation have elapsed, with the prospect of many more days to come. In neonates and children, because of the size of the trachea, the complications of tracheostomy probably outweigh the advantages and are greater than the complications related to prolonged intubations with small uncuffed endotracheal tubes. Tracheostomy is still recognized as a means of securing an airway in certain circumstances such as massive facial trauma, intraoral hemorrhage, laryngotracheal trauma, and acute upper airway obstruction.

Contraindications to tracheostomy are relatively few. Burn patients, because of the risk of spreading sepsis along the tracheostomy tract, pose a relative contraindication to tracheostomy. Tracheostomy following tracheal resection should be avoided whenever possible. Bleeding diatheses may be relative contraindications.

Tracheostomy can be performed under general or local anesthesia. It is best performed with the patient properly positioned with the head extended, thereby delivering the maximum amount of trachea above the sternal notch. A small horizontal incision of 3 to 4 cm in length halfway between the thyroid cartilage and suprasternal notch is generally recommended. The straps are separated in the midline and the thyroid isthmus is divided between clamps, thereby exposing the underlying trachea for accurate counting of tracheal rings. Placement of a traction suture on either side of the second or third cartilaginous ring is helpful in keeping the trachea open while placing a tracheostomy tube. It is ideal to use the second and third tracheal rings. They should be opened in a longitudinal manner parallel to the long axis of the trachea. Once the trachea is opened, the anesthesiologist should withdraw but not remove the endotracheal tube. The opening in the trachea should be spread with the tracheal spreader. The smallest tracheostomy tube that is compatible with adequate ventilation and effective suctioning and does not require excessive balloon pressures to obtain an adequate seal should be inserted. A tracheal hook is sometimes helpful in stabilizing the trachea during placement and also in gaining better exposure of the trachea. Once the tracheostomy tube has been placed, traction sutures are removed and hemostasis achieved. A simple anchoring suture is placed at each end of the incision and tied to the flange of the tracheostomy tube to help hold it in place. The tracheostomy tube is then secured to the flange of the tracheostomy and tightly tied around the patient's neck. Once the airway is secure, the original endotracheal tube can be removed.

Careful attention to detail can eliminate many of the complications associated with tracheostomy. Avoidance of placement of the tracheostomy tube through the first ring lessens the incidence of subglottic stenosis. Avoidance of its placement lower than the fourth tracheal ring lowers the incidence of tracheoinnominate artery fistula. The use of a small tracheostomy tube, the use of a swivel-type adapter, placing minimal traction on the tracheostomy tube, avoiding removal of parts of the tracheal cartilage, and avoiding horizontal incisions in the trachea that over time may enlarge to divide the trachea are ways of preventing stomal stenosis. The use of high-volume, low-pressure cuffs lessens the incidence of cuff stenoses. However, one must be careful—even a low-pressure cuff can be overinflated and cause tracheal damage. The use of low-pressure cuffs and the avoidance of concomitant large, hard, plastic nasogastric tubes will help eliminate tracheoesophageal fistula. Once removed, the overwhelming majority of tracheostomy stomas close on their own. Only a small fraction remain as persistent sinus tracts. If they are bothersome, they can usually be closed using simple surgical techniques.

LARYNGOTRACHEAL TRAUMA

DOUGLAS J. MATHISEN, M.D.

Laryngotracheal trauma is an uncommon problem. All personnel who deal with emergency patients or are involved in airway management should be familiar with the signs and symptoms of laryngotracheal trauma, methods of airway management, and principles of repair.

The majority of these injuries are the result of blunt trauma from the patient's striking his or her neck against the dashboard or steering wheel in an automobile accident. Penetrating trauma is much less common. The signs and symptoms may range from the obvious large laceration of the neck with all the cervical structures exposed to the most subtle injury with only minor complaints of localized pain. Classic signs of hoarseness, stridor, hemoptysis, localized tenderness, and subcutaneous emphysema should alert one to the possibility of a laryngotracheal injury. Radiologic assessment of these injuries is not crucial. In fact, time should never be wasted trying to obtain x-ray studies in a patient who may have a compromised airway, because the status of the airway can change abruptly.

The most crucial aspect of laryngotracheal trauma after its recognition is the management of the airway. Whenever doubt exists as to the status of the airway, emergency tracheostomy should be performed. If the patient has a compromised airway but is still breathing on his or her own, attempts at intubation or inspection of the airway with a flexible bronchoscope should be done in the operating room, with everything set to perform emergency tracheostomy. Repeated attempts at intubation should be avoided and emergency tracheostomy performed without hesitation. This is best done under local anesthesia with the patient breathing on his or her own. In the totally separated trachea, the distal end may have retracted into the mediastinum and may be difficult to locate. It is best found by inserting a finger in the area where the trachea should have been, locating the distal tip by palpation, grasping it with a clamp, and delivering it to the wound. An endotracheal tube can then be inserted and the airway will be secure. If a partially disrupted trachea is found, simply placing an endotracheal tube through the damaged area is the best alternative; it should not, under any circumstances, be placed through noninjured viable trachea. Every attempt should be made to conserve viable trachea, whether securing or repairing an airway.

Careful assessment of associated injuries after the airway has been secured is the next most important aspect of management of these injuries. Because of the type of injury, there is a high incidence of associated injuries to nearby structures. It is important to remember that the cervical spine, spinal cord, esophagus, larynx, and vascular structures are frequently also injured in these patients. Each patient should be carefully assessed for these associated injuries, because failure to recognize any of them could lead to catastrophic complications for the patient. Cervical spine injuries may dictate the course of management of the airway and of the tracheal injury, since extending or flexing the neck would be contraindicated. Disruption of the esophagus must be looked for both by direct inspection and endoscopy. If the esophagus is injured, it should be repaired in two layers and a local strap muscle should be interposed between this suture line and the tracheal suture line. Failure to do so will lead to subsequent tracheoesophageal fistula in a high percentage of cases. Failure to recognize the esophageal injury will lead to obvious sepsis, dehiscence of the tracheal repair, or subsequent stenosis. Injuries to the larynx should be assessed carefully by a competent otolaryngologist if available. Exposed cartilage should be covered by mucosa, and fractures should be set and held in place by stents if necessary. The optimal time to repair any laryngeal injury is at the time of the initial insult. Subsequent repair may not be possible. If the larynx is injured, provision must be made at the end of the case for an airway in the form of a tracheostomy or small endotracheal tube, which is left until the patient's airway can be evaluated postoperatively. Each patient should be carefully assessed for a vascular injury by looking for the presence of bruits, differential pulses, or radiologic signs. These injuries frequently need to be assessed by angiography. Special mention should be made of injuries to the recurrent laryngeal nerves. Recurrent laryngeal nerves may be totally avulsed or divided or simply contused, in which case function will return at a later date. In the case of total transection, it must be assumed that both recurrent nerves have been injured. Never make any attempt to search for the recurrent nerves in these traumatized wounds for fear of dividing one that may be only contused and that may recover function at a later date. Whenever recurrent nerve injury is suspected, provision must be made at the end of the procedure to protect the airway, as for laryngeal trauma.

Repair of laryngotracheal trauma may be one of the few indications for tracheostomy following tracheal surgery. Tracheostomy should never be placed through the tracheal repair, since this will lead to contamination of the suture line and subsequent dehiscence or stenosis. The suture line should be protected with local tissue and separated from the tracheostomy, which should be placed at least two tracheal rings below the level of repair. Local strap muscles or thyroid gland is quite suitable for separating the suture line from the tracheostomy. The only exception to this is the small tracheal injury that may be used as a tracheostomy stoma and the tracheostomy tube placed through it. This, however, should only be done when it seems that the patient either has injury to his recurrent nerves or a long period of ventilation is anticipated. In most cases, even the smallest injury should be simply repaired rather than placing a tracheostomy through it.

The management of simple lacerations or partial tears of the trachea is best accomplished by interrupted suture repair with an absorbable suture such as 4–0 Vicryl. All devitalized tissue should be removed; however, one must try to conserve as much viable trachea as possible at all times. If any length of the trachea has been lost, it is best to put the patient's neck in flexion and hold the position with a stitch from the chin to the chest in order to avoid undue tension on the tracheal repair.

Complex injuries involving a large portion of the trachea or associated with injuries to the esophagus must be handled with great care. Each surgeon must make a decision as to whether or not primary repair should be attempted or whether simply securing the airway is the goal of repair in this situation. If delayed tracheal repair is chosen, esophageal injury should be repaired in all cases and a tracheostomy secured through the injured trachea or simply by bringing out the divided end of trachea as an end stoma. One must be absolutely certain that all viable trachea is preserved for subsequent repair. A tracheostomy should never be placed through normal viable trachea, which may preclude subsequent reconstruction of the airway. The proximal trachea either can be oversewn and a drain placed next to it or it can be brought out as a separate stoma. Subsequent repair should be delayed for a sufficient period of time to allow scarring and inflammation to subside. If primary repair is attempted, it is most important to interpose a viable strap muscle between the esophageal repair and subsequent tracheal repair. Careful inspection of the laryngeal injuries should be made. These should be repaired with the help of an otolaryngologist if at all possible. Fractures should be reduced and held in place by a molded stent. This automatically demands that a tracheostomy be placed after the completed repair. If a large portion of the trachea is injured, it is important to debride devitalized tissue and perform the repair under no tension. This is best accomplished by simply flexing the patient's neck as the repair is completed and mobilizing that space in the pretracheal fascia in front of the trachea down to the level of the carina. No attempt should be made to divide the lateral tissues of the trachea, since this is where the segmental blood supply enters the trachea. Interruption of the lateral blood supply more than 1 to 2 cm from the proposed suture line may lead to ischemia and subsequent stenosis of the repair. End-to-end repair utilizing interrupted 4–0 Vicryl sutures is preferable in all cases. Traction sutures of 2–0 Vicryl placed laterally both proximally and distally and tied prior to tieing the interrupted sutures not only takes tension off the repair but allows the sutures to be tied under minimal tension. These traction sutures can be left in place, as they are of absorbable suture material.

If no attempt was made to primarily repair the airway because of the extent of the injury or paralysis of the larynx, subsequent repair is still possible. A sufficient period of time should be allowed for inflammation and scarring to subside and for resolution of associated problems. Many techniques are available to make a paralyzed larynx functional both from the standpoint of the airway and voice. These procedures should take precedence and be performed prior to any attempted repair of the tracheal stenosis.

SUGGESTED READING

Grillo HC. Surgery of the trachea. In: Current problems in surgery. Chicago: Year Book Medical Publishers, 1970.
Mathisen DJ, Grillo HC. Laryngotracheal trauma. Ann Thorac Surg 1987; 43:254–262.
Montgomery WW. Management of glottic stenosis. Otolaryngol Clin North Am 1979; 12:841–847.
Ogura JH. Management of traumatic injuries of the larynx and trachea including stenosis. J Laryngol Otol 1971; 85:1259–1261.
Sessions DG, Ogura JH, Heeneman H. Surgical management of bilateral vocal cord paralysis. Laryngoscopy 1976; 86:559–566.

TRACHEAL TUMOR

MIKHAIL I. PERELMAN, M.D.

Over the past 23 years we have operated on 165 patients with primary tracheal tumors, including 33 with benign and 132 with malignant tumors.

The radical treatment of tracheal tumors is confined to surgical methods, which we take to include both open operations on the trachea and endoscopic interventions. Radiation therapy in squamous cell and adenoid cystic carcinomas may at times be fairly effective, but the tumors managed in this way tend to recur or metastasize in a year or two. Chemotherapy and immunotherapy for tracheal tumors are as yet devoid of clinical significance.

When tracheobronchoscopy is undertaken in a patient with a suspected or already recognized tracheal tumor, it is important that facilities be available for an endoscopic procedure, specifically laser photocoagulation. After biopsy, this procedure is indicated whenever the tracheal lumen is narrowed and the pulmonary ventilation is compromised.* Our experience shows that after laser photocoagulation emergency surgery for the tracheal tumor is then not required. When benign tumors on a slender pedicle or tracheal polyps are present, one or two laser sessions can evaporate the entire tumor and its base, the equivalent of a radical operation. If the base of a benign tumor is relatively broad, then the feasibility of its radical removal should be gauged from its appearance during endoscopy and by computed tomography (CT). In this way, the presence of extratracheal tumor can be ruled out. In benign tumors with an extratracheal portion and in malignant tumors, tracheal resection is necessary. Indications for tracheal resection depend on its feasibility and on whether or not contraindications are present.

* See chapter *Management of Acute Airway Obstruction* for alternative method.

In a patient with adenoid cystic carcinoma, assessment of tumor spread along the trachea is of primary importance. This can be done most precisely by biopsy of the tracheal mucosa and submucosa. Tissue for microscopic examination is taken 1 cm below and 1 to 2 cm above the bronchoscopically visible tumor. The state of lymph nodes and surrounding organs and tissues is evaluated by palpating the neck and by the use of CT and esophagoscopy. Esophagography and xerotomography are also employed. The latter is better than conventional tomography in demonstrating the tracheal wall and the tumor. However, the actual spread of the tumor can only be established intraoperatively.

In our view, absolute contraindications to attempting a tracheal resection are cervical lymph node involvement, invasion of the esophagus, signs of superior vena cava compression, and Horner's syndrome. Relative contraindications are poor general condition of the patient, old age, severe concomitant disease, and laryngeal hemiparesis. It is advisable to submit such inoperable patients to periodic tracheobronchoscopy with photocoagulation of the tumor, perhaps in combination with radiotherapy. We have not been resorting to tracheostomy in recent years.

The question of operative access for tracheal resection arises mostly with tumors occurring in the midthoracic trachea. We take into consideration the patient's age and the shape of his or her neck and chest. In a young patient with a long neck and sternum, we perform longitudinal-transverse sternotomy, transecting the sternum at the level of the third intercostal space. In an old patient with a sclerotic aorta and a brachiocephalic trunk, we elect to use a posterior approach, with resection of the fifth rib with the patient in the prone position. We also use this approach in patients with tumors in the lower thoracic trachea or in the carina. We consider this route of access more convenient than the standard posterolateral thoracotomy. In cases of doubt as to the operative access to tumors in the midthoracic trachea, we give preference to longitudinal-transverse sternotomy.

During the operation, it is essential to dissect out the involved portion of the trachea together with adjacent fatty tissue and the lymph nodes, taking care not to damage the vagus and recurrent nerves. If the tumor has invaded the nerves, these should of course be divided. If a tracheal tumor has grown into the esophagus, this and the trachea should be carefully separated. True invasion of the esophagus by a tracheal tumor is seldom seen—at any rate much less often than invasion of the trachea by an esophageal tumor. It is much easier and safer to separate the trachea from the esophagus when a thick tube has been passed into the esophagus. Any defects in the esophageal mucosa, which sometimes arise during mobilization of the tumor, should be meticulously sutured. In the typical case, a sleeve resection of the trachea is commenced by transecting it below the tumor, one ring away from its grossly definable border. In a complicated situation, in which the border of a soft tumor cannot be delineated by palpation, intraoperative tracheoscopy and transillumination done in a darkened operating room are very helpful. We make use of this device fairly often. Tracheal resection above the tumor is also performed in such a way as to include one macroscopically unaltered cartilage. We define tumor borders by palpation, visually using transillumination, or else by a longitudinal upward dissection of the tumor-containing tracheal segment. The desire to spare the healthy tracheal wall may be the reason for transecting the trachea obliquely through both its membranous and cartilaginous parts. Such oblique transection does not interfere with the normal healing of a properly performed anastomosis. Immediately after the tumorous tracheal segment is removed, a quick frozen section assessment of both ends is made to ascertain that the resection line has passed within the limits of healthy tissue. If tumor cells are identified in the specimen, the extent of resection should be increased, if possible. However, in patients with adenoid cystic carcinoma, tumor elements in the tracheal submucosa may be detectable far away from the visible tumor. In such cases we forego extended resection in favor of anastomosis within the limits of apparently unaltered tissue in anticipation that postoperative radiotherapy will be beneficial.

Regarding anastomosis in cases of tracheal resection, the following points are worth noting:

1. Tracheal anastomosis from a transsternal approach may be done either through the space between the brachiocephalic trunk and left common carotid artery or to the right of the ascending aorta and brachiocephalic trunk. The more convenient operative field should be determined in each individual case.
2. In operations using a cervical or transsternal route, when the anastomosis would be too tense, we anastomose two-thirds of the tracheal circumference and pass a Silastic T-tube into the tracheal lumen.
3. After a limited sleeve resection of the carina, the medial walls of the main bronchi may be sutured together, then uniting both bronchi with the trachea end-to-end. If the resection has been extensive, we anastomose the trachea to the right bronchus and then completely close the deep-lying stump of the left bronchus, leaving the left lung atelectatic. We agree with H. Grillo that venous blood shunting through the left lung is dangerous. For this reason, the left pulmonary artery should be ligated concomitantly. Anatomic experiments have indicated that this can be done from the same right posterior approach after opening the pericardium and dividing the ligamentum arteriosum.

A dangerous complication after tracheal resection is hemorrhage into the airways from the brachiocephalic trunk, which usually results from the failure of tracheal anastomosis. To prevent this complication, we place a pedicled flap from the pericardium between the anastomosis and the vessel. If hemorrhage has occurred, the trachea must immediately be intubated and an attempt made to close the anastomotic defect by inflating the cuff of the endotracheal tube. Next, the affected segment of the artery should be ligated on both sides or resected.

In cases of late limited tracheal tumor recurrence, a repeat radical operation is occasionally possible. We have performed three such operations with fair success in patients with adenoid cystic carcinoma. In most instances, however, reoperation in those with recurring squamous cell or adenoid cystic carcinoma is unfeasible, too risky, or undesirable for various reasons. One should then be content with treatment with laser photocoagulation and radiotherapy.

SUGGESTED READING

Perelman MI, Koroleva N. Surgery of the trachea. World J Surg 1980; 4:583.

Grillo HC. Tracheal tumors. Surgical management. Ann Thorac Surg 1978; 26:112.

Grillo HC, Zannini P, Michelassi F. Complications of tracheal reconstruction: incidence, treatment and prevention. J Thorac Cardiovasc Surg 1986; 91:322–328.

Pearson FG, Todd TRJ, Cooper JD. Experience with primary neoplasms of the trachea and carina. J Thorac Cardiovasc Surg 1984; 88:511–518.

ACQUIRED TRACHEOESOPHAGEAL FISTULA

HERMES C. GRILLO, M.D.

Nonmalignant tracheoesophageal fistula may arise from a variety of causes. In the 1960s, granulomatous mediastinal infection and trauma were the most important etiologic factors. Since that time, postintubation tracheoesophageal fistulas have loomed large. In a recently reviewed series of patients, fistulas occurred from inlying cuffed tracheal tubes, tracheal laceration during intubation, mediastinal sepsis, laser treatment of tracheal stenosis, inlying tracheostomy tube after laryngectomy, esophageal foreign body, blunt trauma, complication of anterior cervical spine fusion, and perforated esophageal ulcer. The greatest number were due to pressure erosion at the site of a cuffed tracheal tube. Usually this occurs in the presence of an esophageal feeding tube. The "party wall" of esophagus and trachea is compressed between the two foreign bodies, and a fistula results. These fistulas may be large. In most patients there is also circumferential injury to the trachea caused by the pressure of the cuff.

CLINICAL PRESENTATION

If the patient is still on a ventilator when the fistula occurs, there may be a marked increase in tracheal secretions, difficulty in ventilation, and gastric distention. If the patient is taking oral nutrition, coughing will occur following feedings, and the content of the feedings will appear in the tracheal aspirate. Gastric reflux may occur, and this can produce severe pulmonary injury.

DIAGNOSTIC STUDIES

Bronchoscopy demonstrates the fistula quite easily. With small fistulas, such as those due to a small, chronic, foreign body, it may be necessary to instill methylene blue into the esophagus while observing the area of the tracheal inflammation or suspected fistula. Contrast material is rarely necessary. If used it should be in the form of a barium swallow or instillation of barium into the esophagus at an appropriate level. Radiologically, the distal esophagus may be dilated from the air that passes through the fistula.

OPERATION

If a tracheoesophageal fistula appears while the patient is still on the ventilator, reconstruction is deferred. If there is a tube in the esophagus, it is removed. The endotracheal tube is replaced with the gentlest possible sealing cuff, placed, if possible, below the fistula. A gastrostomy is done to keep the stomach empty in order to prevent reflux. A feeding jejunostomy is added. The patient is weaned, and then repair is done (Table 1). Avoid ligating the esophagogastric junction or attempting to divert the cervical esophagus. Usually the latter is not possible because of the high level of the fistula.

Tracheoesophageal fistulas from cuff tubes and other benign acquired tracheoesophageal fistulas in the neck are approached through a collar incision. There is no particular advantage to the less cosmetic oblique incision. If the upper flap of a collar incision is raised sufficiently high, better exposure is obtained than with an oblique slash incision. If the fistula is one that will not require a tracheal resection, it may be approached through the avascular plane anterior to the sternocleidomastoid muscle and medial to the carotid and internal jugular vessels. The thyroid

TABLE 1 Summary of Operative Procedures*

Procedure	*No. of Patients*
Management of tracheal defect	
Resection and anastomosis	14
Direct closure	6
T-tube	1
Management of esophageal defect	
Direct closure	17
End-to-end anastomosis	4
Interposition of muscle flap	16
Esophageal diversion only	1

* From Hilgenberg AD, Grillo HC. Treatment of nonmalignant tracheoesophageal fistula. In: DeMuster TR, Skinner DB, eds. Esophageal disorders: Pathophysiology and therapy. New York: Raven Press, 1985:489.

gland may be reflected forward, and the groove between the esophagus and trachea identified as the dissection is carefully carried to the area of the fistula. If necessary, a bilateral approach may be used through the same incision and planes. The fistula is identified and divided. The tracheal side must be sutured closed, using interrupted 4–0 Vicryl sutures. After excision of the fistula the esophageal side is closed with interrupted 4–0 silk sutures in two layers using the technique of Richard Sweet, inverting the first layer. A sternohyoid muscle is detached at the hyoid bone and sutured between the two prior suture lines to prevent postoperative recurrence of the fistula. The flap must be very carefully fixed in position so that it will provide substantial interposition. If healthy tissue is not interposed, the likelihood of recurrent fistula is great.

When the tracheoesophagus fistula follows a cuff injury, enough circumferential damage of the trachea has occurred in almost every case so that trachea, too, has to be resected. When this has not been done, a later resection of trachea has often been required, since stenosis progressed at the level of cuff injury. A single-stage procedure is optimal. In this case the approach is from the anterior midline through a collar incision. The trachea is dissected close to its wall, reflecting the thyroid laterally. The recurrent laryngeal nerves are not visualized but are reflected laterally with the thyroid by the technique described for resection of tracheal stenosis. Dissection is carried circumferentially around the trachea just inferior to the fistula, and the trachea is transected after placement of lateral traction sutures. Intubation of the distal trachea is carried out across the operative field. The injured segment of trachea is elevated, and the fistula is fully dissected. This is now excised in continuity with the damaged tracheal segment, and finally the upper end of the damaged tracheal segment is transected. The esophageal mucosa is closed with interrupted 4–0 silk sutures, inverting this first layer so that the knots lie inside the lumen. The muscular repair is by mattress sutures of 4–0 silk. The sternohyoid muscle is detached above and sutured over the closure. End-to-end anastomosis of the trachea is next accomplished using 4–0 Vicryl sutures in the usual manner. If a tracheostomy is present, as it usually is, and is adjacent to the area of damage, it, too, is resected with the specimen. If it lies higher and there is an adequate length of good trachea between stoma and stenosis and fistula, then the stoma is left in place and allowed to close, being merely exteriorized at the time of the operation. No tracheostomy tube is left in place. In a rare case in which the trachea does not have to be resected but the fistula is very large so that there would not be enough membranous tracheal wall for tension-free closure, some of the adjacent wall of the esophagus at the margin of the fistula is left with the tracheal side of the fistula. This extra tissue is folded over to form new membranous wall. The slight esophageal narrowing is of no consequence. The membranous wall of trachea, on the other hand, has no spare tissue and cannot be safely pulled together unless this extra tissue is provided (Table 2).

TABLE 2 Results of Operations*†

Result	*No. of operations*
Excellent	16
Permanent tracheostomy	1
Reoperation	2
Death	3

* N=22.
† From Hilgenberg AD, Grillo HC. Treatment of nonmalignant tracheoesophageal fistula. In: DeMuster TR, Skinner DB, eds. Esophageal disorders: Pathophysiology and therapy. New York: Raven Press, 1985:489.

Intrathoracic tracheoesophageal fistulas of an acquired type are even rarer. The best approach for these is usually right thoracotomy. The esophagus and trachea are dissected out carefully. The same principles described above for cervical fistulas apply. Perhaps the safest interposition tissue in the thorax is a pedicled intercostal muscle flap. The flap is raised at an appropriate level, preserving the intercostal vessels. A single flap may be used for both trachea and esophagus if it lies comfortably between the two without traction. Tracheal resection is usually not necessary, since the kind of circumferential injury seen with a cuff does not usually occur at this level. If the fistula is of such inflammatory nature that additional tissue cannot be "stolen" from the esophagus to close a large defect in the membranous wall, the tracheal lesion can be managed by a segmental resection with end-to-end anastomosis. An alternative that I used in a fistula between the left main bronchus and an intrathoracic stomach in a patient who had received prior high-dose irradiation and in whom resection seemed therefore to be unwise was to suture the pleural side of an intercostal muscle flap carefully to the defect, using it alone to seal the defect. An air-tight closure was obtained by using an appropriate number of sutures (4–0 Vicryl). This provided good healing without subsequent stenosis of the bronchus. If a granuloma were to form at the site of the closure, this could be managed later on bronchoscopically. Thus the extremely rare acquired nonmalignant esophagobronchial fistula and the extremely rare congenital ones that are discovered in young adult life may be repaired in the same fashion as tracheoesophageal fistulas.

SUGGESTED READING

Grillo HC. Postintubation tracheo-esophageal fistula. In: Grillo HC, Eschapasse H, eds. International trends in general thoracic surgery, Vol.II. Philadelphia: WB Saunders, 1986:61.

Grillo HC, Moncure AC, McEnany MT. Repair of inflammatory tracheoesophageal fistula. Ann Thorac Surg 1976; 22:113.

Hilgenberg AD, Grillo HC. Acquired non-malignant tracheoesophageal fistula. J Thorac Cardiovasc Surg 1983; 85:492

Wesselhoeft CW, Keshishian JM. Acquired nonmalignant esophagotracheal and esophagobronchial fistulas. Ann Thorac Surg 1968; 6:187.

Wychulis AR, Ellis RH, Anderson HA. Acquired nonmalignant esophagotracheobronchial fistula. JAMA 1966; 196:117.

MALIGNANT TRACHEO-ESOPHAGEAL FISTULA

RONALD C. HILL, M.D.
GORDON F. MURRAY, M.D.

Unfortunately most patients with esophageal carcinoma are seen late in the course of their disease, which is complicated by advanced esophageal obstruction, perforation, or *malignant tracheoesophageal fistula*. Malignant tracheoesophageal fistula is a particularly disastrous consequence of esophageal carcinoma. Although the fistula may be present at the time of original diagnosis of malignant disease, frequently it occurs after radiation therapy for inoperable or recurrent disease. Significant survival is not realistic, and symptomatic relief can be difficult to achieve. The untreated patient, however, faces death by progressive starvation, drowning in his own secretions, without hope or dignity. An aggressive palliative effort is required, focused on early restoration of the patient's ability to swallow without life-threatening aspiration.

NUTRITIONAL SUPPORT

The therapeutic challenge is made more formidable by associated malnutrition and pulmonary complications. Patients with malignant tracheoesophageal fistula are in a dehydrated, debilitated, anemic, and anergic state. Cardiopulmonary reserve is diminished, and resistance to infection is lowered because of impaired antibody production and decreased phagocytic activity of leukocytes. Depression of cell-mediated and humoral immunity is also present. On the other hand, improved total parenteral nutrition and careful attention to the treatment of respiratory infection have enhanced the safety of aggressive palliative intervention. Significant reductions in major wound infections and postoperative complications have been noted when adequate nutritional support is provided in the perioperative period.

Total parenteral nutrition is ideally begun before intervention if the patient has lost greater than 10 percent of his body weight or hypoalbuminemia has occurred. The goal of therapy is to provide intravenously approximately 45 calories per kilogram per day and 1 to 2 g protein per kilogram per day together with essential vitamins and minerals until the patient is able to ingest an adequate amount orally. The percutaneous small cannula jejunostomy is also recognized as an ancillary operative procedure of great value, allowing maintenance of a satisfactory nutritional state by enteral instead of the more hazardous and expensive parenteral route. In any case, nutritional support appears to be an important adjunct to treatment of malignant tracheoesophageal fistula.

PALLIATIVE INTERVENTION

The exact role of various options for palliative intervention in this incurable lesion is hard to define. The surgeon is immediately faced with two disease processes that are potentially and invariably fatal—esophageal carcinoma and pulmonary sepsis. Even when treated, 80 percent of the patients are dead from the cancer within 3 months, 9 percent will live an additional 3 months, and 11 percent survive for more than 6 months. However, the need for adequate treatment planning is emphasized by the fact that all untreated patients die miserably from lung soilage, and the disease is confined to the thorax in as many as one-half of the patients.

Palliative treatment must exclude the site of the fistula from the rest of the digestive tract and must be performed as early as possible before significant aspiration and sepsis occur. Two major treatment methods are available to exclude the esophagorespiratory fistula and restore alimentary tract continuity—esophageal intubation and surgical exclusion with bypass.

ESOPHAGEAL INTUBATION

An endoprosthesis may achieve satisfactory palliation for a limited time by sealing the fistula and relieving the distal obstruction associated with this carcinoma. This approach seems most applicable in elderly or debilitated patients whose general condition precludes more extensive operative procedures. Pulsion intubation through the esophagoscope can be performed after dilation of the malignant stricture, or traction intubation can be performed by laparotomy and oral insertion of a Celestin or Mousseau-Barbin tube. Both methods of intubation have a relatively high initial mortality (about 25 percent) and are complicated by tube obstruction, tube migration, hemorrhage, sepsis, and aspiration. Less often, survivors enjoy a comfortable existence with a soft or liquid diet and good control of their symptoms.

EXTERNAL DIVERSION

Diversion of the cervical esophagus, cervical esophagostomy, and gastrostomy will prevent sepsis from ongoing aspiration of swallowed oral secretions. Interruption of the esophagogastric junction may be necessary to prevent gastroesophageal reflux and retrograde lung soilage. This approach may be the maximal effort the patient will tolerate. In this circumstance an extracorporeal esophagogastric tube developed by Akiyama may permit the patient to swallow and may provide modest palliation.

ESOPHAGEAL EXCLUSION

In suitable patients, esophageal exclusion and bypass afford the best palliation. If possible, the bypass procedure should be accomplished at the time of esophageal exclusion. Colon interposition in this situation is a complex operation with high attendant morbidity and mortality. On the contrary, the transposed stomach in a substernal position is a safe and efficient esophageal substitute. At the time of bypass the esophagus should be excluded and secured at both ends. It is our preference to decompress the distal esophagus into a generous Roux-en-Y jejunal limb to diminish symptoms of persisting aspiration. If both ends of the esophagus are closed, proximal catheter esophagostomy vent should be provided to prevent disruption of the suture lines and mediastinitis in the early postoperative period. This precaution is especially pertinent if the patient requires continued positive pressure ventilation.

RADIATION THERAPY

When a malignant esophagorespiratory fistula occurs de novo, it may be controlled is some instances by radiation therapy. On the other hand, if the fistula occurs after radiotherapy, chances of healing are minimal. Evidence that radiotherapy causes fistula formation is unclear, but our experience suggests that high-dose therapy can lead to tumor lysis and rapid development of a malignant fistula. Early diagnosis of the nonresectable condition before a fistula develops and before aspiration occurs may allow preventive esophageal exclusion and enhance patient comfort and survival. Radiotherapy is indicated to control residual disease once the fistula is excluded.

SUGGESTED READING

Grant JP. Handbook of total parenteral nutrition. Philadelphia: WB Saunders, 1980.

Keagy BA, Loves ME, Murray GF, Starek PJK, Battaglini JW, Wilcox BR. Esophagogastrectomy as palliation treatment for esophageal carcinoma. Ann Thorac Surg 1974; 38:611–616.

Murray GF, Wilcox BR, Starek PJK. The assessment of operability of esophageal carcinoma. Ann Thorac Surg 1977; 23:393–399.

Postlethwait RW. Surgery of the esophagus. New York: Appleton-Century Crofts, 1979.

Sabiston DC Jr, Spencer FC, eds. Gibbon's surgery of the chest. Philadelphia: WB Saunders, 1983.

ACQUIRED TRACHEAL STENOSIS

HERMES C. GRILLO, M.D.

This chapter pertains to postintubation tracheal stenosis, many of the considerations and techniques of which apply to stenosis of other origins. Stenotic lesions of the upper airway resulting from intubation may involve the glottis (edema, ulceration, granulomas, posterior commissural stenosis, anterior commissural stenosis), the subglottic larynx (edema, granulomas, and circumferential stenosis particularly at the cricoidal level, or destruction of the anterior portion of the cricoid cartilage), and the trachea (stomal, cuff lesions, lesions at the location of the tip of a tube, lesions between the level of a stoma and the cuff). Combinations of these lesions occur frequently, particularly lesions in the larynx and the trachea, since many patients have had periods of both endotracheal and tracheostomy intubation. *It is critical that full evaluation be made of the functional and anatomic state of the larynx before embarking on treatment of the trachea.* If the trachea is repaired and it is then discovered that the glottis is incompetent, it may be impossible to perform a tracheostomy without injuring the tracheal anastomosis. Laryngeal repair sometimes requires a temporary tracheostomy. Evaluation of the larynx includes mirror examination by a competent observer, direct laryngoscopy without anesthetic paralysis of the larynx, and fluoroscopic examination of the larynx by a skilled radiologist.

Lesions in the trachea vary greatly. Anterolateral stenosis occurs at the level of the stoma, circumferential stenosis at the level of a cuff injury, malacia at the level of a cuff injury or in a segment between the stoma and the cuff site, and granulomas or ulceration at the level of the tip of a tube. Tracheoesophageal fistula is found in patients who have had a cuff in the trachea and a feeding tube in the esophagus, with erosion having occurred between these pincers. Arterial fistula to the innominate artery occurs either where the tip of the tube or a high-pressure cuff erodes the wall of the trachea anteriorly or, more commonly, when the tracheostomy is made too low and the tube actually rests at a location in the stoma just above the artery. This occurs most commonly in children and young adults. *It is of great importance that the tracheal lesion be defined in specific location (in relation to the cricoid cartilage and the carina), in circumferential extent, in linear extent, and in specific type, and that associated lesions be identified preoperatively.* Observations that are made on careful radiologic studies with fluoroscopy are confirmed at detailed endoscopic examination by means of rigid bronchoscopes with telescopes, and precise measurements are made.

THERAPEUTIC ALTERNATIVES

With few exceptions, tracheal stenosis does not demand a definitive operation either for its emergency or its long-term management. Since resection and primary anastomosis are basically elective procedures, the surgeon should feel that he can guarantee the likelihood of a successful result or he should not undertake the operation. The emergency management of obstruction due to stenosis may require nothing more than humidification and providing a sense of security and tranquilizing medication for the patient while the extent of the lesion is evaluated, or dilation may be performed with general anesthesia under direct vision using rigid bronchoscopes. If the patient cannot maintain an open airway and his medical condition contraindicates early repair, a tracheostomy may be re-established or a new one performed. If the area of stenosis is accessible through the cervical route without endangering the innominate artery, a tracheostomy should be placed directly through the area of already damaged trachea. A tracheostomy should not be established just above or just below an area of stenosis, since it lengthens the extent of the tracheal lesion, potentially complicating future resection. If the area of damage is not accessible through the neck, the tracheostomy may be made at the site of a prior one or at a distance several centimeters away from the lesion to be treated, so that there will be a segment of intervening trachea that permits reconstruction. The stenosis may be dilated through a stoma utilizing common duct dilators (used with great caution) or the tips of Jackson's tracheostomy tube obturators. It is best if dilation is done under direct vision, as described, through rigid bronchoscopes. A tracheostomy tube is then inserted, which passes through the stenosis. If there is any question the level must be checked with a flexible bronchoscope to be certain that the tube does not create an illusion of security when its tip lies above the stenosis.

For the long-term nonsurgical management of a patient with tracheal stenosis, the measures described are taken initially and then, at an appropriate time, a properly measured silicone rubber T-tube (such as that devised by Montgomery) is inserted to maintain the open airway. This permits the patient to breathe and talk by the normal route and may be left in indefinitely with only occasional changes of tube. Extra long T-tubes are available which may be trimmed to needed lengths.*

The question is often raised whether all tracheal stenoses require surgical resection for definitive cure. Injuries to the trachea caused by intubation vary in location, circumferential extent, linear extent, and, most particularly, in depth of damage to the tracheal wall. Granulomas are best treated by bronchoscopic removal either by conventional techniques or laser, with or without injection of triamcinolone into the base where the granuloma has been removed. With lesser degrees of injury to the tracheal wall, prolonged stenting may lead to regression of edema, maturation of scar tissue, and, ultimately, to an adequate if not ideal airway. Stenting may have to be maintained for many months or years before the stent can be permanently removed. Frequently there appears to be an adequate airway but then contraction recurs in the ensuing weeks. Where the lesion is nearly full thickness with destruction of cartilages over a distance, it is not likely that this segment of trachea (especially where the damage is circumferential) will remain open following removal of a stent. In these circumstances, resection is the only definitive treatment possible, which is the usual case.

The role of other modalities for the removal of scar tissue, such as biopsy forceps, cryotherapy, coagulation, laser, and local (as well as systemic) steroids is small. These methods have been applied to a wide variety of lesions. Some success is likely in lesser or partial-thickness lesions. The laser may be effective to a degree in removal of "web-like" stenosis. Such lesions are very rare. Such methods will not, however, correct the severe lesions. Surgery has the advantages, when skillfully applied, of requiring only brief hospitalization (8 to 10 days) and the great likelihood of permanent cure.

Some lesions cannot be treated even by intubation. These include immediately supracarinal lesions. It is not possible to fit a tube that will stay precisely in a single location. Slight movement of a tube through a supracarinal stenosis may permit granulations to close in beneath it and produce obstruction when an illusion of airway control is present. Y tubes may injure the main bronchi if left in place for a time. Trachea-innominate artery fistula obviously requires emergency tamponade and operation. Tracheoesophageal fistula is best managed in its acute phase, when a patient is still on a respirator, by removal of all esophageal tubes, gastrostomy, and jejunostomy, and the insertion of a low-pressure, large-volume cuff. Repair, however, is deferred until the patient is weaned from a respirator, and then a single-stage repair of both esophagus and trachea is accomplished.

SELECTION OF PATIENTS

Systemic contraindications to operative repair are few. Since the approach to be described is extrapleural and involves only a cervical incision or, at most, an upper mediastinal division of the sternum, there is little physiologic stress. If anesthesia is given properly and attention is paid to prevention of seepage of blood and secretions into the tracheobronchial tree and if the patient is extubated immediately after the operation and given first-quality postoperative care, even patients with extremely poor respiratory reserve can have reconstruction done. Contraindications are any disease or circumstances (including lack of experience of the surgeon or lack of skill of the anesthetist) that would lead to placing the patient on a respirator postoperatively. This must be avoided. If the patient has a disease that is almost certain to require repeat tracheostomy within a very short period of time (such as myasthenia gravis with severe and frequent recurrences), there is no point in subjecting him or her to surgical resection. Quadriplegics who are expected to have difficulty in raising their secretions following repair of the trachea should not be subjected to tracheal reconstruction.

Local contraindications include a recent or markedly inflamed tracheostomy that has been performed for the treatment of the stenosis or the presence of florid, easily bleeding granulations and inflammation at the site of the stenosis. If the patient is receiving steroid therapy, he should first be weaned from the medication entirely or have it tapered to low doses. Since there is no need for emergency surgery, it is not justifiable to take the risk of extensive tracheal reconstruction in the presence of high doses of steroids.

SURGICAL TECHNIQUE

General anesthesia should be used for both the initial endoscopic evaluation, often done at the time of a projected resection, and the operation itself. Halothane is preferred. The induction may take a long time if the stenosis is tight.

---

* E. Benson Hood Laboratories, 575 Washington Street, Pembroke, MA. 02359, U.S.A.

The surgeon must be present and be prepared to dilate the stenosis if obstruction develops, using serial pediatric and adult rigid bronchoscopes. If the stenosis is 6 mm in diameter or less, dilation should be done prior to commencing surgery. Otherwise there may be a build-up of carbon dioxide and subsequent arrhythmias prior to the time when the tracheal lumen is accessible through the operative field.

If the lesion is several centimeters or more below the vocal cords, an endotracheal tube may be placed through the cords above the stenosis. It is not necessary in every case to pass the tube through the stenosis. If the stenosis is immediately subglottic, dilation must be done and intubation carried out with a small endotracheal tube.

If the patient is not paralyzed, he will be extubated on the operating table at the conclusion of the procedure. This allows the opportunity to test the adequacy of repair before the patient leaves the operating room. If for any reason ventilation must be carried out for a short period of time, a small endotracheal tube should be put into place and the cuff carefully seated, either above or below the area of anastomosis. Even a low-pressure cuff placed adjacent to an anastomosis may lead to its separation after a period of time.

Approaches. Essentially all postintubation tracheal stenoses can be approached anteriorly either through a cervical incision or a cervicomediastinal incision, even lesions that are immediately above the carina. There are few, if any, indications for a transthoracic approach. If a previous surgeon has mistakenly approached a postintubation stenosis through the thorax, it may be necessary to repeat the approach. The mediastinal portion of the incision usually involves a division of the sternum no more than 1 or 2 cm below the angle of Louis. Since the carina lies at the level of the sternal angle and is posterior to the great vessels at this point, nothing is to be gained by full sternotomy.

The entire neck is prepared, since laryngeal release may be required. Since the cervical incision is short, I prefer to make a second incision directly over the hyoid if a laryngeal release is to be performed, rather than to use a long U-shaped flap. The result is much more cosmetic. Occasionally, when an upper mediastinal division is required, a low, long, curved incision is made at the level of the midmanubrium. This allows for elevation of flaps above into the neck and below to a point below the sternal angle. This incision lies well below the neckline and also avoids the vertical scar of the T-incision.

If a tracheostomy is present, the transverse incision often circumcises it. The site of tracheostomy should not dictate the placement of the collar incision. The tracheostomy can be separately detached as the flap is elevated. The transverse incision should be placed at an optimal point. If the stoma is to be closed rather than excised, in the course of the resection it may be necessary to leave a small amount of skin circumferentially around it to be used in the inversion process.

The upper skin flap is raised with the platysma to a point above the cricoid cartilage. Inferiorly it is raised to the sternal notch. The strap muscles are dissected out of scar tissue and elevated. The anterior surface of the trachea is gradually exposed into the mediastinum.

Technique of Dissection, Resection, and Reconstruction. The anterior surface of the trachea is exposed throughout its length in almost all cases. Dissection is made close to the tracheal surface. The innominate artery often is adherent to an area of cuff stenosis. It is important not to dissect out the artery itself but to keep the dissection close to the tracheal wall. This allows elevation with the artery of scar tissue posterior to it and protects the artery from possible postoperative erosion. In reoperations it may be necessary to isolate the innominate artery proximally and distally with tourniquets. However, this should *not* be a part of the routine procedure.

The level of the lesion is identified, and dissection is carried out carefully circumferentially around the trachea at a point just below the stenosis. The dissection is kept close to the trachea to avoid injury to recurrent laryngeal nerves. No effort is made to identify these nerves, since dissecting them out of scar tissue is likely to lead to injury. Circumferential dissection is done immediately below the lesion because the tissues are less adherent here, and there is less chance of entering the membranous wall of the trachea or the esophageal wall. If the lesion is a distal one, dissection is carried around the trachea just above the lesion. Very little trachea that is to be left in the patient is circumferentially dissected (no more than 1 to 2 cm). Extensive dissection may destroy the blood supply of the trachea and lead to late necrosis and re-stenosis, which may be irreparable.

When circumferential dissection has been made and a tape passed beneath the trachea, traction sutures (2–0 Vicryl) are placed in the midlateral line of the trachea on either side 1 to 2 cm below the projected level of transection of the trachea. These sutures pass vertically through the full-thickness wall of the trachea. A flexible armored endotracheal tube is brought to the field. Appropriate connectors and tubing are passed off to the anesthetist. The trachea is opened anteriorly just below the level of the stenosis. The initial cut is made very close to the disease, since no more trachea than is absolutely necessary should be removed. Once the level of transection has been selected, transection is completed after the anesthetist has withdrawn his tube to a more proximal portion of the trachea. The patient is intubated across the operative field. The lower end of the segment to be removed is lifted upward, dissecting the specimen from the lateral tissues, which contain the recurrent laryngeal nerves, and from the esophagus, to which it may be densely adherent.

Once the upper end of the lesion has been reached, proximal traction sutures are placed and the specimen is excised. The proximal traction sutures may be in the wall of the larynx. The level of transection may lie at the lower border of the cricoid cartilage. At this point, the recurrent laryngeal nerves are within millimeters of the dissection.

Ease of approximation and tension are tested by having the anesthetist flex the patient's neck. The surgeon and assistant pull the traction sutures on their sides of the table to gain a sense of how easily the ends will come together. Obviously judgments about the resectability of the lesion should have been made previously—preoperatively, postendoscopically, or at the initial exploration. It does little good to discover at this point that one has resected more trachea than can possibly be reconstructed. It is unacceptable to do a partial resection of the lesion, since it will almost certainly restenose. Areas of malacia will not be splinted by suturing them to a good segment of trachea below.

If it has been demonstrated that anastomosis can be done without excessive tension, anastomotic sutures are placed. This may be done either by bending the endotracheal tube forward or removing it intermittently. High-frequency ventilation eliminates this problem, if desired.

I use 4–0 coated Vicryl sutures. All sutures are placed prior to completing anastomosis. They are placed so that the knots can be tied on the outside of the tracheal lumen. They are passed through the wall of the trachea 4 mm from the cut edge. They usually pass through cartilages. No effort is made to place them submucosally. Sutures are placed about 4 mm apart. The midline posterior suture is placed first, and each successive suture, first on one side and then on the other, is placed up to the point where the lateral traction sutures reside. Sutures are carefully clipped to the drapes so that their order will not be disturbed. They will be tied front-to-back, although initially they are placed from back-to-front. Sutures anterior to the lateral traction sutures are clipped to the drapes anteriorly.

After placement of all the sutures, the inflatable bag beneath the patient is deflated. The anesthetic tube across the operative field is removed, and the trachea and main bronchi are suctioned to remove blood and secretions. The per oral endotracheal tube is now drawn down across the operative field and slipped into the distal trachea. This original anesthesia tube had been pulled upward at the time of the excision. In order to facilitate placement of the tube if the stenosis is a high one and the tube might slip out through the vocal cords, a rubber catheter was sutured to the tip of the tube, and this is now used to aid the anesthetist in passing the tube downward again. The anesthetist builds up the patient's neck into a flexed position. The lateral traction sutures are then tied simultaneously by the surgeon and his assistant, drawing the ends of the trachea to a point of approximation, but no intussusception. The anastomotic sutures are tied from front-to-back all the way around, and the excess of each suture is cut after it is tied. The lateral traction sutures are next removed.

The thyroid isthmus is resutured across the anastomosis. Otherwise no special concern need be taken to cover the anastomosis. If the suture line lies behind the artery, generally nothing is required. If there has been excessive dissection, a strap muscle may be pedicled between the suture line and the innominate artery. Foreign material is not used. A drain is placed anterior to the trachea. The sternum is wired. The strap muscles are sutured together, and the platysma and skin are closed transversely.

Tracheostomy is not done concomitant with this procedure, since it leads only to the possibility of damage to the anastomosis, inspissation of secretions, and other complications. If the anastomosis is inadequate at this point, a tracheostomy will not salvage it.

One or two heavy sutures are placed from the skin crease just below the point of the chin to the presternal skin. They are kept in for 1 week to remind the patient not to hyperextend the neck suddenly.

Laryngotracheal Stenosis. Lesions in the trachea that have eroded the cricoid cartilage through its entire thickness or lesions produced by an endotracheal tube or cricothyroidostomy involve the subglottic larynx. It is essential that their existence be recognized before the surgery is undertaken. Otherwise the surgeon will be presented with a problem that will not respond to the type of resection just described, and his efforts will compound the problem, perhaps irretrievably. It is not realized by many surgeons that there are 1.5 to 2 cm of subglottic larynx below the vocal cords. Recognition of the level of the cricoid may be made both endoscopically and radiologically. Techniques for the one-stage repair of such stenoses, even when they are circumferential and involve the area anterior to the posterior cricoid plate, have been evolved but are beyond the scope of this brief treatment.

RECONSTRUCTION AFTER EXTENDED RESECTION OF THE TRACHEA

Such reconstruction is a complex problem. The most useful adjunct, although it is not needed for the majority of tracheal stenoses, is laryngeal release. Thyrohyoid release, which attained initial popularity, has the disadvantage of leading, in the majority of cases, to a period of aspiration and difficulty with deglutition. Eventually this responds in most cases, although more slowly in the elderly. The same difficulties are seen, but with much less frequency, following the suprahyoid laryngeal release, as described by Montgomery. It is essential that any surgeon undertaking tracheal reconstruction be familiar with the anatomy and techniques of these releases.

More complex techniques include splinting concomitant malacic segments and intrathoracic releases. It is rarely necessary to do an intrathoracic release for a postintubation stenosis patient undergoing operative correction for the first time. Most extended postintubation lesions I have seen are the result either of inappropriate resectional surgery or of multiple tracheostomies performed for the treatment of a stenosis.

POSTOPERATIVE CARE

Patients are encouraged to cough and clear their secretions with gentle chest physiotherapy. Humidification is provided. If there has been a lot of edema at the laryngeal level, brief use is made of racemic epinephrine and inhaled topical steroids. Systemic steroids may be given for 24 to 48 hours, but these should not be continued because they will inhibit the healing process and increase the chances of postoperative tracheal dehiscence. When a long resection has been performed, particularly if laryngeal release has been done, the patient is cautiously introduced to liquids and foods postoperatively. The chin stitch remains in place for a week, after which the patient is asked not to extend the neck forcefully for another week. Following that the patient may return to normal activities. I

TABLE 1 Results of Massachusetts General Hospital Tracheal Reconstruction for Postintubation Lesions

Results (1964–1982)	
Good	225
Satisfactory	25
Failure	20
Deaths	5
Lost to follow-up	4
	279

TABLE 2 Tracheal Reconstruction, M.G.H.: Results in Early, Late Series

	Case No.	
	1–139	*140–279*
Complications	42	30
Failure	13	7
Deaths	4	1

usually obtain a short series of tracheal x-ray films just prior to patient discharge to check the adequacy of the lumen and the function of the larynx. This is repeated in approximately 3 months to obtain a picture of the late result.

RESULTS

Results and complications in a series extending over 18 years are noted in Tables 1, 2 and 3. The series contains 50 reoperated cases. The incidence of complications, failures, and deaths is reduced from the first to the second half of the series, since in the beginning there were few guidelines to these techniques. At least 200 additional resections for stenosis have since been done, with fewer complications. Granulations, for example, have disappeared with the use of absorbable Vicryl sutures.

TABLE 3 Tracheal Reconstruction, M.G.H.: Complications in the Series

Granulations	26
Dehiscence	4
Re-stenosis	15
Narrowing	6
Residual malacia	3
Innominate arterial hemorrhage	2
Tracheoesophageal fistula	1
Vocal cord dysfunction	5
Aspiration	1
Wound infection	6

SUGGESTED READING

Grillo HC. Surgical treatment of post-intubation tracheal injuries. J Thorac Cardiovasc Surg 1979; 78:860–875.

Grillo HC. Primary reconstruction of airway after resection of subglottic larnygeal and upper tracheal stenosis. Ann Thorac Surg 1982; 33:3–8.

Grillo HC, Zannini P, Michelassi F. Complications of tracheal reconstruction: incidence, treatment and prevention. J Thorac Cardiovasc Surg 1986; 91:322–328.

Grillo HC. Tracheal surgery. In: Ravitch M, Steichen F, eds. Atlas of noncardiac thoracic surgery. Philadelphia: WB Saunders, 1987.

Montgomery WW. Surgery of the upper respiratory system. Vol II. Philadelphia: Lea & Febiger, 1973.

TRACHEAL PROBLEMS IN CHILDREN

MICHAEL R. HARRISON, M.D.
ALFRED A. DELORIMIER, M.D.

Obstructive lesions of the trachea in infants and children are frequently life-threatening because small amounts of secretion or mucosal inflammation can easily obstruct the tiny compromised airway. Aspirated foreign bodies require endoscopic removal. Congenital laryngeal and subglottic lesions such as cysts and lymphangiomas may be resected using an operating laryngoscope and CO_2 laser or those such as hemangiomas may be allowed to involute; tracheostomy is often required during treatment. Acquired subglottic stenosis is preventable by using endotracheal tubes small enough to allow a good air leak in infants. Established subglottic stenosis that does not respond to laser treatment is best managed by anterior cricoid split (Cotton's procedure). We do not use stints or T-tubes.

The focus here is on congenital lesions of the trachea that produce symptoms early in life. Although both tracheal stenosis and malacia may occur primarily in this age group, they are frequently associated with vascular or esophageal anomalies causing compression. In congenital stenosis the tracheal cartilage often forms complete rings.

The infant with a possible distal tracheal obstruction is difficult to manage because diagnostic procedures necessary to formulate treatment may precipitate obstruction that often cannot be corrected, even temporarily, by intubation. Therefore diagnostic and therapeutic procedures must be integrated with plans to manage the airway.

THERAPEUTIC ALTERNATIVES

Severe malacia associated with esophageal atresia may

respond to anterior mediastinal decompression achieved by suspending the aorta to the underside of the sternum. Short segments of refractory tracheal malacia can be resected; long segments of malacia can be stiffened by external splinting with rib which, although it resorbs, provides support while the airway becomes more rigid.

Stenotic lesions of the trachea in infants and children have been managed by tracheal dilation, local injection of steroids, endotracheal stenting, and endoscopic treatment by electroresection, cryotherapy, or laser vaporization. Although the CO_2 laser has proved useful in treating subglottic lesions, none of these endoscopic techniques, including argon and YAG lasers passed through flexible glass rods in the biopsy channel of the bronchoscope, have been useful in the more difficult distal tracheal stenosis. We believe that resection is the treatment of choice for localized lesions involving less than one-half of the tracheal length. Management of longer segments with complete tracheal rings remains an unsolved problem; several surgeons (including ourselves) have attempted to enlarge the lumen by splitting the rings and inserting costal cartilage.

PREFERRED APPROACH

Infants with suspected stenotic and malacic lesions should be managed as conservatively as possible, preferably without intubation. Intubation past the obstruction is often impossible, and 'temporary' stenting of these lesions is seldom temporary because the presence of the tube itself ensures continued trauma, causes irritation, and compromises adequate humidification of gases. Bronchodilators, steroids, and vasoconstrictors may help to shrink edematous mucosa and provide time for transport and evaluation.

Magnified chest x-ray films, flow volume curves, and echocardiography to identify anomalous vessels can all be performed urgently in the intensive care unit. Less critical obstruction may allow time for barium esophagogram and angiography, but all these studies may be replaced by rapid sequence computed tomographic (CT) scan with cine computer reconstruction, a study that delineates dynamic cross-sectional anatomy. Infants with critical airway obstruction are best evaluated in an operating room fully prepared for definitive tracheal reconstruction. A 2.5-mm ventilating bronchoscope is used to visualize the upper trachea. If the length of tracheal involvement cannot be visualized, it can be outlined by bronchogram (with micropaque barium in sterile saline) or by using ray-opaque contrast medium filling a 2-ml Fogarty balloon catheter. An image intensifier and chest x-ray film with the infant on the operating table document the anatomy.

Surgical treatment of congenital tracheal stenosis involves excision of the involved area of narrowing. The stenotic area is rigid and does not dilate. Most tracheal lesions can be exposed by a transverse neck incision with extension by median sternotomy. Bronchial lesions may require a posterolateral thoracotomy on the side opposite the aortic arch. Cardiopulmonary bypass has not proved advantageous. The trachea is divided at the lowest level of stenosis, a sterile endotracheal tube is inserted into the lower trachea or bronchus, and ventilation is established. The trachea is transected at varying levels proximally until a normal caliber is encountered. For short segments of stenosis, up to half the length of a normal trachea can be resected. 4–0 or 5–0 nylon or PDS sutures are placed circumferentially. The distal endotracheal tube is removed and ventilation continued through the original endotracheal tube in the proximal trachea while the ends are approximated and the sutures tied. Lateral traction sutures are sometimes used to relieve tension on the anastomosis.

We prefer to extubate the patient as soon as adequate spontaneous ventilation is achieved. Tracheostomy or prolonged intubation should be avoided. Tubes cause infection, trauma, drying, and inspissation of secretions with plugging of the airway. To minimize tension on the anastomosis, the head and neck are maintained in flexion with a brace fitted about the trunk and extended to the back of the head.

PROS AND CONS OF TREATMENT

Resection has proved to be the treatment of choice in over a dozen infants and children with localized tracheal lesions. The youngest patient was 6 weeks old, and the longest resection was 2.7 cm or approximately half the trachea of a 16-month-old boy. When the lesion could be completely resected, the children did well. Surprisingly, growth of the anastomosis has not been a problem even during the first few years of life. Use of less reactive suture material has decreased the need for endoscopic removal of suture material and granuloma occasionally encountered during the first few postoperative months.

Children with stenoses that are not completely resected either because they are not referred in time or because the extent of the lesion is not defined well enough before or during exploration have not survived. The key to success is expeditious evaluation by an operative team prepared for emergency tracheal reconstruction.

SUGGESTED READING

Harrison MR, Heldt GP, Brasch RC, et al. Resection of distal tracheal stenosis in a baby with agenesis of the lung. J Pediatr Surg 1980; 15:938–943.

Kimura K, Mukohara N, Tsugawa C, et al. Tracheoplasty for congenital stenosis of the entire trachea. J Pediatr Surg 1982; 17:869–871.

Landing BH, Dixon LG. Congenital malformations and genetic disorders of the respiratory tract (larynx, trachea, bronchi, and lungs). Am Rev Respir Dis 1979; 120:151–185.

Nakayama DK, Harrison MR, deLorimier AA, et al. Reconstructive surgery for obstructing lesions of the intrathoracic trachea in infants and small children. J Pediatr Surg 1982; 17:854–868.

Vinograd I, Filler RM, Bahoric A. Long term functional results of prosthetic airway splinting in tracheomalacia and bronchomalacia. J Pediatr Surg 1987; 22:38–41.

ACUTE AIRWAY OBSTRUCTION

DOUGLAS J. MATHISEN, M.D.

Management of acute airway obstruction should be familiar to all thoracic surgeons. The ability to recognize acute airway obstruction and to secure swift control of the airway may be lifesaving maneuvers.

FOREIGN BODIES

Aspiration of a piece of meat in the upper airway is a common cause of acute airway obstruction. If the piece cannot be quickly dislodged by grasping it, the Heimlich maneuver is used. This is performed by standing behind the affected individual wrapping one's arms around him, and grabbing the hands into a ball and thrusting them quickly in an upward direction at the level of the epigastrium. This forces air out of the stomach, clears the esophagus, and thrusts the contents of the abdomen upward against the diaphragm, causing expulsion of air through the airway. Emergency cricothyroidostomy may be necessary if this fails.

Aspiration of foreign bodies below the level of the upper trachea can only be handled with rigid endoscopy. Care must be taken not to impact the foreign body while trying to remove it. A variety of biopsy forceps is available for grasping the foreign body. If the foreign body is too large to be brought out through the endoscope, simply grasping it and removing the bronchoscope with the foreign body pulled against the distal end of it often will remove the object. The use of balloon-tipped catheters is sometimes very helpful. Passing the catheter beyond the foreign body with the balloon deflated, and then inflating it once the catheter has gone beyond the object and gently pulling back will often dislodge it.

TRAUMA

In trauma patients, massive facial fractures may make intubation impossible. The patient may require stabilization of the mandible or maxilla, which would preclude the use of an oral endotracheal tube. In this circumstance, if an emergency airway is required, cricothyroidostomy or emergency tracheostomy should be performed. Massive oral hemorrhage may preclude visualization of the airway and necessitate emergency cricothyroidostomy or tracheostomy to establish an airway. Laryngotracheal trauma may be manifested by acute airway obstruction. The larynx may be crushed and the trachea either partially or totally separated. Attempts at intubation from above may be futile and lead to total loss of the airway. In circumstances involving trauma to the airway, emergency tracheostomy should be performed whenever doubt exists. Attempts to intubate or to examine the airway with a flexible bronchoscope and thread an endotracheal tube over this should be done in the operating room with everthing set up to proceed to an emergency tracheostomy if the airway is lost. If total separation of the airway has occurred, one may find the trachea absent when performing an emergency tracheostomy. The distal end usually retracts into the mediastinum. This can be located by finger exploration in the area where the trachea should have been, by feeling the distal end of the trachea and grasping it with a clamp and pulling it into the wound. An endotracheal tube can then be inserted for control of the airway.

Cricothyroidostomy should be converted to permanent tracheostomy in all situations within 24 hours. Damage to the cricoid cartilage or the larynx by an indwelling tube may be exceedingly difficult or impossible to repair. Repair of the cricothyroid membrane can be attempted or it can be left to close on its own once formal tracheostomy is performed.

TRACHEAL STENOSIS

Critical airway stenosis of less than 6 mm can develop days to months following intubation or tracheostomy. Patients notice increased difficulty in breathing on vigorous exercise and eventually at rest. Patients should be managed initially with bed rest, elevation of the head, application of cool mist, and very gentle sedation. If these measures fail, some provision must be made for providing an airway. Tracheostomy can be performed and is best done using local anesthesia, with the patient awake and breathing on his or her own. It is important to remember that the tracheostomy should be placed through the damaged trachea so as not to utilize viable trachea that might be needed in subsequent reconstruction. Alternatively, dilation can be used to provide an airway. Dilation of the airway demands skill and familiarity with rigid bronchoscopy. It must be done carefully to avoid perforation of the trachea. It is best performed under general anesthesia. Slow induction of anesthesia using a deep halothane technique is the preferred way to anesthetize these patients. This allows the patient to breathe spontaneously at all times. Induction of general anesthesia deep enough to allow rigid bronchoscopy may take as long as 20 minutes. This requires skill and patience on the part of the anesthesiologist. An assortment of rigid bronchoscopes ranging from pediatric to adult sizes should be available to the endoscopist. If the stenosis is located in the subglottic region, a laryngoscope can be utilized to visualize the glottis, and the small pediatric scope can be passed through the stenosis under direct vision. This will then allow control of the airway, and this maneuver can be repeated over and over again until a sufficient airway has been achieved. Steroids and racemic epinephrine may be helpful in the first 48 hours to reduce swelling that may have been induced by multiple passages of the bronchoscope. They should not be continued beyond this point, since they only further complicate reconstructive efforts. Small amounts of bleeding may occur but can be easily controlled with pressure and generally stop without assistance. If the stenosis is farther down the trachea, a larger bronchoscope may be inserted above the stenosis. With the stenotic area under direct vision, a Jackson dilator may then be passed gently through the area. One can usually pass a No. 22 Jackson dilator through a 9 mm rigid bronchoscope. This should then allow a No. 6 rigid bronchoscope through the stenotic area. No. 7 and No. 8 rigid bronchoscopes can be used to further dilate the stenotic area.

It is important to understand that dilation of inflammatory tracheal stenosis is only a temporary measure. Tracheal stenosis usually develops within a week to 10 days.

The laser does not seem to play any role in management of postintubation tracheal stenosis. Its use is tedious, time-consuming, and costly. In addition, it is only a temporary measure and offers no great advantage over simple dilation. The risks of local perforation and increased inflammatory reaction may hinder attempts at ultimate reconstruction. The only exception to this is the very rare weblike tracheal stenosis.

Malignant strictures may lead to acute airway obstruction. Most malignant strictures of the airway can be managed very easily with techniques similar to those previously described for acquired postintubation stenosis. Rigid bronchoscopes can usually be passed beyond the level of the obstructing tumor to gain control of the distal airway. Once this has been accomplished and the patient's ventilation controlled, the rigid bronchoscope can be withdrawn to visualize the area of obstructing tumor. Biopsy forceps may be helpful to remove portions of the tumor initially. The rigid bronchoscope itself can be used to core out the tumor. The beveled tip of the bronchoscope can be used in a corkscrew fashion to actually shave off a large portion of the tumor. This can then be grasped and withdrawn through the bronchoscope. Bleeding is generally minimal and easily controlled with pressure or epinephrine-soaked pledgets or both. Once the majority of tumor has been removed, the biopsy forceps can then be used to remove the remaining bits. We have found this to be a very safe and effective method of providing adequate management of malignant strictures. Bleeding has not been a problem in our cases.

There has been increasingly widespread use of the laser to manage malignant strictures of the airway. We find this method acceptable but feel that it is more costly, more time-consuming, more tedious, and frequently has to be done more than once to achieve a satisfactory airway. We feel that it does not offer any advantages over the use of rigid bronchoscopes and biopsy forceps in managing malignant strictures. The only exception may be the rare carcinoid tumor of the airway, which cannot be removed either because of medical contraindications or distal infection.

SUGGESTED READING

Mathisen DS, Grillo HC. Endoscopic relief of malignant airway obstruction. Ann Thorac Surg (in press).

Mathisen DS, Grillo HC. Management of acute airway obstruction. Int Trends Gen Thorac Surg 1988; 5 (in press).

MEDIASTINAL EXENTERATION

HERMES C. GRILLO, M.D.

I use the term mediastinal exenteration to describe the radical removal of a lesion, usually a malignant neoplasm, which involves both the larynx and the trachea and, in many cases, the esophagus and sometimes the lower pharynx. Adjacent structures may also be involved. Removal of the tumor, therefore, may require excision of the contents of the neck from carotid to carotid and of the upper mediastinum.

INDICATIONS

The principal lesions for which these procedures have been used are (1) adenoidcystic carcinoma that involves so much of the larynx and the trachea that functional airway reconstruction cannot be accomplished, (2) invasive differentiated carcinoma of the thyroid, principally papillary and follicular, usually recurrent, which similarly involves larynx, trachea, and esophagus, (3) undifferentiated thyroid carcinoma that by careful study appears to be localized to the neck and mediastinum, (4) postcricoidal carcinoma of the esophagus invading the organs described, and (5) carcinoma of the larynx that has recurred following prior laryngectomy. Other rare indications have included massive fibrosis due to excessive ^{131}I treatment accompanied by multiple fistulas and hemorrhage.

Patients with invasive differentiated thyroid carcinoma usually have received multiple prior treatment, including thyroidectomy, ^{131}I, and external irradiation, and they now suffer from massive recurrence with obstruction of airway and esophagus. Most patients who have recurrence of laryngeal carcinoma also have had full-dose prior irradiation.

In a few of these patients, the goal may be curative. This applies particularly to patients with localized but extensive adenoidcystic carcinoma and occasionally in an initial approach to thyroid carcinoma or to postcricoidal esophageal carcinoma.

There is a place for palliative resection, extensive as the procedure appears to be. Certain of these patients are in total misery when seen, dying from essentially localized disease with airway obstruction, severe dysphagia, and pain. If the disease is removed, an effective airway established, and swallowing restored, the patient is vastly relieved, and no worse off physiologically or anatomically than a patient who has had a laryngectomy. I thus believe it appropriate to use this approach in some even when there are known pulmonary metastases from slowly progressive tumors such as adenoidcystic carcinoma or differentiated thyroid carcinoma. Balanced against this, however, is recognition that the surgery is of great magnitude and that serious or lethal complications may occur. Radical resection of recurrent laryngeal cancer at the stoma is not often useful if the tumor pervades the paratracheal lymphatics.

In some of these patients, radiotherapy alone can provide palliation initially. This is particularly true with adenoidcystic carcinoma of the airway and, to a lesser extent, postcricoidal squamous carcinoma. Carcinoma of the thyroid, particularly the differentiated type, is less likely to respond well to external irradiation (or to ^{131}I). However, many of these patients when first seen have already received full-dose irradiation. This also complicates a surgical procedure. Combined chemotherapy has provided relatively brief palliation for some patients with squamous carcinoma. It is this lack of satisfactory alternatives in highly symptomatic patients without systemic disease that led to a surgical approach.

PREOPERATIVE EVALUATION

The extent of the disease must be defined precisely. Anteroposterior and lateral radiograms of the neck with and without barium contrast are helpful. Computed tomography (CT) scans of the neck and chest may help to determine the extent of invasion of mediastinal structures, especially blood vessels, and the presence of pulmonary metastases. Aortic arch angiograms will show whether the arteries supplying the brain are involved either by tumor or by degenerative disease, since it may be necessary in some patients to consider elective division of the innominate artery. If esophageal reconstruction with a colon segment is anticipated, superior and inferior mesenteric artery angiograms are helpful to delineate the blood supply of the bowel. Complete bowel preparation should also be done.

A plastic surgery consultation is advisable if a large amount of skin has to be excised around the lesion.

OPERATIVE TECHNIQUE

In the majority of patients, arrangements are made in advance for electroencephalographic monitoring as needed during the operation in the event that it becomes necessary to divide the innominate artery. Electrodes are applied prior to induction of anesthesia so that baseline recordings can be obtained. Intubation is either oral or through an existing tracheostomy. The patient lies supine. The field extends from the chin to the pubis. A thigh is often prepared as a source of split-thickness skin grafts. If a venous graft is required, allowance is made. At least one arm is abducted to be available for arterial or venous access. A warming mattress may be advisable, since the procedure may be lengthly. A nasogastric tube and a Foley catheter are placed.

The operation is best performed by two teams, one for the neck and mediastinum and the other to prepare an esophageal replacement in the abdomen. If intubation has been carried out through an existing tracheostomy, the tube is changed for a sterile flexible Tovell-type endotracheal tube and connected to the anesthesia machine with sterile tubing and connectors, just as in tracheal reconstruction. This tubing may easily be moved and does not hinder the surgeon.

Incisions are individualized, depending on existing stomas, invasion by tumor, or severe radiation change. The usual initial approach is via a curved transverse incision at the level of the clavicles. This permits full exposure of the neck and upper sternum. Exploration is conducted with no irrevocable moves until it is certain that the procedure can be completed. With a bulky lesion such as extensive recurrent thyroid carcinoma, the dissection is carried out just medial to the carotid artery and internal jugular vein on both sides. On very rare occasions one of these vessels may be excised and reconstructed. If the extent of mediastinal involvement cannot be determined adequately through the cervical incision, the inferior flap is raised over the pectoral fascia, and the pectoral muscles are elevated in the midline. The upper sternum may be divided by carrying a vertical split down to the second interspace and cutting across the sternum transversely at that level. Occasionally, depending on the extent of trachea involved, this division may be made through the first interspace. When it has been decided that the lesion will be removed, the abdominal team commences mobilization of that portion of bowel to be used for esophageal reconstruction. Some patients require only laryngotrachiectomy or only removal of the anterior muscular wall or even mucosal wall of the esophagus. Reconstruction is done by narrowing the remaining esophageal tube. If the thyroid is not involved by tumor, one or both lobes may be left intact by dividing the isthmus and turning the lobe back with the lateral blood supply still attached.

When it is clear that the tracheostomy will be mediastinal, a plaque of bony anterior chest wall is removed prior to dividing the trachea. If there is a question about whether or not the lesion can be excised, further dissection is done through the sternotomy prior to removing the plaque of bone. In order to provide for a mediastinal tracheostomy, each clavicle is divided approximately 4 cm from its medial end by passing a Gigli's saw carefully beneath it, avoiding injury to the underlying subclavian vein. The first and second cartilages are also divided on both sides after freeing the intercostal muscles from the junctions of sternum and cartilages. The plaques of clavicle, cartilage, and sternum are removed on both sides. This maneuver is greatly facilitated by the previous division of the sternum, as described. Ideally the pleura should remain intact.

The level of tracheal transection is selected to provide an adequate margin below the level of tumor. Particularly in thyroid carcinoma, lymph nodes lying in the V between the innominate artery and left carotid artery are dissected up with the specimen. Division of the innominate vein is not usually helpful, although it may have to be resected if tumor invades one of these veins. Lateral traction sutures are placed on both sides of the distal trachea, below the expected level of transection. The division is made, and intubation is carried out across the operative field.

The level of esophageal division is selected. As noted, it is not always necessary to resect the esophagus totally. If a narrowed esophagus is left in place, it will serve as an excellent immediate conduit for saliva and nutrition. Indeed, some such patients have not even required dilation but have widened their residual esophagus by swallowing. If the esophagus and upper pharynx are to be removed, distal esophageal transection is carried out, and the entire specimen is elevated away from the prevertebral fascia—assuming colon replacement. I generally close the distal esophagus with a stapler and add a layer of inverting interrupted silk sutures. If the stomach is to be used for reconstruction, the residual esophagus is removed by dissection from above through the exposed mediastinum and completion of dissection from below through the esophageal hiatus. In most of these patients I have personally preferred to use a colon reconstruction and have therefore turned in the esophagus at this point.

When the specimen has been elevated all the way to the pharynx and larynx, proximal transection is done. The suprahyoid musculature is divided with cautery, the superior cornua of the hyoid bone is divided sharply, the muscles attaching to the larynx are divided in the usual manner, the pharynx is circumcised, and the specimen is removed. A substernal tunnel is made bluntly from above and below, pushing more to the left than to the right to avoid entering the right pleura. In the meantime the abdominal team has provided an adequate colon bypass. I usually use the transverse and left colon pedicled on the left colic artery. The middle colic artery is divided at its origin so that the branches will serve as an arcade. A long transplant is required to reach the pharynx. The vascular pedicle is brought up behind the stomach, and the distal end of the colon is anastomosed to the anterior wall of the stomach. Since the vagus nerves have been divided, a pyloromyotomy or pyloroplasty is also done. A draining gastrostomy is placed for ease of postoperative management and a feeding jejunostomy for security.

The proximal colon is anastomosed to the pharynx using two layers of interrupted 4–0 silk sutures. This is done with meticulous care to avoid leakage. Even with prior irradiation, healing can generally be counted on because the colonic tissue has not been irradiated. In addition, in such patients (as in most), a pedicled omental flap is also brought up substernally and placed around the anastomosis. The omental pedicle is generally prepared by dissecting it off the colon and, if needed, off the stomach, leaving the right gastroepiploic artery as the principal blood supply. In patients with a long omentum, it is only necessary to turn the omentum upward and not to pedicle the vessel.

In order to construct a mediastinal tracheostomy, a second transverse incision is made, usually in the submammary line from anterior axillary line to anterior axillary line. With the previous upper transverse incision, a large bipedicled flap is now elevated from the pectoral fascia, taking great care to spare the lateral blood supply. This large flap will now drop down into the mediastinal defect created by removal of the sternal plaque. If it appears that the stoma will reside adjacent to the innominate artery with any degree of tension at all, elective division of the innominate artery is performed. Initially the artery is clamped under electroencephalographic control. If, after a period of time, there is no change in the EEG (and assuming also normal preoperative angiograms), the artery is divided and doubly oversewn proximally and distally. The ends of the artery are carefully buried in healthy tissue, usually the omentum, which is brought up substernally and also placed over the innominate artery and over the aortic arch to interpose its fatty tissue between the tracheal stoma and these vascular structures. Even if the artery is not divided, the omentum is usually brought up concurrently to provide extra security.

A transverse incision is made or a small transverse oval is excised from the middle of the skin flap at an appropriate spot, corresponding to the end of the trachea in the mediastinum. The end of the trachea is anastomosed to the opening in the skin. Four to six absorbable sutures are placed from the subcutaneous tissues to the lateral walls of the trachea distal to the transected end and tied. Anastomosis of the skin to the margin of the trachea is made with 4–0 Vicryl interrupted sutures. This may need intermittent removal and replacement of the endotracheal tube, or high frequency ventilation may be used. Vacuum drains are placed beneath the flaps, and the upper incision is closed. Although with further mobilization of the inferior margin of the submammary incision it would be possible in most cases to pull the skin together, this is avoided in order not to place tension on the tracheal cutaneous anastomosis. Therefore, the defect beneath the lower incision, which overlies the chest wall and not the mediastinal defect, is usually grafted.

POSTOPERATIVE CARE

If ventilation is necessary postoperatively, this is usually done through a Tovell's tube that is carefully taped into position. Because of the anatomic disposition of a mediastinal tracheostomy, a standard tracheotomy tube is usually unsatisfactory. Minimal cuff pressure is used to avoid injury to the stomal suture line. In the past the greatest problem from mediastinal tracheostomy has been separation of the trachea from the skin, with subsequent erosion and massive hemorrhage from the adjacent innominate artery. With placement of omentum over the vessels and sometimes innominate artery division, the complication of major hemorrhage has not been seen. When tracheocutaneous separation has occurred—a particular hazard after preoperative irradiation—subsequent healing has taken place without hemorrhage. When there is extensive cutaneous involvement by tumor or radiation injury, the procedure has been modified to include island myocutaneous flaps. Such problems must be foreseen and reviewed in advance with a plastic surgery consultant. The routine use of myocutaneous flaps is not, however, necessary to accomplish these procedures.

If total thyroidectomy and parathyroidectomy have been necessary, the patient will, of course, require replacement. If there is delayed healing or a tendency to stomal stenosis, a cut-down and carefully sanded proximal end of a Hood's silicone salivary tube serves as an excellent stomal splint.*

* E. Benson Hood Laboratories, 575 Washington Street, Pembroke, MA 02359, U.S.A.

It has been possible for some of these patients to learn a form of esophageal speech despite the colonic replacement. Others have learned to use electronic voice equipment. The loss of pharyngeal muscles may hinder such, however.

SUGGESTED READING

Gomes MN, Krole S, Spear SL. Mediastinal tracheostomy. Ann Thorac Surg 1987; 43:539–543.

Grillo HC. Terminal or mural tracheostomy in the anterior mediastinum. J. Thorac Cardiovasc Surg 1966; 51:422–427.

Krespi YP, Wurster CF, Sisson GA. Immediate reconstruction after total laryngo-pharyngoesophagectomy and mediastinal dissection. Laryngoscope 1985; 95:156–161.

Mathisen DJ, Grillo HC, Vlahakes GJ, Daggett WM. The omentum in the management of complicated cardiothoracic problems. J Thorac Cardiovasc Surg (in press).

Orringer MB, Sloan H. Anterior mediastinal tracheostomy: indications, techniques and clinical experience. J Thorac Cardiovasc Surg 1979; 78:850–859.

CONGENITAL DIAPHRAGMATIC HERNIA

JOSEPH P. VACANTI, M.D.

The management of congenital diaphragmatic hernia (CDH) remains controversial and challenging. The overall mortality rate in newborns presenting with respiratory distress in the first 6 hours of life remains approximately 50 percent. It is now known that the diaphragmatic defect occurs early in gestation and therefore impairs early branching of the tracheobronchial tree and the pulmonary vascular bed. This interruption in branching occurs not only in the lung on the affected side but also in the lung on the contralateral side to a variable degree. The resulting variable pulmonary hypoplasia leads to a pathophysiologic condition termed "persistent pulmonary hypertension" or "persistent fetal circulation." Because of high pulmonary vascular resistance, desaturated blood is shunted through the patent ductus arteriosus and foramen ovale, thereby bypassing the lungs. This persistent right-to-left shunting results in a vicious cycle of hypoxia, hypercarbia, and acidosis and very often leads to the death of the neonate.

We now feel that the high resistance in the pulmonary vascular bed is caused by a combination of spasm in the distal pulmonary arteries and a fixed decrease in the total cross-sectional area of the pulmonary arterial bed secondary to the hypoplasia. The management of these children is aimed at decreasing both the severity and the frequency of episodes of spasm in the pulmonary arterial bed and at allowing the pulmonary vasculature time to increase compliance by remodeling. The pattern of ventilatory support is designed to minimize its undesirable effects on pulmonary blood flow. In the normal newborn, rapid pulmonary growth occurs. Whether this growth is accelerated in the child with CDH is not yet known, but ultimate success in the patients most severely affected hinges upon remodeling of the pulmonary vasculature and true pulmonary growth.

MANAGEMENT PRINCIPLES

A successful outcome requires safe transport, careful anesthetic management during corrective surgery, and meticulous intensive care in the postoperative period. There is considerable controversy as to how to achieve these goals. A multidisciplinary study of infants with CDH has been ongoing at The Children's Hospital, Boston, since October, 1982. We will outline the current management protocol that has evolved from this study.

Infants with CDH who develop respiratory distress within the first 6 hours of life are at highest risk. Those who can achieve a postductal PaO_2 greater than 100 torr are termed "responders" to our standard therapy and most often do not require extracorporeal membrane oxygenation (ECMO) support for survival. Pulmonary arterial spasm is the major component of their respiratory failure, and survival depends on success in managing it. Those infants who were unable to achieve a postductal PaO_2 of 100 torr despite maximal support have uniformly died without the use of ECMO. Pulmonary hypoplasia is more severe, and attempts to break pulmonary arterial spasm are unsuccessful. These patients are termed "nonresponders." Of these children, 80 percent were weaned successfully from ECMO, but 66 percent died later of complications from chronic respiratory failure. We have evidence of true pulmonary growth during this period, but whether it is adequate for long-term survival is still unknown.

We have found that the chronic administration of general anesthesia in the intensive care unit seems to decrease both the frequency and severity of episodes of pulmonary arterial spasm in high risk infants with CDH. Since no vasodilators specific to the pulmonary vascular bed have yet been found, we do not rely upon their use in our management protocol. We routinely minimize administration of fluids in an attempt to decrease total lung water that would adversely affect pulmonary compliance. Finally, we have used a pattern of hyperventilation that results in a low mean airway pressure, reasoning that pulmonary blood flow is compromised to a lesser degree.

OUTLINE OF MANAGEMENT PROTOCOL FOR CDH

Initial Stabilization and Transport

1. Respiratory
   a. Intubation
   b. F_IO_2 of 1.0 at all times
   c. PIP-only enough to move the chest, ideally less than 30 cm H_2O
   d. Positive end-expiratory pressure, 0 to 3.0 cm H_2O

   e. Rate, 60 to 100 breaths per minute by hand bagging
2. Circulatory
   a. Intravenous access—minimize fluids, 10 percent dextrose in water and keep vein open for transport
   b. Arterial access—umbilical arterial line preferable since postductal arterial blood gases are the most important
   c. Maintain systolic blood pressure higher than or equal to 50 mm Hg
3. Arterial blood gases
   a. Maintain postductal PaO_2 higher than 100 torr
   b. Maintain $PaCO_2$ of less than or equal to 30 torr and a pH above 7.50
   c. Use $NaHCO_3$ of 1 to 2 mEq per μg or tris(hydroxymethyl)aminomethane 1 to 2 cc per kilogram to increase pH if hyperventilation is inadequate to maintain alkalemic state
4. Medications
   a. Fentanyl, 10 μg per kilogram per dose every hour
   b. Pancuronium 100 μg per kilogram per dose every hour
5. Other
   a. Careful maintenance of normothermia
   b. Monitor blood glucose and calcium levels (an elevated pH will decrease ionized calcium)

Intraoperative Management

I. Surgical Management

1. Small defect: free posterior lip from retroperitoneal adhesions and close primarily with interrupted permanent sutures
2. Large defect: close with prosthetic material such as Goretex or use a muscular flap of transversus and internal oblique muscle
3. Other
   a. Chest tubes placed both on the affected and the contralateral sides
   b. G-tube placed if no prosthetic material used
   c. Abdominal closure: if too tight, close with skin flaps, and repair fascial defect at 1 week, or use staged mesh closure similar to omphalocele technique

II. Anesthetic Management

1. Respiratory
   a. Maintain hyperventilation with PIP for adequate chest expansion (less than or equal to 30 cm H_2O if possible). Hand ventilate at a rate of 60 to 100 breaths per minute to keep $PaCO_2$ less than or equal to 30 torr
   b. End-expiratory pressure is not necessary
   c. Maintain FiO_2 of 1.0 regardless of arterial blood gases
   d. Do not use nitrous oxide or inhalational anesthetics
2. Circulatory
   a. Ensure good intravenous access
   b. Postductal A-line (umbilical artery line) is preferable
   c. Maintain systolic blood pressure higher than or equal to 50 mm Hg by:
      i. Volume. Try to minimize the fluids the patient receives. Use D_5LR or 5 percent Albumisol or packed cells as 5.0 ml per kilogram push
      ii. Calcium gluconate or chloride. If ionized calcium is less than 1.0, give 10 mg per kilogram (1.0 cc) of calcium gluconate through a well-functioning intravenous line
      iii. Dopamine 10 to 20 μg per kilogram per minute as a last resort
3. Blood Gases
   a. Keep FiO_2 at 1.0 regardless of PaO_2 in full term neonates
   b. Keep pH higher than 7.50 if possible, using hyperventilation ($PaCO_2$ lower than or equal to 35 torr) and systemic alkalinization $NaHCO_3$ at 1 to 2 mEq per kilogram per dose or tris(hydroxymethyl)aminomethane at 1 to 2 cc per kilogram per dose. Both can be repeated until pH is higher than or equal to 7.50—watch serum sodium
   c. Check arterial blood gases every 15 minutes
   d. Use postductal (toe) saturation as a trend monitor
4. Drugs
   a. Fentanyl at higher than or equal to 10 μg per kilogram per hour
   b. Pancuronium at higher than or equal to 100 μg per kilogram per hour
   c. IVs: keep vein open with 10 percent dextrose in water. Supplement with gentle volume pushes of D_5LR, Albumisol, and packed cells as needed
5. Other
   a. Maintain temperature via heated humidifier and warming lights
   b. Check blood glucose and ionized calcium levels every 30 minutes

III. Intensive Care Unit Management in the First 48 Hours

1. Respiratory
   a. Initial ventilator settings:
      Healthdyne Type 3
      Flow 25 to 30 liters per minute
      PIP less than or equal to 30 cm H_2O (if possible)
      Positive end-expiratory pressure 0 to 3 cm
      Rate at 120 to 150 breaths per minute
      Inspiratory time equals 0.2 seconds
      FiO_2 equals 1.0
   b. Wean ventilator rate as systemic alkalinization is effected
2. Circulatory
   a. Two peripheral intravenous or one peripheral and one central line if possible. Avoid

internal or external jugular catheters in case ECMO is necessary

b. Right radial artery catheter (preductal) and umbilical, dorsalis pedis, or posterior tibial artery catheter (postductal). Follow postductal arterial blood gases for ventilator changes

c. Pre- and postductal transcutaneous PO_2 monitors to monitor trends

d. Postductal O_2 saturation monitor for trend back-up. Assess intravascular volume with blood pressure perfusion, and pH. Don't follow urine output in the first 24 hours of life

e. Maintain systolic blood pressure at higher than or equal to 50 mm Hg by:

i. Volume—minimize the fluids if at all possible. Use volume pushes of 5.0 cc per kilogram of packed red blood cells, 5 percent Albumisol of fresh frozen plasma, or D_5RL

ii. Dopamine 10 to 20 μg per kilogram per minute if ongoing volume requirement is excessive

iii. Calcium gluconate 1 cc per kilogram if ionized calcium is less than 1.0

3. Arterial blood gases

a. Keep FIO_2 at 1.0 until the patient is absolutely stable (usually the first 12 to 24 hours). Measure arterial blood gasses at least every hour

b. Maintain alkalosis (pH 7.50 to 7.70) by:

i. Hyperventilation—keep $PaCO_2$ at 20 to 30 torr

ii. Systemic alkalinization

A. $NaHCO_3^-$ Na acetate in maintenance intravenously (1 to 2 ml per kilogram per hour)

1. Maintenance IVs can be D_{5-10} $NaHCO_3^-$ (add 80 mEq of $NaHCO_3^-$ to 500 ml of dextrose in 5 to 10 percent water)

2. Maintenance IVs can also be D_{5-10} normal sodium acetate (add 80 mEq of sodium acetate to 500 ml of dextrose in 5 or 10 percent water)

3. $NaHCO_3^-$ can also be administered by intravenous push, usually 1 to 2 mEq per kilogram

4. Be watchful for hypernatremia and hyperosmolarity

B. Tris(hydroxymethyl)aminomethane

1. Tris buffer can be given by intravenous push at 1 to 2 ml per kilogram. This is probably the buffer of choice for intravenous push in the intensive care unit

C. Potassium acetate

1. For hypokalemia, potassium acetate may be substituted for potassium chloride thereby giving buffer as well as potassium

4. Drugs

a. Fentanyl is continued, usually as a continuous infusion, at a rate of 10 to 100 μg per kilogram per hour. Tachyphylaxis occurs rapidly so that the dose must be increased to high levels, and, occasionally, sufentanil is substituted

b. Pancuronium is continued at 100 μg per kilogram as needed

c. Antibiotics are begun after cultures are obtained, usually ampicillin 100 mg per kilogram per day or gentamicin 2.5 mg per kilogram per day

d. Maintenance IVs: volume kept to an absolute minimum. Use $D_{5-10}/NaHCO_3$ as described

e. Treat with intravenous push of fentanyl before painful procedures or for suctioning and hand ventilation. Dose is 5μg per kilogram intravenous push

f. Dopamine for blood pressure support, as needed

5. Other

a. Laboratory studies:

i. Every one-half to 1 hour: arterial blood gases postductal

ii. Every 4 hours: hematocrit, electrolytes, ionized calcium

iii. Every 8 hours: prothrombin time and partial thromboplastin time

iv. Every 12 hours: complete blood count, platelet count, blood urea nitrogen, creatine, and bilirubin

v. Every 24 hours: liver function studies, culture blood, urine, tracheal aspirate

vi. Clot to the blood bank needs to be continuously updated

b. Stress precautions should be enforced to keep episodes of stress-induced pulmonary arterial spasm to a minimum. Activity in the room should be kept to a minimum. Rounds should be conducted outside of the room. Speakers or TVs should not be allowed in the bed space

This chapter summarizes our current approach to this difficult clinical problem. The use of ECMO in the most severely affected babies has led to an increase in short-term survival, which has been substantial. However, the long-term results have been disappointing. We are now addressing the problem of iatrogenic injury to the lung from prolonged mechanical ventilation. We hope to improve survival by minimizing injury as we allow pulmonary growth to occur.

SUGGESTED READING

Cullen ML, Klein MD, Philippart AI. Congenital diaphragmatic hernia. Surg Clin North Am 1985; 65:1115–1138.

Geggel RL, Murphy JD, Langleben D, Crone RK, Vacanti JP, et al. Congenital diaphragmatic hernia: arterial structural changes and persistant pulmonary hypertension after surgical repair. J Pediatr 1985; 107:457–464.

Vacanti JP, Crone RK, Murphy JD, Smith SD, Black PR, et al. The pulmonary hemodynamic response to perioperative anesthesia in the treatment of high risk infants with congenital diaphragmatic hernia. J Pediatr Surg 1984; 19:672–679.

DIAPHRAGMATIC EVENTRATION— DIAPHRAGMATIC PLICATION

ROBERT M. SADE, M.D.
CHARLES D. SMITH, M.D.

For practical purposes, we define eventration of the diaphragm as an abnormally elevated position of the intact diaphragm caused by paralysis, aplasia, or atrophy of the muscle fibers with varying degrees of fibrosis. This definition includes both developmental abnormalities and disorders of phrenic nerve function. Hernias of the diaphragm are excluded.

Although eventration of the diaphragm may be seen at any age, the most important clinical manifestations occur in newborn infants and in adults beyond the fifth or sixth decade of life. Infants with eventration often have associated malformations, especially of the heart. Focally congenital eventrations may involve part of one or both hemidiaphragms or an entire hemidiaphragm and sometimes are associated with intestinal malrotation. Acquired eventration in infants may be caused by birth injury, or, more frequently, by operative injury of the phrenic nerve, most often after lateral thoracotomy for palliation of congenital heart disease. The overall incidence of operative injury to the phrenic nerve in our series of newborns (younger than 3 months) undergoing lateral thoracotomy for treatment of congenital heart disease was 6 percent, being seen most frequently after Blalock-Taussig shunt. Eventration of the diaphragm of any type rarely is seen in older children and young adults and is almost never symptomatic. Symptoms do not develop in adults with eventration until the fifth or sixth decade of life, and they may include dyspnea and gastrointestinal symptoms such as dysphagia, eructation, heartburn, and epigastric pain. Partial or complete inversion of the stomach may be associated with diaphragmatic elevation.

The therapeutic alternatives for the treatment of symptomatic eventration of the diaphragm are limited to mechanical ventilation in small infants or plication of the diaphragm. No medications can restore diaphragmatic function, and pacing of the phrenic nerve is not useful because when the nerve is normal, there is deficiency of the phrenic muscle, and when the nerve is injured, it degenerates distally. A central nervous system origin of eventration is extremely rare (Table 1).

INDICATIONS AND CONTRAINDICATIONS FOR PLICATION

Localized eventrations in infants are always congenital and do not resolve spontaneously; repair is indicated in symptomatic patients. When an entire hemidiaphragm is involved, it is difficult to distinguish those eventrations that are attributable to birth injury to the nerve and have potential to recover from those that are caused by aplasia and fibrosis of the diaphragm. Therefore, all hemidiaphragmatic eventrations are treated as if they were phrenic nerve injuries. Newborns with eventration of a hemidiaphragm may have severe dyspnea, respiratory distress, and cyanosis, requiring endotracheal intubation and management on a ventilator. Patients who have had an operation in the region of the mediastinum, are found to wean poorly from the ventilator postoperatively, and have an elevated hemidiaphragm on chest x-ray films should be assumed to have an operative injury to the phrenic nerve. Elevation of the hemidiaphragm may not be evident if the patient is receiving positive-pressure ventilation or if there is atelectasis of the ipsilateral lung, so a high level of suspicion of phrenic nerve injury is needed in any newborn who weans poorly from the ventilator after a thoracic operation. Diagnosis is made best by fluoroscopy with the patient off the ventilator. Older children and adults do not require plication unless respiratory or gastrointestinal symptoms are present.

Contraindications to operation in newborns include lethal associated lesions such as chromosomal abnormalities, uncontrolled sepsis, or inoperable congenital heart

TABLE 1 Diaphragmatic Paralysis and Plication

Age Group	*Extent of Involvement*	*Chest X-Ray*	*Fluoroscopy*	*Plication Indication*	*Timing of Operation*	*Risk Factors*	*Expected Outcome*
Newborn	Focal	Elevation of portion of hemidiaphragm	Paradoxical movement of affected portion only	Respiratory distress	When diagnosis made	Associated malformations (especially abdominal viscera)	Very good, mortality rate low
	Hemidiaphragm	Elevation of hemidiaphragm	Paradoxical movement of entire hemidiaphragm	Failure to wean from ventilator	After 1–6 weeks of mechanical ventilation	Associated malformations (especially heart)	Mortality rate high due to associated lesions
Children and adults	Hemidiaphragm	Elevation of hemidiaphragm	Paradoxical or no movement of hemidiaphragm	Symptoms (respiratory and gastrointestinal)	Elective	Respiratory failure	Excellent

disease. Contraindications in adults are the same as those for any thoracotomy.

TIMING OF OPERATION

Focal eventrations will not recover spontaneously, so symptomatic patients are offered operation when the diagnosis is made. Because focal eventrations are seldom symptomatic, however, other causes of symptoms should be sought before surgery is undertaken. When a hemidiaphragm is involved in a newborn, recovery of phrenic nerve function is possible, so these patients are managed by support on the ventilator, with good nutrition provided by a nasojejunal tube for 1 to 6 weeks. Patients with transient phrenic nerve paresis may recover within 6 weeks, but if management on a ventilator is difficult or seems unsafe for any reason, one may wish to ventilate the patient for as brief a time as 1 week. No operation should be carried out until all sources of sepsis have been controlled, heart failure has been treated, and nutrition is adequate.

If a phrenic nerve is known to be cut during the course of a thoracic operation, it should be repaired by careful microscopic anastomosis of the cut ends and the diaphragm plicated. Recovery of diaphragmatic function after such repairs has been reported, but recovery time is measured in months, so prolonged ventilation is not justifiable. Diaphragmatic function may return despite the fact that the diaphragm has been plicated.

TECHNIQUES OF PLICATION

Either a thoracic or an abdominal approach to the diaphragm may be elected. Thoracotomy is preferred because of the excellent anatomic exposure of the hemidiaphragm. Laparotomy may be preferable, however, when there are associated abdominal problems that require surgical correction, such as gastric volvulus, intestinal malrotation, or other congenital anomalies, or in cases of bilateral or central eventrations. The abdominal approach requires mobilization of the liver for plication of the right hemidiaphragm or mobilization of the stomach and spleen for plication of the left hemidiaphragm. In our experience, both approaches have relieved symptoms well and resulted in a low recurrence rate.

Although orientation of the line of plication is not critical, we prefer to place sutures from a lateral to medial direction, resulting in an anteroposteriorly oriented source line. Two or three layers of pledget-reinforced nonabsorbable mattress sutures are placed until the diaphragm is flat. The final row of sutures is placed 2 to 3 cm from the mediastinum medially and from the costophrenic sulcus laterally, depending on the size of the patient. Although it is possible to plicate too tightly, resulting in compromise of the opposite functional hemidiaphragm, the more frequent error is undercorrection, resulting in continuing paradox of the diaphragm and need for reoperation. Care should be taken to avoid injuring major phrenic nerve branches, since recovery of diaphragmatic function may occur later, despite the plication.

Plication of focal eventration of the diaphragm is done in the same way, but only the abnormal portion of the diaphragm is obliterated.

THERAPEUTIC OUTCOME

Among newborns requiring diaphragmatic plication, the mortality rate is very high (67 percent in our series), the most common causes of death being complications due to associated malformations of the heart or abdominal viscera. Deaths resulting from complications of the plication itself are unusual, and deaths caused by residual respiratory malfunction are not common (21 percent in our series). Death should occur only rarely in older children and adults who require plication.

Complications related to the thoracotomy, for example, bleeding or infection, may occur occasionally. Complications of the repair itself include recurrence because of incomplete repair (most commonly), disruption, or stretching of the residual diaphragm. Injury to an adjacent or subjacent abdominal viscus may occur. The relief of symptoms in children and adults undergoing plication is almost always excellent. In newborns who survive, symptomatic relief is usually complete. The operation is durable in the sense that late recurrence of symptoms or of diaphragmatic elevation is unusual. In patients who have operative phrenic nerve injury caused by birth trauma or thoracic operation, follow-up fluoroscopic examination several months later sometimes shows return of movement of the diaphragm, with normal or nearly normal appearance. In most patients, the flattened diaphragm on chest roentgenogram in the early postoperative period often returns in a few months to a relatively normal appearance, with little or no paradoxical movement of the diaphragm.

SUGGESTED READING

Haller JA, Packard LR, Tepas JJ, Rogers MC, et al. Management of diaphragmatic paralysis in infants with special emphasis on selection of patients for operative plication. J. Pediatr Surg 1979; 14:779–785.

Smith CD, Sade RM, Crawford FA Jr, Othersen HB. Diaphragmatic eventration in infants. J Thorac Cardiovasc Surg 1986; 91:937–939.

Symbas PN, Hatcher CR, Waldo W. Diaphragmatic eventration in infancy and childhood. J Thorac Surg 1977; 24:113–119.

Watanabe T, Trusler GA, Williams WG, Edmonds JF, et al. Phrenic nerve paralysis after pediatric cardiac surgery. J Thorac Cardiovasc Surg 1987; 94:383–388.

CONGENITAL TRACHEOESOPHAGEAL FISTULA

KATHRYN D. ANDERSON, M.D.

The most common type of esophageal atresia consists of a blind upper pouch with the lower pouch entering the trachea or right main-stem bronchus. Ten percent of cases of atresia have no fistula. Infrequent are single fistula from the upper pouch, fistula from each pouch, and tracheoesophageal fistula without atresia.

ESOPHAGEAL ATRESIA WITH TRACHEOESOPHAGEAL FISTULA (EA/TEF)

Preoperative Management

The infant is nursed in a propped position, and saliva is aspirated through a sump catheter placed in the upper esophageal pouch. Intravenous fluids are administered. Aspiration pneumonia, common after delay of diagnosis, is treated prior to any major operative intervention. In such cases gastrostomy is performed under local anesthesia to allow gastric drainage and decrease acid reflux and aspiration. Associated problems include imperforate anus, duodenal anomalies, or cardiac defects, and these must be ruled out prior to surgery.

Operative Management

Infants with EA/TEF can usually be separated into three distinct categories according to their birth weight, clinical state, and the presence or absence of associated malformations:

1. Waterston type A: Infant weighs more than 2,500 g and is clinically well with no other obvious anomalies.
2. Waterston type B: Infant weighs between 1,800 and 2,500 g and is clinically well, or weighs more than 2,500 g and has pneumonia.
3. Waterston type C: Infant weighs less than 1,800 g or has severe pneumonia, respiratory distress syndrome, or life-threatening associated anomalies.

Healthy infants categorized as type A can undergo primary surgical repair after a few hours of preoperative preparation. For these infants there are three methods of anastomosis of the esophageal pouch: (1) double-layer end-to-end after the method of Haight; (2) end-to-side upper-to-lower esophageal pouch (Duhamel); or (3) single-layer end-to-end full thickness. The Haight anastomosis is very reliable and rarely leaks, but requires almost routine dilatation because of stricture formation. The Duhamel rarely has stricture formation, but has an unacceptable incidence of recurrent fistula. A single-layer anastomosis is my preference because of a low rate of leakage and rare stricture. Without prior gastrostomy, a right thoracotomy is performed. Low incision in the chest wall will avoid denervation of the latissimus and serratus muscles. The fourth interspace is opened, and injury to the pleura avoided. With a moist applicator tip, the pleura is dissected away from the chest wall posteriorly into the retropleural space. The azygos vein identifies the fistula position, and it is divided between 4-0 silk ties. Structures in this area to be avoided are the vagus nerve adjacent to the esophageal pouches and the thoracic duct along the vertebral bodies. The anesthesiologist then advances a red-rubber catheter (10 or 12F) through the mouth until it can be seen in the upper esophageal pouch. The fistula is dissected between trachea and lower esophageal pouch. The lower pouch is usually flimsy and thin with small segmental aortic blood vessels, and dissection of this pouch is therefore minimized. A stay suture of 4-0 silk is placed below the fistula, which is retracted laterally with a vessel-loop and divided gradually and sutured with interrupted 4-0 silk. The integrity of the suture line is tested by applying 30 cm of sustained airway pressure with the chest filled with saline.

The upper pouch with its thicker muscular wall and good blood supply is placed on tension by the intraluminal catheter and dissected from the trachea as far as necessary to allow a comfortable anastomosis without tension. A small medial blood vessel between esophagus and trachea is constant and can be troublesome. An upper pouch fistula, which occasionally occurs, should be sought entering the side of the pouch unless it has been ruled out by a preoperative contrast esophagram. The upper pouch is opened, and the distal esophagus is "fish-mouthed" to correspond to the circumference of the upper pouch. An anterior row of full-thickness interrupted 4-0 silk sutures is placed with all knots on the outside and then tied. The large rubber catheter is replaced with an 8F catheter and advanced into the stomach. The end sutures are used to twist the esophageal pouches, and the posterior sutures are placed. Following completion of the anastomosis the esophagus is untwisted, and the catheter is used to aspirate the stomach and then withdrawn. If possible, the tracheal and esophageal suture lines are separated by surrounding tissue. A No. 14 clear plastic chest tube is sutured with chromic catgut adjacent to the anastomosis and placed to water-seal drainage.

If a long gap between esophageal pouches is encountered, one or more myotomies can be performed in the upper pouch to increase its length. A gastrostomy should always be performed if a myotomy is necessary or if the anastomosis is under any tension. If the gap is too long to achieve anastomosis, the lower pouch is tacked to the chest wall and the chest closed. Six to 8 weeks later after differential growth has allowed the esophageal pouches to lengthen, a further attempt at anastomosis can be made. be made.

For patients categorized as Waterston type B, primary anastomosis can be delayed for several days until the pneumonia has cleared. A gastrostomy is performed early, antibiotics are administered, and propping, upper pouch suction, and pulmonary toilet are maintained.

The severely premature infant, classified as Waterston Type C, with complicating respiratory distress syndrome or life-threatening cardiac anomalies, is treated with early gastrostomy. After stabilization, retropleural fistula division is accomplished. After a period of growth and resolution of associated problems, delayed primary anastomosis is often possible. In the sickest infants, consideration must be given to abandoning the esophagus. Early fistula division and cervical esophagostomy may be lifesaving and may avoid mortality from chronic lung disease.

Postoperative Management

Antibiotics are given for 72 hours in the healthy infant or for 10 days in the child with previous pneumonia. Fluid administration is increased to 1½ times the maintenance amount after 24 hours. Total parenteral nutrition is administered via peripheral or central vein.

Chest tube drainage is observed for saliva, and barium is given by mouth on the fifth or sixth day. In the absence of a leak the chest tube is removed and gradual oral or gastrostomy feedings begun. Routine esophageal dilatation is not necessary.

Results

At our institution, in type A patients 100 percent survival is achieved; 91 percent of patients survive in whom primary repair is delayed from 1 to 10 days (type B). Prior to staging procedures 57 percent of category C patients died, most from their associated problems. Staging procedures with markedly delayed primary repair or late esophageal substitution increased survival to 80 percent.

Complications

Anastomotic Leak

Leaks are rare, but may occur with anastomotic tension. Even large leaks are tolerated with retropleural dissection and good drainage, and most close spontaneously. Only if the anastomosis is completely disrupted should the esophagus be abandoned.

Central hyperalimentation is required. Oroesophageal suction above the anastomosis is desirable for large leaks, and gastrostomy drainage is mandatory.

Stricture

Conditions that predispose to stricture are Haight anastomosis, anastomotic tension, leak, and gastroesophageal reflux. Persistent narrowing beyond 3 weeks postoperatively or if the infant is choking on oral feedings or refusing to eat usually indicates stricture. Dilatation is performed under general endotracheal anesthesia. Maloney dilators or filiform and followers are used, and dilatation is continued to the point where the esophagus is felt to "grab" the dilator. For a severe stricture, retrograde dilatation over a string and with Tucker dilators is performed as necessary to maintain full oral feedings. If there is no resolution of the stricture after 2 to 3 months, resection of the stricture is considered.

Gastroesophageal Reflux

Gastroesophageal reflux is present in most if not all patients following repair of esophageal atresia. Conditions for reflux are enhanced by poor motility in the lower pouch and decrease of the esophagogastric angle, secondary to anastomotic tension. Most patients are asymptomatic. Most symptomatic patients will respond well to conservative measures such as propping, thickened feedings, and the use of metoclopramide to hasten gastric emptying. Fundoplication is reserved for severe failure to thrive, repeated aspiration, and stricture unresponsive to dilatation.

Esophageal Motility Disorders

Motility of both esophageal pouches is poor with little coordinated peristalsis in the esophagus. In spite of this, most patients eventually swallow well and tolerate oral feedings.

Recurrent Tracheoesophageal Fistula

Recurrent respiratory infections, abdominal distension, and coughing during feeding may indicate a recurrent tracheoesophageal fistula. The fistula is approached transpleurally on the right side. The esophagus is dissected above and below the fistula, which is divided gradually, leaving extra tissue on the tracheal side to avoid narrowing. Both trachea and esophagus are closed in a single layer with 4-0 non-absorbable material; surrounding adventitial tissue is placed between the two suture lines. Postoperatively the child's status is maintained with peripheral parenteral nutrition.

TRACHEOESOPHAGEAL FISTULA WITHOUT ESOPHAGEAL ATRESIA (H-TYPE)

Characteristically in older infants, the symptoms are similar to those of recurrent TE fistula. The fistula is most commonly cervical and is approached through a low right cervical incision. The sternomastoid muscle is divided. The esophagus is identified by an orally placed catheter and dissected circumferentially above and below the fistula at the level of the clavicle. The trachea is cleared above and below the fistula, which is divided, leaving a small cuff of esophagus on the trachea for secure closure without narrowing. Both defects are closed with interrupted 4-0 permanent suture, and muscle tissue is interposed between the two suture lines.

Rarely an isolated fistula will be located too low for a cervical approach, and division is carried out through a right thoracotomy.

ISOLATED ESOPHAGEAL ATRESIA WITHOUT FISTULA

Both esophageal pouches are blind, and the thoracic esophagus is almost entirely absent in isolated esophageal atresia without fistula. Formerly all such infants were treated with cervical esophagostomy, gastrostomy, and later esophageal substitute. There is still a place for such management in the small, sick premature infant, but improvements in neonatal care have enabled delaying until differential growth of the esophagus over 6 to 8 weeks decreases the gap between the two pouches. Stretching of the pouches by bougies is unnecessary. Suction on the upper pouch and gastrostomy feedings are maintained until the two esophageal pouches (evaluated by bougies placed per os and per gastrostomy) are less than 1 cm apart. Anastomosis can usually be accomplished through a right thoracotomy with one or more myotomies performed as necessary. Postoperative management and complications are similar to those in atresia with fistula. Since tension on the anastomosis is the rule rather than the exception, dilatation is usually required.

SUGGESTED READING

Haight C. Some observations on esophageal atresias and tracheoesophageal fistulas of congenital origin. J Thorac Surg 1957; 34:141–172.

Livaditis A, Radberg L, Odensjo G, et al. Esophageal end-to-end anastomosis. J Thorac Cardiovasc Surg 1972; 6:206.

Randolph JG, Altman RP, Anderson KD. Selective surgical management based on clinical status in infants with esophageal atresia. J Thorac Cardiovasc Surg 1977; 74:335–342.

Strodel WE, Coran AG, Kirsh MM, et al. Esophageal atresia: a 41 year experience. Arch Surg 1979; 114:523–527.

Waterston DJ, Bonham-Carter RE, Aberdeen E. Oesophageal atresia, tracheoesophageal fistula—a study of survival in 218 infants. Lancet 1962; 1:819–822.

CAUSTIC BURNS OF THE ESOPHAGUS

J. ALEX HALLER Jr., M.D.

Caustic injuries of the esophagus occur in teenagers and young adults as a result of their ingesting poisonous agents in an attempt at suicide. In children, caustic burns result from accidental ingestion, often of powerful corrosive substances. The goal of initial management in both age groups is to prevent or minimize subsequent esophageal scarring and stricture formation. Limiting the severity of injuries is important because esophageal replacement is not nearly as satisfactory as the retention of an injured and scarred but functional esophagus.

By far the commonest caustic agent ingested by children is concentrated sodium hydroxide in the form of commercial toilet bowl and oven cleaners. Various agents may be ingested in young adults, but weaker alkaline cleaning solutions, such as ammonia, rarely result in stricture formation and therefore do not require aggressive initial therapy. Strong acids are less likely to be ingested but may cause significant injury to the stomach and duodenum. They rarely cause deep injury to the esophageal wall because acid produces a *coagulation* necrosis that limits penetration into the tissue. The opposite is true for caustic agents, which cause a *liquefaction* necrosis, which results in deep penetration and occasionally perforation of the esophagus into the mediastinal structures.

The result of ingestion of all caustic agents is a severe inflammation combined with necrosis, which may lead to varying degrees of stricture formation. In the young child, the inflammatory reaction may be associated with penetration of bacteria through the esophageal wall, and thus antibiotics are an important component of the prophylactic treatment. The former treatment of caustic injuries of the esophagus was based on repeated and continuing esophageal dilation to prevent stricture formation by keeping the lumen open, but this did not prevent ultimate severe strictures and has been largely abandoned in this country. In its place, an indirect treatment was introduced, which consists of systemic steroids to decrease the inflammatory reaction, antibiotics to help prevent secondary infection, and the avoidance of dilation in order to allow for maximal healing of the burn injury during the acute phase of recovery. We have utilized the latter treatment approach for the last 25 years at The Johns Hopkins Hospital and have been satisfied with the immediate response as well as the decrease in long-term complications. This protocol includes early esophagoscopy to identify the presence or absence of an esophageal burn. Those patients with burns who require aggressive treatment of the injury are then selected and those who have no esophageal injury or who require no further intensive management are excluded.

Animal studies have shown that sodium hydroxide destroys the esophageal wall to varying levels both by direct necrosis and by the subsequent intense inflammatory process. This inflammatory reaction extends into the muscle layers and may even involve the surrounding mediastinum. Fibroblast proliferation progresses over the next 2 to 3 weeks, and healing has been completed by the end of that time. Based on these studies, the prophylactic use of steroids and antibiotics is for the first week to 10 days, with a continuation of steroid protection for the full 3 weeks.

On the basis of these laboratory studies and our clinical experience, the following plan of management for acute caustic burns of the esophagus is used in children and adults. The basic ingredients are:

1. A careful history with documentation of caustic ingestion and the agent.
2. Identification of the esophageal burn by esophagoscopy within the first 6 to 12 hours.
3. Immediate initiation of steroid and antibiotic therapy and continuation of steriods for 3 weeks.

4. Immediate and continuing dilation if stenosis is documented by symptoms or by x-ray studies.

The specific protocol for all patients with a history of caustic ingestion in the past 24 hours is as follows:

1. Careful history and identification of the caustic agent.
2. If the agent is a caustic substance likely to cause esophageal injury, the patient is prepared for esophagoscopy.
3. The patient is placed on nothing by mouth, and intravenous fluids are started. The patient is taken to the operating room after appropriate preparation and following general examination of the heart and lungs for general anesthesia. Esophagoscopy is carried out, with careful evaluation of the posterior pharynx. If esophageal injury is noted at entry into the esophagus, no further penetration of the scope is permitted, in order to decrease the chances of perforation. Documentation of the esophageal injury is all that is required, because therapy is based upon the *presence* of the burn and not its *extent*.
4. A chest film is obtained on admission prior to esophagoscopy.

If the patient is found to have an esophageal burn, the following procedure is used:

1. Steroids are begun immediately (dosage of 2 mg per kilogram per day of prednisone or its equivalent for 3 weeks).
2. Antibiotics are instituted (usually ampicillin for 10 days).
3. The patient is continued on nothing by mouth with intravenous fluid management. Fluids may be started when the patient is able to swallow saliva, usually within 48 hours. Then the patient can progress to a soft diet, as tolerated. If secretions or a soft diet is not tolerated, cinefluoroscopy is indicated; if a significant stricture is forming, antibiotics and steroids should be stopped and dilations begun. If no stricture is present, steroids are stopped at 3 weeks, and the patient is followed on a monthly basis as an outpatient.

If no esophageal burn is detected:

1. Institute local mouth care as indicated if there are oropharyngeal burns. The patient is discharged to outpatient follow-up.

Early esophagoscopy is thus the keystone to selection of patients requiring treatment and to the initiation of aggressive, anti-inflammatory medication. All effective therapy is directed toward preventing esophageal strictures and the presence or absence of an esophageal burn is the criterion for initiating any further specific treatment. It must be emphasized that children may have very little evidence of oropharyngeal burns and still have significant esophageal caustic injuries, particularly with ingestion of crystalline lye and some liquid cleaners. It is equally true that severe oropharyngeal burns are not necessarily associated with esophageal injury because the caustic agent may be expectorated, particularly by a child who is surprised that this is not something good to eat!

Emphasis on this preventive therapy results from the serious consequences of a caustic burn, especially in children, with the formation of heavy scar tissue and stenosis that does not respond to dilation. Partial replacement of the esophagus is therefore frequently necessary if such stricture occurs. Replacement entails major thoracic and abdominal operative procedures with either interposition or substitution of colon or small intestine to replace the destroyed esophageal segment. These replacement segments never function as well as the normal esophagus, to say nothing of the morbidity of such operative procedures. This fact underscores the importance of aggressive, initial therapy in preventing the inflammatory reaction and secondary injury.

SUGGESTED READING

Borja AR, Ransdell HT Jr, Thomas TV, et al. Lye injuries of the esophagus. Analysis of 90 cases of lye ingestion. J Thorac Cardiovasc Surg 1969; 57:533–538.

Estrera A, Taylor W, Mills LJ, Platt MR. Corrosive burns of the esophagus and stomach: a recommendation for an agressive surgical approach. Ann Thorac Surg 1986; 41:276–283.

Haller JA, Bachman K. The comparative effect of current therapy on experimental caustic burns of the esophagus. Pediatrics 1964; 34:236–245.

Rothstein FC. Caustic injuries to the esophagus in children. Pediatr Clin North Am 1986; 33:665–674.

HIATAL HERNIA AND ESOPHAGEAL REFLUX

THOMAS M. ROUSE, M.D.
JUDSON RANDOLPH, M.D., F.A.C.S.

Gastroesophageal reflux (GER) has become a frequently recognized entity in children over the past 25 years. Prior to this time it was thought to be an uncommon, self-limited process in infants that resolved when they assumed the upright position. It is now clearly evident that there are life-threatening consequences of pernicious GER in infants and children that demand prompt recognition and treatment.

CLINICAL FEATURES

There are important differences in the clinical presentation of GER in infants and young children as compared to the older child or adolescent. In infants, persistent vomiting from reflux may lead to *failure to thrive*, a term used when growth and development are delayed or stunted. GER should be considered when the infant is consistently below the tenth percentile for weight or if he begins to fall from the growth curve. Babies who have had repairs of esophageal atresia and those with severe brain damage have a predisposition to GER. Growth failure due to reflux also occurs in older children, most often in those with severe neurologic dysfunction.

Aspiration pneumonia and apnea are frequent pulmonary complications in the neonate and young child. Recurrent pneumonia or "dying spells" usually have their onset before 1 year of age, but vomiting is uncommon in these patients. Older children, usually the neurologically compromised, also develop aspiration pneumonia secondary to GER. Occasionally, children with asthma that are resistant to the usual medical regimens have been found to have GER. Some of these patients have shown dramatic improvement when the reflux is eliminated.

Esophagitis and stricture are very uncommon in the infant. In the older child, intractable heartburn and esophagitis are more common presentations of GER, and esophageal stricture may be the initial manifestation of reflux in older children.

An unusual presentation of GER is the Sutcliff-Sandifer syndrome, which is the triad of apparent torticollis, iron deficiency anemia, and gastroesophageal reflux. Affected children show exaggerated contortions of the head and neck, having learned that they can shut off the flow of refluxed material into the mouth with such maneuvers. These motions are sometimes misinterpreted as a neurologic disorder.

MEDICAL MANAGEMENT

Medical therapy is an effective means of controlling gastroesophageal reflux in most infants until the salutary effects of gravity, as the infant stands upright at 10 to 12 months, aid the natural maturation of the lower esophageal sphincter in eliminating reflux. Nonoperative measures have proven successful in approximately 85 percent of those infants we have seen with GER. However, a much higher percentage of children and adolescents require surgical correction.

In infants, small-volume feedings thickened with dry cereal and fortified with glucose polymers can be given every 2 to 3 hours. The baby should be positioned prone with the head elevated 30 degrees. Both metoclopramide and bethanecol have been shown to increase, lower esophageal sphincter (LES) pressure, and the former agent also augments gastric emptying. Drugs that diminish the LES pressure such as morphine, meperidine, diazepam, and theophylline should be avoided. Older children should avoid eating near bedtime, and the head of the bed should be elevated. Antacids or cimetidine may relieve the pain of esophageal irritation.

The infant's response to medical measures must be evaluated daily. If growth failure, pulmonary symptoms, or apnea are relieved within 3 weeks, nonoperative measures can be safely continued. If there has been no progress, the baby should be hospitalized so the same measures can be carried out in a monitored environment. If symptoms continue unabated an operation for control of GER should be recommended.

INDICATIONS FOR SURGERY

Peptic esophageal stricture is an absolute indication for surgery. Also, those rare patients with the Sutcliff-Sandifer syndrome or congenital translocation of the stomach into the chests should undergo prompt operative connection.

Those infants or children with failure to thrive, recurrent pneumonia or apnea, resistant asthma, or esophagitis with proven reflux that is unresponsive to medical management should have antireflux surgery performed. The indications for surgery in 117 infants and children is summarized in Table 1.

OPERATIVE TECHNIQUE

The Nissen fundoplication is the operation we have found most effective in controlling reflux in infants and children. An abdominal approach to the hiatus is used, except in those children with translocation of the stomach into the chest or esophageal stricture. These special problems are best approached through either a left thoracotomy or a thoracoabdominal incision.

TABLE 1 Indications for Nissen Fundoplication in 117 Infants and Children

Infants ≤ 12 mo. (N = 72)			*Children ≥ 1 yr. (N = 45)*		
	Number	*Percent*		*Number*	*Percent*
Failure to Thrive	35	48.6	Failure to Thrive	13	28.8
Pneumonia	24	33.3	Pneumonia	11	24.4
Apnea	8	11.1	Stricture	7	15.5
Esophagitis	4	5.5	Vomiting	6	13.3
Stricture	1	1.4	Pain	5	11.1
			Esophagitis	3	6.1

The abdomen may be adequately opened through a high midline incision or a standard left subcostal approach. The left lobe of the liver is mobilized and retracted to the right to expose the esophagogastric junction. With a nasogastic tube in place, the distal esophagus is mobilized for about 2 inches. The vagal nerve trunks are identified and preserved. The two or three most superior short gastric vessels are divided between silk ligatures, freeing the upper portion of the fundus. The spleen is protected throughout, but if the spleen is accidentally lacerated, all efforts should be made to preserve it. An appropriate-sized Maloney dilator is passed via the mouth into the stomach to act as a stent over which the fundoplication is performed. The crura are brought together posteriorly with 2–0 silk sutures to narrow the hiatus. This in an important maneuver that helps to minimize postoperative migration of the wrap into the chest.

The proximal freed portion of the fundus is pushed superiorly and brought around the gastroesophageal junction posteriorly, then into an anterior position. Ample fundus should be mobilized to allow that fundus remaining on the left of the esophagus to be sutured without tension, first to the anterior esophagus and then to that portion of the stomach that has been wrapped around the gastroesophageal junction. The fundoplication begins just distal to the gastroesophageal junction and extends proximally up the esophagus for a distance of 2 to 4 cm. Three or four interrupted sutures of silk are used to construct and simultaneously anchor the fundic wrap. The esophageal stent is then removed. Next the fundus and the wrap are sutured to the diaphragm adjacent to the esophageal hiatus with strong nonabsorbable sutures.

In infants less than 6 months of age and in neurologically damaged children, a Stamm gastrostomy is created and the mushroom catheter led directly through the anterior abdominal wall via a stab wound. This measure protects against the "gas bloat" syndrome and provides a sure route for adequate caloric intake. Gastrointestinal function usually returns within 3 to 4 days, and the child slowly progresses with feedings over an additional 2 or 3 days. If a gastrostomy is unnecessary then a nasogastic tube should be positioned before abdominal closure is begun.

Peptic esophageal strictures should be dealt with promptly by controlling the GER with a Nissen fundoplication and performing intraoperative esophageal dilatation and calibration. Repetitive dilatations will usually be necessary postoperatively for several months. If the reflux is controlled, resection of the stricture or esophageal replacement is rarely necessary.

RESULTS

Of the 117 patients who required a Nissen fundoplication for control of GER, 104 have had lasting relief of their symptoms. Nine patients developed recurrent symptoms from 30 months to 4 years after surgery, and reflux was documented by esophagogram and pH studies. Eight of these patients have had a repeat Nissen fundoplication with relief of their symptoms. Overall, 112 patients (95.7 percent) have had successful operative control of their reflux symptoms. There have been no operative deaths, but one child died of a strangulated bowel obstruction 18 months after the fundoplication. Our overall results are summarized in Figure 1. Small-bowel obstruction is a complication that occurs more commonly after a Nissen fundoplication than after most other transperitoneal procedures. Four of our patients (3.5 percent) developed adhesive bowel obstructions necessitating laparotomy. Vomiting may not be a prominent early symptom in these patients because

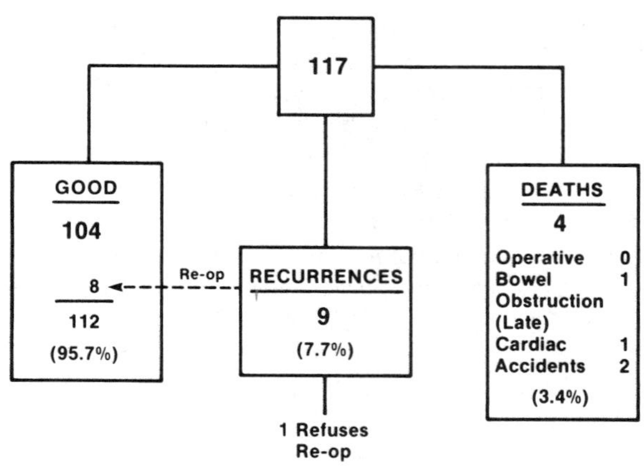

Figure 1 Results of Nissen fundoplication in infants and children.

of the competent fundic wrap. Therefore, any feeding difficulties or abdominal distension should alert the surgeon to a potential intestinal obstruction.

SUGGESTED READING

Foglia RP, Fonkalsrud EW, Ament ME, et al. Gastroesophageal fundoplication for the management of chronic pulmonary disease in children. Am J Surg 1980; 140:72–79.

Hainsberger JK, Corey JJ, Johnson DG, Herbst JJ. Longterm follow-up of surgery for gastroesophageal reflux in infants and children. J Pediatr 1983; 102:505–508.

Jolley SG, Johnson DG, Herbst JJ, et al. An assessment of gastroesophageal reflux in children by extended pH monitoring of the distal esophagus. Surgery 1978; 84:16–24.

Leape LL, Holder TM, Franklin JD, Amoury RA, Ashcraft KW. Respiratory arrest in infants secondary to gastroesophageal reflux. Pediatrics 1977; 60:924–928.

Randolph JG. Experience with the Nissen fundoplication for correction of gastroesophageal reflux in infants. Ann Surg 1983; 198:579–584.

CYSTIC FIBROSIS

SAMUEL R. SCHUSTER, M.D.

PULMONARY RESECTIONS

Cystic fibrosis is an autosomal recessive disease that primarily affects the exocrine glands, resulting in the production of abnormally viscid secretions. These thick secretions obstruct pulmonary bronchi and bronchioles, producing severe pulmonary structural changes. These changes may present as areas of atelectasis, bronchiectasis, and microabscesses, which result in cough, marked mucopurulent sputum production, and febrile episodes. Although most patients have generalized involvement of most areas of the lung, a few present with a localized area of more severe pulmonary involvement. These isolated local areas of more severe disease are likely to result in exacerbation of symptoms and may lead to an accelerated progression of the degenerative changes in the remainder of the lung.

Pulmonary resection in cystic fibrosis is clearly a palliative procedure that can improve the quality of life in a few carefully selected patients.

Patient Selection

Only those patients who show a localized area of pulmonary disease that is advanced far beyond that in the rest of the lung are candidates for local pulmonary resection.

These areas of more severe disease affect the patient's state of well-being and usually markedly alter the quality of life. When it becomes evident that a local area of severe atelectasis or bronchiectasis or both is not responding to the usual nonsurgical measures, surgical resection becomes a consideration. The major question is whether or not the patient can withstand thoracotomy and pulmonary resection.

Preoperative Evaluation

Pulmonary function tests, including ventilation and perfusion xenon lung scans should be done. Although an evaluation of pulmonary function is done preoperatively, these studies have not always been of critical value in providing the necessary information. Most of these studies require the cooperation of the patient and therefore cannot be used in the uncooperative young patient. Furthermore, there is considerable variability in the results of these tests, depending upon the effectiveness of the patient's tracheal toilet on any given day. The most helpful quantitative information is that obtained from the ventilation and perfusion scans. In virtually all instances, the lung to be resected has not been contributing to the patient's overall ventilatory capacity. In the final analysis, the best criterion for determining the patient's capacity to withstand thoracotomy is a clinical evaluation of the level of physical activity that the patient was able to maintain just prior to the immediate acute exacerbation.

Bronchoscopy is not routinely done preoperatively and is rarely helpful in clearing plugged bronchi.

Bronchography also rarely is indicated, although in unusual instances one may wish to evaluate that part of the lung *not* undergoing resection. The magnitude of the disease in the area to be resected clearly is evident on ordinary chest roentgenography, and the ventilation-perfusion scan provides additional quantitative data. Any other information obtained by bronchogram is of little value, and the added morbidity associated with bronchography makes the study undesirable as a routine procedure.

Preoperative Preparation

All patients should be on a vigorous medical program prior to operation. This includes intravenous antibiotics and extensive pulmonary physiotherapy. In those patients with a large amount of thick, mucopurulent sputum, a preoperative tracheostomy 5 to 7 days prior to thoracotomy is extremely helpful.

1. The tracheostomy done well in advance of thoracotomy allows the patient to adjust both physically and psychologically to the presence of the tube prior to the trauma of a thoracotomy.
2. Because of the severe coughing, these patients frequently develop subcutaneous emphysema at the time of tracheostomy. The interval between tracheostomy and thoracotomy allows time for the subcutaneous emphysema to subside.

3. In the interval between operations, the patient can learn to manage the tracheostomy, learn self-suction, and learn to speak with it in place.
4. The tracheostomy enhances preoperative preparation by providing ready access for tracheal toilet.
5. Most important, the tracheostomy provides ready access for postoperative tracheal toilet.

These patients must understand that this is a temporary measure and that the tracheostomy tube will be removed prior to discharge.

Operative Considerations

Since pediatric Carlens' endotracheal tubes are not available and selective bronchial intubation is not accomplished readily, it is best to do pulmonary resections in this group of patients via a posterior thoracotomy with the patient in the prone position. If a standard posterolateral approach is used, the large amount of thick, purulent secretions present may spill into the opposite lung. This is avoided in the prone position. The secretions drain into the trachea, from whence they can be suctioned readily.

These patients all have strikingly hyperplastic peribronchial lymph nodes with increased vascularity of all tissues secondary to the many bronchial artery–pulmonary artery anastomoses. There is foreshortening of the hilar structures and there are numerous vascular adhesions between the parietal and visceral pleurae.

Postoperative Care

Postoperatively, intravenous antibiotics are continued as are vigorous pulmonary physiotherapy, careful tracheal toilet, and early ambulation. Postoperative intermittent positive-pressure breathing is avoided. Assisted respiration should be utilized only when necessary to maintain adequate ventilation, and then only for as brief a time as possible.

MANAGEMENT OF PNEUMOTHORAX AND CONTINUED AIR LEAKS

Pneumothorax is the most frequent complication that occurs as a result of the pulmonary changes in cystic fibrosis. It occurs most frequently in older patients.

The typical cystic fibrosis patient with pneumothorax is a moderately to severely ill teenager with far advanced diffuse bilateral pulmonary disease. The recurrence rate after the first pneumothorax is almost 45 percent. A small number of patients who, in the past, have been treated by chest tube drainage and suction have had persistent air leaks that have been very difficult to manage. The treatment protocol proposed in this chapter has obviated that problem.

Because of the high recurrence rate and persistent air leaks seen in patients treated by observation, needle aspiration, or simple trochar thoracotomy, we have adopted a more aggressive approach.

A review of our results in the treatment of 170 pneumothoraces in patients with cystic fibrosis showed that quinacrine sclerosis and parietal pleurectomy were the most effective methods of management. The recurrence rate for quinacrine sclerosis was 12.5 percent, whereas that for parietal pleurectomy was zero. There has been essentially no discomfort or morbidity associated with the use of quinacrine as a sclerosing agent.

Quinacrine sclerosis is accomplished as follows. After the air leak has been stopped or almost stopped for 24 hours, quinacrine, 100 mg in a 2 percent solution, is instilled via the chest tube in 50 ml of isotonic saline daily for 3 days. Immediately after instillation, the chest tube is clamped for 1 hour. During this time the patient is moved from sitting upright to the right and left lateral decubitus positions and then to a head-down position. The patient remains in each position for 15 minutes to assure exposure of the entire pleural space to the sclerosing agent. After this procedure, drainage and suction are resumed.

Parietal pleurectomy should be done through a small anterior submammary incision of the fifth intercostal space. The only chest wall muscle that needs to be divided is the pectoralis major. The blebs usually found at the apex of the upper lobe and on occasion at the apex of the lower lobe are oversewn. The parietal pleura is removed, extending from the fifth interspace superiorly over the entire apex of the chest. We have not had a problem with postoperative hemorrhage and have found that the discomfort associated with this procedure has been minimal.

Pulmonary function studies that were done prior to and after quinacrine sclerosis or pleurectomy showed no change in pulmonary function.

Quinacrine sclerosis should be utilized for management of the first pneumothorax, and parietal pleurectomy should be done for any recurrence or for a persistent air leak.

MANAGEMENT OF HEMOPTYSIS

Major hemoptysis, a late complication of cystic fibrosis, has increased in frequency because of the current greater longevity of patients with this disease. Hemoptysis occurs as a result of erosion of large, thin-walled bronchial vessels that appear during the course of development of the many bronchial–pulmonary artery anastomoses.

Localization and Treatment

Only rarely is the plain chest x-ray film helpful. Since most of these patients have far advanced bilateral pulmonary disease, there is rarely a specific site of more severe involvement that clearly can be recognized as the source of the hemorrhage.

Bronchoscopy remains the most reliable means of localizing the site of hemoptysis. It should not be done when the patient is bleeding vigorously. It is almost always possible to control early major hemoptysis by sedation and bedrest. Bronchoscopy is best done at the time that the patient still is bringing up small amounts of blood-streaked sputum, but not enough blood to flood the entire bronchial tree at the time of examination. Under these conditions, the bronchus from which the blood is coming can almost always be identified.

We have found it helpful to correlate our bronchoscopic observations with selective bronchial arteriography. There is a striking correlation between the site of hemoptysis and the presence of markedly dilated tortuous and increased number of bronchial vessels and bronchial–pulmonary artery anastomoses.

Modes of Intervention

1. The preferred method is angiographic embolization of the bleeding bronchial artery. This is an effective method of management of massive hemoptysis in these debilitated patients. All the bronchial arteries supplying the area identified as the site of bleeding are embolized.
2. Surgical resection of the pulmonary segment or lobe from which the blood originates is rarely necessary. In the very unusual instance in which hemorrhage is persistent, the surgeon may be forced to proceed with resection. For this reason it is very important to identify the area of lung that is bleeding, in the event that resection becomes necessary as an emergency procedure. In the unlikely event that surgical resection must be done because major hemorrhage is too severe to control by any other method and localization has not yet been possible, on a statistical basis, the right upper lobe is most likely to be the site of such hemorrhage.

SUGGESTED READING

DiSant'Agnese PA, Davis PB. Resection in cystic fibrosis. N Engl J Med 1976; 265:481–485.

Fellows KE, Khaw KT, Schuster S, Shwachman H. Bronchial artery embolization in cystic fibrosis; technique and long term results. J Pediatr 1979; 95:959–963.

Schuster SR, Fellows KE. Management of major hemoptysis in patients with cystic fibrosis. J Pediatr Surg 1977; 12:889–896.

Schuster SR, McLaughlin FJ, Matthews WJ Jr, et al. Management of pneumothorax in cystic fibrosis. J Pediatr Surg 1983; 18:482–497.

Schuster SR, Shwachman H, Harris GBC, Khaw K. Pulmonary surgery for cystic fibrosis. J Thorac Cardiovasc Surg 1964; 48:750–760.

LOBAR EMPHYSEMA

W. HARDY HENDREN, M.D.
JOSEPH P. VACANTI, M.D.

Lobar emphysema is a term that refers to overexpansion of a pulmonary lobe. It is one of the causes for respiratory distress in infants. The overinflated lobe can severely compress the other lobe or lobes on the same side and can cause severe shifting of the mediastinum to the opposite side. Sometimes the emphysematous lobe herniates across the anterior mediastinum into the opposite thorax. Most commonly involved is the left upper lobe, and after that, the right middle lobe. Only rarely is there involvement of a lower lobe or of more than one lobe.

Symptoms of respiratory distress occur most commonly in the first week of life, but in some they develop during the next several months. Males are affected three times more often than females. Symptoms include tachypnea, dyspnea, cyanosis, and cough. They can vary in severity from mild to extremely severe, depending on the degree of hyperinflation of the affected lobe in which there is no air exchange and the degree of compression atelectasis of the other pulmonary lobes. On physical examination there are hyperresonance and diminished breath sounds on the affected side, just as one would see in a child with pneumothorax, with which lobar emphysema must not be confused.

The diagnosis usually can be made by chest films that show an area of hyperlucency with lung markings that are farther apart than usual but with lobar distribution. The most common differential diagnoses are congenital lung cyst, pneumothorax, postpneumonic pneumatocele, and congenital cystic adenomatoid malformation. Lobar emphysema, however, can be differentiated from those conditions by examining the chest roentgenogram carefully, often with a bright light, to note the lobar distribution of the bronchovascular markings that are attenuated. Lung cysts and pneumatoceles have a rounded configuration. The hyperlucency of pneumothorax is the pleural space, quite unlike lobar emphysema, which involves lung parenchyma. Sometimes the overexpanded lung completely fills the ipsilateral chest, compressing the other lobe or lobes into a small, flat, atelectatic disk of lung tissue. When two lobes are involved, they are usually the left upper and right middle lobes. A Xenon ventilation-perfusion lung scan will show delayed uptake, washout of the isotope, and diminished blood flow in the emphysematous lobe. However, the study is not usually necessary. Bronchoscopy and bronchography are usually not necessary and may be dangerous in a desperately ill infant. Usually the infant with lobar emphysema is much younger than the toddler in whom there may be an aspirated foreign body that can cause localized air trapping in one lobe and atelectasis in another. However, we did treat a 4-month-old infant with respiratory distress and lower lobe emphysema who had aspirated a piece of popcorn evidently given to him by an older sibling. Although most infants with lobar emphysema are otherwise healthy babies, 14 percent of these patients have congenital heart disease. Therefore, echocardiography and other cardiac studies should be performed if there is clinical suspicion of a congenital cardiac defect.

The etiology of lobar emphysema cannot be ascribed to a single cause. In about 25 percent of cases microscopic section through the bronchus of the affected lobe will demonstrate cartilaginous dysplasia. This can allow ball valve trapping of air in the bronchus, causing it to overdistend. In nearly half of cases, the cause of emphysema is not certain. It is possible that some of those are also patients with bronchial cartilaginous dysplasia at the root of the affected bronchus, which is not part of the surgical specimen but remains in the patient when the lobe is removed and the bronchial stump is sutured. Extrinsic compression of the bronchus, particularly the right middle lobe, can cause air trapping and lobar emphysema. Intrinsic narrowing of the bronchus is seen occasionally. More recently, it has been shown that polyalveolar lobe is a distinct pathologic entity in about 25 percent of patients with congenital lobar emphysema. In this condition there is a five-fold increase in alveolar number, which can be found on a detailed study of the operative specimen. The airways and arteries of the lobe are normal for age in number, size, and structure, but there are excessive numbers of pulmonary alveoli.

The treatment of congenital lobar emphysema depends on its etiology and the severity of the infant's respiratory distress. In a neonate in severe distress, the diagnosis may rest on a quickly performed chest roentgenogram followed by immediate thoracotomy and lobectomy. During induction of anesthesia, positive pressure ventilation can inflate the affected lobe further, aggravating the infant's distress by greater compression of the good pulmonary lobes. Therefore, the surgeon must be prepared to open the chest immediately, allowing the overinflated lobe to herniate from the thoracotomy incision as a lifesaving measure. In other infants with lobar emphysema, there may be relatively mild symptoms, and a period of observation will be indicated. If there is a background of bronchiolitis, or inspissated mucus, lobar emphysema can be reversible, not requiring operation. In a child of toddler age, bronchoscopy should be performed to rule out a foreign body, extraction of which can result in normal pulmonary ventilation. Although the indications for pulmonary lobectomy are vastly different in infants when compared with adults, the technique and principles of pulmonary lobectomy are the same. The bronchus must be closed securely, without encroaching on the adjacent airway, and it should be covered with a flap of adjacent pleura whenever possible.

Long-term follow-up of patients treated for lobar emphysema during infancy has shown that pulmonary function studies are usually normal, although respiratory flow rate can be somewhat diminished.

SUGGESTED READING

Eigen H, Lemen RJ, Waring WW. Congenital lobar emphysema: Long-term evaluation of surgically and conservatively treated children. Am Rev Respir Dis 1976; 113:823–827.

Hendren WH, McKee DM. Lobar emphysema of infancy. J Pediatr Surg 1966; 1:24–39.

Tapper D, Schuster S, McBride J, et al. Polyalveolar lobe: anatomic and physiologic parameters and their relationship to congenital lobar emphysema. J Pediatr Surg 1980; 15:931–937.

I CONGENITAL ANOMALIES

SEQUESTRATION

THOMAS B. FERGUSON, M.D.

Sequestration is a term first used by Pryce in 1946 to describe an area of embryonic lung tissue supplied by an anomalous systemic artery. Two forms are recognized: extralobar and intralobar. This distinction is important because the clinical presentations are very different.

EXTRALOBAR SEQUESTRATION

Extralobar sequestration is embryonically the more complex anomaly. It is characterized by fetal lung tissue separated from the normal lung by its own pleural investment. In most cases, there is no communication with the tracheobronchial tree, a chief point of differentiation from the intralobar type. Over 90 percent of extralobar sequestrations are found in the left lower thorax. Arterial blood supply is derived from a number of small systemic branches usually arising from the abdominal aorta. The venous drainage is systemic rather than pulmonary, most often into the hemiazygos system.

Extralobar sequestration is rare and usually is recognized in the neonate or infant by its frequent association with other congenital abnormalities, the most common of which is congenital diaphragmatic hernia (30 percent of cases). Other co-anomalies include heart defects, pectus excavatum, and a variety of foregut malformations. Those occurring with diaphragmatic hernia are easily managed, provided that the association is kept in mind and a sequestrum is looked for at the time of hernia repair. Care must be taken on the basis of arterial, venous, and bronchial supply to make certain that one is not dealing with hypoplastic lung, which also often occurs with a congenital hernia but which should never be resected.

In the approximately 50 percent of extralobar sequestrations that are not associated with other anomalies the patients are usually asymptomatic, since there is rarely a bronchial communication with the abnormal lung tissue. The anomaly is detected on routine chest roentgenograms as a dense triangular mass with its apex toward the hilum. No other diagnostic studies are really required. Differentiation from atelectasis or lobar pneumonia is easily made on clinical grounds. A bronchogram shows no filling of the sequestered part. Aortography is not useful because the systemic connections tend to be small and multiple. Operation is recommended in this "silent" variant for confirmation of diagnosis and for removal of the space-occupying lesion that prevents full expansion of the remaining normal lung tissue. Once the vascular supply has been dealt with, excision is a simple matter, since the sequestered lobe is contained in its own pleural envelope, and the hilar stalk is usually small enough to be ligated en masse.

INTRALOBAR SEQUESTRATION

Intralobar sequestration, although still an uncommon lesion, is seen much more frequently than the extralobar type. The sequestered lung shares a common pleural investment with normal pulmonary tissue. The areas most frequently affected are the medial and posterior basilar segments of the lower lobes, with the left side being involved twice as often as the right. The two distinguishing characteristics of this form of sequestration are important both clinically and therapeutically. These are a patent bronchus entering the cripple lung and a large systemic artery supplying the area.

Infection of the fetal lung tissue results in a clinical picture often indistinguishable from pyogenic lung abscess or bronchiectasis, with fever, productive cough, and occasionally hemoptysis. Depending upon the form the infection takes, the chest roentgenogram will show either an infiltrate or an abscess cavity in the lower lobe. Since most pyogenic lung abscesses due to aspiration occur in the midthird of the lung, any cavity in the lower lobe should arouse suspicion of sequestration. Bronchography and bronchoscopy are not helpful in the differentiation, but the latter may aid in identifying the bacterial etiology. The sure way to establish a diagnosis is to visualize the systemic arterial blood supply radiologically. These vessels may arise from the descending thoracic aorta at any level, and even from the abdominal aorta some distance below the diaphragm. In either instance they are of large size and easily seen on contrast injection. In the past the routine use of aortography to obtain a diagnosis seemed unjustified because of procedural risks. However, contrast-enhanced computed tomography (CT) nicely demonstrates these anomalous vessels and should be utilized in every patient with lower lobe inflammatory disease when sequestration might be the cause. Knowledge of the size and location of the anomalous vessels is not critical at the time of surgery, but can be helpful, particularly if the inflammatory response is severe. The other reason for establishing a diagnosis is that excisional surgery is always required for an infected intralobar sequestration. The crippled lung tissue, once infected, will never heal. Therefore, a more direct surgical approach can be taken in these cases than might be advised in other forms of pulmonary inflammatory disease.

Lobectomy is the only form of treatment to be considered, not only because of the presence of infection but also because the sequestered tissue blends imperceptibly into surrounding normal lung without regard for segmental boundaries. The important part of the procedure is identifying and ligating the anomalous artery. The vessel usually courses between the leaves of the inferior pulmonary ligament to reach the lung parenchyma. The remainder of the resection is then no more complicated than the usual lobectomy for inflammatory disease.

SUGGESTED READING

Flye MW, Conley M, Silver D. Spectrum of pulmonary sequestration. Ann Thorac Surg 1976; 22:478–482.

Haller JA Jr, Golladay ES, Pickard LR, et al. Surgical management of lung bud anomalies: lobar emphysema, bronchogenic cyst, cystic adenomatoid malformation, and intralobar pulmonary sequestration. Ann Thorac Surg 1979; 28:33–43.

Sade RM, Clouse M, Ellis FH Jr. The spectrum of pulmonary sequestration. Ann Thorac Surg 1974; 18:644–658.

Zumbro GL, Treasure RL, Seitter G, et al. Pulmonary sequestration. Ann Thorac Surg 1975; 20:161–169.

BRONCHOGENIC CYSTS

ROBERT J. GINSBERG, M.D., F.R.C.S.(C)
THOMAS J. KIRBY, B.Sc. M.D., F.R.C.S.(C)

Bronchogenic cysts are unusual congenital anomalies of lung development arising as a result of a group of cells that break off from the developing lung bud and differentiate on their own. They are therefore most commonly found in close association with the trachea, major bronchi, and esophagus, but they can be found deep in the pulmonary parenchyma as well. A direct communication may exist between the cysts and the tracheobronchial tree. In adults, bronchogenic cysts constitute approximately 10 percent of mediastinal masses reported in surgical series. They usually produce no symptoms, often being discovered incidentally on chest x-ray films. When symptoms do arise, they are most frequently caused by compression of major airways or are a result of secondary infection.

INVESTIGATIONS

Routine chest x-ray films are frequently all that is needed to make a presumptive diagnosis and to initiate treatment. Tomography, both routine and computed (CT), may help in defining the cysts' relationship to the tracheobronchial tree or esophagus. Bronchoscopy and esophagoscopy (or esophagogram) are usually unrewarding other than to confirm the presence of airway or esophageal compression. Percutaneous needle aspiration biopsy under fluoroscopic or CT guidance can cytologically confirm the diagnosis in many cases.

INDICATIONS FOR TREATMENT

Generally cysts that are increasing in size or that are causing symptoms should be operated on. Enlarging cysts have been known to cause compression of major airways (occasionally life-threatening), blood vessels, and the esophagus and should therefore be dealt with. The rare possibility of neoplasm must also be considered. Cysts with air-fluid levels or demonstrating infection require treatment, since their natural history is one of causing recurrent infections, often because of a direct communication with the tracheobronchial tree. Whether asymptomatic, nonenlarging cysts should be treated is a moot point.

THERAPEUTIC ALTERNATIVES

Close Follow-Up

We feel that small, asymptomatic, pulmonary or mediastinal cysts other than those presenting in the subcarinal region can be safely followed by repeat chest x-ray films, reserving treatment for symptomatic or enlarging lesions. Initially, the interval between chest films should be frequent in order to assess growth. Ultimately, yearly chest films will suffice. Any cyst appearing in infancy or childhood, that causes symptoms, has an air-fluid level, or is large is potentially dangerous and should be treated definitively.

Simple Aspiration

Patients who refuse surgery or are too ill to tolerate surgical intervention can be diagnosed and potentially treated by percutaneous transthoracic fine needle aspiration of the cyst. This often confirms the diagnosis, as the aspirate reveals mucoid material and ciliated columnar cells. The procedure may be curative as well if it is possible to completely aspirate the cyst and the epithelial lining has been destroyed by pressure necrosis or previous infection. However, our experience indicates that most cysts managed in this way recur. We limit this technique to diagnose and to deal quickly with life-threatening complications.

Surgery

Mediastinoscopy. Simple mediastinal cysts that have been shown by preoperative investigation (e.g., CT scan) to be within easy reach of a cervical mediastinoscopy can be dealt with by this procedure. At mediastinoscopy the bronchogenic cyst may be palpable; if not, it can be identified visually. The presenting wall is then widely opened using biopsy forceps, and the fluid contents are totally aspirated. The interior of the cyst should be inspected and the wall biopsied to absolutely rule out the possibility of an unsuspecting neoplasm. Prevention of recurrence is predicated on the prior destruction of the secretory epithelium either by pressure or infection. Sclerosing agents or techniques (tetracycline, cauterization, or hypertonic saline) may be used in an attempt to destroy viable lining cells. Theoretically the cyst can be dissected out and removed, but we have found this difficult if not impossible at mediastinoscopy. Since the morbidity and mortality rates for mediastinoscopy are lower than for a thoracotomy, we prefer this approach initially for simple uncomplicated superior mediastinal bronchogenic cysts. Standard thoracotomy is reserved for those patients in whom this technique fails (about 50 percent in our hands).

Thoracotomy. Cysts presenting in infants or children should be removed by thoracotomy to prevent problems in adult life. Those cysts that have air-fluid levels or have had a history of infection are often in direct communication with the tracheobronchial tree and are frequently within the pulmonary parenchyma; they should be excised by thoracotomy. This allows direct closure of any communication between the cyst and the airways. Every attempt should be made to preserve normal functioning pulmonary tissue (cautery dissection technique, wedge excision, or segmentectomy) when possible. Rarely, the cyst is found to communicate with the esophagus. In such cases, careful meticulous closure of the esophageal wall is required. In planning the approach or incision to be used, a preoperative CT scan may be of value, especially in the mediastinal variety of cyst.

Percutaneous Drainage. When superimposed infection occurs, bronchogenic cysts may present much like a lung abscess. Such cysts theoretically could be managed like a lung abscess, with intravenous antibiotics and percutaneous drainage of the cavity, either by catheter or tube thoracostomy. Theoretically, there is an excellent chance of cure with this method, since the cyst's secretory epithelial lining has often been destroyed by the infection. Although we have had unqualified successes treating lung abscesses in this fashion, we have no experience using this technique with bronchogenic cysts.

PREFERRED APPROACH

Simple, small, uncomplicated cysts presenting in adults can be followed closely by chest x-ray films. All others are treated by the simplest method available. We prefer an attempt at ablation by mediastinoscopy when indicated. Thoracotomy is reserved for failures of mediastinoscopy and all other cysts requiring surgery. Every attempt is made to preserve functioning lung tissue. Percutaneous needle aspiration of a cyst may relieve a life-threatening complication quickly prior to surgical removal.

SUGGESTED READING

Eraklis AJ, Griscom NT, McGovern JB. Bronchogenic cysts of the mediastinum in infancy. N Engl J Med 1969; 281:1150–1155.

Ginsberg RJ, Atkins RW, Paulson DL. Case report—a bronchogenic cyst successfully treated by mediastinoscopy. Ann Thorac Surg 1972; 13(3):266–268.

Keerwan WO, Walbaum PR, McCormack RJM. Cystic intrathoracic derivatives of the foregut and their complications. Thorax 1973; 28:424–428.

Nakata H, Nakayama C, Kimoto T, et al. Computed tomography of mediastinal bronchogenic cysts. J Comput Assit Tomogr 1982; 6:733–738.

Rogers LF, Osmer, JC. Bronchogenic cysts: a review of 46 cases. Am J Roentgenol 1971; 91:273–283.

Schwartz DB, Beals TF, Winbis HKJ, Hammersley JR. Transbronchial fine needle aspiration of bronchogenic cysts. Chest 1985; 88:573–575.

Sirivella S, Ford WB, Zikria EA, et al. Foregut cysts of the mediastinum: results of 20 consecutive surgically-treated cases. J Thorac Cardiovasc Surg 1985; 90:776–782.

PULMONARY ARTERIOVENOUS MALFORMATIONS

DOUGLAS J. MATHISEN, M.D.

MANAGEMENT OF ARTERIOVENOUS MALFORMATIONS

Pulmonary arteriovenous malformations (AVMs) are uncommon problems for the cardiothoracic surgeon. To date, only 16 cases have been seen in the last 40 years at the Massachusetts General Hospital. However rare these lesions may be, they are still part of the differential diagnosis of lung masses. Therefore, familiarity with these lesions and their proper management can avoid serious complications related to diagnosis and treatment.

These lesions frequently are seen as asymptomatic abnormalities on routine chest x-ray studies. Certain radiologic features, such as afferent and efferent vessels leading into this mass, may alert the surgeon to the possibility of this lesion. Contrast enhancement by a computed tomography (CT) scan is also diagnostically helpful. When this lesion is suspected, needle biopsy should be avoided.

These lesions are frequently located subpleurally and are composed of thin-walled vessels that pose the threat of significant bleeding if subjected to needle biopsy. When present, symptoms usually consist of the classic triad of dyspnea on exertion, cyanosis, and clubbing, reflecting the arteriovenous shunt that exists in these patients. Extremely large AVMs or multiple AVMs are usually associated with these types of symptoms. Less common symptoms are hemoptysis or spontaneous hemothorax. The association with Osler-Weber-Rendu syndrome in 40 to 60 percent of cases may be the tip-off to a previously undefined lung abnormality on chest x-ray. Paradoxical emboli may be the presenting complaint in a large proportion of patients with AVMs. When an arterial embolus occurs for unexplained reasons, pulmonary AVMs should be considered. Cerebral AVMs are associated in patients with underlying Osler-Weber-Rendu syndrome and may be the reason for their presentation. Brain abscess has also been reported but is now quite uncommon.

Chest x-ray films showing a pulmonary abnormality with an afferent and efferent vessel or enhancement of a pulmonary nodule with contrast by CT scan are typical findings in patients with pulmonary AVMs. The most reliable diagnostic procedure remains pulmonary arteriography. It is important not only in establishing the diagnosis, but also in determining the exact location and number of malformations that may exist. This is most helpful if surgery is to be considered; these lesions often are difficult to identify in the lung, and preoperative knowledge of their location and number is most helpful. The ideal treatment of pulmonary AVMs is surgical excision. Excision should always be conservative and yet compatible with complete removal of the lesion. Simple ligation has proved to be unreliable because of recannulization or development of collateral blood supply. Therefore, total excision of the malformation is desirable. This can usually be accomplished either by local excision or by segmentectomy. In the case of multiple lesions, lung-sparing procedures become even more important. Multiple bilateral lesions can be dealt with by performing staged thoracotomies or, rarely, a median sternotomy and bilateral excision.

Recent attention has been focused on nonoperative management of these lesions. The use of detachable balloons to occlude pulmonary AVMs by angiographers has gained some following in recent years. This option is certainly a possibility in high-risk surgical patients, patients refusing surgery, or patients with multiple lesions and compromised pulmonary function. Theoretical problems do exist with widespread application of this technique, such as balloon migration, propagation of clot, or recannulization of the AVM. We have one case in our own experience in which recannulization did occur some 3½ years following successful balloon embolization of a solitary pulmonary AVM. Long-term follow-up is needed to determine the exact benefit of balloon embolization in this situation before its widespread use is recommended.

SUGGESTED READING

Dines DE, Arms RA, Bernatz PE, Gomes MR. Pulmonary arteriovenous fistuals. Mayo Clin Proc 1974; 49:460–465.

Prager RL, Laws KH, Bender HW. Arteriovenous fistula of the lung. Ann Thorac Surg 1983; 36:231–239.

Terry PB, White RI, Barth KH, et al. Pulmonary arteriovenous malformations. N Engl J Med 1983; 308:1197–1200.

I CHEST WALL

PECTUS EXCAVATUM AND CARINATUM

FRANCIS ROBICSEK, M.D.

Pectus excavatum and pectus carinatum are pathologic conditions in which the exact developmental mechanism is not fully understood, the indication for operative correction is controversial, the surgical technique is debatable, and the postoperative results, except for the cosmetic aspects, are difficult to objectively measure. It is fortunate indeed that at least establishing the diagnosis does not cause undue difficulties. Pectus excavatum and carinatum are the most common anomalies of the anterior chest wall. The proportion of occurrence of excavatum versus carinatum deformities has been reported by different authors to vary between 10:1 and 10:4. In our own surgical experience, these two deformities constituted about 95 percent of 803 patients operated with anterior chest deformities. Males are more commonly affected than females.

PECTUS EXCAVATUM (CHONDROSTERNAL DEPRESSION)

In this anomaly there is a funnel-shaped depression of the sternum and adjacent cartilages. The depression is circular in advanced, and oval in the less accentuated cases. The depression usually begins at the junction of the manubrium and gladiolus and becomes progressively deeper toward the xiphoid process. The costal cartilages are elongated, distorted, and sometimes fused together. The retrosternal space is narrowed, and the heart is more or less displaced into the left hemithorax. In the asymmetric variety there is also an axis deviation of the sternum, such that its anterior surface faces the smaller (usually right) hemithorax.

There is general agreement that if the deformity is severe enough, it should be surgically corrected. More than two dozen different procedures have been recommended for the correction of this deformity. These techniques can be divided roughly into the following groups: (1) operations that do not use special support or fixation; (2) methods in which external support is applied; and (3) procedures using internal support.

Surgical Technique

We have experimented with different methods, and have developed a technique (Fig. 1) that in our experience has offered excellent results. With the patient under endotracheal anesthesia, a slightly upward convex transverse incision is made over the midsternum. The pectoralis muscles are detached on both sides of the sternum, then stripped and retracted laterally, exposing all involved cartilages. The depressed cartilaginous segments are resected subperiosteally.

A transverse cuneiform osteotomy of the sternum at the beginning of its abnormal downward curve is performed next. Care is taken to do the osteotomy in a line that falls to an intercostal space rather than at a chondrosternal junction. The xiphoid process is detached from the sternum and is allowed to retract downward. The tip of the sternum is then lifted with a towel clip, and, with blunt and sharp dissection, the sternum is freed of its mediasti-

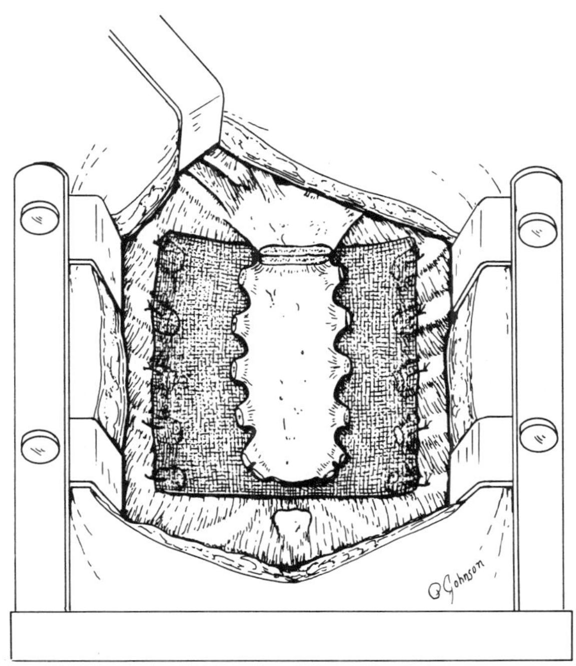

Figure 1 Repair of pectus excavatum: The deformed cartilages are resected bilaterally. A tranverse osteotomy is performed below the angle of Louis, the sternum is bent forward and is supported with a *Marlex* mesh sutured to the distal end of the costal cartilages. The xiphoid process is detached.

nal, perichondrial, and intercostal attachments. The sternum is then bent forward to a slightly overcorrected position. The right pleural cavity is entered deliberately and drained through an intercostal water-sealed catheter to prevent accumulation of blood in the wound itself and to assure undisturbed wound healing.

To stabilize and maintain the sternum in its corrected position, a piece of *Marlex* mesh is cut to approximate size, placed under it, and sutured under slight tension to the distal ends of the divided costal cartilages with nonabsorbable heavy filament sutures. If the pectoralis muscles are well developed, they are joined together in the midline, anterior to the sternum. If they are hypoplastic, they are reattached to the sternal edge. In rare cases in which nodular prominence of the sternocostoclavicular junction is part of the deformity, the dissection is carried around the entire circumference of the sternum. The attachment of the clavicles and the first ribs is cut across with a Gigli saw, and the prominent bone is sculptured off with a chisel. In such cases of extensive mobilization of the sternum, we do not dissect the mediastinal tissue from the upper third of the posterior surface and transect the intercostal muscles lateral to the mammary vessels, leaving the mammary vessels on the posterior surface of the sternal plate. This assures an adequate blood supply. According to our experience, even such an extensive dissection does not lead to flail chest, and the cross-sectioning and partial resection of the sternoclavicular connection do not require special stabilization measures.

Although repair of pectus excavatum is a relatively simple operation occasionally it may create significant technical difficulties. The primary obstacle is not that the operator has to correct the position of the depressed sternum, but that he has to stabilize the breast bone, which is stripped of its cartilaginous support in its new, elevated state. In our experience, this "hammock method" described above has proved to be superior to other forms of pectus excavatum repair.

PECTUS CARINATUM

Besides its generally accepted name, pectus carinatum, protrusion of the anterior chest is known by several other terms, which are chicken breast, pigeon breast, pyramidal chest, thorax cuneiforme, and sternal kyphosis. Anatomically, carinatum deformities may be conveniently divided into four major groups: (1) *keel chest*, (2) *sternum elevatum*, (3) *pouter pigeon breast*, and (4) *asymmetric or lateral pectus carinatum*. The identification of these groups is very important because the appropriate surgical procedure is selected according to these individual subtypes.

Keel Chest. In keel chest the lower third of the sternum arches abnormally forward. Unlike in the elevatum deformity, the xiphoid process is not an axial continuation of the sternum but joins it at an acute angle with the process pointing in the dorsal direction. Keel chest is commonly associated with bilateral symmetric depression of the costal cartilages, mistakenly identified by some as Harrison's grooves.

Sternum Elevatum. In this type of deformity the breast bone is relatively straight; however, its lower end rises significantly above the level of the manubrium. This elevation of the sternum is naturally accompanied by bilateral elongation and protrusion of the costal cartilages.

Pouter Pigeon Breast. Also called arcuate pectus carinatum, pouter pigeon breast is an interesting anterior chest wall anomaly in which upper chondromanubrial prominence is associated with lower chondrosternal depression. This creates a situation in which the manubrium protrudes and the midportion of the sternum arches posteriorly, whereas the tip of the xiphoid process points anteriorly.

Asymmetric or Lateral Pectus Carinatum. This anomaly is characterized by unilateral protrusion of the costal cartilages. The lesion is often associated with contralateral depression of the chest wall as well as hypoplasia, and absence of one of the pectoralis major muscles. The anatomy of lateral pectus carinatum is usually dominated by the deformity of the cartilages, thus the malposition of the sternum appears to be less significant. In the most common variety of the disease, there is marked unilateral prominence of the cartilages from the second one down, with 30- to 45-degree rotation of the sternum around its longitudinal axis toward the sunken opposite side. A less frequently encountered variety of lateral pectus carinatum is the isolated prominence of two or more cartilages with minimal or no sternal involvement.

Surgical Technique

The operation, regardless of the type of the deformity, is performed through a cosmetically suitable upward convex transverse submammary incision in the direction of Langer's lines. The length of the incision is proportional to the degree of the deformity and the planned extent of the procedure. To prevent necrosis of the skin, it is important to carry the incision down to the level of the sternal periosteum in the midline and to the pectoralis fascia on both sides, in order to develop a thick flap of skin and subcutaneous tissue. Using an electrocautery, the pectoralis muscles are detached from the sternum, dissected off the bony chest wall on both sides enough to permit them to be pulled and sutured together later on without undue tension in front of the sternum. A V-shaped transverse osteotomy is now performed on the proximal portion of the sternum at the level of the beginning of the abnormal forward curve, carried to the depth of but not across the posterior lamina in a line corresponding to an intercostal space rather than to a sternocostal junction.

Caudal to the line of the transverse osteotomy, the sternal ends of all costal cartilages are then resected subperiosteally. Shorter segments of the upper with progressively longer segments of the lower cartilages are removed. The extent of the resection in general is more extensive than that performed in pectus excavatum. If a cartilage is protuberant, elongated, or knobby, it is removed in its entire length of involvement because there are instances when postoperative overgrowth of nonresected cartilages can jeopardize otherwise good results. Resection of the medial ends of the bony ribs may become necessary in patients with more advanced deformities. The further course of the operation depends on the anatomic subtype of the deformity.

Keel Chest. In cases of keel chest, also called truly keeled or pyramidal chest, the lower end of the sternum is grabbed with a towel clip, elevated, and the xiphoid process is detached. If the latter appears to be rudimentary, its size is augmented by carrying the line of resection somewhat higher to leave a short portion of the distal sternum in continuity with it, thus "creating" a xiphoid of normal size. The xiphoid is mobilized by severing its connections with the diaphragm, but not those with the rectus muscle. Breaking the posterior lamina of the sternum at the level of the transverse osteotomy, the sternum is pressed posteriorly and brought into a corrected position, thus eliminating the carinatum deformity. Because the pathologic anatomy of the keel chest includes not only protrusion but also elongation of the sternum, the breast bone is shortened by resecting a 2- to 6-cm length of its distal end. The corrected position of the sternum is secured by uniting its distal end with the xiphoid process using wire sutures. Care should be taken that this maneuver is done under tension to assure traction on the sternum by the rectus muscles via the xiphoid, which maintains the sternum permanently in a corrected position. Before the incision is closed, all chondral and bony protuberances are carefully removed using rongeurs and osteotomes. The edges of the pectoralis muscles are united with chromic catgut sutures in front of the sternum to further secure its corrected position and to provide a smooth, soft contour to the anterior chest wall. After presternal approximation of the edges of the pectoralis muscles, there is usually a triangular-shaped hiatus in the lower wound; this may be disturbing to the surgeon's eye, but is filled readily with subcutaneous tissue after the skin is closed. If this defect appears to be significant, it may easily be corrected by a flap of rectus abdominalis muscle. The subcutaneous tissue is closed with interrupted suture and the skin with intracutaneous suture (Fig. 2).

Sternum Elevatum. In patients who have sternum elevatum, an anomaly with sternal protrusion but without sternal elongation, we perform a procedure similar to that used in keel chest but omit sternal shortening. In such patients, the corrected sternal position is maintained primarily by the pectoralis muscles sutured together in front of the sternum.

Pouter Pigeon Breast. The surgical repair of pouter pigeon breast must include elimination of the costomanubrial prominence as well as raising of the lower sternochondral depression. The initial steps of the operation, i.e., transverse skin incision, retraction of the pectoralis muscles, bilateral resection of the cartilages from the second one down, and detachment of the xiphoid process, are identical to those described for the keel chest and pectus elevatum procedures. After these steps are accomplished, however, the operation takes a different course (Fig. 3).

First of all, the tip of the sternum is lifted with a towel clip, and the breast bone is freed with blunt and sharp dissection of both its intercostal and its posterior mediastinal attachments. Attention is then given to elimination of the prominence at the junction of the manubrium and the body of the sternum by chiseling it off with a wide osteotome. After the removal of the protuberant bone, a transverse V-shaped osteotomy is made at the level of the second intercostal space and a second linear osteotomy is done at the deepest point of the midsternal depression. The sternum is fractured at both osteotomy sites and bent

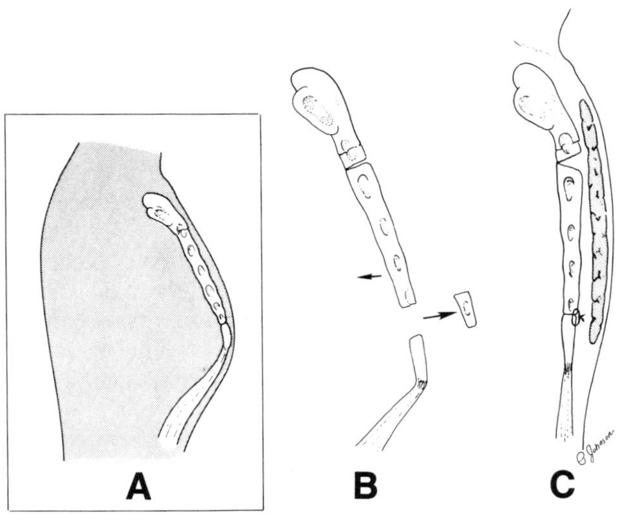

Figure 2 *A*, Repair of pectus carinatum. After bilateral resection of cartilages and performing a tranverse osteotomy the sternum is pushed backward and a segment of its caudal end is resected, *B*. The corrected position of the sternum is secured by using the pulling action of the rectus muscle via the reattached xiphoid process and by tacking the pectoralis major muscles together in the front of the sternum, *C*.

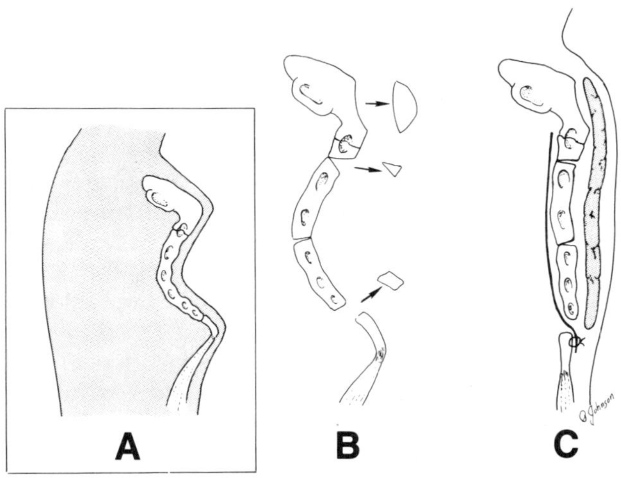

Figure 3 *A*, Repair of pouter pigeon breast. *B*, The manubrial prominence is removed, the axis of the sternum is corrected with a double osteotomy, and the sternum is shortened. *C*, The corrected position of the sternum is maintained with posterior *Marlex* mesh support. The pectoralis muscles are united presternally.

appropriately to bring its axis into a slightly overcorrected position. *Marlex* mesh is cut into proper size and shape, placed behind the sternum, stretched, and sutured in a "drummed-out" position to the distal stump of the resected costal cartilages with heavy nonabsorbable sutures. The sternum that now rests on and is supported by the mesh is covered with the pectoralis muscles tacked together presternally.

The most common wound complication is accumulation of blood or serum under the skin flaps. This may be avoided by entering the right pleural cavity as part of the surgical plan, connecting it widely with the operative field, and draining it through an intercostal water-sealed catheter. This way, even after the chest tube is removed (usually on the second day after surgery), the large pleural surface continues to absorb fluid that otherwise might be collected in the wound.

Lateral or Asymmetric Pectus Carinatum. The operation for the repair of lateral or asymmetric pectus carinatum has to be tailored to the extent and location of the deformity and may be very simple or quite extensive. If the anomaly consists only of unilateral overgrowth of a few cartilages, an incision is made directly over them and the procedure is limited to subperiosteal removal of the unsightly protuberance. More often, however, even in cases in which the deformity is limited, it is advisable to be radical rather than conservative and to remove the neighboring cartilages as well, otherwise, after the closure of the skin, or even worse, at the time of the first postoperative visit, it may become apparent that part of the deformity has been left uncorrected. It is good practice after correction of the bone anomaly to pull the skin edges temporarily together and to critically assess whether additional corrective steps need to be done after permanent closure of the skin is undertaken. Because the cartilages at the sternocostal junction frequently are overgrown, the edge of the sternum on the involved side should be shaved off with an osteotome. If the anomaly also involves the bony portion of the rib, it is advisable to remove the bony protrusion as well. It seems paradoxical, but we have learned that if a unilateral pectus carinatum is severe enough to necessitate extensive resection of the cartilages on one side, a short parasternal segment of the apparently normal cartilages on the opposite side should be removed too. Otherwise, the unbalanced action of these cartilages will tilt the sternum to its side, causing recurrence of the anomaly.

Combined Deformities. Not infrequently it happens that unilateral pectus carinatum is associated with some degree of anterior chest wall depression of the other side, that makes the anomaly even more obvious. This "mixed" form is especially likely to occur in tall asthenic individuals, such as those with Marfan's syndrome. Such combined carinatum-excavatum deformities are invariably accompanied by various degrees of rotation of the sternum toward the depressed side. Interestingly enough, in asymmetric or lateral pectus carinatum, the protrusion is almost always on the left side, and therefore, the rotation of the sternum occurs toward the right. Although Ravitch states that in such cases "the operative attention should always be directed to the depressed side," we believe that both sides should be treated equally and radically. It is our practice to repair such a combined deformity in the following way: The deformed cartilages—prominent on one side, depressed on the other—are bilaterally removed. Care is taken to end up having the peripheral stumps of the resected cartilages on the same level in the anteroposterior plane. Usually the resection needs to be more extensive in length on the prominent rather than on the depressed side. A transverse, wedge-shaped osteotomy is performed high on the sternum, with slightly more bone removed from the lower edge of the osteotomy than from the upper. The sternum is dissected free both laterally and posteriorly. The posterior lamina is fractured, and the abnormal plane of the sternum is corrected by manually twisting the sternum around its longitudinal axis toward the opposite (carinatum) direction. The now horizontal anterior plane of the sternum is secured by placing a figure-of-eight heavy wire suture at the previously depressed edge of the transverse osteotomy.

Marlex mesh is now spread under the sternum and sutured tight to the peripheral stumps of the resected ribs using 1-0 nonabsorbable sutures. The operation is completed by suturing the mobilized pectoralis muscles together presternally.

If pectus carinatum is accompanied by kyphosis, the matter of operative indications as well as the surgery itself should be the common endeavor of the thoracic surgeon and the orthopedist. Simultaneous operations on the anterior chest wall and the spine should be avoided.

Breast augmentation, if needed, can also be more effectively and safely performed after the deformity in the chest wall has been corrected and the rib cage has appropriately stablized.

SUGGESTED READING

Ravitch MM. Congenital deformities of the chest wall and their operative correction. Philadelphia: WB Saunders, 1977.

Robicsek F. Marlex mesh support for the correction of very severe and recurrent pectus excavatum. Ann Thorac Surg 1978; 26:80–83.

Robicsek F, Cook JW, Daugherty HK, Selle JG. Pectus carinatum. J Thorac Cardiovasc Surg 1979; 78:52–61.

Robicsek F, Daugherty HK, Mullen DC, et al. Technical considerations in the surgical management of pectus excavatum and carinatum. Ann Thorac Surg 1974; 18:549–564.

Robicsek F, Sanger PW, Taylor FH, Thomas MJ. The surgical treatment of chondrosternal prominence (pectus carinatum). J Thorac Cardiovasc Surg 1963; 45:691–701.

OPERATIVE MANAGEMENT OF THORACIC OUTLET SYNDROME

DAVID B. ROOS, M.D.

Thoracic outlet syndrome (TOS) is caused by anatomic anomalies that compress the brachial plexus, the subclavian artery, or the subclavian vein. The various anomalies associated with TOS affect the neurologic function of the brachial plexus much more commonly than they alter the flow through the subclavian vessels. The neurologic symptoms arising from brachial plexus involvement may be divided clinically into those of the upper plexus nerves (C5, C6, and C7) and those of the lower plexus nerves (C8 and T1). Upper plexus involvement causes symptoms of pain through the anterolateral aspect of the neck from the clavicle to the ear. This pain sometimes spreads superiorly into the jaw, face, or side of head; anteriorly in the upper chest; posteriorly in the rhomboid region medial to the scapula; laterally across the suprascapular region and outer shoulder and down the outer aspect of the arm through the radial nerve distribution towards the dorsum of the first three digits. Lower plexus involvement causes pain in the supraclavicular region and posteriorly into the scapular or rhomboid area; the pain can occur in the axilla or posterior axillary region and radiate down the medial aspect of the arm through the inner elbow, forearm, and hand to the ring and small fingers in the ulnar nerve distribution. Often upper plexus involvement does not create as much weakness or paresthesia as does involvement with the lower plexus, which may be accompanied by poor grip, arm fatigue, coldness, numbness, and tingling in the ulnar nerve distribution or the entire hand.

Patients with predominantly vascular symptoms are seen much less frequently than those with neurologic complaints. The venous type of TOS is caused by multiple anomalies that compress the subclavian vein extrinsically as it passes through the costoclavicular space. Skeletal anomalies may present as an osteoma of the first rib, a chondroma of the first costal cartilage, or a callous formation from fractured rib or clavicle. Soft tissue anomalies in this region are much more common and include wide insertion of the subclavius muscle tendon, a congenital fibromuscular band from the anterior scalene muscle passing under the vein and attaching to the back of the cartilage or sternum, or fibrous tissue associated with a long cervical rib. Venous symptoms include intermittent venous congestion of the arm with cyanosis, swelling, heaviness, and aching; these symptoms are usually precipitated by arm exertion or elevation and are relieved by rest. If these symptoms are unremitting, the vein probably has thrombosed; however, some patients will suddenly reach a stage of persistent venous congestion without intrinsic occlusion. The diagnosis must be confirmed by venography by means of contrast medium injected into the distal forearm or wrist. The antecubital veins should be avoided because the injection may cause significant artifactual filling. Two-positional venography is recommended, first with the arm dependent and then with it elevated above shoulder level. A persistent filling defect and prominent collaterals are required to substantiate the diagnosis of thrombosis of the axillary subclavian veins as deceptive streaming effects may result from admixture of flow from the deep jugular system and be misinterpreted as fresh or old thrombus.

Arterial symptoms are the least common of all TOS presentations and include peripheral emboli to the fingers, prominent supraclavicular pulsations from an aneurysm, or sudden occlusions with an ischemic, cold, pale, and painful arm and hand. Usually, arterial problems are associated with cervical ribs longer than 4 cm as shorter cervical ribs rarely cause significant arterial compression or disease.

Diagnosis of the neurologic type of TOS is based upon a careful history and physical evaluation of all nerves of the brachial plexus and the muscles they innervate. Electromyography, nerve conduction times, F-wave, and somatosensory evoked potentials are seldom beneficial. Arteriography and venography play no part in diagnosis of the neurologic form of TOS and should be avoided. However, diagnosis of vascular types of TOS requires venography or arteriography.

Conservative treatment of the neurologic type of TOS, by means of physical therapy with hot packs, massage, ultrasonography, and stretching exercises to relieve muscle spasm, and avoidance of heavy exertion or arm elevation may be effective in early and mild cases, but seldom relieves severe symptoms. It may be of slight or temporary benefit in cases of mild vascular involvement, but is ineffective in advanced instances of both venous or arterial involvement.

In the neurologic type of TOS, if symptoms fail to respond to a reasonable course of conservative management, are progressive during such a course of treatment, and cause unacceptable restriction of activities or disability for the patient, surgical relief is indicated. Currently, the most effective procedure for TOS of the upper plexus is supraclavicular neurolysis of the C5, C6, and C7 nerves from abnormal anterior scalene muscle with complete removal of the muscle (total anterior scalenectomy). The antiquated "scalenotomy," in which the anterior scalene muscle is divided or 1 cm of it is resected, often proves ineffective as the significant anomalies affecting the upper three nerves of the plexus remain intact and often resume abnormal pulling and compression of these nerves when the divided muscle, predictably, reattaches by scar formation.

TOTAL ANTERIOR SCALENECTOMY

In performing total anterior scalenectomy, several technical points are of great importance. The patient's head should be turned to the far side, and the head of the operating table should be elevated to increase exposure and reduce venous pressure and bleeding in the neck. The incision, usually about 4 cm long, should be placed in a natural skin crease one or two finger widths above the clavicle so that the upper attachments of the anterior scalene muscle may be reached with good exposure. The clavicular head of the sternocleidomastoid muscle and, usually, the omohyoid muscle are divided to provide safe exposure deep in the neck around the brachial plexus and subclavian artery. The prescalene fat pad should be carefully dissected off the jugular vein, reflected laterally behind a small retractor, and saved for fat coverage of the bare nerves of the brachial plexus after completion of the scalenectomy. The phrenic nerve is located immediately upon exposure of the anterior scalene muscle and carefully protected from instrument manipulation throughout the procedure. The upper trunk of the brachial plexus is then visualized prior to any division of scalene muscle as it may be in an abnormal location, sometimes being found immediately adjacent to the phrenic nerve on the anterior surface of the anterior scalene muscle rather than in its normal position between the anterior and middle scalene muscles.

In patients who develop TOS of the upper plexus, the anterior scalene muscle is usually found to have impressive muscle connections to the neurilemmal sheaths of the upper three nerves of the plexus, which probably cause the upper plexus symptoms from muscle contraction and spasm pulling on these nerves. All of these muscle attachments must be removed carefully along with prominent muscle bundles interdigitating between the nerves connecting the anterior to the middle scalene muscle behind the plexus. The muscle is carefully divided in multiple sections over a hemostat in the middle or lower third—if the muscle is divided all at once the major nerves or vessels may be injured. Under direct vision, the divided ends are then grasped with a hemostat and elevated away from the plexus as the muscles' fibers are dissected off all the nerves and the subclavian artery. The upper segment of the divided muscle is dissected up to its fibrous attachments to the transverse processes of the cervical vertebrae where it is divided and fully removed. The lower end of the divided muscle is dissected inferiorly between the artery and vein to its attachment at the scalene tubercle on the first rib where it is divided and removed. The bed of the anterior scalene muscle is then palpated for taut fibrotic vertical anomalous bands that are often found passing from behind the subclavian artery over the C8 and C7 nerves and attaching to the transverse processes. Since these anomalous bands may cause compression and fixation of the proximal centimeter of these nerves, they should be separated from the nerves and divided over a hemostat; then both ends should be fully excised to prevent them reattaching. Care must be taken to avoid injury to the subclavian artery, which may arch much higher than expected in the supraclavicular region, sometimes as high as three finger widths above the clavicle—a dangerously abnormal position. However, the subclavian vein seems never to be similarly displaced above its usual location below the clavicle.

The C7 and C8 nerves are often covered with a sheath of fibromuscular tissue that may also contribute to nerve compression. This sheath should be split over a hemostat and the reflected edges resected to prevent it from reforming.

After the upper four nerves of the plexus are completely free of all abnormal compression and tissue, they are covered with the prescalene fat, which is passed under the phrenic nerve and tailored to fit over the brachial plexus; the fat is then sutured to the medial aspect of the neck to fill the scalene fossa with normal soft fat in order to cushion and protect the exposed nerves. Each nerve, including the phrenic, should be initially tested with a battery nerve stimulator to confirm recognition of the nerves and, just prior to fat coverage, to prove that they are electrically active and undamaged.

This amount of neck dissection produces a small amount of postoperative drainage for 1 to 2 days, which consists of blood, serum, and perhaps lymph. This drainage should be removed by a small suction catheter, which is placed prior to wound closure. The head is then straightened, the divided ends of the clavicular portion of sternocleidomastoid muscle approximated, the platysma muscle closed with continuous suture, and the skin closed with a continuous absorbable subcuticular suture. Collodion provides an adequate seal and dressing for both the incision and drain site.

FIRST RIB RESECTION

If the patient has TOS predominantly of the lower plexus, the most effective way of decompressing the entire outlet and visualizing all anomalous fibromuscular tissue, which is uniformly found posteriorly near to the T1 nerve and frequently anteriorly near to the vein, is by means of transaxillary first rib resection with removal of the lower aspect of the middle and anterior scalene muscles and any other anomalous tissue in the outlet. To accomplish all these objectives, exposure through a supraclavicular approach is not adequate or safe and usually results in only partial resection of the first rib and soft tissue anomalies.

Safe and successful decompression of the outlet requires careful attention to fine technical details. After intubation, the patient is placed in the lateral thoracotomy position, at about 80 degrees from the horizontal. An assistant holds the arm abducted 90 degrees from the thorax with the elbow flexed 90 degrees at the level of his waist. The double wrist lock of the forearm and wrist of the patient is the most comfortable for the assistant who can periodically elevate the arm and shoulder girdle with light to moderate exertion during the procedure when the surgeon requires deep exposure in the outlet. Excessive, sudden, or prolonged elevation should be carefully avoided to help prevent traction injury to the brachial plexus. A 10 to 12 cm transverse incision is made in the lower aspect of the axilla in the axillomammary crease in females, or over the third rib in males where the skin breaks from the rib cage to cover the axilla. The skin edges are held open with self-retaining retractors, and the axillary tunnel is dissected by blunt dissection to the first rib. A cul-de-sac of fascia is carefully opened with long scissors exposing the thoracic outlet deep to the first rib at that level which separates the axilla from the neck. The subclavian vessels and brachial plexus are dissected from their attachments to the first rib, usually with finger dissection. Firm attachments may require sharp dissection; if this is necessary great care should be taken to avoid injuring these vital structures. The subclavius tendon and anterior scalene muscle are separated from surrounding tissue and carefully divided at their attachments to the first rib after first hooking the anterior scalene with a right-angle hemostat in order to separate it from the artery and avoid arterial injury. The middle scalene and intercostal muscle between the first and second ribs are then pushed off the rib with elevators, care being taken not to strip the periosteum from the rib, and the pleura is dropped to the second rib level. By means of careful visualization and protection of the nerve, the rib is then resected posteriorly behind the T1 nerve. The rib is resected anteriorly near the costal cartilage and removed with muscle fragments still attached, thereby indicating the periosteum is intact, in a deliberate attempt to minimize postoperative scar formation from retained periosteal cells. The remaining stumps of the rib are trimmed with rongeurs, and the posterior stump is left short and smooth well behind the T1 nerve, which again must be carefully visualized and protected with light retraction. The anterior stump is shortened to the costal cartilage and left smooth so that no spicules or bone shelf can affect the subclavian vein.

The redundant and divided lower end of the middle scalene muscle is then pulled down with a long hemostat and 2 to 3 cm more is resected in order to remove the lower part of the muscle to prevent it reattaching to the nerves or other structures of the outlet. After resecting the middle scalene muscle tissue and any abnormal bands posteriorly, this should leave an empty fossa behind the T1 nerve. Similarly, the anterior scalene muscle is pulled down and 1 to 2 cm more is resected to prevent it reattaching. The region is carefully searched for abnormal fibromuscular bands; these are common. They may arise from between the T1 nerve and the artery, or they may form a sling from middle to anterior scalene muscle under the nerve, artery, and vein, thereby attaching to the cartilage or sternum. All taut bands and tissue should be divided and then fully resected to prevent reattachment. If a cervical rib is present, it is removed and rongeured as short as the first rib stump.

The wound is then irrigated twice with sterile saline to cleanse the tissue, remove surgical debris, fat globules, and loose muscle tissue, and to test for pleural integrity. If the pleura has been torn, a chest tube should be placed over the apex of the lung, threaded towards the mediastinum, brought out over the second rib and through the middle of the incision, and then sewn to the lateral chest wall with heavy suture. The shoulder is then lowered and the incision closed with a subcutaneous layer inserted snugly around the chest tube and with an absorbable subcuticular suture around the chest tube as well. Usually, the chest tube may be removed in the recovery room after the patient is awake, when bubbling in the water trap ceases, breath sounds are heard, and a portable upright chest x-ray film documents full expansion of the lung. If the visceral pleura has been torn and bubbles continue, the tube should be left in place until the pleura seals.

As with any major thoracic procedure, postoperative care is directed mainly at achieving good pulmonary function in order to prevent atelectasis. The patient is advised to use the hand normally and to raise the arm straight up alongside the head twice a day, in order to keep the shoulder joint mobile. The patient can use the opposite hand to slowly draw the arm up for support. However, strenuous exercise, reaching, or lifting should be avoided for at least 2 months.

If the patient has both upper and lower plexus involvement, both transaxillary decompression of the outlet for the lower plexus and supraclavicular anterior scalenectomy can be performed as part of the same procedure. I prefer doing the axillary dissection in the lateral position first, then repositioning the patient from his side to his back, turning the head to the opposite direction, elevating the head of the table, and proceeding with the supraclavicular total anterior scalenectomy. Both fields are initially prepared and draped together so that there is minimal interruption between the two stages of the procedure. If the patient has severe bilateral symptoms, bilateral first rib resection may be performed under the same anesthesia, although this requires redraping and positioning the patient. However, if the patient has bilateral upper plexus involvement, I feel strongly that bilateral scalenectomy should not be performed under the same anesthesia since undetected contusion or traction of the phrenic nerve sometimes results in temporary phrenic neuropraxia with resulting paralyzed diaphragm. If involvement is unilateral, serious complications or postoperative problems other than basilar atelectasis are unusual before it gradually resolves. However, bilateral involvement is a serious and complex problem which may require prolonged treatment on the respirator. This occurred once in my experience.

If the patient has intermittent venous compression of significant degree, transaxillary decompression of the entire thoracic outlet is indicated with removal of the first rib, any abnormal cartilage which may be found contributing to venous compression, and all soft tissue anomalies around the vein. This may be a most difficult and exacting operation with the potential of serious injury to the vein that could result in life-threatening hemorrhage or air embolism. Therefore, in such cases blood should be available, and the patient warned of the unusual risks involved. However, careful decompression of the vein usually results in complete and dramatic cure of the problem.

If the vein has thrombosed, clot lysis may be achieved with urokinase (UK) or streptokinase (SK); although these are expensive treatments with potential and serious hemorrhagic complications, especially SK treatment which carries a 25 percent moderate complication rate and a 5 percent serious or fatal complication rate. Urokinase is much safer and requires a briefer course of treatment, usually 12 or 24 hours compared to 72 hours of SK treatment, but UK is 15 times as expensive as SK ($6,000 per

24 hours). If the patient undergoes lytic therapy for a fresh subclavian vein thrombosis, I feel the thoracic outlet should be surgically decompressed before the patient is discharged from the hospital in order to prevent recurrence. Warfarin should be administered during the operation with a protime of 14 to 18 seconds, but the patient should not be sent home on chronic warfarin therapy without the operation as thrombosis may recur even on adequate anticoagulation and the benefits of the expensive thrombolysis are lost. In highly selected patients with early thrombosis, consideration may be given to urgent decompression of the thoracic outlet combined with thrombectomy to reestablish flow through the major vein and eliminate all compressive mechanisms simultaneously. This avoids the risks and expense of fibrinolytic treatment and prolonged hospitalization, but it must be performed only by vascular surgeons experienced in thoracic outlet decompression and management of venous thrombectomy and anticoagulation. Following the procedure, such a patient should be continued on warfarin for several months during the healing stage.

Patients with significant arterial disease in the thoracic outlet usually require surgical correction. The choice of operation depends on the findings of selective arteriography. A fusiform aneurysm, which may accompany a long cervical rib, usually does not require resection and graft replacement, but a sacular aneurysm or any aneurysm that is a source of peripheral emboli does require graft replacement. A significant subclavian artery plaque, with or without emboli, also requires graft replacement with complete decompression of the outlet by first rib and cervical rib resection. Although some surgeons have reported good results resecting the subclavian artery through the axillary approach after the first and cervical ribs are removed, this may require a double operation with transaxillary decompression of the outlet, removal of the rib, and supraclavicular resection of the aneurysm or plaque.

If the patient has a significant associated reflex sympathetic dystrophy, with a cold, pale, swollen arm and hand or causalgia with burning pain and hypersensitive skin, usually through the ulnar nerve distribution, these problems usually respond well to sympathectomy, which may conveniently be performed simultaneously with the transaxillary first rib resection. After the rib has been removed, the mediastinal pleura is carefully stripped down to the third or fourth rib level by finger dissection and the sympathetic chain is located between the first portion of the subclavian artery and the T1 nerve of the brachial plexus. The chain is dissected from surrounding tissue as it passes over the head or neck of the second rib. The stellate ganglion ends at the top of the second rib. The chain may be divided just below the tip of the stellate ganglion, thereby leaving it untouched. The divided lower end of the chain is then elevated and the rami communicantes are divided with long scissors down to the third rib. The chain is then divided again at that level, thus removing approximately 2.5 cm of the sympathetic chain which contains the second thoracic ganglion. That is the ganglion principally involved in providing sympathetic innervation to the upper extremity, predominantly through the T1 nerve of the brachial plexus and the ulnar nerve down the arm. Small sympathetic fibers joining the T1 nerve are then divided. This provides a simple and effective sympathectomy for the arm and hand, which immediately postoperatively results in a hot, dry, pink hand; the procedure minimizes the chance of a Horner's syndrome.

If diagnosis of the thoracic outlet syndrome is made with great care and symptoms are severe enough to be unaffected by conservative management, most patients respond well to appropriate surgical treatment. However, the operations that have been devised demand meticulous surgical technique and full visual exposure in complex and potentially dangerous surgical fields. They require good assistance, excellent lighting, and appropriate special instruments. If all these requirements can be met by careful planning, good to excellent relief may be accomplished in approximately 90 percent of the cases, even in the presence of severe symptoms that fail to respond to all conservative measures. If these requirements are not met, and operations are performed casually with inexperienced technique or assistance, with poor exposure, or with inadequate instruments, disastrous complications with life-threatening hemorrhage or a neurologically crippled shoulder, arm, and hand may result.

SUGGESTED READING

Clagett OT. Presidential address: research and prosearch. J Thorac Cardiovasc Surg 1962; 44:153–166.

Roos DB. Axillary-subclavian vein occlusions. In: Rutherford RB, ed. Vascular surgery. 2nd ed. Philadelphia: WB Saunders, 1984: 1385.

Roos DB. Congenital anomalies associated with thoracic outlet syndrome—anatomy, symptoms, diagnosis and treatment. Am J Surg 1976; 132:771–778.

Roos DB. The place for scalenectomy and first rib resection in thoracic outlet syndrome. Surgery 1982; 92:1077–1084.

Urschel HD Jr, Paulson DI, McNamara JJ. Thoracic outlet syndrome. Ann Thoracic Surg 1968; 6:1–10.

CHEST WALL NEOPLASIA

PETER C. PAIROLERO, M.D.

Chest wall tumors encompass a kaleidoscopic panorama of bone and soft tissue pathology that includes primary neoplasm (both benign and malignant) of the bony skeleton, chest wall metastases, neoplasms that invade the chest wall from lung, pleura, mediastinum, muscle, and breast, and benign non-neoplastic conditions. Nearly all of these disorders have at one time or another been irradiated either as the treatment of choice or in combination with chest wall resection, and it is not uncommon to see patients with a postradiation necrotic chest wall tumor. For these patients, wound hygiene is of major importance, and surgical excision is the only treatment option regardless whether the tumor is a primary neoplasm, metastases, or benign inflammation.

Primary chest wall tumors generally appear as an enlarging mass, many of which are symptomatic. The most common symptom is pain, which often is initially treated as neuritis or musculoskeletal complaint. Malignant tumors are more likely to be associated with signs and symptoms.

The diagnostic evaluation of suspected primary chest wall tumors should include careful history and physical examination, followed by conventional plain and tomographic chest roentgenography. Computed tomography should also be carried out to delineate soft tissue, pleural, mediastinal, and pulmonary involvement.

Chest wall tumors clinically suspected of being primary neoplasms should be diagnosed by excisional rather than incisional or needle biopsy. Likewise, necrotic tumor should be diagnosed by excision. However, if there is a history of known primary neoplasm elsewhere and the chest wall mass is suspected of being a metastasis, then needle or incisional biopsy to establish diagnosis of dissemination is reasonable.

It is well recognized that wide resection of chest wall tumor is essential to successful management. However, the extent of resection should not be compromised because of inability to close the chest wall defect. Consequently the mandatory ingredients for successful management of this problem are adequate resection and dependable reconstruction. This is accomplished most effectively by the joint efforts of a thoracic and a plastic surgeon.

Opinions do differ as to what constitutes adequate resection, the need and method for restoration of the bony thorax, and, finally, the manner of soft tissue reconstruction. For many surgeons a margin of resection grossly free of tumor by several centimeters is considered wide resection. While this may be adequate for chest wall metastases, benign tumor, and certain low-grade malignant primary bone tumors such as chondrosarcoma, more malignant tumors such as osteosarcoma have the potential to spread within the marrow cavity, along the periosteum, or along the parietal pleura, and consequently such an excision would *not* be adequate resection.

All primary malignant neoplasms initially diagnosed by excisional biopsy should have further excision to include all of the involved bone and a 4 cm margin of normal tissue on all sides. For neoplasms of the rib cage, this includes removal of the involved ribs, corresponding anterior costal arches, and several partial ribs above and below the neoplasm. For tumors of the sternum and manubrium, excision of the entire involved bone and corresponding costal arches bilaterally is indicated. Any attached structures such as lung, thymus, pericardium, or chest wall muscles should also be excised.

Metastases, in general, do not need surgical treatment. Occasionally, however, they occur as an indeterminate solitary chest wall mass. In this situation, excisional biopsy is usually adequate.

Desmoid tumor deserves special consideration. Most pathologists consider desmoid as a form of benign fibromatosis. Some, however, consider it a low-grade fibrosarcoma. Whatever the etiology, the tumor tends to be recurrent if inadequately excised, and it should be treated with wide resection similar to primary malignant chest wall neoplasm.

Large chest wall defects frequently can occur as a result of treatment of primary tumors. Historically the thoracic deformity produced after resection of the manubrium and sternum has been the most difficult of all chest wall defects to reconstruct. Not only is there the problem of insufficient soft tissue to bridge this defect, but the reconstruction must also be made sufficiently rigid to maintain adequate pulmonary function and to protect the underlying viscera.

In general, nearly all large bony defects should be reconstructed. The decision not to reconstruct the skeleton depends on the size and location of the defect. Defects less than 5 cm in greatest diameter anywhere on the thorax are usually not reconstructed. Posterior defects less than 10 cm likewise do not require reconstruction because the overlying scapula provides support. Larger defects, however, should be reconstructed. Stabilization of the bony thorax can be accomplished with prosthetic material such as Prolene mesh or 2-mm Gore-Tex Soft-Tissue Patch. Placing either of these materials under tension improves the rigidity of the prosthesis in all directions. The Gore-Tex Soft-Tissue Patch is preferred because this material has the added advantage of preventing movement of fluid and air across the reconstructed chest wall. Marlex mesh is not used, because when placed under tension, this material is rigid in one direction only. Reconstruction with rigid materials such as methylmethacrylate is rarely necessary.

Closure of the soft tissue defect after stability has been achieved may be possible in some patients by direct closure of the remaining skin. In other patients with larger defects, random flaps of chest wall skin and breast tissue may be employed. Soft tissue reconstruction, however, is best accomplished by muscle transposition. The pectoralis major, serratus anterior, latissimus dorsi, and rectus abdominis muscles all have an axial blood supply that permits elevation and rotation of these muscles for a significant distance with or without the overlying skin. Because the omentum by itself contributes no stability to the chest wall, it should not be used initially, but rather it should be reserved as a back-up procedure should muscle transposition fail to totally cover a defect or be unavailable because of a previous operation or radiation.

The key to successful treatment of primary chest wall tumors remains early diagnosis and aggressive surgical resection. This procedure can generally be performed in one operation with minimal respiratory insufficiency and with low operative mortality. In a recent series from the Mayo Clinic, there were no operative deaths, and the overall 1-, 5-, and 10-year survival for patients with primary malignant chest wall neoplasms was

88 percent, 57 percent, and 49 percent respectively. These findings support a continued attitude toward aggressive chest wall resection, which, when combined with current methods of reconstruction, should allow potentially curative resection for most patients with primary chest wall tumor.

SUGGESTED READING

King RM, Pairolero PC, Trastek VF, Piehler JM, Payne WS, Bernatz PE. Primary chest wall tumors: factors affecting survival. Ann Thorac Surg 1986; 41:597–601.

McAfee MK, Pairolero PC, Bergstralh EJ, Piehler JM, Unni KK, McLeod RA, Bernatz PE, Payne WS. Chondrosarcoma of the chest wall: factors affecting survival. Ann Thorac Surg 1985; 40:535–541.

Pairolero PC, Arnold PG. Chest wall tumors: experience with 100 consecutive patients. J Thorac Cardiovasc Surg 1985; 90:367.

Pairolero PC, Arnold PG. Thoracic wall defects: surgical management of 205 consecutive patients. Mayo Clin Proc 1986; 61:557–563.

PROSTHETIC SUBSTITUTES OF THE CHEST WALL

HENRY ESCHAPASSE, M.D.
JACQUES GAILLARD, M.D.

Resection of skeletal structures of the chest wall poses reconstructive problems about which there is considerable controversy among surgeons: Some spurn the use of prostheses while others, we among them, grant them an important but nonexclusive role in tumor resection.

GENERAL PRINCIPLES

Our operative strategy is based on a few simple objectives: very wide, en-bloc resection of the tumor and adjacent tissues with minimal impairment of cardiorespiratory physiology and, if possible, restoration of the normal morphology by a method that is simple, fast, safe, and immediately adaptable to any case. To preserve the respiratory function we avoid useless extensive disinsertion of muscles so as not to divert the muscles from their natural functions. To prevent flail chest while preserving good mobility of the operated area and restore the morphology, we replace the skeletal plan by another solid plan. We repair the diaphragm when it has been resected and avoid pleural complications that might reduce its mobility. We use muscle transplantation as long as it does not interfere with these objectives, but we do not hesitate to implant a prosthesis, sometimes in combination with plastic procedures, to benefit from the advantages of both these techniques, which are not opposed but supplementary to each other.

The theoretic advantages of a prosthesis are obvious, provided it meets the following conditions. It has to be capable of replacing large skeletal defects, it must be adaptable to the coverage needed and then able to be molded during the operation; it should offer solid fixation, fast execution, good anchorage due to good incorporation into adjacent tissues, satisfactory long-term tolerability, adequate resistance to infection, solidity to protect intrathoracic organs, radiotransparency, and abscence of metal components in case later nuclear magnetic resonance (NMR) examination is necessary. Also, it must be possible for the prosthesis to be fixed in such a way as not to interfere with chest wall mobility, and it must not shrink with aging. Certain biomaterials fulfill all these conditions.

The theoretic disadvantages are few. The risk of general toxicity exists during the polymerization when it is done in situ. It can be completely eliminated by fashioning the prosthesis extracorporeally. The second and potential late risk is infection, which always remains possible, even long after the implantation (6 years later in one of our cases).

Experience has taught us that with the modern biomaterials an infection may be cured without removal of the prosthesis, provided the infection occurs during the early postoperative period. After local and general control by antibiotics the tissues can attach themselves to the prosthesis, giving good incorporation. A late infection that appears in association with pyemia, on the other hand, is the consequence of inadequate incorporation. A defect develops around the prosthesis in an organized pocket. Then the patient can be cured only by removing the prosthesis. But this can be done very easily and causes no abnormal mobility of the chest wall because the adjacent tissues are sufficiently fibrous and strong.

Myoplasties admittedly do not entail these risks, but they have other disadvantages: extensive dissections, protracted operation, impossibility of use for very large resections, detachment of respiratory muscles, imperfect stabilization of the chest wall at least during the first days, inadequate protection of the underlying organs, sometimes discomfort, and doubtful cosmetic results. Nevertheless, it has been shown that autoplastic operations may give remarkable results and their association with prosthesis is very useful.

The one indication for use of a prosthesis is in all cases of extensive resection of the bony chest wall. This applies to tumors, particularly cartilaginous ones, which always must be assumed to be malignant. Their potential spread to the bone marrow is macroscopically invisible and inaccessible to preoperative microscopic examination in the boundary zones, which are bony. Excision, therefore, should always be very wide and involve too much rather than too little tissue. The surgeon must resect without caring about the reconstruction. A prosthesis provides a good solution.

Chest wall reconstruction is not necessary in the areas

covered by the scapula and its strong surrounding muscles. Furthermore, after resection of the manubrium, reconstruction with a prosthesis is not justified. For cosmetic purposes, it can easily be achieved with autoplastic techniques. Provided the patient's general condition is good, age is not a major selection factor (ages in our series ranged from 6 to 76 years).

Relative *contraindications* to implantation of a prosthesis are an infected or necrotic field (e.g., after radiotherapy), except when selective antibiotics prove efficacious against specific microorganisms and when the resection extends into healthy, very well vascularized zones. However, in most cases, myoplasties are the safest techniques.

TYPE OF PROSTHESIS

There are many prostheses to choose from. We have abandoned the metal and the nylon mesh appliances because they disrupt under the shearing effect of respiratory movements and poorly resist infection. For the last 20 years we have been using the heavy gauge Marlex mesh, which resists infection, is relatively rigid, easy to shape and to cut to the desired sizes, strong, and readily incorporated. Connective tissue grows through the mesh, anchoring it firmly. We have no personal experience with other materials that also have given good results, such as Silastic, Prolene, and the absorbable materials.

OPERATIVE PROCEDURE

Preoperative embolization of afferent arteries is advisable in hypervascularized tumors (especially thyroid and renal metastases) to reduce operative blood loss.

Meticulous disinfection of the skin and strict perioperative asepsis are indispensable. The surgical approach should be wide and a strategy rapidly worked out, particularly for the incision when superficial planes are to be resected. In such cases, aid from a plastic surgeon is often desirable. Myocutaneous flaps allow wide resections of the skin. We try to be conservative with respect to the skin excision, but to be liberal with regard to resection of underlying muscles and ribs as well as invaded intrathoracic areas, which must be resected en bloc with the wall. In 17 of 42 patients operated on for malignant tumors we have carried out an en-bloc resection, 14 times a part of lung, and/or 5 times the diaphragm. In one patient we resected a part of the pericardium, the spleen, the five last ribs, the upper portion of the abdominal wall, and part of the omentum, of the stomach, and of the diaphragm.

When the osseous defect is of average size (80 to 120 cm^2) we use a sheet of Marlex mesh fixed with separate sutures below the ribs on which it rests. For larger defects we construct a prosthesis in which heavy Marlex mesh is used for the fixation to the edges of the defect, with methyl methacrylate (MMA) in the center to insure good parietal stability and an anatomically normal shape. The prosthesis should be slightly smaller than the defect because the position of the patient on the table during the operation and the retraction of severed and curarized muscles always enlarge the gap. It is better to make a prosthesis too small than too large. As a rule we use one sheet of Marlex, but for covering a very large gap we place a sheet of Marlex below and another above the MMA during the polymerization (sandwich technique that we described in 1972). It is easier to fix the prosthesis with the aid of the Marlex mesh than to do it through the holes made in the MMA or to mold the resin directly around the border of the defect, as do some surgeons. An additional advantage of Marlex is that it allows much better anchorage and preserves relative mobility of the wall.

During the polymerization, which is done extracorporeally, it is very easy to attach Dacron or other soft prosthetic materials to the MMA, for instance, to repair the diaphragm at the same time as a defect of the chest wall. The complex prosthesis is tailored en bloc.

Between the skin and the prosthesis we always interpose muscles or greater omentum. This has a double advantage. It serves as an excellent foundation for the underlying skin, and it provides a means for absorption of the fluid that might collect in the area.

Careful drainage is particularly important in the pleural cavity, to prevent collection of fluid and subsequent costodiaphragmatic adhesions, and also around the prosthesis, to avoid dead spaces. It is essential for good attachment of the patient's tissues and prevention of late sepsis. For this reason we place two to four multiperforated small drains below and above the prosthesis, in addition to the two usual pleural drains.

RESULTS

Results have been regularly good. One patient died in the postoperative period as a result of coronary damage during dissection of an invasive tumor. One patient who had pulmonary insufficiency before a sternochondral resection needed some respiratory support postoperatively, but the chest was perfectly stable. The other patients were extubated immediately, as after standard thoracotomy.

Late complications were very rare and involved infection. We observed one early postoperative infection due to perioperative sepsis. Cure was obtained with antibiotics and drainage without removal of the prosthesis. This patient has been followed-up for 10 years, and there have been no problems. Three late cases of sepsis necessitated removal of the prosthesis 4 to 80 months after the operation. We could remove the prosthesis very easily, and the chest wall remains stable. In two of these three cases, incorporation of the prosthesis was never complete postoperatively; there was an aseptic fluid collection around it. We have no explanation for the third case, in which the sepsis occurred 6 years after the implantation.

We have observed no case of respiratory failure or chest wall deformity or late flail chest. In two of three cases in which epiploplasty was utilized, abdominal eventration occurred at the site of insertion of the omentum and the linea alba. The two patients were treated successfully by cutting the omentum at the level of the abdominal hole and closing it.

Five patients underwent reoperation because of tumor

TABLE 1 Comparison of Results of Use of Autoplastic Procedure and of Prosthesis

	Autoplastic procedure	*Prosthesis*
Mobilization of muscles	−++	-
Adaptability to all cases	-	+++
Facility of modeling	-	+++
Parietal, protection	-	+++
Parietal, stability	+	+++
Incorporation	+++	±
Tolerance	+++	+
Risk of late, infection	-	+
Cosmetic result	±	+

- mediocre; + good; +++ very good; ± variable

TABLE 2 Complications Related to the Technique

Number of cases	27
Sternochondral resection	5
Rib resection	22
Late sepsis	3
Eventration after epiploplasty	2

recurrence. In three cases, the recurrence was at the same place; the resection was completed and the prosthesis replaced with a larger one. In two cases, recurrence was in a distant site, and a second prosthesis was placed. We had no difficulties with these operations.

All the patients had a normal life as a result of the operation. Respiratory function was either unchanged or hardly modified after the widest resections.

Prosthesis in our view reconciles the functional and cosmetic results in case of replacement of large thoracic defects involving the bony wall. Most problems can be resolved simply. Thanks to this technique, a surgeon need not fear performing the extensive resections that certain malignant tumors make necessary. The surgical risk is nil. Late complications of the technique are rare, curable, and have no effect on parietal stability and comfort of the patient.

SUGGESTED READING

Beattie EJ, Kim Y, Fayos J, Sridhar K, Raskin N. Chest wall resection and pulmonary function. In: Grillo HC, Eschapasse H, eds. International trends in general thoracic surgery. Vol II. Philadelphia: WB Saunders, 1986:310.

Eschapasse H, Bonafe M, Taobane M, Brut A, Manelfe C. Intérêt de l'embolisation artérielle pré-opératoire. A propos d'une observation de métastase d'hypernephrome de la paroi thoracique. Ann Chir Thorac Cardiovasc (Paris) 1981; 35:237–240.

Eschapasse H, Gaillard J, Henry E, Vassallo B, Lacheheb M. Chest wall tumors: surgical management. In: Grillo HC, Eschapasse H, eds. International trends in general thoracic surgery. Vol II. Philadelphia: WB Saunders, 1986:297.

McCormack PM, Bains MS, Beattie J Jr, Martini N. New trends in skeletal reconstruction after resection of chest wall tumors. Ann Thorac Surg 1981; 31:45–52.

Paris F, Blasco E, Tarazona V, et al. Total sternectomy for malignant diseases. J Thorac Cardiovasc Surg 1980; 80:459–462.

MUSCLE FLAPS

PETER C. PAIROLERO, M.D.
PHILLIP G. ARNOLD, M.D.

HISTORICAL CONSIDERATIONS

Reconstruction of chest wall defects has been a constant challenge to the surgeon. In 1950, Campbell described transposition of the latissimus dorsi muscle followed immediately by skin grafting for reconstruction of full-thickness defects of the anterior thorax. Unfortunately this excellent method of reconstruction went unnoticed for the next 20 years, until interest in muscle transposition was revived and the technique refined. During the past 15 years, muscle and musculocutaneous flaps of all chest wall muscles have been used with increasing frequency in reconstruction of the thorax.

ETIOLOGY

Defects of the chest wall occur almost always as a result of neoplasm, radiation, infection, or trauma. The chest wall defect produced by resection of most neoplasms involves loss of the skeleton and frequently the overlying soft tissues. Infection, radiation necrosis, and trauma produce partial or full-thickness defects, depending upon their severity.

CONSIDERATION FOR RECONSTRUCTION

The ability to close large chest wall defects is the main consideration in the surgical treatment of most chest wall afflictions. Excision should not be undertaken if the surgeon does not have the confidence and ability to close the defect. The critical questions whether the reconstructed thorax will support respiration and protect the underlying organs must be answered when considering both the extent of resection and the method of reconstruction of the chest wall. Adequate resection and dependable reconstruction are the mandatory ingredients for successful treat-

TABLE 1 Consideration for Reconstruction of Chest Wall Defects

Location
Size
Full thickness vs. partial thickness
General condition of the patient (receiving chemotherapy, steroids, etc.)
Condition of the local tissues (previous irradiation, localized infection, inflammation, scarring, etc.)
Duration of the defect
Lifestyle and type of work
Prognosis

ment. It is our strong belief that these two important items are accomplished most safely by the joint efforts of a thoracic and a plastic surgeon.

Reconstruction of chest wall defects involves consideration of many factors (Table 1). The location and size are of utmost importance, but the past medical history and local conditions of the wound may drastically alter a reconstructive choice. Primary closure, if possible, remains the best option available. If the defect is partial thickness and will accept and support a skin graft, reconstruction in this manner is quite reasonable. If full-thickness reconstruction is required, consideration must be given to both structural stability of the thorax and soft tissue coverage. Reconstruction with prosthetic material and muscle transposition remains our treatment of choice for a noninfected full-thickness defect.

SKELETAL RECONSTRUCTION

Reconstruction of full-thickness defects of the bony thorax is controversial. In some situations, usually small defects, the skeletal component can be ignored and the defect closed with only soft tissues. If structural stability is required, however, either autogenous tissue, such as fascia lata or ribs, or prosthetic material, such as the various meshes, metals, or soft tissue patches, may be used.

It is our opinion that full-thickness skeletal defects resulting from excision of tumors in both the sternum and lateral chest wall should be reconstructed if the wound is not contaminated. We use a 2-mm thick polytetrafluoroethylene soft tissue patch regularly in closing skeletal defects resulting from chest wall involvement of underlying lung cancer or recurrent breast cancer. If the wound is contaminated from previous radiation necrosis or necrotic neoplasm, reconstruction with prosthetic material is not advised as the prosthesis may subsequently become infected, resulting in obligatory removal. In this situation, reconstruction with a musculocutaneous flap alone is preferred.

SOFT TISSUE RECONSTRUCTION

Although both muscle and omental transposition can be utilized to reconstruct soft tissue chest wall defects, muscle is our preferred method and can be transposed as muscle alone or as a musculocutaneous flap. Muscle is also an ideal tissue to place in contaminated wounds. The ability of a muscle flap to contain and eliminate local infection has been demonstrated both clinically and experimentally. Because the omentum lacks structural stability, it should be considered a back-up alternative procedure.

MUSCLE TRANSPOSITION

Latissimus Dorsi

The latissimus dorsi muscle is the largest flat muscle in the thorax. Its dominant thoracodorsal neurovascular leash has an arc of rotation that allows coverage of the lateral and central back as well as the anterolateral and central front of the thorax. Its dependable musculocutaneous vascular connections permit it to be used also as a reliable musculocutaneous flap. This muscle flap can cover huge chest wall defects, since virtually one half of the back can be elevated on the blood supply of a single latissimus dorsi muscle in the uninjured nonirradiated patient. The donor site may have to be skin grafted when large musculocutaneous flaps are elevated.

Pectoralis Major

The pectoralis major muscle is the second largest flat muscle on the chest wall and in many respects is the mirror image of the latissimus dorsi muscle. Its dominant thoracoacromial neurovascular leash, which enters posteriorly about midclavicle, allows both elevation of the muscle and rotation centrally for chest wall reconstruction. It is of major benefit in reconstruction of anterior chest wall defects such as those resulting from sternal tumor excisions and infected median sternotomy wounds.

Serratus Anterior

The serratus anterior muscle has its blood supply from the serratus branch of the thoracodorsal vessels and from the long thoracic artery and vein. Although this muscle can be utilized alone, its main use is as an adjunctive muscle in tandem with the pectoralis major or the latissimus dorsi muscles.

Rectus Abdominis

Utilization of the rectus abdominis muscle for chest wall reconstruction is based on the internal mammary neurovascular leash. The inferior epigastric vessels must be divided to allow rotation to the chest wall. This muscle can be mobilized and moved either as a muscle or as a musculocutaneous flap with the skin component oriented either horizontally or vertically, or both. The vertical skin flap, however, is more reliable, since it is oriented along the long axis of the muscle and thus would maintain more musculocutaneous perforators. The donor site is usually closed primarily. The rectus abdominis muscle is most useful in reconstruction of lower sternal wounds. Either muscle can be utilized, as their arc of rotation is identical.

RESULTS

Several large series have demonstrated that reconstruction of chest wall defects can be performed safely, with minimal deterioration of pulmonary function, and with lasting long-term benefits. Muscle necrosis rarely occurs, and nearly all wounds remain healed. It is our strong belief that the two key ingredients for successful management—namely, adequate, accurate resection of the chest wall lesion and dependable reconstruction—are accomplished most safely by the joint efforts of a thoracic and a plastic surgeon. Muscle or musculocutaneous transposition clearly is the procedure of choice for reconstruction of the thorax.

SUGGESTED READING

Arnold PG, Pairolero PC. Surgical management of the radiated chest wall. Plast Reconstr Surg 1986; 77:605–612.

Arnold PG, Pairolero PC, Waldorf JC. The serratus anterior muscle: Intrathoracic and extrathoracic utilization. Plast Reconstr Surg 1984; 73:240–248.

Pairolero PC, Arnold PG. Management of recalcitrant median sternotomy wounds. J Thorac Cardiovasc Surg 1984; 88:357–364.

Pairolero PC, Arnold PG. Thoracic wall defects: Surgical management of 205 consecutive patients. Mayo Clin Proc 1986; 61:557–563.

THE PLEURA

EMPYEMA AND BRONCHOPLEURAL FISTULA

G. HUGH LAWRENCE, M.D., F.A.C.S.

The degree of maturation of the pleural infection is of primary importance when deciding on alternative modes of treatment in the management of empyema thoracis. The spectrum of therapeutic alternatives extends from thoracentesis through open- and closed-tube drainage to the more extensive procedures of thoracoplasty and decortication of the lung. In addition, muscle flap coverage of a bronchopleural fistula may be necessary. Recently, direct reclosure of the fistulas has been recommended.

The importance of timing in relation to choice of treatment has been painfully relearned since the time of Hippocrates, particularly in postpneumonic cases in which the exact time of onset cannot be determined from the history. The character of the pleural fluid reflects the stage of intrapleural pathology and the stage of maturation of the disease. Thin pus, a pH above 7.2, and sediment of less than 30 percent of an aliquot placed in a test tube reflect absence of pleural symphysis. Open drainage at this time may result in pneumothorax, a serious, occasionally life-threatening, complication.

Rarely in cases in which thoracentesis reveals thin fluid, repeat thoracentesis combined with administration of antibiotics with systemic effects may be sufficient. More often thoracostomy and intercostal closed-tube drainage into an underwater seal device are necessary for continuous drainage. Rib resection and open-tube drainage are reserved for those situations in which the sediment pellicle in the aliquot of pleural aspirate is more than 75 percent and the chest tube is repeatedly plugged with debris from the cavity. Progressive narrowing of the rib interspaces is caused by fibrosis and contraction of the pyogenic membrane. This further prevents insertion of an intercostal tube of adequate size to drain the more solid contents. Particularly in children, open drainage is usually unnecessary, as most cases proceed to complete resolution without more extensive procedures. Irrigation for debridement of residual cavities and enzyme therapy are usually ineffective. Closed-tube drainage may produce complete reexpansion of the lung and closure of early postpneumonic bronchopleural fistulas.

Once tube drainage has achieved maximal lung expansion and a significant pleural space persists, then open drainage or decortication is indicated. In the elderly or debilitated patient or in the patient with a persistent small cavity, resection of a short length of rib (5 cm) under local anesthesia may be all that is necessary to break up loculated fluids, which then drain through an adequate-sized tube placed through the bed of the resected rib.

Two technical points warrant attention. Accurate localization for optimal drainage is often best marked by intracutaneous injection under fluoroscopic control of a solution of methylene blue diluted with a radiopaque medium such as propyliodone (Dionosil). The resultant chest x-ray film will confirm in the operating room the location of the radiopaque marker, which coincides with the readily visible skin tattoo. As a result, an optimum site for drainage is assured, and entering the free pleural space is avoided. Although this is a valuable technique, availability in the operating room of C-arm fluoroscope will make it unnecessary.

Next the neurovascular bundle below the resected rib should be ligated and divided to avoid its delayed erosion by the tube and resultant hemorrhage.

An appropriate drainage tube is often difficult to procure, as gum latex has now been replaced by more rigid plastics. The lumen of the tube should be of adequate size, i.e., large enough to permit insertion of the little finger, and soft enough not to erode the reexpanding lung and its vessels. Two tubes held side by side by a safety pin may be a useful substitute. A skin stitch of monofilament may become less inspissated with drainage and provide a tethering point for the pin during the frequent tube changes over the ensuing weeks. Tube repositioning prevents lung erosion and permits cavity closure. An accurate record should be kept of the length and number of tubes to avoid retention of a tube or a portion of one, resulting in prolonged drainage.

In good-risk patients in whom a large cavity persists after closed-tube drainage, decortication under general anesthesia is advisable. This is particularly true in post-traumatic hemothoracic empyema; it is less often necessary in post pneumonic cases, which usually respond to closed-tube drainage. Careful supervision of introduction, relocation, and replacement of the tube should reduce the necessity for decortication.

Closed-tube drainage does not prevent performance of a subsequent decortication, while open-tube drainage should be avoided if decortication, appears feasible. Empyectomy in the absence of tuberculosis is a technical exercise that my prove unnecessary, for the pleural space once obliterated seldom becomes reinfected. Air leaks should be avoided as one develops a cleavage plane between the pleura and the peel, particularly at the fissures. Air leaks should be controlled by ligature, imbrication of stitches, or cautery.

Resection combined with decortication is indicated when disease persists in the underlying lung, particularly when there has been a bronchopleural fistula or destruction of parenchyma. One must be sure that the remaining lung will be left free of significant disease and will be of sufficient size to prevent persistence of a postoperative pleural space and resultant recurrence of empyema. After decortication, a small residual air space may be obliterated and significant air leak stopped by inducing therapeutic pneumoperitoneum and further elevating the diaphragm with an abdominal binder. With the likelihood of inadequate lung to fill the pleural space, a tailoring thoracoplasty should be carried out in addition to decortication and resection, although, whenever possible, the procedures should not be done at the same time. Primary thoracoplasty is the definitive, but less immediate, solution to this complex problem; resection may then follow at a later stage as necessary.

In some cases it is impossible or inadvisable to reexpand the underlying lung, and as a result thoracoplasty may be necessary to obliterate the residual empyema cavity. Surgical resection and parenchymal fibrosis may have led to markedly reduced lung volume. Such cavities are usually the residual of prolonged open drainage. As a result, the chest wall is no longer pliable after rib resection, and therefore ribs, intercostal muscles, and pariental pleura must be resected to permit collapse of the remaining thoracic parietes into the cavity (Schede thoracoplasty). Packing or prolonged continued tube drainage is necessary until the cavity is completely obliterated. Appropriate physiotherapy and skeletal brace support may help reduce kyphoscoliosis and resultant reduction in respiratory reserve.

In the thoracoplasty it is necessary to close the posterior gutter of the thorax by resecting the rib at its angle, including the tip of the transverse process. This is particularly important in cases with bronchopleural fistula, which usually lies just anterior and lateral to the vertebral body. Closure of the adjacent pleural space is necessary.

The number of ribs resected will depend on the size of the cavity. At times, a tailoring thoracoplasty may be performed to close a small empyema cavity and bronchopleural fistula located peripherally in the upper lobe at the apex. In general, paradox is not a problem, as prolonged infection and fibrosis have stabilized the mediastinum. When in doubt, one should remember the old adage to "peck" at a thoracoplasty in stages.

A difficult situation arises when empyema develops and persists in the left paravertebral space along the aorta. In this location a rubber drainage tube may erode the adjacent vessel. Tube drainage high in the axilla may be extremely uncomfortable. In these and other situations in which prolonged drainage is advisable, an Eloesser flap may be indicated. With marsupialization of the cavity need for a tube is avoided, and the flap enhances the expulsion of air and drainage with each respiration.

When empyema or empyema with bronchopleural fistula follows pneumonectomy for cancer, one is often faced with the prospect of an extensive seven-rib Schede thoracoplasty and closure of the fistual with a pedicle flap of muscle. This disfiguring major procedure is often performed because of expectation of a poor prognosis in the primary disease. The outlook for this complication has improved markedly with the Clagett procedure, which is discussed in the chapter *The Clagett Procedures*. An extended Schede thoracoplasty is usually necessary in cases in which pneumonectomy has been performed for mycotic disease that persists in the pleural space or in which the Clagett procedure has failed repeatedly. In any case with associated bronchopleural fistula a pedicle flap of intercostal muscle may be employed to facilitate its closure.

The treatment of tuberculous empyema, either pure or the more lethal mixed form, requires individualization of surgical procedure, carried out under antimicrobial coverage. When only the pleura is diseased, decortication may be necessary when a residual pleural space persists, particularly after therapeutic pneumothorax. Either resection of a portion of the underlying diseased lung or total pleuropneumonectomy is indicated when the parenchymal involvement is more extensive. In the more lethal situation of mixed empyema, the general condition of the patient is often sufficiently precarious to warrant open drainage and antimicrobial and antibiotic therapy at the outset. After the clinical course has stabilized and the extent of parenchymal involvement has been determined, the need for either Schede thoracoplasty or resection, including pleuropneumonectomy, can be decided upon.

The use of high-velocity jet ventilation has greatly facilitated early management of the subsequent reoperation on bronchopleural fistula. It has been associated with nonoperative closure of some fistulas by markedly reducing tidal volume and lowering peak airway pressures.

In experienced hands, recent attempts at closure of post pneumonectomy fistulas approached through a vertical sternal split incision to gain access to the right bronchus and through the uninfected right chest to close the left bronchus have been associated with success. The bronchus must be redivided between the new line of closure and the old fistula to avoid recurrence. As the choices concerning the method of primary closure, stitch or staple, and also stump reinforcement differ, so do these technical choices vary in reclosure.

When disease persists beneath the area of thoracoplasty and is associated with massive hemoptysis, resection beneath the thoracoplasty area may be necessary after a trial of supportive therapy with blood replacement and oxytocin. Attempts at tamponade with Fogarty catheters followed by catheter embolization of the bronchial artery may be successful in desperate cases. Often resection beneath the thoracoplasty area is technically easier than expected, provided fungal disease does not persist and it is not a reresection. A double-lumen endobronchial tube or blocker of the bleeding bronchus is usually necessary.

SUGGESTED READING

Anderson RP, Lei W. Anterior transpericardial closure of a main bronchus fistula after pneumonectomy. Am J Surg 1983; 145:630–632.
Carlon GC, Ray C, Clain M, McCormack PM. High frequency positive pressure ventilation in management of a patient with bronchopleural fistula. Anesthesiology 1980; 52:160–162.
Lawrence GH. Problems of the pleural space. Philadelphia: WB Saunders, 1983:65.
Lemmer JH, Botham JH, Orringer MB. Modern management of adult thoracic empyema. J Thorac Cardiovasc Surg 1985; 90:849–855.
Stiles QR, Lindesmith G, Tucker BL, Meyer BW, Jones JC. Pleural empyema in children. Ann Thorac Surg 1970; 10:37–44.

OMENTOPLASTY FOR BRONCHOPLEURAL FISTULA

LAURI VIRKKULA, M.D.

Leakage of air from a drained empyema cavity is not dangerous per se, although it usually means a prolonged period of hospitalization for the patient. Adequate drainage may suffice for the treatment in some cases, but patients with persistent empyema cavities require elective operations after a period of drainage. The mode of surgical treatment depends on the location and the size of the cavity. After a pneumonectomy, the empyema cavity constitutes the entire pleural space. Parapulmonary empyema cavities occur in one part of the pleura, and elsewhere the pleural space is usually obliterated by inflammatory pleurodesis.

THE TREATMENT OF SUPRADIAPHRAGMATIC PARAPULMONARY EMPYEMA CAVITY WITH BRONCHIAL FISTULA

Before considering an omentoplasty operation, the treatment for supradiaphragmatic parapulmonary empyema cavity with bronchial fistula is the same as for empyema in general, i.e., early adequate drainage and observation. This type of bronchopleural fistula–empyema combination most often develops as a complication after surgical resection of the lower lobe of the lung. If good expansion of the upper lobe can be achieved, suction drainage through the chest tubes will lead to improvement and recovery of the patient. In the case in which the contents of the cavity do not drain outward via the chest tubes, a second thoracotomy is indicated, with evacuation of the cavity and careful checking of the positioning of the chest drains. Any attempts at resuturing a leaking bronchus that could lead to a pneumonectomy should not be attempted. Signs of inflammation, the size of the cavity, and the presence and type of fluid indicate whether the tube thoracostomy has been adequate. In this context, the amount of air leakage is of less importance. An open-window thoracostomy is the most efficient procedure in treating suppuration. It is done at the earliest when signs of sepsis persist in spite of continuous tube drainage or more usually when an inflammatory pleurodesis has developed in the area of the upper lobe and suppuration continues in the cavity. The chest drains may be disconnected from suction as needed and left open to drain passively, and the condition of the upper lobe may be evaluated with the aid of chest x-ray examination.

After adequate drainage of the contents of the cavity, a reasonable period of observation is in order, because cessation of the process of suppuration takes a certain amount of time; during this time the empyema cavity also decreases in size through healing and sometimes is obliterated. However, a persistent and stabilized supradiaphragmatic empyema cavity is an indication for further surgical management with an omentoplasty.

Because the pedicle of omentum has to fill the entire empyema cavity, it would be ideal if the volume of the pedicle and the volume of the cavity could be assessed preoperatively. However, there is no exact means of determining the volume of the omentum pedicle preoperatively, although the part of the omentum to be drawn into the thoracic space should measure from 150 to 350 cm^3, depending on the fat content of the patient's tissues. If the patient has had an open-window thoracostomy, the volume of the empyema cavity can be assessed by measuring the volume of the moist gauze swabs that were used to fill the cavity. In a patient with a tube thoracostoma, the best evaluation of the size of the cavity is obtained by means of computerized tomography. Contrast roentgenography performed through the drainage tube may be misleading and give the false impression of a sinus tract, even in the case of voluminous empyema cavity.

For the omentoplasty operation, the patient is placed on the operating table in the thoracolaparotomy position. A short upper midline incision is made to expose the greater omentum. It is dissected free from the stomach just along the greater curvature without injuring the gastroepiploic vessels. If the omental pedicle is to be transferred to the left pleural space, the right gastroepiploic vessels are tied and cut close to the gastroduodenal artery. The omentum is freed from the transverse colon and mesocolon. If the pedicle is to be prepared for the right pleural space, the technique is the same, but the right gastroepiploic vessels are left intact at the base of the pedicle and the left gastroepiploic artery is tied and cut. All efforts are made to prepare as large a pedicle as possible.

The empyema cavity is opened through a short thoracotomy incision, or, in the case of an open-window thoracostoma, the edges of the window are prepared for closure. After debridement of the cavity, the surgeon changes his gloves. Placement of the opening is decided by simultaneous examination of both sides of the diaphragm. The right lobe of the liver influences the positioning of the opening. If the lung is fixed onto the diaphragm, it may have to be dissected free. An opening admitting two to four fingers is made through the diaphragm. The opening is usually at the site of the right margin of the spleen on the left and near the sternum anteriorly, in the right side of the diaphragm. The distance of the opening from the bony thorax is usually 2 to 3 cm. The omental pedicle is drawn into the empyema cavity without injuring or twisting it. If necessary, the size of the opening in the diaphragm is reduced with sutures. With a few Dexon sutures the pedicle is then fixed to the edges of the bronchial fistula or near to it, onto the walls of the cavity, and to the edges of the opening in the diaphragm. Compression of the vessels of the pedicle is avoided. No attempt is made to suture close the fistula itself. Drainage tubes are placed in both the abdomen and the thorax. The wounds are closed. The nasogastric tube is left in place.

RESULTS OF OMENTOPLASTY

By using this mode of operative treatment, the empyema cavity and bronchopleural fistula healed in five of our cases out of a total of six. One patient died on the 32nd postoperative day from causes probably not related to the omental pedicle operation. In one case a three-rib thoracoplasty operation was done in conjunction with the pedicle operation, because it was found that the pedicle alone was insufficient to fill up the whole cavity.

In two cases there was a prolonged period of air leakage from the chest drains (16 and 30 days). No complications of an inflammatory nature occurred in the postoperative period, and no problems were experienced due to the opening in the diaphragm or the pedicle.

Advantages and Disadvantages of Omentoplasty for Bronchial Fistula

In the light of our experience gained thus far, it appears that omentoplasty for bronchial fistula produces good operative results. However, part of a few ribs may have to be removed in an open-window thoracostomy, and minor thoracoplasty may have to be done in conjunction with omentoplasty when the volume of the pedicle is found to be too small. No troublesome chest deformities developed, and for this reason it seems as though omentoplasty is of greater benefit than the traditional thoracoplasty. The operation is relatively simple, and it should be noted that no difficult dissection is involved, since the bronchial fistula area does not have to be mobilized and the empyema cavity is not tampered with except when it is opened and the pedicle is tunneled through from the abdomen.

If the volume of the pedicle is sufficient, the air leak ceases at the operation, since the omentum probably immediately obstructs the chest drain as well as the hole in the bronchus. The wall of the cavity as such poses no impediment to healing because of the excellent blood supply it receives via the pedicle. When considering possible complications that may stem from the insertion of the pedicle, it should be borne in mind that, although the abdominal omentum is inaccessible to standard preoperative examinations, the thoracic one may be investigated with the aid of computerized tomography. Also, with omentoplasty, the stomach loses two of its four major blood vessels to the omental pedicle. However, both clinical experience and studies of the collateral circulation of the stomach have shown that such a loss is well tolerated. This situation should be remembered in a case in which a later operation on the stomach has to be performed. In addition, after omentoplasty the stomach can no longer be used for reconstruction of the esophagus.

Editor's Note: Postpneumonectomy empyema and bronchopleural fistula can be managed with initial drainage, closure of the fistula, the use of omentum to cover the bronchus, and performance of a Clagett's procedure at a later date.

The author, however, has had no experience in the use of omental predicle in this way. For the method used by us in postpneumonectomy, empyema patients refer to Dr. Eerola's dissertation.

SUGGESTED READING

Eerola S. Treatment of postpneumonectomy empyema and associated mediastinal fistulae: a clinical study. Academic Dissertation, Helsinki, 1977.

Eloesser L. An operation for tuberculous empyema. Surg Gynecol Obstet 1935; 60:1096–1097.

Estlander JA. Resektion af refben vid kronisk empyema. Nord Med Arkiv 1879; 11:1–14.

Hollender LF, Bur F. Netzplastik. Chirurgie des grossen Netzes. Berlin-Heidelberg: Springer-Verlag, 1985:78.

Schultz RD. Collateral circulation of the stomach. In: Strandness DE Jr, ed. Collateral circulation in clinical surgery. Philadelphia: WB Saunders, 1969:462.

Virkkula L, Eerola S. Use of omental pedicle for treatment of bronchial fistula after lower lobectomy. Scand J Thorac Cardiovasc Surg 1975; 9:287–290.

TRANSSTERNAL TECHNIQUE FOR BRONCHOPLEURAL FISTULA

MIKHAIL I. PERELMAN, M.D.

The first two operations for transsternal closure of bronchial fistulas in pneumonectomized patients were undertaken by us in 1961; one, for a right bronchial fistula, was extrapericardial, and the other, for a left bronchial fistula, was intrapericardial. Both patients recovered. Our further collective experience with the transsternal technique is summarized in Table 1.

Over the past 25 years, the indications for transsternal techniques have varied. At first this approach was considered the best because in empyema of the residual cavity the entire operation could be done aseptically, via uninfected tissue. Later, the indications became somewhat narrow, for in the early 1970s a contralateral approach we had proposed came into use (Chirurgiya 1968; No.4:31–35). This approach is simpler technically than the transsternal one, and it, too, allows the operation to be performed aseptically. In the mid 1970s, the previously employed approach to the fistula through the empyema cavity again became popular. We prefer the posterior route, mainly on the right, with transpleural-transmediastinal dissection of the bronchial stump. On the left, this operation is much more difficult to accomplish because of the location of the aortic arch. Experience has shown that when the pleural cavity has been properly decontaminated, the risk of infection involved in the use of the transpleural-transmediastinal route is low. This route of access has an important advantage over the transsternal one in that it permits removal of the entire bronchial stump; it is also possible to treat and drain the empyema cavity adequately as well as to perform a concurrent thoracoplasty or muscle flap procedure if necessary. Finally, in 1986 we began to use a parasternal approach with resection of the anterior segments of the second and third ribs in patients with chronic empyema whose mediastinums were grossly displaced toward the removed lung. This technique provides a shorter, more direct, and more convenient route of access to the bronchial stump without the risk of pneumothorax formation on the side of the sole lung. Thus, the use of transpleural-transmediastinal technique on the right side and of contralateral or parasternal technique on the left side have limited the indications for the transsternal approach.

Today, we consider the transsternal technique to be indicated in patients with a medial or near-medial disposition of the mediastinum and an empyema that is not amenable to decontamination. Another indication may be a combination of bronchial fistula with arrosional hemorrhage from the pulmonary artery stump—again in patients with a medially disposed mediastinum. One such patient was cured as the result of transpericardial ligation of the right pulmonary artery and bronchial occlusion.

Contraindications to the transsternal technique are a mediastinum that is strongly shifted toward the removed lung, a very short bronchial stump, or its virtual absence (tracheal fistula).

The timing of surgery usually depends on the efficacy of treatment and the clinical course. Conservative treatment includes drainage of the pleural cavity using one or two drainage tubes, continual or systematic lavage of the cavity, cauterization of the fistula via bronchoscope or thoracoscope, and antimicrobial and general supportive therapy. This treatment is continued as long as it is bringing benefit and the hope remains that the fistula will heal.

In the past, we used to perform a complete longitudinal sternotomy, but in recent years we dissect the sternum in an ⊥-shaped manner in patients in whom it is long. First we divide the sternum transversely at the level of the third intercostal space and then dissect the upper portion at the midline. One should always take care to avoid damaging the pleural sac of the sole lung, which in such patients is often contiguous with the entire posterior surface of the sternum. However, it is not always possible to avoid damage. On the right, the bronchial stump can be dissected out without opening the pericardium, via the aortocaval space. This approach is technically difficult, and therefore the transpericardial route is clearly preferable. The pericardium is opened by a vertical incision 7 to 8 cm long as far to the right as possible. The right pulmonary artery is mobilized and sutured with a stapler. The artery is then transected peripheral to the stapler and ligated additionally central to it. The bronchial stump is identified by placing a finger deep inside the wound. In difficult cases, the stump is visualized by transillumination from the inside via bronchoscope in a darkened operating room. Next, the stump is mobilized from the scar by blunt and sharp dissection and sutured with the stapler as close to the trachea as possible. Peripheral to the stapler, the stump is transected and the stapler is removed. The

TABLE 1 Surgery for Postpneumonectomy Bronchial Fistulas

		Results		
Operation	*No. Patients*	*Cured*	*Relapsed*	*Died*
Transsternal	39	29	1	9
Parasternal	2	2	—	—
Thoracopleural	37	35	1	1
Contralateral	25	20	1	4
Total	103	86	3	14

lumen of the peripheral stump is treated with 10 percent tincture of iodine and is resected in as far as possible. In the remaining portion, the mucosa is destroyed by electrocoagulation, 33 percent silver nitrate, or trichloroacetic acid. The lumen of the remaining stump is sutured with several interrupted Vicryl (3–0 to 4–0) sutures. The mechanical suture line on the trachea is covered with a pedicled pericardial flap, which is fixed in place by similar sutures. Myoplastic repair is not usually possible. (It can be effectively done, using the greater pectoral muscle, only from a parasternal approach.) If the fistula is left-sided, we also open the pericardium anterior to the diaphragmatic nerve. To secure a convenient access to the left bronchial stump, it is better to suture, ligate, and divide not only the left pulmonary artery but also the superior pulmonary vein. The bronchus is then treated in the same way as on the right. Before suturing the wound, a drainage tube is passed between the sutured bronchial stumps. A second drainage tube is placed behind the sternum. The two tubes are connected to an aspiration system for 2 or 3 days. Through a separate pleural drainage tube, the empyema cavity is treated with antiseptics or antibiotics and aspirated, in an attempt to obtain a sterile serous exudate. The drainage tube is then removed and the cavity is periodically punctured in order to fill it with plasma containing antibiotics. Subsequently, a fibrothorax should gradually form. If it fails to form, the residual cavity has to be closed by a thoracomyoplastic procedure. The remaining peripheral bronchial stump may persistently secrete mucus or develop a cyst that periodically empties its contents into the pleural cavity. In the former case, coagulating the stump mucus with chemicals through a thoracic fistula may be effective. If not or if a cyst has appeared (as it did in two of our cases), removal of the stump from a transpleural approach is indicated.

The treatment of fistulas recurring after transsternal operations is always difficult.* When it is not feasible to eliminate the fistula by bronchoscopic or thoracoscopic methods, transpleural removal of the dissected-off bronchial stump with concomitant thoracomyoplasty is advisable. During such an operation we usually also remove the pars infraspinate of the shoulder blade.

* Editor's Note: If the fistula has healed, a Clagett procedure can be used to deal with the remaining cavity. The omentum has been particularly helpful in closing recalcitrant BPFs. Mathisen DJ, Grillo HC. The use of the omentum in complicated cardiothoracic problems. J Thorac Cardiosvasc Surg (in press).

SUGGESTED READING

Abruzzini P. Trattamento chirurgico delle fistole del bronco principale consecutive a pneumonectomia per tubercolosie. La Chirurgia Toracica Giugno 1961; 14:3.

Bruni F. Treatment of long stump after pneumonectomy. Int Trends Gen Thorac Surg 1987; 2:413–422.

Mathisen DJ, Grillo HC. The use of the omentum in complicated cardiothoracic problems. J Thorac Cardiovasc Surg (in press).

Perelman MI. Chirurgiya 1968; 4:31–35.

MUSCLE FLAP IN BRONCHOPLEURAL FISTULA

PETER C. PAIROLERO, M.D.
PHILLIP G. ARNOLD, M.D.

Bronchopleural fistula has always been a dreaded complication of pulmonary resection. Many fistulas uncomplicated by underlying pulmonary or pleural disease heal spontaneously or with relatively simple measures. Persistent fistulas, however, are generally associated with pleural empyema and fail to respond to the more common methods of treatment. Among the techniques that have been advocated to control bronchopleural fistula are cauterization, direct suture closure, thoracoplasty, and pulmonary resection. Although all methods of treatment have had some success, failure often can be attributed to a persistent pleural space with continuing empyema and eventual breakdown of repair. To manage empyema in these situations, many thoracic surgeons currently would perform open pleural drainage. We believe that muscle transposition offers an effective alternative method of management because the closed bronchial fistula can be reinforced and the residual pleural space can be obliterated with this technique.

To close a bronchopleural fistula successfully, muscle flaps must have an intact blood supply, a sufficient length to reach the fistula without tension, and a sufficient volume to obliterate the empyema cavity completely. Of the various muscles that have been transposed, the chest wall skeletal muscles (pectoralis major, latissimus dorsi, and serratus anterior) best fulfill these criteria and have been the most satisfactory. In selected situations, however, the rectus abdominis muscle may also be useful.

Chest wall skeletal muscles are ideal to transpose into the thorax. All have a single dominant as well as a secondary blood supply. Complete mobilization of these muscles, which usually includes division of humeral and shoulder attachments and division of the secondary blood supply, has been previously reported and does allow transposition to most intrathoracic locations. The axis of rotation is identical for the latissimus dorsi and serratus anterior muscles, since both are supplied by the thoracodorsal neurovascular leash. The arc of rotation, however, is longer for the latissimus dorsi muscle since the muscle itself is longer. Following complete mobilization, all three muscle flaps are also of sufficient volume that obliteration of most residual pleural spaces is possible. Finally, transposition of the pectoralis major and latissimus dorsi muscles results in minimal functional upper extremity disability. Transposition of the entire serratus anterior muscle, however, does result in winging of the scapula.

All chest wall skeletal muscles require a route of entry when transposed into the thorax. Generally, only a 5- to 7-cm segment of one rib, usually the anterior portion of the second, needs to be resected to provide an adequate entrance into the thorax. The location of this opening is best determined by the muscle's blood supply, and the opening should be selected to avoid kinking of the neurovascular leash and subsequent muscle ischemia.

Although all three skeletal chest wall muscles reach most intrathoracic locations, we generally prefer transposition of the serratus anterior muscle for repair of most bronchopleural fistulas. This muscle is nearly always intact following thoracotomy, and, when completely mobilized, it is a moderate sized, flat, malleable muscle that can be wrapped around structures or inserted into most cavities. When intact, the latissimus dorsi muscle is very similar but much larger and has the added advantage of a longer arc of rotation. In most instances, however, this muscle has been transected during previous thoracotomy, thereby limiting its usefulness to management of apical fistulas or simultaneous transposition with the serratus anterior muscle for additional bulk. The pectoralis major muscle is ideally suited for management of apical bronchopleural fistulas. Fistulas located in this area can frequently be approached through an axillary incision, which readily allows closure of the fistula, mobilization of the muscle, and obliteration of the empyema cavity.

Muscle transposition should be considered in all patients with chronic bronchopleural fistula, especially fistulas secondary to radiation necrosis or destructive lung disease. In these patients, conventional pulmonary resection alone frequently results in a residual pleural space because the remaining lung often has restrictive lung disease that prevents postoperative expansion. In these patients, muscle transposition not only reinforces the closed bronchial stump but also can completely obliterate the residual pleural space.

Bronchopleural fistula associated with postpneumonectomy empyema deserves special consideration. Muscle transposition also should be considered in these patients. However, we make no attempt to obliterate the postpneumonectomy cavity because of its size. Clagett and Geraci, in 1963, demonstrated that the treatment of choice for postpneumonectomy empyema was open pleural drainage without thoracoplasty followed by antibiotic instillation and chest wall closure when the wound was clean several months later. Stafford and Clagett subsequently reported that this method was effective in 88 percent of their patients. We continue to follow this principle. However, we believe that transposition of a well-vascularized muscle to the bronchial stump at the time of open drainage protects the stump from further ischemia and necrosis.

Patients with postpneumonectomy empyema are initially managed with closed thoracostomy tube drainage to control the infection. Open pleural drainage is then performed in the most dependent portion of the thorax, and the pleural cavity is thoroughly debrided. The bronchopleural fistula is simultaneously closed and reinforced with viable chest wall muscle. Wet dressings of a solution of betadine diluted 20:1 are then packed into the thorax and changed several times daily, more frequently if drainage is excessive. Further debridement can be accomplished by placing the patient in a whirlpool tank after several days if his or her condition permits. After 7 to 10 days, the patient can generally be discharged from the hospital, and treatments can be continued at home. Excellent home care can be obtained by a hand-held showerhead followed by wet to dry dressing changes to mechanically debride the wound. After several months, when pink, healthy granulation tissue is present, the pleural cavity is closed following instillation of antibiotic solution.

We have recently reported our experience with intrathoracic transposition of chest wall skeletal muscle in the management of bronchopleural fistula and postpneumonectomy empyema. During a 6-year period, 22 patients (17 males and five females) underwent 35 intrathoracic muscle transpositions. Eleven patients had chronic bronchopleural fistula and 11 had postpneumonectomy empyema. Ten patients had multiple muscle transpositions. Ages ranged from 47 to 80 years, with a mean age of 58.0 years. Thirty-day operative mortality was 9.1 percent (two patients). Follow-up of the 20 operative survivors ranged from 3 to 72 months, with a mean of 17.6 months. Seventeen patients (85 percent) had no further signs or symptoms of bronchopleural fistula or infection. Of the three patients with recurrent infections, two died. We conclude that chest wall skeletal muscle transposition is an excellent method of treatment of persistent bronchopleural fistula.

SUGGESTED READING

Arnold PG, Pairolero PC, Waldorf JC. The serratus anterior muscle: intrathoracic and extrathoracic utilization. Plast Reconstr Surg 1984; 73:240–246.

Clagett OT, Geraci JE. A procedure for the management of postpneumonectomy empyema. J Thorac Cardiovasc Surg 1963; 45:141.

Pairolero PC, Arnold PG. Bronchopleural fistula: treatment by transposition of pectoralis major muscle. J Thorac Cardiovasc Surg 1980; 79:142–145.

Pairolero PC, Arnold PG, Piehler JM. Intrathoracic transposition of extrathoracic skeletal muscle. J Thorac Cardiovasc Surg 1983; 86:809–817.

Stafford EG, Clagett OT. Postpneumonectomy empyema: neomycin instillation and definitive closure. J Thorac Cardiovasc Surg 1972; 63:771–775.

THE CLAGETT PROCEDURE

G. HUGH LAWRENCE, M.D., F.A.C.S.

After pneumonectomy, postresection empyema is immediately treated by closed intercostal tube drainage connected to a waterseal device until the patient has become afebrile and his condition stable. As the majority of pneumonectomies are performed for cancer, which, despite careful preoperative staging, may be associated with a limited prognosis, the surgeon is loathe to subject the patient to a second major and disfiguring procedure, i.e., a Schede thoracoplasty. In the early 1950s James Clagett of the Mayo Clinic faced this problem in a patient in whom two positive lymph nodes were found at pneumonectomy. The empyema was drained with an open tube that was irrigated with neomycin. It seemed illogical that such a large cavity could be closed once infected, yet the tube thoracostomy was closed after the cavity had been irrigated for 6 weeks. This patient survived for more than 20 years after his operation.

The procedure should be performed electively as soon after tube drainage as the patient's condition warrants. It is important to locate the thoracostomy anteriorly, for in this location the patient can carry out his own irrigation and retain it in the hemithorax when reclining. The opening is usually made through the bed of the previous incision. If necessary, a 5-cm length of rib anteriorly should be resected up to but not including the costochondral junction. The skin edges and adjacent subcutaneous tissues are freed so as to marsupialize the wound by sewing them to the thickened peel on the pleura. A biopsy of this peel will yield a meaningful culture on which to base the choice of the antibiotic for irrigation of the empyema cavity. The absorptive surface of the pleura must be recognized when one is considering antibiotic irrigation, for toxicity may result. Ototoxicity has been reported following irrigation with 0.5 percent neomycin solution and may occur with other aminoglycosides. In actuality, as the infection is no longer invasive, it is probable that cavity irrigation twice daily with 0.5 percent acetic acid or Dakin's solution may be as effective and safer. The irrigating solution should be retained for 20 minutes after introduction and then the cavity emptied into a kidney basin.

The timing of the closure may be set empirically at 6 weeks after the start of irrigations, or it may be determined by the appearance of the wound and cavity as well as its drainage. Quantitative wound cultures may be used, with a bacterial count of less than 10^5 of an aliquot of peel biopsy indicating likelihood of successful closure.

There was recurrence in one-third of Clagett's cases, most commonly when the onset of postpneumonectomy empyema was delayed from weeks to 26 years following the initial resection. Five patients consented to a second and, rarely, a third attempt at sterilization of the cavity; all the operations were successful. No single author has a large statistically significant experience with repeated attempts with this procedure. The chance of success in itself warrants a repeat attempt before the surgeon resorts to thoracoplasty.

In closing the thoracostomy wound its edges should be saucerized and the clean surfaces approximated with monofilament retention sutures to be left in place for at least 2 weeks. Most authors feel it important to leave a dose of the antibiotic or other irrigating agent in the cavity at the time of closure. It is probable that optimum nutrition, previous irrigation with reduction in bacteria, and wound closure are more important to final success than is any final topical application.

Cases with a small associated bronchopleural fistula have been managed successfully with this technique provided the cavity has been well drained prior to initiation of irrigations and the fistula is sufficiently small to permit irrigations without aspiration of significant amounts of irrigating solution.

SUGGESTED READING

Clagett OT, Geraci JE. A procedure for the management of postpneumonectomy empyema. J Thorac Cardiovasc Surg 1963; 45:141–145.

Provan JL. The management of postpneumonectomy empyema. J Thorac Cardiovasc Surg 1971; 61:107–109.

Hakim M, Milstein BB. Empyema thoracis and infected pneumonectomy space: case for cyclical irrigation. Ann Thorac Surg 1986; 41:85–88.

SPACE PROBLEMS DURING AND AFTER LUNG RESECTION

EDWARD R. TOWNSEND, M.B., B.S., F.R.C.S.
STEPHEN WESTABY, B.S.,M.S., F.R.C.S.

Traditionally thoracic surgeons have gone to considerable lengths to avoid intrapleural air pockets following lung resection, to such a degree that obliteration of space may mistakenly have become more important than the preservation of lung tissue in patients with poor respiratory reserve. In the era of tuberculosis and before the prophylactic (and therapeutic) use of antibiotics, an air space between the lung and the chest wall was synonymous with empyema. In today's surgical practice in areas in which atypical tuberculosis is prevalent, the space may need to be obliterated. Thoracoplasty, plombage, and open drainage have been used to eradicate chronic sepsis and patient debilitation. But does this now necessarily apply? Our experience would suggest that this is not the case.

PREVENTION OF SPACES DURING LUNG RESECTION—THE "EXPECTED SPACE"

After lobectomy, segmental resection, decortication, or drainage of pneumothorax, we expect healthy lung to expand to fill the pleural cavity. Elevation of the ipsilateral diaphragm, together with shift of the mediastinum; usually compensates effectively for resection of a single lobe, especially when an air leak is minimal or absent. Circumstances that predispose to residual air pockets are as follows:

1. Extended resections, for instance, right-sided upper or lower lobe, together with the middle lobe.
2. A fixed mediastinum or diaphragm after empyema.
3. A large air leak from the surface of the residual lung tissue.
4. Poor compliance of the residual lung tissue.

Under these circumstances, a residual air space may be expected. Undoubtedly the best opportunity to eliminate this space is before chest closure. A number of procedures have been advocated for this purpose, including thoracoplasty, pleural tent (which leaves an extrapleural space), and phrenic nerve crush. The authors suggest the following approach.

First, ask the question, "Is preservation of the residual lobe necessary for a satisfactory functional outcome?" One must balance the risks of prolonged intercostal drainage and restriction of activity in the postoperative period against the benefits of the residual lung tissue in terms of respiratory function and limitation of activity. If the patient has adequate respiratory reserve, then it may be better both in terms of rate of recovery and eradication of disease to resect the entire lung.

When the residual lung must be preserved, it is important to minimize air leak so that negative pressure may be applied to the space.* This is best done by diathermy coagulation of multiple small areas or by suture of large raw areas. However, the latter technique may further reduce the volume of residual lung tissue and must be performed with care. In the future surgical glues (fibrin-based) will play an increasingly important role in sealing leaks. Intercostal drains must be carefully placed and hemostasis must be meticulous so as to avoid an intrapleural hematoma. Suction is used to oppose the visceral pleura to the chest wall over as great an area as possible, thereby encouraging the two surfaces to adhere. On occasion pleurectomy or talc pleurodesis may be used to expedite this process. The authors have successfully used phrenic nerve crush in patients with considerable mismatch between lung volume and pleural space, but we avoid this following pneumonectomy. Diaphragmatic function usually recovers between 6 weeks and 3 months after operation.

After lung resection, it is imperative to maintain full expansion of the residual lobe by breathing exercises, physiotherapy, and careful airway toilet. In patients with excess secretions or infections, a mini-tracheostomy may be required. Collapse of a small residual lobe is difficult to reverse, produces a space, and predisposes to intrapleural and pulmonary infections. Prophylactic antibiotics are given routinely to all our patients, and in the presence of a space, this administration is prolonged. Suction on the drains is continued until the space is obliterated. Normally the air leak ceases within 6 to 8 days. After this the risks of intrapleural infection via the drain track, or (rarely) as a result of hemorrhage from an intercostal drain, or, more particularly, from immobilization of the patient, become unacceptably high. The drains are therefore withdrawn, and the patient is observed carefully to determine the outcome. In the majority of patients the lung remains expanded or a small and acceptable air space forms and persists. In the absence of infection and as long as the lobe remains functional, we consider such a space acceptable and do not advocate further drainage. Daily clinical examination and chest x-ray studies are required to determine the progress of the space. The majority slowly reduce in size or become filled with fluid that either slowly absorbs or persists.

THE PERSISTENT AIR LEAK

In the majority of patients air leaks progressively decrease and then stop. In a small proportion, however, usually those with emphysema, a large volume air leak may persist. This situation is often found in association with a fully expanded residual lobe or a small apical air pocket. Suction on the intercostal drain potentiates the air leak in these patients and should be discontinued, unless the lobe collapses completely as a result. After 6 to 8 days the visceral pleura is usually adherent to the chest wall and the lung will not totally collapse. In such circumstances we recommend clamping the drain or drains ear-

* Editor's note: We would agree with the authors in recommending the use of a generous apical pleural tent to cover any raw surface of lung in order to facilitate stoppage of air leaks and simplify the management of spaces.

ly in the day, followed by an x-ray taken 1 to 2 hours later. Provided there is no significant change in the air space, reconfirmed by a repeat x-ray 6 hours later, the drains remain clamped. A further x-ray study is performed the next day. If the pneumothorax is unchanged, the drains are removed, or if the air space has increased, drainage is reestablished and the procedure repeated in 4 to 5 days. In the authors' experience, it is nearly always successful.

APPEARANCE OF A SPACE IN THE EARLY POSTOPERATIVE PERIOD

A postoperative space may be filled with air, blood, lymph, or pus. A hemothorax is caused by inadequate hemostasis, reactionary hemorrhage, or inadequate drainage. These are all preventable and should be managed by surgical evacuation at an early stage to prevent empyema or fibrothorax. The authors advocate suction on all intercostal drains in the early postoperative period in order to prevent hemothorax. When the residual lung has initially filled the hemithorax, an air space may form if the drains are removed prematurely (from a delayed air leak) or if air is allowed to enter the pleural cavity accidentally. Both circumstances are preventable. A small apical space may prove acceptable and disappear completely in a few days. Larger spaces should be eliminated immediately by needle aspiration or preferably by further intercostal drainage and suction until the visceral and parietal pleurae adhere. Again, experience has shown that small residual air pockets are harmless in the absence of infection and preferable to the undoubted morbidity associated with prolonged intercostal drainage. (Thoracoplasty is seldom justified in such circumstances.) However, in the presence of a large space with persistent air leak, artificial pneumoperitoneum has proved effective in elevating the diaphragm and allowing the residual lobe to fill the space. This must be performed with extreme care, preferably using a peritoneal dialysis catheter and not a needle, which may easily lacerate the viscera. Up to 1 L of air may be used to inflate the peritoneal cavity, while carefully observing vital signs. This is best done within the first 24 hours postoperatively with the patient kept in the upright position. The authors favor thoracoscopy and talc (plain or iodized) in recurring pneumothoraces, when the residual lung can be shown to fully inflate and fill the space.

THE INFECTED RESIDUAL SPACE

The incidence of intrapleural infection following lung resection has been dramatically reduced by modern antibiotic prophylaxis. Predisposing surgical factors such as contamination of the pleural space, prolonged duration of surgery, excessive use of diathermy, and autoinfection may be avoided by appropriate preoperative preparation and good surgical techniques. Diabetics and immunosuppressed patients are at higher risk for infections. An infected space suspected in the febrile patient is confirmed by needle aspiration and culture.

It is imperative to drain an infected space and initially attempt to obliterate it by negative pressure. Appropriate antibiotic treatment and physiotherapy are essential to limit the spread of infection and preserve respiratory function.

The authors have successfully used space irrigation through an intravenous catheter in conjunction with dependent intercostal drainage. A long venous catheter is inserted into the apex of the space, which is irrigated with normal saline, or dilute betadine, or an antibiotic solution such as gentamicin or neomycin. Underwater seal drainage applies negative pressure to the space and may eventually obliterate it. After a series of six negative cultures on 3 successive days, the drain may be removed, or if a space persists, then fill the space with the appropriate antibiotic and remove the drain and close the drain site (Clagett's procedure). If this approach proves unsuccessful, further management is directed to the treatment of empyema as discussed elsewhere.

SUGGESTED READING

Barker WL, Langston HT, Naffah P. Postresection spaces. Ann Thorac Surg 1966; 2:299–326.

Rainer WG, Newby JP. Prevention of residual space problems after pulmonary resection. Am J Surg 1967; 744–747.

Weisel W, Thimming KF, Watson RR. The fate of the residual pleural space following small resections for pulmonary tuberculosis. J Thorac Surg 1957; 33:390–398.

MALIGNANT PLEURAL EFFUSION

M. WAYNE FLYE, M.D., Ph.D.

Recurrent pleural effusions are prevalent and vexing problems in patients with advanced malignant disease. Many of these patients experience marked respiratory discomfort, although other aspects of the disease would allow them to lead active and productive lives. Frequent thoracenteses inconvenience both patient and physician, can cause the complications of pneumothorax and protein depletion, and at best provide only temporary symptomatic relief. More satisfactory methods for controlling these effusion have been developed.

Malignant pleural effusions are most commonly secondary to lung cancer, breast cancer, or lymphoma (Hodgkin's or nonHodgkin's). Metastases from malignant ovarian, genitourinary, and gastrointestinal tumors as well as less common malignant tumors such as mesothelioma, sarcomas, and melanoma also can cause pleural effusion. The primary mechanisms of pathogenesis of neoplastic effusion are thought to be pleural involvement or lymphatic obstruction by tumor.

The development of shortness of breath, cough, or chest pain in a patient with known malignant disease should raise the suspicion of pleural effusion. While physical findings, such as dullness or egophony, often pick up only the larger effusions, a chest roentgenogram will detect as little as 100 ml of pleural fluid if obtained in the lateral decubitus position. Pleural effusion seen on an upright chest roentgenogram represents at least 300 ml of fluid. Development of a pleural effusion in a patient with malignant disease probably, but not always, represents progression of the tumor. However, careful evaluation of the effusion is warranted in all patients without regard to a previous history of malignant disease.

An accurate distinction between exudative and transudative pleural effusion is important. If it can be established with certainty that an effusion is secondary to a transudative process (specific gravity <1.018), pleural disease as such can be ruled out, and appropriate therapy can be directed at the altered hydrostatic or colloid osmotic pressure. If an effusion is clearly secondary to an exudative process, further diagnostic efforts, including cytopathology and pleural biopsy, must be undertaken to establish the exact nature of the pleural disease. An exudate is present if one or more of the following criteria exist: (1) pleural fluid protein–serum protein ratio greater than 0.5; (2) pleural fluid (lactic dehydrogenase or LDH)–serum LDH ratio greater than 0.6; or (3) pleural fluid LDH greater than 200 IU. Once the exudative nature of the effusion has been established, cytologic examination of the pleural fluid is part of routine evaluation. Since the absence of malignant cells in the pleural fluid does not rule out malignant disease, a pleural biopsy may be diagnostic.

In some patients, treatment of the underlying tumor may result in objective improvement of the pleural effusion. Unfortunately, despite recent advances in chemotherapy and radiation therapy, there are still many patients who are disabled by persistent effusions. Despite their lack of direct effect on tumor growth, other techniques have been developed to provide local control of pleural fluid accumulation and alleviate the associated respiratory distress.

THORACENTESIS

Thoracentesis is clearly the first technique to employ in a patient with an effusion. Of course, it must be done initially for diagnostic purposes, but it is also important for determining the effect of removal of the effusion on the patient's respiratory symptoms. Symptoms of some patients are relieved after the first thoracentesis, and they require no further local therapy. For the many patients who rapidly have recurrence, further thoracenteses are unlikely to give lasting relief. In addition, repeated and frequent thoracenteses are not without complications. Hypoproteinemia often results and even contributes to an increasing rate of effusion reaccumulation. Pneumothorax, empyema, and fluid loculation also threaten each aspiration. For these reasons, thoracentesis has a limited role in the continuing treatment of recurrent malignant effusions.

PLEURODESIS

The ideal treatment of a recurrent pleural effusion should be 100 percent effective, safe, and convenient. The intrapleural administration of isotopes, nitrogen mustard, or chest tube drainage alone should no longer have a role in the local therapy of recurrent malignant effusion because of the difficulties of administration or their ineffectiveness.

Because of its minimal inconvenience and toxicity, I favor tetracycline as the intrapleural sclerotic agent of choice. Although intrapleural instillation of a talc suspension is almost as convenient as that of a tetracycline solution, sterile talc is not as readily available, and the side effects are not as well documented. Because of its frequent side effects and occasional serious complications, we do not recommend intrapleural use of quinacrine.

Whichever agent is used, the effectiveness of local therapy is correlated with the degree of pleurodesis achieved. To maximize the chance of this obliterative process, concomitant thoracostomy drainage is mandatory. For the intrapleural agent to be most effective in producing the necessary chemical pleuritis, the pleural space must be fully evacuated before the agent is instilled. After the agent has been allowed to be fully distributed over the pleural surfaces, any subsequent effusion must be immediately removed so that both pleural surfaces remain opposed.

I advocate the following technique for tube thoracostomy and chemical pleurodesis: The lightly sedated patient is placed on his side, and the eighth intercostal space is identified at the midaxillary line. After several milliliters of local anesthesia have been injected, a 24 F thoracic catheter is inserted at this point and advanced until the last hole in the tube (an extra hole cut before insertion) is inside the pleural space. The tube is sutured in place, and the chest cavity is drained into a waterseal suction device. Complete evacuation of fluid and full lung expansion should be verified by chest roentgenography before proceeding with the intrapleural agent. Because instillation of either tetracycline or talc may be painful, an injection of meperidine or morphine is administered 1 hour before instillation to minimize this discomfort. If tetracycline is to be used, 500 mg is diluted in 30 to 50 ml of saline solution. For talc, 20 g of USP talc powder previously gas sterilized and aerated is suspended in 250 ml of sterile saline solution. Just before instillation the chest tube is clamped. Tetracycline is administered by needle directly into the chest tube. Ten to 20 ml of saline solution are then injected to clear the tube. The talc suspension is instilled with a catheter-tipped syringe directly into the temporarily disconnected chest tube. Regardless of the agent used, the chest tube is then left clamped for 2 hours. During this period the patient is placed in several positions, including supine and prone, to distribute the agent over the entire pleural surface. The tube is then unclamped and left on low suction. After instillation is completed, pleural drainage is carefully monitored. Only when drainage ceases (usually 3 or 4 days) and the pleural space is obliterated is the chest tube removed. Occasionally a second course of treatment is needed for inadequate pleurodesis.

PLEURECTOMY

Since many surgeons consider parietal pleurectomy to be far more effective than chemical pleurodesis in the treatment of recurrent pneumothorax, pleurectomy should also be more effective in controlling recurrent malignant pleural effusion. Although there is 99 percent improvement in the control of the effusion, these patients in general are poor operative risks. The mortality is 6 to 10 percent, and the incidence of postoperative complications is about 25 percent. Therefore, pleurectomy should not be considered for most patients. In the occasional patient, however, one or both lungs may have become trapped in an underexpanded state. After evacuation of the pleural fluid, the patient may still have impairment of respiratory effort. The surgeon may then be tempted to decorticate the lung to allow both reexpansion and pleurodesis. However, the trapped lung has usually resulted from extensive intrapleural tumor, and the results of thoracotomy generally are not satisfactory.

Occasionally, prolonged thorocostomy drainage may result, thereby limiting the patient's activities, contributing to protein loss, and confining the patient to the hospital. The use of a pleuroperitoneal shunt should be considered for these cases. Although normally the intraperitoneal pressure exceeds the negative intrapleural pressure, continued production of the pleural effusion will generate a pressure gradient with drainage into the peritoneal cavity.

Although the prompt and efficient management of the malignant pleural effusion generally does not contribute to the patient's longevity, it usually greatly contributes to his comfort and well-being.

SUGGESTED READING

Austin EH, Flye MW. The treatment of recurrent malignant pleural effusion. Ann Thorac Surg 1979; 28:190–203.

Anderson CB, Philpott GW, Ferguson TB. The treatment of malignant pleural effusions. Cancer 1974; 33:916–922.

Light RW. Pleural effusions. Med Clin North Am 1977; 61:1339.

Martini N, Bains MS, Beattie EJ Jr. Indications for pleurectomy in malignant effusion. Cancer 1975; 35:734–738.

Shedbalkar AR, Head JM, Head LR, et al. Evaluation of talc pleural symphysis in the management of malignant pleural effusion. J Thorac Cardiovasc Surg 1971; 61:492–497.

SPONTANEOUS PNEUMOTHORAX

BLAIR A. KEAGY, M.D.
BENSON R. WILCOX, M.D.

Tuberculosis was thought to be the cause of pneumothorax until 1932, when Kjaergaard established a nontuberculous etiology for the majority of patients with this problem. He recognized that spontaneous pneumothorax most often occurs in young, otherwise healthy individuals following rupture of a subpleural bleb. Bleb formation is most likely due to dissection of air from the rupture of an alveolus. The air then passes through interstitial tissue planes into the fibrous layer of the visceral pleura, where it accumulates to form a bleb. This sequence may result from partial obstruction of a peripheral airway.

The reported incidence of spontaneous pneumothorax depends on the population reviewed and has ranged from 6 to 15 cases per 100,000 population, with a male preponderance of three or four to one. In addition, there is an increased frequency in tall people and individuals with long narrow chests. The usual age for the occurrence of a spontaneous pneumothorax is from 20 to 30 years.

Pneumothorax tends to occur most often while the patient is sedentary rather than during a period of heavy exercise. There is a slight predilection for the right lung. The predominant symptom associated with a pneumothorax is chest pain, which occurs in 95 percent of patients. Less common symptoms include shortness of breath, present in about half of the patients, and cough, found in approximately 10 percent.

Various etiologic relationships have been established. Smoking is clearly associated with the development of a pneumothorax, and meconium staining at birth has been seen in neonates who subsequently developed both pneumothorax and pneumomediastinum. There is a slight familial association with pneumothorax, and abnormalities of the first or second rib have been seen in some patients with pneumothorax.

Other causes of pneumothorax include malignancy, chronic obstructive pulmonary disease, cystic fibrosis, trauma, and esophageal perforation. Infrequently, pneumothorax is associated with the menstrual period. At one time it was felt that air entered the peritoneal cavity through the female genital tract and then entered the chest through a diaphragmatic defect. More recently, however, operative findings have suggested that the cause is a defect in the pleura secondary to endometrial implants.

Reports on the incidence of recurrent spontaneous pneumothorax following an initial episode are variable, generally falling in the range of 50 percent, although recurrence rates as high as 70 percent have been reported to occur in individuals treated without a chest catheter. The rate of recurrence increases after the second or third event and may be as high as 70 to 80 percent.

The rate of complications associated with pneumothorax is higher in patients older than 40 years and the risk of operation is greater. Rather than the usual apical location seen in younger patients, older individuals tend to have a more diffuse cystic disease, and all blebs cannot be removed. Thus in many cases recurrences in patients with chronic obstructive pulmonary disease may be best treated with repeated chest tube insertions. This approach avoids the higher risk of surgery, although many chest tube insertions may be required over a period of months or years.

TREATMENT

Observation and Bed Rest

Historically, pneumothorax was treated with bed rest and observation. The main disadvantage associated with this approach was the time required for resolution of the problem. In some cases a hospital stay of 10 days to 2 weeks was necessary, with even longer times required for complete reexpansion of the lung. Only rarely is it acceptable to treat pneumothorax noninvasively. Certainly, intervention is indicated if there is a circumferential lung collapse of 1 cm or an apical deflation of 3 to 4 cm.

Oxygen Therapy

Oxygen therapy was endorsed for a brief period in the past, based on the idea that inhalation of a high concentration of oxygen might increase the rate of absorption of gas from the pleural cavity. Although the mean rate of absorption of the pneumothorax may increase with the use of oxygen, this mode of therapy has not achieved widespread endorsement.

Aspiration

Aspiration of the pneumothorax is still advocated by some clinicians as a simple means of resolving the problem. The negative features inherent in this technique are the inability to evacuate the entire pneumothorax with failure to approximate the visceral and parietal pleurae, and the lack of pleural scarring that is associated with placing a foreign body such as a chest catheter in the thoracic cavity. In addition, the underlying cause of the pneumothorax, pleural blebs, is not addressed. Several reports on this technique cite a success rate of less than 50 percent, so aspiration has a limited applicability.

Thoracostomy Tube

The most successful treatment for a pneumothorax is insertion of a chest catheter. The Argyle tube is the type most commonly used, although many surgeons prefer the soft rubber variety, feeling that it is more likely to promote pleural symphysis. A chest tube allows complete evacuation of the pleural air with expansion of the lung, even in the face of a continuing air leak. This lung expansion permits adherence between the visceral and parietal layers of the pleura, and the tube itself may promote some degree of pleural symphysis. The catheter is often placed in the fifth or sixth intercostal space in the anterior axillary line, although some surgeons prefer to use the second intercostal space in the midclavicular line as the site of insertion. Although this location may leave a small scar in a prominent location, the apical tube is particularly useful when treating a loculated apical pneumothorax.

Complications may be associated with insertion of a chest catheter if proper technique is not employed. An air leak may occur around the entrance site if an adequate subcutaneous tunnel is not created before penetration into the pleural space. Also, care must be taken to place the tube directly over the top of the chosen rib to avoid laceration of the intercostal artery and/or vein that runs along the inferior surface of the rib. If such an injury occurs, it may be useful to insert a Foley catheter through the tube site so that when it is inflated and pulled snugly against the chest wall, tamponade is achieved. Rarely, operative intervention may be necessary to control such bleeding.

Another problem occasionally associated with chest tube insertion is perforation of the diaphragm. The dome of the diaphragm may be much higher than the tube's site of insertion on the thoracic cage, and the diaphragm may lie directly against the chest wall. If a trocar is used in the procedure, the diaphragm may be pierced, resulting in laceration of the liver or spleen.

Other complications associated with chest tube insertion include disruption of adhesions with intrathoracic bleeding, and kinking of the chest tube with failure to evacuate air from the thorax. One unusual but difficult to manage problem associated with chest tube insertion is unilateral pulmonary edema. The mechanism for this phenomenon is not well understood. It has been suggested that pulmonary reactive hyperemia may play a part in this process; however, studies using lung scans revealed that when the lung is reexpanded, the flow to that organ actually remains below normal for several days. An alternative theory is that unilateral pulmonary edema may be caused by anoxic damage to the pulmonary capillaries.

Some controversy exists with regard to the management of the patient following chest tube placement. Most physicians admit these individuals to the hospital and connect the catheter to underwater seal drainage; 10 to 15 cm of suction is usually sufficient. Some clinicians have advocated connecting the chest tube to a flutter valve and treating the patient without hospital admission. In an otherwise healthy, responsible individual with a simple pneumothorax, this approach may have some merit, but its use should be the exception rather than the rule. Certainly, admission to the hospital is mandatory in those individuals with recurrent pneumothorax, hemothorax, or incomplete expansion of the lung after chest tube insertion.

Scar Producing Agents

The injection of scar producing agents into the thorax to promote pleural symphysis has been suggested by many investigators. The drugs that have been used most often are quinacrine and tetracycline. Some series have shown that there have been fewer recurrent pneumothoraces with a thoracostomy tube and a scar producing agent than with a chest catheter alone. The procedure is generally without risk, although it may be associated with chest discomfort that may be partially relieved by mixing a topical anesthetic with the solution. Because the results obtained with this technique are not clearly superior to those obtained with chest tube insertion alone, it is not worth the added discomfort and expense in the usual case of spontaneous pneumothorax.

Operation

Nine to 25 percent of otherwise healthy patients with spontaneous pneumothorax require thoracotomy. Individual surgeons differ regarding the indications for operation, but the following conditions have been used to justify surgical intervention in patients with this problem: (1) history of a previous pneumothorax, (2) continuing air leak and/or failure of complete lung reexpansion after 1 week, (3) massive air leak with incomplete reexpansion of the lung after 1 day, (4) presence of a significant pneumohemothorax, (5) history of right and left pneumothoraces occurring either simultaneously or on separate occasions, and (6) possible lack of access to adequate medical care in the future.

Incisions that can be used in the operative treatment of a pneumothorax include an anterior thoracotomy, a lateral thoracotomy, a transaxillary thoracotomy, and a median sternotomy. The approach that provides the best cosmetic result and is associated with the least postoperative morbidity is the transaxillary incision. This is a 2.5- to 4-inch incision made across the lower axilla. Care is taken to avoid the intercostobrachial nerve. The third intercostal space is exposed by dividing only a small portion of the serratus anterior muscle. After the thorax is entered, the lung and pleura are inspected and any blebs that are easily accessible are stapled. This is followed by pleural abrasion using a gauze pad. The location and size of the incision slightly limit accessibility to all areas of the pleura, but, because of the usual apical location of the blebs in these patients, adequate treatment is possible. A chest tube is inserted to allow reexpansion of the lung. The recurrence rate associated with surgery is less than 1 percent.

It is preferable to use a larger and more traditional thoracotomy when there is some complicating feature of the pneumothorax, such as a previous chest operation or a pneumothorax in a patient with other underlying lung pathology such as chronic obstructive pulmonary disease and blebs in locations other than the apex. If there is a need to treat bilateral disease, a median sternotomy may be useful. The blebs in both apices can be stapled and bilateral pleural abrasions readily performed through this approach.

There is general agreement that a vital part of the operation for treatment of a pneumothorax is excision of the apical blebs. In the past, some surgeons advocated pleurectomy as a way of ensuring symphysis of the lung and chest wall, but this was often accompanied by postoperative complications including hemothorax, Horner's syndrome, and fibrothorax. In general, dry sponge pleural abrasion is quite effective and it is certainly less traumatic than pleurectomy.

SUGGESTED READING

Brooks JW. Open thoracotomy in the management of spontaneous pneumothorax. Ann Surg 1973; 177:798–805.

Deslauriers J, Beaulieu M, Despres J-P. Transaxillary pleurectomy for treatment of spontaneous pneumothorax. Ann Thorac Surg 1980; 30:569–573.

Kalnins I, Torda TA, Wright JS. Bilateral simultaneous pleurodesis by median sternotomy for spontaneous pneumothorax. Ann Thorac Surg 1973; 15:202–206.

Saha S, Arrants JE, Kosa A, et al. Management of spontaneous pneumothorax. Ann Thorac Surg 1975; 19:561–564.

Wied U, Halkier E, Hoeier-Madsen K, et al. Tetracycline versus silver nitrate pleurodesis in spontaneous pneumothorax. J Thorac Cardiovasc Surg 1983; 86:591–593.

PLEURAL MESOTHELIOMA

C. FREDERICK KITTLE, D.B., M.S., M.D.

The management of diffuse (malignant) pleural mesothelioma is perhaps the most frustrating and challenging problem in thoracic surgery. The incidence of mesothelioma is increasing and, despite many ingenious therapeutic efforts, at the present there is no reported instance of a cure. Malignant pleural mesothelioma varies in the rate of its relentless course between diagnosis and death from a rapid progression of only several months to many months or several years.

The most frequent symptoms of diffuse pleural mesothelioma are dyspnea from the associated pleural effusion and chest wall pain caused by tumor invasion. Other localized symptoms are uncommon. Since mesothelioma is a tumor of the parietal pleura, pulmonary symptoms are rare.

Preoperative assessment of a patient with mesothelioma should consider whether or not the disease has extended into the peritoneal cavity and whether or not it is present in the opposite pleural cavity. The natural growth of the tumor extends inferiorly more than superiorly. CT scans of the chest and upper abdomen provide the best evaluation of the extent of disease and whether or not it is localized to one hemithorax. Bilaterality of pleural mesothelioma is seen in about 10 percent of patients at initial presentation.

The likelihood of this diagnosis is suggested by the radiologic features of the chest film or a chronic recurring effusion or both. It is sufficient reason to warrant performing thoracotomy, unless some definite contraindication to the operation exists. The difficulty in differentiating chronic pleuritis and particularly adenocarcinoma involving the pleura from mesothelioma cannot be overcome by current pathologic techniques. Since this difficulty is further compounded by the small amount of material obtained when a needle pleural biopsy is done, this is not recommended as an initial or a separate procedure.

Distant metastases rarely occur, and procedures for

determining bone and brain involvement are not carried out unless clinically indicated.

EXTRAPLEURAL PNEUMONECTOMY IN CONTINUITY WITH DIAPHRAGM

Initially this operation was done utilizing a posterolateral incision (fifth or sixth interspace) to enter the extrapleural region. However, in order to excise the diaphragm, a second, more inferiorly situated lateral incision was needed (seventh or eighth interspace). This could also be accomplished by mobilizing the skin flap inferiorly and entering the thoracic cavity through the seventh or eighth interspace. Complete excision of the diaphragm is difficult with a posterolateral approach. Most recently, a thoracoabdominal incision centered over the seventh interspace has been used and provides excellent exposure. The patient is placed in a supine position, with the shoulder and hip rotated about 45 degrees.

Dissection is begun laterally in the extrapleural plane, and this space is developed posteriorly and then medially to the hilus, superiorly to the apex of the hemithorax, and anteriorly to the retrosternal space. When the mediastinum is reached retrosternally, the pericardium is opened. The phrenic nerve is transected superior to the hilus, and the pericardial incision is continued inferiorly to the diaphragm. The pulmonary artery and the pulmonary vein or its tributaries are then divided by stapling. The main stem bronchus is identified at its origin by extending the pericardial incision posteriorly, and it is divided after stapling. Attention is then turned to the peritoneal dissection.

The diaphragm is incised within the pericardial cavity to enter either the peritoneal cavity or the "bare" space above the liver. The peritoneum is incised anteriorly, and the anatomic boundaries of the diaphragm can be appreciated by palpation and inspection from the peritoneal side. The medial side of the diaphragm is incised anteroposteriorly to the esophagus or the cava, leaving the diaphragm attached posteriorly, laterally, and anteriorly. By developing the extrapleural plane circumferentially for the remaining 270 degrees, the crus and the lateral origins of the diaphragm can be followed to their origin and transected.

The specimen is then removed en bloc—the parietal pleura, the pericardium, the diaphragm with its peritoneum, and the lung.

Care must be taken to avoid damage to the superior vena cava and to the recurrent laryngeal nerve unless it is involved grossly by tumor.

The pericardial defect is considerable and must be covered on the right to prevent torsion or herniation of the heart into the pleural space. Similarly, the diaphragm must be reconstituted by a watertight prosthesis. Our preference is Goretex or Dacron velour. Mediastinal nodes—carinal, superior, and inferior—are excised for staging tests.

PLEURECTOMY

In those patients in whom pleural effusion is symptomatic and palliation is desired, or in whom extrapleural pneumonectomy is not considered worthwhile, parietal pleurectomy can be done through a lateral sixth interspace thoracotomy incision. After the incision has passed through the intercostal muscles, the extrapleural space is developed by blunt dissection. The space is readily freed posteriorly, anteriorly, and superiorly. It is developed to the hilus, care being taken to preserve the recurrent laryngeal nerve and to avoid entering the superior vena cava. After this space is mobilized, the pleural space is entered and the parietal pleura as well as the mediastinal pleura incised around the hilus. The pleura does not strip from the diaphragm, but as much as possible of the mesothelioma in this area should be removed. In many instances the mesothelioma does not involve the visceral pleura. However, in patients with extensive disease, it may be necessary to decorticate the lung and remove the mesothelioma from the visceral pleura and its extension along the fissures. The mesothelioma seldom invades the lung parenchyma.

The question arises as to whether or not the pleurectomy is superior to some type of less invasive pleurodesis such as the injection of tetracycline or the insufflation of talc. Both of these therapies have been used, but the reports are so few that no conclusion can be reached regarding them. In view of the inexorable progress of diffuse pleural mesothelioma and the patient's limited life span, it is conceivable that such therapy may be as effective as operative pleurectomy for relieving the effusion.

COMPLICATIONS AND RESULTS

In patients undergoing operative procedures for mesothelioma, more complications and decreased pulmonary function have been noted with extrapleural pneumonectomy than with pleurectomy. In our group of 33 patients operated on, there were three deaths (9.1 percent) related to operation: one due to uncontrollable bleeding from the superior vena cava, one from pulmonary embolism, and one from myocardial infarction. Major postoperative complications were noted in eight patients: bronchopleural fistula (two), chylothorax (one), contralateral pleural effusion (one), severe cardiac arrhythmia (one), and respiratory failure necessitating tracheostomy (one).

In the 28 patients who underwent pleurectomy, there were three deaths (10.7 percent): one from a myocardial infarction; one from postoperative renal failure; and one, who previously had been treated for a lymphoma, from empyema and renal failure.

The complications after pleurectomy were fewer than with the extrapleural pneumonectomy. One patient who had a completely collapsed lung with massive hemothorax developed empyema postoperatively that responded to tube drainage. A second patient developed contralateral pleural effusion that subsequently was shown to be contralateral disease, although preoperative CT imaging had not disclosed tumor on that side.

The survival rates for these two groups of patients have been calculated (as of January 1, 1987). The median survival time for those undergoing pneumonectomy is 13.3 months and for pleurectomy, 10.9 months, but the variance among the patients is so great that no statistical significance is present. Another way of expressing survival is that among the extrapleural pneumonectomy patients eight survived 2 years or longer, six survived for 3 years, five for 4 years, and two for 5 years; among those undergoing pleurectomy, four survived 2 years or more, two for 3 years, two for 4 years, and two for 5 years. The longest survivors lived for 82 months after extrapleural pneumonectomy and 79 months after pleurectomy, both with recurrent disease.

Most of our patients received postoperative adjuvant therapy, chemotherapy (multidrug therapy, particularly with doxorasicin [Adriamycin]) and/or radiation. However, the extreme variability in the extent and type of disease precludes any definitive comments regarding the effect of these treatment modalities in our patients.

Our present philosophy regarding diffuse pleural mesothelioma consists of a high index of suspicion based on the chest imaging and the clinical history, followed by open biopsy and pleurectomy. Adjuvant therapy remains a subject for continuing clinical investigation.

SUGGESTED READING

Antman K, Aisner J. Asbestos-related malignancy. Orlando, FL; Grune & Stratton, 1987.

Faber LP. Malignant pleural mesothelioma: operative treatment by extrapleural pneumonectomy. In: Kittle CF, ed. Controversies in thoracic surgery. Philadelphia: WB Saunders, 1986:80.

Ginsberg RJ. Diffuse malignant mesothelioma: a therapeutic dilemma. Ann Thorac Surg 1986; 42:608.

Kittle CF. Mesothelioma: diagnosis and management. Chicago: Year Book Medical Publishers, 1987.

McCormack P, Martini N. Malignant pleural mesothelioma: operative treatment by pleurectomy. In: Kittle CF, ed. Controversies in thoracic surgery. Philadelphia: WB Saunders, 1986:76.

THE MEDIASTINUM

THYMUS: MYASTHENIA GRAVIS AND THYMOMA

EARLE W. WILKINS Jr., M.D.

MYASTHENIA GRAVIS

Rationale for Thymectomy

The association between the thymus gland and myasthenia gravis remains unclear. Indirect evidence suggests that myasthenia gravis is an autoimmune disease, but whether the mechanism is one resulting from circulating antibodies (muscle shares a cross-reacting antigen with epithelial cells of the thymus) or the result of cellular immune responses mediated by sensitized lymphocytes has not been settled. A controlled prospective study of thymectomy for myasthenia gravis has never been reported. Nevertheless, there is reasonable statistical evidence to support the rationale of thymectomy in selected patients. Remissions following surgical thymectomy, when they do occur, are almost always permanent.

Since the exact relationship between the gland and the disease is unclear, when thymectomy is attempted, it should be complete. Despite growing interest in transcervical thymectomy, transsternal exposure provides a surer prospect for totality of gland removal. Jaretzki has demonstrated, by careful anatomic dissection, a remarkable variation in the extent of the gland.

Indications for Thymectomy

Experience with thymectomy for myasthenia gravis at the Massachusetts General Hospital has involved patients of either sex, most commonly those under age 40. The procedure has not been carried out, as in some clinics, upon diagnosis but has been reserved for those with moderate to severe symptoms not adequately controlled by medical measures, including anticholinesterase drugs, steroids, and plasmapheresis. However, the results of thymectomy, in the form of total remission or definite improvement, have been sufficiently promising to permit a move toward early thymectomy in the younger patient, particularly in the female. Patients with pure ocular myasthenia have not been offered thymectomy at the Massachusetts General Hospital.

Preoperative Preparation

This requires the collaborative efforts of the neurologist, anesthesiologist, and thoracic surgeon. Appropriate dosage and frequency of anticholinesterase medication are determined to achieve stability of the disease before embarking on the operation.

In the more severe cases of disease, plasmapheresis is a useful preoperative adjunct. The apparent basis of its beneficial effect is a reduction in circulating levels of acetylcholine receptor antibody. This reduction is best accomplished by a program of three plasma exchanges on alternate days in the week preceding thymectomy. Each run provides an exchange up to 4 L, depending primarily on the size and tolerance of the patient. The blood cells are returned to the patient suspended in an equal volume of 5 percent albumin, normal saline, or lactated Ringer's solution with supplements of potassium, calcium, and magnesium ions as physiologically necessary.

Corticosteroids are avoided in stabilization of the preoperative myasthenia gravis patient. Although it has been reported that high doses of corticosteroids, both before and after thymectomy, provide a smoother postoperative course, the risks of delayed wound healing, susceptibility to sepsis, and gastrointestinal bleeding contraindicate its use in all thymectomy patients except a few with very special indications.

Preoperative radiation of the mediastinal bed of the thymus gland, once practiced under study conditions at the Massachusetts General Hospital, is *not* indicated in the nonthymomatous myasthenic patient. It, too, enhances the risk of postoperative complications related to wound healing and infection.

Radiologic evaluation is helpful in delineation of the possibility of a thymoma. The minimal study includes four-view chest films and either conventional plasma tomography or computed tomography (CT). The latter seems to provide the most useful information in terms of the possible presence and extent of a thymic tumor.

It is useful to obtain a baseline determination of respiratory function, including the vital capacity and the one-second forced expiratory volume (FEV_1). Measurement of these parameters, both under conditions of maximal anticholinesterase medication and under its deprivation, is ideal.

In the female, the timing of thymectomy is best planned at a point avoiding the immediate premenstrual period when general body fluid retention may compromise the process of postoperative weaning from ventilatory support. It must be remembered that, although they are used infrequently in the present era, enemas in the myasthenic patient may be complicated by a phenomenon of circulatory collapse.

In the immediate preoperative preparation, no anticholinesterase medication is administered after the last usual evening dose prior to the day of surgery. Most anesthesiologists avoid the routine use of atropine prior to anesthesia.

Anesthesia

Endotracheal general anesthesia is essential. After several minutes of preoxygenation, induction is accomplished with thiopental sodium. Halothane (Fluothane) is the usual agent of choice for maintenance of anesthesia; it permits maximal oxygenation and avoids peripheral effects at the myoneural junction, such as occur with ether compounds.

Muscle-relaxing drugs are contraindicated during surgery on myasthenic patients. If one proves necessary, as during difficult intubation, succinylcholine may be used cautiously. It is a depolarizing rather than a competitive blocking agent. Its removal from the myoneural junction area is a function of cholinesterase activity, which is assumed to be unimpaired in patients with myasthenia gravis. Anticholinesterase drugs are never administered during the surgery.

Surgical Technique

The thymus gland is a cervicothoracic structure, extending from the inferior border of the thyroid gland to the level of the fourth costal cartilages. The direct, most revealing surgical approach is, therefore, a cervicothoracic incision. A median sternotomy provides the essential ingredients of this approach. A partial upper sternotomy provides adequate access to the anterior superior mediastinum.

The patient is placed supine, without a lift under the upper dorsal spine but with 15 degrees' flexion of the table, permitting the thorax and head to be slightly elevated. A vertical midline incision is made from the suprasternal notch to the level of the fourth cartilages. It is a preoperative refinement to mark the midline with the patient standing, so that operating table positioning, especially when one arm is extended on an arm board, does not result in a skewed direction of the scar. The superior mediastinum is entered by dissection in the midline above the manubrium and blunt finger separation of areolar mediastinal tissue away from the posterior surface of the sternum. A tough transverse tendinous band must be divided at the posterosuperior border of the manubrium. Cortical bone of the manubrium is most easily divided with Lebsche's shears. This permits easy placement of the sternum-splitting knife. Careful visual sighting is used to guide the sternal knife in the midline as it is struck with the mallet. The sternum is divided to approximately a three-quarter sternotomy. The maneuver of sternotomy can also be accomplished with the Stryker compressed-air or electric-powered saw from above downward.

The thymus gland is exposed by identification of its characteristic gray-ink color, which distinguishes it from the yellow fat of the mediastinum. Grasping with a Duval's type forceps permits appropriate elevating tension for easy dissection of the gland from the underlying pericardium. The dissection is begun from below upward in the extracapsular plane. An effort is made to push the mediastinal extension of each pleural membrane laterally. If either pleural space is inadvertently entered, no attempt is made to suture and close the defect. In the absence of trauma to the surface of the lung, positive-pressure ventilation by the anesthesiologist at the time of sternal closure permits full expansion of the lungs. The principal arterial supply laterally on either side from the internal mammary arteries is identified and divided. In the posterolateral dissection of the thymus toward the lung roots, care is taken not to damage the phrenic nerves. Even a transient unilateral diaphragmatic palsy may present major post-thymectomy management problems. The venous drainage from the thymus into the inferior aspect of the left innominate vein via one or two sizable tributaries is identified and divided. The two upper poles, extending into the base of the neck, are dissected, identifying and dividing small arterial branches from the inferior thyroid arteries. One or both upper poles may pass posterior to the innominate vein. The inferior parathyroid glands may be apparent at this point in the dissection and should be preserved.

The anterior mediastinal thymic bed is then carefully inspected to be certain of both hemostasis and totality of thymectomy. The sternum is approximated with three stainless steel wires (monofilament No. 6 surgical steel wire with Tapercut V-40 needle) placed either through the sternum or around the sternum in each intercostal space. In either circumstance, caution is exercised not to lacerate the internal mammary arteries. Posterior compression of the sternal edges permits twisting of the wire and accurate anatomic approximation. Mediastinal drainage, if necessary, is managed with a suprasternal suction catheter of the Jackson-Pratt or Hemovac type. In the female, a brassiere or breast binder is immediately applied. Breast support, by avoiding lateral sagging, helps prevent possible keloid formation.

Alternative surgical approaches are available. (1) A limited median sternotomy can also be accomplished by elevation of the lower flap of a wide collar incision, thus exposing the upper 10 cm of sternum. Partial sternotomy is then carried out through this incision. Its aim is cosmetic in that midline anterior chest incisions sometimes heal with unattractive scars. (2) The strict transcervical approach with elevation of the sternum by the so-called "upper-hand" retractor has achieved popular use. It is said to result in easier postoperative patient recovery and shorter hospital stays. It does require a more particular technical skill, which includes a steeper learning curve for the surgeon. Thoroughness of thymic gland removal may be compromised, if not precluded, by this limited access. It is the author's bias, therefore, that until it is scientifically proved that total removal of thymic tissue is unnecessary, transsternal exposure provides a more certain prospect for total gland excision. In this regard, Jaretzki's, demonstrations are pertinent. They show a remarkable variation in the extent of anatomic location of the thymus gland. Application of this knowledge suggests that wider, and not more limited, exposure of the anterior mediastinum is in order. The transcervical approach must not be used for a thymoma.

Postoperative Management

The care of the postoperative thymectomy patient, for all but those with mild myasthenia gravis, should take place in the intensive care unit, preferably under the supervision of nurses who are experienced in care of the myasthenic patient. The keys to immediate postoperative intensive care are (a) monitoring of arterial blood gases, (b) estimates of ventilatory function, (c) evaluation of the chest x-ray film for pneumothorax, atelectasis, frank collapse, or pleural fluid, (d) oropharyngeal and tracheal suctioning, and (e) chest physiotherapy support. Anticholinesterase medication is *not* resumed before 48 hours after the operation.

Perhaps the most critical decision is the timing of tracheal extubation. For the patient with mild myasthenia and for the patient with more severe disease who has been ideally prepared with plasmapheresis, this often can be accomplished while the patient is still on the operating table. That patient, however, needs to go to the intensive care unit for the first 48 hours when there is the greatest danger of development of complications or decompensation of the myasthenia gravis. If the patient is to remain intubated, comfort dictates that a transnasal endotracheal tube should be employed. Tracheostomy is avoided because of its proximity to a freshly healing sternotomy incision.

When pyridostigmine bromide (Mestinon), the commonly used anticholinesterase, is resumed, it should be initiated slowly in low doses. There frequently is a transient sensitivity during which time anticholinesterase drugs produce side effects of excessive salivation, bronchial secretions, and even abdominal cramps simulating overdose. Pyridostigmine is available for intramuscular administration, or it may be given via a small nasogastric feeding tube if the patient cannot swallow. When the vital capacity is consistently in excess of 1 L, the endotracheal tube can be safely removed.

Complications

The most frightening complications are myasthenic or cholinergic crises. In the postoperative patient managed by careful titration with intravenous neostigmine bromide, it is frequently clinically impossible to distinguish excessive tracheobronchial secretions resulting from too much anticholinesterase medication and the motor weakness of myasthenia with an inability to cough normal postoperative secretions. This dilemma is best avoided by the withdrawal of all such medications in the immediate postoperative period in the intubated patient.

The remainder of possible complications is principally respiratory: atelectasis, pneumonia, persisting pneumothorax, pleural effusion, aspiration, phrenic nerve palsy, and, very rarely, pulmonary embolism.

THYMOMA

The differences in the management of the patient with a thymoma require emphasis. The thymoma is a tumor with overt or potential malignant characteristics, and its radiologic demonstration mandates treatment as a malignant tumor.

1. If the patient has accompanying myasthenia gravis, prompt stabilization of the myasthenia under hospital conditions and not by a slower outpatient process is in order.
2. Radiologic evaluation must be more precise, requiring CT search for evidence of local invasion or pleural implantation. Vessel enhancement during CT study is helpful in this regard. Direct angiographic study by superior vena caval injection may be necessary. If contrast injection is employed, it should be directed from the left to provide opacification of the left innominate vein.
3. Preoperative radiation therapy may be considered if the thymoma is huge or unusually bulky, or if radiologic evaluation suggests vascular invasion. The dosage usually is 4,000 rads in 4 weeks followed by surgical exploration within another 4 weeks.
4. The surgical exposure is always accomplished by a full median sternotomy, accompanied by wide opening of both pleural spaces, to permit complete search for extent of the tumor and for pleural implants.
5. If the patient is myasthenic, it is better not to attempt extubation on the operating table. These myasthenic patients can be more difficult to manage in the intensive care unit.

Pathology

Next to lymphoma, thymoma is the most frequent tumor of the anterior mediastinum. It occurs in any decade from the teen years onward and is equally divided in incidence between the sexes. If it occurs in adolescence, it may be aggressively malignant. The actual malignant nature of a thymoma is not easily assessed by direct microscopic pathologic evaluation. In clinical terms, malignancy is more often related to gross characteristics determined at the time of operation. Lack of an enveloping capsule or local invasion of adjacent tissues, including pericardium, pleura, great veins, or phrenic nerve, is a better indication of malignancy than strictly cellular characteristics. They may indeed be prognostic of possible later recurrence. The thymoma does not usually metastasize by embolic hematogenous or lymphatic pathways, but it does metastasize to pleural surfaces, perhaps by droplet implantation. The thymoma may also recur locally if its capsular integrity is violated. For this reason, biopsy is best avoided either postoperatively or during surgery.

Pathologic staging of thymoma has not been addressed by the American Joint Committee for Cancer Staging and End Results Reporting Task Forces. Bergh has provided a useful scale for such staging: Stage I: intact capsule or tumor growth only within the capsule; Stage II: pericapsular growth, into mediastinal fat or adjacent pleura or pericardium; and Stage III: invasive growth into surrounding organs, intrathoracic pleural metastases, or both.

Surgical Technique

If the tumor seems confined to the thymus gland, it is removed with *total* thymectomy. There have been five patients in the Massachusetts General Hospital series who developed myasthenia after the removal of a thymoma, usually by a posterolateral approach, without removal of all thymic tissue.

If the tumor appears invasive, radical excision is attempted utilizing the following maneuvers: identification of the phrenic nerves through the open pleural spaces, opening the pericardium low on its surface, removal of adherent mediastinal pleural membranes, wedge excision of areas of invaded lung, exposure of the superior vena cava with excision of the left innominate vein if involved, and excision by pleural stripping of any implants on the parietal surfaces. Invasion of the vena cava requires special consideration. Small areas of involvement may be removed with a side-biting vascular clamp and primary closure, or patching may be carried out with pericardium or harvested saphenous vein. Major involvement may necessitate temporary venovenous shunting with the careful placement of an interpositioned graft using autologous vein fashioned to provide comparable size and lumen.

Every effort should be made to preserve phrenic nerve function if the patient is myasthenic. Sacrifice of one nerve under these circumstances is reasonable; sacrifice of two is usually disastrous in terms of postoperative ventilatory weaning.

Results

Careful records and follow-up of all patients have been maintained at the Massachusetts General Hospital since the first thymus operation in 1941. Results are tabulated for patients with myasthenia gravis and no tumor and for those with thymoma with or without myasthenia (Tables 1 through 5).

There is a distribution of cases in all decades from the second through the eighth. The peak incidence for thymoma patients with myasthenia is between 40 and 49 (22 cases, 30 percent); without myasthenia, between 60 and 69 (20 cases, 29 percent).

TABLE 1 Classification of 196 Myasthenics Without Thymoma 1941–1986 (Osserman Classification)*

Osserman Group	*Female*	*Male*
I		1
IIA	10	4
IIB	104	24
III	23	4
IV	24	2
Totals	161	35

* This reflects two principles followed at Massachusetts General Hospital: not to operate on patients with mild myasthenia (IIA) or on severe cases that are acute (III).

TABLE 2 Operative Mortality for Nonthymomatous Patients by Decade*

	Operations	*Deaths*	*%*
1941–49	36	4	11
1950–59	69	4	6
1960–69	45	1†	2
1970–79	23	0	0
1980–86	23 (196)	0	0

* The hospital mortality since the establishment of the Massachusetts General Hospital respiratory intensive care unit was one patient in 95 thymectomies (1%).
† pulmonary embolus

TABLE 3 Response of Myasthenia Without Thymoma to Thymectomy

Osserman Group A (total remission)	39%
Osserman Group B (full activity on some medication)	44%
No improvement	17%

TABLE 4 Thymoma by Sex and the Presence of Myasthenia (1942–86)

	Male	*Female*	*Totals*	*%*
Myasthenia	38	35	(73)	51%
No myasthenia	32	38	(70)	49%
Totals	70	73	(143)	

TABLE 5 Thymoma by Age, Sex, and the Presence of Myasthenia

	Myasthenia Gravis		*No Myasthenia Gravis*	
Decade Age	*Male*	*Female*	*Male*	*Female*
10–19	1	2	3	2
20–29	5	4	3	3
30–39	8	9	3	3
40–49	12	10	7	5
50–59	7	5	3	4
60–69	4	2	7	13
70–79	1	3	6	7
80–				1
Totals	38	35	32	38

TABLE 6 Thymoma Hospital Mortality

Decade	*Operations*	*No. Deaths*	*%*
1942–49	17	2	12
1950–59	33	3	9
1960–69	25	1	4
1970–79	33	1	3
1980–86	35	0	0
Totals	143	7	5

TABLE 7 Thymoma Staging (Bergh Classification)

1964–86	
Myasthenia (35):	
Stages I	15
II	15
III	5
(Male 21, Female 14)	
No Myasthenia (45):	
Stages I	23
II	14
III	7
(Not explored)	1
(Male 19, Female 26)	

All patients were subjected to surgery, 119 undergoing total excision of the thymoma, seven subtotal removal, and 17 biopsy only. The hospital mortality rate is presented in Table 6.

There have been no deaths in the last 67 patients operated (since the death in 1970).

At the time of the last formal, detailed follow-up of patients with resected thymomas operated on before 1983, the 10-year cumulative survival was 67 percent. (This varied from 84 percent in Stage I thymoma patients without myasthenia to 22 percent in Stages II and III thymoma patients with myasthenia.) In terms of impact on myasthenia gravis, there were 21 percent Osserman group A results (total remission) and 39 percent group B results (patients returned to full activity but taking either pyridostigmine or corticosteroids).

SUGGESTED READING

Bergh NP, Gatzinsky P, Larsson S, et al. Tumors of the thymus and thymic region: I. Clinicopathologic studies on thymomas. Ann Thorac Surg 1978; 25:91–98.

Jaretzki A III, Bethea M, Wolff M, et al. A rational approach to total thymectomy in the treatment of myasthenia gravis. Ann Thorac Surg 1977; 24:120–130.

Lisak RP, Barchi RL. Myasthenia gravis. Vol. 11. Major problems in neurology. Philadelphia: WB Saunders, 1982.

Wilkins EW Jr. Thymectomy. In: Cohn LH, ed. Modern techniques in surgery (cardiac/thoracic surgery). Mount Kisco, NY; Futura Publishing, 1981; 38:1–13.

Wilkins EW Jr, Edmunds LH Jr, Castleman B. Cases of thymoma at the Massachusetts General Hospital. J Thorac Cardiovasc Surg 1966; 52:322–330.

MEDIASTINAL TUMOR

EARLE W. WILKINS Jr., M.D.

Consideration of the subject of mediastinal tumors begins with (1) a definition of mediastinal compartments; and (2) a categorization of the variety of neoplasia encountered in them.

An arbitrary although practical and generally accepted division of the mediastinum includes the superior, anterior, middle, and posterior components. (1) The superior mediastinum lies above a plane extending from the sternal angle of Louis to the fourth thoracic vertebral body. The mediastinum inferior to this compartment is thus subdivided into (2) the anterior—in front of the anterior pericardium, (3) the middle—the space occupied by the heart and great vessels, the tracheobronchi and their related lymph nodes, and (4) the posterior—behind the posterior pericardium and including the paravertebral gutters.

In conventional tabulation of mediastinal tumors, neoplasia of the heart, tracheobronchi, and esophagus are considered under their respective body systems. Thus, tumors of the mediastinum are grouped as follows, in rough order of frequency of incidence: (1) neurogenic, (2) thymic, (3) lymphomatous, (4) germ cell, (5) mesenchymal, (6) endocrine, and (7) primary carcinoma. In addition, usually indistinguishable clinically and radiologically, are the various cysts of the mediastinum: pericardial, bronchogenic, enteric, and mesothelial or pleural. It has been speculated that there is an incidence of one mediastinal tumor per 100,000 population, a frequency that is three times that of a bronchial carcinoid tumor, but one-seventh the incidence of gastroesophageal neoplasms and one-thirtieth that of bronchial carcinomas. The latter fraction may be decreasing even further because there is no evidence of an increased incidence of mediastinal tumors, whereas the incidence of bronchogenic carcinoma continues to soar.

DIAGNOSIS

Radiology. Study of the mediastinum and its tumors is primarily radiologic. In the interest of cost containment, the planning of particular studies is carried out with the consultative collaboration of the thoracic radiologist. The specific techniques that may be utilized include (1) the four-view chest films, (2) fluoroscopy, (3) linear or planar tomography, (4) computed tomography (CT), and (5) magnetic resonance imaging (MRI). Fluoroscopy, underutilized in the era of modern imaging, permits dynamic assessment of vocal cord function and integrity of the recurrent laryngeal nerves, intrinsic/transmitted arterial pulsations, diaphragmatic excursion and functional impairment of the phrenic nerves, and shows evidence of any distortion of the esophageal outline. CT has become, with appropriately employed contrast, the basic tool for evaluation of the mediastinal tumor; its cross-sectional imaging and high contrast resolution help in the definition of the size, shape, density, and vascularity of specific tumors. MRI is still in an evolving status, but it does provide coronal and sagittal planar views with particular definition of vascular structures and without radiation exposure.

Ultrasonography and radionuclide scanning have limited utility. The former may be helpful in differentiating a cyst from a solid tumor and the latter in assessing a mediastinal thyroid mass with ^{131}I or sometimes mediastinal adenopathy with ^{67}Ga.

Under certain circumstances, angiography is enormously important in evaluating the mediastinum and its tumors. Aortography is particularly helpful in the differentiation of vascular structures, such as aneurysms or congenital anomalies, and in the selective catheterization of specific arteries, such as a bronchial vessel feeding a paraganglioma. Digital subtraction angiography is a further refinement that may provide substantive but adequate information without the risk of percutaneous aortography.

Biopsy. There are three approaches for tissue assessment of a mediastinal tumor: (1) percutaneous needle aspiration biopsy, (2) mediastinoscopy, and (3) mediastinotomy, usually by the parasternal or so-called Chamberlain's technique.

Percutaneous needle aspiration biopsy under video guidance permits the radiologist a low-risk opportunity to obtain tumor aspirate for cytologic evaluation. It usually does not provide sufficient tissue for histologic study. There is little evidence that tumor is disseminated by this technique. Its principal hazards lie in the development of pneumothorax and in hemorrhage from unrecognized highly vascular tumors. Larger needle biopsy by Vim-Silverman or Tru-Cut needle techniques is not advised for seeking histologic as opposed to cytologic specimens. Needle biopsy of thymomas is *contraindicated* because of the possibility of mediastinal seeding or pleural droplet dissemination of tumor.

Mediastinoscopy enjoys its principal role in the assessment of adenopathy in the mediastinum and, thus, in the definition of a lymphoma. Its limitations are anatomic because of the inaccessibility of three particular areas: the anterior mediastinum, the subaortic region or "aortic window," and the posterior subcarinal location of lymph nodes.

The anterior mediastinotomy provides access to two of these areas, the anterior mediastinum and the aortic window. Its limitation lies in its unilateral, ipsilateral approach. In certain circumstances, therefore, mediastinoscopy and anterior mediastinotomy are combined.

THERAPY

The application of appropriate therapy for a given mediastinal tumor requires both specific and generalized considerations, largely related to the pathologic nature of the tumor being treated. A limited pathologic classification is therefore helpful (Table 1).

General Guidelines

1. All mediastinal tumors are investigated by CT for evidence of invasion of adjacent structures, for suggestive

TABLE 1 Classification of Mediastinal Tumors

Neural Tumors
Neurilemoma
Neurofibroma
Neurofibromatosis
Ganglioneuroma
Neuroblastoma
Paraganglioma
Pheochromocytoma
Granular cell tumor
Thymic Tumors
Thymoma
Carcinoid
Thymolipoma
Carcinoma (primary)
Hodgkin's disease of thymus
Nonthymic Lymphomas
Hodgkin's disease
NonHodgkin's lymphomas (e.g., lymphocytic, histiocytic)
Germ Cell Tumors
Teratoma, including dermoid cyst
Dysgerminoma (seminoma)
Embryonal carcinoma
Endodermal sinus tumor
Choriocarcinoma
Mesenchymal Tumors
Lipoma/liposarcoma
Lymphangioma
Hemangiopericytoma
Primary Carcinoma
Cysts
Thymic
Bronchogenic
Pericardial
Mesothelial
Enteric (duplications)

evidence of vascularity indicating the need for additional study, and for the presence of lymphadenopathy.

2. Patients with lymphomas are candidates for multimodal therapy: surgery, radiation, and chemotherapy. The principal diagnostic evidence for lymphoma is the finding of regional lymphadenopathy by CT examination. Under these circumstances, lymph node biopsy is indicated when accessible.
3. The primary therapy for almost all other mediastinal tumors is surgical extirpation, usually without the need for biopsy.
4. Mediastinal cysts, even when suggested by CT or ultrasonography, are best removed surgically because of concern regarding underlying tumor, or the threat of subsequent secondary infection. The only exception is a pericardial cyst, which, if correctly diagnosed, can be managed by aspiration.

Specific Considerations

1. The neural tumor, which may be found in all mediastinal compartments, is most common posteriorly. In this location, special attention must be given the possibility of a dumbbell-shaped tumor, partly paravertebral and partly intraspinous. These are usually neurilemomas and require simultaneous combined laminectomy and thoracotomy, by a neurosurgeon and a thoracic surgeon, for safe removal. When it is suspected by the finding of an enlarged intervertebral foramen on CT or polytome radiography, the possibility of this tumor is assessed by myelography or, if subsequent experience confirms its accuracy, by MRI.
2. Tumors confined to the thymus gland are best approached by median sternotomy and excision without biopsy (see chapter on *Myasthenia Gravis and Thymoma*). The occasional patient with Hodgkin's disease or other lymphoma confined to the thymus is then a candidate for further staging and adjuvant therapy. Mediastinal lymphadenopathy found in association with a thymic tumor on CT is not likely to indicate a thymoma.
3. Germ cell tumors occur primarily in the anterior mediastinum. Tumor markers—human chorionic gonadotropin, alphafetoprotein, and carcinoembryonic antigen—may be helpful in making the specific diagnosis. Patients with these tumors, except for the mature teratoma, are candidates for multimodal treatment.

Surgical Technique

Approach to the anterior mediastinal tumor is presented in steps as an example of surgical technique.

A total median sternotomy is used in all cases. Unless the tumor is small, encapsulated, and obviously confined, both pleural spaces are opened widely to assist in determining the anatomic extent of tumor. This is especially important for the malignant thymoma, which metastasizes by droplet implantation on visceral and parietal pleural surfaces.

Vascular margins are then assessed. The pericardial sac may be opened, again unless tumor is grossly free, to assess the posterior extent of invasion. The pulmonary vessels are also inspected intrapericardially. The superior vena cava is identified through the opened right pleural sac and dissected to identify the confluence of right and left innominate veins. An impression is usually gained at this point of whether the left innominate vein is free or involved by tumor. The exact determination of this situation must await further dissection of the tumor. The left innominate vein, however, may be removed with relative impunity if it is invaded.

The two phrenic nerves are identified by dissection posteriorly between the pericardium and lungs. If tumor occludes these spaces, the nerves usually can be identified distally on the lateral pericardium or at the point of diaphragmatic insertion, and then traced cephalad. Except in patients with myasthenia gravis, one phrenic nerve may be sacrificed for total removal of tumor. Sacrifice of two nerves raises the serious question of postoperative respiratory dysfunction and possible respirator dependency.

Lung involvement is determined, although this may be necessary before dissection of the phrenic nerves. Lung involvement usually occurs by direct extension into the anterior segments of either upper lobe, the middle lobe, or occasionally the anterior portion of the lower lobes. Direct extension to the lung is best removed by wedge excision using the GIA stapler, once the proximal pulmonary vessels are determined to be free. From this anterior approach, the pulmonary arteries may be dissected to isolate and divide segmental arteries if a segmentectomy or even a lobectomy is necessary.

If the tumor lies within the thymus gland, a total thymectomy is necessary; this requires cephalad dissection into the base of the neck for removal of the upper poles of the thymus.

Once these steps are completed, the tumor, with the entire contents of the anterior mediastinum, can be readily extracted. The bed is carefully inspected for hemostasis, for residual tumor, and for evidence of lymphadenopathy. The pleural cavities are each drained with a No. 28 Argyle catheter. The sternotomy is closed with heavy wire circumferential sutures. Particular care is necessary to avoid puncture of the internal mammary vessels.

MGH EXPERIENCE

A 20-year experience at the Massachusetts General Hospital from 1963 through 1982 includes 155 patients with proven mediastinal tumors (Table 2).

TABLE 2 Mediastinal Tumors from the Massachusetts General Hospital (1963–1982)

Thymomas		42
Encapsulated	21	
Invasive	19	
Hyperplasia	2	
Neural Tumors		27
Ganglioneuroma	9	
Neurofibroma	6	
Schwannoma	5	
Neuroblastoma	5	
Paraganglioma	1	
Neurofibromatosis	1	
Germ Cell Tumors		23
Mature teratoma (including dermoid)	7	
Endodermal sinus	5	
Dysgerminoma	4	
Embryonal carcinoma	4	
Teratocarcinoma	3	
Lymphomas		21
Hodgkin's	8	
Histiocytic	7	
Lymphocytic	2	
Reticulum cell	2	
Large cell	1	
Undifferentiated	1	
Cysts		15
Thymic	6	
Pericardial	4	
Bronchogenic	2	
Pleural	2	
Parathyroid	1	
Mesenchymal Tumors		13
Liposarcoma	4	
Lymphangioma	3	
Hemangioma	1	
Hemangiopericytoma	1	
Other sarcomas	4	
Thyroid Tumors		5
Substernal goiter	3	
Follicular adenoma	1	
Papillary carcinoma	1	
Lymph Nodes		5
Sarcoid	3	
Angiofollicular hyperplasia	2	
Miscellaneous		4
Primary carcinoma	2	
Multiple myeloma	1	
Fibrosing mediastinitis	1	
Total		155

Special Problems

The general thoracic surgeon must be aware of certain special problems and particular pitfalls in the surgical management of mediastinal tumors. Each of the following has been personally encountered at the Massachusetts General Hospital.

Size. The size of an anterior mediastinal tumor, especially without incontrovertible evidence of invasion of adjacent structures, is not a contraindication to surgical exploration and attempted resection. A 3.1-kg well-differentiated liposarcoma with distortion and compression of the superior vena cava has been successfully and completely removed. Conversely, a huge thymoma, treated by preoperative radiation to promote ease of resectability, resulted in severe and incapacitating pulmonary radiation fibrosis.

Vascularity. A mediastinal tumor, particularly in the middle or posterior compartments lying adjacent to a great vessel, should be investigated with angiography and selective arterial catheterization to delineate exact vascular anatomy before any attempt at removal. A posterior mediastinal paraganglioma was preoperatively not recognized to have a 1-cm feeding artery arising directly beneath it from the descending thoracic aorta. Prohibitive blood loss necessitated staging the ultimately successful procedure until percutaneous, transaortic embolization of the feeding artery was accomplished. In a similar case, a parabronchial mass proved to be an aneurysm of the right bronchial artery in the midst of extensive mediastinal vascular malformation. This was appropriately managed by angiographic placement of an embolizing detachable balloon.

Mediastinoscopy. Biopsy of apparent mediastinal lymph nodes through the mediastinoscope is carried out only after as careful preoperative radiologic verification as possible *and* after mediastinoscopic needle aspiration to exclude a vessel simulating a node. For instance, the bronchial artery aneurysm mentioned previously was initially considered by radiologic evaluation to be a large bronchial lymph node. A similarly located mass in another patient proved to be a fibrous histiocytoma of the right pulmonary artery.

SUGGESTED READING

Berg HNP, Gatzinsky P, Larsson S, et al. Tumors of the thymus and thymic region: I. Clinicopathological studies on thymoma. Ann Thorac Surg 1978; 25:91–98.

Grillo HC, Ojemann RG, Scannell JG, et al. Combined approach to "dumbbell" intrathoracic and intraspinal neurogenic tumors. Ann Thorac Surg 1983; 36:402–407.

Marchevsky AM, Kaneko M. Surgical pathology of the mediastinum. New York: Raven Press, 1984.

Wychulis AR, Payne WS, Clagett OT, Woolner LB. Surgical treatment of mediastinal tumors. A 40-year experience. J Thorac Cardiovasc Surg 1971; 62:379–392.

SUBSTERNAL GOITER

MARK R. KATLIC, M.D.
HERMES C. GRILLO, M.D.

Substernal extension of a goiter into the unyielding thoracic inlet enhances the potential of this generally benign neck mass to cause stridor, dysphagia, or even asphyxiation. Such a substernal goiter, defined as any thyroid enlargement that has its greater mass inferior to the thoracic inlet, can be expected in 2 to 14 percent of all patients undergoing thyroid surgical procedures. Virtually all substernal goiters arise from and maintain some attachment to the cervical thyroid gland. Mediastinal goiters developing from truly ectopic thyroid tissue are rare. Substernal goiters arise equally from the right and left lobes of the thyroid gland and generally reside in the anterolateral mediastinum, although 10 to 15 percent are limited to the posterior mediastinum. Patients are usually in the fifth decade of life and frequency of occurrence is higher in women.

Symptoms of dyspnea, stridor, and dysphagia occur and may be positional, but 15 to 50 percent of patients have no symptoms whatsoever. A smaller group of patients (2 to 3 percent) experience the acute onset of stridor from incarceration of the mass in the thoracic inlet or from hemorrhage. Most patients have a palpable neck mass or tracheal deviation, though 10 to 20 percent manifest no such abnormality. Substernal goiters are adenomatous by nature, being multinodular or having one or more follicular adenomas. Carcinoma occurs in 2 to 3 percent and is often occult.

DIAGNOSIS

Measurements of thyroid function are rarely helpful, as these patients are nearly always euthyroid. The standard chest roentgenogram is the only study routinely required for the diagnosis of substernal goiter; computerized tomography with contrast will show characteristic nonhomogeneous enhancement and may occasionally be helpful. We have found radioisotope thyroid scanning less useful, since there may be little or no functioning thyroid tissue in the substernal component. Needle biopsy carries increased risk in substernal goiters and is rarely necessary, since the indications for resection involve the need to relieve the mechanical rather than the cytopathologic effects of the mass. If necessary, the palpable cervical portion of the goiter can be safely biopsied.

TREATMENT

The treatment of substernal goiter is surgical. There is little evidence that medical treatment is effective in relieving mechanical symptoms or even in halting progressive growth. Radioactive iodine treatment may be useful for the very rare hyperfunctioning nodule in a substernal goiter, but is less successful for the more common diffuse multinodular goiters. These respond poorly to prolonged thyroid suppression with levothyroxine, with signs and symptoms remaining stable or progressing despite documented suppression of thyroid-stimulating hormone. The presence of a substernal goiter, therefore, in all but the highest risk patient is an indication for resection. Asymptomatic patients benefit from removal of the small but present risk of acute stridor or occult thyroid carcinoma and symptomatic patients experience relief of dyspnea and dysphagia.

OPERATION

A standard operative approach is used for each patient with substernal goiter. The patient rests supine on the operating table with a roll beneath the shoulders and with the back elevated to decrease engorgement of the cervical veins. The neck and anterior chest are prepared and draped. A midcervical collar incision allows access to the goiter inferiorly and the superior pole vessels superiorly and may be extended in T fashion if a partial or complete sternotomy is needed. Subplatysmal flaps are elevated superiorly and inferiorly, and the strap muscles are divided. Individual ligation of the upper pole vessels is first performed, after which the goiter is mobilized in a subcapsular manner, thereby minimizing injury to the pleural apices, the inferior thyroid veins, and the recurrent laryngeal nerve. The substernal mass is then delivered into the neck by traction, a sweeping motion of the surgeon's finger, patience, and occasionally sponge-holding clamps or other instruments. Intentional fragmentation of the mass is not performed, since it could result in increased bleeding or incomplete removal of the rare occult carcinoma. In the unusual instance in which the goiter cannot be delivered, an upper partial sternotomy may be performed. Following mobilization of the goiter, the recurrent laryngeal nerve is identified and the attachments of the lobe and isthmus to the trachea are divided. For the occasional patient with a bilateral goiter, a bilateral subtotal resection or a lobectomy plus subtotal contralateral lobe resection is performed. Removal of goiters located in the posterior mediastinum may be more difficult, but even these generally can be removed through a cervical incision only. A small rubber drain is brought through the incision and removed on the first postoperative day. The patient is generally discharged on the third or fourth postoperative day.

No single operative approach is perfect for every patient, for goiters vary greatly in size and position, but the vast majority are approachable through a standard cervical collar incision. In 80 recent patients at the Massachusetts General Hospital and 20 at the Wilkes-Barre General Hospital, 98 required only this incision. Other options, in decreasing order of probable need, include upper sternotomy, upper sternotomy plus anterior thoracotomy, complete sternotomy, or posterolateral thoracotomy with or without cervical resection through a second incision. We attempt to identify the recurrent laryngeal nerve and at least one parathyroid gland, often the superior one, in each case. Intraoperative or postoperative problems with the trachea, such as tracheomalacia or tracheal "collapse," have been alluded to throughout the history of goiter surgery, but rarely occur. The most reasonable course upon recognition of tracheomalacia is endotracheal intubation for 24 to 48 hours or longer. In the rare patient in whom the problem persists beyond this time, tracheostomy or tracheal T-tube placement may be considered.

RESULTS

There are no available data relating to deaths from untreated substernal goiter. A death or major complication from resection of substernal goiter, however, should be rare. Problems related to bleeding, pneumonia, recurrent laryngeal nerve palsy, myocardial infarction, and pulmonary embolism have been reported but are unusual. An occasional patient may experience transient recurrent nerve dysfunction, transient hypocalcemia, atelectasis, or wound seroma. Patients can be expected to do well and to be relieved of upper respiratory and esophageal obstruction. Those with occult carcinoma are likely to be cured. All patients should be examined for potential recurrence of goiter over their remaining lifetimes; since up to 20 to 25 percent may experience such recurrence. Although most surgeons place patients on levothyroxine (0.1 to 0.2 mg per day) indefinitely after resection of substernal goiter, it may be unnecessary, and there is little evidence that it will prevent recurrence of the goiter.

Surgery should therefore be recommended for all but the highest risk patient with substernal goiter. With a minimum of preoperative evaluation and a maximum of careful operative technique, the surgeon can offer the patient freedom from dyspnea, dysphagia, possible occult malignancy, and the threat of acute asphyxiation.

SUGGESTED READING

Allo MD, Thompson NW. Rationale for the operative management of substernal goiters. Surgery 1983; 94:969–977.

DeAndrade MA. A review of one hundred twenty-eight cases of posterior mediastinal goiter. World J Surg 1977; 1:789–797.

Johnston JH Jr, Twente GE. Surgical approach to intrathoracic (mediastinal) goiter. Ann Surg 1956; 143:572–579.

Katlic MR, Grillo HC, Wang CA. Substernal goiter: analysis of eighty patients from Massachusetts General Hospital. Am J Surg 1985; 149:283–287.

Katlic MR, Wang CA, Grillo HC. Substernal goiter: a collective review. Ann Thorac Surg 1985; 39:391–399.

LUNG NEOPLASIA

SMALL-CELL CARCINOMA

JOHN A. MEYER, M.D.

Small-cell carcinoma is a tumor of extreme biologic malignancy, characterized by early and widespread dissemination, rapid growth, and relatively short patient survival. The original TNM criteria for staging of lung cancer specified that all cases of small-cell carcinoma be classified as stage III, because survival was uniformly poor and seemed to bear no relation to anatomic extent of disease. Medical oncologists from the beginning classified patients with small-cell carcinoma only by the scheme of the VA Lung Group as having limited disease if identifiable tumor involvement was limited to one hemithorax plus the ipsilateral supraclavicular nodes; this represents the area that could be encompassed by a single radiation field. Any more distant involvement was classified as extensive disease. Recently, however, improved patient survival resulting from aggressive combined treatment has revived consideration of TNM staging for small-cell carcinoma.

Histologic classifications of this tumor have led to much confusion. We should disregard talk of small-cell adenocarcinoma, small-cell squamous carcinoma, and the like. Present consensus divides pure small-cell carcinoma into two histologic subtypes: (1) classic oat cell carcinoma, made up of small round cells with scanty cytoplasm and closest to lymphocytes in appearance; (2) intermediate-cell carcinoma, comprising those cell types previously called polygonal, fusiform, and spindle cell. Several reviews have found no differences in clinical behavior or prognosis among these types. A third category, admixture of small-cell carcinoma with another cell type (generally large-cell anaplastic) tends to respond poorly to treatment, is rarely seen on initial biopsies, but is found commonly after prolonged treatment or at autopsy.

Several studies have claimed prognostic significance for ultrastructural features of the tumor cells, but these dealt only with survival after surgical resection. Another study found that the presence of ultrastructural features thought indicative of squamous differentiation paradoxically was associated with *better* response to chemotherapy. The final criterion of small-cell carcinoma is a deletion of sites 14 to 23 on the p (short) arm of chromosome 3, known as the 3p deletion; this has correlated well with identification of small-cell carcinoma by light microscopy. More recent studies relate excessively malignant biologic behavior to the degree of amplification of the c-*myc* oncogene; the most malignant "variant" cell lines showed greatest amplification, as much as 20- to 60-fold. Again the variant line was found more frequently at autopsy. Accelerating expression of the particularly malignant phenotype may be a natural consequence of genetic instability in tumor cell populations; the variants, being more malignant, tend to have a selective growth advantage over the earlier cell lines.

THERAPEUTIC CONSIDERATIONS

The same biologic characteristics that distinguish small-cell carcinoma have made it virtually incurable by surgical resection, except for a few of the earliest and most minimal lesions. Very sensitive to radiotherapy, it seldom can be controlled or eradicated because of the tendency to dissemination outside the treatment field. Rapid growth rate, short doubling time, and high labeling index favor its responsiveness to chemotherapy, which has the advantage besides of being a systemic treatment method. The concept of combined methods has influenced treatment strategy for the past 15 years; the large bulk of tumor at the primary site and the mediastinal nodes can be treated effectively by irradiation, and the disseminated component by intensive chemotherapy. Treated in this way, almost all patients with "limited" disease will respond, with complete remission in as many as 70 to 90 percent and median survival of 12 to 15 months. Patients with "extensive" disease do much less well; approximately 20 to 30 percent achieve clinically complete remission, and median survival averages perhaps 7 to 8 months.

Chemotherapy regimens utilize three or even four drugs concurrently to maximum reasonable tolerance. Highly active agents include cyclophosphamide (Cytoxan), cis-diamminedichloroplatinum (cisplatin), chloroethyl-cyclohexyl-nitrosoureal (CCNU or lomustine), the epipodophyllotoxin VP-16-213 (etoposide), doxorubicin (Adriamycin), amethopterin (methotrexate), and the plant alkaloid vincristine. Treatment cycles generally are 3 to 4 weeks in length, except that 6- to 8-week cycles are necessary with the nitrosoureas because of delayed marrow toxicity. When treatment is properly managed by a skilled oncologist, life-threatening toxicity is rare.

Careful diagnostic studies and staging are prerequisite to treatment. Cytologic specimens often are misleading, and a histologic biopsy specimen is required. Computed tomography (CT) of the brain and isotope scanning of the liver and skeletal system are done even in the absence of symptoms, as are bilateral iliac crest bone marrow aspiration and biopsies. Initial studies of renal function must be done if the treatment regimen is to include cisplatin, and the left ventricular ejection fraction must be determined if Adriamycin is to be used. CT of the chest is useful and I do mediastinoscopy in all patients not showing the M_1 factor, to identify N_2 if present. While medical oncologists divide patients before treatment only into categories of limited or extensive disease, I have sought to do careful staging in those patients with apparently early or localized disease.

If the initial diagnosis of small cell carcinoma has been made by resection of a pulmonary nodule, the same studies are carried out in the postoperative period for dissemination, before the course of treatment is determined.

TREATMENT: STRATEGIES AND RESULTS

Intensive combination chemotherapy is the key to all treatment programs. Patients presenting initially with extensive disease (M_1) are treated by chemotherapy only; radiotherapy may be added for palliation if brain metastases are present, or if bone pain and other severe symptoms are unresponsive to chemotherapy. There is no evidence that radiation therapy prolongs life in this group. Only a very few patients, less than 1 percent in all, have achieved long disease-free survival.

Patients with limited disease generally do much better. Almost all respond, by standard criteria, when both chemotherapy and irradiation of the primary site are used, and the majority achieve complete remission. Radiation therapy appears to increase the response rate, but it is not clear whether it actually prolongs survival. Patients who quit smoking, even if only from the time of diagnosis, have a better chance of long survival. Relapse in the brain is common; prophylactic cranial irradiation (PCI) is given to those patients who achieve complete remission, even though some investigators doubt that it benefits survival. Without PCI, cumulative failure rate in the central nervous system approaches 80 percent by 2 years after the start of treatment. Empirically, most patients are treated for a year or until progression; no guidelines are known that indicate when treatment may safely be discontinued. Perhaps 15 percent of limited-disease patients have prolonged remission and presumably have had their disease eradicated. Relapse more than 30 months after start of treatment is most unusual, almost nonexistent. Long survivors, however, are subject to many late complications of treatment such as optic atrophy, neurologic deterioration, acute leukemia, and prolonged bone marrow suppression.

SURGICAL RESECTION IN SELECTED CASES

A key attribute of chemotherapy is that no matter how successful, it reduces tumor burden by a pattern of first-order kinetics. In a logarithmic calculation of growth or regression, the same chemotherapeutic effect is required to reduce a tumor mass 10 cm in diameter to 1 cm as to reduce the last surviving 1,000 cells to one cell. Both effects represent a "three-log" or thousandfold reduction of tumor burden; a three-log reduction means that chemotherapy has killed 999 of every 1,000 tumor cells. Considering that a far-advanced 10-cm tumor mass amounts roughly to 10^{12} cells, and a residual tumor 1 cm in diameter to 10^9 cells, it is clear that complete remission is not remotely equivalent to cure. Treatment failure after complete remission results from regrowth of an unknown residual fraction of cells, now resistant to the chemotherapy.

The question arose whether clean surgical resection of apparently localized disease would help subsequent chemotherapy to eradicate the residual before losing effect.

In phase II trials of chemotherapy and surgical resection, we found that a biopsy from the mediastinal nodes showing tumor (N_2 disease) was associated with eventual relapse in all cases. Relapses for the most part were at distant sites and were very late in several cases, but it was clear that surgical resection did not add a potentially curative factor in this group.

Conversely, patients with TNM Stages I and II who underwent initial clean surgical resection and the full course of chemotherapy on an adjuvant basis have done very well. Only one of 10 such patients suffered relapse, while two others died of unrelated causes before 5 years. Seven of 10 (70 percent) remained well 5 years after treatment. We cannot prove that surgical resection was a factor in this good survival; the patients may have done well simply because they had early-stage disease. Conversely, however, accurate staging is not possible without resection, and proof of Stage I or II is a highly favorable prognostic sign. Useful criteria for initial surgical resection are that the tumor be peripheral, surrounded by clear lung, and that results of all studies for dissemination, including mediastinoscopy, be normal. The patients must receive the full course of chemotherapy postoperatively; relapse at a distant site will be incurable.

Most of these patients with Stage I or II, however, did not receive prophylactic cranial irradiation; reliable data proving that it would be beneficial are not available. There is at least some risk of relapse in the brain if PCI is omitted, but there also is some risk of late neurologic sequelae if it is given. Until the question can be resolved for early lesions, we would recommend PCI for Stage II disease, if the patient agrees, but suggest omission for those with Stage I.

SUGGESTED READING

Aisner J, Alberto P, Bitran J, et al. Role of chemotherapy in small cell lung cancer: a consensus report of the International Association for the Study of Lung Cancer workshop. Cancer Treat Rep 1983; 67:37–43.

Johnson BE, Nau MN, Gazdar AF, et al. Oncogene amplification of c-*myc* and N-*myc* in cell lines established from patients with small cell lung cancer is associated with shorter survival. Proceedings of the American Society for Clinical Oncology (ASCO) 1985; 4:186.

Meyer JA. Effect of histologically verified TNM stage on disease control in treated small cell carcinoma of the lung. Cancer 1985; 55:1747–1752.
Meyer JA. Five-year survival in treated stage I and II small cell carcinoma of the lung. Ann Thorac Surg 1986; 42:668–669.
Meyer JA, Comis RL, Ginsberg SJ, et al. Phase II trial of extended indications for resection in small cell carcinoma of the lung. J Thorac Cardiovasc Surg 1982; 83:12–19.

N_2 DISEASE IN NON–SMALL-CELL LUNG CANCER

F. GRIFFITH PEARSON, M.D., B.Sc.(Med), F.R.C.S.(C), F.A.C.S.

DEFINITION OF N_2 DISEASE

N_2 disease, as defined by the new American Joint Committee staging system, identifies metastases to ipsilateral mediastinal lymph nodes or subcarinal lymph nodes. Using the new AJC staging, N_3 disease is present when metastases occur in contralateral mediastinal lymph nodes, contralateral hilar lymph nodes, or in the prescalene nodes on either side. At the present time, patients with N_3 disease are not considered operable. Resection is recommended in carefully selected patients with N_2 non–small-cell lung cancer.

INDICATIONS FOR RESECTION

As with other malignancies, the N status is of major prognostic importance. When lymph node metastases do occur, the prognosis is further influenced by the level of nodal station involved, the number of nodes, and the extent of involvement (microscopic and intranodal versus gross or extranodal spread). Multiple levels of involvement, spread to stations distant from the primary tumor, and extranodal spread all adversely affect survival. Surgical treatment is recommended for those patients in whom a complete resection is deemed possible. There is now convincing data from published reports that surgery is the *best* treatment for N_2 disease when a complete resection is possible. There is no indication for palliative resection in patients with lung cancer, and the potential for cure in N_2 tumors managed by nonsurgical means such as radiotherapy or chemotherapy is negligible. Unfortunately, most N_2 tumors are inoperable at the time of discovery either because of hematogenous spread or of extension to nodal locations that preclude a complete and potentially curative operation. A challenging goal for the thoracic surgeon is to minimize the number of patients with N_2 disease who undergo thoracotomy and whose lesions cannot be completely resected. Prethoracotomy and intraoperative staging of the disease are critically important to achieving this objective.

PRETHORACOTOMY STAGING

It is widely accepted that neither plain chest films nor conventional mediastinal tomography can accurately define the N_2 status. Computed tomography (CT) is the procedure of choice for the noninvasive imaging of abnormal mediastinal lymph nodes. In a recent prospective study, we compared the accuracy of CT scanning and nuclear magnetic resonance imaging (MRI) and were unable to identify any significant benefit from using MRI. Using standardized CT scans, reasonably accurate projections of nodal diameter are possible. If any of the superior mediastinal nodes identified in the CT scan exceed 1 cm in diameter, mediastinoscopy is recommended for confirmation. A proportion of these "enlarged" nodes will prove to be benign at the time of mediastinoscopy, since mediastinal nodes frequently enlarge because of benign reactive changes associated with the tumor or because of pneumonitis in association with the primary lung cancer. Using a 1-cm diameter as the upper limit of normal, we still employ invasive staging with mediastinoscopy, since 10 to 15 percent of these "negative" nodes are found to harbor metastatic tumor. It is true, however, that most of these small nodes that contain metastatic tumor prove to be completely resectable, and many centers favor proceeding to thoracotomy without mediastinoscopy if the CT scan is negative, i.e., all nodes less than 1 cm in diameter.

Cervical mediastinoscopy is recommended as a staging procedure for most cases of presumably operable lung cancer in our institution. Mediastinoscopy more clearly defines cell type, identifies contralateral spread in some cases (which precludes complete resection), and may clearly demonstrate spread of tumor beyond the capsule of the node with fixation to mediastinal structures such as the trachea or great vessels to a degree that obviates complete removal of the tumor.

In patients with primary tumors in the left upper lobe or hilus of the left lung, standard cervical mediastinoscopy is done initially. If, on frozen section assessment, the nodes biopsied at cervical mediastinoscopy are negative for tumor, a left anterior or extended cervical mediastinoscopy is done to evaluate nodes in the subaortic anterior mediastinal locations. When the diagnosis of N_2 disease is established by mediastinoscopy in patients with non–small-cell tumors that otherwise appear operable, there are some cases in which complete resection is judged possible. These are cases in which the nodal involvement is ipsilateral and without extracapsular spread and fixation to unresectable mediastinal structures such as the trachea or great vessels. These more favorable mediastinoscopy positive cases constitute approximately 5 percent of all our resections for lung cancer. Another 5 percent are added when N_2 disease is encountered at thoracotomy at locations that are inaccessible at mediastinoscopy or mediastinotomy.

MANAGEMENT OF N_2 DISEASE AT THORACOTOMY

When N_2 disease is encountered, a radical lymphadenectomy is recommended with the objective of extending resection beyond the highest level of nodal involvement. Intraoperative frozen section facilities are essential in these cases in order to assure the surgeon, where possible, that all recognizable tumor has been removed. The nodal map described by Naruke in Japan is recommended for labeling nodal location and is in current use by the Lung Cancer Study Group for the multicenter North American trials of adjuvant therapy in resected lung cancer.

En bloc resection of the superior mediastinal lymph nodes is relatively straightforward on the right side. The mediastinal pleura is incised vertically from the hilus of the lung to the apex of the mediastinum. The right vagus nerve is identified, and care is taken to preserve the right recurrent laryngeal nerve that loops under the subclavian artery near the apex of the right hemithorax. The entire packet of fatty tissue that lies along the right and anterior aspects of the mediastinal trachea is removed; some mobilization of the posterior aspects of the superior vena cava and ascending aorta is required to provide adequate exposure. The azygos vein may be divided to further facilitate exposure. The subcarinal compartment of nodes is initially mobilized inferiorly, just anterior to the esophagus and posterior to the bronchus intermedius. The lowest of these subcarinal nodes lies posterolateral to the pericardium; which is easily identified as the nodes are mobilized. As this subcarinal dissection is carried more superiorly, the medial wall of the left main bronchus is exposed and cleared to the level of the carina itself. En bloc removal of the superior mediastinal nodes on the left side is technically very difficult or impossible. Dissection and mobilization are carried up under the aortic arch to the left lateral wall of the trachea, taking care to identify and preserve the left recurrent laryngeal nerve that is always at significant risk during this part of the operation. The highest nodes on the left side of the superior mediastinum are not accessible through this subaortic exposure. Fortunately, a high left paratracheal station is an unusual site for metastases.

Finally, it is noted that certain specific circumstances make this mediastinal lymphadenectomy considerably more difficult. If thoracotomy is delayed for more than 7 to 10 days after mediastinoscopy, significant vascular adhesions will be encountered in the peritracheal tissues. Similar dense adhesions may be encountered in cases receiving preoperative irradiation or chemotherapy or both.

An en bloc mediastinal lymphadenectomy will skeletonize the anterior and lateral aspects of the trachea and carinal regions. As a result, tracheobronchial blood supply may be significantly diminished and will be further impaired if the patient has received preoperative radiotherapy. In such cases, it is essential to protect the main bronchial stump following pneumonectomy on either side. On the right side, there may be difficulty in developing a good vascularized flap if the azygos vein, adjacent mediastinal pleura; and underlying fat have been resected. An intercostal muscle bundle may be used in such cases. My own choice is to obtain cover using a flap of pericardium developed from the right lateral and anterior aspects of the ascending aorta. This flap is thicker and has a more substantial circulation than a flap of parietal pleura developed from the adjacent chest wall. Following left pneumonectomy, it is almost always possible to obtain a good vascularized cover by suturing the anterior wall of the esophagus to the posterior pericardium at the level of the bronchial closure, which buries the left main bronchus deeply in the mediastinum.

ROLE OF ADJUVANT THERAPY IN THE MANAGEMENT OF RESECTED N_2 DISEASE

There is still no evidence that adjuvant radiotherapy or chemotherapy improves survival in patients with non-small-cell N_2 tumors that have been resected. If the resection is judged to be complete following the final pathology report, I would recommend that the patient receive no additional therapy unless he or she has been entered in a prospective trial evaluating some adjunctive modality.

SUGGESTED READING

Martini N, Flehinger BJ, Zaman MB, et al. Prospective study of 445 lung carcinomas with mediastinal lymph node metastases. J Thorac Cardiovasc Surg 1980; 80:390–399.

Naruke T. Staging of N_2 disease. Chest (Suppl) 1986; 89:3385–3395.

Pearson FG, Delarue NC, Ilves R, et al. Significance of positive superior mediastinal nodes identified at mediastinoscopy in patients with resectable cancer of the lung. J Thorac Cardiovasc Surg 1982; 83:1–11.

Pearson FG, Nelems JM, Henderson RD. et al. The role of mediastinoscopy in the selection of treatment for bronchial carcinoma with involvement of superior mediastinal lymph nodes. J Thorac Cardiovasc Surg 1972; 64:382–390.

SUPERIOR SULCUS TUMOR

DONALD L. PAULSON, M.D., Ph.D.

Tumors in the superior pulmonary sulcus are usually bronchogenic carcinomas that evoke a characteristic clinical syndrome because of their location at the extreme apex of the upper lobes of the lungs. Situated in the narrow confines of the thoracic inlet, these tumors extend locally to involve adjacent structures, including the lower roots of the brachial plexus, intercostal nerves, the sympathetic chain, more or less rib destruction, and vertebral infiltration, causing constant and characteristic pain in the distribution of the eighth cervical and first and second thoracic nerve roots and often Horner's syndrome.

Other tumors that may produce a similar clinical syndrome by invasion of the thoracic inlet, such as more extensive carcinomas that extend to the inlet from another primary location in the remainder of the upper lobes, are excluded as apical chest tumors and are not pertinent to a discussion of the management of tumors in the superior pulmonary sulcus as described by Pancoast.

Thirty years ago, tumors in the superior pulmonary sulcus were widely held to be resistant to irradiation and inaccessible to complete and curative resection. Average survival time of untreated patients after diagnosis was 10 to 14 months. Radiation therapy alone or following resection left few survivors after 1 year. During the last 25 years, results have been improving. Irradiation used alone has been reported to relieve pain, prolong survival, and in some instances effect a cure. Irradiation combined with incomplete resection has been reported to be encouraging, although the results are not always comparable, as frequently less extensive apical chest tumors are confused with typical superior pulmonary sulcus tumors. Preoperative irradiation combined with extended resection has improved survival dramatically.

PRETREATMENT STUDIES

A tumor in the superior pulmonary sulcus is usually suspected by the characteristic history of pain in the shoulder and down the arm along dermatomes corresponding to T1 and C8 nerve roots and by radiographic evidence of a small shadow at the extreme apex of the chest in the thoracic inlet. Planigraphy, bone scanning, and computed tomography (CT) are used to delineate the location of the tumor and extent of involvement of ribs, paraspinal region, and vertebrae. Magnetic resonance and vascular imaging may be indicated.

Cytohistologic proof of the tumor has been obtained in a small percentage of cases by sputum examination, flexible bronchoscopic aspiration, brush biopsies, and transbronchial needle biopsy. Percutaneous fine-needle biopsy through the posterior cervical triangle just anterior to the trapezius fold and the posterior portion of the first rib, using CT and biplane fluoroscopy for localization, has been effective in obtaining cytohistologic proof in 95 percent of the patients in whom it was used.

Open biopsy of the cupola of the pleura through a supraclavicular scalenotomy incision may be necessary for histologic diagnosis, particularly when the diagnosis is in doubt.

Mediastinoscopy and scalene node biopsy of palpable nodes are helpful for establishing the histologic diagnosis and for staging and determining the extent of involvement.

PREOPERATIVE IRRADIATION AND EXTENDED RESECTION

The results of preoperative irradiation combined with extended resection for proven carcinomas in the superior pulmonary sulcus during the last 30 years are significant in that in 63 percent of the patients the disease was considered operable and 30 percent of all patients who completed combined treatment survived 5 years or longer, including 45 percent of those patients having T^3N^0 lesions.

The purpose of preoperative irradiation is to limit the extent of the tumor so that it is better localized and thus more completely resectable. With megavoltage equipment, a tumor dose of 3,000 rads, given in 10 fractions over 12 elapsed days, is delivered over the tumor in the superior pulmonary sulcus, the chest wall, and the superior mediastinum beyond the midline.

The pathologic effects of irradiation of the tumor are related to the length of survival after extended resection. Those patients (without nodal involvement) in whom no residual viable carcinoma could be found in the chest wall or margins of resection did well and were long-term survivors. However, those patients in whom viable tumor was found in the chest wall, the margins of the resection, the perineural lymphatics, or the nerve roots at the intervertebral foramen did poorly and died in less than 2 years, mainly from distant metastases, but also with local recurrence of carcinoma, regardless of postoperative external beam radiotherapy.

Clinical and experimental observations indicate that preoperative irradiation in doses not sufficient to cause gross regression of tumor will decrease local recurrence, prevent growth of disseminated tumor cells, and increase survival when compared with irradiation or operation alone.

The theoretic advantages of preoperative over postoperative irradiation depend on the treatment being administered prior to surgical interference and its attendant risks of dissemination, implantation, or inflammation, together with violation of the vascular bed of the tumor resulting in reduced oxygen tension and consequent diminished radiosensitivity. The use of additional postoperative radiation in patients who have had preoperative radiation and resection increases the risk of radiation fibrosis and nerve entrapment of the brachial plexus because the increased cumulative dose exceeds the tolerance of normal tissues.

Two to 3 weeks after completion of preoperative irradiation, a complete extended en-bloc resection is performed, usually including the entire first rib and the posterior portions of the second and third ribs, portions of the first three thoracic vertebrae (including the transverse processes and portions of the bodies as indicated), the intercostal nerves together with the eighth cervical nerve root (if involved), the lower trunk of the brachial plexus, and a portion of the stellate ganglion and dorsal sympathetic chain. The involved lung is resected by either lobectomy or segmentectomy, and radical dissection of regional hilar and mediastinal lymph nodes is carried out.

In the absence of nodal involvement, there has been no significant difference in survival among patients with squamous cell carcinoma, large-cell undifferentiated carcinoma, or adenocarcinoma. None of the patients with hilar or mediastinal nodal involvement survived 2 years, whereas 45 percent of those without nodal metastases survived 5 years or longer.

Bone destruction, involving mainly ribs or transverse processes, was present in half of the patients; in the absence of vascular or nodal involvement, 30 percent survived more than 5 years.

Permanent neurologic deficits involving the ulnar nerve, resulting from resection of the lower trunk of the brachial plexus, are not incapacitating. If the extent of the tumor permits preservation of the eighth cervical nerve, the defect secondary to resection of the first and second nerve roots is not severe. Horner's syndrome if not present preoperatively develops postoperatively secondary to dorsal sympathectomy of at least a portion of the stellate ganglion. None of these defects is disabling, and all patients surviving more than 3 years are relieved of their original pain.

Absolute contraindications to surgical intervention, in addition to the usual cardiopulmonary limitations, include more extensive involvement of the brachial plexus or bodies or laminae of the vertebrae, mediastinal perinodal involvement, and distant metastases. Venous obstruction, although not typical of carcinoma in the superior pulmonary sulcus, is another contraindication to operation, if present. In some instances, patients with ipsilaterally involved mediastinal nodes have undergone resection for palliation of pain, but survival has been limited to 2 years. Similarly, resection of an extensively involved subclavian artery with grafting, may rarely be necessary, although these patients usually do not survive 2 years.

SUGGESTED READING

Pancoast HK. Importance of careful roentgen-ray investigations of apical chest tumors. JAMA 1924; 83:1407–1411.

Pancoast HK. Superior pulmonary sulcus tumor: tumor characterized by pain, Horner's syndrome, destruction of bone and atrophy of hand muscles. JAMA 1932; 99:1391–1396.

Paulson DL. Extended resection of bronchogenic carcinomas in the superior pulmonary sulcus. Surg Rounds 1980; 3:10–21.

Paulson DL. Superior sulcus carcinomas. In: Sabiston DC Jr, Spencer FC, eds. Gibbon's surgery of the chest. 4th ed. Philadelphia: WB Saunders, 1983:506.

Paulson DL. The importance of defining location and staging of superior pulmonary sulcus tumors. Ann Thorac Surg 1973; 15:549–551.

CHEST WALL INVASION IN NON–SMALL-CELL CARCINOMA

PHILIP E. BERNATZ, M.D.

Invasion of the chest wall by non–small-cell bronchogenic carcinoma occurs in approximately 5 percent of lung cancers. Although such extension implies unresectability, this conclusion may be difficult to confirm preoperatively and, in the absence of distant metastases, surgical resection is the treatment of choice with hope of a comfortable prolonged survival in up to 50 percent of patients.

PREOPERATIVE CONSIDERATIONS

When extrapulmonary invasion of lung cancer occurs, two-thirds of patients will be harassed by significant persistent, progressive, and relentless chest wall discomfort. This history, plus an appropriate abnormal chest roentgenogram, sets the stage for surgical treatment, although age and clinical picture otherwise must raise suspicions of metastatic cancer, primary chest wall tumors, lymphoma, desmoids, or inflammatory lesions such as actinomycosis that are prone to involve chest wall and lung and may or may not be best treated by resection. Bone scans are of little diagnostic aid locally, but are effective in focusing attention on other areas in the skeleton that would modify surgical attack on the primary lung lesion. From a local standpoint in the thorax, plain chest films, special views, including tomography, computed tomography, and magnetic resonance imaging, in that order, may depict the degree of extrapulmonary malignant invasion. But even the best of these modalities, alone or in combination, falls short in 25 to 35 percent of cases of providing evidence that precludes exploration or even justifies preoperative radiotherapy or chemotherapy for an ominous lesion in the hope that a successful resection may follow. The effectiveness of such adjuvant therapy has not been shown to improve resectability or prolong survival, but we have seen marked subsidence of visible and palpably proven chest wall involvement by lung cancer following radiation therapy. We utilize it preoperatively if apparent tumor extension is near the vertebral column. A tissue diagnosis of malignancy must precede such a treatment program and is usually obtained by percutaneous needle biopsy.

Bronchoscopy is performed even with these peripheral lesions, and especially if the sputum is positive for malignant cells. A multicentric bronchogenic carcinoma (usually squamous cell type) must be excluded. If computed tomography reveals no enlarged mediastinal lymph nodes, mediastinoscopy is not done. When there is mediastinal lymph node (N2) enlargement (1 cm), mediastinoscopy is done just prior to thoracotomy. With positive mediastinal lymph nodes we are inclined to avoid resection, because long-term survival (5 years) in our resected patients with $T_3N_2M_0$ has been limited to one patient. This reluctance to proceed with radical surgery is reinforced by a surgical mortality rate of 12 percent in our most recent surgical series (73 patients).*

SURGERY

The standard posterolateral skin incision is modified by the level of thoracic wall involvement but permits good access to the hilus of the lung. The serratus anterior muscle is preserved intact by retracting it either medially or, laterally, unless tumor invasion interferes. The transaxillary or midline sternal approaches are reserved for selected patients with very limited local disease, or the sternal approach for the presence of bilateral abnormalities. The site of the chest wall invasion may be evident exterior to the ribs and dictates the interspace entrance into the pleural space, usually at a distance anteriorly. Specimens of pleural washings are obtained for cytologic study, and this is repeated following the resection. With limited exposure, the mediastinum is assessed, lymph nodes dissected if exposure permits, and the definitive plan of resection formulated. Palliative resection, especially with pneumonectomy, is not acceptable, but may be forced as a compromise. If there is obvious tumor invasion of the chest wall and resection appears possible, biopsy is done if histologic diagnosis has not been established preoperatively. A needle biopsy usually suffices, and there is minimal threat of contamination. If simple adherence of the visceral and parietal pleurae is suspected from palpation (e.g., mobility of the lung), an extrapleural plane is developed with finger dissection. If the layers separate easily, the lung is freed completely, but, if not, mobilization of the involved portion of the chest wall is done before malignant contamination of the pleural space can occur. Compromise procedures that leave tumor on the chest wall to be managed by postoperative radiation therapy have been disappointing in controlling the malignancy, and can be rationalized only in high-risk patients with borderline cardiorespiratory function.

If vertebral body involvement by tumor is evident, except in the case of minimal invasion, we would usually not proceed with resection, because we have had virtually no surviving patients with vertebral column invasion.

Resection of the involved chest wall is usually done initially, utilizing cutting cautery on soft tissue and obtaining a 4-cm, apparently free margin around the tumor. A normal rib and interspace above and below guide the dissection. Intercostal vessels are secured with suture ligatures. The extent of chest wall resection need not be compromised by concerns of reconstruction. The hilar structures may be secured initially in the procedure, but often the chest wall invasion dictates that this mobilization be done before good hilar exposure is obtained. Conservative pulmonary resection is usually possible with these peripheral lung cancers, so a segmental or wedge resection can suffice for those patients whose respiratory reserve is often compromised, and when chest wall resection further compromises function. The pulmonary veins are invariably interrupted first to decrease chances of malignant cell dissemination. Larger vessels are stapled (2.5-mm length) and bronchi similarly closed (3.5- to 4.8-mm length). Dissection of mediastinal lymph nodes for staging and therapy accompanies each procedure.

If the chest wall defect is covered by the scapula and attached muscles, we usually close the soft tissue with no additional attention to the site of resection. However, a surgical mortality of 12 percent in the past has motivated us to maximize efficiency of respiratory mechanics. The defect is usually closed using a Goretex film sutured tautly, but Marlex, Dacron, or Dexon mesh is also satisfactory. Rarely do we use autogenous ribs or steel strips to reinforce such a defect. Pedicled muscle transplants are employed over prostheses only if local muscle invasion and resection justify such coverage. Appropriate antibiotics are used in the perioperative period (48 hours), or as long as chest tubes are in place. Continuous epidural analgesia is used for 48 to 96 hours postoperatively, and ventilatory support is continued only if tidal volumes are ineffective in the immediate postoperative assessment.

RESULTS

Actuarial overall 5-year survival (Kaplan-Meier) of 73 patients following resection of a non–small-cell bronchogenic carcinoma with chest wall invasion was 39 percent. In the absence of lymph node metastasis, 50 percent of patients enjoyed long-term survival (5 years). Variables examined, including age, sex, location of tumor, extent of pulmonary resection, tumor size, cell type, and postoperative adjuvant therapy, did not singularly affect the survival adversely. Postoperative radiotherapy (12 patients) and chemotherapy (three patients) were used so sparingly that we cannot assess their value, except to say that in this experience they added nothing of benefit with respect to prolongation of survival. Others have advocated postoperative radiotherapy, noting it improved the survival of patients with $T_3N_0M_0$ lesions from 28 percent to 78 percent for a period of 5 years, but these data were derived from only 23 patients, so more experience is needed before deriving any final conclusions about the value of this adjuvant therapy. We do employ postoperative radiotherapy when the margins around the chest wall invasion have been compromised for one reason or another. Although current results discourage the use of adjuvant chemotherapy after resection, more effective combinations of drugs are likely to emerge and deserve clinical trials.

Recurrent cancer is usually metastatic in multiple sites and not amenable to resection. The time of recurrence averaged about 1 year following surgery in our series. We

* Editor's note: Many would argue that mediastinoscopy should be done in all patients with chest wall involvement because of the stated low cure rate and high mortality.

think it logical to advise resection of a localized recurrence in some instances. The local resection is usually diagnostic as well as therapeutic, and advisable if the tumor-free interval is reasonable (more than 6 months).

SUGGESTED READING

Grillo HC. Pleural and chest wall involvement. Int Trends Gen Thorac Surg 1985; 1:134–138.

Patterson GA, et al. The value of adjuvant radiotherapy in pulmonary and chest wall resection for bronchogenic carcinoma. Ann Thorac Surg 1982; 34:692–697.

Piehler JM, et al. Bronchogenic carcinoma with chest wall invasion. Ann Thorac Surg 1982; 34:684–692.

CARINAL NEOPLASIA

HERMES C. GRILLO, M.D.

Tumors of the carina fall into two groups. First are those that are primary in the airway. The greatest number of these are adenoid cystic carinomas, followed by a wide variety of benign and malignant lesions, including carcinoid tumors, squamous cell carcinoma, mucoepidermoid carcinoma, sarcomas of various types, and granular cell tumors. The second group is composed of bronchogenic carcinomas that have presumably originated in the main bronchi and extended to involve the carina. These include squamous cell carcinoma, adenocarcinoma, and large cell undifferentiated carcinoma. Oat cell carcinoma obviously may be seen but is usually so extensive that it is not a surgical problem. Surgical resection of the carina presents problems in the management of anesthesia during the reconstruction, in adequate access, in the anatomic techniques of reconstruction, and in the possibility for serious postoperative complications. Experience is limited. Eschapasse reported 19 cases from France in 1974, I reported 36 carinal resections in 1982 (although the number is now much increased), and Perelman reported 34 cases in 1986.

CLINICAL PRESENTATION

Patients primarily present with cough, dyspnea on exertion, hemoptysis, and stridor. A high degree of carinal obstruction may be present bilaterally, with a normal-appearing chest x-ray—at least on first examination. If hemoptysis does not occur, diagnosis may be delayed while patients are treated for "adult-onset asthma."

DIAGNOSTIC STUDIES

Tomograms of the carina are of most use in assessing the extent of the lesion, its location, and the amount of the apparently uninvolved airway above and below. CT scan with contrast is primarily useful to show extraluminal tumor. Bronchoscopy shows the extent of the intraluminal involvement and permits biopsy. If borderline obstruction is present, the bronchoscopist must be cautious about biopsy unless he is prepared to open up the airway on an emergency basis. In bronchogenic carcinoma, the usual considerations about distant disease apply. Thus the CT scan should include the liver and adrenals. In the case of bronchogenic carcinoma, it is better to defer mediastinoscopy until the time of proposed possible surgery in order not to confuse the mediastinal field.

EMERGENCY MANAGEMENT

Patients with carinal tumors may have nearly total obstruction on one side and subtotal obstruction on the other. In preparation for resection or as a temporizing maneuver, if the patient requires further study, the airway may be opened endoscopically. Bronchoscopy is done under general inhalation anesthesia without respiratory paralysis, using a ventilating rigid bronchoscope. The carina is assessed with Hopkins' telescope. The side with the lesser obstruction is first opened using the tip of the rigid bronchoscope as a coring device, a large-bore suction tube, and biopsy forceps. Manipulations are done intermittently to permit adequate ventilation. The opposite side is cleaned out in the same fashion. The YAG laser may be used through a rigid bronchoscope to accomplish the same goal, but generally this takes longer and is no more efficient. Its presumed advantage is that it avoids bleeding. However, in no case have I found bleeding to be such that it interfered with the procedure or caused any hazard.

ANESTHESIA

Anesthesia for carinal resection is by inhalation. A long, single-lumen tube with a flexible end is utilized so that it may later be advanced and reach from the patient's mouth into a main bronchus. High-frequency, "jet" ventilation is an alternative system that is particularly applicable for carinal reconstruction in that it eliminates the need for tubes across the operative field.

Cardiopulmonary bypass seems to be attractive for this type of surgery on first appraisal. In practice in difficult dissections it presents great danger, since manipulation of the lung in the presence of heparin will lead to parenchymal hemorrhage. Thus, in the simple cases in which it can be used safely, it is not needed, and in those cases in which it could theoretically facilitate operation, it is too dangerous. In some complex cases I have used two anesthesia machines with two small endotracheal tubes to ventilate two portions of the tracheobronchial tree simultaneously, or a bifid catheter for high-frequency ventilation.

APPROACHES

Right posterolateral thoracotomy in the fourth interspace usually provides the best exposure to the carina for difficult dissection or complex reconstruction. An earlier approach that I utilized was a "trap door" incision, consisting of a collar incision, a vertical sternotomy with angulation into a thoracotomy in the fourth right interspace. Although this allows access to the entire trachea, it has no particular advantage for carinal exposure. Median sternotomy allows for bilateral hilar mobilization and left pneumonectomy if it is required, but access is much less adequate for extensive dissection, as, for example, when tumor involves the esophagus. Perelman described this modification of the Abruzzini approach between the superior vena cava and aortic arch to the carina. Left thoracotomy is used when a tumor involves a large extent of left main bronchus and only a limited amount of carina. Where more extensive carinal resection with left pneumonectomy is necessary, the aortic arch interferes with access whether one attempts to approach the carina from the right or the left. Bilateral thoracotomy in the fourth interspace has been employed in such cases. Although this provides excellent access to both hili, it creates postoperative ventilatory problems.

OPERATION

In bronchogenic carcinoma involving the carina, mediastinoscopy with frozen sections is done at the time of proposed thoracotomy. The procedure is of greater magnitude than simple pneumonectomy, and therefore I do not proceed unless the patient is N2 negative. I do not, however, perform mediastinoscopy in patients with adenoid cystic carcinoma, since experience has demonstrated that even with positive nodes the biologic behavior of the tumor is such that the patient is far better off having resection done (with postoperative irradiation).

The carina is exposed and tapes passed around the trachea proximal to the tumor and around the right and left main bronchi. The left main bronchus is easily accessible through the right side of the chest just anterior to the esophagus and vertebrae. Dissection is usually done gently while ventilating both lungs, retracting the right lung. It is possible to guide the endotracheal tube into the left lung. I avoid skeletonizing the bronchial tree much proximal or distal to the area of planned resection, in order to preserve blood supply.

The right pulmonary ligament is divided. If it appears that hilar mobilization will be required, it is more convenient to do this prior to dividing the tracheobronchial tree. Initial mobilization consists of making a U-shaped incision in the pericardium inferior to the right pulmonary vein. This allows considerable upward movement of the carina. If necessary, the pericardium may be circumcised all the way around the hilus to provide further elevation. If complete circumcision of the pericardium is done, the vascular and lymphatic pedicle to the right main bronchus is preserved behind the pericardium to maintain lymphatic and vascular supply. Laryngeal release does not translate any useful mobility to the level of the carina.

The order of division of the tracheobronchial structures varies. I usually divide the left main bronchus and intubate it directly or, often, I have divided the trachea above the tumor and then passed an endotracheal tube through the distal tracheal segment into the left main bronchus. Either procedure allows the right lung to collapse, facilitating further dissection of the tumor-containing segment. The left recurrent laryngeal nerve lies on the aortic arch just on the other side of the trachea. As the specimen is taken up, including its lymph nodes, one must search for the nerve to be certain that it is not injured. The right recurrent nerve lies high in the chest, taking off beneath the subclavian artery. However, it, too, can be endangered. Lateral traction sutures are placed in the left and right main bronchi and the trachea. This allows for easier handling of these structures and also helps to hold the anesthesia tube in the left main bronchus.

If during dissection and manipulation the patient's oxygenation falls, the shunt through the unventilated right lung may be eliminated by slipping a gentle vascular clamp on the right pulmonary artery. Another alternative is to periodically inflate the right lung with oxygen. High-frequency ventilation may also be used, since it does not maintain the lung in its fully expanded state and is easier to work around.

Methods of reconstruction are varied and depend on the extent of resection and the patient's individual anatomy. Absorbable 4–0 Vicryl sutures are used for anastomosis, without complications.

When the lesion is a small one and located just at the carina, it is possible to reapproximate the medial walls of the right and left main bronchi to create a new carina, which is then sutured to the distal end of the trachea. This technique is rarely applicable because the left main bronchus is held distally by the aortic arch, and when one sutures the right main bronchus to the left main bronchus, the carina cannot be elevated. The only way that anastomosis can therefore be done is to bring the trachea down. This will devolve only to the extent that cervical flexion permits. I dissect bluntly in the anterior pretracheal plane to provide maximum mobility.

If the tumor is somewhat more extensive, I have usually found that end-to-end anastomosis of either the left main bronchus or the right main bronchus to the trachea must be done first. If it is possible to approximate the left main bronchus and the trachea end-to-end initially, this is preferable. Having once established that connection, the right main bronchus is elevated after intrapericardial mobilization and implanted into a right lateral wall opening in the trachea approximately 0.5 cm above the previous end-to-end anastomosis. The aperture in the trachea is made in the lateral cartilaginous wall as an ovoid opening, taking care to leave cartilage all the way around.

When a greater length of trachea has to be removed, there is no way in which the trachea and left main bronchus can be approximated. Therefore, the right main bronchus is anastomosed end-to-end to the trachea. The left main bronchus is sutured into the medial side of the bronchus intermedius.

Some lesions at the carina, including bronchogenic carcinoma of the proximal right main bronchus, may require removal of the right upper lobe as well as the carina. In some patients the bronchus intermedius and middle lobe must also be removed. In these cases the bronchus intermedius or the lower lobe bronchus may be elevated and implanted into the lateral wall of the trachea, as described. However, in some patients this is not possible, and the lobar or bilobar bronchus is implanted into the medial wall of the left main bronchus where a limited amount of trachea had been removed and end-to-end anastomosis of trachea to left main bronchus has been possible. Individual solutions are worked out for special cases.

A most difficult problem is presented by the occasional patient who has tumor involving a considerable amount of the left main bronchus and of the lower trachea as well. Once resection has been performed, there is no way in which the distal left main bronchus can be brought across the mediastinum and attached either to the lateral side of the right main bronchus or to the trachea. Perelman solved the problem by stapling the left main bronchus distally and ligating the left pulmonary artery to prevent shunting in an unventilated lung. Anastomosis is carried out between the trachea and right main bronchus, and the left lung is left in place as a nonfunctional organ. A transverse bilateral thoracotomy or median sternotomy allows sufficient access to perform left pneumonectomy at the same time as the carinal resection and reconstruction of right main bronchus to trachea.

If a tumor involves most of the left main bronchus but only a limited amount of carina, left pneumonectomy with carinal resection can be done from the left side. If tapes are placed about the lower trachea and the right main bronchus and around the aortic arch itself, it is possible to bring the carina up into the field on the left sufficiently to perform a direct anastomosis of the right main bronchus end-to-end to the trachea.

Right pneumonectomy for bronchogenic carcinoma involving the carina is easily enough done from the right side. Usually the extent of trachea to be removed is not great, and end-to-end anastomosis of the trachea to the left main bronchus is feasible. In a few of these patients the tumor is so limited that it is possible to salvage the right lower lobe and reimplant it as described.

In a number of patients who have had prior left pneumonectomy and who have required carinal resection, the operation has been done through the right chest, maintaining ventilation in the right lung throughout, never collapsing it completely. This has worked out very satisfactorily.

It is essential that all of these anastomoses be covered by viable tissue. This is principally to prevent the possibility of bronchovascular fistula. Usually I use broad pedicled pleural flaps and occasionally Brewer's pericardial fat pedicle. On infrequent occasions I have used pedicled intercostal flaps. If one wraps an airway of any type circumferentially with an intercostal flap, it is essential to remove the periosteum from it beforehand in order to prevent the occurrence of a ring of new bone formation that can obstruct the airway.

These methods have been used not only for carinal neoplasms but also for inflammatory and idiopathic stenoses of the carina. I have not used carinal prostheses because the potential for complications is too great; e.g., granulations particularly at the bronchial ends despite the intussuscepted prosthesis currently in use and hemorrhage from erosion of mediastinal vessels with or without preceding sepsis. Similar problems have attended the attempt to perform staged resections, although some of these have succeeded, as have prostheses. The concept of staged reconstruction consists largely of devolving cervical trachea down into the mediastinum to permit completion of the mediastinal reconstruction with later reconstruction of the cervical airway to reconnect it to the larynx. When tumor cannot be resected and primary reconstruction effected, it would seem to the patient's benefit at the present time to treat him or her with radiotherapy.

COMPLICATIONS

Complications and mortality after carinal resection have been higher than after sleeve resection of the trachea. My earlier reported mortality rate was 13 percent. Two other series reported 17 percent and 31 percent. This is undoubtedly because of the magnitude and complexity of the procedures. As time has gone on, the complications have been fewer. Deaths were seen from one bronchovascular fistula in a patient who did not have tissue interposed between the vessel and the anastomosis, and in patients who required postoperative ventilation and died of respiratory failure. Particularly following pneumonectomy with carinal resection, congestion of the remaining lung progressing to fatal respiratory failure has occurred. The etiology is not completely known, but is it suspected by Peters and his associates to be caused by overhydration intraoperatively, with failure of the capillary bed to handle the fluid load and resulting interstitial edema. This problem may be accentuated after carinal resection by interference with the lymphatic drainage of the residual lung if an extensive lymphadenectomy has also been done.

Nonfatal complications have included rare anastomotic stenosis, formation of granulation tissue prior to use of absorbable sutures, and one stenosis due to calcification in an intercostal flap with residual periosteum. Restenoses were successfully reconstructed at a later date.

SUGGESTED READING

Eschapasse H. Les tumeurs trachéales primitives. Traitment chirurgical. Rev Fr Mal Respir 1974; 2:425.

Grillo HC. Carinal reconstruction. Ann Thorac Surg 1982; 34:356–373.

Grillo HC, Zannini P, Michelassi F. Complications of tracheal reconstruction: incidence, treatment and prevention. J Thorac Cardiovasc Surg 1986; 91:322–328.

Pearson FG, Todd TRJ, Cooper JD. Experience with primary neoplasms of the trachea and carina. J Thorac Cardiovasc Surg 1984; 88:511–518.

Perelman MI, Koroleva NS. Primary tumors of the trachea. In: Grillo HC, Eschapasse H, eds. International trends in general thoracic surgery. Vol. II. Philadelphia: WB Saunders, 1987:91.

Peters RM. Postpneumonectomy pulmonary edema. In: Grillo HC, Eschapasse H, eds. International trends in general thoracic surgery. Vol. II. Philadelphia: WB Saunders, 1987:460.

Wilson RS. Anesthetic management for tracheal reconstruction. In: Grillo HC, Eschapasse H, eds. International trends in general thoracic surgery. Vol. II. Philadelphia: WB Saunders, 1987:3.

OCCULT NEOPLASIA

PETER C. PAIROLERO, M.D.
VICTOR F. TRASTEK, M.D.
W. SPENCER PAYNE, M.D.

Lung cancer is the most common malignant disease in the United States today. More than 99 percent of these cancers are eventually diagnosed and localized because of an abnormal chest roentgenogram. A few patients, however, have a normal chest roentgenogram and microscopic studies indicating malignant cells in the sputum. Although this combination of findings has been referred to as occult cancer, it does not specifically imply occult lung cancer, since approximately 10 percent of these patients will have cancer of the upper airway. Localization of these tumors can at times be difficult.

All patients with occult cancer (normal chest roentgenogram and abnormal cytologic findings in sputum) should first have complete examination of the head and neck, including the nose, sinuses, mouth, oropharynx, hypopharynx, and larynx. Biopsy should be done of any suspicious areas. Patients in whom results of head and neck examination are normal should then be considered to have occult lung cancer and should undergo bronchoscopic localization.

Nearly always, occult lung cancer is in situ or early invasive squamous cell carcinoma. Consequently, only minimal mucosal abnormalities are present, and routine visual bronchoscopic examination often may not show any abnormality. Nonetheless, initial bronchoscopy, utilizing a flexible fiberoptic bronchoscope, is done in the conventional manner with the patient awake.

Each bronchopulmonary segment is visualized. A biopsy is done of any abnormal areas. In two-thirds of these patients, occult lung cancer can be localized with a single bronchoscopic procedure using this technique. In the past, for those patients in whom initial results of bronchoscopy were entirely normal, a second bronchoscopic procedure was performed 4 to 6 weeks later under general anesthesia. Each bronchopulmonary segment was again examined and then brushed. This latter type of bronchoscopic procedure was then repeated at 2-month intervals as many times as necessary to localize the lung cancer. In the Mayo Clinic's experience more than 98 percent of occult lung cancers were localized with four bronchoscopic procedures.

More recently, however, attempts have been made to preferentially mark cancer cells with the intention of improving identification during bronchoscopy. The most promising marker is hematoporphyrin. Not only has hematoporphyrin been shown to be selectively concentrated by neoplastic tissue, but when activated by violet light of wavelengths between 400 nm and 407 nm, hematoporphyrin also exhibits strong reddish fluorescence. Hematoporphyrin derivative, a specially prepared recrystallized form of hematoporphyrin, has been the most extensively studied preparation to detect early lung cancer.

Past attempts to visualize hematoporphyrin fluorescence with the rigid open-tube bronchoscope or the standard flexible fiberoptic bronchoscope have proved disappointing. Occult squamous cell carcinoma usually arises within the proximal four divisions of the tracheobronchial tree. Half of these tumors are located in the upper lobe bronchi. Thus most occult neoplasms are beyond the range of the rigid bronchoscope. Although the flexible fiberoptic bronchoscope is ideal to evaluate upper lobe tumors, transmission of violet light through a fiberoptic bronchoscope of sufficient intensity to produce tumor fluorescence detectable by the eye alone is difficult. Moreover, white illumination is required for visual examination, and this tends to mask any faint red fluorescence.

Kinsey and co-workers at the Mayo Clinic have developed a photoelectric hematoporphyrin detector that is used simultaneously with a conventional flexible fiberoptic bronchoscope. The illuminating light source for the bronchoscope alternates between white and violet light. Because of the high-frequency oscillation, the endoscopist does not visualize either the exciting violet light or the hematoporphyrin fluorescence. Instead, fluorescence is detected photoelectrically. Once detected, an audiosignal is generated that is proportional to the intensity of fluorescence. A biopsy is then done at the site of maximum audiosignal.

With utilization of hematoporphyrin, localization is now usually successful with one bronchoscopic procedure. Nonetheless, conventional bronchoscopic examination with the patient awake is still done initially, because two-thirds of all cases of occult lung cancer will be diagnosed in this manner. For those patients, then, in whom localization is not possible, hematoporphyrin is utilized.

An individual carcinoma is considered localized when it is visible at the time of biopsy or, if not visible, when a single diagnostic biopsy specimen is obtained at bronchoscopy or when diagnostic bronchial brushings are collected from the same bronchopulmonary segment at two separate bronchoscopic examinations.

Once it is localized, patients should undergo conventional pulmonary resection of the lung cancer. In a recent report from the Mayo Clinic, 54 patients (all men) were found to have roentgenographically occult lung cancer. The mean age was 61 years and ranged from 45 to 76 years. All patients had abnormal cytologic findings in sputum and normal chest x-ray findings. The cancer was localized by bronchoscopy in all patients; the number of examinations ranged from one to five, with a mean of one and one-half. Seventy-five percent of cancers were localized within 169 days of the abnormal results of cytologic examination of sputum. Pulmonary resection for cure was performed in all patients. Lobectomy was done in 38 patients, pneumonectomy in nine, and bilobectomy in seven. Operative mortality was 5.6 percent.

Fifty-eight cancers were detected in these 54 patients. All 58 cancers were resected, and all were squamous cell carcinoma. TNM classification was T in situ (TIS) N_0 M_0 in 19 patients, T_1 N_0 M_0 in 25, T_1 N_1 M_0 in five, T_2 N_0 M_0 in four, and T_3 N_0 M_0 in one. The bronchoscopic examination also correlated well with the extent of tumor. All patients in whom the lung cancer was not endoscopically visible at the time of localization had no evidence of extrabronchial tumor invasion or metastatic involvement of lymph nodes. Overall 5-year lung cancer survival was 90 percent. Five-year survival for the 44 patients with TIS N_0 M_0 and T_1 N_0 M_0 neoplasms was 91 percent. Lung cancer developed subsequently in 12 patients (22 percent). Eleven of these patients had a second primary squamous cell carcinoma of the lung, six of which again were occult. Thus it appears that patients with occult lung cancer have a strong likelihood of long-term survival if treated early. Close surveillance is indicated because of the high incidence of a second primary lung cancer.

SUGGESTED READING

Cortese DA, Kinsey JH, Woolner LB, et al. Clinical application of a new endoscopic technique for detection of in situ bronchial carcinoma. Mayo Clin Proc 1979; 54:635–640.

Cortese DA, Pairolero PC, Bergstralh EJ, et al. Roentgenographically occult lung cancer: a ten-year experience. J Thorac Cardiovasc Surg 1983; 86:373–380.

Kinsey JH, Cortese DA, Sanderson DR. Detection of hematoporphyrin fluorescence during fiberoptic bronchoscopy to localize early bronchogenic carcinoma. Mayo Clin Proc 1978; 53:594–600.

Sanderson DR, Fontana RS. Early lung cancer detection and localization. Ann Otol Rhinol Laryngol 1975; 84:583–588.

Woolner LB, Fontana RS, Cortese DA, et al. Roentgenographically occult lung cancer: pathologic findings and frequency of multicentricity during a 10-year period. Mayo Clin Proc 1984; 59:453–466.

UNRESECTABLE NEOPLASMS OF THE LUNG

NAEL MARTINI, M.D.

Whereas small-cell carcinoma is now viewed as a systemic disease, the prognosis and outcome in the non–small-cell variants currently are dependent on effective local treatments. Fifteen to 30 percent of patients with carcinoma of the lung present for medical care relatively early, and at present surgery for this group of patients is the most effective treatment.

However, not every patient with operable disease has a tumor that is resectable. Reasons for unresectability range from extension of the tumor to vital structures such as the vena cava, trachea, or major vessels to restricted lung reserve that precludes adequate resection even if feasible. Most of these patients are treated by external radiation therapy, since radiation, like surgery, contributes to local-regional control. A course of 6,000 rads reportedly offers the best local control, with a 25 percent survival rate at 2 years. However, the complications are more severe than in patients with lower dosage schedules.

Alternative methods explored today include combining external radiation therapy with hypoxic sensitizers or hyperthermia. Still other methods include intraoperative electron beam irradiation and intraoperative interstitial radiation or brachytherapy. This latter treatment is extensively used at our center and we consider it to be the treatment of choice for localized unresectable cancers.

The advantages of interstitial implantation over conventional external radiation therapy are mainly attributable to its ability to deliver high doses of radiation to the tumor itself while limiting damage to the surrounding normal tissues. Localization is more precise because the seeds are inserted into the tumor only, and doses as high as 16,000 to 25,000 rads may be delivered with little damage to the surrounding tissues.

Our indications for implantation include several groups of patients:

1. Patients with limited pulmonary reserve and in whom adequate resection would necessitate the removal of lung tissue beyond their tolerance (an example is a patient with a 5-cm perihilar tumor without mediastinal involvement, necessitating a pneumonectomy that he or she could not tolerate).
2. Patients with hilar tumors adherent to the major vessels with no clearance for safe dissection or division of hilar structures.
3. Patients with tumors extending to the mediastinum or attached to the trachea, esophagus, aorta, or superior vena cava.
4. Patients with extensive involvement of the chest wall or spine, in whom complete tumor excision is not possible.

Implantation is generally not used for highly anaplastic tumors such as small-cell cancers, and it is also not used when there are distant metastases.

When the decision is made at thoracotomy that the tumor is unresectable, the radiotherapist is asked to assess and perform the implantation. Considerable time is first spent to expose and mobilize the tumor and make it accessible to implantation. This is the responsibility of the surgeon. Pleural adhesions are lysed, and hilar vessels and major structures are identified and their positions clearly noted. For centrally located tumors, the pericardium frequently is opened to allow assessment of the medial aspect of the disease and to allow adequate implantation without injury to the major vessels.

Intraoperative implantation has been particulary useful in treating superior sulcus tumors. The majority of these are unresectable by reason of their extension to the brachial plexus and the spine. The technique of implantation in superior sulcus tumors is as follows. The posterolateral thoracotomy incision is extended to the base of the neck. The scapula is mobilized to allow access to the tumor from within the rib cage as well as through the intercostal spaces. The pleural cavity is entered through the third or fourth interspace. Often it becomes necessary to detach the lung apex from the thoracic inlet to permit access to the paraspinal tissues. A palliative resection by wedge excision of the lung lesion is often carried out to reduce the tumor bulk and facilitate adequate intraoperative implantation. The implantation itself is then performed by the brachytherapist.

The main disadvantage of implantation is the need for surgical intervention. However, if the patient can tolerate a thoracotomy, the morbidity and mortality attendant upon implantation are the same as for exploratory thoracotomy and biopsy without resection, considerably less than for major resections.

Formerly this type of treatment was restricted to very few institutions because it utilized high-energy radionuclides, i.e., radon, gold, or iridium, posing problems of radiation exposure to operators and patients and to personnel in contact with patients. Since 1965, we have been using low-energy idodine sources, which have been equally effective. Radioiodine is a low-energy gamma emittor and has a long half-life of 60 days. This long half-life allows it to be stored in the hospital and makes implants available on short notice. Radiation exposure is also substantially reduced.

Currently there are two available methods of implantation. The first is the placement of permanent iodine-125 seeds into the tumor. The dimensions of the tumor to be implanted are measured with a caliper. The number of seeds required for implantation is based on the radioactivity of each seed and the volume of tumor and is calculated with the use of a nomogram (Fig. 1).

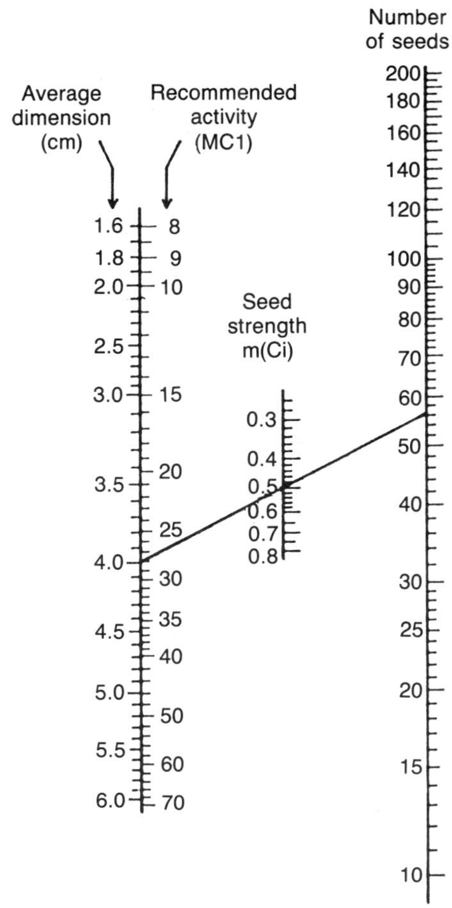

Figure 1 Nomogram for determination the of number of radioactive sources required to be implanted into a tumor. (Reprinted with permission of Anderson LL. Memorial Sloan-Kettering Cancer Center.)

The second method of implantation is referred to as temporary implantation. It consists of the placement of several small catheters along the mediastinum, chest wall, or diaphragm, where the disease is less well defined, for subsequent implantation of iridium-192. These catheters are inserted through the chest wall, advanced into the desired position, and secured in place with absorbable sutures. Iridium-192 is then afterloaded into the catheters 3 to 5 days after surgery. These are temporary sources of irradiation, since both the iridium and the catheters are removed after 3 or 4 days.

Postoperative external radiation therapy to the mediastinum or the primary tumor or both is given only if there are positive hilar or mediastinal lymph nodes or if all gross tumor could not be implanted.

With the introduction of computer analysis, it has become possible to accurately determine the dose distribution within the implanted tumor and hence evaluate the adequacy of the treatment.

When postoperative external radiation therapy is given, tumor doses of 3,000 to 4,000 rads are given in 3 to 4 weeks, and as a rule the external radiation dose does not exceed 4,500 rads.

In stage I or II disease, the reasons for unresectability are attributable to the location of the tumor and the patient's limited cardiopulmonary reserve. In stage III disease, reasons for unresectability are extension into the mediastinum with fixation to major vessels, trachea, or esophagus, extensive chest wall involvement precluding complete resection, and unresectable N_2 disease.

On the average, interstitial brachytherapy adds from 45 minutes to an hour to operating time, does not increase hospital stay, and often converts an exploratory thoracotomy into a therapeutic procedure.

Because of the satisfactory results obtained by implantation, our criteria for operability have been expanded, and patients who ordinarily would not be offered surgery undergo thoracotomy because of the availability of this alternative. Despite our expanded surgical indications, very few patients are explored for diagnosis only without the benefit of treatment by resection or implantation.

In our experience to date with over 1,000 patients treated by implantation for unresectable disease, we have observed that local and regional control of the tumor is achieved in 70 percent of all patients. In a small group of 55 patients with stage I or II disease treated by implantation, the 5-year survival rate attained is 32 percent. Implantation has been particularly useful in unresectable tumors of the superior sulcus, with a resultant 5-year survival rate of 20 percent. However, the vast majority of the patients treated by implantation have stage III disease.

Although prolonged survival into 5 or more years is rarely seen, the 2-year survival rate of this large group of patients is 40 percent. Most succumb to distant metastases despite effective locoregional control.

There are several protocols currently in progress assessing the merits of adjuvant chemotherapy in locally advanced lung carcinoma, but as yet there is no evidence that the regimens used reduce the incidence of recurrence or prolonged survival in these patients.

SUGGESTED READING

Hilaris BS, Gomez J, Nori D, et al. Combined surgery, intraoperative brachy-therapy and postoperative external radiation in stage III non-small cell lung cancer. Cancer 1985; 55:1226–1231.

Hilaris BS, Martini N. Interstitial brachytherapy in cancer of the lung: a 20-year experience. Int J Rad Oncol Biol Phys 1979; 5:1951–1956.

Hilaris BS, Martini N, Wong GY, Nori D. Treatment of superior sulcus tumor (pancoast tumor). Surg Clin N Amer 1987; 67:965–971.

Hilaris BS, Nori D. The role of external radiation and brachytherapy in unresectable non-small cell lung cancer. Surg Clin N Amer 1987; 67:1061–1071.

Hilaris BS, Nori D, Beattie EJ, et al. Value of perioperative brachytherapy in the management of non-oat cell carcinoma of the lung. Int J Oncol Biol Phys 1983; 9:1161–1166.

Hilaris BS, Nori D, Martini N. Results of radiation therapy in stage I and II unresectable non-small cell lung cancer. Endocuriether Hypertherm Oncol 1986; 2:15–21.

SUPERIOR VENA CAVA SYNDROME

ALEX G. LITTLE, M.D.

Superior vena cava (SVC) syndrome is clinically manifested by swelling of the face, head, and neck without swelling of the trunk or lower extremities. One or both upper extremities may be swollen as well. These phenomena are caused by mechanical obstruction of the SVC. Our focus is on therapy, but the basis of appropriate treatment strategies is a knowledge of the possible etiologies. In approximately 10 percent of cases the cause is benign, mediastinal infections or granulomatous diseases or both or thrombosis due to indwelling catheters. In the remaining 90 percent the etiology is malignant, most commonly lung cancer. However, other malignancies such as lymphoma and metastatic carcinoma from other organs are responsible in approximately 15 percent of patients by involvement of mediastinal lymph nodes. And finally, although lung cancer is responsible for approximately 75 percent of patients with SVC obstruction, the actual prevalence of cell type is fairly evenly divided among the common histologic types, so that approximately two-thirds of cases are due to non–small-cell lung cancer and one-third are due to small-cell carcinoma. The point is that the causes of SVC syndrome are varied, and this is important, as will be outlined further on.

Treatment of patients with SVC syndrome involves two considerations: treatment of the effects of the venous obstruction itself and treatment of the underlying cause. Until recent years there was widespread acceptance of the clinical tenet that SVC obstruction was a medical emergency and mandated immediate mediastinal irradiation for therapy. This has been shown to rarely be the case and in my experience occurs in no more than a small minority of patients. Patients must be individualized, and when life-threatening cerebral edema or laryngeal edema of an extent sufficient to cause significant respiratory distress is present, then urgent and immediate mediastinal irradiation on a presumptive diagnosis of malignancy is warranted. However, even when the swelling is quite dramatic, most patients can be managed by measures such as elevation of the arms, head, and neck to maximize venous drainage, diuresis to promote fluid loss, and oxygen supplementation if required. In fact, the signs of SVC obstruction tend to spontaneously improve over a period of a week to 10 days, even without treatment of the underlying cause, because collateral venous channels develop in the chest wall and mediastinum. This also serves to diminish any sense of urgency about instituting early radiotherapy.

DIAGNOSIS

The next step in management is to establish the histologic diagnosis of the underlying cause because of the variable diagnoses that produce this syndrome. Although most cases respond to some extent to mediastinal irradiation, SVC syndrome of benign etiology obviously requires no irradiation and some malignancies, such as small-cell lung cancer and lymphoma, may be more appropriately treated initially with chemotherapeutic agents. The diagnosis should be obtained expeditiously so that it is known if the patient suddenly decompensates. The approach should be guided by physical examination, chest roentgenogram, and computed tomographic (CT) scan of the chest and mediastinum. When palpable lymph nodes are present in the supraclavicular, cervical, or scalene areas, then biopsy under local anesthesia is very likely to be diagnostic and should be the first procedure performed. "Blind" scalene node biopsy is much less likely to yield diagnostic tissue. When lymph nodes are not enlarged or biopsy results are negative, alternative approaches are required. Despite theoretical concerns about the danger of flexible bronchoscopy, we have had no complications when performing this procedure in these patients. Therefore, when in addition to mediastinal pathology chest x-ray study shows a lung mass that is amenable to bronchoscopic access, bronchoscopy is a safe and frequently successful diagnostic maneuver.

If no lung mass is demonstrated, if the lung mass is

too peripheral to allow visualization and biopsy, or if bronchoscopy is not diagnostic, then further intervention should still be guided by the anatomy demonstrated by the chest film and CT scan. If mediastinal lymphadenopathy is documented on CT scan, then operative sampling of the mediastinal nodes should be performed next. The choice between cervical or parasternal mediastinoscopy depends upon the location of the mediastinal adenopathy. The procedure most likely to provide a direct approach should be chosen, since both are safe to perform even when enlarged venous collaterals are present. If a chest CT scan has been obtained, it should be used as a guide. Otherwise, the transcervical approach is chosen, unless the chest x-ray shows a left upper lobe carcinoma or adenopathy in the aortopulmonary window. In these situations, parasternal mediastinoscopy, e.g., the Chamberlain procedure, is preferable. Care is required in carrying out the appropriate dissections, and clearly one needs to pay even more attention than usual to the policy of aspirating mediastinal structures with a long needle to document their nonvascular nature prior to obtaining a biopsy. When proper precautions are utilized, there is no greater morbidity in performing mediastinoscopy via either approach in these patients than in patients without SVC obstruction. These patients do have impaired wound healing because of the edematous tissues, but this is not a serious problem and is not a contraindication to diagnostic intervention.

Percutaneous needle biopsy or aspiration can be considered for either lung lesions or mediastinal masses. Particularly when sampling the mediastinum, a thin-bore needle should be used for obvious reasons. This means that one is limited to a cytologic analysis of aspirated cellular material rather than histologic examination of tissue. This may make positive identification of the malignancy impossible.

THERAPY

Treatment of the underlying malignancy producing the SVC obstruction is based on a firm, histologic diagnosis. For most patients with non–small-cell lung cancer, the appropriate treatment is radiation therapy directed to the mediastinum. I have, however, treated one patient with localized involvement of the SVC by a squamous cell, T_3 primary tumor with en bloc resection of the right upper lobe and superior vena cava. Final, pathologic staging was $T_3N_0M_0$. The patient is alive and without evidence of disease 3½ years later. This is obviously an unusual patient, but the occasional possibility of curative resection should be kept in mind when the syndrome is caused by direct invasion of the primary tumor rather than by mediastinal nodal metastases.

Initial treatment for patients with small-cell lung cancer can be either mediastinal irradiation or chemotherapy, with the latter being preferred by most thoracic oncologists at this time. Treatment for lymphoma is also variable, and precedence may be given to irradiation or chemotherapy. The treatment for carcinoma metastatic to the mediastinum from organs other than the lung is dependent upon responsiveness to alternative therapeutic modalities.

On occasion, surgical bypass of the obstructed venous segment is appropriate. Doty has identified a group of patients with nearly complete SVC obstruction and reversed flow through the azygos vein as those most likely to benefit from bypass from the innominate vein to the right atrium. These patients typically have more pronounced cerebral or airway symptoms than most patients. Venacavography is required to define the vascular anatomy. When bypass is required, it is performed through a median sternotomy, and use of a spiral vein graft fashioned from saphenous vein is the ideal conduit, since prosthetic grafts tend to thrombose.

SUGGESTED READING

Lewis RJ, Sisler GE, MacKenzie JW. Mediastinoscopy in advanced superior vena cava obstruction. Ann Thorac Surg 1981; 32:458–462.
Little AG, Golomb HM, Ferguson MK, Skosey C, Skinner DB. Malignant superior vena cava obstruction reconsidered: the role of diagnostic surgical intervention. Ann Thorac Surg 1985; 40:285–288.
Schraufnagel DE, Hill R, Leech JA, Pare JA. Superior vena caval obstruction. Is it a medical emergency? Am J Med 1981; 70:1169–1174.
Skinner DB, Salzman EW, Scannell JG. The challenge of superior vena caval obstruction. J Thorac Cardiovasc Surg 1965; 49:824–833.
Stanford W, Doty DB. The role of venography and surgery in the management of patients with superior vena cava obstruction. Ann Thorac Surg 1986; 41:158–163.

SPIRAL VEIN GRAFT

DONALD B. DOTY, M.D.

Composite vein grafts constructed from the saphenous vein have been used clinically for bypass or replacement of the vena cava. In 1974, Chiu, Terzis, and MacRae reported construction of a composite vein graft from the external jugular vein in dogs that was matched to the size of the superior vena cava. The donor vein was opened longitudinally and wrapped in spiral fashion around a tubular stent. The edges of the vein were sutured together to form the conduit. This report stimulated the successful application of this technique in humans by Doty and Baker in 1976. At present, composite vein grafts constructed from the saphenous vein appear to be the most useful conduits for bypass or replacement of the superior vena cava.

Of all the options available for bypass of the superior vena cava, the most logical seems to be that of a graft interposed between the innominate or jugular vein on the left side and the right atrial appendage. A midsternal incision provides ready access to these large veins and the right atrium and interrupts few collateral venous channels in the chest wall. Because of the intracranial sinus venous connections in the skull, it is possible to achieve adequate venous drainage of the head through one internal jugular vein, so that the innominate or jugular vein to right atrium route should reliably decompress the head and the ipsilateral arm. Decompression of the contralateral arm should be improved by the usual collateral channels, which will be more available once the venous competition in the head and opposite arm is eliminated by the bypass graft.

End-to-end anastomosis of the innominate vein to the bypass conduit is probably best in order to assure obligatory flow into the graft. A graft of exactly the same size as the vein to which it is connected is preferred so that there will be slight outflow resistance to assure adequate venous distending pressure along with obligatory flow into the graft. Larger or smaller grafts offer no advantage.

PATIENT SELECTION

Patients selected for operation to bypass the obstructed superior vena cava should be those in whom venography shows complete obstruction of the superior vena cava associated with thrombosis of caval tributaries and distention of the veins of the upper compartment due to inadequate collateral circulation.

Contrary to popular belief, operative intervention may be very beneficial for patients with benign processes causing obstruction of the superior vena cava. Operation may be offered to these patients, provided that significant symptoms persist after sufficient time has passed to allow for development of collateral venous circulation (6 to 12 months). More urgent intervention may be required for acute thrombosis of the superior vena cava attributable to benign causes. For some patients in whom a malignant process is causing obstruction of the superior vena cava, bypass of the superior vena cava may be an important aspect of palliative treatment. Patients appropriate for palliative bypass of the superior vena cava should be those in whom the onset of the syndrome is acute and severe, especially those with signs of cerebral or laryngeal edema. These signs, in association with obstruction of the superior vena cava, indicate that life expectancy without operative intervention is on the order of 6 weeks. Thus surgery should be performed without delay so that definitive and orderly treatment of the primary disease process may proceed in a comfortable patient. When this treatment plan is followed, the natural palliated life course is followed, with patients surviving an average of 1 year without recurrence of superior vena cava syndrome.

Patients who should not be offered operation are those in whom collateral circulation has adequately decompressed the upper compartment veins so that there are only mild symptoms and signs of superior vena cava syndrome. Patients who have bulky tumors in the anterior mediastinum that may compress the thoracic inlet are not suitable for venous bypass because the veins are either not accessible or the route of the bypass graft is blocked.

PREPARATION FOR OPERATION

Medical measures such as bed rest with the head of the bed elevated and the administration of diuretics provide patient comfort and bring the patient to the operating room in better condition. Patients requiring exploratory thoracotomy for diagnosis should be considered for the midsternal approach with biopsy and operative bypass of the superior vena cava. Administration of intravenous fluids and medications through the upper extremity veins would seem to be contraindicated, but remarkably, these veins can be used, and the substances infused get into the systemic circulation without undue delay. Lower extremity venous infusion sites, however, are probably preferable, and patients coming to surgery should have at least one large-bore catheter inserted in a leg vein opposite to that selected for removal of the saphenous vein for the bypass graft.

CONSTRUCTION OF COMPOSITE SPIRAL SAPHENOUS VEIN GRAFT

The spiral vein graft should be precisely the same diameter as the vein to which it is to be anastomosed and exactly long enough to span between the vein and the right atrial appendage. There is no advantage to extra length, which may cause the graft to kink or buckle. As a practical matter, the saphenous vein excised from groin to knee will be just about right for a graft 12 mm in diameter, which will span between the innominate vein and right atrial appendage.

The saphenous vein is distended with heparinized saline solution and all side branches are ligated. The vein is opened longitudinally through its entire length. An Argyle thoracostomy catheter, which is exactly the same size as the vein to which the graft will be anastomosed, is chosen to form the stent on which the composite graft will be constructed. The opened saphenous vein is then wrapped around the stent catheter in spiral fashion, with the intimal surface against the stent and maintaining orientation of the direction of the valves. The edges of the saphenous vein are joined by continuous sutures of 7–0 polypropylene, forming a spiral anastomosis the length of the graft.

BYPASS OF THE SUPERIOR VENA CAVA

A midsternal incision is made. The incision may be extended into the neck, with division of the strap muscles on either side to obtain access to the internal jugular vein if necessary. Chest wall collateral circulation is controlled by electrocautery. An autotransfusion device (Cell Saver, Haemonetics Corp., Natick, MA) is helpful in reducing blood replacement requirement. A biopsy of the obstructing process in the mediastinum is taken. The upper portion of the pericardium is opened in the midline to expose the right atrial appendage. The thymic remnant is removed, and the innominate vein is completely mobilized. When the internal jugular veins are used as the input site, the strap muscles on that side should be removed to open up the thoracic inlet as much as possible.

Heparin, 100 to 300 units per kilogram, is administered intravenously to the patient. The innominate vein is ligated as close to the superior vena cava as possible. A soft jaw vascular clamp (Fogarty) is applied at the jugular-subclavian vein confluence, and the innominate vein is divided so that as much length as possible is preserved.

The end of the composite graft is pushed slightly off the end of the stent. An end-to-end anastomosis of the graft to the innominate vein is constructed with continuous stitches of 7-0 polypropylene suture. When the anastomosis is complete, the stent is removed.

The entire right atrial appendage is excluded by vascular clamp, the tip of the appendage excised, and all trabeculae within the appendage are removed. The end of the vein graft is anastomosed to the right atrial appendage with 5-0 polypropylene suture. The completed graft lies anterior to the aorta. The pericardium is left open; wound closure is routine.

POSTOPERATIVE CARE

Postoperatively, the condition of the patient may temporarily appear worse, with more facial and periorbital edema owing to the supine body position and extended neck during the operation. The patient should be placed in bed with the head elevated to 30 to 45 degrees. The endotracheal tube should be removed cautiously in case of some laryngeal edema. The upper compartment venous system will rapidly decompress so that facial edema will largely disappear within 24 to 48 hours. Persistence or worsening of facial edema suggests early failure of the graft and is an indication for reoperation. Aspirin, 650 mg, and dipyridamole (Persantine), 75 mg, should be given twice daily for approximately 6 months to reduce platelet adhesiveness while the graft is becoming fully established. Patency of the graft is usually obvious, with regression of symptoms and signs of superior vena cava obstruction, but it may be objectively assessed by Doppler ultrasound examination of the internal jugular veins. On the side of the graft, increased flow velocity will be detected. Confirmation of patency of the graft may be obtained by contrast venography.

SUGGESTED READING

Ahmann FR. A reassessment of the clinical implications of superior vena cava syndrome. J Clin Oncol 1984; 2:961–969.

Doty DB. Bypass of superior vena cava: six years experience with spiral vein graft for obstruction of superior vena cava due to benign and malignant disease. J Thorac Cardiovasc Surg 1982; 83:326–338.

Doty DB, Baker WH. Bypass of superior vena cava with spiral vein graft. Ann Thorac Surg 1976; 22:490–493.

Nieto AF, Doty DB. Superior vena cava obstruction: clinical syndrome, etiology and treatment. Current Prob Cancer 1986; 10:441–484.

Stanford W, Doty DB. The role of venography and surgery in the management of patients with superior vena cava obstruction. Ann Thorac Surg 1986; 41:158–163.

SOLITARY PULMONARY NODULE

EARLE W. WILKINS Jr., M.D.

The solitary pulmonary nodule must not be neglected. A useful maxim is that a reasonable diagnosis for every such nodule should be sought, even if this requires surgical excision. The only exception would be an incidental finding in a patient so physically infirm or physiologically impaired as to be not capable of tolerating a definitive procedure.

Logic entails the pursuit of certain guidelines, such as that patients should not be subjected to unnecessary operation, but also that the opportunity for cure should not be missed in patients with early carcinoma of the lung. The goals, therefore, are (1) to avoid life-threatening or function-limiting complications in pursuit of a diagnosis that proves benign, and (2) to offer permanent respite from the insidious development of primary lung carcinoma.

DIAGNOSIS

Techniques useful in providing diagnostic information, some of which are very recent in development and application, include (1) computed tomography (CT), (2) magnetic resonance imaging (MRI), (3) fiberoptic bronchoscopy, including transbronchial biopsy, (4) radiologically guided brush biopsy, utilizing flexible brush catheters, and (5) percutaneous needle aspiration biopsy. Refinement of skills in cytodiagnosis of specimens obtained from early morning sputum collection, from postdiagnostic procedural sputum, and from the diagnostic techniques just mentioned permits an increased rate of accurate diagnosis.

In the effort to substantiate a diagnosis of malignant disease, it is important not to omit procedures or techniques for making a diagnosis of an inflammatory process. These include:

1. a careful history, including places of residence, exposure to tuberculosis, travel experience, occupational exposure, and evidence of prior malignant disease,
2. a complete physical examination, including not only the routine search for lymphadenopathy and hepatomegaly, but also the often neglected areas of anorectum, nasopharynx, and larynx,
3. a search for and review of earlier chest roentgenograms, even if previously read as negative,
4. skin testing (tuberculin, histoplasmin, coccidioidin) where indicated,

5. serum titer evaluation, especially for coccidioidomycosis, and
6. culture (regular, tuberculous, and fungal) of specimens obtained from invasive procedures.

Parallel with these diagnostic measurements must come an assessment of pulmonary function and general physical evaluation, which may preclude an attempt at ultimate surgical excision and, from a practical point of view, perhaps even negate the need for diagnosis at all.

THERAPY

If CT suggests the presence of enlarged mediastinal lymph nodes (greater than 1 cm in diameter), *mediastinoscopy* is indicated. It provides access to mediastinal nodes in the paratracheal, anterior subcarinal, and proximal bronchial loci; it does not provide access to anterior mediastinal, subaortic, or posterior subcarinal nodes. *Mediastinotomy* permits a direct approach to the first two of these inaccessible areas, with concomitant mediastinoscopy when necessary. These techniques not only provide the possibility of direct diagnosis but offer staging information in the event that the ultimate diagnosis is malignant.

Thoracotomy is the ultimate diagnostic tool and also the means for definitive management. The initial two essentials are (1) placement of the incision, and (2) performing as limited a local excision as technically possible.

For the peripheral nodule, a properly placed minithoracotomy incision permits the necessary wedge excision; it must be large enough to permit application of the facilitating stapling devices. For example, (1) an anterior thoracotomy, even of the Chamberlain type extended transpleurally, provides an approach to an anterior segment nodule. (2) A lower short anterolateral incision is an acceptable approach to a nodule in the middle lobe or the lingula. (3) A low lateral incision is often applicable to the nodule lying on the diaphragmatic surface of either lung. (4) A high axillary incision may be designed for excision of a nodule in proximity to the major fissure. However, posterior or apical nodules are not accessible in a minithoracotomy incision and require the full conventional posterolateral thoracotomy.

Unless the wedge excision is all that the pulmonary physiologic status of the patient will permit, which is often the case in patients with chronic obstructive pulmonary disease, prompt frozen section pathologic assessment is essential. If the frozen section confirms a primary carcinoma of the lung, the need for further resection should be determined at this time. A second thoracotomy is never wise, unless the patient insists on personal participation in the decision for greater resection.

It is the general preference of thoracic surgeons at the Massachusetts General Hospital to perform primary lobectomy if the solitary nodule is deeply located within a lobe. Such a location significantly increases the likelihood that it is a primary carcinoma. A hamartoma, on the other hand (unless endobronchial), is always subpleural.

The inappropriate placement of a minithoracotomy may tax the ingenuity of the surgeon when the frozen section findings dictate the need for extension of the incision for further resection. Careful planning and thoughtful anticipation are therefore essential.

THE MASSACHUSETTS GENERAL HOSPITAL EXPERIENCE

Time has altered neither the findings nor the applications of a survey of the "asymptomatic isolated pulmonary nodule" conducted some three decades ago at the Massachusetts General Hospital. In an analysis of 77 patients over a 7-year period, all of whom presented with a finding of an unsuspected pulmonary nodule on routine chest roentgenogram and all of whose diagnoses proved pathologic following surgical removal, the findings were as shown in Table 1.

One might expect a decreased incidence of tuberculosis as the only real change from this decade. In an analysis subsequent to the prior report, 42 percent of patients presenting with an asymptomatic primary lung carcinoma survived 5 years, a finding *not* sufficiently encouraging to warrant mass chest film screening.

The striking statistic from the survey was that in those 50 patients over age 50, 58 percent proved to have carcinoma of the lung. The conclusion still pertains: (1) "exploration of the thorax for diagnosis presents a negligible morbidity," and (2) "the results of expectant management may be tragic."

A RECOMMENDED PLAN

These facts lead to a recommended protocol for management.

1. Check history for relevant clues to a possible diagnosis.
2. Do a *complete* physical examination; palpate for regional lymph node enlargement including in particular the supraclavicular fossae.
3. Retrieve all prior chest films for comparison.
4. Assess for pulmonary ventilatory function, including arterial blood gases. Measurement of the FEV_1 is a minimum.
5. Plant intradermal antigens for skin testing only if time is not of the essence *and* there is a suggestion, particularly from the history, that a particular granuloma should be suspected.

TABLE 1 Postsurgical Analysis of 77 Patients over a 7-Year Period with Asymptomatic Pulmonary Nodule

Finding	*No.*	*(%)*
Primary carcinoma	27	35
Tuberculosis	18	23
Hamartoma	11	14
Other benign tumor	10	13
Secondary carcinoma	6	8
Other inflammatory lesions	5	7

6. Check an early morning or a 24-hour sputum collection for malignant cells and for tubercle bacilli.
7. Consider invasive diagnostic testing, especially fiberoptic bronchoscopy or percutaneous needle aspiration biopsy or both.
8. If no diagnosis is obtained *or* if the diagnosis is carcinoma, operate.

CAVEATS

The experience of the 33 years since the Massachusetts General Hospital study cited has been accompanied by a number of pitfalls that seem to have been especially laid for the unwary and the unwise.

1. The exact and final diagnosis is not always what it seems. A lung nodule, stationary for as long as 5 years, may still be carcinoma. A nodule with calcification is not always a granuloma. The diagnosis of a prior carcinoma in another organ does not make the lung nodule a metastasis. A double diagnosis is always possible.
2. Informed consent mandates the provision to the patient of both all possible diagnoses and every method of therapy. Such information must include the essential need for a precise diagnosis. The teaching axiom that "appropriate management requires accurate diagnosis" is nowhere more important. However, if the modern patient wants the nodule taken out, consider this possibility right away.
3. Beware of the situation of watching and waiting, particularly if it does not coincide with surgical insight. If forced into this stance, insist on a second opinion. The second opinion is not always only for advice to the patient; it may also be a protection for the advisor.
4. When in doubt, take it out.

SUGGESTED READING

Wilkins EW Jr. The asymptomatic isolated pulmonary nodule. N Engl J Med 1955; 52:515–520.

Wilkins EW Jr. The management of the indeterminate solitary pulmonary nodule. Surg Rounds 1984; March:82–86.

SLEEVE LOBECTOMY

INGOLF VOGT-MOYKOPF, M.D.
GÜNTHER MEYER, M.D.
HEINRICH BÜLZEBRUCK, Ph.D.

Bronchoplastic and angioplastic techniques are the best means of avoiding the need for pneumonectomy and are employed in benign and malignant lung diseases (Table 1). In benign diseases, the entire pulmonary parenchyma may be preserved. The precondition for performance of a parenchyma-conserving operation is preoperative tumor staging, which has to be as precise as possible. The endobronchial extent of the tumor and the stage of lymph node involvement are of pre-eminent importance. The findings obtained intraoperatively determine the choice of the definitive surgical procedure.

In principle, the histologic tumor type does not influence the choice between an organ-conserving operation and other resection techniques. The proportion of pneumonectomies for lung disease could be lowered to 20 percent by the development of organ-conserving resection techniques. These procedures often are equally radical and carry an equally good chance of cure, and they place a much smaller burden on the patient because healthy regions of the lung are preserved.

Pneumonectomy is still indicated in lung cancer patients with healthy function (especially younger patients) who have central tumor at or around the upper lobe ostium (right T_3, left T_2), mostly in combination with involvement of the lymph nodes surrounding the main bronchus (N_1). Whether the hilar lymph nodes on the main bronchus (N_1) are affected by contiguous spread of tumor or via lymphogenic metastatic spread can often be demonstrated unequivocally only on the resected specimen.

If we decide to operate on N_2 tumors, and if the N_2 involvement has been established by preoperative or intraoperative histologic examination, we attempt to carry out limited resection as well in patients with healthy respiratory function and do not perform pneumonectomy. The precondition is that local tumor growth can be controlled by lobectomy or sleeve lobectomy. Since the long-term prognosis may depend above all on the stage of lymph node involvement, the quality of life of the patient can be improved with the same degree of radicality as in pneumonectomy. In addition, a more favorable point of departure for the adjuvant follow-up treatment (radiotherapy or chemotherapy) necessary in the N_2 stage can be attained.

The possible development of a second primary lung cancer is another indication for lung-sparing procedures such as sleeve lobectomy to be carried out initially. Surgical resection might be possible in this situation, which would be precluded if a more extensive procedure had been carried out initially.

We observe the rule that pneumonectomy is not carried out in patients with nonmalignant tumors and other benign conditions (e.g., cicatrical strictures or injury sequelae) as long as it can be confirmed that the pathologic process has not led to irreversible damage of the bronchi or pulmonary parenchyma in the sense of poststenotic complication. Such a "destroyed lung" or severe interstitial fibrosis of the parenchyma is an indication for pneumonectomy. Such poststenotic damage can mostly be demonstrated unequivocally prior to operation with the subtle diagnostic procedures available today.

TABLE 1 Frequency of Broncho- and Angioplastic Procedures Compared With Total Number of Resections (Without Resection of Bifurcation)

Pathology	*Time (years)*	*Total Number of Resections*	*Number of Plastic Procedures*	*Percent*
Bronchial carcinoma	1973–1983	1,332	248	19
Benign lung tumors	1980–1985	93	5	5

INDICATIONS

Bronchoplastic Techniques

In benign diseases of the central bronchial tree (e.g., cicatricial stenosis, bronchial adenoma), the affected bronchial region can frequently be removed without resection of parenchyma. If this is no longer possible because of the involvement of lobe and segment bronchial branch points, the corresponding lobes or segments must be resected along with the affected bronchial region.

In malignant diseases of the central bronchial tree, the most radical tumor resection is a fundamental stipulation. The pertinent lobe must always be resected along with the tumor. The indications are local (endobronchial) tumor spread, the extent of metastatic lymph node involvement, the respiratory reserves, and the presence of risk factors. The following groups fall into these categories:

1. Patients without increased surgical risk who have central circumscribed tumors of the upper lobe (group 1) are a group in whom the indications for organ-conserving operation are controversial. This applies especially when there is metastatic involvement of one or several lymph nodes at the upper lobe and/or main bronchus (N_1). Whereas we formerly established the option for organ-conserving surgery only in patients with healthy respiratory function and no involvement of the lymph nodes (right T_3 N_0 M_0; left T_2 N_0 M_0), we consider today that a sleeve resection of upper lobe tumors is justifiable also in those with isolated or circumscribed lymph node involvement with intranodal growth at the main bronchus (right T_3 N_1 M_0; left T_2 N_1 M_0).

Since the operation is elective, sufficient resection must be ensured both in the direction of the trachea and in the distal direction (intraoperative examination by rapid section), and the indication for organ-conserving surgery must be established very strictly with regard to the danger of recurrence and risk of complications. As soon as doubts are present as to sufficient extent of resection, the more radical pneumonectomy must be preferred. Pneumonectomy is still the oncologically safest and most frequently applied procedure in central tumors when there is a choice. Where there is lymph node involvement in the fissure, pneumonectomy is always more radical, but it cannot be more radical than sleeve lobectomy in mediastinal lymph node involvement (N_2).

2. The second group of patients (group 2) are those at increased surgical risk (restricted pulmonary function, other risk factors), which no longer permits pneumonectomy. Limit values of pulmonary function are just second capacity forced expiratory volume of about 1.2 L per second and a maximum ventilation volume of less than 45 L per minute. However, these values must always be related to the overall clinical impression of the patient. Three categories of such patients can be distinguished, depending on tumor involvement in the upper lobe: (1) Those with isolated tumor involvement in the upper lobe and/or main bronchus without lymph node involvement (see group 1). (2) Those with a conglomerate tumor with involvement of the regional lymph nodes (per continuitatem or metastatic) and infiltration of the main bronchus from the outside. (3) Those with a peripherally localized primary tumor with metastatic involvement of the lymph nodes at the upper lobe and/or main bronchus that infiltrates the bronchus from the outside. In this case, the lumen can be endobronchially free of tumor. The affected lung region with its lymph node metastases can be radically resected by a sleeve operation with a potential for cure.

3. The last group of patients (group 3) are those in whom the indications for surgery are palliative, such as avoiding or eliminating complications of hemorrhage or suppuration caused by the tumor.

Angioplastic Procedures

Tangential resection of the pulmonary artery is indicated when malignant tumors of the central bronchial tree have invaded in the direction of the pulmonary artery to an extent that the corresponding segmental arteries are involved by tumor and the usual application of ligatures is technically no longer possible or would result in stenosis of the main trunk of the pulmonary artery.

The infiltration of the main trunk of the pulmonary artery already entails a T_3 stage in direct tumor spreading and an N_1 stage in infiltration of a metastatically affected lymph node in the hilus. This entails a more advanced stage, the prognostic relevance of which cannot be precisely established at present. As long as this is technically feasible, we avoid pneumonectomy by segmental resection of varying extent at the trunk of the pulmonary artery when the involvement of the artery is similarly circumscribed to the tumor situation at the bronchial tree: (1) A central tumor has directly infiltrated the main trunk of the pulmonary artery and can be removed, together with a segment of the pulmonary artery. (2) The hilar lymph node metastasis of a peripherally localized primary tumor has infiltrated the main trunk of the pulmonary artery and can be radically removed via a segment resection of the pulmonary artery. (3) An operation necessary for palliative reasons can be limited by means of a pulmonary arterial sleeve.

SURGICAL TECHNIQUE

Ventilation is always carried out via a double-lumen tube in order to ensure adequate ventilation of the patient, even when the bronchial system is open. In anastomosis at the bifurcation region, such a tube may occasionally be inconvenient. In such cases, we use one-sided high frequency jet ventilation. The localization and extent of the underlying disease are decisive factors in the choice of the plastic surgery technique. Surgical techniques for the bronchus, the pulmonary artery, and a combination of both (combined sleeve resection) can be distinguished (Table 2).

Bronchoplastic Techniques

Bronchoplastic operations extend from segment resection of a bronchial region without removal of the parenchyma via sleeve segment resection to sleeve lobectomy (bifurcation resection). The extensions in the region of the bifurcation cannot be considered here, nor can all the various techniques. We will describe the principle of a sleeve resection of the upper lobe.

After resection of the involved bronchial segment and severance of the pulmonary ligament to mobilize the lower lobe, the corresponding ends of the bronchi can mostly be readily juxtaposed. In longer resections, e.g., an upper bilobectomy with complete main bronchus resection and reanastomosis into the bifurcation part of the trachea, an additional mobilization of the bifurcation may become necessary in order to avoid excessive tension of the anastomosis and thus the danger of complete suture dehiscence.

The blood supply is of crucial importance for the process of healing at the anastomosis. In the dissection of the bronchial tree, an overly radical skeletization of the bronchi with suppression of the blood supply therefore should be avoided. Especially in terms of radical tumor surgery and the lymphadenectomy necessary for postoperative staging, the bronchial arteries cannot always be conserved. Before anastomosis, the resection ends are checked for adequate blood flow, and at least fine petechial bleedings should be visible at the two edges. With 2.5-fold lens magnification, one can avoid error. If the resection ends appear to have deficient blood flow, secondary resection can be carried out. Projecting parts of severed cartilage bridges should be carefully excised in order to obtain anastomosis margins that are as smooth as possible and that have good blood flow.

For the anastomosis suture, we use monofilament absorbable suture material (PDS) No. 4 or 5 , which is well tolerated. The suture is carried out in single-button technique (no U sutures). Sufficient bronchial wall must always be gripped in order to prevent the stitches from tearing out. The membranous part is only adapted and finally knotted in order to prevent the stitches from cutting into it. The stitches should not be placed too close together so as not to endanger the blood supply of the resection margins. Possible differences in caliber of the bronchus ends to be anastomosed can be compensated for by oblique cutting of the smaller part or (better) by gathering the membranous part of the larger end of the anastomosis.

After finishing the anastomosis, a check for leaks is performed by a water test under ventilation (P_{max} = 40 cm H_2O). Additional protection against anastomosis insufficiency is afforded by covering the anastomosis with a pedicule of fat-free pleural or pericardial flap as well as azygos flaps on the right side. In addition, we place a Redon drainage beside the anastomosis in order to avoid development of encapsulated hematomas, which may lead to suture insufficiency in the case of infection.

TABLE 2 Frequency of Broncho- and Angioplastic Procedures (Without Resections of Bifurcation) for Bronchial Carcinoma (1973–1983)

Procedure	*Bronchial Carcinoma*	
	*No.**	*Percent*
Bronchial Sleeve resection	93	38
Smaller bronchoplastic procedures	75	30
Sleeve resection of pulmonary artery	8	3
Smaller angioplastic procedures	43	17
Combined sleeve resection (bronchus and pulmonary artery)	29	12

* No. = 248

Angioplastic Techniques

If the tumor has already reached the pulmonary arterial trunk, the affected part can be removed by segment resection similar to that used in the bronchus. We carry out more than 90 percent of these vasoplastic operations in the region of the upper lobe, where they have mostly been combined with bronchoplasty techniques ("double sleeve").

Before segment resection, the main trunk of the pulmonary artery must be exposed up to its point of origin in order to have sufficient space for anastomosis with a ligated vessel. Proximal and distal control of the pulmonary artery is mandatory to avoid excessive blood loss. It is unknown what intravascular alterations of the lungs occur from an activation of blood clotting by central stasis or absence of flow brought about in the periphery. Therefore we administer 5,000 to 7,500 IU of heparin systemically before ligation. In addition, we open the vessel every 3 minutes in order to start the circulation again. The follow-up investigations (pulmonary arterial angiography, perfusion and ventilation scintigrams) carried out so far have shown good functional results. If the pulmonary artery cannot be ligated in the lobe cleft for technical reasons, clipping of the lower lobe vein is possible as an alternative, thus avoiding reflux into the pulmonary artery.

We perform vascular anastomosis continuously with a nonabsorbable monofilament suture material (Prolene) No. 5 or 6 in the end-to-end procedure. Although appreciable fluctuations in vessel caliber are frequently present, these can be readily compensated for by oblique cutting or additional incision of the smaller section of the vessel. However, large variations in caliber necessitate a single-button suture technique. According to our experience, the results of segment resection with wide anastomosis are better than those of long tangential resection, which carries the danger of a substantial narrowing of the lumen and subsequent thrombotic occlusion.

Combined Sleeve Resection of Bronchus and Pulmonary Artery

Most combined sleeve resections are carried out together with an upper lobectomy. Bronchial anastomosis is always carried out first. After its completion and that of lymphadenectomy, the vascular suture is carried out last in order to avoid damage to the vulnerable vascular anastomosis by further surgical manipulation. We always separate the vascular anastomosis from the bronchial anastomosis. Otherwise, an insufficiency at the bronchial anastomosis can have catastrophic consequences at the vascular anastomosis. For this purpose, the bronchial anastomosis is covered especially carefully with a broad-stemmed fat-free pleural, pericardial, or azygos patch. We decide in each individual case whether this covering can be completed before or after completion of the vascular anastomosis.

POSTOPERATIVE CARE

Immediately after completing the bronchial anastomosis, the surgeon carries out the first bronchoscopic inspection of the anastomosis intraoperatively. Intraluminally located sutures (carrying the danger of incrustation), protruding "naked" cartilage bridges (carrying the danger of necrosis), and the formation of bulges or kinks that may block the lumen can then be corrected immediately.

The subsequent course of the patient depends on careful surveillance and treatment in the intensive care unit. Even where the patient demonstrates adequate spontaneous breathing, during the first 12 hours we prefer to leave in a tube with a single lumen even distal to the anastomosis in order to ensure sufficient bronchial toilet. The staff that carries out the aspiration of the tubes or occasionally may have to perform a mini-tracheotomy must be experienced. If necessary, aspiration may have to be carried out bronchoscopically. Postoperative coughing up with the aid of physiotherapy, which has been practiced preoperatively, is very important where there is mucus retention owing to disturbed mucociliary function. Even in an apparently uncomplicated course, we carry out a further bronchoscopic check at the latest on the sixth to eighth postoperative day on the basis of our own experience. Depending on the local findings, radiologic results, clinical course, and condition of the patient, further bronchoscopy may be carried out in order to forestall possible deleterious complications. By consistently using this procedure, we were able to attain a marked lowering in the rate of complications in recent years.

COMPLICATIONS

The bronchoplastic and angioplastic operations on the lungs are subject to several typical complications. The most feared complications are circumscribed fistulization and total dehiscence of the anastomosis owing to necrosis. The latter complication can mostly be diagnosed in good time by bronchoscopy. It is often difficult to distinguish between a mucosal or total wall necrosis. Only the experienced surgeon can decide whether one should continue to wait and observe in the hope of spontaneous healing or whether secondary pneumonectomy must be carried out. When local findings are doubtful, we are guided by the clinical symptoms (general conditon, fever, leukocytosis, severe halitosis, and detection of bacteria in the pleural exudate). If small leaks in the anastomosis are noticed as a result of corresponding auscultation phenomenon (whistling sound or lack of expansion of the pulmonary lobe), and these are confirmed bronchoscopically, then we proceed in a manner similar to that for treating small bronchial stump fistulas after standard lobectomies.

On the other hand, silent small fistulas or suppuration on the perforation canal that also cannot be detected endoscopically and that can lead by erosion to abrupt and then lethal hemorrhages can be insidious both at the site of conservatively treated arterial stumps and of continuous vascular sutures of the pulmonary artery. In the last 2 years, we succeeded twice in forestalling by secondary pneumonectomy this impending event, suspected from the seventh postoperative day because of the appearance of small dark-red hemoptyses. If at all possible, living tissue with good blood flow should be placed between the bronchial sleeve and the pulmonary artery, depending on the situation. Redon drainage is left in situ at least until after the first postoperative bronchoscopic check, i.e., for about 8 to 10 days. If necroses or small fistulas occur, we leave in the Redon drainage until healing has taken place. Application of these principles has led to the occurrence of a mass hemorrhage only once in the last 50 operations performed, including an increasing number of plastic operations.

In the last 3 years, we have no longer observed the other typical complications, i.e., cicatricial stricture, suture granuloma, and kink stenosis. Improved suture materials have led to a decrease in the number of foreign-body granulomas and the cicatricial strictures associated with them. If granulomas develop, they can be resected endoscopically. On the other hand, relevant stenoses necessitate resection with reanastomosis. We no longer carry out bronchial wedge excisions or partial sleeves. We regard a complete sleeve resection as more radical and subject to fewer complications, since bronchial kinking with subsequent retention of secretions, atelectasis, and retention pneumonia are avoided. In major edema of the mucosa with stenosis, we administer antiedematous drugs (diclofenac, dexpanthenol) parenterally or by inhalation. Preparations containing cortisone should be dispensed with if possible (except for an asthmatic attack) in order to avoid impairment of wound healing at the bronchial tree.

The problem of local regional recurrence can be decreased but not avoided at the bronchus by intraoperative rapid-section examination of the resection margins. The final histologic work-up on the resection preparation often provides the first indication of lymphangitic involve-

TABLE 3 Thirty-Day Mortality Rate for Various Diseases Following Broncho-Angioplastic Procedures

	Bronchial Carcinoma			*Benign Tumors*		
	No.	*Deaths*	*Percent*	*No.*	*Deaths*	*Percent*
Bronchoplastic procedures	168	23	14	5	0	0
Angioplastic procedures	51	7	14	—	—	—
Combined sleeve resection, (bronchus and pulmonary artery)	29	3	10	—	—	—
Total	248	33	13	5	0	0

ment. Additional procedures and the therapeutic consequences in this case correspond to those in the same situation after standard operations (radiotherapy or secondary pneumonectomy). However, the tendency to suture dehiscence appears to be markedly greater in such a situation. The more frequent local occurrence owing to regionally invading lymph node metastases is noticed clinically at a much later time and then is often no longer suitable for surgical reintervention. In the literature, the data on the frequency of local recurrence after bronchoplastic operations fluctuate between 2 percent and 51 percent. A rate of 16 percent was found in our own patients.

Thrombosis at the suture site of the pulmonary artery (pulmonary embolism) after tangential or segmental resection can be manifested in two forms: first, acutely, with dramatic deterioration of the patient's general condition, clinical signs of severe infection, and radiologic rarification of the vascular structures and increasing shadow in the area. The diagnosis is confirmed most rapidly and certainly by pulmonary angiography. Secondary pneumonectomy is mandatory. In the second form, the thrombosis can be manifested chronically by symptoms that are hardly detectable clinically and by a discrepancy between the perfusion and ventilation scintigrams. A secondary pneumonectomy is not necessary, since the lung can be left behind as a "plug." We have not seen this latter complication for the past 3 years.

RESULTS

The results are shown in Tables 3 and 4. The 30-day mortality rate (Table 3) of the 248 plastic operations (from 1973 to 1983) totals 13 percent. The surgical risk is thus found to be in the same range in the angioplastic and bronchoplastic operations as in extended pneumonectomies, with a rate of 16 percent in our own patients in the same period. It must be taken into consideration that the high risk patient constitutes our main indication for sleeve resection. Since 1980, we have been able to lower the mortality of pneumonectomies and plastic operations to 8 and 9 percent.

Causes of death in sleeve resections were right ventricular failure (six times), acute hemoptysis (five times), pulmonary embolism (four times), anastomosis insufficiency (three times), and sepsis (once).

In accordance with the indications, 97 percent of our patients had T_2 and T_3 tumors and 32 percent had N_2 tumors. According to the TNM (tumors, nodes, and metastases) classification of the International Union Against Cancer (UICC) of 1979, 44 percent of the patients were in stages I and II, but 46 percent were already in stage III. The 5-year survival rate (Table 4) is also not affected negatively by the methods of reconstructive operation. Patients with stages I-II and III disease have similar long-term results, with 32 percent and 13 percent 5-year

TABLE 4 Thirty-Day Mortality and Survival Rates by Stage* Following Broncho- and Angioplastic Procedures for Resection of Lung Cancer†.

		Stages I and II				*Stage III*			
		No.	*30-Day Mortality (Percent)*	*3-Year Survival (Percent)*	*5-Year Survival (Percent)*	*No.*	*30-Day Mortality (Percent)*	*3-Year Survival (Percent)*	*5-Year Survival (Percent)*
Bronchoplastic procedures	(No. = 168)	80	14	40	33	70	13	20	13
Angioplastic procedures	(No. = 51)	21	9	37	12	25	20	9	3
Combined sleeve resection (bronchus and pulmonary artery)	(No. = 29)	9	0	67	44	17	18	25	15
All plastic procedures	(No. = 248)	110	13	40	32	112	16	20	13

* Stage IV excluded.
† Stage grouping according to UICC, 1978.

survival as compared with 35 percent and 17 percent in the standard resections. Whereas the difference between those with N_0 and N_1 tumors was not significant (37 percent and 30 percent 5-year survival time, so far no patient with an N_2 tumor has survived for 5 years. However, even after standard resections, only 8 percent of the patients with mediastinal lymph node metastases are still alive after 5 years. Compared with pneumonectomy, there is a distinct advantage to sleeve lobectomy, with a 25 percent as compared to a 13 percent probability of 5-year survival. When there is strict determination of the indications and comparable lymph node involvement, sleeve lobectomy provides similar results to those of standard lobectomy for the same stage tumors.

SUGGESTED READING

Allison PR. Course of thoracic surgery in Groningen. Quoted by Jones PW. Ann R Coll Surg 1954; 25:20–22.

Faber LP, Jensik RJ, Kittle CF. Results of sleeve lobectomy for bronchogenic carcinoma in 101 patients. Ann Thorac Surg 1984; 37:279–285.

Pichlmaier H, Spelsberg F. Organerhaltende Operation des Bronchialcarcinomas. Langenbecks Arch Chir 1971; 328:221–234.

Vogt-Moykopf I. Gefäßplastiken bei Bronchusmanschettenresektion. Prax Klin Pneumol 1974; 28:1030–1035.

Vogt-Moykopf I, Fritz TH, Meyer G, Bülzebruck H, Daskos G. Bronchoplastic and angioplastic operation in bronchial carcinoma: Long-term results of a retrospective analysis from 1973 to 1983. Int Surg 1986; 71:211–220.

LUNG-SPARING PROCEDURES: SEGMENTAL RESECTION

L. PENFIELD FABER, M.D.

The removal of one or more segments of the lung can be an appropriate resection for patients with inflammatory disease, primary lung cancer, or metastatic lung cancer. Preservation of lung tissue does provide a better quality of life for the elderly patient as well as those with chronic obstructive pulmonary disease, and segmentectomy should always be considered when doing a resection for a second or third primary bronchogenic carcinoma. The alternative procedure, lobectomy, is a less difficult resection, but the advantages of sparing lung tissue make segmentectomy the operation of choice in selected patients.

TECHNIQUE OF SEGMENTECTOMY

Bronchoscopy is indicated to view the segmental anatomy and also to be certain that the bronchus is not diseased. It can be accomplished as a part of the preoperative evaluation or at the time of thoracotomy. The inflamed bronchus may not heal satisfactorily, and cancer at the segmental orifice requires a lobectomy.

A lateral incision through the fourth or fifth intercostal space provides adequate exposure, and rarely is the more standard posterolateral thoracotomy incision required.

Segments commonly resected on the right are the posterior, apical, and anterior segments of the right upper lobe; superior and medial basal segments of the right lower lobe; the posterior segment of the right upper lobe and superior segment of the right lower lobe in continuity; and the four basal segments of the right lower lobe in one unit. Segmentectomy of the right middle lobe is rarely carried out, since the remaining lung tissue is minimal. Segmental resections of the left lung include the apicoposterior, anterior, and lingular segments of the left upper lobe; superior, anteromedial basal segment of the left lower lobe; and the basal segments of the left lower lobe. The superior segment of the left lower lobe and posterior segment of the left upper lobe can be resected as a unit when disease crosses the major fissure. The lateral, posterior, and anterior basal segments of either of the lower lobes are technically difficult resections and are only done when it is mandatory to conserve as much lung tissue as possible.

Careful assessment of disease in the lung tissue and hilus is initially carried out to determine if segmentectomy is a proper resection. Parenchymal margins of resection can be close in inflammatory disease when drug control is optimal, but a minimal margin may be inappropriate when dealing with primary lung cancer. Decision for segmentectomy is also affected by the general condition and age of the patient.

The dissection begins with identification of the pulmonary artery to the segment to be removed, and it is ligated and transected. Because the pulmonary artery is in close proximity to the segmental bronchus, this latter structure is then dissected free. Segmental bronchial anatomy is not constant, and the thoracic surgeon should be familiar with its many variations. Preoperative bronchoscopy helps to identify any unusual anatomy. The bronchus is transected and can be closed with either stapling techniques or interrupted fine absorbable sutures. The 3.5-mm leg-length staple is usually indicated for segmental bronchial closure. It can sometimes be difficult to place the stapling instrument around a segmental bronchus because of adjacent pulmonary structures, and stapling may also leave a long segmental stump due to difficulty in positioning the instrument.

It is important to remember that the bronchus and pulmonary artery are in the center of the anatomic segment, and the pulmonary vein defines the peripheral anatomic boundary of the segment. The dissection of the pulmonary vein must be precise to be certain that venous drainage to the remaining lung tissue is not compromised.

Removal of a segment following ligation of the hilar structures requires experience, and it is not done by forcibly pulling on the clamped segmental bronchus. The proper anatomic plane is along the venous pathway, and the adjacent segmental veins will be seen when the proper dissection plane has been completed. Traction is placed on the clamps holding the bronchus, pulmonary artery, and, particularly, the segmental vein, and the other hand is used to gently and bluntly free the parenchyma by a rolling together of the thumb and forefinger. Small bronchi and vessels that transect segmental planes must be individually clamped, transected, and ligated. The proper segmental plane cannot be identified by inflation and deflation of the lung, since collateral ventilation negates this technique. My preference is to perform a segmentectomy with the lung inflated rather than deflated during one-lung anesthesia. Excessive lung tissue is not removed, and the proper segmental plane is more easily identified.

After the segment has been removed, the raw surface of the remaining lung is carefully inspected for bleeding points, which are cauterized, and small bronchi are individually ligated or transfixed with absorbable suture. The remaining segments of the lobe must inflate and deflate easily, and if they do not, the bronchus should be inspected to be certain that inappropriate bronchi were not transected. Boggy and edematous residual lung tissue may indicate compromise of pulmonary venous drainage. In these instances, it may be necessary to complete the lobectomy to prevent serious postoperative complications.

There are several ways to manage the raw surface of the remaining lung tissue to minimize postoperative air leaks, and the surgeon should be familiar with them all. It may appear simple to approximate the edges of the visceral pleura, but this can defeat the purpose of the segmentectomy, as this technique compromises inflation of the remaining lung tissue. However, it may be necessary when a parenchymal air leak is large, and it is also effective following resection of the superior or inferior division of the left upper lobe. A raw surface can frequently be approximated to the surface of the adjacent lobe along the major fissure and is best accomplished by using interrupted absorbable sutures. A running suture may pull out of the lung tissue when it expands, and more air leak and bleeding are created. This method of approximation is well suited for superior segmentectomy of either lower lobe as well as posterior segmentectomy of either upper lobe. After anterior segmentectomy of the right upper lobe, the raw surface lays flat on the adjacent mediastinum, and following anterior segmentectomy of the left upper lobe, the two surfaces of the lingula and apicoposterior segment can be approximated. A pleural flap can be used to cover the raw surface and is reserved for those cases in which the parenchymal air leak appears to be excessive.

Chest tube placement is critical in order to minimize postoperative complications, and the anterior tube must be placed to the apex and well anteriorly to evacuate all of the air and permit full expansion of the lung. The basal tube is inserted dependently and posteriorly to evacuate blood and fluid. Suction at 20 cm of water pressure is begun in the operating room and is usually maintained until the air leak stops.

Stapling of the lung parenchyma can be done to minimize postoperative air leaks, but there are shortcomings with this technique. The lung tissue is compressed at the staple line and expansion is compromised. It is best to staple the lung tissue after the artery, bronchus, and vein have been transected in order to better define the proper segmental plane. A significant amount of lung tissue is brought together by the staples, and the closure may disrupt when the lung is forcibly inflated. The staple line should be reinforced with a running absorbable suture to prevent this complication.

SEGMENTECTOMY FOR INFLAMMATORY DISEASE

Segmental resection for inflammatory disease of the lung is indicated when medical management has failed to control the disease. Segmentectomy is applicable to bronchiectasis, a small lung abscess, pulmonary tuberculosis, and fungal diseases. On occasion, a benign inflammatory process is identified when exploratory thoracotomy is carried out for a suspected diagnosis of carcinoma, and segmentectomy can encompass the pathologic process. Precise anatomic definition of the involved lung can be accomplished by computed tomographic scans, lateral tomograms, and bronchograms. These methods of assessment provide better delineation of adjacent diseased lung tissue than does palpation or inspection of the lung at the time of surgery.

Bronchiectasis frequently involves the basal segments of either lower lobe, and it is important to preserve the large and well-functioning superior lower lobe segment. Bilateral bronchograms are indicated to define all diseased segments of the lung and to be certain that surgery is indicated in the presence of bilateral disease. Bronchiectasis can also be localized to one particular segment of any lobe and is usually due to prior pulmonary infection.

A lung abscess that fails to resolve with medical management is frequently large, and segmentectomy will not remove all of the diseased lung. If an abscess is small and the margin of resection by segmentectomy is adequate, then it would be the procedure of choice. This is particularly true when an aspiration abscess involves the superior segment of a lower lobe.

Surgical resection for pulmonary tuberculosis is rarely indicated as a result of improved chemotherapy. Bronchiectasis, bronchial stenosis, secondarily infected cavities, and a persistent positive sputum finding may all be indications for resection. If the disease is localized to the apicoposterior segment of an upper lobe, then segmentectomy is the procedure of choice, but the extent of disease frequently requires lobectomy. An adequate margin of resection is necessary in the patient with resistant organisms and also in patients with atypical pulmonary tuberculosis.

A thoracotomy may be done for the presumptive diagnosis of bronchogenic carcinoma but benign inflammatory disease is found instead. In this instance, segmental resection can remove the pathologic process and preserve adjacent lung tissue. Wedge resections using stapling techniques in this situation should be avoided as they are not anatomic and residual inflammatory disease in the staple line may lead to postoperative complications.

SEGMENTECTOMY FOR CANCER

Segmentectomy is a valid operation for primary lung cancer. It can be particularly applicable to patients over the age of 70 and in those with decreased cardiopulmonary function. A surgical mortality of 2 percent and 5-year survival rate of 55 percent in reported series indicate the merit of the procedure.

Segmentectomy can be the procedure of choice when the cancer is 3 cm or less in diameter, is located in the periphery of the anatomic segment, and the regional lymph nodes are free of metastatic disease.

If the diagnosis has not been established preoperatively, needle aspiration cytology is carried out after the chest is opened. Diagnostic accuracy approaches 100 percent, and incisional biopsy or wedge resection is avoided. After the clinical diagnosis of carcinoma is confirmed, dissection is started in the area of the pulmonary artery and segmental bronchus. An appropriate lobar or segmental lymph node is removed and sent for frozen section analysis. If microscopic cancer is identified in the lymph node, lobectomy is carried out. If the lymph node is negative for cancer, segmentectomy becomes the operation of choice. If any positive lymph nodes are encountered during the procedure, or the margin of resection is questionable, additional lung tissue is removed. This may be an additional segment or the entire lobe.

Approximately 6 percent of patients with lung cancer will develop a second primary, and these patients are ideal candidates for a limited pulmonary resection. Despite a large lesion or positive lymph nodes, a segmentectomy may still be preferred because of marginal pulmonary function or a prior pulmonary resection. Wedge resection is usually indicated for metastatic carcinoma to the lung, but a larger lesion may require a more anatomic resection. Peripheral carcinoids and localized bronchoalveolar carcinomas are tumors particularly well suited for segmental resection.

The incidence of local recurrence in either the same lobe or the ipsilateral mediastinum is approximately 12 percent, and the surgeon must weigh this risk of recurrence with the low mortality and reported cure rate in making the final decision for segmentectomy or lobectomy.

COMPLICATIONS OF SEGMENTECTOMY

Prolonged air leak, bronchopleural fistula, pleural space problems, and empyema are all interrelated complications of segmentectomy. The key words that minimize these complications are "no space, no problem." Preventive measures can be done to ensure that the lung expands fully following segmentectomy, and these will minimize complications. Chest tube placement is important, and the anterior tube must be positioned up to the apex. Suction is used at 20 cm of water pressure and can be increased if a pleural space remains. Good pain control is necessary to ensure that the patient breathes deeply and coughs vigorously to clear secretions. The lung must expand fully to obliterate any space, and nasotracheal aspiration and bedside fiberoptic bronchoscopy are indicated at the first sign of atelectasis.

Pneumoperitoneum can be helpful to elevate the diaphragm and assist in space obliteration, but it should be used in the first few days after surgery to achieve satisfactory results. Intraoperative maneuvers such as phrenic crush, transplantation of the diaphragm, pleural tents, and osteoplastic thoracoplasties are not required following segmental resection. Space complication and prolonged air leak relate to failure of the lung to expand adequately or an air leak from a larger bronchus that was not transfixed at the time of resection.

Suction is maintained for a minimum of 7 days and if at this time air leak is significant, then reoperation can be considered. This is entirely dependent on the course of the air leak (whether or not it is diminishing in amount), the general condition of the patient, and the surgeon's estimation of the cause of the leak. It is appropriate to maintain suction for 12 to 14 days, and if the air leak still persists, then discontinue suction. If a pleural space does not develop or enlarge, the patient is connected to a one-way valve and discharged from the hospital. Small alveolar air leaks will heal and the chest tube(s) can be removed in 2 to 3 weeks. The presence of a benign pleural air space is usually not a serious problem, as it will be obliterated within several weeks. If an empyema does develop, it must be treated in the standard fashion.

If the air leak persists through the one-way valve 4 weeks after discharge from the hospital, the patient most likely has a fistula, and the tube is converted to open drainage. A small space or small air leak will close in time, and then the tube can be slowly backed out. An infected pleural space that does not obliterate itself must be treated with either thoracoplasty or myoplasty.

SUGGESTED READING

Bennett WF, Smith RA. Segmental resection for bronchial carcinoma. A surgical alternative for the compromised patient. Ann Thorac Surg 1979; 27:169–172.

Errett LE, Wilson J, Chiu RC, et al. Wedge resection as an alternative procedure for peripheral bronchogenic carcinoma in poor-risk patients. J Thorac Cardiovasc Surg 1985; 90:656–661.

Jensik RJ, Faber LP, Kittle CF. Segmental resection for bronchogenic carcinoma. Ann Thorac Surg 1979; 29:475–483.

Stair JM, Wombie J, Schaefer RF, et al. Segmental pulmonary resection for cancer. Am J Surg 1985; 150:659–664.

CAUTERY EXCISION

JOEL D. COOPER, M.D., F.R.C.S., F.A.C.S.(C)

Limited pulmonary resection is frequently used for excision of lung lesions, especially benign tumors, inflammatory lesions, metastatic tumors to lung, and, at times, primary lung carcinoma, especially when it occurs as small peripheral lesion or when the patient's limited pulmonary reserve precludes a more standard excision. Most limited resections are done in a nonanatomic fashion, preserving as much lung tissue as possible. Such resections are usually accomplished by application of stapling devices or clamps to the lung tissue. This technique causes deformity of the remaining lung and may be difficult if not impossible to apply in the case of a deep-seated lesion.

Electrocautery techniques have been used in the past to excise portions of lung tissue. We have been particularly impressed with the technique described by Mikhail Perelman from Moscow. This technique is applied to inflated lung and allows precise nonanatomic excision of a portion of the lung without blood loss. Furthermore, following removal of the lesion, a dry cavity with a black charred surface is left in the lung with very little or no air leak whatsoever.

For this technique, which Perelman calls precision cautery excision, the lung must be inflated. Two fine pairs of forceps are used by the surgeon. With one pair of forceps in the left hand, the surgeon holds lung tissue adjacent to the pathologic structure. In the right hand the surgeon holds the forceps for electrocoagulation, with which he grips a very small portion of tissue at a time and coagulates it. The coagulated tissue is then pulled apart with the forceps or incised with scissors. Visible branches of the bronchial tree and large vascular branches are isolated, ligated, and divided rather than coagulated.

Because the excision is done while the lung is expanded, it is possible to achieve a far more precise excision of the lesion than is obtained by resecting a wedge from a collapsed lung.

Initially we utilized standard ventilation of the lung through an endotracheal tube. More recently we have utilized a double-lumen tube that permits ventilation of the contralateral lung while the operated side is statically inflated with 5 cm of positive end-expiratory pressure. This eliminates movements in the operative field during the dissection and facilitates the procedure.

Our experience with the technique has been quite satisfactory. In most patients there has been no air leak from the raw surface of the lung at the end of the procedure, and in others the air leak was minor, lasting only a day or two. There have been no instances of postoperative hemorrhage or prolonged air leak.

The use of the limited resection is generally accepted for certain benign or inflammatory lesions, for diagnostic excision, or for excision of single or multiple metastatic lesions to the lung. When dealing with primary lung carcinoma, of course, the rationale for limited resection remains a subject of some debate. If the evaluation of the regional lymph nodes reveals no tumor involvement, then a limited resection may be appropriate for small peripheral lesions, even in patients with a pulmonary status that would permit a more extensive resection. However, for patients in whom limited pulmonary reserve prohibits a major resection, or for patients who have undergone previous pneumonectomy and present with a new primary lesion in the contralateral lung, the precision cautery technique permits safe, nonanatomic resection through inflated lung without compression or injury to surrounding lung tissue. Because there is no bleeding or air leakage during the procedure, the field is not obscured, and precise dissection is possible even in the vicinity of major bronchi or blood vessels.

The major disadvantage of the technique is its tedious nature, because only very small bits of lung tissue can be cauterized and divided at one time. We, and others, have explored the possibility of utilizing laser dissection as a substitute for cautery dissection of the lung. To date, however, the laser techniques have not proved sufficiently precise or expeditious. Though infrequently used, we feel that the precision cautery technique is a useful addition to the existing techniques for limited pulmonary resection.

SUGGESTED READING

Cooper JD. Complications of tracheostomy: pathogenesis, treatment and prevention. In: Delarue NC, Eschapasse H. eds. International trends in general thoracic surgery. Vol. 2. Philadelphia: WB Saunders, 1987:21.

Cooper JD, Perelman M, Todd TRJ, et al. Precision cautery excision of pulmonary lesions. Ann Thorac Surg 1986; 41:51–53.

CHEMOTHERAPY FOR NON–SMALL-CELL CARCINOMA

E. CARMACK HOLMES, M.D.

The results with chemotherapy in advanced lung cancer have not been as dramatic as those in breast cancer, small-cell carcinoma of the lung, testicular carcinoma, and many other solid tumors. In the past, a few premature reports of encouraging response rates with chemotherapy have been difficult to corroborate, and a general pessimism regarding chemotherapy in lung cancer has developed. However, with the development of combined chemotherapeutic agents, especially those that include cisplatin (cisplatinum), response rates of 35 to 40 percent have been obtained in patients with advanced metastatic non–small-cell carcinoma of the lung. The agents that are most commonly employed include the combination of cyclophosphamide, doxorubicin (Adriamycin), and cisplatin (CAP); cisplatin and vindesine or cisplatin with etopside (VP-16); and cyclophosphamide, doxorubicin, methotrexate, and procarbazine (CAMP). In general, the response rates are inversely proportional to the extent of disease and the performance status. It is also true that responders live longer than nonresponders. However, there is continuing controversy over the overall benefit derived from chemotherapy in patients with advanced non–small-cell carcinoma of the lung.

Since patients with smaller tumor burdens have higher response rates to chemotherapy, it seems logical that in the adjuvant setting, when the tumor burden is microscopic, chemotherapy should have its maximum effect. Since we as surgeons do not treat patients with disseminated non–small-cell carcinoma of the lung, we are primarily interested in the possibility of chemotherapy enhancing the surgical effect. Patients who have non–small-cell lung cancer that is confined to the thorax and who have no evidence of dissemination beyond the thorax have a much better response to chemotherapy than patients with disseminated disease. The response rates to chemotherapy in these patients with localized disease are 60 to 70 percent. With this very high response rate it would certainly seem logical that the combination of surgery and chemotherapy should be better than surgery alone. It is this logic that has led to the clinical investigation of the possibilities of combining surgery and chemotherapy. Certainly not all patients with non–small-cell carcinoma of the lung are candidates for experimental adjuvant therapy. Patients with T_1N_0 disease have a 5-year survival rate of higher than 80 percent, and therefore surgery alone is indicated in these patients. Patients with stage II disease and patients with limited mediastinal nodal involvement are most likely to benefit from the combination of surgery and chemotherapy.

Chemotherapy has been used both preoperatively and postoperatively. When used postoperatively it is assumed that the surgical procedure has eliminated the local disease and that adjuvant chemotherapy is directed toward the microscopic systemic disease. Since the vast majority of patients with resected lung cancer develop systemic disease as the first site of recurrence, chemotherapy is the logical choice in this setting. Chemotherapy can also be used in a "neoadjuvant" or induction way when given prior to surgery. To date, this has been used predominantly in patients who have advanced local disease. It is used to decrease the tumor burden and increase resectability in patients whose disease would otherwise be technically unresectable. Thus preoperative chemotherapy may convert unresectable to resectable disease.

There have been numerous studies evaluating chemotherapy following surgical resection. Unfortunately most of these studies were done in the past 15 to 20 years, when effective combination chemotherapy was not available. A variety of chemotherapeutic agents have been evaluated following surgery, with no improvement in survival rates found. These include cyclophosphamide (Cytoxan), nitrogen mustard, methotrexate, lomustine (CCNU), and hydroxyurea. More recently, surgical adjuvant studies using cyclophosphamide, doxorubicin, methotrexate, and procarbazine (CAMP), and cyclophosphamide, doxorubicin, and cisplatin (CAP); have demonstrated improved patient survival. The Lung Cancer Study Group is a group of university-based surgeons, medical oncologists, pathologists, radiation oncologists, and statisticians which has performed a number of studies evaluating adjuvant therapy. In one study, patients with stages II and III adenocarcinoma and large cell carcinoma of the lung were randomized to receive immunotherapy or combination chemotherapy consisting of cyclophosphamide, doxorubicin, and cisplatin in the postoperative period. Patients received cyclophosphamide (400 mg per square meter of body surface), doxorubicin (40 mg per square meter of body surface), and cisplatin (40 mg per square meter of body surface). They received six monthly treatments. In general, the therapy was extremely well tolerated. All patients were treated on an outpatient basis, and most continued to be very active. In this study over 90 percent of the patients had positive nodes, and half of the patients had positive mediastinal nodes. The median disease-free survival time in these patients treated with surgery alone is only 6 to 7 months. One hundred thirty patients were randomized into this study, and they were carefully stratified for the pertinent prognostic factors. After a median follow-up of almost 2 years, there was a statistically significant improvement in disease-free survival in the patients receiving the adjuvant chemotherapy.

In a second study, patients with non–small-cell carcinoma of the lung who had extensive intrathoracic disease and who had microscopic residual disease following surgery were randomized to receive radiation therapy alone or radiation therapy plus CAP chemotherapy. Again the treatment group receiving the CAP chemotherapy had a significantly prolonged disease-free survival compared with the group receiving radiation therapy alone. Therefore, in two independent studies use of combination chemotherapy demonstrated a prolongation in survival time in patients with advanced resectable lung cancer. It appears that these agents have an effect on microscopic residual disease and are capable of prolonging survival following surgery.

There has been considerable interest in the recent past in the use of preoperative chemotherapy, either alone or in combination with radiation therapy, in patients with locally advanced, unresectable non-small-cell lung cancer. Studies have shown response rates of 70 percent and resection rates as high as 90 percent in patients with disease that was considered technically unresectable prior to the preoperative therapy. In some of these studies as many as 20 to 25 percent of the patients were histologically free of disease at the time of surgical resection. The Lung Cancer Study Group has evaluated CAP chemotherapy in combination with radiation therapy in a group of patients with locally advanced disease. Fifty percent of these patients responded to the preoperative chemotherapy and proceeded to surgery. Two-thirds of these patients had complete resections. The median survival in the patients undergoing complete resection was 15 months, which was significantly better than in those patients who did not undergo surgery or who underwent incomplete resections. In a second study, patients with apparently unresectable disease were treated preoperatively with cisplatin, continuous 5-fluorouracil, and 3,000 rads of radiation therapy. This study is currently in progress; however, this regimen is better tolerated than the CAP + radiation therapy regimen and the response rates are in the same range.

All of these studies clearly indicate that preoperative chemotherapy in combination with radiation therapy can have a dramatic effect on the tumor. The response rates are considerably higher than in patients with advanced disease, and there are a significant number of patients in whom no viable disease was found at the time of surgery. All of these studies are highly experimental and no prospective randomized phase III trials have tested the ability of preoperative chemotherapy to improve survival time over surgery alone, or chemotherapy alone.

SUGGESTED READING

Holmes EC. Surgical adjuvant therapy of non-small cell lung cancer. Chest 1986; 89:295S–300S.
Holmes EC, Gail M. The Lung Cancer Study Group. Surgical adjuvant therapy for stage II and stage III adenocarcinoma and large cell undifferentiated carcinoma. J Clin Oncol 1986; 4:710–715.
Mountain CM, Gail M, The Lung Cancer Study Group. Surgical adjuvant intrapleural BCG treatment for stage I non-small cell lung cancer. J Thorac Cardiovasc Surg 1981; 82:649–657.
Taylor SG, Trybula M, Bonomi PD, et al. Simultaneous cisplatin-fluorouracil infusion and radiation followed by surgical resection in regionally localized stage III non-small cell lung cancer. Ann Thorac Surg 1987; 43:87–91.

RADIATION THERAPY

NOAH C. CHOI, M.D.

Radiation is capable of sterilizing carcinoma of the lung at the primary site and the regional lymph node when a sufficient dose, i.e., 5,000 to 6,000 cGy (TDF 82–99) is delivered. The role of radiation therapy for lung carcinoma can be categorized as follows: (1) curative radiation therapy in unresectable non–small-cell lung carcinoma (NSCLC); (2) postoperative radiation therapy in non–small-cell lung carcinoma; (3) combined preoperative radiation and extended en-bloc resection in superior pulmonary sulcus tumor.

CURATIVE RADIATION THERAPY FOR UNRESECTABLE NON–SMALL-CELL LUNG CARCINOMA

Of the many patients for whom curative surgery is not possible, only those with disease still limited to the chest are suitable for curative radiation therapy aimed at eradication of the tumor, a form of local and regional treatment capable of sterilizing both the primary carcinoma and the metastases in the regional lymph nodes. When radiation therapy is carefully designed for each patient, it is feasible that an unresectable carcinoma of the lung that is still limited within the regional lymphatics can be sterilized by high doses of radiation delivered to the tumor-bearing areas, while adjacent normal vital structures, such as the spinal cord, a large volume of the normal lung tissue, and the heart, are spared from excessive doses of radiation. Careful screening for distant metastases is essential in those patients considered for curative radiation.

Indications

Indications for curative radiation therapy are (1) locally advanced, stage T3 or N2 carcinoma without distant metastasis and (2) early-stage (T1–2N0M0 or T1–2N1M0) resectable, but medically inoperable, carcinoma. The patient's general condition should be good enough to tolerate a course of radiation therapy that lasts for 5.5 to 7 weeks (70 or greater on the Karnofsky scale). Definitive radiation aimed at a long-term control of locoregional carcinoma is also indicated for patients with the following conditions: (1) minimal involvement (lymph node smaller than 2.5 cm) of the ipsilateral supraclavicular lymph node group; (2) early stage of superior vena cava syndrome without distant metastasis; (3) paralyzed vocal cord secondary to involvement of the recurrent laryngeal nerve; (4) centrally located carcinoma involving the carina.

Selection of Patients

Careful assessment of a patient's cardiopulmonary status is essential in general evaluation of the suitability of curative radiation therapy. It is necessary to compromise radiation doses and target volume for patients with either poor pulmonary or cardiac reserve. Conversely, patients with estimated postradiation therapy pulmonary function that is judged to be sufficient for normal activity can be aggressively treated to the maximum and optimal level of radiation doses and treatment volume.

Radiotherapeutic Techniques

Three important radiotherapeutic factors consist of target volume, radiation dose and fractionation schedule, and radiation portal arrangements. For locally advanced unresectable lung carcinoma (T3 or N2 tumor), the target volume includes the primary lesion with a 2-cm margin of clinically uninvolved lung, the entire mediastinum, and the medial halves of both supraclavicular fossae. Patients with surgically resectable but medically inoperable carcinoma require a target volume smaller than that for unresectable carcinoma. There is a reasonable correlation between radiation dose and response of lung carcinoma. With the currently available data, an optimum schedule of radiation therapy seems to be in the range of a total dose of 5,600 to 6,400 cGy, given in 180 to 200 cGy of daily fractions, 5 days a week over a period of 5.6 to 7.4 weeks.

The arrangement of the radiation portals is dependent on the planned total dose, the type of radiation, and the shape of the target volume. An arrangement of two parallel opposing portals (POP) applied anteriorly (AP) and posteriorly (PA) to the chest is simple and accurate with the least risk of a geographic miss. However, the maximum dose that can be delivered with this technique is in the range of 4,400 to 4,500 cGy because of the tolerance of the spinal cord. An outright three-field arrangement of an anteroposterior (AP), a right posterior oblique (RPO), and left posterior oblique (LPO) is a reasonable technique to deliver the dose to a small target volume located centrally. The drawbacks of this technique are a relatively high radiation dose (50 percent of total dose) to the pulmonary tissue in the path of the oblique beams, the potential risk for an inadequate dose along the paravertebral regions, and the difficulty of dealing with a large target volume because of the poor pulmonary tolerance.

A treatment technique that I have developed is a combination of AP–PA POP with a three-field of AP-RPO-LPO arrangement, with which one can deliver a high radiation dose (5,600 to 6,400 cGy) to the target volume while normal vital structures are kept below the threshold dose that will cause permanent radiation injuries (spinal cord dose less than 4,400 cGy and pulmonary dose in the path of the oblique beams less than 1,200 to 1,400 cGy). With this technique the total dose of 6,400 cGy is delivered by an arrangement of AP-PA POP for the initial 3,600 to 3,800 cGy and then by the three-field (AP-RPO-LPO) arrangement for the remaining 2,600 to 2,800 cGy, using daily fractions of 180 to 200 cGy. Any target volume away from the main-stem bronchus and mediastinum requires a supplemental dose of 400 to 600 cGy to increase the minimum tumor dose to 6,000 to 6,400 cGy. For this technique to be successful, individually tailored cerrobend blocks are essential for protection of the uninvolved pulmonary tissue from the AP-PA portals and the spinal cord from the oblique beams.

Results

For patients with unresectable lung carcinoma subjected to high-dose radiation therapy, the 5-year cure rates are of the order of 5 to 10 percent across the country. With carefully designed radiation therapy employing a modern sophisticated technique and careful selection of patients, a 5-year cure rate of 10 to 15 percent is expected. The rate of control of local and regional tumors is probably the best criterion for effectiveness of various radiotherapeutic approaches using different dose levels and target volume. This rate, which is a function of radiation dose, tumor size, and other less well understood systemic factors, has been achieved in 50 to 70 percent of the patients with the current high-dose radiation therapy.

Relief of distressing symptoms is another goal in addition to cure in thoracic radiation therapy. Hemoptysis, which is alarming to patients and their families, is well relieved in more than 90 percent of patients with a moderate dose (3,000 to 4,000 cGy) of radiation. Dyspnea associated with obstruction of the trachea, carina, or lobar bronchi is also well relieved in more than 80 percent of patients by 4,500 to 5,000 cGy of radiation. Cough associated with carcinoma located in the main-stem bronchus or carina is more likely to be relieved than that associated with peripheral carcinoma of the lung. Local pain associated with direct spread of carcinoma to the surrounding normal structures, such as the chest wall, vertebrae, brachial plexus, and mediastinum, has also been well relieved by irradiation. Superior vena cava syndrome is a common complication of locally advanced lung carcinoma. The more recent the onset of the symptoms caused by the obstruction of venous drainage, the faster the relief of the distressing symptoms by irradiation. Radiation has been effective in relieving the presenting symptoms in more than 80 percent of patients. Relief of the hoarseness by irradiation depends on the degree of injury to the recurrent laryngeal nerve by metastatic carcinoma and its duration. Hoarseness alone without distant metastasis should not preclude high-dose radiation therapy, inasmuch as some of these patients can live normal lives for many years. Complete recovery from the hoarseness is, however, rare even with high-dose radiation therapy, implying that recovery of the damaged recurrent laryngeal nerve is exceptional.

POSTOPERATIVE RADIATION THERAPY IN NON–SMALL-CELL LUNG CARCINOMA

The fate of patients with positive regional lymph nodes or margins of an incomplete surgical resection has been very poor, with a 5-year survival rate of 0 to 20 percent.

This rate is far lower than the cure rate of 30 to 40 percent when there is no involvement of the regional lymph nodes or when the resection margins are free of tumor. Carefully planned radiation therapy with a moderately high dose (5,400 to 5,600 cGy, TDF 89–92) of radiation should be able to convert a surgical resection from incomplete to complete by sterilizing residual microscopic carcinoma at the tumor bed and the regional lymph nodes.

Indications

Postoperative radiation therapy is recommended for patients with positive regional lymph nodes (stages N1 and unforeseen N2 lesions) or with incomplete resection of the tumor margins because of the invasion of the tumor beyond the pulmonary parenchyma and visceral pleura to the chest wall, mediastinal structures, carina, or diaphragm (T3 lesions). The category of stage N1 of the current TNM system consists of a wide spectrum of regional lymph node involvement ranging from an intrapulmonary lymph node to multiple lymph nodes at the hilum. One may choose a policy of close surveillance for patients with a single metastasis to the intrapulmonary lymph node. However, postoperative radiation is a reasonable and safe choice for patients with metastases to multiple hilar lymph nodes. Because of the possible potential pulmonary injury associated with this treatment, patients should be carefully screened for adequate pulmonary function reserve before they are subjected to a course of 5.5 to 6 weeks of radiation.

Radiotherapeutic Techniques

The importance of radiotherapeutic techniques cannot be overemphasized inasmuch as the outcome of the treatment depends heavily on the success or failure of the sterilization of the residual tumor at the target volume selected and the relative frequency of serious complications associated with the adopted techniques. The target volume should include the tumor bed and the areas of the entire regional lymphatic drainage, which consists of the ipsilateral hilum, including the bronchial stump, with a 2- to 2.5-cm margin of uninvolved pulmonary tissue, the entire mediastinum, and the medial halves of both supraclavicular fossae. The optimum dose-fractionation schedule seems to be in the range of 5,400 cGy, given in daily fractions of 180 to 200 cGy, 5 days a week over a period of 5.4 to 6 weeks (TDF 89).

The radiotherapeutic techniques I use give consideration to the amount of pulmonary tissue remaining after lobectomy or pneumonectomy. For patients who have had a lobectomy, a total tumor dose of 5,400 cGy is delivered to the target volume by a sequential combination of AP-PA POP for the initial 3,600 cGy and a three-field arrangement of AP-RPO-LPO for the remaining 1,800 cGy. For patients who have had a pneumonectomy, a total tumor dose of 5,400 cGy is delivered by a sequential combination of AP-PA POP for the initial 4,200 cGy and an arrangement of anterior and posterior oblique opposing portals for the additional 1,200 cGy: right anterior (RAO) and left posterior oblique (LPO) opposing portals for the left-sided lesion and left anterior oblique (LAO) and right posterior oblique (RPO) opposing portals for the right-sided lesion.

Results

For patients with locally advanced carcinoma of the lung (N1, unforeseen N2 or T3 lesion), carefully administered postoperative radiation therapy has been able to improve survival. The cure rate of patients with N2 lesion has been improved from 3 to 10 percent after surgery alone to 10 to 30 percent after treatment with aggressive postoperative radiation. The benefit of postoperative radiation seems to be more conspicuous for patients with adenocarcinoma than for patients with squamous cell carcinoma. The role of postoperative radiation for stage N1 squamous cell carcinoma is a subject for further study. It is interesting to note that the pattern of failure seems dependent on the histologic type of the tumor. The most common site of failure for patients with squamous cell carcinoma is the tumor bed and the regional lymphatics. For patients with adenocarcinoma the brain seems the most common site of failure.

SUPERIOR PULMONARY SULCUS TUMOR

Paulson and colleagues pioneered a combined approach of preoperative radiation followed by extended en-bloc resection of the tumor, the chest wall, and the involved adjacent structures. The target volume for preoperative radiation includes the ipsilateral hilum and the upper two-thirds of the entire mediastinum, including the thoracic inlet and the subcarinal region in addition to a generous margin of 5 cm around the primary lesion. The apex of the ipsilateral axilla is also included. The dose-fractionation schedule that I employ delivers daily fractions of 180 to 200 cGy, 5 days a week for a total dose of 3,600 cGy in 3.6 to 4 weeks. An extended en-bloc resection is performed 3 weeks after irradiation, and this is supplemented with an additional dose of 1,400 to 2,000 cGy given in daily fractions of 180 to 200 cGy, 5 days a week to either the tumor bed for positive resection margins or the regional lymphatics for involved lymph nodes, starting approximately 4 weeks after surgery. This combined approach achieved a 5-year cure rate of 25 to 35 percent. Other radiotherapeutic options include use of an accelerated fractionation schedule as preoperative radiation that delivers 150 cGy twice daily for a total dose of 3,000 to 3,600 cGy and employment of an interstitial implant of radioactive sources at the site of residual tumor.

Radiation therapy alone has been used for superior pulmonary sulcus tumor if surgery is not to be performed because of the underlying medical conditions or extensive invasion of the surrounding structures by the tumor, i.e., the brachial plexus, subclavian arteries, vertebral bodies, and the mediastinum. Because of these unfavorable factors the long-term survival rate after radical radiation therapy alone is poor, with a 5-year cure rate of 5 to 10 percent. For the same reason the local failure rate after radiotherapy alone is as high as 45 to 50 percent, with tumor spread to the spinal canal being a common final event for carcinoma invading the vertebrae.

SUGGESTED READING

Choi NC, Carey RW, Kaufman SD, et al. Small cell carcinoma of the lung: a progress report of 15 years' experience. Cancer 1987; 59:6–14.
Choi NC, Doucette JA. Improved survival of patients with unresectable non-small-cell brochogenic carcinoma by an innovated high-dose en-bloc radiotherapeutic approach. Cancer 1981; 48:101–109.
Choi NC, Grillo HC, Gardiello M, et al. Basis for new strategies in postoperative radiotherapy of bronchogenic carcinoma. Int J Radiat Oncol Biol Phys 1980; 6:31–35.
Choi NC, Kanarek DJ, Kazemi H. Physiologic changes in pulmonary function after thoracic radiotherapy for patients with lung cancer and role of regional pulmonary function studies in predicting postradiotherapy pulmonary function before radiotherapy. Cancer Treat Symp 1985; 2:119–130.
The Lung Cancer Study Group. Effects of postoperative mediastinal radiation on completely resected stage II and stage III epidermoid cancer of the lung. N Engl J Med 1986; 315:1377–1381.

BENIGN AND LOW GRADE MALIGNANT TUMORS

JOHN R. BENFIELD, M.D.
JOHN C. WAIN Jr., M.D.

Pulmonary neoplasms include an aggregate of benign and low grade tumors of the lung that account for 5 percent or less of all lung neoplasms. There is enough diversity and heterogeneity among the unusual lung tumors so that accurate diagnosis and appreciation of tumor biology are essential for optimal treatment planning.

Carcinoid tumors are the most frequent of the low grade cancers. To emphasize the apparently common cell of origin for typical and atypical carcinoids and small-cell undifferentiated lung cancers (SCLC), we prefer to call this family of tumors the Kulchitsky cell carcinomas (KCC) of various grades: grade I is synonymous with typical carcinoids; grade II denotes atypical carcinoids; grade III is SCLC. In our experience with over 300 patients, the differentiation among grades of KCC is best made by light microscopy. KCC-II and KCC-III may be difficult to differentiate if only small tissue samples or suboptimal cytologic specimens are available. Nearly 10 percent of our patients with KCC-II eventually developed SCLC.

Among carcinoids, about 75 percent are central endobronchial tumors. Approximately 90 percent are KCC-I (typical carcinoids), which are slow-growing, and no lymph node metastasis occurs in over 90 percent of these. Patients with KCC-II tumors have lymphatic metastases up to 70 percent of the time; 25 to 50 percent of them can be expected to die of their cancers within 5 years of the time of diagnosis.

Adenocystic carcinomas are the second most frequently occurring low grade pulmonary malignancy.

Mucoepidermoid carcinomas, the least prevalent of the low grade lung cancers, include variants of low grade and high grade malignant behavior. These neoplasms have a tendency to perineural and submucosal infiltration; they frequently cause death, but the time span for doing so may be over many years. Low grade and localized tumors are slow-growing and usually without metastases; high grade lesions are rapidly fatal.

Pulmonary fibrochondrolipomas (hamartomas) are the most common true benign neoplasms of the pulmonary interstitium that do not metastasize. They entrap bronchial and alveolar epithelium during their inexorable growth, and thus they may compromise vital structures if left untreated.

Mesenchymal tumors are rare benign neoplasms that include chondromas, lipomas, xanthomas, and granular cell myoblastomas. Except for granular myoblastomas, which occur more commonly in the upper airway than in the bronchi, mesenchymal tumors generally occur as localized endobronchial lesions. These tumors are benign; complete excision is curative.

Localized pulmonary lymphomas (previously termed pseudolymphomas) are clonal lymphoid proliferations. Supplementary to morphologic studies, the use of immunohistochemical methods to study surface markers has resulted in the definition of lymphomas according to criteria of clonal lymphoid proliferation. To permit immunohistochemical studies, fresh tissues must either be quick-frozen at −150 °C or preserved in non-cross-linking fixatives such as Bouin-Hollande solution. The prognosis for patients with pulmonary lymphomas is generally good, including 10-year survivor rates of 70 percent for some monoclonal lesions. The presence of a polyclonal cell population is often associated with aggressive lymphomas and poor prognosis. Paraproteinemia, especially of IgM, has been associated with an increased likelihood of development of disseminated lymphomas.

The clinical presentation of unusual pulmonary neoplasms depends whether the lesions are endobronchial or parenchymal in location. In general, the endobronchial lesions are KCC, adenocystic carcinomas, mucoepidermoid carcinomas, or benign mesenchymal neoplasms. Laminar tomography (not computed tomographic scanning) remains the most accurate and useful method for radiologic demonstration of the anatomy of the major airways. Bronchoscopy is the definitive diagnostic test; biopsies can usually be obtained without causing significant hemorrhage, but rigid bronchoscopes and general anesthesia should be immediately available in preparation for the possibility of massive bleeding.

Unusual pulmonary neoplasms in the parenchyma typically present as asymptomatic, isolated, peripherally located masses. As seen on tomography, they are smoothly circumscribed lesions with regular borders. Percutaneous transthoracic needle biopsies have usually not provided a definitive diagnosis.

TREATMENT

The following selected case histories illustrate current therapeutic issues regarding each of the lesions described above.

KCC-I (Typical Carcinoid). A 27-year-old man who was a nonsmoker had a 1-year history of intermittent hemoptysis. The chest roentgenogram was normal. Bronchoscopy without biopsy by the referring pulmonologist revealed a smooth, light red lesion in the left main bronchus. Biopsies during repeat bronchoscopy were inconclusive. Without definitive histologic diagnosis, the lesion was removed by a sleeve resection of the left main stem bronchus. The margins of resection were free of tumor by frozen and permanent sections that confirmed the diagnosis of KCC-1.

This case illustrates removal of KCC-I with maximal preservation of pulmonary tissue. The lesion originated within submucosal glands. We believe that endobronchial resection, e.g., by laser methodology, would have placed the patient at risk for local recurrence. Lymph node sampling at operation was done to establish the stage of disease (T_1N_0).

KCC-II (Atypical Carcinoid). A 69-year-old man with a history of smoking was found to have an asymptomatic left upper lobe pulmonary nodule. Tomography revealed nodularity of the left hilus. The cytologic features of specimens obtained with percutaneous needle aspirates were considered compatible with KCC-III (SCLC) prior to referral to us. We considered the cytologic material inadequate for firm diagnosis. The diagnosis of KCC-II was made by biopsy through a limited anterior thoracotomy. A left pneumonectomy was done to remove the tumor, which involved the upper and lower lobes. Focal pleural invasion and N_1 metastases in one of seven hilar nodes were found; mediastinal nodes were free of cancer. The patient has remained free of disease for 4 years.

This case illustrates that KCC-II and KCC-III cannot reliably be differentiated if cytologic specimens are suboptimum, and that the presence of regional lymphatic metastases does not preclude long survival time following resection. The operative approach to KCC-II should include complete resection and lymphadenectomy. Neither routine postoperative irradiation nor adjuvant chemotherapy is indicated.

Commentary about KCC. Differential diagnosis includes lymphoproliferative lesions and SCLC. Proper diagnosis requires adequate sampling and permanent sections; immunohistochemical studies may be helpful. Ablation with bronchoscopic methods generally cannot be recommended because of the deep intramural origin of KCC. Excision is the recommended treatment. The treatment methods of our choice are bronchial sleeve resections or segmentectomies. Whereas lobectomies or pneumonectomies are sometimes needed to encompass the tumors, more conservative resections usually suffice, because local recurrences are rare. The role of lymphadenectomy in the treatment of KCC-II (atypical carcinoids) is controversial; we recommend lymphadenectomy, believing it to be primarily valuable for staging purposes. The role of chemotherapy in the treatment of KCC-II remains unclear. When KCC-II could not be completely excised, we have recommended systemic therapy such as that employed for control of KCC-III (SCLC).

Adenoid Cystic Carcinomas. A 78-year-old man with a history of smoking and a productive cough had a right hilar and lower lobe mass. Bronchoscopic biopsy of a right lower lobe endobronchial lesion revealed adenoid cystic carcinoma. Resection required a right pneumonectomy. Frozen sections of the margins of the resection were negative, but final histologic examination revealed peribronchial lymphatic infiltration and submucosal involvement at the bronchial margin. Postoperative radiation therapy was recommended but refused by the patient, who is free of apparent disease 6 months after resection.

This case illustrates the propensity of adenocystic carcinomas for perineural or lymphatic infiltration and for submucosal spread. Removal of adenoid cystic carcinomas may require more extended resections than other cancers with similar appearance on radiologic studies. Frozen sections may incompletely evaluate the adequacy of resection.

Commentary about Adenocystic and Mucoepidermoid Carcinomas. Complete excision is the treatment of choice. Bronchoplastic or tracheoplastic reconstructions are advisable when indicated, but the propensity of these lesions for local invasion and to submucosal spread must always be recalled. The margins of resection should be carefully evaluated by extensive use of frozen sections. Radiotherapy has been an effective, useful method for local control of unresectable cancers. We have encountered recurrences up to 20 years after apparently curative resections.

Endobronchial Mesenchymal Lesions. A 72-year-old man with a history of smoking had a productive cough. His chest roentgenogram was unremarkable, but bronchoscopy revealed a smooth, polypoid lesion that partially obstructed the left main bronchus. Biopsy revealed foamy, spindle-shaped cells. The lesion was excised with a sleeve resection of the left main stem bronchus. The final histologic diagnosis was fibrous xanthoma, and the patient is free of disease 12 years after resection.

Commentary about Mesenchymal Lesions. These neoplasms are all benign, but complete excision is required to establish an accurate diagnosis and to ensure local control. A sleeve resection with bronchoplastic reconstruction is typically done. An anatomic pulmonary resection is rarely required, and lymph node dissection is unnecessary.

Pulmonary Fibrochondrolipoma (Hamartoma). A 52-year-old man with a history of smoking had an asymptomatic new .5-cm left lower lobe nodule. Because the lesion could not be felt at thoracotomy, it was resected by lobectomy 6 years ago. Histologic examination revealed a fibrochondrolipoma, and the patient is now free of disease.

This case illustrates that on rare occasions, lobectomy may be needed to remove a nonpalpable radiologically apparent lesion that would normally be excised by a lesser resection.

Commentary about Hamartomas. Presumptive diagnosis can often be made on the basis of the radiologic appearance of a mass with remarkably smooth and well-delineated outlines. Hamartomas characteristically deflect percutaneous needle punctures, and definitive preoperative diagnosis is usually lacking. We proceed directly with wedge excisions of peripherally located lesions; smooth masses in central locations that require consideration of lobectomy as compared with segmentectomy are managed with intraoperative needle aspirates that are immediately examined after rapid staining methods. If no evidence of cancer is found, the most conservative possible resection (usually segmentectomy) is undertaken; completion lobectomy because of an unexpected diagnosis of carcinoma has rarely been required.

Localized Pulmonary Lymphomas. An asymptomatic 50-year-old woman with a history of smoking had excision of a malignant melanoma of her shoulder in 1972. In 1979, several pulmonary nodules defied diagnosis from specimens obtained by needle aspirations. After excisional biopsies, the lesions were considered to be pseudolymphoma. After review in 1983, the lesions were reclassified as well-differentiated lymphocytic lymphoma. Serum protein electrophoresis at that time confirmed the diagnosis of typically associated Waldenström's macroglobulinemia with a monoclonal IgM gammopathy and marrow involvement.

This case illustrates that (1) pulmonary mass lesions should be biopsied and not presumed to be metastases; (2) studies of surface markers in pulmonary lymphocytic infiltrates are needed to establish an accurate diagnosis; (3) wedge excision is generally required for diagnosis in patients with lymphoproliferative lesions of the lung.

Commentary about Lymphomas. Often the lesion is a solitary mass, thus demanding differentiation from bronchogenic carcinoma. Characteristically, preoperative percutaneous needle aspirates have revealed nonspecific aggregates of lymphocytes. After conservative excision, the fresh tissues should be prepared for immunohistochemical studies.

Supported in part by PHS Grant number CA09477 awarded by the National Cancer Institute, DHHS.

SUGGESTED READING

Arrigoni MG, Woolner LB, Bernatz PE. Atypical carcinoid tumors of the lung. J Thorac Cardiovasc Surg 1972; 64:413–421.

Carter D, Eggleston JC. Tumors of the lower respiratory tract. Armed Forces Institute of Pathology, Fascicle 17. Hartmann W, ed. 1980 (reprint 1983).

Kennedy JL, Nathwani BN, Burke JS, et al. Pulmonary lymphomas and other pulmonary lymphoid lesions. Cancer 1985; 56:539–552.

Paladugu RR, Benfield JR, Pak HY, Ross RK, Teplitz RL. Bronchopulmonary Kulchitsky cell carcinomas I and II alias typical and atypical carcinoids. Cancer 1985; 55:1303–1311.

LUNG INFECTION

FUNGAL INFECTION

TIMOTHY TAKARO, M.D.

Clinically significant cases of fungal infections of the lung of interest to thoracic surgeons are uncommon because most fungal infections can be managed effectively medically. Nevertheless, from time to time, chest surgeons are called upon either to assist in the diagnosis of an unknown lesion or to provide definitive treatment. Often the surgical procedure provides both the diagnosis and the treatment.

This chapter is limited to a discussion of the five most common fungal infections, with brief additional remarks. The management of moniliasis (*Candida* infections) is described elsewhere.

Some of these infections occur in the clinical setting of compromised or lowered host immunity. This is observed when immunosuppressive therapy has been used, as in organ transplantation, or when antimetabolites for the treatment of malignancies or the use of corticosteroids for a variety of conditions has resulted in immunosuppression. The acquired immunodeficiency syndrome (AIDS) is a newcomer to this group of diseases, involving a lowering of the host's immunologic defenses. As a general rule, therefore, pulmonary biopsy specimens from patients in these categories should be evaluated for multiple opportunistic pathogens, including the mycoses.

ASPERGILLOSIS

The treatment of aspergillomas (fungus balls) is controversial because of the wide range of severity of the underlying pulmonary disease, the unpredictability of the course of the disease, and the lack of controlled studies of the relative merits of surgical, nonsurgical, or expectant treatment.

Medical therapy is generally conceded to be unsatisfactory for aspergillomas, but most centers, including ours, would use amphotericin B (possibly in combination with 5-fluorocytosine) in a sick symptomatic individual in whom resectional surgery was not appropriate. We do not resect aspergillomas routinely. Our indication for surgery is severe hemoptysis. We are wary of patients with compromised pulmonary function or evidence of widespread fibrocystic pulmonary damage or both resulting from such diseases as sarcoidosis, bullous emphysema, tuberculosis, or bronchiectasis. It is difficult to manage the complications of bronchopleural fistula and of empyema following resectional surgery in patients with evidence of chronic parenchymal disease beyond the confines of the cavity containing the aspergilloma. Thin-walled isolated cysts containing aspergillomas with no evidence of gross disease in the remaining lung do not often cause such problems.

Alternatively, some surgeons advocate prophylactic resection of all aspergillomas, to forestall the possibility of severe life-threatening hemoptysis. Since evidence from controlled studies about the efficacy of this approach (many aspergillomas spontaneously regress, and others remain unchanged for years) is lacking, it is difficult for us to recommend this course. *Aspergillus* empyemas require drainage and sometimes thoracoplasty to obliterate the pleural space. The use of amphotericin B locally can be helpful. Removal of a nidus of infection (such as a suture) can also be important.

NORTH AMERICAN BLASTOMYCOSIS

Three forms of this disease are encountered: pulmonary, cutaneous, and disseminated. Pulmonary blastomycosis is not primarily a surgical condition. Indeed, self-limited disease requiring no treatment is not uncommon. However, blastomycotic infection of the lung can imitate bronchogenic carcinoma exactly, and herein lies its challenge for the thoracic surgeon. Strong efforts to accurately diagnose this disease should be made, especially in academic areas (in the southeastern, southcentral, and midwestern states, particularly Arkansas, Kentucky, Mississippi, and Wisconsin), to avoid an unnecessarily radical pulmonary resection under the mistaken assumption that the underlying disease is carcinoma.

The treatment of choice for a known infection is drug therapy. For mild or moderately severe cases, ketoconazole is the drug of choice over amphotericin B because of its lower toxicity and greater ease of administration by the oral route. The drug is ordinarily administered in doses of 400 to 600 mg per day. Because of poor absorption by the gastrointestinal tract when gastric acidity is insufficient, it is not given to patients with achlorhydria or together with antacids and cimetidine. For severe or life-threatening infections, amphotericin B must be used (see the section on histoplasmosis).

Ordinarily, neither known cavitary nor nodular disease is an indication for resection.

COCCIDIOMYCOSIS

Most patients with coccidiomycosis come to the attention of thoracic surgeons either because of a solitary nodule of undiagnosed etiology or because of the complications of a coccidioidal cavity. Our management of solitary pulmonary nodules of undiagnosed etiology is described in the section on histoplasmosis. While most such nodules occur as a result of exposure in the clear-cut endemic areas in the southwestern part of the United States, the disease is not confined to these areas, since extensive travel has allowed it to become widespread.

Resection for cavitary disease is indicated if the cavity appears to be enlarging (presumably to avert the danger of rupture, with subsequent pyopneumothorax) or if it is thick-walled or secondarily infected. If the cavity *has* ruptured or is causing severe or recurrent hemoptysis, or if the patient has or is suspected of having coexisting pulmonary tuberculosis, these are also indications for resection. A sero-positive patient with a peripheral cavity who has a negative skin test (indicating severely compromised immunity) should probably also have the lesion resected.

Since coccidioidal cavities are often located in an intersegmental plane, sometimes crossing a major fissure, they are best handled by wedge resection, multiple segmentectomy, lobectomy, or a combination of these. The postoperative complication rate of bronchopleural fistula, empyema, or recurrence is relatively high and calls for adjunctive drug therapy.

Until recently, the only antifungal agent with proven efficacy against coccidiomycosis was amphotericin B. This drug should be used in conjunction with surgery (both pre- and postoperatively) in all patients with diabetes, significant other medical problems, bilateral disease, or following rupture of the cavity when operation has been delayed. The drug should be used postoperatively if a complication such as bronchopleural fistula has developed or if residual disease is suspected. Recently ketoconazole has been shown to be effective and a newer agent, itraconazole, is showing promise as well.

CRYPTOCOCCOSIS

Although cryptococcosis is said to be the second most important cause of death from a fungal infection (after histoplasmosis), the fatal forms of the disease, including meningeal and pulmonary manifestations, occur most commonly in patients with compromised immune defenses. The form most usually seen by the thoracic surgeon is that of the chronic granuloma, presenting as a mass lesion or solitary pulmonary nodule. Sometimes central cavitation or necrosis is observed. The diagnosis is usually made histologically at transbronchial or open lung biopsy. If the diagnosis is made prior to surgery, we recommend treatment with amphotericin B (0.3 mg per kilogram per day), combined with 5-fluorocytosine (150 mg per kilogram per day in 6-hour doses). This combination may be additive, permits a lower dose of amphotericin B to be used, may inhibit the emergence of resistance to 5-fluorocytosine, and may obviate the need for surgery. There is no unanimity of opinion regarding the need for drug treatment if the diagnosis is made at thoracotomy in a nonimmunocompromised patient. We would nevertheless treat such a patient with both drugs, since *no* patients receiving drug treatment later developed cryptococcal meningitis, whereas 10 percent of surgically treated patients with apparently inactive disease later *did* develop cryptococcal meningitis.

HISTOPLASMOSIS

Although in endemic areas almost everyone shows evidence by skin testing of having been infected by *Histoplasma capsulatum*, thoracic surgeons see this disease primarily in three forms: the chronic granuloma (presenting as a solitary pulmonary nodule), chronic cavitary disease, and mediastinal granulomatous disease.

Our approach to the solitary pulmonary nodule is as follows: if the roentgenologic appearance of the nodule (plain films or conventional tomograms) shows dense calcification, especially with a central nidus or with concentric lamellations, it is considered to be benign and requires no treatment. If there is eccentric or scarce calcification, or none, further study is required. A peripherally located nodule in a reasonably low risk patient over the age of 40 who is a smoker is regarded as an indication for removal by wedge resection. If the nodule has been unchanged for at least 2 years, however, it is likely to be benign and will be observed on x-ray films at 6 and 12 months to assure stability.

In a patient under 40 years of age or in a high risk patient, a needle aspiration biopsy may be done in an effort to arrive at a diagnosis without surgery. If the biopsy is technically adequate and shows no malignancy but also no specific benign disease, it is reasonable to temporize, relying on further observation. These can be difficult problems at times and the patient's wishes are also taken into account. In any event, if a histoplasmoma is found on the resected specimen, no further treatment is required because this is a healed lesion.

Cavitary histoplasmosis is a different matter. We would treat a patient with sputum-positive cavitary histoplasmosis with a course of amphotericin B therapy and not surgery because there is no evidence in controlled studies that resection prolongs life or lessens relapses. If an undiagnosed cavitary lesion is resected and found to demonstrate active histoplasmosis, the patient should receive the same drug treatment. Some surgeons advocate resecting known cavitary lesions of histoplasmosis. In this instance, a month of drug therapy prior to and following surgery should be instituted.

Treatment with amphotericin B is not simple. Before embarking on a course of treatment and in order to avoid anaphylaxis, the patient is given a test dose of 1 mg of amphotericin B slowly (30 to 60 min) intravenously, and renal function is assessed by blood chemistries. The drug is then administered in gradually increasing increments of 5 mg each day until a daily dose of 1.0 mg per kilogram body weight is reached. The usual curative total dose is considered to be 2.0 to 2.5 g. Because of the nephrotoxicity of the drug, the development of azotemia must be monitored by obtaining daily serum creatinine concentrations; levels up to 3 mg per deciliter can be accepted before reducing the dosage or lengthening the dosage interval (i.e., every other day). Other blood cellular and serum components are also monitored.

Ketoconazole represents an alternative form of drug therapy with reported effectiveness.

The indications for surgery for the variety of mediastinal manifestations of histoplasmosis depend upon the complications induced by the intense granulomatous and fibrous reaction that histoplasmosis can produce in some patients. These include the middle lobe syndrome, a bronchiectatic airless middle lobe produced by compressive lymph nodes surrounding the bronchus, which may require lobectomy; esophagotracheal fistula, which requires division; and pericarditis, which may require a pericardial window procedure or pericardiectomy. Management of the superior vena caval syndrome is beyond the scope of this presentation.

SPOROTRICHOSIS

The rare pulmonary cavitary disease caused by *Sporothrix schenckii* is best managed by a combination of amphotericin B and resective surgery. Alternative treatment with a saturated solution of potassium iodide is less effective.

SUGGESTED READING

Cunningham RT, Einstein H. Coccidioidal pulmonary cavities with rupture. J Thorac Cardiovasc Surg 1982; 84:172–177.

Med Lett Drugs Ther. Drugs for treatment of systemic fungal infections. 1986; 28:41–44.

National Institute of Allergy and Infectious Diseases Mycoses Study Group. Treatment of blastomycosis and histoplasmosis with ketoconazole. Ann Intern Med 1985; 103:861–872.

Rohatgi PK, Rohatgi NB. Clinical spectrum of pulmonary aspergillosis. South Med J 1984; 77:1291–1301.

Takaro T. Pulmonary infections. In: Sabiston DC, ed. Textbook of surgery: the biological basis of modern surgical practice. Philadelphia: WB Saunders, 1985:2007.

HYDATID DISEASE

BERNARD T. LE ROUX, Ch.M., F.R.C.S.(Edin)
DAVID F. BLYTH, F.R.C.S.(Edin)

In areas where hydatid disease is endemic, the thoracic surgeon is more likely to be aware of the radiographic features of pulmonary hydatid disease than is his counterpart in a nonendemic area, who is likely to encounter pulmonary hydatid disease only among patients who have traveled.

Pulmonary hydatid disease poses a radiologic problem when the hydatid is small, single, and symptomless, since it must be differentiated from numerous other causes of isolated, peripheral, pulmonary lesions. The technique of delivery favored is different from the management of other single peripheral lesions, and this makes preoperative recognition of hydatid disease important. Uncomplicated pulmonary hydatid cysts are seldom completely circular, because they are so soft that they are dented and disfigured by adjacent structures. Sharp definition, without adjacent pulmonary reaction, is typical of the solitary, small, uncomplicated hydatid cyst. Close proximity to a pleural surface is common, but by no means invariable. Abutment on the chest wall further modifies shape, but if the hydatid lies remote from the pleural surface, it is usually ovoid in shape, the long axis of the egg coincident with that of bronchi and vessels. The diagnosis can then confidently be made on the basis of the dented, often folded shape of the lesion. Multiplicity of cysts, even when some are effete, is radiologically unmistakable.

The radiologic features of an effete hydatid are often diagnostic—lack of clarity of outline, an air-containing crescent within the opacity, sometimes with a level, occasionally the classic "water-lily" sign, and multiplicity further serve to facilitate the diagnosis. The radiologic appearances may be simulated by a mycetoma and by gangrenous lung in cavitated chronic destructive pneumonia. A mycetoma is often mobile and a pulmonary slough rarely convincingly so.

If the diagnosis of pulmonary hydatid disease is suspected, a search by computed tomography (CT) for hydatids elsewhere, particularly in the liver, is a wise precaution despite the fact that evidence of widely disseminated hydatid disease with pulmonary hydatid is rare. Density measurements with CT have not served to consistently identify a pulmonary hydatid on the basis of its liquid content.

A variety of techniques for the management of pulmonary hydatids have been described. The one favored as offering the opportunity for delivery of an intact cyst involves close collaboration with the anesthetist. After formal thoracotomy and identification of the cyst (most cysts suitable for this form of management are immediately subpleural), the patient is well oxygenated by the anesthetist while the pleural space is packed with large sponges. For a brief period ventilation by the anesthetist is held in abeyance, and the adventitious capsule of compressed lung is incised without damage to the cyst wall. Distinction between the two is unmistakable, and the uncomplicated cyst is not adherent to the adventitious capsule. A receiver is then appropriately placed, and the anesthetist gently inflates the lung, a maneuver that usually delivers the cyst into the receiver. Some cysts burst. Contamination of the pleural space is obviated by the packs. When cysts have burst, later pleural recurrence of hydatid disease, even when mebendazole is not given is not known to have occurred.

There is always an open bronchus, usually 2 or 3 mm in diameter, in the adventitious capsule, which is closed by suturing. Some favor obliteration of the space left by evacuation of the cyst by a series of pursestring sutures; others do not use this technique and leave the space unmodified. With either technique, ultimate radiologic appearances are satisfactory, with the patient having a normal chest film usually within 10 days of thoracotomy.

After preliminary thoracotomy, some surgeons prefer to aspirate an uncomplicated cyst as completely as possible through its adventitious capsule before incising this capsule to ensure that the pleural space is not contaminated by rupture.

Bilateral anteriorly placed hydatids are managed simultaneously through a bilateral anterior thoracotomy. Those inconveniently placed for an anterior approach are managed through separate lateral thoracotomies during the same period of anesthesia.

Cysts complicated by infection lie crumpled within the adventitious capsule, which has in effect become the wall of the chronic lung abscess. It may yet be possible to identify the open end of a bronchus in the floor of this abscess, but it may not accept suturing. One satisfactory technique of management, after evacuation of the abscess content, is to close the incision in the abscess wall with a pursestring suture snugged around a Pezzer's catheter, the end of which is trimmed to leave a wide flange. The catheter is pulled through the chest wall at a distance from the thoracotomy, and the pleural space is drained separately. Gentle traction on the Pezzer's catheter pulls the lung against the chest wall and the flange of the catheter against the inner aspect of the abscess wall. There is usually good radiologic evidence of healing within very few days, without residual air leak, and the catheter is then simply pulled out, the flange easily collapsing as it passes through the chest wall.

In some rare instances, very large uncomplicated hydatid cysts may so completely occupy the whole of a pulmonary lobe that the best management may be judged to be lobectomy. Large complicated hydatids are also occasionally most satisfactorily managed by lobectomy. If this is likely to be the operation undertaken, it is wise to perform preliminary bronchography to map the extent of bronchial damage.

An uncomplicated subpleural hydatid cyst may occasionally rupture into the pleural space, usually as the result of strenuous effort on the part of the patient, such as during labor at term. In these circumstances, a tension pneumothorax develops. Initial management of this is by closed tube thoracostomy. The bronchopleural fistula does not close, and occasionally the crumpled hydatid, lying at the bottom of the pleural space, is radiologically recognizable. Management is by formal thoracotomy and closure by suture of the bronchopleural fistula and evacuation of the hydatid skin. It is in these circumstances that postoperative use of drugs such as mebendazole or albendazole, may be recommended.

SUGGESTED READING

Barrett NR, Thomas D. Pulmonary hydatid disease. Br J Surg 1952; 40:222–244.

Elhassani NB. Pulmonary hydatid disease in childhood. J R Coll Surg Edin 1983; 28:112–115.

Le Roux BT. Pulmonary hydatid disease. Thorax 1972; 27:365–367.

Shanks SC, Kerley P. A textbook of x-ray diagnosis. 3rd ed. Vol. 2. London: HK Lewis, 1962.

LUNG AMEBIASIS

BERNARD T. LE ROUX, Ch.M., F.R.C.S.(Edin)
CIRO CAMPANELLA, M.D.

Except in unusual circumstances, pulmonary amebiasis is not a surgical disease. Metronidazole is the treatment of choice for invasive amebiasis, with tinidazole as alternative therapy.

Of the world's population 10 percent is infested with *Entamoeba histolytica* (WHO estimate), but in only a small number does the parasite invade body tissues—for reasons not entirely clear. With tissue invasion the organism increases in size and ingests erythrocytes (hematophagous *E. histolytica*). Isoenzyme differentiation between pathogenic and nonpathogenic *E. histolytica* enables the identification of several different zymodemes (strains determined on the basis of the isoenzyme electrophorectic mobilities of hexokinase and phosphoglucomutase), only some of which are characteristic of pathogenic varieties. Either there are strains of *E. histolytica* only some of which are pathogenic or, when the ameba becomes pathogenic, the isoenzyme pattern changes to enable red cell ingestion. The amebic gel diffusion test is reliable evidence of active or past amebiasis and is especially sensitive in nonendemic areas. In endemic areas its value lies mainly in the fact that a negative result usually means illness is not caused by invasive amebiasis; a positive result in the same population group, since the test remains positive for a long time after healing has occurred, is less significant of invasive amebiasis as the cause of present illness.

Extension of amebiasis from the liver to the lungs and pleura is well documented. Pleuropulmonary amebiasis may develop as a consequence of *direct extension* from the liver through the diaphragm, or *hematogenous dissemination* may occur to the lung from bowel.

With regard to direct extension from the liver into the pleural space or lung, it is common to hear a pleural rub in a patient with an amebic liver abscess. Such a rub may disappear with specific antiamebic treatment, or it may be a prelude to the development of a serous pleural effusion or amebic empyema, the consequence of rupture of an amebic abscess of the liver or subphrenic space into the pleural space. Rub and serous effusion are not inevitable precursors to the development of empyema. Amebic empyema thoracis may also result from direct extension of an amebic lung abscess to the pleura. The development of amebic empyema may be abrupt or insidious; an insidious onset is more usual, but sometimes the onset is acute, with severe pain and shock, followed quickly by death. The right pleural cavity is more often involved, but occasionally left-sided amebic empyema is found. There are well-documented cases of left amebic empyema that has developed as a complication of amebic pericarditis, itself the manifestation of direct extension of hepatic amebiasis through the diaphragm into the pericardium.

Pus obtained at thoracentesis in a patient with amebic empyema is usually "anchovy" in color, but may be yellow or green, and in 5 percent of cases bile may be identified macroscopically. It must be examined for both pathogenic bacteria and, by appropriate techniques, amebae. Drug therapy for amebiasis, in conjunction with intermittent closed drainage (by thoracentesis), is more often successful in amebic empyema thoracis than in any other forms of empyema; continuous closed (tube thoracostomy) drainage may be necessary; occasionally open drainage is required, sometimes with drainage also of the subphrenic lesions, particularly when the amebic pus is contaminated with pathogenic bacteria, especially *E. coli*.

While transdiaphragmatic migration of amebae may occur from the liver to the lung in lymphatic channels, without macroscopic evidence of rupture through the diaphragm, the usual manner of extension is by perforation of a subphrenic or hepatic abscess through the diaphragm, across an obliterated pleural space, with pulmonary consolidation or abscess. Direct extension to a bronchus with little involvement of the pulmonary parenchyma and evacuation of the subphrenic lesion by coughing may also occur. There is, in these circumstances, a hepatobronchial fistula. Pulmonary lesions are most common in either the middle or the right lower lobe, often with abscess formation. The left lower lobe or the lingular segment of the left upper lobe may be the site of amebic lung abscess; pulmonary involvement is occasionally bilateral.

Repeated small hemoptyses may precede expectoration of characteristic dark, reddish brown sputum in which *E. histolytica* may be found. Radiographically there is usually some evidence of a pulmonary lesion, and the diaphragm is elevated; a triangular shadow with its base on the diaphragm is, in circumstances of known hepatic amebiasis, characteristic. Prognosis is good. With appropriate drug therapy, recovery is rapid in the patient with a hepatobronchial fistula and not noticeably more protracted if there is a related pulmonary abscess.

Complications such as empyema, metastatic abscess, and residual pulmonary fibrosis may occur. Surgical drainage is required only when the condition of the patient, to whom adequate medical treatment has been administered, deteriorates or fails to progress, and the decision to embark on a surgical procedure must not be made prematurely. The administration of metronidazole, 800 mg thrice daily, and postural drainage will cure most amebic lung abscesses; secondary bacterial contamination of the lung abscess may require appropriate chemotherapy. Resolution is the rule; very occasionally, irreversibly damaged lung, with symptomatic bronchiectasis or a chronic cavity, may require resection. Since an amebic liver abscess is occasionally in communication with the biliary system, it sometimes happens that rupture of an abscess into the bronchus is followed by formation of a bronchobiliary fistula, which is recognized by the expectoration of bile-stained sputum. Recovery with conservative management is again the rule.

In the management of a patient in an area in which amebiasis is endemic and in a patient exposed by travel to the possibility of infestation by *E. histolytica*, it is important to keep in mind the possibility of pulmonary or pleural amebiasis when faced with the need to treat a right lower pulmonary or pleural lesion that resists standard management of acute infection. Ultrasonography and computed tomography often serve to demonstrate the liver lesions, which are almost always related to the supraphrenic amebic extensions, most often through the bare area into the middle lobe. The surgeon who embarks prematurely on exploration of an unexplained pleuropulmonary lesion inseparable radiographically from a diaphragmatic dome, who finds that the supraphrenic lesion communicates through a ragged hole in the diaphragm with either a subphrenic space or the liver, should withdraw after no more than appropriate biopsy, and not embark on pulmonary resection, so likely is the diagnosis to be amebiasis, and so complete is resolution with appropriate drug therapy.

There is both clinical and necropsy evidence of the occurrence of pulmonary amebiasis in the absence of hepatic amebiasis. A lesion may develop in an area of lung remote from the diaphragm, and this may reflect hematogenous spread or transbronchial spread by aspiration or "bronchial embolism" where there is a bronchohepatic fistula. Reports of pulmonary lesions attributed to amebiasis are sometimes based on the association of bowel infestation with *E. histolytica*, the disappearance of radiologic opacities following antiamebic therapy, and the demonstration of degenerate ameba in the sputum. The validity of such accounts must be accepted with caution. Bowel infestation with *E. histolytica* is common in endemic areas and may coexist with many other diseases; when infestation with *E. histolytica* coexists with areas of pulmonary consolidation, the etiology of which is never established, the apparent therapeutic effect of metronidazole may be no more than coincidental; and particular care is needed in the identification of amebae in the sputum, since, unless morphologic characteristics are unequivocal or the organism contains red blood cells, the parasite may easily be confused with *E. gingivalis*, a common oral commensal. Single pulmonary lesions that may be hematogenous are more commonly described than are multiple lesions, and multiple lesions attributable to pulmonary amebiasis are probably very uncommon.

SUGGESTED READING

Adams EB, MacCleod IN. Invasive amebiasis: amebic liver abscess and its complications. Medicine 1977; 56:325–334.

Kokhani RC, Garud AD. Treatment of amoebic liver abscess with tinidazole and metronidazole. Drugs 1978; 15 (Suppl 1):23–25.

LeRoux BT, Mohlala ML. Odell JA, Whitton ID. Pleuropulmonary amoebiasis in suppurative diseases of the lung and pleural space. Part 1: Empyema thoracis and lung abscess. Curr Probl Surg 1986; 22:73–80.

Maddison SE. Characterization of an entamoeba histolytica antigen-antibody reaction by gel diffusion. Exp Parasitol 1965; 16:224–235.

Wilmot AJ. Clinical amoebiasis. Oxford: Blackwell, 1962.

TUBERCULOSIS

J. GORDON SCANNELL, M.D.

The healing or elimination of the tubercular cavity is the historical objective of surgery in pulmonary tuberculosis. Elaborate strategies were worked out to promote fibrous healing by collapse or, alternatively, elimination by resection with proper timing.

All these procedures have now been changed. Tuberculosis has become an outpatient disease in which effective antibiotics and chemotherapy are of critical importance. Since the disease has not been eradicated, there are a few residual indications, and for surgical management, the whole pace of tuberculosis treatment has been profoundly altered. It remains a chronic disease that is profoundly affected by environment, and rules of management that apply in a medically sophisticated setting may be totally inappropriate under conditions of war, famine, or limited resources.

Collapse therapy became obsolete in the early 1950s with the advent of streptomycin, its derivatives, and subsequently chemotherapy. It is unlikely that collapse therapy will again find a place in our surgical handbooks. For the student of history and for an understanding of tuberculosis, the reader is referred to John Alexander's classic volume on collapse therapy.

Resection of focal pulmonary tuberculosis and residual cavitary disease was admittedly more selective and, if the infecting organism could be controlled, more certain than collapse therapy even before streptomycin appeared on the scene. E.D. Churchill, a pioneer in this as in other fields of thoracic surgery, and Robert Klopstock, a pathologist turned surgeon, discussed the problem with great clarity in 1943. Limited resections became increasingly safe under the protection of streptomycin, later isoniazid (INH) and ethambutol, and so on down the litany of agents. Even now a small residuum of cavities remains in which resection is preferable to an "open negative," particularly when atypical organisms are present, but the great number of segmental resections for tomographic demonstration of residual cavities after an arbitrary period of therapy vanished along with Max Chamberlain and the world of sanitoria, so brilliantly described by Robert Taylor in *Saranac, America's Magic Mountain*.

Two clear indications for surgery in tuberculosis remain: (1) destroyed lung, usually beyond irreversible major bronchial damage, and (2) tuberculous empyema with bronchopleural fistula. In both cases segmental resection, so applicable in the small residual cavity, has little place. Resection of destroyed lung in tuberculosis depends on bacteriologic control of both the original tuberculous infection and the invasive potential of any secondary organism. So far as possible, acute inflammatory changes must be controlled at the level of bronchial resection. The contralateral lung or the lobes that are to be preserved must have a reasonable reserve. A period of intensive chest physiotherapy is essential. Urgent indications for surgical intervention in large residual cavities are (1) ongoing or repeated infections, (2) hemoptysis, (3) seeding of the contralateral lung, and (4) inability to exclude carcinoma. Many individuals with a destroyed lung have extensive contralateral disease so that it becomes a fine point in judgment between the immediate risk of operation and long-term protection. Since healing of the bronchial stump is paramount, strategies to reinforce its healing by intercostal pedicle grafts, omental grafts, or other modifications must be strongly considered. Bronchial stump blowout can be disastrous or at the very least extremely difficult to handle. Revision requires closure in relatively flexible tissue with reinforcement by normal vascularized tissue. Extrapleural approaches by way of anterior mediastinotomy can be considered if one is dealing with a long bronchial stump on the right. A staged approach, with drainage of the empyema followed by repeat thoracotomy, is the usual course.

Bronchopleural fistula and a destroyed lung or lobe with tuberculous or mixed empyema are the second indications for surgery in pulmonary tuberculosis. Pleuropneumonectomy or pleurolobectomy, sometimes referred to as empyemectomy, is the procedure of choice. Sarot defined the rationale and technique in 1949 just as bacteriologic control became a reality.

The concept of excision plus primary closure is a long-established principle in tuberculosis surgery. Appropriate timing is of key importance with a first-stage dependent drainage of the empyema to control secondary invaders. All the principles of good hygiene, namely nutrition, rest, and elimination of stress, are essential. The formidable operative procedure is surprisingly well tolerated when there is reasonable reserve on the contralateral side and the patient is in reasonable balance with the disease.

The practical problems of the surgery of tuberculosis still revolve around supportive long-term care, particularly if complications occur. Since sanitoria are no longer available, long-term facilities for chronic care must be developed.

SUGGESTED READING

Alexander J. The collapse therapy of pulmonary tuberculosis. Springfield, IL: Charles C Thomas, 1937.

Chamberlain JM, Klopstock R. Further experiences with segmental resection in pulmonary tuberculosis. J Thor Surg 1950; 20:843–853.

Churchill ED, Klopstock R. Lobectomy for pulmonary tuberculosis. Ann Surg 1943; 117:641–669.

Sarot IA. Extrapleural pneumonectomy and pleurectomy in pulmonary tuberculosis. Thorax 1949; 4:173–223.

OPEN LUNG BIOPSY

BENEDICT D. T. DALY, M.D.

Open lung biopsy is an important diagnostic procedure for evaluating diffuse or focal pulmonary parenchymal disease. This procedure usually is performed through a small anterior thoracotomy incision (Klassen's) in the second through fifth intercostal spaces or through a larger posterolateral thoracotomy incision. These techniques rely on visual inspection and palpation of the lung to select the area of abnormality to be biopsied. To minimize the invasiveness of these open lung biopsy techniques while preserving or improving their high diagnostic yield, computed tomography (CT) of the thorax may be used to define the surface localization of three types of pulmonary parenchymal lesions: small subpleural nodules (often noted only on chest CT), pulmonary infiltrates in those patients who are immunocompromised, and chronic diffuse infiltrative lung disease. This procedure is called a CT-guided minithoracotomy.

Patients are scanned initially in the standard supine position. Examinations are carried out at total lung capacity with a slice thickness of 8 to 10 mm, with the examination extending from the thoracoabdominal junction through the lung apices. In patients with chronic diffuse infiltrative lung disease, an area of minimal abnormality is selected in order to obtain tissue from active and hence more characteristic disease. Areas of dense opacity are avoided. In patients who are immunocompromised and in whom infection is suspected, an area of maximal disease is selected to obtain tissue that may have identifiable pathogens on histologic section or tissue culture. Generous samples of tissue are obtainable most easily from areas of lung that are adjacent to the fissures so that disease that abuts the fifth or sixth intercostal space is selected preferentially. Subpleural nodules that abut the parietal chest wall also are suitable for biopsy by this technique. Subscapular and paraspinal nodules may be biopsied but are more difficult to approach. Paramediastinal or juxtadiaphragmatic lesions are not reachable by this technique.

Once the disease area to be biopsied has been identified on the standard supine CT images, the patient is placed back in the CT gantry in the exact position in which he or she would be placed on the operating table. The abnormal area then is rescanned at total lung capacity. A series of barium markers is placed on the chest wall to mark the site of the lesion on the body surface. A select scan then is repeated to assure the accuracy of these markers. Radiotherapy dye is used to replace the barium markers in order to identify the planned incisional site.

At thoracotomy, the radiotherapy dye marker is replaced with a scratch prior to prepping the chest. A 5-cm incision is made over the interspace closest to the skin mark. When the mark approximates the base, apex, or anterior margin of the lung, the incision is made 1 to 2 cm from the mark in the direction of the hilus because the lung retracts once the chest is opened. The underlying chest wall musculature is incised and spread with a self-retaining retractor. The intercostal muscles and pleura then are incised *only* over the 5-cm length of the incision, and the ribs are separated with two McBurney's retractors. The pulmonary abnormality is identified by palpation or inspection, and the area to be biopsied is brought to the interspace by the anesthesiologist's adjusting lung volume. Ventilation is interrupted briefly during biopsy. For peripheral nodules, mattress sutures are utilized to obliterate the parenchymal defect and are placed prior to excision. In the case of diffuse or patchy infiltrative lung disease, a 2 to 3 cm deep portion of lung may be excised using a TA-30 stapler or two angled rows of staples placed with the GIA stapler. The biopsy is carried out with the lung inflated in order to preserve normal microscopic pulmonary architecture. When staples are not used, Allen's clamps are placed on the wedge of lung to be removed and kept in place while the lung is fixed. A No. 24 chest tube is left in the pleural space, and the lung is tested for an air leak. The intercostal muscles are reattached to the rib below by passing sutures either around the rib or into its periosteum in order to avoid creating a lung hernia. The remainder of the chest is closed with running absorbable sutures.

The use of CT in this procedure obviates the need to visually or manually explore the chest to locate the appropriate pathologic condition. Hence, the need for operative exposure of the lung is small. Chest wall mechanics are affected only minimally. Even patients who are severely dyspneic at rest have been extubated within 24 hours of biopsy. Of the 66 patients operated on using this technique, only three have died. All were immunocompromised and died from their underlying disease. A specific diagnosis has been made in every patient. In deciding to employ a CT-guided minithoracotomy, the high diagnostic specificity and minimum morbidity of this procedure must be weighed against less invasive but less specific biopsy techniques such as transbronchoscopic or percutaneous needle lung biopsy.

SUGGESTED READING

Daly B, Faling L, Pugatch R, et al. The usefulness of computed tomography (CT) in guiding open lung biopsy. Chest 1985; 895:4485.
Daly BDT, Pugatch RD, Faling LJ, et al. Computed tomography minithoracotomy: a preliminary report of a new approach to open lung biopsy. Radiology 1983; 146:543–544.
Gaensler EA, Carrington CB. Open biopsy for chronic diffuse infiltrative lung disease: clinical, roentgenographic, and physiologic correlations in 502 patients. Ann Thorac Surg 1980; 30:411–426.
Klassan KP, Anlyan AJ, Curtis CM. Biopsy of diffuse pulmonary lesions. Arch Surg 1949; 59:694–704.

BRONCHOLITHIASIS

L. PENFIELD FABER, M.D.

The most common cause of broncholithiasis is calcification in hilar lymph nodes that has developed in areas of necrosis from a prior granulomatous infection, most commonly histoplasmosis or tuberculosis. The continuous motion of ventilation causes erosion of the bronchial wall by the calcified lymph node, or the dense fibrous reaction around these enlarged lymph nodes causes compression or distortion of adjacent bronchi.

Cough and hemoptysis are the most common symptoms of broncholithiasis, and both are directly related to erosion or compression of a bronchus. The coughing up of calcified lymph nodes (lithoptosis) is an infrequent complaint of these patients but can recur, since there may be several calcified lymph nodes in close proximity to the eroded bronchus.

It is important for the thoracic surgeon to have a critical awareness of the manifestations of broncholithiasis in order to make an early diagnosis. The presence of mediastinal and hilar lymph node calcification associated with bronchial symptoms and radiologic changes should suggest the possible diagnosis of broncholithiasis.

BRONCHOSCOPY

It is important for the endoscopist to be aware of the subtleties of bronchial pathology associated with eroding calcified lymph nodes. Granulation tissue and stenosis can have the appearance of carcinoma and broncholithiasis should be considered when biopsy and brushing procedures produce negative findings. Dysplastic cells may be reported by the pathologist and are caused by the longstanding bronchial irritation. In this instance, it is important for the thoracic surgeon to be aware of the differential diagnosis of broncholithiasis and to not just assume that cancer is present. The calcified lymph node can sometimes be seen through the bronchoscope, and its gritty characteristics will be clearly identified when biopsy is attempted. It is necessary to critically assess the extent of the bronchial erosion in order to appropriately plan the type of pulmonary resection. Bronchoplastic procedures particularly, will be required to conserve a maximum amount of lung tissue.

It can be difficult to identify a bronchoesophageal fistula on the bronchial side of the fistula because granulation tissue and secretions frequently obscure the opening. The esophagogram or esophagoscopy confirms the presence of a fistula into a main bronchus.

THERAPEUTIC ALTERNATIVES

Treatment should be directed toward the removal of the calcified lymph nodes and all the damaged bronchial or lung tissue, and it is best accomplished by thoracotomy and resection.

Bronchoscopic removal of a broncholith can be attempted, but the stone must be visible and somewhat loose. Endoscopic removal of a broncholith with a flexible fiberoptic bronchoscope is contraindicated, because it is not possible to safely dislodge and remove the stone with baskets, balloon catheters, or small biopsy forceps passed through the small channel of the flexible instrument. Any attempt at bronchoscopic removal requires the use of the open-tube bronchoscope. The broncholith is usually firmly imbedded in the bronchus, and forceful manipulation can result in hemorrhage or bronchoesophageal fistula. Frequently only a portion of the calcified lymph node is removed through the bronchoscope, and symptoms will then recur. Endoscopic broncholithectomy is only indicated for patients who cannot tolerate or refuse thoracotomy.

The neodynium YAG laser has been used for the dissolution and removal of a large broncholith. The technique should only be attempted by an endoscopist who is experienced in the use of the YAG laser, since fatal hemorrhage could result from destruction of the bronchus or pulmonary artery.

So-called conservative management consisting of antibiotics and watchful expectancy is contraindicated because the offending calcification will continue to cause symptoms, and fatal hemoptysis could occur.

INDICATIONS FOR SURGERY

The indications for thoracotomy are (1) recurrent or massive hemoptysis, (2) recurrent pulmonary infection, (3) bronchoesophageal fistula, and (4) suspected bronchogenic carcinoma. Hemoptysis will recur as long as the offending broncholith is present, and several hundred cubic centimeters of blood loss would necessitate urgent surgical therapy. Chronic pulmonary suppuration can only be resolved by removal of the calcified lymph node, diseased bronchus, and damaged lung tissue. A fistula between the esophagus and bronchus will not close unless the fistulous tract and calcified lymph node are removed and the defects in the esophagus and bronchus are repaired. Despite negative biopsy findings, the clinician may still believe that carcinoma is present, and thoracotomy is then indicated to establish the diagnosis and carry out the proper resection.

Nonsurgical therapy is entirely dependent upon the severity of the patient's symptoms and his willingness to accept recurrent symptoms if the broncholith is not removed. The patient must be made aware that follow-up by observation alone could result in significant complications of massive hemoptysis, lung abscess, and bronchoesophageal fistula. Some patients have minimal symptoms, and in this instance, the recommendation for thoracotomy is dependent upon the experience and judgment of the thoracic surgeon. Any decision for surgery is always affected by the age and general condition of the patient.

If the patient has coughed up the broncholith or it has been removed endoscopically, then nonsurgical management may be appropriate. Repeat bronchoscopic examination is necessary to be certain that bronchial obstruction is no longer present and the bronchus is free of recurrent granulation tissue.

Broncholiths are frequently multiple, and the removal of one stone does not necessarily mean that the problem is resolved. Nonsurgical management includes the periodic use of antibiotics, as related to bacterial sensitivity, and the use of cough suppressants, but the persistence of symptoms makes the patient a candidate for surgery.

TECHNIQUE OF SURGERY

The thoracic surgeon must be aware that surgery for the removal of a broncholith may be technically difficult. He must carefully plan what type of resection will maximize the conservation of lung tissue and also plan with the anesthesiologist the management of airway during the procedure. Although the morbidity and mortality rates of surgery for broncholithiasis are no higher than for most resections, the patient and family must be made aware of the complexity and possible technical difficulty of the operation. The resection must be as conservative as possible. Proper planning should include the options of segmentectomy and bronchoplastic resection as alternatives to lobectomy and pneumonectomy.

Anesthetic management of the airway includes preparation for one-lung anesthesia. This can be accomplished with a double-lumen endotracheal tube or a long single-lumen endotracheal tube properly positioned in either the right or left main stem bronchus. If the anesthesiologist is familiar with methods of high frequency ventilation, they should be available in case oxygenation becomes a problem during the operation. The anesthesiologist and thoracic surgeon should use techniques with which they are both familiar. Preoperative discussion is helpful.

Intraoperative bronchoscopy with the flexible fiberoptic bronchoscope can be of benefit in clearing the airway of blood or secretions during the procedure, and the bronchoscope and appropriate adaptor should be available. A bronchoplastic anastomosis can also be visualized by bronchoscopy upon its completion.

A posterolateral thoracotomy is recommended to provide wide exposure and access to the anterior and posterior hilar structures. The pleural space may be obliterated by adhesions from the prior granulomatous infection, and good visualization of the esophagus and subcarinal area is required on the right side. The lateral thoracotomy is reserved for patients with localized distal segmental obstruction.

Dissection of the hilar structures and pulmonary artery can be difficult and hazardous because of obliteration of the normal tissue planes by a dense fibrous reaction. If these findings are confirmed in the early aspect of the dissection, proximal control of the main pulmonary artery is advisable.

If a main stem or lobar bronchus has been compressed or eroded, it is appropriate to begin the dissection by attempting to free the tissue around the calcified lymph node and remove it from the adjacent bronchus. This is particularly true when the broncholith has eroded the bronchus intermedius or the posterior aspect of the right upper or lower lobes. It may be possible to remove a broncholith that has caused only bronchial distortion without erosion, but some type of resection is usually necessary. Initial removal of the broncholith may not be possible when it involves the middle lobe or the left upper and lower lobes, and in this instance it is necessary to isolate and transect the vessels prior to removal of the broncholith and diseased bronchus.

The broncholith may have eroded only a small portion of the bronchus, and after it is removed, the edges of the bronchus can be resected and a primary closure with interrupted sutures can be accomplished. It is recommended that 4–0 polyglycolic sutures be used for bronchotomy and bronchoplastic procedures. The surgeon must be certain that the closure is not under tension and that viable bronchial tissue has been approximated.

If a segmental bronchus is obstructed by the broncholith, then segmentectomy is the procedure of choice. It is difficult to free the pulmonary arterial branches to the segment, but cautious persistence will result in their isolation and ligation. The bronchus may be severely damaged by the broncholith, and it must be resected back to viable tissue before it is closed. If good bronchial tissue cannot be identified when doing a segmentectomy, then lobectomy becomes the resection of choice. The use of staples or sutures to close the bronchus depends on the length of viable bronchial tissue available for transection and also the personal preference of the surgeon.

Stapling is contraindicated when the broncholith and granulation tissue are close to the point of origin of the anatomic bronchus to be removed.

Broncholiths that have eroded the main stem bronchus, the bronchus intermedius, or the posterior wall of the right or left upper lobe bronchus provide the opportunity for bronchoplastic procedures. A sleeve of the bronchus intermedius can also be accomplished with preservation of all three lobes of the right lung. Upper lobe sleeve lobectomy is an alternative to pneumonectomy, and middle lobe sleeve lobectomy is the alternative to bilobectomy. A broncholith that has eroded the right or left main stem bronchus can usually be removed with subsequent bronchoplastic repair of the bronchus, and pneumonectomy can be avoided.

When a bronchoesophageal fistula is present, it is helpful to have a nasogastric tube or bougie in the esophagus to assist in its identification. The fistulous tract is usually found in the center of the calcific and fibrotic peribronchial lymph nodes and is frequently encountered when the fibrous tissue is transected. Once identified, the fistula is dissected back to the wall of the esophagus, which is then repaired in two layers. All of the abnormal lymph nodes must be removed, and the proper bronchial and pulmonary resection is carried out. If diseased lymph nodes are permitted to remain, the pathologic process will recur, and the second operation will be even more difficult than the first.

Calcified lymph nodes in the carina frequently create traction diverticula of the esophagus, and caution should be used when these nodes are removed. A small diverticulum can be transected; if it is not recognized and repaired, a postoperative esophageal fistula can be catastrophic.

Versatility is required not only in the approach to any single procedure but also in the application of a variety of possible techniques, that may provide the definitive resection. The surgeon must be prepared for node removal, bronchotomy, segmentectomy, lobectomy, bronchoplasty resection, and possible pneumonectomy.

Pleural flaps are used to reinforce bronchoplastic closure and are always placed between the esophagus and bronchus when a fistula has been repaired. Retained secretions may be a problem in these patients, and vigorous supportive care and early bronchoscopy are indicated.

RESULTS

If all of the calcified lymph nodes are removed in the area of the offending broncholith and a satisfactory resection of chronically infected lung tissue and bronchus has been accomplished, these patients do well. Clinical awareness of the manifestations of broncholithiasis permits early diagnosis by the thoracic surgeon and initiates the proper recommendation for therapy. The avoidance of the complications of observation can thus be avoided. Long-term follow-up of these patients is important, since cancer has been noted to develop in an area of prior broncholithiasis.

SUGGESTED READING

Arrigoni MG, Bernatz PE, Donoghue FE. Broncholithiasis. J Thorac Cardiovasc Surg 1971; 62:231–237.

Cole FH, Cole FH Jr, Khandekar A, Watson DC. Management of broncholithiasis: is thoracotomy necessary? Ann Thorac Surg 1986; 42:255–257.

Dixon GF, Donnerberg RL, Schonfeld SA, et al. Advances in the diagnosis and treatment of broncholithiasis. Am Rev Respir Dis 1984; 129:1028–1030.

Faber LP, Jensik RJ, Chawla SK, et al. The surgical implication of broncholithiasis. J Thorac Cardiovasc Surg 1975; 70:779–789.

Trastek VF, Pairolero PC, Ceithaml EI, et al. Surgical management of broncholithiasis. J Thorac Cardiovasc Surg 1985; 90:842–848.

LUNG ABSCESS

J. GORDON SCANNELL, M.D.

Acute and chronic lung abscesses today are treated medically, but certain surgical indications remain for external drainage or resection under the protection of antibiotics. For example, a residual cavity or foci of chronic infection with recurrent hemoptysis may be sufficient threat to warrant resection. Failure of the abscess to clear poses the threat of concealed malignancy. The very old or debilitated patient may require early external drainage; this is not necessarily a poor compromise as long as adequate long-term medical and nursing care is available. In the future, the threat of immune deficiency disease may force us to rethink our drainage sequences.

Of chief importance in lung abscess (or segmental pneumonitis) is exclusion of bronchogenic carcinoma. Even if there is an obvious history of aspiration, early bronchoscopy is usually indicated both for diagnosis (including biopsy and cytologic examination) and therapy (endobronchial drainage, aspiration for identification of invasive organisms, and retrieval of a foreign body, if present). Adequate radiologic evaluation, including CT if available, should precede endoscopy, but radiologic methods deal with shadows and endoscopy deals with reality.

If adequate anesthetic support is available, most surgeons prefer rigid bronchoscopy with its optimal fiberoptic and biopsy capability, but the point is arguable by those who opt for the convenience of flexible bronchoscopy and reasonable visualization. The responsible surgeon must be skilled in both methods. The argument that flexible endoscopy extends the field of vision is tenuous, at least in an acute, inflammatory process. Again, cancer must be excluded beyond reasonable doubt.

If the acute lung abscess is the result of septic embolization or infarction (as occurs in bacterial endocarditis, septic endophlebitis, or intravenous narcotics) medical clearing is the rule. Only those where disease progresses to widespread destruction or real or threatened extension into the pleural cavity require drainage or resection.

Pneumonia following an alcoholic spree, a coughing fit, extensive intraoral operations, or ongoing "bronchial" infection in a debilitated patient should respond promptly to intensive antibiotic therapy, with response measured in weeks, not days. During the period of observation, steady though not necessarily rapid progress should be expected. Such patients should be hospitalized, at least in the initial phases of their management.

Extension of an intrapulmonary abscess into the pleural space is a major complication. A complicating empyema is suggested by failure to respond to antibiotics, confirmed by x-ray films and CT study if available, and established by thoracentesis. The source of the aspirated pus—pleura or lung—is the dilemma. In either case, external drainage is necessary, for intrabronchial drainage is rarely adequate. Closed thoracotomy, i.e., the insertion of a chest tube into the cavity or space, may be sufficient in rare cases; this procedure is similar to the so-called Monaldi treatment of tuberculous cavities, fortunately a thing of the past. Conventional rib resection and open drainage may be necessary. The surgeon should be well advised that an intrapulmonary abscess is a vascular process. If the surgeon is determined to proceed with early thoracotomy and decortication, he must be prepared to deal with the diseased lung, which is not, at this stage at least, a candidate for re-expansion to obliterate the pleural space. Combined decortication and segmental or lobar resection may be the procedure of choice in the subacute or chronic state, since the formidable vascularity of the acute phase has partially subsided. At any stage, the technical demands are great, since the inflammatory process involves the bronchial artery rather than the low pressure pulmonary arterial system.

Multiple-stage drainage of lung abscess is now rarely necessary. If early drainage is elected, it should be carried out where pleural surfaces are adherent, so as to prevent conversion of a local process into a total empyema. Chest wall tenderness and radiologic evidence are helpful in planning the approach.

Finally, it should be noted that the superior segment of either lobe is the classic site of an aspiration abscess. It is also commonly the site of destructive abscesses in geriatric patients in whom there is an unproved assumption of some associated pulmonary infarction. In any event, a patient who is not a candidate for aggressive resection may do surprisingly well with external drainage.

Lung abscess or a complicating empyema has by definition, a major bronchial communication, usually evident immediately upon drainage. All irrigations must be done cautiously. When properly drained, the abscess cavity slowly obliterates while the bronchopleural cutaneous fistula closes. Persistent leak raises the possibility of malignant disease, tuberculosis, or other granulomatous disease. Primary drainage of an otherwise nonresectable malignant abscess is inadvisable, unless it is clear that external drainage will relieve a distressing, productive cough. External drainage of a tubercular abscess is rarely indicated, although it is a curious phenomenon that external drainage of tuberculosis in earlier times often allowed conversion of a positive to a negative sputum. This was the basis of the Monaldi procedure in order to salvage an otherwise intolerable situation.

Hemorrhage is an ever-present hazard of drainage. It may be of major, even fatal, proportions. Readjustment of the drainage tube may control the bleeding, and gauze packing of the cavity is a last resort. Presumably, the reason for open drainage precludes resection in the geriatric or debilitated patient, but a few basically low-risk patients may be candidates for a second-stage resection for a persistent bronchopleural fistula. Resection back to normal lung or bronchial stump is indicated, with careful bronchial closure and re-expansion of the normal lung.

SUGGESTED READING

Monaldi V. Endocavitary aspiration: its practical applications. Tubercle 1947; 28:223.

Sweet RH. Analysis of Massachusetts General Hospital. Cases of lung abscess from 1938 through 1942. Surg Gynecol Obstet 1945; 80:568–574.

BRONCHIECTASIS

WILL C. SEALY, M.D.

Bronchiectasis literally means dilatation of the bronchi, but in the disease bronchiectasis the bronchi, including their muscular coat and ciliated epithelium, are not just dilated, but are partially destroyed. The process usually extends to the fifth order of bronchi, which end blindly with cystic or saccular configuration. The pathogenesis of the process, simply stated, is the triad of infection, obstruction, and destruction.

Most patients with bronchiectasis can be considered as having either localized or multisegmental bronchiectasis. The localized form of bronchiectasis results from one event, which in most patients is an obstructive one, such as a retained foreign body, a slow-growing intrabronchial tumor, bronchial stenosis, or bronchial obstruction secondary to external compression. Occasionally the localized type follows one episode of pneumonia.

The symptoms of the localized form of bronchiectasis include cough and sputum production with repeated episodes of acute pneumonitis and hemoptysis. The diagnosis in most patients can be made on the basis of the history, physical examination, radiography, and bronchoscopy. Bronchograms may be needed only if the cause cannot be demonstrated by bronchoscopy. The treatment is surgical and is nearly always accomplished by lobectomy or pneumonectomy. Segmental resection is rarely indicated. Medical treatment has little if any part to play in this easily corrected surgical problem.

In the multisegmental group there is a characteristic, but bizarre, distribution pattern of the bronchiectasis, as well as other clinical similarities. The onset of the disease is usually insidious, with the first manifestation of bronchiectasis at the age of 4 to 6 years. The patients have had a long history of upper and lower respiratory infections. Sputum production may be profuse and foul. Hemoptysis is common and sometimes may be profuse. Many patients have a history of pansinusitis, and in years past an occasional patient would develop a brain abscess. These patients seem to have "poor resistance to infection," but certainly in the past, only a few had any specific immunologic defect. Now the latter is more frequently the case. At the time the surgeon sees the patient the disease has reached its limits, and there is usually no further progression. Although once a common problem, multisegmental bronchiectasis is now quite rare, a tribute to empiricism and what might be considered by some as the indiscriminate use of antibiotics in children with respiratory infections.

The lung segments involved in multisegmental disease in various combinations include the following: the basilar segments on both sides, the lingula, and the middle lobe. An occasional patient may have only basilar segment involvement, but would otherwise belong to the multisegmental group. These are dependent areas of the lung in the upright position and are not the common sites for aspiration infections.

The diagnosis of multisegmental bronchiectasis can be made from the history, physical examination, radiography of the chest, including posteroanterior and lateral views, with a bronchoscopic examination used to exclude the presence of bronchial obstruction. Bronchograms are needed only if there is to be an operation. It is imperative that the bronchi of all lobes be outlined with the iodized oil. Since topical anesthesia is used in most patients, the success of the examination depends upon completing it before the anesthesia wears off. The best bronchograms are made with the contrast medium introduced into the trachea by nasotracheal tube, the worst involved side being outlined first. This can be done without the use of the fluoroscope, for this lengthens the study. The bronchi of one lung can be quickly and successfully outlined by proper positioning of the patient as the iodized oil is instilled. Then lateral and oblique films of the chest are obtained, with a right oblique view for outline of the left side, and the opposite for the right. Following this the less involved side can be filled, and another oblique view and a posteroanterior film obtained. Some thoracic surgeons like to fill one side and wait for 2 to 3 weeks before filling the other side. The need for instillation of the contrast agent through the bronchoscope frequently results in alveolar filling and retention of oil within the lung. Children must be under anesthesia when bronchography is carried out. Operation should never be done until at least 3 weeks after the bronchography.

Medical treatment of multisegmental bronchiectasis can be effective when involvement is minimal. It may be mandatory if the disease is extensive and the patient's pulmonary function is poor. The most important part of conservative management is the use of postural drainage, 2 to 4 times per day, and repeated every day even when there is little or no sputum production. A fixed plan of continuous or intermittent administration of a broad-spectrum antibiotic is frequently used. During acute infections and episodes of hemoptysis, a large dose of the appropriate antibiotics should be used for 7 to 10 days. In some patients with a severe bilateral multisegmental form, operation is occasionally done for the worst side, followed by medical treatment, which may then effectively control the disease on the less-involved side.

Operations for multisegmental disease nearly always include one or more segmental resections. Even when resection is extensive the results can be good, because nearly all of the excised lung is nonfunctioning. Occasionally one or two normal basilar segments have to be removed, as it is not practical to preserve them when the other basilar segments are involved. Successful operation depends on careful evaluation of the bronchogram and pulmonary function as well as painstaking preoperative preparation. The latter includes vigorous breathing exercises, postural drainage, and antibiotics. I have found that intrabronchial medications are not helpful. In bilateral disease, 6 months should elapse between the operations, allowing time for good mobility to develop on the side operated upon first.

The technical problems at operation include abundant adhesions that are vascular. There is an increase in the size of the bronchial arteries to the involved segments, which must be looked for and controlled. Segmental resection requires careful isolation and identification of the appropriate pulmonary artery and vein before interruption. The surgeon takes advantage of the fact that pulmonary veins course between segments and serve as a guide to the blunt separation of the segments. Staplers are rarely used, as this technique compromises some of the functioning lung. When used on the bronchus it tends to leave too much length.

Anesthesia can be a problem because of the excess secretions even after careful preoperative preparation. A Carlens type intratracheal tube is not indicated, even though the patient is operated on in the lateral position. During segmental resection the lung has to be kept inflated. When the segmental bronchus is occluded, in carrying out a resection, the segment may become smaller, but still will remain partially inflated. This is due to collateral ventilation supplying any remaining normal alveoli in the diseased segment.

As an example of the operative approach, I will use the worst surgical case situation, a patient with disease in both basilar segments, the lingula, and the middle lobe.

The left side is frequently the most severely involved. The approach to this side will be described first. A posterior lateral intercostal incision through the left fifth or sixth interspace is needed for good exposure. After the adhesions are divided, the inferior pulmonary ligament and the mediastinal pleura are incised, the inferior pulmonary vein is identified. These steps mobilize the lung. The major fissure is developed completely, exposing the left pulmonary artery. The superior segmental, lingular, and basilar arteries are identified and the latter two divided. The next step is to lift the lung upward and then divide the basilar segmental branches of the inferior pulmonary vein. Following this the basilar segmental bronchus is divided, and a clamp is left on the distal end, leaving the bronchial stump as short as possible. It may be necessary to divide the first two branches of the basilar bronchi in order not to encroach upon the lumen of the superior segmental bronchus. The bronchi are closed with absorbable sutures. A long stump can be the site of secretion collection and cause cough and sputum production after operation. The superior segment is quite large, sometimes making up more than half of the lower lobe, and sits on the basilar segments like a hat on a head. The surgeon immediately looks for the intersegmental veins and follows this guide. With traction on the clamp in the distal basilar bronchus, he begins the dissection, keeping the index finger as close as possible to the bunched nodular and diseased bronchi. If the surgeon keeps these two facts in mind, the basilar segments can be peeled away from the superior segment by blunt dissection with a minimum number of air leaks and very little bleeding.

After removal of the basilar segments the lingula is grasped, and by superior and anterior traction on the tip of the lingula the bronchus can be easily found. The lingular artery was divided when the pulmonary artery was first isolated. The inferior branches of the superior pulmonary vein supplying the lingula are then divided. The separation of the lingula is completed with the blunt dissection, as just described for the basilar segments.

There is one problem that may occur on the left side, even when the lingular segment is normal. When the basilar segments are removed the lingula drops inferiorly and is deflected posteriorly. In this position the bronchus is kinked, and bronchiectasis may develop. For this reason many have advised that the lingula always be removed when the basilar segments are excised. I believe that only the inferior lingula need be excised when the segment is normal. This can easily be done by identifying the inferior lingular bronchus by palpation and isolating it with a right-angle clamp. Then it can be easily removed by subsegmental resection. The vessels are divided as they are encountered.

Another problem somewhat like this needs to be watched for. Occasionally the anterior segment of the upper lobe may be involved in its most distal portion because of involvement by continuity with the diseased middle lobe or lingula. This area frequently appears poorly filled on the bronchogram. When the lobe drops inferiorly to fill some of the space occupied by the basilar segments, even a small area of bronchiectasis can become symptomatic. Occasionally a subsegment of this segment has to be removed.

The superior segment, after its isolation, is then sutured by a subpleural running stitch to the posterior segment of the upper lobe to prevent kinking of the bronchus. Chest tubes are carefully placed, one laterally going to the apex of the chest and another more posteriorly going directly into the space left by removal of the basilar segments. Active suction is applied to both tubes. Air leaks may be profuse for several days.

The operation on the right is not greatly different from that on the left. Six months should elapse before it is done. It is not practical to remove only part of the middle lobe, even if only the lateral segment alone is involved. Many times the middle and upper lobe are adherent. The middle lobe can be separated from the anterior segments of the upper lobe just as was done for basilar segmental resection.

Postoperatively the patient should be observed closely and airways should be kept open. The superior segment particularly should be kept free of secretions and aerated. This may require daily lateral roentgenograms. If the superior segment becomes atelectatic, bronchoscopic aspiration should be carried out. Antibiotics should be continued for 5 to 7 days.

The results of surgery in multisegmental disease can be excellent, the mortality low, and complications minimal. Recurrences usually mean that an overlooked diseased area becomes significant as a result of the area becoming dependent after operation. Fortunately, multisegmental bronchiectasis, as in most suppurative diseases of the respiratory tract, has nearly disappeared. When found, it can be successfully treated by operation, but requires that the surgeon be able to evaluate the bronchogram, conduct a meticulous operation, and then carefully supervise the postoperative care. The operation truly tries the mettle of the surgeon.

SUGGESTED READING

Bradham RR, Sealy WC, Young WG Jr. Chronic middle lobe infection and factors responsible for its localization. Ann Thorac Surg 1966; 2:612–616.

Churchill ED. Lobectomy and pneumonectomy for bronchiectasis and cystic disease. J Thorac Surg 1937; 6:286–311.

Lindskog GE, Hubbell DS. An analysis of 215 cases of bronchiectasis. Surg Gynecol Obstet 1955; 100:643–650.

Overholt RH, Langer LA. A new technique for pulmonary segmental resection, its application in the treatment of bronchiectasis. Surg Gynecol Obstet 1947; 84:257–268.

Sealy WC, Bradham RR, Young WG Jr. Surgical treatment of multisegmental and localized bronchiectasis. Surg Gynecol Obstet 1966; 123:80–90.

MASSIVE HEMOPTYSIS

SURGICAL AND TAMPONADE THERAPY

ANTONIO A. GARZON, M.D.

Hemoptysis is a common symptom of cardiopulmonary disease. In the majority of cases, hemoptysis is self-limited and does not threaten the life of the patient. However, in a few cases, the bleeding may be extensive enough to produce aspiration of blood and asphyxiation of the patient. Rarely, the amount of blood lost is such that life is threatened not only by the risk of aspiration but also by the risk of exsanguination.

A number of years ago we defined massive hemoptysis as the loss of 600 ml of blood in 24 hours and exsanguinating hemorrhage as the loss of 1,000 ml at a rate of 150 ml per hour. This figure has been accepted by a number of authors who have reported on this subject. Crocco and colleagues, by carefully measuring expectorated blood, were able to correlate the mortality rate of the hemoptysis patients with the amount of blood lost. Patients who bled 600 ml in a 16-hour period had a mortality of 75 percent when managed conservatively.

The incidence of massive hemoptysis is not known. We estimate on the basis of our early experience that less than 1 percent of patients with hemoptysis bleed massively; however, recently other authors have estimated a higher incidence. The most common cause of massive hemoptysis is tuberculosis, followed by neoplasm and bronchiectasis (Table 1).

TABLE 1 Etiology of Massive Hemoptysis in 74 Pulmonary Resections

Diagnosis		Total	Patients Exsanguinating	Massive
Tuberculosis		48	13	36
Bronchiectasis		8	4	4
Lung abscess		5	2	3
Neoplasm		9	4	4
Bronchogenic	7			
Metastatic	1			
Sarcoma	1			
Others		4	3	1
Actinomycosis	1			
Fibrosing mediastinitis	1			
Unknown	2			
		74	24	50

MANAGEMENT OF MASSIVE HEMOPTYSIS

Although massive hemoptysis is a frightening experience for the patient and the physician, it can be controlled if a logical plan of action is carried out. The first thing to do is localize the site of bleeding. This is necessary even before any other treatment can be started. At times bleeding from the nasopharynx and aspiration of blood into the trachea may recreate conditions that seem to be produced by hemoptysis, or expectorated blood may go into the nasopharynx and be interpreted as coming from the area. Blood may be swallowed and vomited, mimicking upper gastrointestinal bleeding. A few patients can tell the physician which lung is bleeding because they notice a gurgling sensation on the side of the chest the blood is coming from. A chest x-ray film may be helpful when the hemoptysis first appears, but later, with aspiration, it is difficult to determine which is the original lesion and which is the aspiration pneumonitis. For these reasons, it is absolutely necessary that all patients with massive hemoptysis undergo bronchoscopy.

The endoscopic procedure should be performed during the time of active bleeding. Bronchoscopy may increase the amount of bleeding, and the surgeon must be prepared to deal with this contingency. A few suggestions are helpful in controlling bronchial bleeding at the time of endoscopy. All bronchoscopies should be performed in the operating room, patients' blood should be typed and cross-matched, consent for possible pulmonary resection should be available, and endotracheal tubes of different sizes, venous Fogarty balloon catheters, and suction equipment should be ready and tested (two suctions are of great help in case one becomes occluded by blood clots).

We use a rigid ventilating bronchoscope and prefer general anesthesia. If a high-frequency jet ventilator is available, it is very useful because it keeps the end of the bronchoscope open all the time and allows the surgeon to perform the endoscopic examination without having to worry about the ventilation of the patient. Suction channels of fiberoptic scopes are too small to remove the blood quickly, and the lenses become coated with blood, making it difficult to see. Besides providing an airway, the rigid ventilating bronchoscope allows isolation of the site of the bleeding and performance of the necessary maneuvers to control it.

We have successfully used two methods to stop bleeding: either we tamponade the site of the bleeding bronchus with a large Fogarty venous balloon catheter (size 8 or 9), or we put an endotracheal tube in the nonbleeding lung and perform one-lung ventilation. The second maneuver does not control the blood loss but provides an adequate airway. The choice of one method over the other depends on the location of the bleeding. Tamponade with a balloon catheter can be used in bleeding coming from the left lung, the right lower lobe, and the middle lobe but not the right upper lobe, since the right main stem bronchus is too short, and the catheter tends to slip into the trachea. If possible, a smaller balloon catheter should be placed into the right upper lobe bronchus to stop the bleeding. Balloon catheters are useful because they allow direct vision of the area that has to be blocked.

One of the problems in the use of the Fogarty catheter is that the hub at its end is too large to pass through the lumen of the bronchoscope. This can be solved by placing the catheter into the trachea outside the bronchoscope and then manipulating it into the proper place under direct vision. If the balloon catheter is introduced through the lumen of the scope, we have detached the hub and connected the rest of the catheter to a 50-cm piece of rubber tubing (tourniquet tubing). With this arrangement, the balloon can be inflated under direct vision and the scope removed without deflating the balloon. A regular endobronchial tube should be carefully positioned in the trachea 2 or 3 cm above the carina and the balloon inflated. This will help to stabilize the Fogarty catheter against the tracheal wall and prevent dislodgement. We strongly recommend that a small amount of contrast material be placed in the balloon and a chest x-ray taken to check its position. The alternative solution is to intubate the left main bronchus and perform a thoracotomy with one-lung ventilation. If it is difficult to position the endotracheal tube, it can be guided with a fiberoptic bronchoscope. The proper location of the tube in the left main stem bronchus should be checked with a chest x-ray film after the patient has been put in the lateral position for thoracotomy. A common pitfall is to introduce the tube too deeply into the left main stem bronchus and occlude the left upper lobe.

In a number of patients who have been bleeding actively, we have done the pulmonary resection without blockage or single-lung ventilation. The secret to this successful procedure is to have an experienced anesthesiologist who can keep the endotracheal tube and the trachea free of blood and ventilate the patient at the same time. Under these circumstances, it is mandatory that the bleeding bronchus is clamped as soon as possible. Early in our experience, we used double-lumen tubes. We were disappointed with these tubes because they were difficult to place under bleeding conditions and easily become clogged with blood.

RESULTS OF SURGICAL THERAPY IN PATIENTS WITH MASSIVE HEMOPTYSIS

When the site of massive hemoptysis has been identified and temporarily controlled, a decision about operability must be made. Our criteria of inoperability include patients with unresectable bronchogenic carcinoma, patients with metatastic carcinoma who are in terminal stages of the disease, and those with impairments of pulmonary function to such a degree that the vital capacity is less than 40 percent of the predicted value, or a force expiratory volume of less than 40 percent in the first second. Using these criteria, we rejected fewer than 10 percent of our patients. If the patient is considered to be operable, surgery should proceed without delay because the incidence of a second bleeding episode is high (80 percent). As soon as the chest is opened, the bronchus should be dissected and temporarily occluded with a vascular clamp. The pulmonary resection should then proceed without haste. Lobectomy is preferred to pneumonectomy, unless the lung is completely destroyed.

The results of our experience in pulmonary resection for massive bleeding are shown in Table 2. The main factors in the occurrence of mortality were the presence of active bleeding at the time of the resection and the rate of bleeding before the operation. Our total 30-day mortality was 13.5 percent (10 patients out of 74). Twenty-four patients had exsanguinating hemoptysis. They bled an average of 1,250 ml of blood before the operation, at a rate of 500 ml per hour. In this group, six patients died (25 percent), two of them on the operating table from exsanguination and asphyxiation and the other four during the postoperative period. Only four patients of the 50 with massive hemoptysis died.

In our experience, pulmonary resection is the treatment of choice for massive hemoptysis because of the high rate of recurrence of bleeding (80 percent). For those patients who are not candidates for pulmonary resection, tamponade of the bleeding bronchus can be used. Our personal experience with this method is rather limited; however, others have indicated satisfactory results with at least temporary control of the bleeding. The use of irrigation of cold saline through the bronchoscope to stop the bleeding has been reported, and we do have a limited positive experience. In our cases it was effective in controlling the bleeding from massive hemoptysis, at least temporarily. Embolization of the bronchial and intercostal arteries has been reported, but because of the risk of neurologic complications, this method has not achieved great popularity. It should be reserved for those individuals who are not candidates for pulmonary resection.

TABLE 2 Surgical Mortality in Massive Hemoptysis

			Mortality	
Procedure	*Number*	*Diagnosis*	*Operative*	*Post Op*
Pneumonectomy	10	Tuberculosis	2	1
	3	Other	1	1
Lobectomy	33	Tuberculosis	0	2
	24	Other	1	1
Cavernostomy	3	Tuberculosis	0	1
	74 (24)*		10 (6)*	

*Patients with exsanguinating hemoptysis

SUGGESTED READING

Conlan AA, Hurwitz SS. Management of massive hemoptysis with rigid bronchoscopy and cold saline lavage. Thorax 1980; 35:901–904.
Crocco JA, Rooney JJ, Fankuahen DS, et al. Massive hemoptysis. Arch Intern Med 1968; 121:495–498.
Garzon AA, Gourin A. Surgical management of massive hemoptysis. A ten year experience. Ann Surg 1978; 187:267–271.
Gourin A, Garzon AA. Control of hemorrhage in emergency pulmonary resection for massive hemoptysis. Chest 1975; 68:120–121.
Saw EC, Gottlieb LS, Yokoyama T, Lee BC. Flexible fiberoptic bronchoscopy and endobronchial tamponade in the management of massive hemoptysis. Chest 1976; 70:581–589.

MASSIVE HEMOPTYSIS: CONTROL WITH TRANSCATHETER VESSEL EMBOLIZATION

JANETTE S. DENHAM, M.D.
CHRISTOS A. ATHANASOULIS, M.D.

Life-threatening hemoptysis has a bronchial artery source in 95 percent of cases. Surgical resection is the primary mode of therapy. In those patients who are poor surgical candidates, bronchial artery embolization (BAE) may be used preoperatively for stabilization or as an alternative to surgery for definitive therapy.

INDICATIONS

BAE has been used to treat both acute massive and chronic intermittent hemoptysis. Common etiologies for pulmonary hemorrhage include cystic fibrosis, bronchiectasis, pneumoconiosis, abscess, neoplasm, and tuberculosis. BAE is indicated in patients with conditions that increase the morbidity of surgical therapy, such as (1) diffuse bilateral pulmonary disease, (2) a vital capacity less than 40 percent of that predicted, (3) recurrent bleeding following surgery, (4) nonresectable bronchogenic carcinoma, and (5) an occult bleeding site.

PREPROCEDURE EVALUATION

Prolonged delay prior to therapy cannot be tolerated by these seriously compromised patients. Initial attention is directed toward cardiovascular and ventilatory stabilization, with administration of the necessary fluids, blood products, and oxygen. Continuous blood pressure readings and cardiac monitoring are initiated. Because asphyxiation is the leading cause of death, it is crucial to establish a secure airway, usually under the supervision of an anesthesiologist. Temporary occlusion of the involved bronchus with a balloon catheter may be required. A peripheral pulse examination and a baseline neurologic assessment are also performed.

Preprocedure localization of the involved bronchial segment is attempted in order to expedite the embolization procedure. Chest radiography may reveal a likely lesion, but it is often misleading because of aspiration of blood into adjacent lung segments and the contralateral lung. The principal means of localization is bronchoscopy. Unless the patient has diffuse pulmonary disease and bilateral embolization is anticipated, a bronchoscopic examination is performed prior to transfer to the angiographic suite.

BRONCHIAL ARTERY ANATOMY

A clear understanding of the visceral and parietal branches of the descending thoracic aorta is necessary prior to performing embolization. Parietal branches include intercostal, subcostal, and superior phrenic arteries. Visceral branches include pericardial, esophageal, mediastinal, and bronchial arteries.

The distribution of the bronchial arteries is variable. Generally there are two or three bronchial arteries that arise at the fifth or sixth thoracic vertebral level cephalad to the left main stem bronchus. The superior right bronchial artery most commonly arises as a common trunk with an intercostal artery. Left bronchial arteries may arise directly from the aorta or from a common right-left bronchial trunk. Aberrant bronchial arteries can arise from the subclavian, innominate, thyrocervical, internal mammary, and inferior phrenic arteries. In patients who continue to bleed following BAE, an aberrant bronchial or pulmonary artery source must be considered.

The anterior and posterior spinal arteries receive contributions from the thoracic aorta. The posterior spinal artery receives segmental contributions from the dorsal rami of the intercostal arteries. The anterior spinal artery most commonly anastomoses with a thoracic aortic branch arising between the third to seventh thoracic level on the right and a large thoracolumbar branch arising between the ninth thoracic to the second lumbar level on the left. In addition, spinal branches may arise from the bronchial arteries. Uflacker found spinal arterial supply originating from a right common intercostal bronchial trunk in 42 of 72 patients. These branches are small and must be diligently sought prior to occlusion of any thoracic aortic branch.

METHOD

A transfemoral approach is preferred for the selective catheterization of bronchial arteries. A variety of 5 to 7 French tapered catheters may be required, depending on the configuration of the vessel being studied. A femoral introducer sheath is used to facilitate exchange.

In the past, 60 percent meglumine iothalamate was considered to be the least neurotoxic of the available ionic intravascular contrast agents. The newer nonionic media, iohexol and iopamidol, have even less neurotoxicity and have become the preferred contrast media for bronchial arteriography. Concentrations of iodine of 300 mg per milliliter are adequate. Injection and filming rate depend on the flow characteristics of the selected vessel. Generally, hand injections of 1 to 2 ml per second for a total of 10 ml, with filming at two frames per second, are performed. Magnification and subtraction images enhance visualization. Digital subtraction capability is useful because of the multiplicity of injections required. In addition, the improved contrast resolution of digital filming aids in identifying small spinal artery contributions.

The angiographer is directed to the bleeding lung segment by the results of the bronchoscopic examination. Contrast extravasation is rarely identified during bronchial arteriography. Bronchial artery hypertrophy, hypervascularity, bronchial artery to pulmonary artery shunting, and aneurysm formation are secondary angiographic signs of bleeding. Generally bronchial arteries are embolized regardless of angiographic confirmation of bleeding.

A variety of particulate embolic agents have been successfully used for BAE; however, surgical gelatin pledgets and polyvinyl alcohol are the most common. Whatever the agent, several general principles are followed. The catheter must be securely seated in the bronchial artery so that delivery of the embolic material does not result in catheter dislodgement and inadvertent embolization. Throughout the procedure, attention should be directed toward warning signs of inadvertent embolization such as the development of abdominal tenderness or acute changes in peripheral pulses or neurologic status. Small particles approximately 250 microns in size are initially injected to embolize distal branch arteries, followed by larger particles to occlude the artery proximally. Only small aliquots of embolic material are injected, followed by frequent contrast injection to assess progress. Spinal contributions not visualized prior to embolization of the distal bronchial artery may become apparent on repeat injection as the peripheral vascular resistance increases. Embolization is stopped before complete occlusion of the vessel to avoid reflux of embolic particles into the aorta. The use of a balloon occlusion catheter at the vessel origin provides an additional safety factor.

CONTRAINDICATIONS

In the past, the demonstration of a spinal branch arising from the bronchial trunk was considered a contraindication to embolization. Uflacker, however, reported no complications following proximal embolization of 42 common intercostal-bronchial arteries with spinal branches. The alternative to proximal embolization is superselective catheter placement past the spinal artery branch. With the aid of somatosensory evoked potential monitoring, selection and embolization can be performed safely. Failure to obtain secure catheter positioning remains the only absolute contraindication to BAE.

POSTPROCEDURE CARE

Following the procedure, patient care includes vital sign monitoring, ensuring hemostasis at the puncture site, frequent evaluation of extremity pulses, and vigorous hydration. Analgesics may be required to relieve postembolization pain. If pulmonary hemorrhage recurs, embolization may be repeated.

RESULTS AND COMPLICATIONS

Three large patient series have been published. The results of these studies are listed in Table 1. Overall initial success is in the 85 percent range, with recurrent late bleeding occurring in 25 percent.

Frequent minor complications of BAE include temporary postprocedural retrosternal or intercostal pain, dysphagia, and fever. These symptoms usually resolve within 72 hours following embolization. Serious complications are infrequent. Inadvertent embolization to the gastrointestinal tract and extremities has been described. There is one reported case of spinal cord infarction following intercostal artery embolization. Bronchial infarction and bronchopleural fistula formation uncommonly result from BAE.

These results suggest that bronchial artery embolization is both a safe and effective therapy for life-threatening hemoptysis. In addition to its use as a definitive therapy in patients who are poor surgical candidates, it may be

TABLE 1 Results of Bronchial Artery Embolization

Author	*Patients Embolized*	*Initial Success*	*Follow-up Time*	*Bleeding Recurrence*
Remy	49	41/49 (83.7%)	2–30 months	6/41 (14.6%)
Uflacker	64	49/64 (76.6%)	1–47 months	10/33 (30.3%)
Rabkin	306	278/30 (90.8%)	24–96 hours	39/278 (14.0%)
			36–60 months	36/158 (22.8%)

employed prior to surgery in an attempt to stabilize a compromised patient and improve the surgical outcome.

SUGGESTED READING

Olson R, Athanasoulis C. Hemoptysis: treatment with transcatheter embolization of the bronchial arteries. In: Athanasoulis C, Pfister R, Greene R, Roberson G, eds. Interventional radiology. Philadelphia: WB Saunders, 1982:196.

Rabkin J, Astafjev V, Gothman L, Grigorjev Y. Transcatheter embolization in the management of pulmonary hemorrhage. Radiology 1987; 163:361–365.

Remy J, Arnaud A, Fardou H, Giraud R, Voisin C. Treatment of hemoptysis by embolization of bronchial arteries. Radiology 1977; 122:33–37.

Schrodt J, Becker G, Scott J, Warren C, Benenati S. Bronchial artery embolization: monitoring with somatosensory evoked potentials. Work in progress. Radiology 1987; 164:135–139.

Uflacker R, Kaemmerer A, Picon P, et al. Bronchial artery embolization in the management of hemoptysis: technical aspects and long-term results. Radiology 1985; 157:637-644.

EMPHYSEMA

THE SURGICAL MANAGEMENT OF GIANT BULLAE

HUGOE R. MATTHEWS, F.R.C.S.

Definitions

When alveolar walls are destroyed or disrupted by degenerative lung disease (usually emphysema), an increasingly large air space is formed within the confines of the lung substance and the visceral pleura. Such spaces are called bullae, and they are therefore by definition distinct from air cysts of congenital or other origin. The nonspecific term bleb is used loosely to describe bullae that are visible but very small (less than 1 to 2 cm in diameter) and has little if any value.

Bullae should be classified by their number, size, and location and whether they are associated with local or generalized lung disease. In the lower range, bullae should be described by their actual size (e.g., 5 cm), but with larger bullae it is more practical to relate them to the size of the lung fields on the chest film. They are then described as occupying less than half of one hemithorax, more than half of one hemithorax, or more than one hemithorax (which necessarily implies mediastinal shift or herniation of the bulla to the contralateral side). The term "giant" bulla has no generally agreed upon definition.

Pathophysiology

When a bulla is opened it is seen to contain trabeculae of attenuated lung tissue and one or more fistulous communications with the tracheobronchial tree. Air can therefore pass into or out of the bulla, but it does so only slowly, and bullae rarely ventilate with each breath. To demonstrate this by ventilation scanning requires the use of an inhaled radioisotope with a relatively long half-life (e.g., xenon-133); activity is seen to appear later and persist longer in the area of the bulla than elsewhere in the lung fields.

It is commonly believed that large bullae compress the surrounding lung, but this is almost certainly not the case. It is more probable that their size and poor elasticity prevent the inspiratory expansion of the chest wall from being transmitted to the rest of the lung, with resulting passive atelectasis. Enlargement occurs partly through a tearing of the lung parenchyma. Radiologically the lung appears to vanish, but only a small proportion is actually destroyed; most of it is merely collapsed and can be relied upon to expand and provide useful gas exchange if the bulla is removed or obliterated. To the surgeon, bullae are important as a cause of spontaneous pneumothorax, as a remediable cause of dyspnea, and as an associated disease or incidental finding at thoracotomy for other conditions.

SYMPTOMATIC BULLAE

Indications

The removal or obliteration of large bullae (i.e., occupying one half of one hemithorax or more) allows room for the remaining lung to expand and results in an improvement of dyspnea that is roughly proportional to the size of the bulla. In other words, the larger the bulla, the better the result. Selection of the patient for surgery is therefore based on the severity of symptoms, with reference to the patient's personal exercise requirements, and the size of the bulla. Patients with smaller bullae and mild symptoms are treated medically (e.g., with bronchodilators, cessation of smoking), but large bullae causing moderate or severe disability require surgery. Pulmonary function studies serve to document the respiratory state before and after treatment, but the absolute values do not help in selection for surgery. The postoperative improvement that occurs does, however, affect selection, since it means that high-risk patients (even those with preoperative carbon dioxide retention) can undergo surgery for bullous disease even though they would be quite unsuitable for most other forms of pulmonary surgery. Investigations designed to identify compression of the remaining lung (e.g., bronchography or angiography) are unnecessary, as results are always positive if the bulla is large enough.

If a large bulla is mistaken for a pneumothorax and intubated an iatrogenic bronchopleural fistula is produced, with an air leak that may be of considerable magnitude. Conservative treatment is unlikely to be successful, and early operation is required to close the leak and eradicate the bulla.

Operative Treatment

Intracavity Drainage. This technique aims to obliterate the bulla by a combination of sclerosis of the associated fistulas and suction collapse of the bullous cavity. Surgery is performed through a small intercostal incision over the site of the bulla. A nonabsorbable pursestring suture is placed in the wall of the bulla, which is then opened so that iodized talc can be insufflated around the internal fistulas under direct vision. A large Foley catheter is inserted into the bulla and the pursestring tied. Additional talc is insufflated into the pleural space to promote pleurodesis, an intercostal drain is inserted, and the chest is closed. Both tubes are then placed on suction. This method is simple and relatively noninvasive, but it is not always successful, particularly with multilocular bullae, as the fistulas may not close or the lung may fail to expand. It is reasonable, therefore, to use this as the first line of treatment in suitable cases, but if prolonged drainage is required, it is better to proceed to bullectomy, which if properly performed will offer the patient a speedier discharge from the hospital and a more complete result.

Bullectomy. Unlike the previous method, complete excision of the bullous area ensures immediate and optimal expansion of the affected lung, provided that postoperative air leaks are avoided by a reinforced suture technique of the type described below. Functional lung is not removed, and the procedure is suitable for all bullae, whether single or multiple, small or large. In patients with bilateral large bullae, a unilateral staged approach is preferred to median sternotomy, since bilateral air leaks, if they were to occur, might be fatal. An additional reason is that if the worst side is done first, the improvement may be so dramatic that a contralateral operation is not required.

The operation is performed through a routine thoracotomy incision in the fifth intercostal space. When the chest is opened the lung is deflated, using a double-lumen endotracheal tube, and the bulla is opened in order to identify the boundary between the bulla and the remaining lung tissue, which forms the desired line of resection. Two strips of Teflon felt approximately 1 cm wide are applied on either side of the line of resection, and a series of interrupted horizontal mattress sutures of 2–0 silk is inserted through all four layers (i.e., both layers of felt and both walls of the bulla). These sutures are then tied and the bulla is excised, the cut surface of the lung being further oversewn with a continuous over-and-over 2–0 silk suture, again incorporating all four layers. This technique plugs the suture holes and also prevents the sutures from tearing out, so that only a short period of postoperative drainage is required. If additional bullae are present, they are resected or ligated as appropriate. Pleurectomy is not performed. When pneumostasis is secured, the chest is closed with a No. 32 Argyle drain, without suction. In some cases lobectomy may appear to be an attractive option, but it should be positively avoided because it inevitably removes some functional lung tissue and is likely to cause prolonged air leaks from even small communications with the adjoining lobes.

Results. With correct selection, the symptomatic results of surgery are very gratifying, and even high-risk patients can be expected to recover promptly without the need for respiratory support. In the long term the underlying degenerative lung disease tends to get worse, but recurrent bulla formation is very rare.

INCIDENTAL BULLAE

In some patients who require thoracotomy for another condition, bullae may be known to exist prior to operation, usually as seen on a chest film, or they may be discovered during the course of the procedure. A decision then has to be made as to whether anything should be done about them at the time of operation, either to treat them or to prevent a spontaneous pneumothorax during anesthesia or the recovery phase. In general, ipsilateral large bullae should be resected as already described in order to improve lung function, whereas ipsilateral small bullae may be ligated but should not be sutured. Contralateral bullae are left undisturbed, but a second chest drain may be inserted across the mediastinum into the opposite side of the chest to protect against a possible postoperative pneumothorax.

SUGGESTED READING

MacArthur AM, Fountain SW. Intracavitary suction and drainage in the treatment of emphysematous bullae. Thorax 1977; 32:668–672.

Parmar JM, Hubbard WG, Matthews HR. Teflon strip pneumostasis for excision of giant emphysematous bullae. Thorax 1987; 42:144–148.

Pearson MG, Ogilvie C. Surgical treatment of emphysematous bullae: late outcome. Thorax 1983; 38:134–137.

Potgieter PD, Benator SR, Hewitson RP, Ferguson AD. Surgical treatment of bullous lung disease. Thorax 1981; 36:885–890.

FISTULA

BRONCHOBILIARY FISTULA

DAVID P. BOYD, M.D., F.R.C.S.(C)

Fistulas between the bronchial tree and the biliary system result from trauma to the extrahepatic bile ducts during cholecystectomy. Fortunately, their occurrence is rare. In our total experience with more than 2,500 operations for repair of postoperative strictures of the bile ducts, only 50 fistulas involving the bile duct were seen. As in all cases of true subphrenic infection, both the surgical treatment and the pathogenesis of bronchobiliary fistula can be understood completely only after a careful look at the normal anatomy.

In contrast to traditional teaching from the time of Barnard, experience has taught that two spaces are present above the liver. Separated by the falciform ligament, these spaces are extremely large. Anterior and posterior subphrenic spaces on both sides, separated by the coronary ligament referred to so frequently in the literature, simply do not exist. They are anatomic myths unless artificially created by pyogenic membranes.

The crux of the confusion lies in the position of the coronary ligament. The mistake is that the ligament is not superior but posterior in common with other ligaments and mesenteries of the viscera. When the position of the ligament is drawn correctly, it becomes apparent that a true subphrenic collection can be drained only by a transpleural approach. Bile under pressure, like exudate, seeks to escape. The soft diaphragm and lung may yield before the more rigid liver.

If the pleura is free, a massive bile empyema occurs. The change in the patient's condition is apparent, and urgent correction of the intrathoracic dynamic findings is required. Water seal drainage is temporarily sufficient, but the patient will not get well until the subphrenic space is thoroughly drained and the lesion in the biliary tract is repaired. In the presence of pleural symphysis, a true bronchobiliary fistula occurs, with copious expectoration of bile. Cure has uniformly been achieved by the steps outlined here. It has never been necessary to resect a pulmonary lobe or segment.

As indicated, these two events, massive bile empyema or profuse coughing of bile, are sudden and dramatic and thus make diagnosis obvious. One prodromal sign of an impending problem may be pleural effusion. If this occurs after an upper abdominal operation in the absence of heart failure, subphrenic infection is strongly indicated. This finding was present in 35 percent of our patients and was always ipsilateral and unilateral.

New nuclear radiologic procedures have rendered identification and localization of collections in body cavities more precise. While percutaneous therapeutic

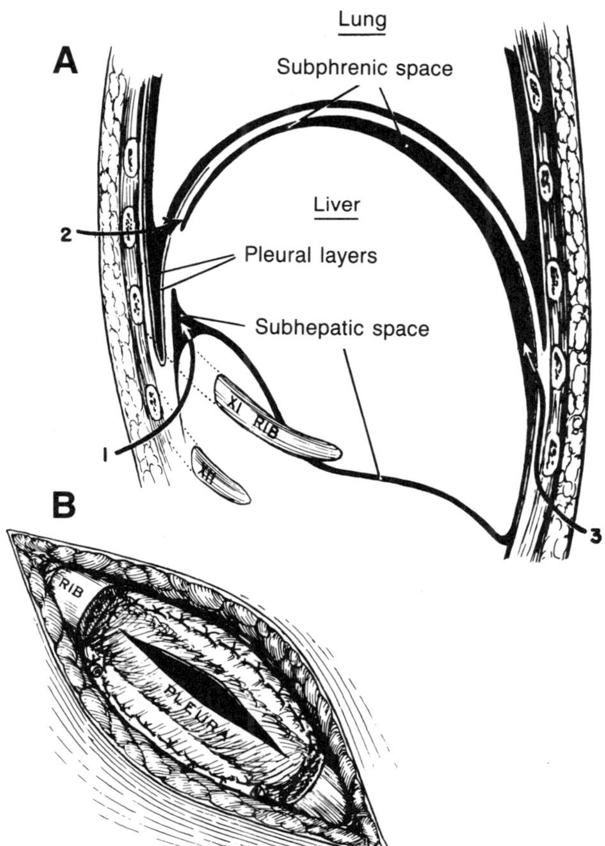

Figure 1 *A*, Position of the ligament is correctly drawn. As noted, a truly subphrenic collection can be drained only by a transpleural approach. (1) Approaches to the subhepatic and subphrenic spaces are indicated: one-twelfth rib extraserous route (Ochsner); (2) Trendelenburg transpleural route. *B*, After appropriate rib resection, the pleura is sutured to the diaphragm. This provides adequate, safe, direct and dependent access to the subphrenic space. (From Boyd DP. The anatomy and pathology of the subphrenic spaces. Surg Clin North Am 1958; 38:621, with permission.)

drainage techniques have met with some success, we do not believe they have a place in the management of bronchobiliary fistula. The surgical treatment is detailed in Figure 1. Proper drainage and correction of the biliary pathology will result in resolution of bronchobiliary fistulas without need for pulmonary resection.

SUGGESTED READING

Barnard HL. Surgical aspects of subphrenic abscess. An address delivered before the surgical section of the Royal Society of Medicine, January 14, 1907. Br Med J 1908; 1:371–377 and 429–436.

Boyd DP. Annual oration, Massachusetts Medical Society 1966. The subphrenic spaces and the emperor's new robes. N Engl J Med 1966; 275:911–917.

Boyd DP. Bronchobiliary and pleurobiliary fistulas. Ann Thorac Surg 1977; 24:481–487.

Boyd DP. Intrathoracic complications of subphrenic abscess. J Thorac Cardiovasc Surg 1959; 38:771–777.

Harley HRS. Hunterian lecture: Royal College of Surgeons of England. Subphrenic abscess, with particular reference to spread of infection. Ann R Coll Surg Engl 1955; 17:201–224.

LUNG TRANSPLANTATION

JOEL D. COOPER, M.D., F.R.C.S., F.A.C.S.(C)

Organ transplantation is recognized as appropriate therapy for patients with end-stage renal, cardiac, or hepatic failure. Progress in transplantation for end-stage lung disease has lagged behind. The first unilateral human lung transplant was performed in 1963, and in the ensuing 20 years, more than 40 transplants were attempted without long-term clinical success. Most recipients died within days or weeks from respiratory failure, lung infection, rejection, or failure to heal the bronchial anastomosis. Our initial attempt at human lung transplant in 1978 ended in failure as a result of bronchial dehiscence in the third week. We subsequently began a series of laboratory investigations in animals, designed to study factors affecting bronchial healing following transplantation. From these experiments we concluded that the routine use of prednisone for immunosuppression in the early postoperative period adversely affected bronchial healing and contributed to bronchial complications. Cyclosporine, on the other hand, caused no adverse effects on bronchial healing. It was also demonstrated that wrapping the bronchial anastomosis with a pedicle of omentum provided prompt reestablishment of blood flow to the bronchial arteries by means of collateral circulation from the omentum, which developed within days.

On the basis of these laboratory developments, we decided to resume clinical lung transplantation. In November of 1983, a 58-year-old man with end-stage pulmonary fibrosis underwent single lung transplantation at the Toronto General Hospital. The transplant proved successful; the patient was able to resume a normal lifestyle and continues to do well 3 years later.

We now have performed a total of seven lung transplants for patients with end-stage pulmonary fibrosis. Five of these transplants have been successful, and all five recipients have returned to a normal life and regular employment. The mean survival time is now 16 months, and there have been no late complications or deterioration of lung function.

We have utilized only donors with a normal-appearing chest roentgenogram, no purulent secretions on bronchoscopy, and a PaO_2 greater than 300 mm Hg when measured on 100 percent oxygen.

For the initial five transplants, the donors were brought to our hospital so that the organ removal procedure and the transplant operation could be done in adjacent operating rooms. For the last two lung transplants, we obtained the lungs from distant centers.

The procedure is done with cardiopulmonary bypass available. However, bypass has been required for only one of the seven transplants. The omentum has been utilized in all cases. Following induction of anesthesia, with the patient in the supine position, a small upper midline abdominal incision is performed. Through this the omentum is mobilized and its tip is placed in the retrosternal position, following which the abdominal incision is closed. The patient is then turned to the lateral thoracotomy position. The nondependent groin is prepped and draped in case partial venoarterial bypass is required. The pulmonary artery is encircled as proximally as possible and temporarily occluded with a tourniquet. If the patient tolerates this satisfactorily, the lung is removed. If not, then the tourniquet is released and partial venoarterial bypass instituted by the groin vessels, after which the extraction of the lung proceeds. The superior and inferior pulmonary veins are ligated and divided extrapericardially. The pulmonary artery is clamped as centrally as possible. The recipient bronchus is divided a few rings above the upper lobe take-off. Following removal of the lung, the pericardium is opened around the stumps of the pulmonary veins. A clamp is placed on the left atrium proximal to the veins. The ties then are removed from the veins, and the veins are joined with an incision, creating a generous atrial cuff. The donor lung, which is deflated and cooled by immersion, then is placed in the chest, and the atrial anastomosis is performed with running polyethylene suture. The pulmonary artery is anastomosed similarly. Prior to completion of the pulmonary artery anastomosis, the atrial clamp is removed, allowing back bleeding through the lungs and out the pulmonary artery anastomosis. The anastomosis then is completed and the pulmonary artery clamp is removed, restoring flow to the deflated lung. If the shunt produced by this maneuver causes a fall in the oxygen saturation, intermittent ventilation of the transplant lung is instituted until the bronchial anastomosis has been performed. Such ventilation can be carried out using a jet ventilator with a catheter placed across the field, or with a sterile endotracheal tube inserted intermittently into the transplant bronchus. The donor bronchus has been divided into two rings above the upper lobe take-off. It is anastomosed in end-to-end fashion with the recipient bronchus, using either interrupted sutures or a running suture to the cartilaginous portion and interrupted sutures to the membranous portion. The omentum then is drawn up through the retrosternal tunnel and wrapped completely around the bronchial anastomosis. We also leave a generous apron of pericardium attached to the hilus of the donor lung. Part of this pericardium can be used to wrap the pulmonary artery anastomosis if desired. The free edge of the pericardium also is tacked to the omentum, since this may aid in the development of collateral circulation through the hilus of the lung to the bronchial circulation.

Patients with pulmonary fibrosis are ideally suited for lung transplantation. In general, there is no chronic infection in the lungs, and cardiac function usually is well maintained. The poor compliance and the increased pulmonary vascular resistance in the remaining native lung ensure that following transplant, ventilation and perfusion will be directed preferentially toward the transplant lung. We have published our experience with the intitial two successful lung transplant recipients.

Unfortunately, a large number of patients with end-stage lung disease are not ideal candidates for single lung transplantation. These include patients with emphysema, chronic pulmonary infection, or end-stage lung disease associated with severe right-sided heart failure.

Unilateral lung transplantation for emphysema has been attempted in the past with poor results. The native lung becomes hyperinflated, progressively pushing the mediastinum toward the transplant side with progressive crowding of the transplanted lung. Ventilation preferentially goes to the hyperinflated emphysematous lung while perfusion is directed to the transplant lung, which has a lower vascular resistance than the diseased native lung. This is clearly an unsatisfactory situation.

For patients with chronic sepsis, such as those with cystic fibrosis or advanced bronchiectasis, single lung transplant is similarly inappropriate. The chronic residual infection in the contralateral, native lung would be a serious liability, particularly in the face of postoperative immunosuppression.

For patients with combined end-stage lung disease and right-sided heart failure, both the heart and lungs require replacement. This includes patients with primary pulmonary hypertension and patients with Eisenmenger's syndrome. In 1981, the Stanford group demonstrated long-term clinical success with combined cardiopulmonary transplantation for such patients. Since that time, more than 100 heart and lung transplants have been performed, with a one-year survival rate of 54 percent. The majority of these transplants have been performed for pulmonary vascular disease in association with right-sided heart failure. Because of our interest in transplantation for end-stage interstitial lung disease, we have developed a heart-lung transplant program to complement the single lung transplant program. We, and several other centers, have achieved success in applying this operation to patients with end-stage lung disease secondary to emphysema or chronic infection. We like to refer to such operations as "lung-heart" transplantations, to emphasize their use for respiratory failure rather than for the cardiac failure that requires their use in patients with pulmonary hypertension and Eisenmenger's syndrome.

Candidates for lung-heart transplantation generally are oxygen-dependent, chronically ill, and have abnormal chest wall mechanics, including increased chest diameter and flattened diaphragms. In this type of patient, lung-heart transplantation has been less successful than has combined heart-lung transplantation for individuals with right-sided failure secondary to pulmonary vascular disease. Nonetheless, we feel that increasingly the combined operation will be successful in selected individuals with end-stage lung disease.

Many individuals with end-stage emphysema, cystic fibrosis, and certain other conditions still may have a normal functioning heart. Though as noted, single lung transplantation is not appropriate for such individuals, it seems unnecessary to discard their hearts in order to perform a combined lung-heart transplant. In this situation the heart transplant is included strictly for technical considerations and subjects the recipient to all the risks and complications associated with cardiac transplantation, in addition to the problems associated with the lung portion of the lung transplantation. We have developed, in the laboratory, a procedure for simultaneous bilateral lung transplantation, without including the heart, for such individuals. With this procedure, the two lungs are left attached to each other by the trachea, the common pulmonary artery, and the left atrium. We have achieved preliminary success with this operation in animals and anticipate its use in patients in the near future.

If this procedure proves satisfactory, we anticipate utilizing single lung transplantation for patients with end-stage pulmonary fibrosis, double lung transplantation for patients with emphysema or chronic pulmonary infection in the presence of normal cardiac function, and combined lung-heart transplantation for patients with end-stage lung disease in association with poor right ventricular function.

Many problems remain to be solved. Chief among them is the ability to obtain a greater number of satisfactory donors. At the present time, very few donors have suitable lungs for transplantation. Pulmonary injury, infection, and edema commonly occur in brain-dead patients; therefore, not one organ in ten available donors is suitable for use in lung or lung-heart transplantation. Furthermore, size matching is more important for lung and lung-heart transplantation than for other organs, because problems arise when donor lungs are either too small or too large for the recipient's chest. This further restricts the pool of donors available for any particular recipient. Finally, reliable methods for lung preservation have not been developed, as they have been for kidney, heart, and liver preservation. Thus in most instances, permission must be obtained from the donor's family to bring the donor to the transplant center, further restricting the number of available donors. There has been some recent progress with lung preservation using both topical cooling, and flushing of the lungs with various cold solutions. Using topical cooling, we have successfully procured and transplanted a lung obtained from another city, with a total ischemic time of 4 hours. By flushing the pulmonary circulation with cold electrolyte solution, other centers have successfully performed distant procurement of lungs with ischemic times up to several hours. If techniques can be developed to provide for safe ischemic periods of 6 to 10 hours, this would be an important advance.

SUGGESTED READING

Solis E, Kaye MP. The Registry of the International Society for Heart Transplantation: Third Official Report—June 1986. J Heart Transplant 1986; 5.

Toronto Lung Transplant Group. Unilateral lung transplantation for pulmonary fibrosis. N Engl J Med 1986; 314:1140–1145.

ESOPHAGEAL NEOPLASIA

BENIGN TUMOR

ROBERT A. GUSTAFSON, M.D.
GORDON F. MURRAY, M.D.

Benign neoplasms of the esophagus, while rare, are of concern because most tumors continue to grow slowly, eventually producing symptoms. Elective removal prior to the onset of disabling pulmonary or swallowing problems is indicated with the vast majority of benign esophageal tumors. The need for adequate treatment planning is emphasized by the fact that obstruction and pulmonary complications may lead to the death of the patient, and early recognition with surgical removal is nearly always curative.

Benign tumors of the esophagus are far less common than their malignant counter parts. Overall the lesion appears to be about 1/50th as frequent as esophageal carcinoma. Leiomyoma, an *intramural* muscular tissue tumor, is the most frequently encountered benign neoplasm. Although esophageal leiomyomas represent only about 0.5 percent of all benign smooth muscle tumors of the alimentary tract, they account for 75 percent of all benign esophageal neoplasms. *Intraluminal* tumors are very rare. The majority of these lesions originated in the upper third of the esophagus; they are benign polypoid tumors composed of vascular fibrous tissue, adipose tissue, and myxomatous material. They are best described as fibrolipomas.

INTRAMURAL TUMOR

Although confusion with a malignant tumor, achalasia, or stricture may exist, classic radiologic and endoscopic findings usually provide an accurate diagnosis of the intramural leiomyoma. Appropriate surgical therapy should then result in minimal morbidity and rare mortality. The majority of leiomyomas occur in the lower two-thirds of the esophagus, where the smooth muscle predominates. Various extensions of growth are noted, the most common being a horseshoe configuration. Multiple tumors have been reported, and they may become very large. In addition, calcification, cystic change, mucosal ulceration and malignant degeneration may occur. Rarely an epidermoid carcinoma is seen in association with a leiomyoma.

Preoperative Investigation

Study after a barium swallow is the primary diagnostic tool in the identification of a leiomyoma. A smooth, crescent-shaped tumor that produces significant compromise of the esophageal lumen without delaying passage of the barium column is classically seen. The mass obliterates the mucosal folds overlying it and meets the normal esophageal wall at an abrupt angle proximally and distally. A forked-stream appearance is created by the passage of barium to either side of the lesion. Computed tomography may aid further in establishing the extent of the lesion. The possibility of multiple leiomyomas should be considered, both on examining the contrast study and at the time of surgical exploration.

Esophagoscopy should be performed in all cases to examine the status of the overlying mucosa. A mobile mass with normal overlying mucosa and a variable amount of luminal narrowing will be demonstrated. With the exception of the annular lesion, there is little resistance to the passage of the esophagoscope. Ulceration of the mucosa is an unusual finding and suggests sarcomatous degeneration of the neoplasm. Histologic confirmation of the diagnosis by biopsy through the intact mucosa is unnecessary and undesirable, since the effort will violate the operative site and complicate later enucleation of the mass. Endoscopic removal of the rare pedunculated leiomyoma is mentioned only to be condemned because of the risk of esophageal perforation and compromise of later surgical excision.

Surgical Management

Excision is required in most patients to confirm the diagnosis and to prevent progressive growth. Malignant degeneration of a leiomyoma is rare, but its possibility may be considered another reason for excision. As noted, leiomyomas are most common in the distal esophagus; therefore a standard thoracotomy incision is usually applied. A left thoracotomy through the sixth or seventh intercostal space provides excellent exposure of the distal esophagus, while a right thoracotomy is preferred for more proximal lesions. The well-circumscribed intramural nature of the leiomyoma allows surgical enucleation without mucosal disruption. Reconstitution of the muscle wall is not mandatory, and even large defects can be left without complication. On the contrary, mucosal tears should be carefully repaired with interrupted suture without narrowing the lumen. Esophageal resection may be necessary for extensive or annular lesions. Ulceration of the esophageal mucosa may also make enucleation of the tumor impossible. Conservative resection of the involved esophagus and end-to-end anastomosis are the treatment of choice. Gastroesophageal competence should be restored with one of the fundoplication procedures if the lower esophageal sphincter is destroyed.

The cervical approach to the proximal thoracic esophageal leiomyoma deserves consideration in the treatment of all accessible lesions. The well-defined intramural nature of the leiomyoma favors the limited transcervical exposure. The advantages of the technique are simplicity and safety. The well-recognized morbidity of a standard thoracotomy is avoided, without compromise of the excisional effort.

It is notable that there has been no recent report of death as a complication of the removal of a leiomyoma. However, when resection is necessary, an incidence of mortality must be expected. No report of tumor recurrence following simple enucleation has been recorded. Morbidity is also low and is related primarily to the development of esophageal stricture, which is usually responsive to bougienage.

INTRALUMINAL TUMOR

Fibrolipomas are polypoid and attached to the wall of the esophagus with a stalk. The mobile polyp may occur in a sensational manner with regurgitation. Aspiration of even a small tumor may lead to death from asphyxiation. In low-lying lesions, trauma or peptic digestion may lead to surface ulceration and hemorrhage. Awareness of fatal complications and the obstructive liability of these benign polyps should lead to early surgical intervention.

Preoperative Investigation

In most cases a definite diagnosis may be made only at surgery. The greatest diagnostic aid is offered by careful radiographic examination, especially by cine-esophagography. The diagnosis is suggested by a smooth, sharply demarcated outline of an ovoid filling defect that moves about in the lumen of the esophagus. Because normal mucosa may overlie the tumor, esophagoscopy is notoriously fraught with incomplete or false negative information. Moreover, the polyps are poorly fixed, and attempts at biopsy may produce perforation and mediastinitis. Endoscopic removal is decried, as the elongated pedicle may contain large blood vessels.

Surgical Management

The treatment of choice is early surgical intervention. Admittedly difficult, the exact site of origin must be determined by careful roentgenologic and esophagoscopic examinations. Almost all of these tumors originated in the cervical esophagus, and an incision anterior to the sternomastoid muscle is appropriate. The incision may be made on the right or left side opposite the origin of the tumor. An axial esophagotomy on the contralateral wall allows the surgeon to clearly view the pedicle and secure the vascular base. A frozen section examination should be performed in every case, as there have been several reported instances of squamous carcinoma adjacent to the benign lesion. The surgeon must also be aware of the rare carcinosarcoma, which may appear grossly to be a benign polypoid neoplasm.

SUGGESTED READING

Leand PM, Murray GF, Zuidema GF, Shelley WM. Obstructing esophageal polyp with eosinophilic infiltration. Am J Surg 1968; 116:93–96.

Plachta A. Benign tumors of the esophagus. Review of literature and report of 99 cases. Am J Gastroenterol 1962; 38:639.

Schorlemmer GR, Battaglini JW, Murray GF. The cervical approach to esophageal leiomyomas. Ann Thorac Surg 1983; 35:469–471.

Seremetis MG, Lyons WS, DeGuzman VC, Peabody JW Jr. Leiomyomata of the esophagus. An analysis of 838 cases. Cancer 1976; 38:2166.

Smith CW, Murray GF, Wilcox BR. Intramural esophageal hamartoma. An unusual cause of progressive stricture in a child. J Thorac Cardiovasc Surg 1976; 72:315–318.

MALIGNANT TUMOR OF THE LOWER THIRD OF THE ESOPHAGUS

EARLE W. WILKINS Jr., M.D.

Resection of malignant tumors of the distal esophagus is a standardized operation with low morbidity and reasonable salvage, both in terms of palliation and potential cure. The "modern" era of its use dates from a half century ago to the work of Adams and Phemister. At the Massachusetts General Hospital the procedure has been performed since 1939, as reported in the initial work of Churchill and Sweet. The basic principles of their technique—wide resection with regional lymphadenectomy, preservation of blood supply to the replacing stomach, and a meticulous layered inverting anastomosis—constitute the essentials of a successful resection even today. The refinement of details and the application of supportive measures, including endotracheal anesthesia, intravenous volume replacement, appropriately applied antibiotics, and postoperative respiratory intensive care, have permitted extraordinarily low morbidity and mortality, as reported by Mathisen and his colleagues.

Resection of malignant tumors of the lower third of the esophagus consists of an esophagogastrectomy and is done primarily for carcinoma. It includes removal of the distal esophagus and proximal stomach with grossly normal margins of at least 5 cm at either end, and resection in continuity with paraesophageal, paracardial, left gastric, and celiac lymph nodes. When required for removal of gross disease, extended resections include removal of the spleen, body and tail of the pancreas, the diaphragm, and the left lobe of the liver.

DIAGNOSIS

The preoperative work-up for establishing the diagnosis and the extent of disease is standard. It includes (1) an upper gastrointestinal barium series (UGIS), (2) endoscopy, and (3) computed tomography (CT) of the thorax and upper abdomen.

The UGIS, in addition to indicating proximal extent of gross disease and degree of circumferential esophageal involvement, is useful in the fluoroscopic assessment of vocal cord paresis, tracheobronchial aspiration or fistula formation, diaphragmatic excursion, and concomitant esophageal motility disorder.

Esophagoscopy is essential for biopsy or cytologic confirmation of the type of malignant tumor, for a more accurate determination of the extent of tumor both grossly by inspection and microscopically by mucosal biopsy, for detection of a Barrett's mucosal pattern including its proximal extent, and sometimes for determining the distal extent of the tumor and extent of gastric involvement. The latter necessitates using the flexible fiberoptic esophagogastroscope, which occasionally may be coaxed through the tumor, but never with force. If it can be so passed, the status of the pylorus is also determined.

CT imaging is the least important of the diagnostic tools but does provide information regarding mediastinal lymph nodes, the bulk of tumor, and possible pulmonary involvement either by direct invasion or by metastasis. It is not accurate in determining aortic or pericardial extension, apparently because of the inconsistent presence of fat planes. Below the diaphragm, it is less useful. It is peculiarly incapable of accurate assessment of celiac-left gastric lymph node involvement, even of the extent of gastric wall involvement. It may be helpful in the detection of hepatic metastasis.

SURGICAL PREPARATION

Assessment of physiologic "operability" involves evaluation primarily of both respiratory and cardiovascular function.

The former is measured by standard pulmonary function tests, stressing the one-second vital capacity (FEV_1) and maximum breathing capacity, by arterial blood gases, or by gross but reliably helpful stair-walking. In these tests, an FEV_1 less than 1 L, an elevated Pco_2, or a doubling of respiratory rate on climbing two flights of stairs deserve special consideration.

Cardiovascular evaluation is directed at assessment of coronary blood flow, ventricular contractility, and the presence of dysrhythmia. Here, past history, physical examination of the heart, and the electrocardiogram determine the need for cardiology consultation and special methods of testing, including thallium myocardial scanning, coronary arteriography, pulmonary artery pressure measurement, and the need for preoperative digitalization.

THE OPERATION

Anesthesia

Light general anesthesia is used with endotracheal intubation. A double-lumen tube is preferred, permitting deflation of the left lung during dissection of the esophagus and particularly during the meticulous conduct of the anastomosis. Overload with intravenous fluid is avoided because of the threat of the "down-lung" syndrome postoperatively, especially if one-lung gaseous exchange is utilized. Routine broad-spectrum antibiotics, always initiated preoperatively, may need repeating during the procedure if it exceeds 4 hours. A sump nasogastric tube is placed in the esophagus prior to initiation of surgery.

Approach

A left transthoracic or thoracoabdominal incision is always used for a lower third esophageal neoplasm. It is planned with the level of anastomosis in mind. This technically most demanding part of the operation requires the optimal field exposure. Thus the higher the anticipated anastomosis, the higher the initial incision in the chest wall. In general, a rib resection facilitates both the expeditious opening of the chest and the extent of operative exposure. The seventh rib is more commonly removed. Extension of the incision across the costal arch is usually necessary for careful dissection of the stomach, celiac node removal, and pyloromyotomy, although not infrequently the abdominal portion of the operation may be carried out entirely through the diaphragm. Therefore, the upper abdomen is prepared and draped into the field, permitting an initial posterolateral incision from costal arch to paraspinal scapular level, which then can be subsequently extended across the costal cartilaginous arch if needed.

Exploration

Upon opening the pleura, the left lung, diaphragm, and pericardium are carefully assessed. The mediastinal pleura is opened just anterior to the aorta from the esophageal hiatus to the aortic arch, permitting determination of the extent of the lower third tumor, possible invasion of either lung or the aorta, and the presence of metastasis to paraesophageal, aortic, or even subcarinal lymph nodes. Before further dissection of the esophagus, the diaphragm is opened, usually circumferentially 2 cm from the chest wall (but radially if the hiatus or diaphragm itself is involved by direct extension of tumor). Thorough abdominal exploration is then possible, with particular attention to (1) lymph nodes in the left gastric–celiac axis region, (2) hepatic metastases, (3) involvement of the stomach wall, and (4) mobility of the stomach sufficient to permit its intrathoracic replacement of the esophagus. The pylorus is examined for evidence of scarring or hypertrophic stenosis.

Decision

With appropriate preoperative evaluation, the finding of categorical unresectability is seldom encountered. The nature of the disease is such and the morbidity of a distal resection so limited that palliative resection is both possible and desirable at this stage, even in the face of nodal or hepatic metastases. If gastric extension of the tumor prevents mobilization of the stomach, an intraluminal esophageal tube is a graceful method for accepting defeat in attempted resection and yet providing palliation for dysphagia.

Dissection

The actual resection is begun in the mediastinum, freeing the esophagus and its draining lymph nodes in continuity. The pulmonary ligament is divided close to the lung to permit removal of its nodes. The dissection is carried out medially along the back of the pericardium and the inferior pulmonary vein up to the level of the left main bronchus. The esophagus is encircled with first the fingers and then a Penrose tape, at a point well away from tumor. This permits gentle traction and facilitates dissection of mediastinal nodes and fat with the esophagus. Two to five direct aortic arterial branches to the esophagus are ligated immediately against the adventitial aortic wall. The tumor itself is freed last. Tumor is left behind if there is definite aortic invasion. The vagus nerves are divided on the wall of the esophagus just below the aortic arch. The thoracic duct is seldom seen from the left thoracotomy incision and is not routinely removed or ligated. If it is encountered, it may be ligated with impunity just above its entry into the mediastinum through the aortic hiatus.

The abdominal dissection includes four components: (1) separation of the greater omentum with preservation of the gastroepiploic arcade, (2) removal of the left gastric lymph nodes with division of the left gastric artery as it arises from the celiac axis, (3) pyloromyotomy, and (4) transection of the stomach.

The lesser omental sac is entered at a convenient level and the omentum divided from pylorus to spleen. Use of the stomach to replace the esophagus hinges on preservation of both the right gastroepiploic and the right gastric arteries. Thus the omental gastroepiploic branches are divided 5 to 10 mm from the arcade, allowing accurate ligature without compromise of the arcade itself. Cautery coagulation is avoided because of the threat of thrombosis of the arcade. Greater curvature dissection is carried to the esophageal hiatus by division of the gastrosplenic or so-called short gastric vessels and with them the left gastroepiploic artery as it arises from the splenic artery.

The approach to the left gastric lymph nodes is facilitated by division of the gastrohepatic omentum well away from the stomach wall, placing an encircling Penrose tape for traction. Actual access is from behind the stomach. Care is taken with division of a uniformly present branch of the splenic artery to the back of the proximal gastric wall. With upward traction on the stomach, the left gastric artery and vein are identified, doubly ligated at their origins, and divided. All adjacent tissue, including nodes along the celiac axis itself, is then swept toward the stomach.

The need for a gastric drainage procedure has never been scientifically settled. Because of an inevitable vagotomy effect resulting frequently in diminished gastric motility, a pyloromyotomy has been routinely and arbitrarily performed. A pyloroplasty is not used because of the enhanced possibility of alkaline reflux. Pyloroplasty (a two-layered Heineke-Mikulicz type) is actually carried out only if substantial peptic ulcer scarring compromises the pyloric channel or if duodenal entry occurs during myotomy. The duodenum is mobilized with a Kocher's maneuver to facilitate the drainage procedure and the mobility of the stomach into the thorax.

Points are chosen and marked with sutures on both the lesser and greater curvatures. On the lesser side, this is usually just distal to the left gastric, node-containing tissue; on the greater side, it is at the upper extent of the gastroepiploic arcade. These points should be at a minimum of 5 cm from the gastric extent of gross tumor. The stomach is then divided between a distal row of TA-90 staples and a long proximal clamp that is later used for traction of the specimen as the anastomosis is being accomplished. The stapled gastric resection line is inverted with interrupted No. 4–0 silk sutures.

Adequacy of Resection

In all cases, except perhaps in the purely palliative procedure in which gross disease is known to have been left behind, the resection margin should be carefully checked. This is done by both the surgeon with direct inspection and the pathologist with frozen section. The latter is particularly necessary in the esophageal margin in cases of adenocarcinoma, in which submucosal extension of tumor is not uncommon. When such extension is found, an additional resection of the esophagus must be carried out, often with the need for a supra-aortic anastomosis. This added dissection is facilitated by resection of a higher rib, the fourth or even the third, through a paravertebral extension of the same incision. When the esophagus is thus exposed above the aortic arch, the thoracic duct is at particular risk for injury and usually must be ligated. For this extended procedure, the stomach is brought through the posterior mediastinum to the right of or behind the aortic arch prior to supra-aortic anastomosis.

The Anastomosis

Basic Principles. The integrity of an esophagogastric anastomosis following resection of an esophageal carcinoma is predicated on the observation of a set of specific principles. Careful concurrence with the details involved in these principles assures a successful anastomosis.

Blood Supply. Maintenance of an adequate arterial supply and of venous drainage of the gastric segment is mandatory and is the single most important essential. The right gastric and right gastroepiploic arteries with their respective arcades are *both* necessary for viability of the stomach. Venous return is rarely discussed, but its interruption could result in venous infarction. The esophagus is not dissected out of its proximal bed more than is necessary to perform the anastomosis, usually no more than 2 cm.

Lack of Tension. The mobility of the two ends for the anastomosis is obtained *entirely* from the stomach. The esophagus cannot and must not be dissected proximally to gain length. The stomach, on the other hand, can be easily advanced its necessary length by freeing it from the omentum to the level of the pylorus and by a thorough duodenal release with a Kocher's maneuver. To prevent postoperative tension on the anastomosis by a full stomach, four to six sutures are placed tacking the gastric wall to the mediastinal pleura or prevertebral fascia for appropriate suspension.

Atraumatic Tissue Handling. Clamps are not applied to the edges of portions of esophagus and stomach to be anastomosed. Cautery is not used. The placement of sutures is guided by holding the previous stitch rather than by grasping with even the most atraumatic of tissue forceps.

Inversion of Tissue. The esophagus is void of an outer mesothelial layer, such as the peritoneum covering the abdominal viscera. Its strongest layer is its mucosa; it must be completely inverted and covered by esophageal muscle as the anastomosis is completed.

Gastric Decompression. Egress for gastric contents under pressure must be provided, especially in the event that gastric amotility results in retention. Vomiting exerts undue force against the suture line and must be avoided.

A two-layer sutured anastomosis is always carried out. The general thoracic resident must learn this technique during training. The use of the mechanical stapler, although it produces a satisfactory anastomosis, does not actually save real time. Upon thorough review of literature statistics, it is evident that the one-layer anastomosis results in an unnecessarily high rate of leakage. The particular suture material is perhaps the least important detail. However, use of interrupted sutures is important in providing capillary flow to the healing and sealing edges and in permitting an adequate anastomotic orifice. Purse-string sutures are avoided. Fine silk is easily handled, inexpensive, and provides no untoward, foreign-body complication.

An end-to-side anastomosis is preferred. This is accomplished, after inversion closure of the transection line of the stomach, by excising a circular button of stomach from its anterior surface. The exact placement of this button must be precise: no closer than 2 cm to the gastric turn-in and near the greater curve where maximal length is obtained and where arterial inflow is the greatest. A posterior row of No. 4–0 silk mattress sutures is first placed through muscle of the esophagus and the combined serosa and muscle wall of the stomach. Appropriate placement of these four to six sutures is satisfied before they are tied; when they are tied, the stomach is brought up to the esophagus, with the finger securing the knot placed above the anastomosis. Approximating only the posterior one-third of the circumference of the anastomosis with this row facilitates exposure of the mucosal layer. This second layer, also of No. 4–0 silk, approximates the mucosa of the stomach to the mucosa of the esophagus. Interrupted technique in simple inverting fashion is used; these sutures are tied as they are placed, permitting gentle upward traction to expose the proper placement of the ensuing suture. The posterior layer is carried out from both directions around to the anterior aspect, taking particular care to invert this layer with knots tied on the inside. The final suture in this layer is a Connell's mattress suture. The outer anterior row is completed in its residual two-thirds with interrupted mattress sutures, again lifting the stomach upward to the esophagus. If there is omentum available, it is sutured over the anterior suture line.

This anastomosis, so placed in end-side fashion, has gastric serosal coverage supporting its posterior aspect. It provides a mucosal flap-valve that helps to minimize postoperative reflux.

RESULTS

Results are presented first for the technical aspects of the procedure. These have been most recently assessed for the years 1980 to 1986 by Mathisen. In this period 104 esophageal resections were carried out in which the stomach was used to replace the esophagus. Not all were lower third tumors, but the technical aspect under consideration pertained to all. The critical measure of success in this operation is the anastomotic leakage rate. In these 104 resections, there was none. The overall morbidity is presented in Table 1.

In 30 years of experience with esophagectomy and

TABLE 1 Data for 104 Esophageal Resections, 1980–1986

	No. of Patients
Operative approach	
Left thoracoabdominal (lower third)	64
Abdominal-right thoracic	40
Mortality (hospital or 30-day)	2
Anastomotic leaks	0
Transfusions	31
(Average blood loss)	(650 ml)
Morbidity-major	
Pneumonia	12
Re-exploration for bleeding	2
Morbidity-minor	
Atelectasis	71
Atrial fibrillation	9
Ventricular arrhythmias	8
Urinary tract infection	3
Wound infection	2
Posthospital dilation	5

esophagogastric anastomosis, both in personally conducted operations and in assisting thoracic residents, the author has not had an anastomotic leak. The possibility of such a leak is defined by an UGIS that is carried out in all patients at days 7 to 10.

Actuarial survival for the years 1980 to 1986 indicates an 8 percent 5-year (anticipated) rate for the adenocarcinoma group but a 34 percent rate for squamous cell carcinoma patients. This dichotomy is explained, to a certain extent, at least, by the ongoing protocol study utilizing adjuvant chemotherapy and radiation for the latter group.

Esophagogastrectomy for lower third esophageal carcinoma is a safe operation that provides the best palliation for dysphagia. Its effectiveness is best measured by the success of the anastomosis.

SUGGESTED READING

Adams WE, Phemister DB. Carcinoma of lower thoracic esophagus: report of successful resection and esophagogastrostomy. J Thorac Surg 1938; 7:620–621.

Churchill ED, Sweet RH. Transthoracic resection of tumors of the stomach and esophagus. Ann Surg 1942; 115:897–920.

Churchill ED, Sweet RH. Transthoracic resection of the stomach and esophagus. (Case reports). Ann Surg 1942; 116:566–573.

Mathisen DJ, Grillo HC,Hilgenberg AD, Moncure AC, Wilkins EW Jr. Transthoracic esophagogastrectomy: a safe approach to carcinoma of the esophagus. Ann Thorac Surg 1988; 45:137–143.

UPPER THORACIC ESOPHAGEAL CANCER

DAVID M. SHAHIAN, M.D.
F. HENRY ELLIS Jr., M.D., Ph.D.

Cancer of the esophagus is an uncommon malignancy. The 9,400 cases diagnosed in 1985 represent 1 percent of all new cancer cases for the year. Although the anatomic locations of intrathoracic esophageal tumors have traditionally been divided into thirds, there is no practical difference in diagnosis, treatment, or prognosis between middle and upper third lesions. We regard all tumors requiring anastomosis at or above the level of the aortic arch as upper thoracic esophageal lesions. Resection requires either a combined abdominothoracic approach or transhiatal blunt esophagectomy, whereas lesions of the lower thoracic esophagus or gastric cardia are best approached through a left thoracotomy.

GENERAL CONSIDERATIONS

Intrathoracic esophageal tumors are epidermoid carcinomas in over 70 percent of patients. Approximately 25 percent of tumors are adenocarcinomas arising in a Barrett's esophagus. Less common tumors include sarcomas, mucoepidermoid or adenoid cystic carcinomas, adenocarcinoma without associated Barrett's esophagus, melanoma, and small-cell carcinoma. At the time of diagnosis, at least two-thirds of patients with esophageal carcinoma have stage III or IV disease because of full-thickness penetration of the esophageal wall, lymph node involvement, metastatic disease, or a combination of these. Most such patients are incurable using current treatment programs, but those with stage I or II disease have a 30 to 40 percent chance of surviving 5 years after resection.

For most patients with esophageal carcinoma, esophagogastrectomy without preoperative adjuncts offers the best opportunity for prompt, effective, and sustained palliation. In many institutions, including our own, the hospital mortality is less than 5 percent, and most patients are discharged from the hospital within 2 weeks after operation with an effective swallowing mechanism. Most alternative therapies have been less successful in providing both palliation and a chance for cure.

THERAPEUTIC OPTIONS

External beam radiation has its proponents, but in most series the 5-year survival rate is low, and palliation is less effective and sustained than after resection. Preoperative radiation, chemotherapy, or both prior to esophagogastrectomy may increase the resectability rate, sometimes causing regression or complete eradication of viable tumor. However, combined therapy prolongs the overall duration of treatment by 2 to 3 months and has not yet been shown to increase long-term survival. For a disease in which the median survival time after resection is less than 2 years, we prefer to maximize the enjoyable, symptom-free, and productive time for each patient by simple esophagectomy.

Patients with diffuse systemic metastases, a locally unresectable tumor, or malignant tracheoesophageal fistula may require other methods for palliation. Palliative substernal colon or gastric bypass without resection is one option, but this is a formidable procedure in a patient whose life expectancy is short. Laser therapy offers relief of dysphagia with far less morbidity. Esophageal intubation using "traction" tubes has been associated with a hospital mortality as high as 20 to 25 percent due to erosion, bleeding, perforation, proximal migration, cricopharyngeal dysfunction, and aspiration. The latter complications increase in incidence according to how proximally the tumor is located. Endoscopic peroral intubation may provide greater safety and ease of insertion.

ESOPHAGOGASTRECTOMY

With the exceptions noted, esophagogastrectomy is our preferred treatment both for the palliation and cure of upper thoracic esophageal carcinoma requiring anastomosis at or above the level of the aortic arch. This may be accomplished using either the combined abdominal and right thoracic approach, occasionally with anastomosis to the cervical esophagus, or the transhiatal approach.

Preoperative Evaluation

Some patients are debilitated when first seen, and for them preoperative hyperalimentation may be of value. Otherwise, prompt resection without prolonged preoperative testing or preparation is preferred. A computed tomographic (CT) scan of the thorax is useful in determining the presence of extensive hepatic or nodal metastases as well as the extent of mediastinal invasion. A patient is rarely denied surgical exploration solely because of positive findings on CT scan, but the study may help in planning the operative procedure. Bronchoscopy is advisable for most patients with upper thoracic esophageal tumors, and the presence of tracheal or bronchial invasion is a contraindication to aggressive surgical therapy.

Ivor Lewis Approach

If a CT scan suggests considerable mediastinal invasion, an initial thoracotomy may be performed to assess resectability. In most instances, however, exploratory laparotomy is performed first through an upper abdominal midline incision. Diffuse hepatic or peritoneal metastases contraindicate resection, but isolated metastases do not. Rarely, dense left gastric nodal metastases may make safe division of the left gastric artery impossible. If there are no intra-abdominal contraindications, the stomach is mobilized, preserving the right gastroepiploic and right gastric arteries. The omentum is not removed, since this does not affect regional recurrence or survival. The short gastric vessels are divided preserving the spleen, unless it is obviously involved by tumor. The peritoneum over the distal esophagus is incised, the left lobe of the liver is mobilized, and the esophagus is freed circumferentially at the hiatus. Dissection of the esophagus is extended bluntly into the lower thorax, and the hiatus is widened. The left gastric artery and vein are doubly ligated and divided. Kocher's maneuver and pyloroplasty or pyloromyotomy complete the abdominal exploration.

The patient is then turned to the lateral position, and a right thoracotomy is performed through the bed of the nonresected sixth rib. The tumor is mobilized from the mediastinum, and the azygos vein is divided. The stomach is withdrawn through the hiatus, taking care to avoid rotation or excessive mobilization. The stomach is transected at the cardia, and an end-to-side esophagogastric anastomosis several inches proximal to the growth is carried out using two layers of interrupted silk (DMS) or an inner layer of running chromic catgut and another layer of interrupted silk sutures (FHE). The specimen is removed, a nasogastric tube is placed across the anastomosis into the gastric pouch for postoperative drainage, and the chest is closed with intercostal tube drainage.

Despite a grossly free margin of over 5 cm, microscopic tumor may be found at the proximal margin. This requires reresection. If insufficient intrathoracic esophagus remains thereafter, the thoracotomy is closed and the cervical esophagus exposed through an oblique or transverse cervical incision, through which a cervical esophagogastric anastomosis is performed. If high intrathoracic or cervical anastomosis is required and previous gastric operation or anatomic considerations make gastric transposition impossible, a cervical esophagostomy and feeding gastrostomy are performed. Substernal colon bypass is done as a secondary procedure.

Transhiatal Esophagectomy

Lesions that are easily dissected from the mediastinal, vascular, and tracheobronchial structures may be removed using the transhiatal approach. Its purported advantages include the avoidance of a thoracotomy, the ease of managing cervical anastomotic leaks, and the removal of the entire thoracic esophagus, thereby encompassing skin lesions and lymphatics. Its disadvantages include possible injury to contiguous tracheobronchial and vascular structures and its violation of traditional principles of cancer resection. In our experience transhiatal esophagectomy does not diminish morbidity, mortality, or hospital stay. Actuarial analysis has demonstrated no difference in long-term survival between transhiatal and transthoracic esophagectomy, suggesting that less radical periesophageal dissection is not detrimental. We have limited the use of transhiatal esophagectomy to small and easily mobilized lesions of the upper thoracic esophagus that would otherwise require the Ivor Lewis approach.

Abdominal exploration proceeds as outlined for the initial stages of the Ivor Lewis procedure. An incision is made along the anterior border of the sternocleidomastoid muscle, and the cervical esophagus is exposed, taking care to avoid injury to the recurrent laryngeal nerve in the tracheoesophageal groove. The esophagus is bluntly mobilized down to the level of the carina. Further transhiatal mobilization from the abdomen is performed. The esophagus and stomach are divided at the cardia, and a Penrose drain is sutured to both to facilitate their subsequent transthoracic delivery. The stomach and esophagus are delivered through the cervical wound taking care to avoid rotation, and the anastomosis is performed. A Penrose drain is left in the cervical wound.

Postoperative Management

Postoperatively, the patient is placed in a reverse Trendelenburg position. On postoperative day 4 or 5, a contrast esophagogram is obtained. If no leak or obstruction is observed and if intestinal motility is noted clinically, the nasogastric tube is removed and oral feedings are begun. If this is tolerated, the pleural drainage tubes are removed. The patient is usually discharged from the hospital within 7 to 14 days with an admonition to eat small and frequent meals, to keep the head of the bed elevated, and to avoid eating for several hours before retiring at night.

Complications

Intrathoracic anastomotic leakage is an uncommon but life-threatening complication. Occasionally a small leak may be contained by the surrounding mediastinal structures and inflammatory reaction. In such a case, the nasogastric tube and pleural tubes are kept on suction, and intravenous hyperalimentation is begun. Contrast esophagography is repeated in 5 to 7 days, at which time the leak is often resolved. A major disruption can be resutured if recognized easily, but otherwise drainage and diversion as well as hyperalimentation are required.

Gastric obstruction may occur at several levels. Redundant stomach in the right chest results in a J or "drainpipe" deformity with functional obstruction. Axial rotation of the stomach may also lead to obstruction. Both require reexploration and derotation or replacement of excess stomach into the abdomen. Obstruction at the hiatus is possible because of inadequate hiatal enlargement at the time of operation and requires laparotomy for correction.

If pyloromyotomy or pyloroplasty has not been performed, obstruction at this level may be expected in 10 percent of patients and requires a gastric drainage procedure. The appearance of a chylous effusion in the right chest implies operative injury to the thoracic duct. Medical management is usually unsuccessful. The most effective treatment is right thoracotomy with bulk ligation of the prevertebral para-aortic tissues just cephalad to the hiatus.

Immediate complications of transhiatal esophagectomy include membranous tracheobronchial injury or hemorrhage from the azygos vein or esophageal or bronchial artery, each of which requires right thoracotomy for control. Entry into either pleural space is common and presents no problem if recognized and treated by tube thoracostomy. Recurrent nerve dysfunction may arise from direct injury in the tracheoesophageal groove or from the blunt para-aortic dissection of the esophagus. In our experience, the incidence of anastomotic leaks is greater with transhiatal esophagectomy than after transthoracic resection, presumably because the stomach is maximally stretched and its blood supply is marginal. Cervical anastomotic leaks are easily treated by hyperalimentation and prolonged cervical drainage, and they heal spontaneously. An anastomotic stricture is usually a late occurrence and requires dilation.

Results

The wide variation of reported results necessitates reliance on personal experience. At the Lahey Clinic, the overall operability rate from 1970 to 1986 was 80 percent. Of the 272 operations performed for carcinoma of the esophagus and cardia, 70 were for lesions of the upper thoracic esophagus, of which 65 (92.9 percent) were resections. Three deaths occurred within 30 days of operation, for a hospital mortality rate of 4.6 percent. The 5-year actuarial survival rate was 15.6 percent. There was no difference in survival between patients with squamous cell cancer versus those with adenocarcinoma in Barrett's esophagus or between patients having transthoracic resection as compared with resection via the transhiatal route.

SUGGESTED READING

Ellis FH Jr, Gibb SP, Watkins E Jr. Esophagogastrectomy: a safe, widely applicable, and expeditious form of palliation for patients with carcinoma of the esophagus and cardia. Ann Surg 1983; 198:531–540.

Lewis I. The surgical treatment of carcinoma of the oesophagus, with special reference to a new operation for growths of the middle third. Br J Surg 1946; 34:18–31.

Orringer MB. Transhiatal esophagectomy without thoracotomy for carcinoma of the thoracic esophagus. Ann Surg 1984; 200:282–288.

Shahian DM, Neptune WB, Ellis FH Jr, Watkins E Jr. Transthoracic versus extrathoracic esophagectomy: mortality, morbidity, and long-term survival. Ann Thorac Surg 1986; 41:237–246.

Tryzelaar JF, Neptune WB, Ellis FH Jr. Esophagectomy without thoracotomy for carcinoma of the esophagus. Am J Surg 1982; 143:486–489.

CARCINOMA OF THE CERVICAL ESOPHAGUS

HERMES C. GRILLO, M.D.

Squamous cell carcinoma of the esophagus is least common in the cervical region. Its management may be difficult; it may involve the larynx and trachea, it may metastasize to cervical lymph nodes, and if surgically manageable, it may require extensive procedures.

EVALUATION

The extent of disease is assessed by careful palpation of the neck, barium contrast x-ray films with fluoroscopy, computed tomographic scan of the neck and mediastinum (and upper abdomen), and careful endoscopy of the larynx, trachea, and esophagus. Particular attention must be paid to laryngeal function, to the possibility of airway involvement, and to the distance, if any, between the cricopharyngeus and the proximal extent of the tumor. The usual attention must be paid to the possibility of distant metastases.

Superior and inferior mesenteric artery angiograms are done to determine the blood supply of the colon in the event that it is used for reconstruction of the esophagus.

SELECTION OF PATIENTS AND THERAPEUTIC ALTERNATIVES

If there is extensive disease, either locally in the neck with a large fixed mass or multiple cervical metastases, or if other metastatic disease is evident, the likelihood of obtaining prolonged palliation by any modality of treatment is small and the scale of surgery that would be required for removal of the lesion is such that operation is usually not justified. Chemotherapy, irradiation, or both may be utilized, although without much likelihood of prolonged regression. Placement of an endoesophageal prosthesis is usually impossible to accomplish satisfactorily at this level.

More limited lesions are categorized into those that involve the larynx and those that do not. Localized postcricoidal carcinoma of the esophagus may be cured in a small number of patients by laryngotracheal pharyngoesophagectomy. This mutilating operation leaves the patient without a larynx. It is justified only when there is a possibility of cure.

A small number of patients present with localized carcinoma of the cervical esophagus that is distant enough from the cricopharyngeus so that an attempt at extirpation with laryngeal preservation is possible.

In either case we believe that at present it is reasonable to subject the patient to two cycles of combined chemotherapy and then proceed to an attempt at surgical extirpation. Previously, we used to expose these patients to preoperative radiotherapy to the extent of 4,500 rads. We now reserve radiotherapy for postoperative adjunctive treatment if the pathologic findings indicate it.

OPERATIVE TREATMENT

Postcricoidal Carcinoma

When the carcinoma invades the posterior cricoid, it is not possible to salvage a functional larynx. Resection must therefore include the larynx, enough trachea to provide a margin below the tumor, and removal of the entire cervical esophagus, including the upper mediastinal esophagus as well as the lower portion of the pharynx. Usually the length of trachea to be removed is small enough so that the postoperative end tracheostomy lies at the base of the neck. Sometimes a mediastinal tracheostomy is required (see the chapter *Mediastinal Exenteration*). A generous collar incision provides excellent access to both sides of the esophagus. If the flap is raised high enough on the side of the major exposure (or on both sides), just as good an exposure can be obtained as through an oblique incision anterior to the sternocleidomastoid muscle. The incision may be tailored by dropping it so that an end tracheostomy will not lie in the middle of the incision. Exposure initially is made on the side of major involvement, dissecting in the prevascular plane to the prevertebral fascia. The extent of involvement is completely assessed before definitive resection is performed. If one or both lobes of the thyroid gland are uninvolved, as frequently is the case, the isthmus is divided and the lobes turned back, saving their blood supply and the parathyroid glands. If the tumor involves the thyroid gland or is too close to it for a safe margin, one or both lobes are sacrificed. The trachea is transected at a point low enough to provide a margin of normal tissue. Intubation is carried out across the operative field. The esophagus is dissected for some distance down into the mediastinum and divided arbitrarily using the stapler. The stump is further inverted with 4–0 silk sutures. If total esophagectomy is elected, the dissection can be carried down to the carina from the cervical approach and completed transhiatally from below. The specimen is elevated, and the lateral attachments of the larynx on either side are divided. The pharynx is entered through an incision above the hyoid bone and carried laterally. The tumor can be visualized directly and adequate margin obtained above it posteriorly. The epiglottis is removed with the hyoid.

Since cervical esophageal cancer rarely spreads distally, total esophagectomy is not required but is a matter of preference. If total esophagectomy is done, it is simplest to mobilize the stomach for replacement and bring it up either in the posterior channel of the esophagus or through a substernal tunnel. This is prepared by pushing the hand upward substernally, more to the left than to the right to avoid a pleural tear. The tunnel is completed from above. I prefer to use the transverse and left colon pedicled on the left colic artery, taking a generous length, and using the middle colic artery where it branches to right and left as part of the arcade that will carry the colonic blood supply. Division is usually made at the hepatic flexure so that there is an adequate length to reach all the way to the pharynx. The vascular pedicle of the bypass is brought up retrogastrically, and the distal end of the colonic segment is brought onto the anterior wall of the stomach for a two-layer anastomosis. The replacement is isoperistaltic. The thoracic inlet is often too restrictive for the colon or gastric replacement, causing venous engorgement. For this reason, I frequently remove the head of one clavicle and an arc of sternum. Bringing the colon up in this fashion does not cause any difficulty in subsequently fashioning the tracheostomy. The colon is simply moved a little to one side of the tracheostomy. A colon bypass is made as straight as possible. Care is taken not to twist it. Excess bowel is removed. Direct end-to-end anastomosis is usually made, although end-to-side is acceptable. Two layers of interrupted 4–0 silk sutures are used, inverting the knots of the first layer into the lumen.

A reversed gastric tube may also be employed for esophageal replacement. Leakage appears to be more common with this technique, especially when used infrequently by a surgeon. Pedicled jejunum does not easily reach the cricoid level unless the proximal portion has its blood supply augmented by microvascular anastomosis. Free jejunal segments may also be employed, but the length of operation is much increased, and special skills are required. Cutaneous tubed esophageal replacements are fraught with complications of leakage and stenosis and have the initial disadvantage of being multistaged procedures. Although myocutaneous flaps may be single-staged, multiple problems remain when they are used for esophageal replacement.

If metastatic lymph nodes are found in the neck, appropriate cervical lymph node dissection may be done at the same time.

Cervical Lesions Not Involving the Larynx

When the esophageal lesion does not involve the larynx, initial dissection and exploration of the lesion are more difficult. The esophagus is encircled below the lesion at a reasonable point that will provide a satisfactory distal margin. Proximal dissection is carried out with great care to avoid entering the tumor or injuring the recurrent laryngeal nerves, which at this level lie in the grooves between trachea and esophagus. The advantage of a collar incision is more evident in this case, since dissection may be effected bilaterally with greater ease, doing each portion from the appropriate side. When the lesion is high, it is mandatory to obtain the patient's prior permission to perform laryngectomy in the event that it is required. Esophageal resection in these cases is usually carried up to the level of the cricopharyngeus muscle. Division of the esophagus, therefore, is at the point where it essentially fuses to the back of the larynx at the cricoid level. In a small number of patients in whom the trachea has proved to be involved in a limited area, I have done concurrent sleeve resection of the trachea. Special care must be taken not to devascularize the distal end of the trachea in the process of dissecting the esophagus, if the trachea is to be divided. Although the undivided trachea can tolerate division of some of these vessels, the divided one may not. Recurrent laryngeal nerves should be spared unless one is involved by tumor.

If the lesion extends to the thoracic inlet, partial vertical sternotomy allows proper exposure for dissection. In addition, if transhiatal esophagectomy is elected, dissection of esophagus to or below the carina is possible under direct vision, lessening blood loss and minimizing injuries to thoracic duct, azygos vein, and trachea that have so often been reported with "blunt esophagectomy."

Reconstruction in these patients is done in the same way as in patients with postcricoidal lesions. The colon pedicled on the left colic artery is advanced substernally, and direct anastomosis is performed in the cricopharyngeal region. Access for anastomosis at this level is difficult, since the proximal end is fixed to the back of the larynx, which, in turn, is not very movable. With a tape around the trachea (and recurrent nerves), however, drawing it forward and to one side and then to the other, it is possible to perform the anastomosis quite satisfactorily. I prefer to do part of the anastomosis from the right side and part from the left side through the already described bilateral approach. This vastly improves access for what otherwise would be the far side of the anastomosis. A gastrostomy tube provides postoperative decompression until peristalsis returns.

When cylindrical tracheal resection is done—only in rare cases—direct end-to-end anastomosis is performed in the usual manner. Prior to tracheal anastomosis, a strap muscle, usually the sternohyoid, is divided at its proximal end and sutured across the esophageal anastomosis to prevent fistula. The neck and upper mediastinum are drained.

POSTOPERATIVE CARE

The cervical and upper mediastinal drains are removed early, depending on the amount of drainage. With careful anastomosis, leakage is a very rare occurrence. If a small leak should develop, it requires drainage and generally closes with conservative management. With preoperative mesenteric angiography and close attention to the blood supply of the colon and its handling during surgery, colonic necrosis should not occur. Gastric drainage through the gastrostomy tube is continued until peristalsis returns, and the patient is then placed on a progressive diet. As a matter of protocol patients receive two further cycles of chemotherapy. Radiation is given in accordance with the pathology found at operation.

Even in patients who have developed remote metastases at a later date, far better palliation has been provided by surgery than by irradiation alone.

SUGGESTED READING

Grillo HO. Mural tracheostomy in the anterior mediastinum. J Thorac Cardiovasc Surg 1966; 51:422.

Moores DW, et al. One stage reconstruction for pharyngolaryngectomy. J Thorac Cardiovasc Surg 1983; 85:330–336.

CHEMOTHERAPY, RADIATION, AND SURGERY IN ESOPHAGEAL NEOPLASIA

ZWI STEIGER, M.D., F.A.C.S.

When treated by surgery or radiation alone, patients with carcinoma of the esophagus have a poor prognosis. The resectability rate for cure is low, the operative mortality is high, and the long-term survival rate is in the single digit figures. Still there is a need for a therapeutic intervention to attempt elimination of the tumor when the disease appears localized or to achieve palliation to afford the patient adequate swallowing. To accomplish this we have been combining chemotherapy, radiation, and surgery, the currently available and accepted three modalities utilized in cancer therapy.

Surgery and radiation are the traditional methods used to control the primary tumor. They have no effect on metastatic disease, which is commonly the cause of the patient's death. In addition to its own local effect chemotherapy potentiates the local effects of radiation and is aimed at controlling metastatic disease.

The majority of patients with carcinoma of the esophagus have lost a large amount of weight and are in poor physical condition. Preoperative hydration and hyperalimentation are accomplished prior to surgery either via a Hickman's catheter placed in the superior vena cava or a jejunostomy. If the esophagus is not completely obstructed, a feeding tube is passed into the jejunum through the nose.

The chemotherapy utilized at present is 5-fluorouracil, 1,000 mg per square meter of body surface per day for 4 days as a continuous infusion and cisplatin, 100 mg per square meter of body surface as a bolus injection on day 1. These agents have proven activity against esophageal carcinoma. Although the toxicity level of these drugs is acceptable, careful monitoring of kidney function and for possible myelosuppression is essential. Prior to instituting chemotherapy, a complete patient work-up is carried out.

Two hundred rads a day five times a week are directed to the primary lesion, including 5 cm above and 5 cm below the lower level of the tumor. The width of the port is 8 cm. Radiation is given for 3 weeks, for a total dose of 3,000 rads. On completion of the radiotherapy, the 5-fluorouracil and cisplatin are repeated. The second dose may have to be postponed or the dose modified pending the severity of myelosuppression or impaired kidney function.

In many instances at this point the dysphagia is relieved and the patient can resume oral alimentation.

If there are no contraindications (advanced patient age, poor general condition), esophagectomy is performed 3 weeks after completion of the second chemotherapy dose. Occasionally, the operation has to be delayed when myelosuppression is present.

At surgery, the stomach is mobilized through an upper midline incision. The gastroepiploic and right gastric vessels are preserved. The left gastric vessels are ligated and divided. The gastrocolic ligament is divided. The duodenum is mobilized, and a Heinecke-Mikulicz pyloroplasty is performed. The distal esophagus is mobilized bluntly through the stretched hiatus or after dividing the right crus. The resectability of the tumor is assessed. We have commonly encountered dysrrhythmias while trying to mobilize the esophagus through the hiatal route. If the patient tolerates mobilization of the esophagus via the transhiatal route and the tumor is not invading the surrounding structures, then this is accomplished. The cervical esophagus is then exposed through an incision along the left sternocleidomastoid, and the mobilization of the upper third of the thoracic esophagus is completed. The esophagogastric junction is now divided between staples and the gastric side reinforced with a continuous serosal suture of 3–0 silk. The esophagus is then resected and the stomach advanced in the posterior mediastinum until the fundus can be seen in the lower neck and further pulled up in the neck incision. The cervical esophagus is anastomosed to the fundus. We use 3–0 silk in an interrupted fashion for the anastomosis and "ink-well" the anastomosis with another interrupted row of 3–0 silk sutures. A jejunostomy is also performed. This is done for hyperalimentation in the immediate postoperative period. If during the transhiatal exploration of the chest the mobilization of the esophagus cannot be accomplished, the abdomen is closed. The patient is then turned on the left side, and the right side of the chest is entered through the bed of the fourth or fifth rib. The esophagus is resected and the previously mobilized stomach delivered into the chest. The proximal esophagus is then anastomosed to the fundus using the EEA stapler with a size 28-mm cartridge. If the tumor is in the upper third of the thoracic esophagus, a separate incision is made in the neck, and the anastomosis between the cervical esophagus and the fundus is performed in the neck. A feeding jejunostomy is also done prior to closure of the abdomen.

The patient is kept overnight on the respirator and then weaned. The stomach is kept decompressed with a nasogastric tube. An intravenous solution supplemented with jejunal alimentation is maintained until oral feeding is resumed. When residual tumor is present in the resected esophagus, radiotherapy is resumed 3 to 4 weeks after the operation, for a total dose of 5,000 to 6,000 rads.

The same treatment plan is applied for adenocarcinoma of the esophagus as for squamous cell carcinoma. The effect of chemotherapy and radiation therapy on the primary tumor is less pronounced in adenocarcinoma.

In advanced disease, chemotherapy and radiation therapy are given for palliation in the manner described. If no relief of dysphagia is achieved, a palliative esophagectomy or bypass of the tumor using the stomach or colon is carried out.

Some of the drawbacks of this combined therapeutic approach are the prolonged hospitalization, the delay in the surgical intervention in the patient who does not respond to the combined therapy, and the occasional postoperative occurrence of the adult respiratory distress syndrome.

The advantages are the increased number of patients whose tumors become resectable, the effect of the chemotherapeutic agents on metastatic and occult disease, and in a number of patients avoidance of surgery.

As new chemotherapeutic agents are developed, new protocols are being designed that will supplant our present one.

SUGGESTED READING

Franklin R, Steiger Z, Vaishampayan G, et al. Combined modality therapy for esophageal squamous cell carcinoma. Cancer 1983; 51:1062–1071.

Kelsen DP, Ahuja R, Hopfan S, et al. Combined modality therapy of esophageal carcinoma. Cancer 1981; 48:31–37.

Leichman L, Herskovic A, Leichman CG. Non-operative therapy for squamous cell cancer of the esophagus. J Clin Oncol 1987; 5(3):365–370.

Leichman L, Steiger Z, Seydel HG, et al. Preoperative chemotherapy and radiation therapy for patients with cancer of the esophagus. A potentially curative approach. J Clin Oncol 1984; 2:75–79.

Rosenberg JC, Franklin R, Steiger Z. Squamous cell carcinoma of the thoracic esophagus: an interdisciplinary approach. Curr Probl Cancer 1981; 5:1-51.

RADIATION THERAPY IN ESOPHAGEAL NEOPLASIA

NOAH C. CHOI, M.D.

The natural history of carcinoma of the esophagus has been altered very little by current therapeutic methods, and therefore any reported cure rate over 10 percent is a reflection of patient selection rather than improved therapeutic factors. It has not been a simple matter to achieve even a sustained palliation of dysphagia that will last more than 6 months by either surgery or radiation. The death of a patient as a result of palliative procedures becomes acceptable only if it is balanced by a very appreciable expectation of gain in survival.

Surgery for esophageal carcinoma is judged incomplete, according to the definition of an operation of cancer, if there are nonresectable vital structures in immediate contact with the esophageal wall, thus precluding the resection of enough normal tissue to make a clean margin. This anatomic restriction for a radical cancer operation, coupled with a high operative mortality rate of 10 to 20 percent, has resulted in radiation being a better therapeutic alternative for carcinoma of the upper two-thirds of the esophagus.

Radiotherapy, however, has its own limitations. The long-term survival rate ($\geq$ 5 years) has been only 5 to 10 percent, even with the maximal tolerable dose of radiation of about 6,000 to 6,600 cGy, although a resulting sustained palliation of dysphagia has been appreciated by the majority of patients. Approximately 50 percent of these patients, even after definitive radiotherapy, continue to have persistent uncontrolled or recurrent locoregional carcinoma leading to recurrent dysphagia. Biologic reasons for this poor control of locoregional carcinoma with radiation include the fact that the carcinoma usually is large and contains a significant component of hypoxic tumor cells, intrathoracic vital structures have a limited tolerance to radiation, and the patient's general condition is poor.

Recent advances in the frontier of preoperative therapy with a combination of multidrug chemotherapy and radiation or multidrug chemotherapy alone have been encouraging, and improved survival for even advanced locoregional carcinoma may be attainable in the near future. The management of esophageal carcinoma will undergo a major revision over the next 5 to 10 years, and therefore a brief discussion on the role of radiation is timely and necessary.

The role of radiation therapy in the management of esophageal carcinoma can be discussed under the following headings: (1) radiation therapy for resectable but medically inoperable or unresectable esophageal carcinoma; (2) radiation therapy in combination with multidrug chemotherapy as preoperative therapy for resectable esophageal carcinoma; (3) postoperative radiation therapy for positive margins or involved regional lymph nodes after preoperative chemotherapy and surgery; (4) surgical salvage for local failure after definitive radiotherapy; (5) management of adenocarcinoma of the esophagus; and (6) new trends in prospect.

RADIATION THERAPY FOR RESECTABLE BUT MEDICALLY INOPERABLE OR UNRESECTABLE ESOPHAGEAL CARCINOMA

It has been well demonstrated that radiation alone is capable of achieving a long-term cure of patients with this type of tumor. With carefully designed radiation therapy, a long-term cure rate of 5 to 10 percent has been achieved with a radiation dose of 5,600 to 6,000 cGy (time, dose, and fractionation [TDF] 92 to 99). The majority of patients with unresectable esophageal cancer suffer greatly from dysphagia, and palliation is another important goal of the overall management. It is usually not necessary to separate the goals of management into palliation and cure in patients who have no demonstrable distant metastases, inasmuch as these two objectives can be integrated into a total plan that may accomplish both without one's compromising the other. Preferred management of patients with esophageal carcinoma should be organized in such a way that palliative measures are a part of the sequence leading to cure rather than a separate route of treatment. Radiation therapy can achieve both goals without one's compromising the other by tailoring the radiation dose and treatment volume according to the patient's tolerance.

Important radiotherapeutic factors to achieve the goals include a clear definition of target volume, optimal radiation dose and fractionation schedules, and proper arrangements of radiation portals to secure optimal dose distribution within the target volume.

The target volume adopted by the author includes margins of at least 5 to 6 cm in the cephalad-caudad directions beyond the radiologic extent of the tumor and a lateral margin of 3 cm beyond the lateral border of the tumor outlined by the esophagogram to secure an adequate lateral coverage of the mediastinum. A typical field size for a tumor 6 cm in length is 18×9 cm^2. For lesions in the lower third of the esophagus, the radiation field is extended into the upper abdomen to cover celiac and gastric lymph nodes. Both supraclavicular regions are also included for lesions involving the upper two-thirds of the esophagus.

Several fractionation schedules have similar biologic effects on both normal and neoplastic tissues. For an intended cure by radiation therapy, the fractionation schedule employed by the author delivers a total dose of 6,000 to 6,400 cGy in 180 to 200 cGy of daily fractions, 5 days a week, over a period of 6 to 7 weeks. Patients who are judged incurable because of either their poor general condition or the presence of distant metastases can be treated by speedy fractionation schedules. A total dose of 4,000 to 4,500 cGy in 220 to 250 cGy of daily fractions, 5 days a week, is a reasonable schedule for speedy palliation of dysphagia.

The arrangement of the radiation portals depends on the planned total dose and types of radiation. To deliver a curative dose of radiation to the mediastinum, it is necessary to combine anteroposterior-posteroanterior parallel opposing portals with right posterior oblique and left posterior oblique or right and left lateral opposing portals. A treatment technique employed by the author delivers the initial 3,600 to 3,800 cGy by anteroposterior-posteroanterior parallel opposing portals and the remaining 2,200 to 2,400 cGy by a 3-field arrangement of anteroposterior-right posterior oblique-left posterior oblique for a total dose of 6,000 cGy in 180 to 200 cGy of daily fractions, 5 days a week, over a period of 6 to 7 weeks.

A wide range of long-term cure rates by radiation therapy has been reported, and the current cure rate of 5 to 10 percent is a reflection of patient selection and therapeutic factors. It has been a common practice that patients with small resectable lesions (stage T_1) are usually treated by surgery, with radiation therapy being used for those with unresectable (stage T_3) or medically inoperable lesions. There has been no controlled trial of radiation therapy versus surgery for squamous cell carcinoma of the esophagus. It is, however, most likely that radiation therapy can be as effective as surgery for stage T_1 lesions. The study from Edinburgh by Pearson and associates demonstrated that radiation therapy is as effective as surgery at all three anatomic levels of the esophagus. The long-term cure rate tends to be better for females than males. Radiation therapy is more successful than surgery for lesions in the upper two-thirds of the esophagus, and vice versa for the lower one-third of the esophagus.

Relief of malignant esophageal obstruction is another important goal of therapy. Radiation therapy offers improved quality of life by providing sustained relief of malignant esophageal obstruction in the majority of patients (60 to 70 percent), even when attempted cure fails. Of 51 patients who received definitive radiation therapy for unresectable carcinoma at the Massachusetts General Hospital, 60 percent were able to enjoy improved swallowing for two-thirds of the duration of their lives.

RADIATION THERAPY IN COMBINATION WITH MULTIDRUG CHEMOTHERAPY AS PREOPERATIVE THERAPY FOR RESECTABLE ESOPHAGEAL CARCINOMA

The concurrent use of radiation and multidrug chemotherapy is advantageous in achieving the maximal tumor control when the combined antitumor effect from both methods is more than just the additive of each. Cis-platinum and 5-fluorouracil are known to enhance the effects of radiation. The pilot study from the Wayne State University and the expanded trial of the same study design by the Southwest Oncology Group and Radiation Therapy Oncology Group showed that concurrent chemotherapy and radiation can be given with an acceptable toxicity (9.3 percent of surgical mortality) and that no residual carcinoma was found in 25 percent (22 out of 86) of patients. Although the results of this study represent a significant improvement over the results of previous preoperative therapy employing either radiation alone or a combination of radiation and other less effective chemotherapeutic agents, residual tumor is still found in a large number of patients. It is certain that both drug and radiation programs can be improved to achieve a better result.

POSTOPERATIVE RADIATION THERAPY FOR POSITIVE MARGINS OR INVOLVED REGIONAL LYMPH NODES AFTER PREOPERATIVE CHEMOTHERAPY AND SURGERY

Postoperative radiation has recently been explored as an element of a combined approach of chemotherapy, surgery, and radiation for positive resection margins or involved regional lymph nodes in an attempt to improve local tumor control and long-term survival. One example is a pilot study from the Massachusetts General Hospital that consists of two preoperative cycles of cis-platinum plus 5-fluorouracil, esophagectomy, and postoperative radiation employing 5,000 cGy in 180 to 200 cGy of daily fractions, 5 days a week to the tumor bed and adjacent mediastinum for involved regional lymph nodes or positive resection margins. Complete clinical remission as evaluated by the esophagogram, computed tomography of the chest, and inspection at the time of the surgery was achieved in 45 percent of patients. The tumor was resected in 81 percent of patients, and operative mortality was 10 percent. Only 5 percent of patients showed no evidence of residual tumor on microscopic examination. A projected median survival time is 16.5 months, but the long-term survival rate remains to be determined. Kelsen and associates at the Memorial Hospital also explored the role of preoperative chemotherapy by employing cis-platinum plus bleomycin initially and cis-platinum plus bleomycin plus vindesine later. Postoperative radiation therapy was delivered at 400 cGy twice a week for a period of 4 weeks for patients with stage T_3 or N_1 disease. The overall treatment-related mortality was 9 percent. The median survival time for the entire group was 16.2 months, and 2-year survival was 26 percent.

SURGICAL SALVAGE FOR LOCAL FAILURE AFTER DEFINITIVE RADIOTHERAPY

When the failure rate is as high as 60 percent with current definitive radiotherapy for locoregional carcinoma of the esophagus, surgical salvage is an appropriate alternative for recurrent esophageal obstruction. If such a procedure is contemplated, no demonstrable distant metastases should be present, and the patient's general condition should be adequate. A patient who has the potential to withstand operation should be followed closely with a view to salvage by resection in the event that local recurrence develops. Such surgery is technically more difficult than esophageal resection in a patient who has not received radiation therapy. The majority of patients who suffer local recurrence after definitive radiotherapy for unresectable carcinoma are not suitable for surgery. Indeed, in a large series of patients treated by Pearson and associates, only a few patients were salvaged by surgery.

MANAGEMENT OF ADENOCARCINOMA OF THE ESOPHAGUS

Adenocarcinoma of the esophagus represents less than 5 percent of all esophageal carcinomas. Because of its tendency to occur in the lower one-third of the esophagus, surgery has become the primary form of treatment. Postoperative radiation therapy has been used for either positive resection margins, involved regional lymph nodes, or both. However, the impact of this postoperative radiation therapy for long-term cure remains to be determined. Adenocarcinoma involving the mid one-third of the esophagus can be managed by preoperative radiation and surgery if the lesion is potentially resectable (stages T_2 and early T_3). Even when subsequent surgery cannot be employed because of the development of distant metastases or steady deterioration of the patient's general condition, preoperative radiation can often offer improved quality of life by providing relief from esophageal obstruction.

NEW TRENDS IN PROSPECT

Innovative approaches are being sought to improve the dismal outcome of the current treatment for patients with more advanced esophageal carcinoma (stages T_2, T_3, or N_1). An exploration of concurrent radiation and chemotherapy for a potential synergism is an interesting and potentially rewarding approach. The combined modality of drugs (cis-platinum and 5-fluorouracil) and radiation as preoperative therapy is such an example.

Accelerated or hyperfractionated radiation therapy has a potential for better local tumor control, although the reaction of the esophageal mucosa to radiation is expected to be more marked by this approach than by the conventional once a day schedule. Accelerated radiation therapy is also an attractive way to combine radiation with drugs.

Intraluminal therapy by means of intracavitary application of ^{192}Ir or ^{60}Co has been used either for palliation of esophageal obstruction or as a supplement to the primary tumor after external beam irradiation. Although this approach has not had any significant impact on the management of advanced esophageal carcinoma, it might be of benefit for patients with early stage carcinoma.

Other approaches, which have been studied without positive results, include hypoxic cell sensitizer (misonidazole) and particle-beam irradiation (neutron, helium ion).

SUGGESTED READING

Carey RW, Hilgenberg AD, Wilkins EW, et al. Preoperative chemotherapy followed by surgery with possible postoperative radiotherapy in squamous cell carcinoma of the esophagus: Evaluation of the chemotherapy component. J Clin Oncol 1986; 4:697–701.

Earlam R, Cunha-Melo JR. Esophageal squamous cell carcinoma: I. A critical review of surgery. Br J Surg 1980; 67:381–390.

Katlic M, Grillo HC. Carcinoma of the esophagus. In: Choi NC, Grillo HC, eds. Thoracic oncology. New York: Raven Press, 1983:279.

Kelsen D, Bains M, Hilaris B, Martini N. Combined modality therapy of esophageal cancer. Semin Oncol 1984; 11:169–177.

Langer M, Choi NC, Orlow E, Grillo HC, Wilkins EW Jr. Radiation therapy alone or in combination with surgery in the treatment of carcinoma of the esophagus. Cancer 1986; 58:1208–1213.

Leichman L, Steiger Z, Seydel HG, et al. Preoperative chemotherapy and radiation therapy for patients with cancer of the esophagus: a potentially curative approach. J Clin Oncol 1984; 2:75–79.

Pearson JG. Radiation therapy for carcinoma of the esophagus. In: Choi NC, Grillo HC, eds. Thoracic oncology. New York: Raven Press, 1983:303.

ESOPHAGEAL NEOPLASM: PALLIATION WITH SALIVARY TUBES

ALAN D. HILGENBERG, M.D.

In patients with obstructive esophageal neoplasms, palliation of dysphagia is the most important goal of therapy. Although more patients now have the potential for cure since the advent of aggressive multimodality treatment for esophageal carcinoma, many patients are encountered who are not candidates for chemotherapy or esophageal resection. These include patients who are very elderly, those with severe cardiac, respiratory, or renal diseases, and patients with widely disseminated metastatic disease.

Although resection undoubtedly offers the best palliation, several alternatives are available for patients who are unsuitable operative candidates. These include radiation and/or chemotherapy, laser ablation of intraluminal tumor, and dilation of the esophageal tumor and stenting with an intraluminal tube. Laser ablation is popular and attractive because a prosthesis within the esophagus is not necessary and gastroesophageal reflux can be avoided if the lower esophageal high-pressure zone remains intact. The laser's disadvantages include the need for several treatment sessions, regrowth of the neoplasm with recurrent esophageal obstruction, and the risk of esophageal perforation.

Esophageal intubation can usually be carried out by the peroral method, and this is preferable to the older approach utilizing a laparotomy and pulling the tube into position. Advantages of the peroral method include a choice of local or general anesthesia, gentle and progressive dilation of the esophageal tumor, a wide variety in the choice of diameters and lengths of esophageal tubes, which can be tailored to the patients' specific anatomic needs, and avoidance of a laparotomy. The indication for insertion of a peroral esophageal tube is palliation of the dysphagia associated with severe obstruction of the esophagus due to a biopsy-proven malignancy in patients who are unsuitable for surgical exploration and resection. Typical patients include those with medical contraindications to resection, those with extensive metastatic disease, those who have local invasion of mediastinal structures preventing resection, those with malignant tracheoesophageal fistulas, those who were treated primarily with radiation therapy and have recurrent esophageal obstruction, and those with local recurrence following previous esophageal resection.

Our technique of peroral esophageal intubation includes careful dilation of the tumor followed by insertion of a Silastic salivary bypass tube manufactured by Hood Laboratories of Pembroke, MA. General endotracheal anesthesia is usually used, although local anesthesia is possible. Initial esophagoscopy is done with the flexible esophagoscope, and a careful measurement is made of the distance between the upper incisors and the top of the esophageal tumor. This distance is then marked on a length of plastic tubing three-eighths inch or one-half inch in diameter; this tube serves as a "pusher tube." Dilation of the tumor is then carried out, and this can be done very nicely with the Savary dilators, which are passed over a wire inserted through the tumor, or with Maloney's bougies. When maximum dilatation has been achieved, a tube diameter approximately equal to the largest bougie is selected for insertion. This size is usually between 10 mm and 16 mm in diameter. The tube length is shortened so that, if possible, the distal end of the tube will lie beyond the tumor but not through the gastroesophageal junction. For those tumors located at the gastroesophageal junction, the tube necessarily traverses the junction into the stomach. The well-lubricated and tailored esophageal tube and the pusher tube are loaded on a small flexible endoscope or a bougie that will fit through the lumen of both of these tubes, and this composite is inserted through the patient's mouth and passed into the esophagus to the length previously measured on the pusher tube. The bougie and pusher tube are then removed, and repeat esophagoscopy is carried out in order to confirm satisfactory positioning of the Salivary bypass tube above the tumor.

Our experience includes placement of prosthetic tubes in 47 patients between 1979 and 1984. The median patient age was 67 years, and all but two tumors were located in the middle and distal thirds of the esophagus. Squamous cell and adenocarcinomas were represented in equal numbers.There was one hospital death (2.1 percent) and one perforation which the patient survived. All patients with prostheses experienced improved swallowing, although full liquids was the typical diet. Only one tube migrated after a course of radiation therapy resulted in tumor regression. Reflux and aspiration were noted in four patients. The average survival period was 3.5 months after tube insertion.

The peroral insertion of a tailored Silastic prosthetic tube can be accomplished with a low mortality and low risk of perforation in patients with advanced unresectable or recurrent esophageal carcinoma. Such tubes reliably improve dysphagia and increase patients' comfort during their remaining short life span.

SUGGESTED READING

Den Hartog Jager FCA, Bartelsman JFWM, Tytgat GNJ. Palliative treatment of obstructing esophagogastric malignancy by endoscopic positioning of a plastic prosthesis. Gastroenterology 1979; 77:1008-1014.

Montgomery WW. Salivary bypass tube. Ann Otol Rhinol Laryngol 1978; 87:159-162.

Richter JM, Hilgenberg AD, et al. Endoscopic palliation of obstructive esophagogastric malignancy. Gastrointest Endosc (in press).

Watson A. A study of the quality and duration of survival following resection, endoscopic intubation in esophageal carcinoma. Br J Surg 1982; 69:585-588.

I ESOPHAGEAL REPLACEMENT

ESOPHAGEAL REPLACEMENT

EARLE W. WILKINS Jr., M.D.

The surgical clinician must be thoroughly grounded in the technical considerations in the use of the various visceral esophageal substitutes but also, perhaps even more important, in the proper judgmental selection of which replacement to use under specific circumstances.

CHOICES

This discussion does not take into consideration (1) prosthetic replacement or (2) extrathoracic skin tube construction. The first of these has never reached the status of safe, leak-free use, merely because of sepsis at the replacement suture line; the second is essentially of historical interest.

This leaves three visceral substitutes for replacement of the esophagus: (1) stomach (transpositioned or reversed greater curvature tube), (2) colon, and (3) jejunum (transpositioned or autografted with microvascular anastomoses).

Specific factors that come into play in the ultimate selection include availability, anomalous anatomic variants, pathology in the substituting viscus, technical reliability in vascular supply and anastomotic healing, and experience of the operating surgeon.

PRINCIPLES

Particularly in malignant disease, the stomach is the most reliable substitute for the esophagus. This is because of its remarkable intrinsic blood supply, which permits its viability with only two of its original five arterial sources, and to its innate spatial pliability, which permits elongation with use of a point high on the greater curvature for anastomosis.

In nonmalignant disease, particularly peptic stricture in which a short replacement only is necessary, an interposed segment of either jejunum or transverse colon provides a mechanism for avoiding further gastroesophageal reflux. For a long replacement, however, when the substituting viscus must reach the neck, the colon is preferred because of its reliable marginal arterial supply, which is less complex and more easily prepared in dissection than the series of mesenteric vascular arcades of the jejunum.

There are special considerations at the extremes of patient age. In children still in the physiologic growth years, the stomach is better left in its normal anatomic and functional position and replacement effected by colon or jejunum (the latter reaches to higher levels more easily in children than in adults). In the older patient, i.e., beyond age 70, the stomach is preferred even in patients with nonmalignant disease because of less frequent atherosclerotic interference with its supplying arteries than with those of the colon and because there is need for only one anastomosis instead of the three required in intestinal replacement.

In general, the higher an esophagogastric anastomosis, the less likely the development of reflux peptic esophagitis. On the other hand, a full stomach lying at the apex of the thorax or reaching into the neck is a nocturnal risk for tracheobronchial aspiration of gastric contents.

STUDIES

Care must be taken that the replacement organ is actually usable anatomically and pathologically free of disease. Diagnostic methodology to clarify these points is limited to three procedures: endoscopy, arteriography, and contrast radiology.

The first of these provides the most useful information. If an esophageal carcinoma permits passage of an endoscope beyond the tumor, the interior of the stomach and duodenum should be carefully inspected with the flexible esophagogastroduodenoscope for (1) evidence of a second carcinoma, (2) peptic ulceration or scarring, and (3) adequacy of the pyloric channel. If the colon is to be utilized, it should be totally inspected by colonoscopy.

Arteriography is listed second because, when necessary, prior radiologic contrast studies may obscure its interpretation or delay its performance. The role of arteriography is in the assessment of colonic blood supply. Anomalous variations have been reported in over 10 percent of patients in whom the colon has been studied in this fashion. The point of particular interest is the marginal arterial communication between the left branch of the middle colic artery and the left colic artery, on which the successful employment of the left colon for replacement of the esophagus depends. The arterial vascular distribution to the right colon is less consistent. The great benefit of colonic arteriography is the clear anatomic road map it provides, with elimination of any surprise and/or confusion at the operating table. It further defines the presence of compromising atheromatous occlusion, especially at the origin of the inferior mesenteric artery. The complete arteriographic study includes catheter opacification of the celiac axis and superior and inferior mesenteric arteries.

Contrast radiology is the conventional method, by barium enema or upper gastrointestinal series, for outlining the extent of mucosal disease, diverticulosis, or diverticulitis. It requires no special comment. Computed tomography, ultrasonography, and magnetic resonance imaging in general are not helpful.

DRAWBACKS

There is no perfect esophageal replacement. Each viscus has some limitation, the details of which the surgeon must understand. The ultimate selection of the viscus to replace the stomach is a matter of judgmental balance of its pros and cons.

In the case of the stomach, when it is transpositioned into the chest utilizing the right gastroepiploic and right gastric arteries as its vascularizing source, its principal drawback is the loss of its physiologic function in nutrition. It becomes a conduit rather than a digestive organ. Other limitations are a potential for reflux acid-peptic esophagitis and a threat of nocturnal tracheal aspiration. When a reversed gastric tube is utilized, splenic loss results from obligatory splenectomy. When the colon is selected, the ultimate reliability of its marginal arteries *and* veins comes into question. The need for arteriography raises the possibility of technical complications in performance of the procedure, particularly of raising an intimal vascular flap or the development of coagulation compromise of an atherosclerotically narrowed femoral artery. An added drawback in the use of the colon is the requirement for three anastomoses: esophagocolic, cologastric, and colocolic.

MASSACHUSETTS GENERAL HOSPITAL EXPERIENCE: STOMACH AND COLON

The effectiveness of the choice of esophageal replacement is measured by (1) freedom from operative complications, (2) physiologic function, and (3) durability of the substituting viscus in its unaccustomed location.

Stomach

A review of 104 esophagectomies for carcinoma of the esophagus was conducted for the period 1980 to 1986. The resection was carried out by standard surgical approaches: left thoracoabdominal in 64, combined abdominal-right thoracic in 40. In each case the esophagectomy was accompanied by mediastinal and left gastric lymph node dissections. The hospital mortality was two (1.9 percent). The tumors were advanced, 78 patients (75 percent) having lymph node metastases. The striking finding was an anastomotic leakage rate of *zero*. All these patients underwent routine postoperative barium contrast study. The technique of anastomosis was standard in all 104, an inverting two-layer suture employing interrupted fine silk in both layers. Over 90 percent of the procedures were performed by senior cardiothoracic residents. The principal conclusion from this study is that the stomach is indeed a most reliable replacement for the esophagus. Blood supply for the two organs to be joined is the paramount requirement in the prevention of suture-line leakage. The stomach provides this vascularity with its right gastroepiploic and right gastric arteries intact.

Five patients have required one to three postoperative dilations for suture-line stricture. Late peptic stricture has not been a problem. Massachusetts General Hospital experience with use of the stomach to replace the esophagus dates back to 1940. It is known that the stomach provides a durable, lifetime replacement for the esophagus.

The stomach may also be utilized as an esophageal bypass via the anterior mediastinal route. Attention then must be addressed to the possible need for drainage of the esophagus by (1) Roux-en-Y esophagojejunal anastomosis or (2) external cervical drainage of the distal end of the transected cervical esophagus.

Colon

In an earlier study, the first 100 patients undergoing esophageal replacement or bypass by colon were evaluated, representing the period 1955 to 1978. The diagnostic indications are presented in Table 1.

The colon was used as a *replacement* for the esophagus in 34 patients; as a *bypass*, in 66. The route of colon placement for esophageal substitution is presented in Table 2.

There was a hospital mortality of nine, with the primary cause listed in Table 3.

There were three additional instances of nonfatal colon necrosis and seven transient cervical anastomotic leaks.

TABLE 1 Esophageal Diagnoses in 100 Consecutive Patients Undergoing Replacement or Bypass by Colon

Carcinoma	72
Caustic stricture	13
Congenital atresia	8
Peptic stricture	5
Achalasia	1
Postlaryngectomy stricture	1

TABLE 2 Anatomic Route of Colon Replacement

Anterior mediastinal	86
Left thoracic (Waterston)	10
Posterior mediastinal	2
Antethoracic subcutaneous	2

TABLE 3 Hospital Deaths

Colon necrosis	4
Pneumonia	2
Cardiovascular failure	2
Hepatic failure	1

The latter all healed spontaneously with local drainage only. The seven cases of colon necrosis are further broken down in Table 4 according to the side of colon utilized for the replacement. It seems clear that the left colon, retaining its source of blood supply from the left colic artery via its marginal communication with the midcolic artery, is the more reliable replacement. All colon placements in this series were isoperistaltic. Since preoperative analysis of the total mesenteric vascular pattern has been studied by angiographic techniques, there has been just one example of postoperative colon necrosis.

The late results verify the durability of the colon. The longest survivor has been swallowing normally through her esophagus-colon for 32 years. Eight patients have required proximal anastomotic dilation. Vomiting, when necessary, is normally possible through the interposed colon.

A disturbing late complication has been the development of atonic redundancy of the colon. This phenomenon can be minimized by avoiding excessive length of the colon replacement and by keeping the colon in the anterior mediastinum by avoiding wide opening of the right pleural membrane. Peptic ulceration has not occurred in the colon in this series.

TECHNIQUE

The operative details for replacement of the esophagus by the stomach are presented in the chapter *Malignant Tumor of the Lower Third of the Esophagus*.

Use of the colon for replacement of the esophagus requires attention to a specific set of principles and details. The left colon is the preferred segment for advancement into the thorax.

Principles

1. A preliminary vascular mapping is a requisite for the choice of colon and for definition of not uncommon anomalies.
2. The colon must be free of any disease, best determined by colonoscopy and barium enema study. These are carried out in this order, the colonoscopy defining mucosal abnormalities and the barium enema anatomic arrangement and extramucosal changes, such as diverticulosis.
3. Isoperistaltic placement of the colon in the thorax is superior to antiperistaltic.
4. A two-team approach is optimal, especially for the abdominal phase of colon preparation while the esophageal dissection is being conducted via a cervicomediastinal approach or while the cervical esophagus is being prepared in case of bypass only.

TABLE 4 Side of Colon Selected

	Uses	*Leaks*	*%*
Right	32	5	15.6
Left	68	2	2.9

Details (For a Bypass Procedure)

Abdominal. A long left paramedian incision is used extending to the xiphoid process. The colon is inspected for any unsuspected pathology, and its blood supply is verified.

1. The entire omentum is detached.
2. The posterior peritoneum is opened lateral to the descending colon. Careful blunt dissection is used to free its mesentery from retroperitoneal structures.
3. These two steps aid in the taking down of the splenic flexure. The spleen may usually be preserved undamaged; if it is damaged, every effort is made to control bleeding and avoid splenectomy.
4. The middle colic artery and vein are doubly ligated and divided near their origin at the superior mesenteric vessels.
5. Needed length of colon is measured and plotted along its axis as it is held cephalad from its left colic arterial source. The higher the proposed anastomosis, the longer the length of colon required and the farther to the right the point of colon transection.
6. The transverse colon is transected using the GIA stapler.
7. The mesentery of the sigmoid colon is transilluminated in identifying the left colic artery and electing the point of appropriate sigmoid transection.
8. The descending or sigmoid colon is transected using the GIA stapler.
9. The colon segment to be used, now attached only to its supplying artery and vein, is passed posterior to the stomach through a rent in the gastrohepatic omentum. This permits the most direct alignment of its artery and avoids any subsequent postsurgical pressure displacement downward by a full stomach.
10. A retrosternal tunnel is constructed by blunt dissection, separating the diaphragmatic attachments from the back of the xiphoid process and passing two fingers, and then the whole hand, into this avascular compartment. Entry into the pleural sacs is minimized by sweeping the supinated hand gently from the midline to the left. At this point particular attention is directed to cardiac dysrhythmia or hypotension. Should either of these occur, the hand must intermittently be withdrawn until such cardiovascular abnormalities have been corrected.
11. After retrosternal placement of the colon has been carried out (see Cervical below), the cologastric

anastomosis is made to the anterior aspect of the midbody of the stomach, or to the proximal jejunum if the stomach has been removed, using a two-layer anastomosis—inner fine running catgut and outer interrupted silk sutures.

12. The colocolic anastomosis completes the establishment of recontinuity—two layers of interrupted silk. This may be actually carried out as the initial anastomosis.
13. The colon mesentery is meticulously closed, to itself or to the retroperitoneum, leaving no aperture for small bowel herniation.

Cervical. A left oblique presternocleidomastoid incision is preferred, extending from the tip of the mastoid process to the suprasternal notch. Broad exposure is essential. The lower pretracheal muscle insertions are detached.

1. The prevertebral fascial plane is exposed by dividing the omohyoid muscle and bluntly dissecting the tissues in the space anterior to the carotid sheath.
2. The cervical esophagus is identified from behind, just on the prevertebral fascia, and is encircled cautiously, immediately upon its muscular coat, to avoid damage to either recurrent nerve. It is then gently retracted with a Penrose tape. Recurrent nerve palsy, even unilateral, enhances the likelihood of postoperative aspiration.
3. The upper portion of the retrosternal tunnel is bluntly dissected with fingers, in conjunction with step 10 above.
4. If the entrance to this plane does not accept four fingers comfortably, it is enlarged by removing 2 to 3 cm of the anterior ends of the left clavicle and the left first rib. In the bypass procedure particularly, adding a structure emerging from the thoracic inlet requires sufficient room to avoid vascular compromise of the transpositioned colon and its anastomosis.
5. The cervical esophagus is transected 2 to 3 cm below the cricopharyngeus muscle border, turning in the stapled distal end with interrupted silk sutures and marking the proximal end with identifying long stitches.
6. The colon is passed through the tunnel with attention to three details. A long, heavy thread attached to the proximal colon end is first brought through a glove or sheet of plastic covering its end and then upward through the tunnel. The "gloved" end is guided upward through the retrosternal space, avoiding contamination. Care is taken to allow the colon mesentery containing its sustaining vessels to lie on the right posterior aspect of the colon; it should be checked that there is no possibility of twist.
7. Once placed, the end of the colon is carefully inspected for arterial pulsations; if none are visible or palpable, they are checked by incising the colon, where the stapled closure end is actually excised. A Doppler probe is often helpful. If the blood supply is inadequate, the colon segment is withdrawn into the abdomen, reassessed, and carefully replaced. Rarely, blood supply is totally insufficient, and the colon must be discarded. A nonviable colon segment is a tragic life-threatening postoperative complication. Arterial enhancement by a cervical microvascular anastomosis from an inferior thyroid or internal mammary artery is an alternative procedure for consideration.
8. A two-layer inverting interrupted silk anastomosis between esophagus and colon completes the procedure (see the chapter *Malignant Tumor of the Lower Third of the Esophagus* for details). The larger colon lumen requires wider spacing of sutures on its side in comparison to those placed in the esophagus.
9. Closure is accomplished without drainage.
10. Simple interrupted platysma and skin closure permits easy "second-look" exposure under local anesthesia if there is any postoperative concern about viability of the colon. If a necrotic colon is encountered postoperatively, it must be completely removed early.

Miscellany. 1. A gastrostomy provides early decompression of the stomach, particularly to avoid vomiting, and later is useful for feeding. 2. A sump nasogastric tube is placed through the upper anastomosis to prevent gaseous distention of the colon segment in the mediastinum. 3. A portable chest film is obtained immediately upon completion of the operation while the patient is still on the operating table. Single or bilateral chest tubes are inserted if pneumothorax is discovered. 4. Oral feedings, except for sips of water, are not begun until a barium swallow study shows intact anastomoses on days 7 through 10.

SUGGESTED READING

Mathisen DJ, Grillo HC, Hilgenberg AD, Moncure AC, Wilkins EW Jr. Transthoracic esophagogastrectomy: a safe approach to carcinoma of the esophagus. Ann Thorac Surg (in press).

Nebesar RA, Kornblith PL, Pollard JJ, Michels NA. Celiac and superior mesenteric arteries. Boston: Little, Brown, 1969.

Wilkins EW Jr. Long-segment colon substitution for the esophagus. Ann Surg 1980; 192:722–725.

SHORT SEGMENT JEJUNAL INTERPOSITION

HIRAM C. POLK Jr., M.D.

By definition, when one faces the issue of esophageal replacement for benign diseases, one is usually dealing with a sequence of judgment errors, treatment failures, or, worse still, technical misadventures.

The patient with benign disease who has been allowed to progress to a need for esophageal replacement as part of his primary operation has either neglected him- or herself or been medically mismanaged. These situations are increasingly avoided by knowledgeable internists who are now often more sophisticated in matters of gastroesophageal reflux.

As we have stated elsewhere, the need for esophageal replacement is primarily determined by the presence of an undilatable stricture, which is increasingly infrequent, and the more frequent and common cause today, failure of previous operative therapy of gastroesophageal reflux. The frequency with which such failure is identified is in no measure an expression of a general lack of efficacy of antireflux operations. It simply is an inevitable spin-off of the frequency with which antireflux operations are being carried out across the country, with failure rates on the order of 4 to 10 percent.

There are no specific indications for selection of jejunal interposition. On the other hand, it has been my general preference for its use in the face of the nondilatable stricture, and I find its greatest value in those patients who have continuing reflux that has not responded to multiple previous operations. It is this "locked in the open position" situation that I think is most amenable to jejunal interposition. The only specific contraindication would be the presence of disease in the small bowel, such as diverticula or Crohn's disease, and the problems of length. Although Ong and others have shown the capacity to take long jejunal loops to the posterior pharynx, in general this is technically fraught with difficulty. Under those sets of circumstances, we usually prefer to use the colon. Angiography is almost never needed in preparation for the fashioning of a jejunal segment, since the blood supply is predictable and, if the upper segment is indeed diseased, one can easily shift to a slightly lower portion of jejunum.

Certain technical details are worthy of emphasis. The surgeon should choose a segment of jejunum well distal to the ligament of Treitz with as wide a mesenteric base as is feasible, and the length of the segment should be more than sufficient to replace the segment of esophagus to be resected. The blood supply to the jejunum can best be seen by transillumination in all but the most obese patients. The most important technical maneuver in this undertaking is to place notches just as a seamstress might to lengthen the peritoneal covering of the mesentery. The mesentery and its blood vessels are quite elastic. On the other hand, the fan-shaped peritoneum overlying the mesentery can be sharply restrictive of length, and notches of this sort are very useful, particularly when the segment must be carried well up into the chest.

As previously described, we pass the segment through the transverse mesocolon, behind the stomach, and well up into the chest. We had a brief experience using endoesophagus to the side of the jejunum, but we have one patient in whom the proximal jejunal pouch has become a nuisance. We think that we would not do that again, although it will occasionally allow you to take the segment a little higher than if you use the end of the jejunum exclusively.

We also have erred in one case in doing the jejunogastrostomy too low in the stomach; it is very important that it be well up in the fundus of the stomach, since if it is placed in the antral area, vigorous antral contractions may lead to bowel reflux in all of these patients.

The other details of the procedure, including the relative desirability of a pyloroplasty or pyloromyotomy, are noted in detail elsewhere.

The reason for preference for jejunum over colon or stomach when esophageal replacement is required is largely a theoretic one and based on a sequence of experiments done by Henry Harkins more than 3 decades ago, indicating that the jejunum was somewhat more tolerant of gastric secretions than the colon. Clearly, the decision to use low esophagogastric anastomosis after resection for benign disease is usually associated with persistent symptoms no matter to what extent one pursues "ink-welling" or a fundoplasty kind of procedure. The exception to this may well be the reversed gastric tube of Gavrilu, although this procedure has been used so sporadically as to make it difficult to define its real utility. My own preference for jejunal interposition is based on an experience that now dates to 22 years. It is the long-term utility of this method that reassures me as to its value. We have now performed 35 procedures for gastroesophageal junction replacement with jejunum in a group of patients who had an intimidating series of previously failed operations. More than half of these patients have had follow-up barium studies of the proximal alimentary tract more than 10 years after their operation, indicating the long-term durability of the procedure. The test of method is, of course, the fact that no patient among the 34 survivors has seen a physician for anything that was interpreted clinically or radiographically as complications of gastroesophageal reflux. We do have two patients who represent failures of the method of substitution, both manifesting imprecisely defined arrays of gastrointestinal dysfunction, one being an overt upper alimentary tract cripple with severe dumping syndrome. In one case, this dysfunction was due to placement of the *jejunogastric* anastomosis well into the antrum so that when reflux occurred with antral contraction, this was immediately corrected by moving the jejunogastrostomy into the upper stomach with an excellent intermediate term result. The other long-term failure has not yet been assessed, but it is thought to represent a patient whose physiologic disability is accentuated by her psychiatric abnormalities. In addition, Cuschieri and associate recently reported similar good results using the same method.

The technical details of the operation are demanding,

particularly as pertains to protection of the blood supply to the jejunum, especially its venous limb, and the need for a secure and now preferred end-to-end esophagojejunal anastomosis.

SUGGESTED READING

Jones EL, Skinner DB, DeMeester TR, Elkins RC, Zuidema GD. Response of the interposed human colonic segment to an acid challenge. Ann Surg 1973; 177:75–78.

Merendino KA, Dillard DH. The concept of sphincter substitution by an interposed jejunal segment for anatomic and physiologic abnormalities at the esophagogastric junction. Ann Surg 1955; 142:486.

Plazk LF Jr, Fried W, Woodward ER. Relative susceptibility of the gastrointestinal tract to experimental acute peptic ulceration. Surg Forum 1956; 7:389–393.

Polk HC Jr. Jejunal interposition for reflux esophagitis and esophageal stricture unresponsive to valvuloplasty. World J Surg 1980; 4:731–736.

Wright C, Cuschieri A. Jejunal interposition for benign esophageal disease: technical considerations and long-term results. Ann Surg 1987; 54–60.

FREE JEJUNAL GRAFT

M. J. JURKIEWICZ, M.D., F.A.C.S.
CHRISTIAN E. PALETTA, M.D.

Reconstruction of the cervical esophagus using transplanted intestine dates back to 1906 when Alexis Carrel reported his successful transplantation of intestine to the neck in a dog. Longmire in 1946 successfully anastomosed an ischemic jejunal segment to the internal mammary vessels. The first immediate free jejunal transfer was performed by Seidenberg in 1959 for cervical esophageal replacement.

With the development of microsurgical techniques in the early and mid 1970s, free tissue transfer became introduced into the operative theater. A wide variety of tissues was available for distant transfer. Each had its own advantage and utility. Such tissues include muscle (such as the latissimus dorsi, the gracilis, the rectus abdominis), cutaneous flaps (groin flap, scapular flap), the great or second toe for thumb reconstruction, iliac crest and fibula for bony reconstruction, the omentum, and the jejunum. With increasing experience in microvascular surgery, the successful transfer of these tissues approaches 90 to 95 percent. The procedure can be accomplished in one stage and provides the patient who has had an extensive pharyngeal and upper esophageal resection with an intact functioning cervical conduit.

INDICATIONS AND CONTRAINDICATIONS

The indications for free jejunal transfer in cervical esophageal reconstruction are listed in Table 1. In the overwhelming majority of instances, free jejunal reconstruction follows surgical removal of a malignant pharyngeal or laryngeal neoplasm. This may be done either immediately following the pharyngectomy, laryngectomy, or both, or several months or years later following operation for local recurrence or stricture due to radiation and scarring.

Contraindications to free jejunal transfer are listed in Table 2. Previous or subsequent irradiation is not a contraindication. While irradiation usually makes dissection of the recipient vessels more difficult, it does not usually prevent the successful microvascular transfer. If irradiation has been particularly damaging, occasionally the contralateral neck vessels will be utilized as recipient vessels.

ALTERNATIVE FORMS OF TREATMENT

Various forms of cervical esophageal replacement have been used over the past 40 years. Free skin grafts are advantageous in their simplicity. Unfortunately they are not applicable in the complex wounds often seen following extensive tumor resection and irradiation. A high incidence of orocutaneous fistula and recurrent stricture follows use of this technique. Various neck flaps have been utilized that require tubing of neck skin. While this may be applicable in lye stricture, this tissue is not usually available in the tumor patient who has undergone irradiation. Employment of the deltopectoral flap remains a useful technique in a selected patient with complications. Unfortunately it is usually a two-stage procedure. Replacement with the pectoralis major myocutaneous flap is a

TABLE 1 Indications for Free Jejunal Grafts

Full circumferential resection of pharynx, larynx, and cervical esophagus
Partial resection of pharynx, larynx, and cervical esophagus when residual tissue insufficient for safe closure
Fixed cervical stricture following resection and primary closure
Cervical stricture following caustic ingestion
Adequate stomach and colon not available for reconstruction

TABLE 2 Contraindications to Free Jejunal Transfer

Child less than 2 to 3 years of age
Significant atherosclerotic carotid disease
Absence of adequately trained microvascular team
History of small-bowel obstruction with significant adhesions
History of inflammatory bowel disease or Gardner's syndrome

reliable one-stage method. It is useful for a less than circumferential resection. It is usually too bulky when the skin island is tubed for total cervical esophageal replacement.

Gastric or colon interposition is preferred by some surgeons for cervical esophageal reconstruction. Each has the advantage of being a single-stage procedure with a reliable blood supply and is more applicable for middle and lower esophageal replacement. When used in the middle and upper neck, it often results in excessive tension at the proximal suture line.*

ADVANTAGES OF THE FREE JEJUNAL GRAFT

The advantages of the free jejunal graft are listed in Table 3. The jejunum represents an excellent substitute for the cervical esophagus. A segment up to 20 cm can be transferred based on a single pedicle. The integrity of the gastrointestinal tract is preserved, thereby avoiding complications related to the disruption or loss of the gastroesophageal junction or pylorus. The chief disadvantage of the free jejunal graft is that it requires a surgical team skilled in microsurgical techniques. Such a team, however, is now available in most centers.

SURGICAL TECHNIQUE

When used in immediate reconstruction following pharyngolaryngectomy, a two-team approach is the most expeditious. Care must be taken during the extirpative procedure to identify and preserve branches of the external carotid artery. The superior thyroid, lingual, and facial arteries are all usually sufficient with respect to location, adequate vessel diameter, and blood flow. In addition, the transverse cervical artery at the base of the neck can be preserved during neck dissection and utilized if the external carotid artery branches are too scarred or fragile from irradiation. Occasionally, contralateral vessels may be used when ipsilateral vessels are inadequate. For venous drainage the external jugular vein or a branch of the internal jugular vein is utilized.

Once it has been established that an adequate recipient artery and vein are available, laparotomy is performed. An upper midline incision is utilized. The ligament of Treitz is identified. A segment of jejunum, usually 15 to 30 cm from the ligament of Treitz, is chosen for transfer. Typically 10 to 14 cm of bowel is necessary in most cases. The vascular arcade is identified. The segment of bowel is then isolated in its vascular pedicle. Care must be taken not to injure the superior mesenteric artery. The two ends of bowel are then divided. The segment of jejunum to be transferred is then left only on its pedicle, while the jejunal anastomosis is formed in a two-layer fashion. This allows the surgeon to observe the viability of the entire free jejunal segment over a 10- to 20- minute period of blood flow from its isolated pedicle (Fig. 1). A feeding jejunostomy is usually created at the end of the abdominal procedure to provide for immediate postoperative nutritional support. In addition, should a problem develop with the flap or a fistula occur, the jejunostomy will maintain enteral support.

Once the recipient vessels are prepared for microscopic anastomosis, the jejunal pedicle is divided and irrigated with heparin. The graft is then transferred to the neck. The jejunum is placed in an isoperistaltic fashion. The proximal anastomosis is often at the level of the nasopharynx and is best carried out prior to the microsurgical anastomosis. A single layer of 3-0 Dexon is used for the proximal anastomosis. The vascular anastomosis is then accomplished using 9-0 or 10-0 prolene or nylon (Fig. 2). Peristalsis is usually seen within 15 minutes of the completion of the vascular anastomosis. A 16 F tube is placed via the nose through the jejunum and into the thoracic esophagus. This serves as a stent to allow the flow of saliva and mucus through the graft for the first week. The distal anastomosis is completed, and the neck flaps

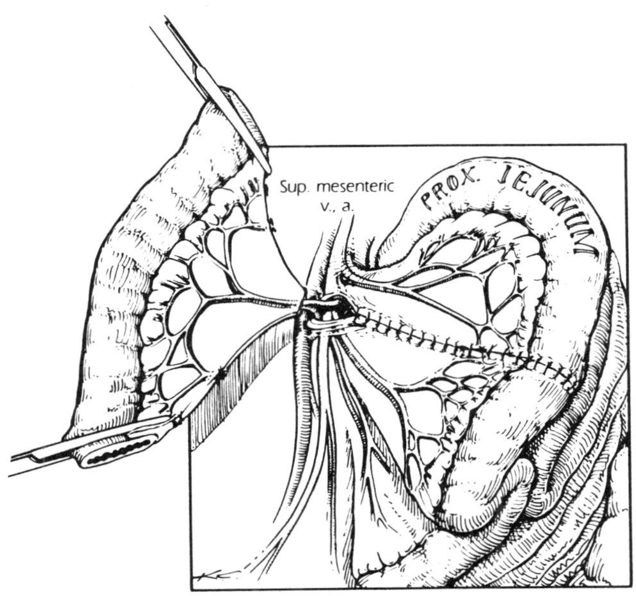

Figure 1 A segment of jejunum has been dissected with its vascular pedicle. Bowel continuity is reestablished with an end-to-end anastomosis. (Courtesy of Kip Carter in Athens, Georgia.)

* Editor's Note: The authors would disagree except for the use of the stomach to the base of the tongue. At all other levels the stomach and colon can be used without tension, especially when the left colon is used and incorporates the right and left branch of the middle colic artery so that the hepatic flexure can also be used for additional length.

TABLE 3 Advantages of Free Jejunal Graft

Dependable, consistent donor site
One-stage procedure
Transfer reliability rate > 90%
Low mortality—5%
Low incidence of postoperative stricture
Successful transfer independent of preoperative or postoperative radiation treatment
Less bulky compared with regional myocutaneous flaps
Continuity of gastroesophageal junction and pylorus not disturbed

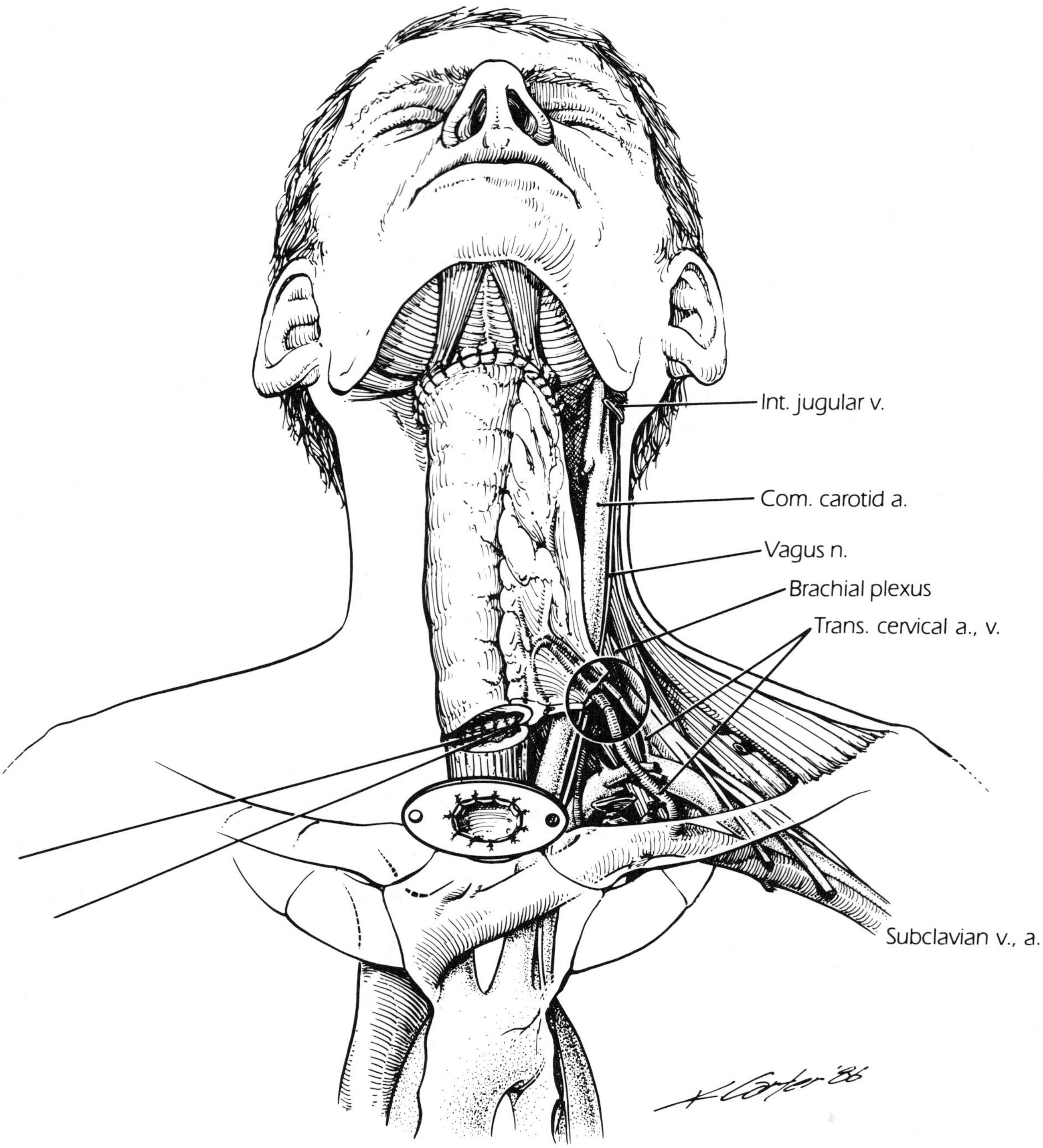

Figure 2 The segment of free jejunal graft is sutured in an isoperistaltic manner. The proximal anastomosis is carried out first. An adjacent artery and vein (here the transverse cervical vessels) are anastomosed to the jejunal vessels in a microvascular fashion. A portion of the jejunum is then covered with a split thickness skin graft in order to monitor the flap in the postoperative period. (Courtesy of Kip Carter in Athens, Georgia.)

are closed. A small segment of the jejunum is left exposed or covered with a split skin graft. This allows the surgeon to check the viability of the flap.

Five to seven days following surgery, gastrografin is given orally, and radiographic examination is carried out. If no leak is present, administration of clear liquids is begun and the diet advanced as tolerated.

RESULTS

We have carried out more than 90 free jejunal grafts for cervical esophageal reconstruction since 1978. The results of our first 55 are listed in Table 4. We have achieved a 90 percent success rate in free graft transfer with mortality of 5 percent.

TABLE 4 Results of Free Jejunal Graft in 55 Patients (1978–1984)

	No.	*%*
Successful graft viability	49	90
Perioperative mortality	3	5

TABLE 5 Complications

Recipient Site
- Microvascular thrombosis
- Jejunal graft necrosis
- Esophagocutaneous fistula
- Anastomotic stricture
- Anastomotic aneurysm
- Dysphagia
- Revascularization mucorrhea
- Aspiration

Donor Site
- Anastomotic leak
- Small-bowel obstruction
- Feeding jejunostomy problems
- Abdominal dehiscence

COMPLICATIONS

There is a wide variety of complications that can be encountered from free jejunal transfer. Complications can occur at both the recipient site and the donor site (Table 5). While these complications are infrequent, when they do occur they can be devastating to the patient.

SUGGESTED READING

Hester TR, McConnell F, Nahai F, Cunningham S, Jurkiewicz MJ. Pharyngoesophageal stricture and fistula: treatment by free jejunal graft. Ann Surg 1984; 199:762–769.

Hester TR, McConnell F, Nahai F, Jurkiewicz M, Brown R. Reconstruction of cervical esophagus, hypopharynx and oral cavity using free jejunal transfer. Am J Surg 1980; 140:487–491.

Jurkiewicz MJ. Reconstructive surgery of the cervical esophagus. J Thorac Cardiovasc Surg 1984; 88:893–897.

Jurkiewicz MJ. Vascularized intestinal graft for reconstruction of the cervical esophagus and pharynx. Plast Reconstr Surg 1965; 36:509–517.

Sasaki TM, Baker HW, McConnell DB, Vetto RM. Free jejunal graft reconstruction after extensive head and neck surgery. Am J Surg 1980; 139:650–653.

REVERSED GASTRIC TUBE GRAFT

HENRY J. HEIMLICH, M.D., D.Sc.(Hon), F.A.C.S., F.C.C.P.
GERSON C. CARR, M.D., S.B.

The reversed gastric tube (RGT) is the most physiologic substitute for the esophagus. The stomach enjoys an excellent blood supply and tolerates its own secretions. The upper end of the pedicled tube graft that is anastomosed to the cervical esophagus or hypopharynx is fashioned from gastric antrum. The antral portion of the stomach contains no acid-secreting parietal cells; therefore the esophagus proximal to the one and only anastomosis is not subject to acid peptic digestion. The operation is indicated whenever replacement of the esophagus is warranted.

THERAPEUTIC ALTERNATIVES

The stomach is technically suitable for esophageal replacement. Its anatomic site is close to the organ to be replaced. Preoperative cleansing or bacterial suppression is not required. Adequate graft length is always available when there has been no prior gastric resection. No vascular anastomosis is required because the graft pedicle provides augmented perfusion via its own intact blood supply. The thick, serosa-invested stomach wall adapts well to stapling and suture techniques, and the muscle tone maintains a resilient conduit without haustra or mucosal valves to impede the passage of a food bolus.

The RGT usually traverses an intrathoracic route, but functions equally well when circumstances dictate placing it in a subcutaneous antesternal tunnel. The intestinal tract remains intact, avoiding obstruction, compression, or internal herniation about abdominal anastomoses or displaced mesenteric pedicles.

For all the reasons mentioned above, we believe that the use of jejunal or colonic interposition to replace the esophagus is less desirable than the reversed gastric tube.

TECHNIQUE

The RGT procedure uses splenectomy to augment blood supply to the gastric tube. In 1955 the senior author published experimental work demonstrating that splenectomy performed with ligation and division of the splenic artery and vein distal to the origin of the left gastroepiploic vessels enables survival of the gastric tube, whereas the older Beck-Jianu operation that preserves the spleen was never successful for esophageal replacement. In recent years it has been demonstrated that splenectomy may not be required in young children, presumably because of the adaptability of the circulation and mobility of the lienorenal ligament.

Because of the cardinal importance of augmenting graft perfusion via the left gastroepiploic vessels in the adult patient, the hilus of the spleen must not be treated in the usual manner employed for splenectomy. Rather than dividing the splenic pedicle between clamps, the technique here requires leaving the splenic vessels intact until exposure permits dissection and individual ligation of their branches. Preliminary steps include division of the full length of the gastrocolic ligament; sharp dissection to free the gastric fundus and cardia from any tether to the diaphragm; division of adhesions between the spleen and parietes with care to avoid injury or premature stripping of its peritoneum; division of the short gastric vessels; and freeing of the pancreatic tail from its bed until the spleen and its vessels can be delivered intact to the level of the anterior abdominal wall. Only then should the operator proceed to incise the peritoneum overlying the anterior hilus of the spleen where the branches of the splenic vessels may be clamped and divided.

A gastrostomy is provided for postoperative care. As a general rule, gastrostomies function best when placed high on the anterior wall of the stomach near the lesser curvature, whether in anticipation of or during esophageal reconstruction. Should a preexisting gastrostomy impinge upon the greater curvature, it can be closed and incorporated in either the tube or the gastric remnant.

The open upper end of the RGT is created 4 cm proximal to the pylorus by dividing the greater curvature between two rows of staples placed obliquely. This angle increases the diameter of the orifice at the upper end of the tube, facilitating the subsequent anastomosis in the neck. Staples should be long enough to securely approximate the thick walls of the antrum.

The row of staples that close what will become the upper end of the RGT is cut away, and a 28 F (9.3 mm diameter) rectal tube is inserted to be held against the greater curvature while staples are being inserted to form the RGT. The staples that would otherwise be included in the anastomosis are removed and replaced with interrupted sutures. Using a continuous seromuscular suture, the surgeon oversews and inverts the long row of staples that close the gastric remnant and the side of the tube. To accommodate growth in children, the sutures must be interrupted or absorbable. The tube is wrapped in the omentum to protect both the longitudinal suture line and the anastomosis in the neck.

COMPLICATIONS

After splenectomy performed as outlined above, the potentially fatal complication of graft necrosis will not occur; we have not had a case. Should there be any reason to doubt either the viability of the RGT or the integrity of the splenic and gastroepiploic vessels in the graft pedicle, the closed end of the RGT can be brought up into the neck, with the anastomosis deferred for a second-stage operation.

Performance of the operation in two stages is recommended for patients who might not tolerate the hours of general anesthesia required for a one-stage procedure. Furthermore, after a delay of 2 to 4 weeks, adhesions about the tube will seal it off so that spillage from an anastomotic leak will be confined to the region of the neck. This delay is an especially valuable safeguard in patients previously subjected to radiotherapy for cancer of the cervical or upper thoracic esophagus, since they are at high risk for leaks at the anastomosis.

Drainage may be omitted when there is a secure anastomosis between an RGT with an adequate blood supply and a normal or hypertrophic cervical esophagus. Leakage is most likely at the T-shaped junction where the suture line in the tube meets the two-layer anastomosis to the cervical esophagus or hypopharynx. A small leak usually heals spontaneously.

Angulation or stricture is possible where the lower end of the RGT enters the gastric remnant. A few properly placed interrupted sutures between the stomach and the right anterior parietal peritoneum will usually prevent this problem. Should dysphagia occur later because of angulation where the RGT enters the stomach, it can be overcome by means of a longitudinal incision with transverse closure.

SUGGESTED READING

Heimlich HJ. Esophageal replacement with a reversed gastric tube. Dis Chest 1959; 36:478–493.

Heimlich HJ. Esophagitis: complications treated by total bypass without esophageal resection. Ann Thorac Surg 1970: 10:203–212.

Heimlich HJ. Reversed gastric tube (RGT) esophagoplasty for failure of colon, jejunum and prosthetic interpositions. Ann Surg 1975; 182:154–160.

Heimlich HJ. Heimlich operation for esophageal replacement. In: Nyhus LM, Baker RJ, eds. Mastery of surgery. Boston: Little, Brown, 1984:440.

Heimlich HJ, Winfield JM. The use of a gastric tube to replace or bypass the esophagus. Surgery 1955; 37:549–559.

TRANSHIATAL ESOPHAGECTOMY

MARK B. ORRINGER, M.D.

Despite improvements in preoperative evaluation, anesthetic and operative techniques, and postoperative care, esophageal resection and reconstruction remain a formidable undertaking in patients whose nutritional and pulmonary status have been compromised by impaired swallowing. Transhiatal esophagectomy without thoracotomy eliminates the morbidity of a thoracotomy in these patients as well as the hazards of an intrathoracic anastomotic disruption, since the routine performance of a *cervical* esophageal anastomosis minimizes the likelihood of fatal sepsis resulting from anastomotic disruption. My personal experience with more than 300 patients undergoing transhiatal esophagectomy without thoracotomy has led to my current belief that there are few indications for opening the thorax in patients requiring esophageal resection and reconstruction, either for benign or malignant disease.

INDICATIONS AND CONTRAINDICATIONS

Virtually every patient who is a candidate for esophageal resection is regarded as a candidate for transhiatal esophagectomy without thoracotomy. This method of esophageal resection has been possible in patients who have had prior mediastinal irradiation, mediastinitis from perforation, multiple prior esophageal operations, or a megaesophagus of achalasia. I have performed transhiatal resections in patients who have undergone multiple prior esophagomyotomies, repair of perforations, repair of esophageal atresia, and repair of hiatal hernias. It is neither the number nor types of prior esophageal operations that determine whether transhiatal resection is possible, but rather the degree of periesophageal fibrosis and adhesions encountered at the time of resection. Virtually all of my patients with esophageal carcinoma who have received preoperative chemotherapy and radiation therapy have had an esophagus that could be resected without opening the thorax.

My primary indication for transthoracic esophagectomy is an inability to perform a transhiatal resection. In 175 patients with carcinoma of the intrathoracic esophagus, transhiatal esophageal resection has been possible in all but six; these six required either a thoracotomy or an esophageal bypass because of adherence of the diseased esophagus to contiguous intrathoracic structures. In 84 patients with benign disease requiring esophageal resection, the transhiatal approach has been utilized successfully in 80. In the remainder, because of dense periesophageal adhesions appreciated on palpation and inspection of the esophagus through the diaphragmatic hiatus, the transhiatal route was abandoned and a transthoracic resection performed. In patients with esophageal carcinoma, endoscopic evidence of tracheobronchial *invasion* (not contiguity) is an absolute contraindication to transhiatal esophagectomy without thoracotomy. Because patients with hepatic, supraclavicular lymph node, or distant metastatic disease have such a limited life expectancy, they are not regarded as candidates for esophagectomy. Above all, it must be realized that the major contraindication to transhiatal esophagectomy is the surgeon's determination on palpation of the esophagus through the diaphragmatic hiatus and the cervical incision that transhiatal resection is unsafe. Thus, tumor fixation to the aorta, the pericardium, or the tracheobronchial tree discovered during transhiatal exploration should be regarded as warning signals, and persistent attempts to resect the esophagus through the hiatus should be abandoned lest a catastrophe occur. If the esophagus containing a tumor is grasped through the diaphragmatic hiatus and "rocked" so that the surgeon can be reasonably confident that there is no fixation to contiguous structures, transhiatal resection will almost inevitably be possible.

PREOPERATIVE PREPARATION

Abstinence from cigarette smoking for at least 2 weeks before surgery and the use of an incentive spirometer on an outpatient basis are consistently rewarded by fewer postoperative respiratory complications. When severe esophageal obstruction precludes adequate caloric intake, placement of a nasogastric feeding tube through the endoscopically dilated stricture allows an intake of 2,000 to 3,000 calories per day and avoids the need for intravenous hyperalimentation, which I virtually never utilize. Oral hygiene must not be neglected, since virulent bacteria in carious teeth may greatly increase the severity of infection should an anastomotic leak occur. Therefore dental consultation and repair or extraction of carious teeth are routine. If there is a history of previous gastric surgery, adequate gastric length for esophageal substitution may not be available. In such cases, a barium enema study is obtained to evaluate the suitability of the colon as an esophageal substitute, and the colon is prepared preoperatively in the event that colonic interposition is required.

TECHNICAL ASPECTS

The patient is positioned supine, with the neck extended and the head turned toward the right. The operative field extends from the mandible to the pubis and from midaxillary line to midaxillary line. The arms are padded and placed at the patient's side after insertion of a radial artery catheter for monitoring of intra-arterial blood pressure during the transhiatal resection.

A self-retaining, table-mounted upper-abdominal ("upper-hand") retractor facilitates exposure. The operation is performed through an upper-midline supraumbilical abdominal incision and a 5 to 8-cm oblique cervical incision paralleling the anterior border of the left sternocleidomastoid muscle.

The stomach is mobilized by dividing the left gastroepiploic and short gastric vessels along the high greater curvature and then the left gastric artery and its branches along the high lesser curvature. The spleen is protected. The right gastroepiploic artery is preserved as the greater omentum is divided between clamps and ligated at least 1.5 cm away. A Kocher maneuver, pyloromyotomy, and feeding jejunosotomy are routine. After encircling of the esophagogastric junction the diaphragmatic hiatus is progressively dilated, one finger at a time, until the surgeon's hand can reach into the posterior mediastinum through the diaphragmatic hiatus. A surgeon whose glove size is larger than 7 may be unable to fit his hand safely into the mediastinum without inordinate displacement of the heart and secondary hypotension. Transhiatal esophagectomy is performed as a midline dissection, with the volar aspects of the fingers applied to the esophagus to minimize injury to adjacent structures. Five to ten cm of distal thoracic esophagus are mobilized through the diaphragmatic hiatus prior to turning attention to the neck.

Through the neck incision the sternocleidomastoid muscle and carotid sheath are retracted laterally, and the trachea and thyroid gland medially, avoiding injury to the recurrent laryngeal nerve. The cervical esophagus is encircled with a Penrose drain, and as upward traction is applied to this drain, blunt dissection of the cervical esophagus from the superior mediastinum is performed by advancing the index and middle fingers alongside the esophagus into the chest.

The esophageal mobilization is performed in an orderly fashion through the diaphragmatic hiatus and the cervical incision. First, the esophagus is dissected away from the prevertebral fascia posteriorly. Anteriorly the esophagus is mobilized away from the tracheobronchial tree. The remaining lateral attachments are then gently avulsed by a downward raking motion of the fingers trapping the esophagus against the prevertebral fascia. When the entire esophagus is mobile the cervical esophagus is divided with a GIA surgical stapler, and the thoracic esophagus is delivered downward through the diaphragmatic hiatus into the abdominal wound. The entire stomach and attached esophagus are placed on the anterior thorax, and the distal esophagus or proximal stomach is separated from the specimen with the surgical stapler. This technique of esophagectomy can also be utilized for tumors limited to the esophagogastric junction, since division of the stomach along the lesser curvature 4 to 6 cm distal to the tumor preserves the entire greater curvature and that point that reaches most cephalad to the neck. After removal of the esophagus, both pleurae are inspected visually and by palpation, and if indicated, a chest tube is inserted. A Penrose drain is then positioned in the esophageal bed in the posterior mediastinum so that one end emerges from the cervical incision and one end from the diaphragmatic hiatus. The most cephaled-reaching point of the gastric fundus is sutured to the Penrose drain in the abdomen. Traction on the cervical end of the Penrose drain and gentle manipulation of the stomach from below through the diaphragmatic hiatus are used to position the stomach into the chest in the original esophageal bed until the gastric fundus is visible in the neck incision. The stomach is then suspended in the neck by suturing it to the prevertebral fascia. In virtually every normal patient the gastric fundus easily reaches several centimeters above the level of the clavicles and permits a tension-free cervical esophagogastric anastomosis. If inadequate length of stomach is left because of prior resection or injury, a colon interposition procedure is performed by mobilizing an isoperistaltic segment of colon and positioning it into the posterior mediastinum in the original esophageal bed. The jejunostomy tube is secured to the anterior abdominal wall, the abdominal incision is closed, and an end-to-side anastomosis between the cervical esophagus and gastric fundus is performed with a single layer of 4-0 interrupted absorbable (polyglycolic acid) suture.

DISCUSSION

Based upon my experience with more than 300 transhiatal esophageal resections, I can categorically state that the normal stomach will reach to the neck in virtually every patient. The stomach has been used as the esophageal substitute in 96 percent of my patients, colon being utilized only in those patients who had undergone prior gastric resection for peptic ulcer disease.

When gastric outlet obstruction due to pylorospasm complicates esophageal resection and reconstruction, the result may be disastrous. I therefore *always* perform a gastric drainage procedure in these patients. My preference is pyloromyotomy, which not only eliminates the intraabdominal suture line of a pyloroplasty, but also avoids a suture line at right angles to the axis of the elongated stomach, which is pulled upward as it is positioned through the posterior mediastinum. When utilizing the posterior mediastinum (the original esophageal bed) for visceral esophageal substitution, it is not necessary to enlarge the thoracic inlet. In contrast, resection of the medial clavical and adjacent manubrium to enlarge the superior opening into the anterior mediastinum is routine when *retrosternal* gastric or colonic interposition is carried out.

The operative mortality in my patients with carcinoma has been 6 percent, and 88 percent have left the hospital able to swallow within 3 weeks of operation. Measured intraoperative blood loss has averaged approximately 1,000 cc. A chest tube has been required in two-thirds of our patients undergoing transthoracic esophagectomy. In patients with esophageal carcinoma the actuarial survival following transhiatal esophageal resection has been similiar to that achieved in the majority of large series of transthoracic esophagectomies.

I believe that anastomosis of the stomach to the cervical esophagus will emerge as the best means of reconstructing the esophagus for both benign and malignant disease. The stomach is an upper gastrointestinal organ that is thick walled and resilient and not subject to redundancy and tortuosity, which occur with colon interposition. Occasional outpatient dilation is required in approximately 15 percent of patients following a cervical esophagogastric anastomosis. More importantly, clinically significant gastroesophageal reflux in these patients is the exception rather than the rule. This approach is therefore an excellent option in patients who have had multiple failed antireflux operations as well as those with neuromotor esophageal dysfunction that has failed to respond to standard esophagomyotomy.

I emphasize that a sound knowledge of thoracic anatomy and surgical complications and their management is essential when performing esophagectomy and esophageal reconstruction, regardless of the technique used. My experience with transhiatal esophagectomy without thoracotomy indicates that this is a safe, well-tolerated operation, the "hazards" of which can be minimized by careful technique, experience, and clinical judgment.

SUGGESTED READING

Orringer MB. Technical aids in performing transhiatal esophagectomy without thoracotomy. Ann Thorac Surg 1984; 38:128–132.

Orringer MB. Transhiatal esophagectomy without thoracotomy for carcinoma of the thoracic esophagus. Ann Surg 1984; 200:282–288.

Orringer MB. Transhiatal esophagectomy for benign disease. J Thorac Cardiovasc Surg 1985; 90:649–655.
Orringer MB, Orringer JS. Transhiatal esophagectomy without thoracotomy—a dangerous operation? J Thorac Cardiovasc Surg 1983; 85:72–80.
Orringer MB, Sloan H. Esophagectomy without thoracotomy. J Thorac Cardiovasc Surg 1978; 76:643–654.

ANASTOMOTIC LEAK

JOHN R. BENFIELD, M.D.
JOHN C. WAIN Jr., M.D.

Currently mortality after esophageal resections is 8 to 12 percent. Although anastomotic leaks occur in less than 10 percent of patients after esophagectomy by experienced surgeons, leaks are primarily responsible for at least 50 percent of the deaths. When anastomotic disruptions are successfully managed, patients are often hospitalized for *at least* 3 to 4 weeks longer than would have been required after an uncomplicated operation; the goal of achieving normal swallowing with a reasonable quality life is usually delayed by at least another month. Since most patients with esophageal cancer can look forward only to approximately 1 year of palliation, the management of an anastomotic disruption consumes a significant portion of the patient's residual life.

Why are esophageal anastomoses subject to leakage? Tension upon suture lines, suboptimum exposure during the accomplishment of anastomoses, and compromise of the blood supply as a result of technical considerations account for most anastomotic disruptions. The absence of a serosal layer in the esophagus, the relatively poor blood supply of the midthoracic esophagus, and nutritional depletion are factors that predispose to poor healing.*

PREVENTION

Although its efficacy in preventing anastomotic disruptions is not entirely clear, preoperative total parenteral alimentation (TPN) is usually utilized in preparing patients for esophagogastrectomy. Anastomotic leakage can best be prevented if risk factors specific to particular operations are fully appreciated. Hence, we shall address selected preventive aspects of esophagogastrectomies and interposition operations.

Esophagogastrectomy requires anastomosis of the esophagus, a relatively fixed viscus, to the stomach, essentially a pedicle graft dependent upon the right gastric and gastroepiploic arteries for its blood supply. During mobilization of the stomach, the gastric arcades must be well preserved to maintain collateral channels. A *generous* Kocher maneuver must be done to avoid tension upon the anastomosis, and the diaphragmatic hiatus must be adequately enlarged so that the elevated stomach can lie comfortably within it.

We recommend that the site for anastomosis to the stomach be separate from the closure of the line of resection. In the chest or in the neck, our preference is to avoid the use of intestinal clamps on the esophagus. We place a row of interrupted sutures between the muscularis of the esophagus and the serosa of the viscus to be anastomosed to it, often utilizing a residual cuff of the specimen to be resected to facilitate exposure during the placement of a second row of interrupted sutures between an additional full thickness of the stomach and the esophagus. After completion of the posterior row of the anastomosis, excess tissue is excised, and the anterior row of the anastomosis is completed. To insure good visibility, we utilize a head light and suction tip of the type customarily used in neurosurgery. We prefer hand-sewn anastomoses, but stapled anastomoses can be safely and expeditiously used. After completion of an anastomosis with the stomach, there should be enough gastric mobility to permit at least partial plication of the fundus of the residual stomach to surround the anastomosis. The stomach is anchored to the parietal pleura to minimize tension on the anastomosis.

Left thoracotomy is recommended only for resection of the most distally located esophageal lesions. We avoid thoracoabdominal incision, instead relying primarily upon a left lateral thoracotomy with circumferential division of the diaphragm; a separate abdominal incision is made if needed. We avoid anastomosis at the level of the aortic arch through the left chest, preferring instead to utilize right thoracotomy for anastomosis at this level.

Right thoracotomy is recommended for extensive lesions of the lower esophagus or for midesophageal lesions. Anastomoses are made in the chest above the level of the azygous vein, or in the neck. When we anticipate making an intrathoracic anastomosis, the abdominal portion of the procedure is accomplished first; thereafter the stomach is drawn into the chest after closure of the abdomen and right posterolateral thoracotomy. When preoperative information indicates that resectability of the esophagus is in doubt or that the cervical anastomosis is required, esophageal mobilization via right thoracotomy is accomplished first. Thereafter the patient is placed in the recumbent position so that abdominal mobilization of the stomach and cervical incision can be accomplished.

Colon interposition can be accomplished either through the posterior mediastinum in the bed of the resected esophagus or substernally. There are two keys to the prevention of anastomotic disruption from colon interposition operations: (1) the vascular pedicle from the abdomen must be free of tension, (2) the colon must be free of constriction at the thoracic inlet. In occasional cases

* Editor's Note: We feel that single-layered anastomoses are more prone to leak than two-layered anastomoses.

it is advisable to resect a portion of the manubrium, and rarely we have excised the medial segment of the clavicle.

DIAGNOSIS

Anastomotic disruption is suspected when there is clinical evidence of sepsis, usually including pneumonia and atelectasis. In 11 years of our compiled experience with 19 patients who had anastomotic leaks, 18 occurred after palliative resection, thus indicating that patients with far-advanced disease are at higher risk for anastomotic leaks than individuals whose resections are potentially curative. During operation, a nasogastric tube is positioned through the anastomosis with the intent of leaving it in place until an esophageal radiograph has been obtained between the 5th and 7th postoperative day after ingestion of water-soluble contrast material. Should the nasogastric tube have been prematurely removed, we believe it best not to reinsert a tube; instructions to this effect are made part of the postoperative orders.

Anastomotic disruptions are characterized according to increasing severity: (1) leaks in the neck, (2) minor intrathoracic anastomotic defects, (3) significant intrathoracic leaks. Management of anastomotic disruptions should be according to the severity of the problem.

MANAGEMENT

Cervical leaks usually respond well to simple, adequate drainage, and such leaks are normally healed within 1 month of drainage. Unless there is radiographic evidence of distal obstruction, we do not undertake esophageal dilatation during the healing phase of the fistula. Repeat esophagograms are obtained when clinical criteria indicate that the fistula has healed. In occasional patients who may have clinically significant strictures, we usually proceed directly with the use of Maloney dilators, having found no regular need for esophagoscopy prior to initial dilatation and the first feeding.

Minor intrathoracic anastomotic defects are those that are recognized primarily and perhaps exclusively as a result of the routine use of esophagograms prior to feeding. By definition, patients with leaks in this category are clinically asymptomatic; subtle signs such as low-grade fever or leukocytosis may exist. Sinus tracts into the mediastinum are limited in scope in this group of individuals. Our recommendation is to continue the use of nasogastric suction and to refrain from oral feedings. Antibiotics need not be given, except when there may be clinical evidence of sepsis. Chest tubes need not be reinserted unless there is evidence of pleural fluid accumulation. Esophagography should be repeated at approximately weekly intervals after the sinus tract was demonstrated, and in most instances one can expect to find no further evidence of leakage from the anastomosis after a single week has elapsed.

Significant intrathoracic leaks are accompanied by intrathoracic fluid collection, esophageal-pleurocutaneous fistula, abscess formation, or a combination of these findings. These patients are at high risk of death, and aggressive management is indicated before clinical criteria indicate the appearance of grave signs of sepsis. The important principles of management are: (1) The abscess(es) must be drained completely, even if repeat thoracotomy or laparotomy is required; percutaneous drainage procedures are usually inadequate. In most instances the combination of establishing adequate drainage with a secondary operation and appropriate nutritional and antibiotic management is sufficient treatment. (2) If operative drainage does not promptly result in an improved clinical course, the response should be prompt and vigorous. Proximal diversion with cervical esophagostomy may be necessary, or reoperation to close the fistula with the use of a muscle pedicle flap may be required. If a tertiary operation is required, we recommend proximal diversion of the esophagus with division of the esophagus and creation of a cervical esophagostomy, usually with gastrostomy and without closure of the distal esophagus; one can expect subsequent reconstruction to require an interposition operation. We have not had occasion to use a jejunal free graft with blood supply from microvascular anastomoses for this purpose, but we anticipate that this may become the method of choice for cervical reconstructions.

Nutritional management begins with the placement of a feeding jejunostomy at the time of the esophagectomy. Feeding through this tube begins as soon as ileus has subsided, in recognition of the fact that at least a further week will elapse before the patient is able to achieve adequate nutrition orally. Total parenteral nutrition plays a crucial role in modern management of anastomotic disruption. When a leak is found, a cuffed silicon rubber catheter is placed into the right atrium. The goal is to provide patients with 35 to 45 kcal per kilogram per day and 1.5 g protein per day.

Through the use of supplementary nutrition and adequate drainage of esophageal anastomotic leaks, approximately 80 percent or more of patients who suffer this complication can be expected to survive.

Supported in part by grant CA09477-02 from the National Cancer Institute of the National Institutes of Health, Bethesda, Maryland.

SUGGESTED READING

Stabile B. Nutritional support in intra-abdominal sepsis. In: Wilson SE, Finegold SH, Williams RA, eds. Intra-abdominal infection, New York: McGraw-Hill, 1982:410.

Wilson SE, Stone R, Scully M, Ozeran L, Benfield JR. Modern management of anastomotic leak after esophagogastrectomy. Am J Surg 1982; 133:95–101.

SHORT-SEGMENT COLON INTERPOSITION

DOUGLAS J. MATHISEN, M.D.

The ideal esophageal substitute should possess the following qualities: (1) its use should be associated with minimal mortality and morbidity, (2) it should be long enough to be suitable for the variable lengths of the esophagus that need to be substituted, (3) it should serve as a reliable conduit for food and secretions, (4) it should be refractory to acid, and (5) it should provide good long-term functional results. The use of short-segment colon interposition fulfills many of these requirements. Short-segment colon is generally defined as a portion of the splenic flexure of the large intestine encompassing variable amounts of the transverse and descending colon and has as its main vascular pedicle the ascending branch of the left colic artery and the marginal artery of Drummond. Other segments of the colon can be used in short-segment interposition, but we have found this to be the most reliable.

Indications for the use of short-segment colon interposition encompass any situation in which the distal esophagus is no longer suitable to allow for proper nutrition and handling of saliva. Such situations include patients with nondilatable peptic strictures, failed operations for achalasia, complications resulting from multiple failed antireflux procedures and rarely esophageal malignancy. Contraindications to its use include patients with advanced atherosclerosis and inadequate left colonic blood supply or inherent disease within the colon, such as ulcerative colitis or diverticulitis. When consideration is given to the use of short-segment colon interposition, each patient should undergo a thorough mechanical bowel preparation. The use of angiography in young, otherwise healthy patients is probably not necessary but certainly is helpful in identifying anomalies of the vascular tree. In older patients short-segment colon interposition should be an indication for arteriography in order to look for complications of atherosclerosis. The use of arteriography in these situations eliminates potential complications and inordinate operative time spent trying to assess the adequacy of the vessels.

The technique we have preferred utilizes a generous thoracoabdominal incision in order to allow adequate exposure of the esophagogastric junction, removal of the diseased portion of the esophagus, and mobilization of a segment of colon based on the left colic artery. If it can be determined that the diseased esophagus can be removed and there is a need for interposition, the first step should be to mobilize the segment of colon to be used. The segment of colon used is an isoperistaltic segment based on the ascending branch of the left colic artery and marginal artery of Drummond. Once the length of colon is determined, the segment of bowel is isolated by identifying the ascending branch of the left colic artery; care is taken to preserve it and its venous drainage at all times. Collateral vessels are identified and isolated. Fine, noncrushing vascular clips are then placed on these collateral vessels to assess the adequacy of arterial and venous supply to the proposed segment prior to actual division of the vessels. Once these clips have been applied, attention can be turned to removing the diseased segment of esophagus and preparing for the colonic interposition. Division of the colonic segment is then commenced with the use of the GIA stapler both proximally and distally. It is important to avoid inserting excess amounts of colon in the thoracic cavity because of the problem of redundant loops that may develop long term. The proximal anastomosis is fashioned first. We prefer a two-layer interrupted silk end-to-end anastomosis. To prevent reflux, it is important to have at least 12 cm of colon intra-abdominally and ideally to place the cologastric anastomosis posterior on the body of the stomach to allow for compression of the colonic segment by the stomach. Excess distal colon is carefully removed. The cologastric anastomosis is accomplished using the same two-layer, 4–0 silk interrupted technique as described previously for the proximal anastomosis. We have generally not passed a nasogastric tube through the colon segment but preferred to withdraw the nasogastric tube above the proximal anastomosis. Gastric distention is avoided by the use of a gastrostomy tube. In most cases the vagus nerve cannot be preserved in these operations, and pyloromyotomy or pyloroplasty is indicated. Continuity is restored in the large bowel and the trap in the mesentery closed. Patients are allowed nothing by mouth until peristalsis returns and flatus passes. We routinely obtain barium contrast studies prior to feeding the patients to ensure an intact anastomosis and no mechanical problems related to the colon segment.

The most devastating complication of short-segment colon interposition is necrosis of the segment. Signs of sepsis, peritonitis, pneumothorax, or free air under the diaphragm are all possible indications of this devastating complication. Water-soluble contrast studies may show anastomotic leaks, and gentle flexible endoscopy with a pediatric gastroscope may reveal necrosis of the colonic segment. Depending upon the degree of soilage present, this problem should be handled by removal of the necrotic segment and proximal diversion of the esophagus, and appropriate measures taken to drain the stomach and provide for jejunal feeding. If soilage is at a minimum, reconstitution of the alimentary tract may be considered by direct esophagogastric anastomosis or jejunal interposition. If anastomotic leaks occur and a viable segment of colon remains, individual consideration should be given to each patient as to the best course of action. If adequate pleural drainage already exists, this may be all that is necessary, along with maintaining the patient on nothing by mouth and intravenous antibiotics. Consideration should be given, however, to exploring and possibly repairing the leak by resuturing the area and reinforcing with either omentum or local muscle flaps. Proximal diversion of the esophagus and removal of the colonic segment may be necessary. Anastomotic leaks require prompt recognition, because failure to do so may lead to death of the patient.

Long-term problems of colonic interposition are related to localized stenosis of the proximal or distal anastomosis or the development of redundant segments of colon intrathoracically. Anastomotic strictures can sometimes be dealt with by simple dilation. When this fails, revision of the anastomosis can be accomplished either by total resection and reanastomosis or by a plastic type procedure of the Heineke-Mikulicz variety. Redundant segments should be infrequent if care is taken to avoid placing excess colon in the chest. If they do occur and the patient becomes symptomatic, segmental excision may have to be performed. Great care must be taken in these situations to preserve the marginal artery of Drummond for fear of jeopardizing the entire segment of colon.

Careful attention to technical detail and proper selection of patients can lead to a successful outcome in the overwhelming majority of patients. The colon provides a passive conduit for food and is generally refractory to the adverse effects of acid reflux. Its main advantage over jejunum for short-segment interposition is the availability of suitable length to reach any level for esophageal replacement.

SUGGESTED READING

Belsey R. Reconstruction of the esophagus with left colon. J Thorac Cardiovasc Surg 1965; 49:33.

Keenan DJM, et al. Surgery for benign esophageal stricture. J Thorac Cardiovasc Surg 1984; 88: 182–188.

Postlethwaite RW, et al. Colon interposition for esophageal substitution. Ann Thorac Surg 1971; 12:89–109.

HIATAL HERNIA

PREOPERATIVE EVALUATION OF GASTROESOPHAGEAL REFLUX

TOM R. DEMEESTER, M.D.
KARL H. FUCHS, M.D.

Medicine advances by retrospective analysis relating symptoms to anatomic lesions and then using this relationship prospectively to clinically diagnose the presence of a lesion. There are, however, abnormalities that cause symptoms without anatomic lesions. For the most part, these are abnormalities of organ function that give rise to symptoms prior to the development of an anatomic lesion. The lesion occurs as a consequence of the abnormal function. To identify such abnormalities requires detecting the abnormal function which, if allowed to persist, causes the anatomic lesion. Gastroesophageal reflux disease is such an abnormality and accounts for more than 70 percent of esophageal pathology.

Gastroesophageal reflux is a common disease with a prevalence assumed to be as high as 0.36 percent or 360 cases per 100,000 population. Despite this prevalence, its exact diagnosis is difficult to establish because of the difficulty in defining the disease. In essence, gastroesophageal reflux disease is increased esophageal exposure to gastric juice. After a latency period this causes a variety of symptoms, some of which are specific, such as heartburn and regurgitation, whereas others are nonspecific, such as chest pain, cough, choking, dysphagia, and wheezing. Consequently, diagnostic testing is necessary to confirm the presence of the disease prior to proceeding with surgical therapy. Tests used to evaluate patients suspected of having gastroesophageal reflux disease are upper gastrointestinal roentgenographic barium studies, esophagoscopy, standard acid reflux, motility of the lower esophageal sphincter, and 24-hour esophageal pH monitoring.

UPPER GASTROINTESTINAL ROENTGENOGRAPHIC BARIUM STUDY

This is the most common test used in current medical practice to evaluate upper gastrointestinal symptoms. In the past a roentgenographic hiatal hernia was thought to indicate the presence of an incompetent cardia. This, fortunately, is no longer true. Currently, the flow of barium from the stomach into the esophagus occurring spontaneously in an upright patient is considered the only dependable roentgenographic sign of gastroesophageal reflux. When this flow is induced by a variety of maneuvers it is less dependable, since under these conditions the reflux of barium into the esophagus can be observed in 25 percent of normal subjects. The inability to demonstrate reflux in the upright position does not exclude the presence of the disease.

ESOPHAGOSCOPY

Esophagoscopy detects the presence of gastroesophageal reflux by observing mucosal changes in the esophagus associated with increased esophageal exposure to gastric juice. In essence it is a test to detect the complications of gastroesophageal reflux and when the above changes are observed, the presence of the disease is inferred. Today, most endoscopic examinations are performed with a flexible fiberoptic scope. Esophagitis is scored as grade 1 for an erythematous and friable mucosa, grade 2 for linear erosions, grade 3 for deeper, wider, and interlacing linear erosions with islands of edematous mucosa between erosive furrows (the so-called cobblestone mucosa), and grade 4 for the presence of a fibrous stricture. When a stricture is observed, the endoscopist should assess the grade of esophagitis associated with it and whether Barrett's mucosa is present. Occasionally, Barrett's mucosa can occur without a stricture. Gastroesophageal reflux disease is considered present when any grade of esophagitis is observed, although some physicians do not accept grade 1 as indicative of disease.

THE STANDARD ACID REFLUX TEST

The standard acid reflux test attempts to induce reflux by loading the stomach with acid and having the patient perform exaggerated physiologic maneuvers. The test is performed by placing 300 ml of 0.1 normal hydrochloric acid in the patient's stomach and a pH electrode 5 cm above the upper border of the distal esophageal sphincter, which has been previously located by manometry. The pH of the esophagus is then monitored while the patient performs four maneuvers in the supine position: deep breathing, Valsalva's, Müller's (inspiration against a closed glottis), and cough. These maneuvers are repeated in the right and left lateral decubitus positions and with the head down 20 degrees. This provides 16 possibilities for acid reflux to occur. A decrease in esophageal pH to less than 4.0 is considered evidence of reflux. At the beginning of the test, before the patient is placed in the supine position, the distal esophagus must have a pH greater than 4.0. This may require the patient to stand erect and to swallow repeatedly to clear the esophagus of acid. Patients in the erect position who fail to clear the esophagus after 20 effective swallows are considered abnormal in all positions and maneuvers and are scored as 16. If reflux occurs on positioning or after a maneuver, the esophagus is cleared according to the flow diagram in Figure 1. Two or more reflux episodes out of 16 challenges constitute an abnormal finding or a positive test.

ESOPHAGEAL MANOMETRY

Esophageal manometry is used to measure abnormalities of the distal esophageal sphincter associated with incompetency and increased esophageal exposure to gastric juice. It is performed by using a catheter consisting of five fluid-filled polyethylene tubes bonded together, each with a lateral opening of 0.8 mm in diameter. The openings are sequentially placed at 5.0-cm intervals from the distal end of the catheter and radially oriented 45 to 90 degrees. A constant infusion of distilled water is delivered to each tube by a pneumohydraulic low compliance system at a rate of 0.6 ml per minute. The sphincter occludes the outflow of water from the lateral openings of the tubes, resulting in a rise in pressure in the system equal to the occlusive force. Five pressure recordings of the lower esophageal sphincter are obtained by withdrawing the catheter in 1-cm increments from the stomach through the sphincter into the esophagus.

A typical pressure recording is shown in Figure 2. The end respiratory gastric baseline pressure is used as a zero reference for pressure measurements. A persistent rise in pressure exceeding 2 mm Hg above the gastric baseline marks the distal border of the sphincter. The proximal border is marked by the point where sphincter pressure drops to inspiratory esophageal baseline pressure. The five measurements of the distance in centimeters between these two points are averaged and represent the overall length of the sphincter.

The point at which the end-expiratory pressure changes from a positive to a negative deflection represents the respiratory inversion point. The five measurements of the distance in centimeters between the respiratory inversion

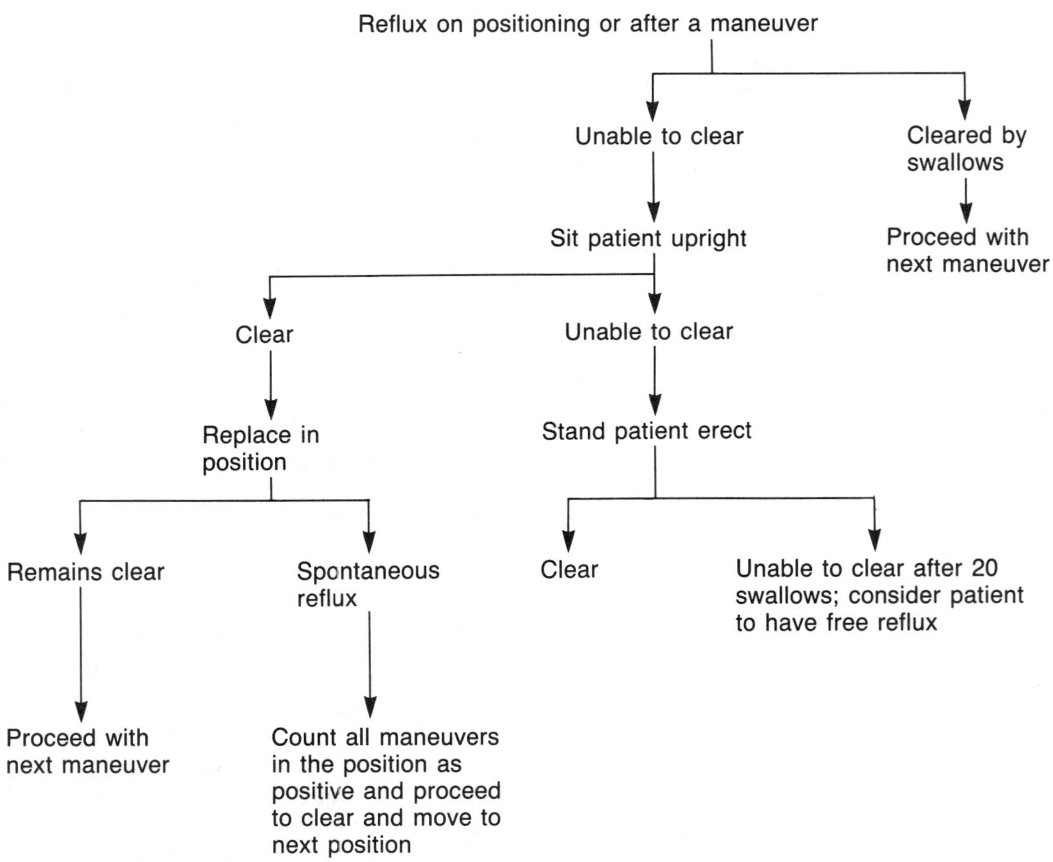

Figure 1 Procedure for performing the standard acid reflux test.

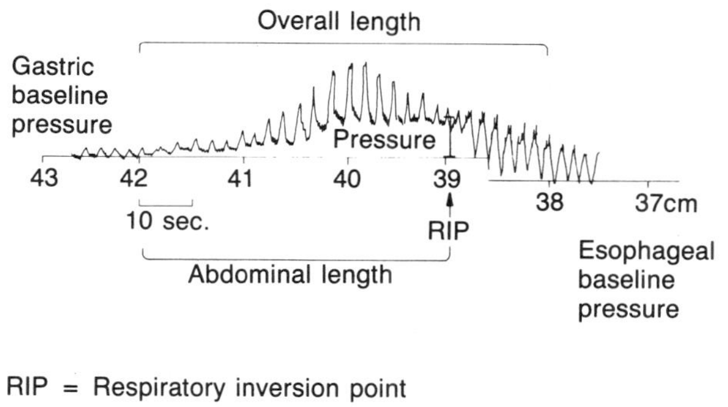

Figure 2 Manometric pressure recording of lower esophageal sphincter.

point and the distal part of the sphincter, that is, the length of the pressure wave that reflects positive excursions with respiration, are averaged. This represents the length of sphincter exposed to the positive pressure environment of the abdomen or the abdominal length of the sphincter.

The amplitude of the sphincter pressure is measured as the difference in millimeters of mercury between the gastric baseline and the pressure at the respiratory inversion point during the middle of the respiratory cycle. The five measurements of pressure are averaged and represent the sphincter pressure.

The criteria for a mechanically defective sphincter are a pressure of 6 mm Hg or less, an overall length less than 2 cm, or an abdominal length less than 1 cm. These values are below the fifth percentile of those measured in 50 normal subjects.

TWENTY-FOUR HOUR ESOPHAGEAL pH MONITORING

Esophageal pH monitoring directly measures the esophageal exposure to gastric acid by recording the pH continuously over a 24-hour period. The test is performed by placing a pH electrode 5 cm above the upper border of the distal esophageal sphincter as measured by manometry. The pH monitoring system is standardized at pH values of 4.0 and 7.0 prior to beginning the test period. A normal diet is served, unique only in the absence of food and beverages having a pH value of less than 5.0 or greater than 7.0. At the completion of the monitored period, the probe is advanced into the stomach to document the pH of the gastric contents, and the calibration procedure is repeated to determine the amount of drift by the pH electrode during the study. Patients are instructed to record their symptoms, such as heartburn, regurgitation, dysphagia, chest pain, cough, and wheezing in a diary and asked to press an event marker on the recorder when symptoms occur. They are asked to remain upright when awake and to lie flat only when retiring for the night.

Acid reflux is identified whenever the pH in the esophagus drops to 4.0 or below. The esophageal exposure to gastric juice is measured by a composite mathematical score that incorporates six components of the 24-hour record: percent of time the esophageal pH is 4.0 or less (1) for the total 24-hour period, (2) for the time in the upright position, and (3) for the time in the supine position; (4) the total number of reflux episodes, (5) the number of episodes lasting 5 minutes or longer, and (6) the duration of the longest episode in minutes. Patients who accumulate a score that exceeds the mean score of normal subjects by more than two standard deviations are considered to have abnormal esophageal exposure to gastric juice and a positive test result. Currently most 24-hour pH monitoring tests are done on an ambulatory basis with a recorder that samples and records esophageal pH at 4- to 6-second intervals. The data are then analyzed by a computer and provide the user with a numerical and graphic report of the values for each of the above-listed components (Fig. 3) as well as the overall score for the test.

COMMENTS ON TESTS DESIGNED TO DOCUMENT THE PRESENCE OF GASTROESOPHAGEAL REFLUX

Several studies have been performed comparing the accuracy of diagnostic tests for gastroesophageal reflux.

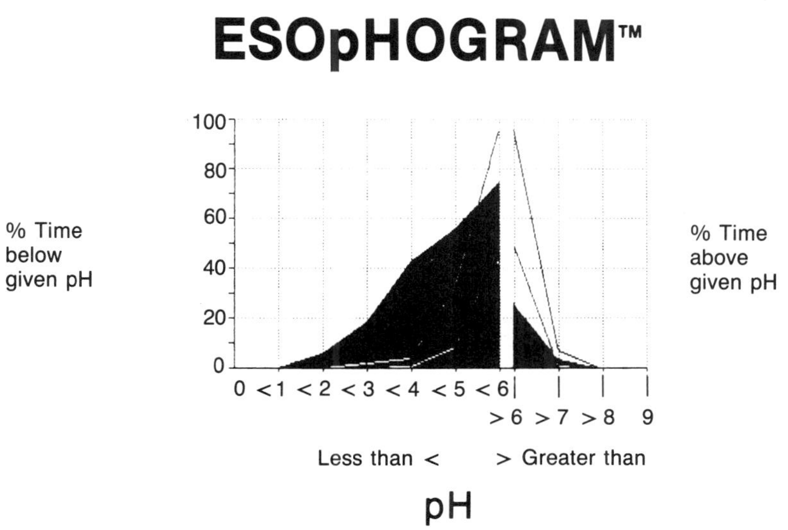

Figure 3 Example of computerized pH data display. Graph shows patient data (solid black area) compared with normal median values (lower white line) and the 95 percentile value above the median values (top white line) at various pH levels.

These studies have shown that the standard acid reflux test is a highly specific test; that is, it is normal in the absence of disease, but its sensitivity or ability to detect patients with the disease is too low to use in practice. A similar situation exists for endoscopy. Only about 60 percent of patients with classic symptoms of heartburn and regurgitation and documented gastroesophageal reflux disease have evidence of mucosal damage on endoscopy; the remainder have a normal endoscopic examination. Consequently, the diagnosis of gastroesophageal reflux disease can be a problem when a test is used that requires a morphologic change to be positive. Esophagoscopy is a test used to detect the complications of gastroesophageal reflux disease. It should not be regarded as a test for the presence of the disease. Esophagoscopy can even be misleading in symptomatic patients in whom a disease complication is visualized. In approximately 90 percent of the patients who have endoscopic esophagitis, acid reflux can be documented objectively by 24-hour pH monitoring. The cause of esophagitis in the remaining 10 percent is usually drug-induced mucosal damage or, in a small number of patients, the reflux of alkaline gastrointestinal contents.

The measurement of a profoundly inadequate distal esophageal sphincter, based on the criteria of a pressure of 6 mm Hg or below, an overall length of less than 2 cm, or an abdominal length of less than 1 cm, can be used as an indicator for the presence of gastroesophageal reflux. The presence of any one of the criteria is associated with an 80 percent incidence of increased esophageal exposure to gastric juice documented on 24-hour esophageal pH monitoring. In the remaining 20 percent of patients, the deficiency is compensated for by effective clearance function of the esophageal body. If all three criteria are abnormal, the incidence increases to 92 percent. The most common mechanical cause of an incompetent sphincter is inadequate pressure. The efficiency of a sphincter with normal pressure, however, can be nullified by an inadequate abdominal length or an abnormally short overall length. In practical terms this means that patients with low distal esophageal sphincter pressure or those with normal pressure but short abdominal length are unable to prevent reflux caused by fluctuations of intra-abdominal pressure that occur with daily activities such as changing body position. Similarly, patients with low distal esophageal pressure, or those with normal pressure but short overall length, are unable to prevent reflux caused by independent increases in intragastric pressure above intra-abdominal pressure. In addition, patients who have a short overall sphincter length on a resting esophageal motility study are also less able to protect against reflux caused by progressive gastric dilation. This is because further shortening of the sphincter occurs with gastric dilations, in a manner similar to the shortening of the neck of a balloon on inflation. Reflux occurs in these individuals when the overall sphincter length shortens below that necessary for the sphincter pressure present to maintain competency. These criteria do not document the presence of gastroesophageal reflux disease; rather, the disease is inferred by the presence of a mechanically defective sphincter.

Most studies have shown that 24-hour esophageal pH monitoring is the most accurate way to measure abnormal esophageal exposure to gastric juice and, therefore, the presence of gastroesophageal reflux disease. In essence gastroesophageal reflux disease is a condition in which the esophagus is exposed to an increased amount of gastric juice. Twenty-four hour pH monitoring measures pH changes in the esophagus as they occur spontaneously. It does not depend on performing maneuvers designed to induce reflux. It simply measures reflux as it occurs over a 24-hour period and relates the event to the symptoms experienced by the patient. It is important to emphasize that a positive test only indicates that the esophagus is exposed to increased gastric juice. It does not identify the cause of the increased acid exposure. Shorter 8-hour pH monitoring studies have less sensitivity, and with the advent of ambulatory technology, they have no particular advantage. Occasionally 24-hour pH monitoring is touted as being another form of the Bernstein test; however, this is not true. The Bernstein test detects an acid-sensitive esophagus or the presence of symptoms when the esophagus is perfused with exogenous acid. When the test results are positive, it assumes the presence of reflux. It is not a direct measurement of endogenous reflux and, therefore, lacks the sensitivity and specificity of 24-hour esophageal pH monitoring.

SUGGESTED READING

DeMeester TR. Definition, detection and pathophysiology of gastroesophageal reflux disease. In: DeMeester TR, Matthews H, eds. International trends in general thoracic surgery, vol III: benign esophageal disease. St. Louis: CV Mosby, 1987:99–127.

DeMeester TR, Johnson LF. The evaluation of objective measurements of gastroesophageal reflux and their contribution to patient management. Surg Clin North Am 1976; 56:39–53.

DeMeester TR, Wang CI, Wernly JA, et al. Technique, indications, and clinical use of 24-hour esophageal pH monitoring. J Thorac Cardiovasc Surg 1980; 79:651–670.

Fuchs KH, DeMeester TR, Albertucci M. Specificity and sensitivity of objective diagnosis of gastroesophageal reflux disease. Surgery 1987; 102:575–580.

Zaninotto G, DeMeester TR, Schwizer W, et al. The lower esophageal sphincter in health and disease. Am J Surg 1988; 155:104–111.

HILL PROCEDURE FOR GASTROESOPHAGEAL REFLUX

KJELL THOR, M.D.
LUCIUS D. HILL, M.D.

One of the most common abnormalities of the upper gastrointestinal tract is a malfunctioning gastroesophageal (GE) junction, with its attendant esophagitis, heartburn, and dysphagia. The frequency of GE reflux calls for strict indications for surgery. Operations should be founded on sound rationale and aided by modern technology to be effective.

In 1967 our group reported a procedure consisting of posterior fixation of the GE junction with calibration of the lower esophageal sphincter. The goal of this procedure is to restore the function and anatomy of the GE junction to as near normal as possible. To understand the rationale of the operation, we will recount the important features of the normal antireflux barrier.

The GE junction is a highly efficient and complex mechanism that allows for swallowing of a bolus and yet maintains a resting pressure that prevents reflux of gastric content. The main components of this complex mechanism that can be assessed by objective measurements are (1) the lower esophageal sphincter, (2) the GE valve created by the angle of His, (3) esophageal clearance, and (4) posterior fixation of the dorsal mesentery. The diaphragm needs further study to determine its importance. Failure of any of these components can impair the antireflux barrier. Formerly, measurement of the lower esophageal sphincter pressure focused attention on the lower esophageal sphincter, almost to the exclusion of the other factors. The role of the diaphragm was downplayed, and the GE valve created by the acute angle of His as part of the antireflux barrier was almost overlooked. We have recently shown in cadavers without hiatal hernia or esophageal disease that there is a measurable pressure gradient across the GE junction that requires from 7 to 15 cm of water pressure in the stomach before reflux occurs. By simply depressing the fundus to approximately 45 degrees, the angle of His becomes more obtuse, the valve is eliminated, and the osteum of the esophagus is converted into a funnel, allowing free reflux and elimination of gradient. Since there is no sphincter function in the cadaver, the presence of a gradient across the GE junction and the maneuver of depressing the cardia eliminate the valve, and the gradient indicates that the flap valve contributes to the competence of the GE junction in an in-situ preparation. In addition to those factors in the normal individual, reflux produces an instantaneous and powerful peristaltic wave that rapidly cleanses the lower esophagus of refluxed material. Furthermore, the entire gastrointestinal tract, including the hollow as well as the solid viscera in humans and most vertebrate animals, is suspended by the dorsal mesentery to the posterior body wall. The esophagus is no exception to this rule. Extensive cadaver dissections demonstrate that the esophagus is primarily fixed posteriorly by a dense plate of fibroareolar tissue extending from the median arcuate ligament all the way above the aortic arch. When this posterior attachment becomes lengthened or attenuated, the GE junction then slides cephalad into the posterior mediastinum, with the consequent development of a hiatal hernia.

In a patient with hiatal hernia or GE reflux, the components of the antireflux barrier are lost. The GE junction loses its posterior attachment and slides into the posterior mediastinum, thereby converting the flap valve to a funnel, which eliminates the gradient created by the flap valve. In addition, the sphincter may be distracted by the phrenoesophageal membrane. The diaphragm, instead of supporting the GE junction, now actually impinges on the stomach and increases intragastric pressure, which further serves to overcome the lower esophageal sphincter. The net result of all these forces is reflux.

In the past, hiatal hernia was considered a synonym for GE reflux. This mechanistic and simplistic belief misled clinicians into attaching a multitude of symptoms to a common radiologic finding. Reflux may occur without a hiatal hernia. The cause for failure of the GE junction in these cases is not yet known. Loss of the angle of His and of the GE valve may well be important factors in these patients.

From the preceding discussion it becomes clear that the aim of an antireflux surgical procedure should be to restore the posterior attachment of the esophagus to aid in the restoration of the valve, in esophageal clearance, and in sphincter function. The mature view is one recognizing the importance of each of these features. To focus attention only on the sphincter, esophageal clearance, or the valve is to ignore the importance of the necessary components.

INDICATIONS

Because the symptoms of esophagitis, including heartburn and dysphagia, are so common, it is important that the indications for surgery remain strict. It can be argued that the patient with intractable heartburn, reflux, and dysphagia does not need sophisticated tests to determine that surgery is indicated. Even in these patients, however, it is important to know the status of the lower esophageal sphincter, the presence of reflux, the level of gastric acid, and if the patient has esophagitis or Barrett's esophagus. It is mandatory to rule out cancer. Only by measuring these baselines will the surgeon know over the long term whether there has been improvement in the patient's problems.

Intractability. The most common indication for operation is failure to respond to medical management or intractability under the guidance of a physician specializing in gastrointestinal disease.

Esophagitis. The second most common indication for operation is esophagitis. This may vary from edema and erythema of the mucosa accompanied by spasm to severe forms of ulcerative esophagitis with stricture.

Stricture and Ulceration. Approximately 14 percent of patients in our series were operated on for stricture. The presence of a stricture usually indicates that refractory esophagitis has been allowed to proceed too long. Effective antireflux surgery with dilation provides excellent therapy for patients with peptic esophageal stricture. There is no indication for an esophageal resection.

Bleeding. Bleeding from the esophagus is usually chronic and low grade, producing persistent anemia. Approximately 10 percent of patients operated on in our series had chronic anemia.

Respiratory Complications. Pulmonary complications are often overlooked by physicians. We have operated on a number of patients under long-term treatment for asthma in whom the history indicated that the so-called "asthma" occurred when the patient was lying down or following episodes of reflux. In these individuals, surgery is rewarding because it not only clears the symptoms of reflux but eliminates the symptoms related to aspiration or overflow into the tracheobronchial tree.

Large Hernias. In a small group of patients with sliding hiatal hernia, operation is required because the hernia is large enough to produce pressure symptoms in the chest with cardiorespiratory embarrassment. In these individuals, episodes of incarceration may cause pain that is so severe that it is misinterpreted as a myocardial infarction.

Finally, there is a group of patients in whom inflammation can be seen both at endoscopy and biopsy, but in whom other standard tests will fail to show reflux. The patient who shows good sphincter pressure and no reflux during the single pull-through examination on pH and pressure study may be found on more intensive study to have transient relaxation or to have reflux mainly in the upright position. The introduction of 24-hour pH monitoring serves to point out those patients who do not have reflux in the recumbent position but have severe reflux in the upright position. In this small group of patients, operation may be required because of persisting symptoms.

Of the 1,640 patients operated upon in our series, 11 percent underwent surgery because of coexisting problems associated with hiatal hernia. Gallbladder disease was the most common coexisting problem. In these individuals, it is very important that a hiatal hernia be diagnosed and assessed before operation. It is unwise to add a hiatal hernia repair to routine cholecystectomy or ulcer operation if the patient does not have GE reflux severe enough to warrant the procedure. Hiatal hernia is so common that the surgeon may find it in a number of patients with other upper abdominal disease. In many of these cases, the hiatal hernia is asymptomatic. To subject a patient to formal repair of an asymptomatic hiatal hernia invites the complications of the procedure with no benefit to the patient. If a hiatal hernia is suspected in a patient with gallbladder or upper abdominal disease, its evaluation should be done before operation so that the surgeon can judge whether repair is indicated.

TECHNIQUE

Gastroesophageal restoration (Hill's operation) is accomplished through an upper midline abdominal incision. The abdomen is explored. The pylorus in particular is examined carefully for any evidence of pyloric stenosis that might impede gastric emptying. The triangular ligament of the left lobe of the liver is divided and the liver retracted to the patient's right. The upper hand retractor is placed to facilitate exposure. The phrenoesophageal membrane is divided on the diaphragm, removing as much of the fibroareolar tissue as possible. These bundles are used in the repair. The lesser omentum is divided, and the esophageal hiatus is exposed. The esophagus is gently diverted to the patient's right, and the attachment of the cardia to the diaphragm is divided. As few short gastric arteries as possible are divided. This dissection must be done with care so as not to tear the spleen. Division of the phrenogastric and superior portions of the gastrosplenic ligament mobilizes the upper part of the gastric fundus. The fundus can then be rotated so that the posterior part of the stomach can be visualized. This allows the GE junction to be retracted down, and the hernia is reduced. By retracting the anterior and posterior phrenoesophageal bundles, an intra-abdominal segment of esophagus becomes visible. The anterior and posterior vagus nerves are visualized and kept in view so they will not be damaged. Retracting the stomach to the patient's left exposes the preaortic fascia. The median arcuate ligament lies immediately above the celiac trunk. It can be exposed by careful blunt dissection at the midpoint of the aorta. The celiac artery usually arises cephalad to the median arcuate ligament. Dissection of the celiac axis has been a deterrent to performing this operation in many hands. If it is difficult to locate the ligament, or if the surgeon is not familiar with vascular surgery and is uncomfortable with dissecting out the celiac axis, a safer alternative procedure is recommended. By retracting the esophagus to the patient's left, the surgeon can expose the esophageal hiatus. The fibroareolar tissue overlying the aorta and the esophageal hiatus can be simply divided by sharp dissection, thereby exposing the aorta. A finger is then passed gently beneath the preaortic fascia, down the celiac artery, and the preaortic fascia is lifted off the aorta. This can then be grasped with the Babcock clamp, and the sutures simply placed through the fascia. Care must be taken not to damage the short branches that pass from the aorta to the crura. By staying in the midline, these branches are avoided. If a branch of the celiac or the aorta is avulsed, brisk bleeding may occur. This may be dealt with simply by gentle pressure with a finger, exposure of the branch, and ligation with a vascular suture.

The crura of the esophageal hiatus are loosely approximated behind the esophagus with nonabsorbable sutures. The stomach is then rotated in a clockwise direction to expose the posterior part, thereby clearly displaying the anterior and posterior bundles of tissue that previously held the GE junction in the diaphragm. The bundles are grasped with special Babcock clamps well above the left gastric artery. Strong nonabsorbable sutures, either 0-silk or 0-synthetic material, are used for the repair. Usually five sutures are placed in the anterior and posterior phrenoesophageal bundles are carried through the preaortic fascia. These sutures are placed with the vagus nerves in full view in order not to damage them (Fig. 1). A single

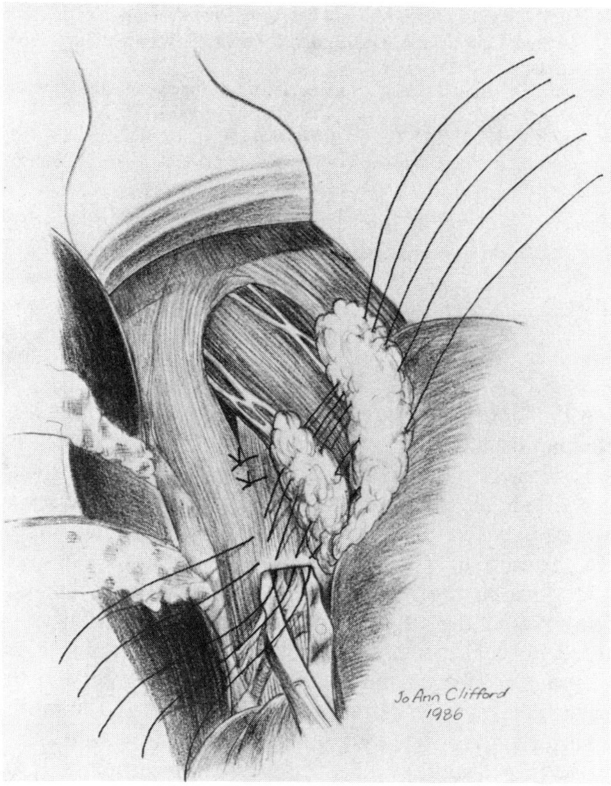

Figure 1 The diaphragm is closed loosely behind the esophagus. Five sutures are placed through the phrenoesophageal bundles and the median arcuate ligament, with the vagus nerves in full view.

knot is placed in the top three sutures, which are then clamped with long hemostats. Measurement of the sphincter pressure is obtained by passing the side hole of the modified nasogastric tube through the GE sphincter. If the pressure is above 55 mm Hg, the sutures are loosened. If it is below 30 mm Hg, the sutures are tightened, depending on the problem at hand. After the proper pressure is obtained, all five sutures are tied, and a final pressure measurement is taken. The barrier is about 3 to 4 cm in length. In addition to measuring the sphincter, the valve of His is accentuated by this procedure and can be readily palpated through the wall of the stomach. In patients who have had previous operations that have resulted in scarring and destruction of the GE junction, the valve may be destroyed or inadequate. In these cases, a gastrostomy is performed, and the valve is secured with sutures in the anterior and posterior edges, thereby lengthening it to 3 to 4 cm. Attempts to calibrate the cardia with a bougie are unsatisfactory because it is difficult to determine whether the wrap around the bougie is tight or loose.

INTRAOPERATIVE MANOMETRY

In 1977 our group first reported the use of a simplified method of measuring the pressure in the sphincter during operation to yield an objective determination of whether an adequate barrier had been created. The restoration of sphincter function is aided materially by intraoperative manometrics. Many studies have shown that the most important component of the antireflux barrier is the lower esophageal sphincter. We use a number of sophisticated tests before and after both medical and surgical therapy to determine what results are achieved. It is reasonable, therefore, that we should assess what is being achieved during surgery itself. Unless sphincter function is restored during surgery, all of the pre- and postoperative results are invalid. If an adequate antireflux barrier is not established, the operation is a total failure. Calibration of the cardia aided by intraoperative measurement of the lower esophageal sphincter is a direct and purposeful effort to preserve and enhance the sphincter.

RESULTS

The most important criterion of success is patient satisfaction. If a patient is free of heartburn, can eat a full meal, and can resume normal activity, including bending over in the garden and indulging in strenuous exercise without reflux or heartburn, then the operation should be considered a success. On the other hand, we have been particularly meticulous in our follow-up using pH and pressure studies 2 to 3 months after surgery whenever possible. In those patients who refuse pH and pressure studies, we obtain a GE tract scintiscan series to test the effectiveness of the operation designed to curtain reflux.

Three major retrospective studies of the long-term effect of surgical treatment with the Hill repair have been performed by us in more than 1,300 patients out of 1,685 patients operated upon over a 24-year period. The results are summarized as follows: excellent or good results have been obtained in over 95 percent, with a failure and recurrence rate of 1.5 to 5 percent. The complication and mortality rates have been very low, 0.2 percent, with one death in the last 500 operations for primary repairs. In 114 redo operations (mainly failed Nissen's repairs), the mortality rate has been 1.7 percent, and for strictures 0.5 percent. A complication of the Hill repair has been dysphagia, usually transient and present in 5 to 20 percent of patients. Less than 5 percent of patients have required dilation. In one of our series, 48 percent had dysphagia before surgery compared with about 20 percent postoperatively. It should be emphasized that the majority of those patients had no reflux and tolerated this new situation without dilation. Whether postoperative dysphagia is caused by persistent motility disorders which were present preoperatively in 41 percent of patients has not yet been evaluated. In over 1,600 operations we have had brisk bleeding from branches from the aorta or celiac artery in only eight instances. Ligation of these vessels has produced no discernible complications. In one series 28 percent of our patients had pulmonary symptoms before surgery and 6 percent postoperatively. There have been four fistulas from the esophagus. Two of these were treated with drainage, and both patients expired. These were treated early in our experience, before Celestin's tubes were available. The two other patients were treated with insertion of Celestin's tube and survived. Only one of the fistulas occurred in a primary repair. We have not encountered the devastating gastrobronchial, gastroaortic, gastropericardial, and gastrocutaneous fistulas that we have seen with the Nissen procedure.

SUGGESTED READING

Hill LD. An effective operation for hiatal hernia: an eight year appraisal. Ann Surg 1967; 166:681–692.

Hill LD. Progress in the surgical management of hiatal hernia. World J Surg 1977; 1:425–438.

Hill LD. Intraoperative measurement of lower esophageal sphincter pressure. J Thorac Cardiovasc Surg 1978; 75:378–382.

Hill LD, Chapman KW, Morgan EH. Objective evaluation of surgery for hiatal hernia and esophagitis. J Thorac Cardiovasc Surg 1961; 41:60–74.

Mercer CD, Hill LD. Gastroesophageal reflux disease. What to do when conservative measures fail. Postgrad Med 1984; 76:77–80.

Russell COH, Hill LD. Gastroesophageal reflux. In: Ravitch MM, ed. Current problems in surgery. Chicago: Year Book Medical Publishers, 1982:1.

BELSEY MARK IV HIATAL HERNIORRHAPHY

MARK K. FERGUSON, M.D.
DAVID B. SKINNER, M.D.

The Belsey Mark IV operation is designed to create an effective antireflux mechanism at the esophagogastric junction. It was first performed in 1955 and is currently in widespread use throughout the world. The usual indication for the Belsey Mark IV operation is the same as that for any antireflux procedure, namely, symptomatic and complicated gastroesophageal acid reflux that is refractory to medical management. The Belsey operation is particularly suited for those patients in whom a transthoracic approach is preferable. Indications for a transthoracic approach include the presence of other thoracic disease requiring exploration, a peptic esophageal stricture, and the necessity for reoperation in patients who have had previous esophageal surgery. Relative indications for a transthoracic approach are obesity, Barrett's esophagus, and previous abdominal surgery. Although the Belsey Mark IV operation may be used routinely for most patients, we select it particularly for patients with impaired esophageal motility, as it results in comparable control of reflux with a less dramatic rise in lower esophageal sphincter pressure than other fundoplications. Such patients typically include those with severe reflux esophagitis and transmural fibrosis and those with smooth muscle disorders, such as scleroderma. This nonobstructing wrap is also valuable in prophylaxis against reflux following extended myotomy for achalasia and diffuse esophageal spasm.

Techniques for performing the Belsey Mark IV operation have remained unchanged since its original description 30 years ago. A lateral thoracotomy incision is performed through the left sixth interspace. In adults a 1-cm segment of seventh rib underlying the paraspinous muscles is excised to avoid uncontrolled fracture. The intercostal neurovascular bundle may be divided to minimize postoperative pain. The esophagus is mobilized out of its bed from the level of the hiatus to the carina. The phrenoesophageal membrane and the peritoneum are incised around the margin of the esophageal hiatus, allowing the stomach to be drawn up into the pleural cavity. It is not usually necessary to divide the short gastric vessels. Posteriorly, it is important to incise the lesser sac and divide the communicating artery, known as Belsey's artery, between the left gastric and inferior phrenic arteries. Failure to do so may lead to unfortunate intra-abdominal hemorrhage. The lower esophagus is prepared by removing the fat pad and connective tissue at the gastroesophageal junction. This allows apposition of gastric serosa to esophageal muscle. Care is taken to preserve both vagus nerves. After retracting the esophagus and stomach anteriorly, the decussating fibers of the right crus are identified in preparation for placement of the posterior buttress sutures. This is facilitated by placing tension on the central tendon of the diaphragm with an Allis forceps. It is helpful to dissect the pericardium off the diaphragm medially to permit adequate bites of tendinous diaphragm. Number 0 silk sutures on an atraumatic needle are passed through the two halves of the right crus beginning just anterior to the aorta and continuing anteriorly at 1-cm increments. Normally three to five sutures are placed but are not tied at this stage.

The fundoplication stitches are placed to create a 270-degree anterolateral wrap of the esophageal circumference. Two rows of mattress sutures, with three stitches in each row, are placed through the seromuscular layer of the stomach and the muscular layers of the esophagus to effect this. A single hemoclip is first placed to mark the gastroesophageal junction, facilitating identification of this location in plain chest films used in postoperative follow-up. Felt pledgets are not necessary for an optimal repair and may result in excessive fibrosis or erode into the esophagus or stomach. The first row sutures enter through the seromuscular layer of the stomach 2 cm below the gastroesophageal junction and are passed through the two muscle layers of the esophagus 2 cm above the junction. The direction of the sutures is then reversed, passing through the esophagus and stomach to create a mattress effect. Following placement of the first row sutures, they are tied gently to avoid damage to the esophageal muscle. The second row sutures pass first through the diaphragm at the junction of the central tendon and the muscular ring of the hiatus. This is facilitated by use of a spoon retractor to avoid unseen injury below the diaphragm. The sutures are passed through the seromuscular layer of the stomach 4 cm below the gastroesophageal junction and through the muscular layers of the esophagus 4 cm above the junction. Their direction is reversed, passing through the esophagus, stomach, and the diaphragm. The stomach and gastroesophageal junction are manually reduced below the diaphragm, and the second row sutures are tied gently, again to avoid damage to the esophageal muscle. Finally the posterior buttress sutures are tied starting with the most posterior stitch, firmly approximating the halves of the crus. Adequate space must remain to easily admit one finger following closure of the hiatus. A nasogastric tube is placed, as is an intercostal drain. The incision is closed in a standard fashion. Alimentation can normally begin in 1 or 2 days and a baseline postoperative barium swallow test is obtained prior to discharge.

Postoperative complications are infrequent and minor. The procedure can routinely be performed with an operative mortality of less than 1 percent. Some patients experience early mild postoperative dysphagia, which is due to edema in the region of dissection. More severe dysphagia, when present, may be due to an excessively tight closure of the hiatus with the posterior buttress sutures. Recent data show that partial esophageal obstruction caused by a fundoplication can, at least transiently, result in esophageal dysmotility, which may also contribute to dysphagia. In most cases these symptoms resolve spontaneously with time, and dilation is rarely necessary. Because the gastrointestinal tract is not entered, the incidence of serious complications, including wound infection, gastric perforation, esophageal leak, and empyema, is less than 5 percent. If a leak is diagnosed postoperatively, it is usually well contained and may be observed. More serious leaks should be treated by appropriate drainage of the affected space. Gastric dilatation may occur, but is much less frequent than following a Nissen procedure because patients usually retain the ability to belch following a Belsey procedure. When gastric dilatation does occur, it is often secondary to vagus nerve injury. Treatment with metoclopramide improves symptoms in most cases.

As with the other commonly performed antireflux operations, the Belsey antireflux procedure carries a success rate of about 85 percent for patients followed 5 years or more. Operator experience is a significant determinant of surgical outcome, as operations performed by a surgeon experienced in this technique have a failure rate less than half that of the overall group. Many patients with recurrences have onset of symptoms within months of their operation. However, there is an incidence of recurrence up to 15 years postoperatively, making long-term follow-up of these patients mandatory. When symptoms recur, it is important to investigate their source. Over 20 percent of patients with symptom recurrence following technically successful antireflux surgery have problems unrelated to reflux or the previous operation. Investigations should routinely include a barium swallow study to document the anatomy of the repair, endoscopy to assess the presence of esophagitis, manometry to evaluate esophageal body function and adequacy of the reconstructed sphincter, and extended esophageal pH monitoring to quantitate reflux. Half of the patients with recurrent symptoms following antireflux surgery require reoperation (5 to 8 percent overall). When reoperation is performed, it is often a simple matter to document the source of the recurrent symptoms. In most cases recurrence can be attributed to one or more technical problems. The most common technical errors include inadequate mobilization of the esophagus or stomach resulting in tension on the repair; less than adequate circumference of wrap; and inappropriate depth of the sutures, either too shallow or too deep, leading in the first case to breakdown of the repair and in the second case to localized perforation. Anatomic factors may also predispose to recurrence, as in type II hernias with a very large hiatal defect or esophageal foreshortening due to peptic stricture. Symptomatic hernia recurrence may be corrected successfully with a second Belsey Mark IV antireflux operation, particularly when one or more of the above technical problems are found and can be corrected. A complete dissection of the hiatus and mobilization of the esophagus are performed to determine whether the tissues remain suitable for reconstruction. If the presence of fibrosis, esophageal shortening, or perforation is prohibitive, resection and reconstruction with colon interposition should strongly be considered. Otherwise, the standard repair as described above is performed by the most experienced member of the surgical team.

SUGGESTED READING

Baue AE, Belsey RHR. The treatment of sliding hiatus hernia and reflux esophagitis by the Mark IV technique. Surgery 1967; 62:396–404.

Little AG, Ferguson MK, Skinner DB. Reoperation for failed antireflux operations. J Thorac Cardiovasc Surg 1986; 91:511–517.

Orringer MB, Skinner DB, Belsey RHR. Long-term results of the Mark IV operation for hiatal hernia and analyses of recurrences and their treatment. J Thorac Cardiovasc Surg 1972; 63:25–34.

Skinner DB. Pathophysiology of gastroesophageal reflux. Ann Surg 1985; 202:546–556.

Skinner DB, Belsey RHR. Surgical management of esophageal reflux and hiatus hernia. J Thorac Cardiovasc Surg 1967; 53:33–54.

NISSEN FUNDOPLICATION FOR GASTROESOPHAGEAL REFLUX

F. HENRY ELLIS Jr., M.D., Ph.D.

Modern surgery of the esophagogastric junction reflects a major change in attitude on the part of surgeons. The former emphasis on restoration of normal anatomy has been replaced by emphasis on physiologically directed surgical procedures, and thus antireflux operations have supplanted anatomic repairs of hiatus hernia. Furthermore, gastroesophageal reflux is now believed to result from a hypotensive lower esophageal sphincter (LES) rather than a hiatus hernia.

Most patients with gastroesophageal reflux secondary to a hypotensive LES also have a sliding esophageal hiatus hernia, but whether the hernia is the cause or the result of the reflux is unclear. In addition, several other conditions can lead to a hypotensive LES and reflux. Reflux symptoms are being recognized in increasing numbers of patients who do not have hiatus hernia or systemic disease and who have not undergone previous operation. This suggests that a defect in the antireflux mechanism rather than the anatomic defect may be at fault. In my opinion, the Nissen fundoplication discussed in this chapter surpasses all other antireflux procedures in achieving successful and long-lasting control of gastroesophageal reflux.

ANTIREFLUX OPERATIONS

Basically four antireflux procedures—the Nissen fundoplication, the Belsey Mark IV, the Hill posterior gastropexy, and the Angelchik prosthesis—are currently used by the majority of surgeons. The Nissen fundoplication is most commonly performed for a variety of reasons, not the least of which is that both clinical and experimental studies have shown it to be the most effective operation for long-term control of gastroesophageal reflux. The Belsey Mark IV, which requires thoracotomy and relies on sutures through the esophageal musculature, is essentially a partial fundoplication that envelops 240 degrees of the circumference of the distal esophagus. The reported incidence of recurrent reflux after its use is about twice that after the Nissen procedure. The Hill posterior gastropexy, a fundoplication of even lesser degree, may have specific indications, but it is less effective in the prevention of reflux than the Nissen or Belsey Mark IV procedure. The Angelchik prosthesis has attracted wide attention because of the simplicity of insertion. Its effects are mechanical rather than physiologic. Despite some evidence that the Angelchik device prevents reflux, many complications have necessitated its removal. These complications coupled with insertion of a foreign body have discouraged most thoughtful esophageal surgeons from its use.

In my opinion, the Nissen fundoplication is the most effective antireflux maneuver available. It provides the surgeon with the greatest degree of flexibility in application, and when it is applied properly, complications are relatively few.

NISSEN FUNDOPLICATION

For the Nissen fundoplication to achieve satisfactory results the surgeon must be aware of its proper indications and contraindications and familiar with certain aspects of its performance. Medical treatment of gastroesophageal reflux controls symptoms in the majority of patients. Operation should be undertaken only when symptoms persist after a prolonged period (i.e., 3 to 6 months) of medical therapy or when significant endoscopic evidence of esophageal ulceration persists despite some amelioration of symptoms. Some surgeons might adopt a more aggressive approach in the presence of the complication of replacement of the lower esophageal mucosa with columnar epithelium (Barrett's esophagus). Nevertheless, I have used the same indications for operation in patients with Barrett's esophagus as in other patients with reflux disease because antireflux operations have failed to achieve predictable regression of abnormal mucosa and do not protect against malignant degeneration. The sole exception might be in a patient with severe dysplasia, in which case consideration should be given to resection.

The lack of success after fundoplication encircling a distal esophageal stricture has influenced me to avoid the application of this technique in patients with strictures. In such circumstances I prefer an esophageal lengthening procedure (Collis gastroplasty) with the Nissen wrap performed over the newly formed gastric tube rather than around the firm fibrous strictured area of the distal esophagus. This modification is also preferred after the esophagus is shortened to avoid leaving the wrap in the chest, a potentially dangerous maneuver. The Nissen total wrap should be avoided in patients with poor peristaltic activity of the esophagus, particularly those with achalasia and scleroderma, because it usually leads to obstructive symptoms postoperatively. Lesser wraps of the Belsey or Hill variety are more appropriate for patients who do not have esophageal peristalsis. I disagree with those who advocate performance of an antireflux procedure whenever a paraesophageal hiatus hernia is repaired. Mixed varieties of sliding and paraesophageal hernias certainly exist, but the symptoms are usually the result of mechanical factors related to the paraesophageal element, and only rarely is the LES hypotensive, thus necessitating a wrap.

Adherence to four major principles minimizes postoperative problems and maximizes the chances of success after a Nissen fundoplication: (1) The abdominal approach is preferred, the thoracic approach being reserved for those patients with a previous thoracotomy or those in whom some shortening of the esophagus is suspected. (2) The entire gastric fundus should be freed by division of the short gastric and posterior gastric vessels, thus allowing easy wrapping of the distal esophagus. (3) The fundoplication should be applied loosely, a goal facilitated by use of a large-bore indwelling stent. (4) A relatively short wrap of the distal esophagus, which is currently preferred to the longer wrap advocated originally, facilitates the ability to belch postoperatively and minimizes the risk of "gas bloat" syndrome.

Surgical Technique

Through an upper midline abdominal incision the left lobe of the liver is mobilized, and the phrenoesophageal membrane is divided to permit mobilization of the distal esophagus into the abdomen where it is encircled with a Penrose drain for traction. The short gastric vessels are ligated and divided, and the posterior part of the gastric fundus is freed by dividing the posterior gastric vessels. The freed gastric fundus is then passed behind the distal esophagus where it envelops the lower 1.5 to 2 cm of this structure by approximating the adjacent seromuscular margins of the anterior and posterior gastric wall with interrupted heavy nonabsorbable sutures. Two sutures are used, one of which incorporates a small portion of the anterior esophageal wall. Care is taken to avoid injury to the vagus nerves. A few fine interrupted nonabsorbable sutures are used to reinforce the fundoplication and to secure the collar of the wrap around the esophagus. All of the maneuvers are carried out with a temporary indwelling Maloney dilator of large caliber (42 F to 46 F). The hiatus is narrowed behind the wrap of the distal esophagus with one or two heavy nonabsorbable sutures, and only then is the stent removed. Nasogastric drainage is necessary in patients undergoing reoperation in whom consideration should be given to performance of concomitant pyloromyotomy or pyloroplasty because of the increased hazard of vagal injury when reoperative procedures are undertaken. The surgical incision is closed in the traditional fashion. Oral feeding is resumed with the return of intestinal function. Patients are usually discharged from the hospital within 1 week to 10 days of operation.

Results of Operation

The reported results of the Nissen fundoplication are difficult to analyze because of the many variations of the operation that are now used. Anterior plication, posterior plication, anchoring of the plication to the preaortic fascia, addition of selective vagotomy, and incomplete and double plication are only some of the many variations. The procedure has usually been reported as successful in the permanent relief of reflux in about 90 percent of patients.

From January 1970 to January 1987, I performed a total of 121 Nissen fundoplications for reflux. The technique used was as described earlier, and the mortality was zero. A review of the results of some of these operations, more than one fourth of which were reoperative procedures, disclosed that permanent control of reflux was achieved in 90 percent of patients. However, an entirely satisfactory result was achieved in only 82 percent of these patients. The primary reason for this was that too tight a wrap in earlier years had resulted in recurrent reflux, dysphagia, or "gas bloat" syndrome in some patients. During the last 10 years the use of a larger stent has minimized these problems. About 85 percent of the patients are able to belch postoperatively, and recurrent reflux or "gas bloat" symptoms are extraordinarily uncommon. Transient dysphagia, which may be noted 7 to 10 days postoperatively, usually resolves spontaneously. Postoperative dysphagia is more apt to occur if the esophagus lacks peristalsis or if the wrap is too long and too tight.

MANAGEMENT OF COMPLICATIONS

Complications that require treatment usually result from a wrap that is too tight. Recurrent reflux, "gas bloat" syndrome, and postoperative dysphagia are most common. Reoperation is usually required for relief of symptoms, although the incidence of the "gas bloat" syndrome usually decreases with time. Resuture of the fundoplication in the case of recurrent reflux or takedown of the wrap and refashioning it as a "floppy" fundoplication in the case of "gas bloat" or dysphagia is the recommended reoperative technique. In my experience, another common cause of postoperative dysphagia is the misinterpretation of regurgitation as reflux in patients whose main problem is an esophageal motor abnormality. The "slipped" Nissen is a rare complication; rather than true migration of the wrap, this usually represents a fundoplication that initially was improperly placed around the proximal stomach instead of the distal esophagus. Reoperation with proper positioning of the wrap is indicated. More serious complications, including fistulas, perforations, and gastric ulcerations, have been described but fortunately are extraordinarily uncommon. When encountered, such complications may necessitate heroic surgical measures, usually involving resection, for control.

SUGGESTED READING

DeMeester TR, Bonavina L, Albertucci M. Nissen fundoplication for gastroesophageal reflux disease: evaluation of primary repair in 100 consecutive patients. Ann Surg 1986; 204:9–20.

Ellis FH Jr, Crozier RE. Reflux control by fundoplication: a clinical and manometric assessment of the Nissen operation. Ann Thorac Surg 1984; 38:387–392.

Leonardi HK, Ellis FH Jr. Complications of the Nissen fundoplication. Surg Clin North Am 1983; 63:1155–1165.

Leonardi HK, Lee MK, El-Kurd MF, Ellis FH Jr. An experimental study of the effectiveness of various antireflux operations. Ann Thorac Surg 1977; 24:215–222.

Nissen R. Eine einfache Operation zur Beeinflussung der Refluxoesophagitis. Schweiz Med Wochenschr 1956; 86:590–592.

COLLIS-BELSEY HIATAL HERNIORRHAPHY

F. GRIFFITH PEARSON, M.D., B.Sc.(Med), F.R.C.S.(C), F.A.C.S.

The concept of "gastroplasty" combined with an antireflux hiatal repair was introduced by Collis in Great Britain in 1957. This procedure was devised as an operation for patients with peptic esophagitis and acquired short esophagus in whom the more radical operation of resection and replacement was the commonly recommended surgical therapy. We adopted this approach for similar cases of acquired short esophagus beginning in 1964 with some modifications; a transthoracic rather than thoracoabdominal exposure was employed, and a Belsey-type partial fundoplication was used for the antireflux reconstruction as an alternative to Collis' original repair. Following this early experience we have extended the indications for the application of this technique and reviewed the incidence of complications and the functional results with long-term follow-up. The following commentary is based on our experience between 1964 and 1984 in 430 patients with complex reflux problems that were managed by a modified gastroplasty and partial fundoplication.

INDICATIONS FOR GASTROPLASTY AND FUNDOPLICATION

The rationale for the addition of gastroplasty to an antireflux operation is to eliminate tension on the repair. In the presence of obvious acquired esophageal shortening, the use of any of the standard repairs (Nissen, Belsey, Hill) inevitably results in some tension and an increased risk of failure due to some degree of anatomic recurrence. Our current indications for the addition of gastroplasty include:

1. obvious acquired shortening due to peptic esophagitis and stricture,
2. subtler degrees of acquired shortening that are frequently encountered in cases that require reoperation and in cases of massive, sliding hiatal hernia with intrathoracic stomach. In this latter group of patients, the subtler degrees of shortening may be difficult to evaluate before operation with the usual techniques of contrast radiology and endoscopy. If a standard repair is selected in such cases, these lesser degrees of shortening may only become evident when the repair is completed and some degree of tension is noted.

OPERATIVE TECHNIQUE

Exposure is obtained with a left posterolateral thoracotomy through the sixth intercostal space. The incision is carried well forward to within a few centimeters of the diaphragmatic attachment at the anterior end of the sixth interspace in order to provide optimal access for dissection at the level of the diaphragmatic hiatus. The level of this incision is also optimal for application of the GIA stapler for contruction of the gastric tube.

A left endobronchial blocker is used in order to permit collapse of the left lung and facilitate the operative exposure. The inferior pulmonary ligament is divided, and the mediastinal pleura is incised from the diaphragmatic hiatus below to the posterior aspect of the pulmonary hilus above. The esophagus is mobilized circumferentially between these levels with careful identification of both vagus nerves, which are carried with the mobilized esophagus. The technique for mobilization of the cardia and gastric fundus is identical to that described in the original Belsey Mark IV procedure. With the exception of redo cases, I have *never* found it necessary to divide any of the short gastric vessels. The addition of gastroplasty requires a more extensive clearance of the esophagogastric fat pad from the anterior and lesser curvature aspects of the cardia.

The gastric tube is created on the lesser curvature side of the stomach, in continuity with the distal esophagus over a length of 4 to 5 cm. This can be accomplished with a single application of the GIA stapler. The gastric tube should be of uniform diameter throughout its length and closely approximate the diameter of an indwelling No. 48 F Maloney's bougie. The subsequent 270-degree fundoplication is fashioned with three tiers of sutures placed between esophagus and stomach and extends for a length of 4 to 5 cm. The Belsey Mark IV repair uses only two tiers of these fundoplicating sutures.

ALTERNATIVE TECHNIQUES

Acquired Short Esophagus

In patients with obvious acquired shortening, a number of intrathoracic antireflux reconstructions have been used: intrathoracic Nissen fundoplication, Thal procedure, and Woodward's modification of the Thal procedure. These intrathoracic reconstructions predispose to symptoms because of retention of air and fluid in the intrathoracic stomach and a significant incidence of gastric ulceration with perforation or massive hemorrhage, which has been identified with long-term follow-up. Progressive herniation of the intrathoracic stomach is another reported complication.

The combination of a complete, 360-degree fundoplication with gastroplasty has been popularized by Henderson and by Orringer. A Nissen-type fundoplication is undoubtedly more effective than a partial fundoplication in the prevention of subsequent reflux. Complete fundoplication, however, may prevent normal or physiologic gastroesophageal reflux and result in an inability of the patient to belch or vomit when necessary. Such adverse functional side effects rarely result after a Belsey-type partial fundoplication. The incidence of significant dysphagia is also greater after a complete fundoplication.

Severe Peptic Stricture

In cases of severe peptic stenosis, there are still proponents of resection and bowel interposition, even though the stricture may be dilatable using current techniques. Resection and interposition do result in immediate resolution of the dysphagia and obviate the need for any postoperative dilations. Jejunum or colon is the bowel segment most commonly used as a replacement for the distal esophagus. These reconstructions are technically more difficult than gastroplasty and result in a significantly greater morbidity and mortality rate regardless of experience.

COMPLICATIONS OF GASTROPLASTY AND FUNDOPLICATION

The complications of this operation are the same as those for any of the standard antireflux repairs except for the increased potential for leakage from the lines of gastric division and closure. In our experience, the leak rate is less than 1 percent (which is not dissimilar to the leak rate reported in standard repairs) in patients who are being operated on for the first time. The leak rate is higher in redo cases but not significantly different from the leak rate reported using other techniques of reconstruction in patients who have undergone prior antireflux surgery. Several authors have reported actual necrosis of the gastric tube. This complication has not occurred in any of our cases possibly because we never divide short, gastric vessels during "first-time repairs." The regular division of these short gastric vessels described by some authors may impair the circulation to the gastric tube and suture lines in some cases.

RESULTS AND MANAGEMENT OF FAILURES

In our patients with acquired short esophagus due to esophagitis and dilatable peptic stricture, good results were obtained in 90 percent of patients who did not have an underlying primary motor disorder or a history of previous antireflux surgery. This high proportion of good results has been sustained over long periods of follow-up and was achieved with a low operative mortality and a morbidity that was no greater than that anticipated following any standard hiatal repair.

Reoperation after unsuccessful previous antireflux surgery has achieved good results in 80 percent of patients on long-term follow-up. The higher incidence of failure in these redo cases is undoubtedly related to the increased technical difficulty associated with reoperation, and the potential for a good result diminishes progressively with the number of reoperations. In such cases, the region of the distal esophagus and cardia may be severely damaged, warranting the decision to manage the failure by resection and bowel interposition.

Long-term results have been least favorable in those patients who have developed severe degrees of peptic esophagitis in association with a primary motor disorder (achalasia, scleroderma, diffuse spasm). When followed beyond 5 to 10 years, the failure rate in this group of patients has approached 50 percent. When ulcerative reflux esophagitis and stenosis develop following esophagomyotomy for achalasia or diffuse spasm, there appears to be no conservative operation that will predictably control both reflux and dysphagia in the face of an aperistaltic esophagus and an absent distal sphincter. As a result of these observations, we currently recommend serious consideration of resection in any patient with achalasia who has endoscopic confirmation of gross ulcerative peptic esophagitis or peptic stricture.

SUGGESTED READING

Pearson JG. Collis-Belsey procedure for peptic strictures: five to fifteen year follow-up. In: DeMeester TR, Skinner DB, eds. Esophageal disorders: pathophysiology and therapy. New York: Raven Press, 1985:257.

Pearson FG. Surgical treatment of a peptic stricture. In: Stipa S, Belsey RHR, Moraldi A, eds. Medical and surgical problems of the esophagus. New York: Academic Press, 1981:159.

PARAESOPHAGEAL HERNIA

ASHBY C. MONCURE, M.D.

CLASSIFICATION

The commonly occurring sliding hiatal hernia (type I), in which the esophagogastric junction is displaced cephalad, has clinical significance when productive of gastroesophageal reflux. In contrast, the rarer paraesophageal rolling hiatal hernia (type II), in which the esophagogastric junction is in its normal location and the stomach ascends into the mediastinum through the esophageal hiatus paralleling the esophagus, has clinical importance because of the more acute devastating complications associated with it, such as hemorrhage, incarceration, and strangulation. When the esophagogastric junction ascends into the mediastinum in association with the paraesophageal component, termed a combined or type III hiatal hernia, patients may have both gastroesophageal reflux and the classic complications associated with a paraesophageal hiatal hernia.

When the colon, omentum, or small intestine is within the hiatal hernia sac, the hernia is termed a multiorgan or type IV hernia. Some experts believe that type III and type IV hiatal hernias merely represent advanced degrees of a type I sliding hiatal hernia.

CLINICAL PRESENTATION

The paraesophageal hiatal hernia (type II) will hereafter be grouped with type III and type IV hiatal hernias for discussion of their clinical presentation, diagnosis, and management. These hiatal hernias are most frequently encountered in asymptomatic patients who undergo radiologic examination of the chest for other reasons. Those patients, usually in an elderly population, who are symptomatic present with symptoms representative of esophageal or gastric obstruction, gastrointestinal hemorrhage, respiratory embarrassment, or gastroesophageal reflux.

Obstructive symptoms are those most frequently encountered and range from postprandial discomfort in the precordium, left anterior chest, or low thoracic back, to dysphagia, nausea, and vomiting. Occasionally patients may develop complete obstruction usually associated with organoaxial volvulus. Severe unrelenting pain suggests an incarceration and impending strangulation of the entrapped mediastinal stomach.

Upper gastrointestinal hemorrhage associated with these hiatal hernias usually occurs within the incarcerated proximal stomach, either from mucosal congestion or occasionally from frank ulceration. Patients with this complication may present with iron deficiency anemia reflective of occult hemorrhage or with frank strident acute upper gastrointestinal hemorrhage.

Respiratory embarrassment usually becomes evident with the symptom of dyspnea, probably reflective of encroachment of the gas- and fluid-filled stomach on the intrathoracic lung volume.

Symptomatic gastroesophageal reflux, productive of heartburn and acid regurgitation and occasionally of nocturnal regurgitation and aspiration, may also be present, primarily in the type III and type IV hiatal hernias.

DIAGNOSIS

In the asymptomatic patient, these varieties of hiatal hernia are discovered by the presence of an air-fluid level seen behind the heart on plain chest films. They may also be discovered by upper gastrointestinal barium contrast examinations accomplished for reasons other than diagnosing the hiatal hernia, and a barium enema study may demonstrate transverse colon within the mediastinum.

In the acutely symptomatic patient, the diagnostic approach is dictated by the clinical presentation. In those patients with acute upper gastrointestinal hemorrhage, the chest x-ray film may alert the upper gastrointestinal endoscopist to the probable diagnosis. In those patients presenting with obstruction, barium examination of the upper gastrointestinal tract will demonstrate the hernia and also provide information regarding the probable site of obstruction, either esophageal or gastric. In those patients with symptoms of gastroesophageal reflux, esophagoscopy and esophageal manometry and pH testing usually confirm the suspected diagnosis of associated lower esophageal sphincter incompetence and esophagitis.

MANAGEMENT

The exact incidence of major complications associated with these hiatal hernias is not known but probably is on the order of 10 to 25 percent. Because of the catastrophic nature of these complications, elective repair in medically low risk patients is generally advised. In symptomatic patients, surgical repair is indicated after the diagnosis is established and the patient is properly prepared. In those patients presenting with obstruction, initial nasogastric tube drainage is advisable, if the tube can be placed into the stomach. Upon placement of the tube, a rush of air and retained gastric contents may occur. When acute hemorrhage is the presenting symptom, initial management with histamine-2 antagonists and antacid therapy is appropriate if the hemorrhage is not massive, in which case emergency repair is needed. Pulmonary aspiration is managed with pulmonary physical therapy, postural drainage, and appropriate antibiotics. Esophagitis is initially managed with antacids, histamine-2 antagonists, and elevation of the head of the bed.

In those patients with severe unrelenting pain, total unrelieved obstruction, and massive ongoing hemorrhage, urgent repair is indicated.

Types II, III, and IV hiatal hernias may be repaired from either the transabdominal or transthoracic route (left thoracotomy). Patients with massive obesity, those with type IV hiatal hernias and those with esophageal shortening are best approached transthoracically because the exposure problems related to obesity are less prevalent with posterolateral thoracotomy incisions and greater flexibility of dissection within the chest and management of a short esophagus are afforded by the thoracic approach. Patients with upper gastrointestinal hemorrhage distal to the esophagus or with concomitant major intra-abdominal disease processes or patients who have undergone a previous left thoracotomy or have significant pleural disease in the left hemithorax (such as previous left empyema) should be approached transabdominally.

The contents of the hernia are carefully mobilized, care being taken to preserve the intact vagus nerves. Thereafter, a standard antireflux procedure such as the Belsey Mark IV procedure if the approach is transthoracic or the Hill or Nissen procedure if it is transabdominal should be carried out, accomplishing the common denominators of these procedures, i.e., crural repair, fundoplication of variable extent, and with the Belsey or Hill procedure, intra-abdominal fixation of the lower end of the esophagus.

Occasionally, the surgeon may have difficulty in reducing the contents of the hernia back into the abdominal cavity when approaching the hernia through a left thoracotomy approach. This may be facilitated by using a peripheral counterincision in the diaphragm through which the surgeon can pull down the contents of the hernia with the left hand into the abdominal cavity while the right hand pushes down from above.

In patients with significant esophageal shortening, after Hurst-Maloney mercury-filled tapered rubber dilators are passed to assure that any lower esophageal stricture can be successfully dilated intraoperatively, a Collis-Belsey gastroplasty-antireflux procedure is carried out. The necessity for subsequent interval lower esophageal dilations should be anticipated.

Because gastric outlet obstruction is often a problem postoperatively in these all too frequently elderly patients, placement of a gastrostomy tube for gastric decompression facilitates postoperative care.

Cardiorespiratory complications are those most frequently encountered postoperatively, and the surgeon should be mindful of measures to prevent them, such as avoidance of fluid overload, assiduous control of tachycardias and severe hypertension, and use of positive-pressure ventilation, if needed, in the early postoperative period.

SUGGESTED READING

Malt RA. Hiatal herniorrhaphy. In: Malt RA, ed. Surgical techniques illustrated; a comparative atlas. Philadelphia: Ardmore Medical Books, 1985.

Pearson FG, Cooper JD, Ilver R, et al. Massive hiatal hernia with incarceration: a report of 53 cases. Ann Thorac Surg 1983; 35:45–51.

Skinner DB, Belsey RHR, Hendrix TR, Zuidema GD, eds. Gastroesophageal reflux and hiatal hernia. Boston: Little, Brown, 1972.

RECURRENT HIATAL HERNIA

ROBERT D. HENDERSON, M.B., F.R.C.S.(C), F.A.C.S.

Despite extensive literature on the surgical management of hiatal hernia, very little is written about the management of recurrent hernias. Although recurrence is recognized as an important problem, many of these cases are not accurately diagnosed and frequently are labeled functional, and patients often are regarded as gastrointestinal cripples who will not benefit from further surgery.

It is important to examine the specific problems inherent in various primary hernia repairs, to look at the diagnostic accuracy of our investigative techniques, and to evaluate the effectiveness of revision surgery.

The three most commonly performed primary hernia repairs are the Belsey, the Hill, and the Nissen. All three procedures incorporate an intra-abdominal segment of esophagus and add a fundoplication. Proponents of the Nissen have noted that it may work equally well in the chest if the fundoplication is intact.

With the Belsey procedure, a 270-degree partial fundoplication is used, and with the Nissen, a 360-degree total fundoplication; the Hill repair fixes the esophagogastric junction to the median arcuate ligament with an added short-length total fundoplication.

In patients with partial fundoplication the anatomic recurrence rate is 15 to 20 percent; however, at least 50 percent will have continued reflux as documented radiologically, by nuclear scan, or by pH monitoring. Despite the presence of continued reflux, most of these patients are much improved and many are asymptomatic.

In total fundoplication procedures the anatomic recurrence rate is similar; however, in some, even with the fundoplication in the chest, there is effective reflux control. While continued or recurrent reflux symptoms are the most common problem with partial fundoplication procedures, overcompetence is the more typical presentation in patients with total fundoplication. Overcompetence can occur with inability to eructate or vomit or with early satiety and bloating. Generally the most severe symptom of overcompetence is dysphagia.

In the presence of total fundoplication, dysphagia may occur immediately after surgery, or there may be an interval of normal swallowing followed by dysphagia. The most common presentation is immediate dysphagia, and this is produced by too tight or too long a fundoplication and occasionally by too narrow a diaphragmatic hiatus. In my experience, too long a fundoplication is the most common cause of dysphagia.

In those with late dysphagia, this may be caused by a variety of factors; however, intussusception of stomach through an intact fundoplication occurs only in those with a total fundoplication.

PREOPERATIVE INVESTIGATION

The management of recurrent hiatal hernia is highly specialized and should be reserved for those with experience in this area. Preoperative evaluation should be detailed. History is important not only in determining the present symptoms but also in examining the symptom complex before each previous operation. Some of the presenting symptoms may be operatively induced.

Because of operative distortion, radiologic studies are less accurate following surgery. However, they are an essential part of evaluation, often showing anatomic recurrence, reflux, stricture, and occasionally traumatic diverticula or other evidence of surgical injury.

Esophageal manometric studies are usually indicated to exclude the presence of primary motor disorders, such as achalasia, DES, and scleroderma. They are also of value in determining the extent of operative and reflux-induced motor damage. Manometry can be combined with a Bernstein test and common cavity pH testing.

Reflux testing using 8-, 12- or 24-hour studies is helpful, particularly if symptoms can be correlated with an episode of low pH. Other methods include nuclear studies.

Esophagogastroduodenoscopy is mandatory to exclude gastric and duodenal disease and to determine high pressure zone (HPZ) tone and the extent of esophageal reflux injury. When this detailed study is completed a decision has to be made whether further surgery is indicated or will be beneficial. The major factors in this decision are the extent of reflux damage, the severity of symptoms, and the disruption of the patient's life style. Counterbalancing these factors should be the experience of the surgeon and the anticipated chance of success.

SURGICAL MANAGEMENT

There are three possible approaches to surgical management:

1. Revision and standard repair (Belsey, Hill, and Nissen)
2. Resection and interposition
3. Gastroplasty

Other methods such as a Thal-Woodward have been described, but have not obtained general acceptance. In my view, esophageal shortening and poor-quality tissue make the standard repair less likely to succeed; however, good results have been reported by experienced surgeons.

Resection and interposition have been advocated by some others after three failed repairs. I would disagree with this approach and would reserve resection for the very rare patient with an esophagus destroyed by fistulas or myotomy or by other cause of unusually severe esophageal injury.

My approach has been standard for the past 10 years. All patients requiring surgical revision have had a thoracoabdominal total fundoplication gastroplasty and pyloromyotomy.

A short incision is used crossing the rib margin just below the xiphoid. The esophagus and gastric fundus can be mobilized under direct vision, avoiding major muscle injury. Posterior crural sutures are placed for later approximation. A 5-cm gastroplasty tube is cut over a 60 F bougie. The completion fundoplication is sutured to the gastroplasty suture line and distal 1.5 cm of esophagus to create an intra-abdominal segment of 6.5 cm (5 cm tube and 1.5 cm esophagus). The fundoplication is approximated at the level of the HPZ and upper gastroplasty tube over a distance of 1 cm. This tailored fundoplication supplies stability, uses only 1.5 cm of esophageal length, and avoids problems of overcompetence by its reduced length (Fig. 1).

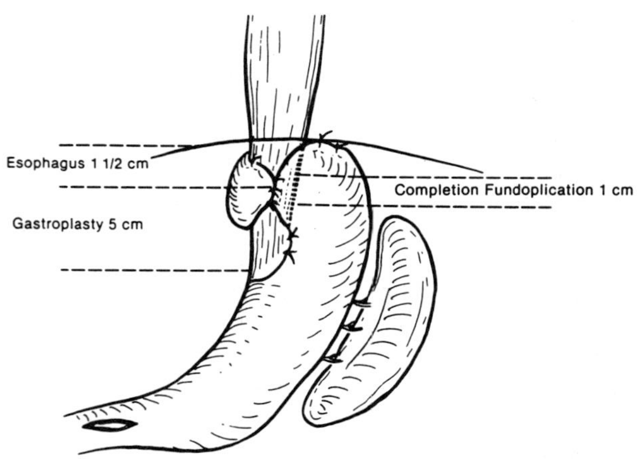

Figure 1 The gastroplasty tube is 5 cm in length and 60 Fr. in circumference. With this method of fundoplication 5 cm of tube and 1.5 cm of esophagus are sutured to the fundus to create 6.5 cm of intra-abdominal esophagus. The tailored completion fundoplication is 1 cm in length and lies at the junction of the gastroplasty tube and HPZ.

Pyloromyotomy is routinely added, since even with intact vagi, function is presumed to be decreased by scar and manipulation.

In a series of 335 consecutive patients who underwent total fundoplication gastroplasty and who were observed for 5 to 10½ years, 93.1 percent were asymptomatic, 3.9 percent had minor residual symptoms, and in 3 percent results were poor.

In a series of 190 patients with recurrent hiatal hernia who required revision gastroplasty and who were followed for 5 to 10½ years, 86.5 percent were asymptomatic, minor residual symptoms were present in 8.1 percent, results were poor in 4.9 percent, and there was one postoperative death (0.5 percent). When these data were analyzed further it was found that of patients with recurrent hernia alone, 90 percent were asymptomatic; however after gastric surgery 80 percent were asymptomatic. Most patients with mild persistent symptoms had gastritis.

Careful preoperative evaluation is essential so that the exact cause of failure can be determined. The thoracoabdominal approach allows dissection under direct vision in both chest and abdomen and avoids injury to the esophagus and gastric fundus. Gastroplasty is used to give a tension-free repair, and a tailored fundoplication allows optimal reflux control while avoiding the problems of overcompetence. Pyloromyotomy is added because of vagal scar and to avoid delayed gastric emptying.

With 10 years' experience this surgical approach to recurrent hiatal hernia has proved to be effective.

SUGGESTED READING

Dilling EW, Peyton MD, Cannon JP, Kanaly PJ, Elkins RC. Comparison of Nissen fundoplication and Belsey Mark IV in the management of gastroesophageal reflux. Am J Surg 1977; 134:730–733.
Henderson RD. Nissen hiatal hernia repair: problems of recurrence and continued symptoms. Ann Thorac Surg 1979; 28:587–593.
Henderson RD. The esophagus: reflux and primary motor disorders. Baltimore:Williams & Wilkins, 1980.
Henderson RD. Surgical management of the failed gastroplasty. J Thorac Cardiovasc Surg 1986; 91:46–52.
Polk HC Jr, Zeppa R. Fundoplication for complicated hiatal hernia: rationale and results. Ann Thorac Surg 1969; 7:202–211.

MANAGEMENT OF PEPTIC STRICTURE OF THE ESOPHAGUS

F. GRIFFITH PEARSON, M.D., B.Sc.(Med), F.R.C.S.(C), F.A.C.S.

DEFINITION

Peptic stricture of the esophagus is caused by scarring and cicatricial contracture following ulceration of the squamous mucosa with inflammation of the underlying wall of the distal esophagus. The damage is secondary to abnormal reflux of gastric contents that may, in some cases, include bile and other digestive enzymes attributable to duodenogastric reflux. Peptic strictures are commonly associated with acquired shortening of the intrathoracic esophagus caused by vertical scar contracture. Strictures may be categorized as (1) severe—longer than 3 cm and requiring forceful dilation; (2) moderate—less than 3 cm but still requiring forceful dilation; and (3) mild—usually short in length and easily dilated with minimal resistance on bougienage.

Abnormal esophageal reflux occurs when there is failure of the physiologic protective mechanisms in the esophagus and cardia. An intra-abdominal location of the lower esophageal sphincter is an important component of this mechanism, and reflux strictures are almost always associated with a sliding hiatal hernia. The severity of stricture may be modified through loss of the normal peristaltic function in the body of the esophagus. This function deteriorates with age, and peptic strictures are most common in the elderly population. The peristaltic pump that clears refluxed material from the esophagus is altogether missing in patients with achalasia and in some with scleroderma. Recognition of these underlying motor disorders is of critical importance for the appropriate selection of therapy.

OPTIONS IN MANAGEMENT

Medical Treatment and Interval Dilation

Many patients with peptic stricture may be judged as unsuitable risks for corrective surgery. As mentioned, this condition is common in the frail and very elderly, and such patients can almost always be managed conservatively. In most instances, dilation can be done as an outpatient procedure using indirect bougienage with the taper-tipped, mercury-weighted Maloney's dilators. The interval between dilations varies greatly among individual patients, who are instructed to return for dilation with each recurrence of significant dysphagia.

Antireflux Surgery

It is now generally accepted that the majority of *dilatable* peptic strictures will resolve with satisfactory resolution of dysphagia provided that further reflux is effectively prevented. In patients with little or no acquired esophageal shortening, the standard hiatal repairs (Nissen, Belsey Mark IV, Hill) may give satisfactory and enduring results. Subtle degrees of shortening, however, are difficult to evaluate even at the time of operation, and the resultant tension on a standard repair predisposes to a higher incidence of failure and continuing reflux. Of these three standard repairs, the Hill procedure is designed to tolerate best some degree of tension.

A variety of intrathoracic reconstructions has been described for the management of patients with peptic stricture and obvious acquired shortening: Thal procedure, Woodward's modification of the Thal operation, and intrathoracic Nissen fundoplication. Although these operations may effectively prevent reflux and permit resolution of the stricture, they are frequently associated with undesirable side effects, including postprandial distress caused by air and fluid retention in the intrathoracic stomach, ulceration with hemorrhage or perforation in the intrathoracic stomach, and some cases of progressive herniation.

My choice of procedure in patients with stricture and acquired shortening is a modified Collis' gastroplasty and fundoplication. In this operation, the stomach and antireflux repair lie within the abdomen, and all tension on the repair is eliminated. Anatomic recurrence of herniation is exceedingly rare following this operation.

Distal Esophageal Resection and Bowel Interposition

In patients at acceptable risk, nondilatable strictures may be managed by resection of the distal esophagus and interposition of a segment of jejunum or colon. My personal choice is to use a short segment of left colon pedicled on the left colic artery, as originally described by Belsey. During the last 20 years, however, the need for this operation has been rare. Using the currently available techniques of bougienage, almost all peptic strictures can be dilated and managed by a more conservative antireflux repair in patients who are surgical candidates. Indeed, at the present time resection is reserved for those patients who suffer disruption or perforation of the esophagus following forceful dilation. Such disruption or perforation is rarely encountered preoperatively and has usually been observed at the time of intraoperative dilation using the Hegar dilators passed retrograde through a small gastrotomy incision. If the stricture cannot be adequately dilated before operation, the patient should be advised that a resection may be necessary and the colon suitably prepared.

TECHNIQUES OF DILATION

The techniques and protocol for stricture dilation are of critical importance if optimal results are to be obtained.

Preoperative Dilation

In most cases this can be accomplished using topical anesthesia (20 to 30 ml of 2 percent viscus lidocaine) and short-acting sedation such as intravenous diazepam. The dose of diazepam must be titrated with particular attention to the patient's size and age. In the average adult under 70 years of age and in otherwise satisfactory health, I use a rapidly injected intravenous bolus of 10 mg of diazepam. Ideally, the stricture should be dilated at least to a size 50, and Maloney's bougies are used for the initial effort. Since the tapered tip of all of these bougies is of the same shape and diameter, I have found it most effective to begin the dilation with a No. 50 Maloney's dilator. The tip of this larger bougie enters the top of the stricture just as easily as a much smaller size, and it is a much more effective dilator because of its relatively greater weight and rigidity. Dilators under size 40 tend to buckle in the pharynx when resistance in the stricture is encountered. During bougienage, I stand on the right side of the patient and support the bougie at the back of the tongue with my left index finger to prevent buckling at this level while exerting some pressure to advance the bougie, which is held in the right hand. In cases of severe stricture, the bougie may be tightly gripped in the stenotic segment, and if the first attempt at passage of a size No. 50 French fails, subsequent attempts are made with progressively smaller diameter bougies, e.g., No. 48 or 46.

If it is not possible to achieve dilation with the Maloney bougies, a more forceful and controlled dilation can be done using the Savary, Puestow, or Plummer dilators, all of which are passed over a string or wire. The indwelling string or wire will prevent perforation by the tip of the bougie but will not preclude splitting the stricture if the dilation is sufficiently forceful. I prefer the Savary dilators passed over a guidewire that has been accurately positioned using a flexible esophagoscope.

Postoperative Dilation

Mild strictures are identified by easy passage of a No. 50 French Maloney's bougie at the first attempt. These cases rarely require postoperative dilation, which is only done if patients present with recurrent dysphagia. Moderate strictures are deliberately brought back for dilation within 1 to 3 weeks of operation. This can be done on an outpatient basis using the same technique described for preoperative dilation with the Maloney bougies. If no resistance is encountered at this first postoperative bougienage, the patient is instructed to return for dilation only if dysphagia recurs.

Long, severe strictures always require one or more postoperative dilations. Again, using a size No. 50 Maloney's dilator, the bougienage is repeated at approximately monthly intervals until there is no longer any resistance to its passage. Thereafter, the patient is instructed to return if there is any recurrence of dysphagia. On occasion, patients with the most severe stages of dilatable stricture have required interval dilation for up to 18 months following repair.

SPECIAL PROBLEMS

Achalasia

Following esophagomyotomy or balloon dilation, some patients with achalasia may develop pathologic reflux with ulcerative esophagitis and stricture. The experience of many surgeons has shown that there is no conservative antireflux operation that predictably prevents reflux on the one hand and avoids significant dysphagia on the other. Assuming that the operative risk is appropriate, the recommendation in these patients is for thoracic esophagectomy and replacement. The entire thoracic esophagus is abnormal in these cases, and I favor a transhiatal esophagectomy and elevation of the stomach through the mediastinal bed of the resected esophagus with an anastomosis in the neck. In patients with achalasia, the functional results of these reconstructions have been almost uniformly good.

Stricture Secondary to Nasogastric Intubation

A severe stricture may rapidly develop at the lower end of the esophagus in association with a period of nasogastric intubation. This complication usually follows a period of severe, postoperative illness and ileus. Once the patient recovers, there may be no further pathologic reflux, and healing occurs with a mature scar that is no longer associated with edema and thickening of the adjacent esophageal wall so characteristic of the usual active peptic stricture. These strictures are usually short, appear clean and uninflamed at endoscopy, and are devoid of thickening and inflammation in the muscular wall. Indirect dilation of these thin-walled strictures is much more likely to result in perforation caused by a vertical splint in the strictured but thin-walled segment of esophagus.

SUGGESTED READING

Belsey RHR. Esophageal reconstruction with colon for benign disease. In: Stipa S, Belsey RHR, Moraldi A, eds. Medical and surgical problems of the esophagus. New York: Academic Press, 1981:195.

Ellis FH. The surgical management of esophageal stricture. In: Stipa S, Belsey RHR, Moraldi A, eds. Medical and surgical problems of the esophagus. New York: Academic Press, 1981:181.

Henderson RD. Management of the patient with benign esophageal stricture. Surg Clin North Am 1983; 63:885–903.

Orringer MB. Surgical treatment of esophageal strictures resulting from gastroesophageal reflux. In: Stipa S, Belsey RHR, Moraldi A, eds. Medical and surgical problems of the esophagus. New York: Academic Press, 1987:165.

Pearson FG. Surgical treatment of a peptic stricture. In: Stipa S, Belsey RHR, Moraldi A, eds. Medical and surgical problems of the esophagus. New York: Academic Press, 1981:159.

Pearson JG. Collis-Belsey procedure for peptic strictures: five to fifteen year follow-up. In: DeMeester TR, Skinner DB, eds. Esophageal disorders: pathophysiology and therapy. New York: Raven Press, 1985:257.

Skinner DB. Benign esophageal strictures. Adv Surg 1976; 10:177–196.

ESOPHAGEAL DILATION

JOEL D. COOPER, M.D., F.R.C.S., F.A.C.S.(C)

"The most dangerous procedure in thoracic surgery," that's how one of my mentors used to describe esophageal dilation, especially for chronic stricture. A wide variety of techniques and equipment have been designed for esophageal dilation, and while a limited number of these suffices for most situations, it is necessary to maintain familiarity with different techniques in order to deal safely and effectively with some of the more difficult problems that arise in a specialized practice.

Among the types of dilators I consider essential are the Maloney bougies, the gum elastic bougies mounted on a thin metal shaft, the Eder-Puestow bougie, the Savary bougies, and the Grundzig-type of balloon dilators. Essential esophagoscopes include the flexible pediatric-sized esophagoscope (7.9 mm), the standard flexible esophagoscope (11 mm), the rigid oval esophagoscope (12 × 16 × 50), the short rigid esophagoscope (12 × 18 × 35), and the large Negus esophagoscope (15.6 × 17.6).

The most common indications for esophageal dilation are peptic esophageal stricture secondary to gastroesophageal reflux; malignant esophageal tumor, prior to insertion of an endoesophageal tube; Schatzki's ring; anastomotic stricture following esophageal resection; and more rarely, stricture caused by ingestion of caustic material, monilial esophagitis, and a variety of other unusual causes. Rarely, esophageal dilation may be of temporary benefit for certain types of motor disorders, including achalasia and diffuse esophageal spasm.

INDIRECT DILATION

When dilation is being performed for the first time on a patient with the recent onset of dysphagia, it may be performed as a therapeutic adjunct to diagnostic endoscopy. In this situation a barium swallow is mandatory prior to endoscopy. For subsequent therapeutic dilations, radiologic and endoscopic assessment of the esophagus is not required each time, but should be repeated at intervals in order to rule out significant changes in the esophageal pathology.

I usually prefer general anesthesia for the initial dilation, since both rigid and flexible endoscopy might be utilized and several different types of dilators employed. An exception to this is in the patient presenting with a radiologically demonstrated Schatzki's ring together with a consistent clinical history. For such individuals, flexible endoscopy and subsequent passage of Maloney's dilators may be accomplished quite satisfactorily under local anesthesia with or without the use of intravenously administered sedation. Patients undergoing repeated dilation for peptic stricture are generally seen on an outpatient basis, without antecedent endoscopy and without the need for sedation.

TECHNIQUE OF DIRECT DILATION

When a tight inflammatory stricture is dilated initially, the rigid esophagoscope is inserted prior to any attempted dilation. After the esophagoscope is advanced to the strictured area, dilators are passed through it. The smaller-sized Maloney's bougies, up to size 28, can be accommodated through the lumen of the rigid esophagoscope. When passing the dilators through the esophagoscope, one can feel the exact amount of force being applied to the stricture. This is not the case when the dilators are passed indirectly, because the friction between the bougie and the pharynx and esophagus do not allow one to "feel" the exact amount of force applied to the stricture.

If the stricture is tight, such that the small flexible Maloney's bougies passed through the esophagoscope do not easily traverse it, then the gum elastic–tipped bougies are utilized through the rigid esophagoscope, under direct vision. With these gum elastic bougies, the tip of the bougie can be angled to help find the passage of an eccentrically placed stricture. After the gum elastic bougies, up to size 28, have been employed through the rigid esophagoscope, the esophagoscope is withdrawn, and indirect bougienage is carried out using Maloney's bougies, preferably up to size 50. However, with some tight strictures, I prefer to limit dilation to size 40 or 44 initially, then repeat it several days later with the larger sizes.

In some cases of rigid or eccentrically placed strictures, the indirect use of Maloney's bougies may be unsatisfactory, since it is difficult to determine exactly how much force is being placed on the stricture for the reasons noted previously. In this case, I would use the Negus esophagoscope, which has a considerably larger diameter than the standard esophagoscope. This scope allows passage of gum elastic–tipped bougies or Maloney's bougies up to size 46.

At times, the lumen of the esophagus may be virtually obliterated by a severe stricture, so that the passage cannot be found. I have found it helpful, on occasion, to insufflate air down the esophagoscope through the stricture and into the stomach. When pressure is applied to the upper abdomen, some of the air may be forced back up through the strictured area, and the bubbling produced by such air can be visualized through the esophagoscope, aiding in the localization of the lumen. If the lumen cannot be found or will not accept even a fine gum elastic–tipped bougie, a flexible guidewire may be placed through the strictured area into the stomach. A Grundzig-type dilating balloon can be inserted over the guidewire and used for the initial dilation. Such a dilating balloon, up to 1.8 cm in diameter, can be obtained from the vascular angiography department, where they are used for balloon dilation of large vessels.

After this initial balloon dilation has been performed, standard dilation techniques, as described before, may be utilized.

For very long or irregular strictures, the passage of a flexible guidewire under fluoroscopic control may greatly facilitate dilation using the Eder-Puestow system. While this type of dilation is seldom utilized, it can be very helpful on occasion. Recently we have found the Savary dilators to be particularly useful over a guidewire. These are firm, smoothly tapered radiopaque bougies with a small hollow core that allows them to be passed over a guidewire. The use of a guidewire, of course, does not exclude esophageal perforation, because the majority of perforations produced at the time of dilation are caused not by penetration of the wall of the esophagus by the tip of the bougie but rather by a split of the esophageal wall resulting from excessive dilation.*

For strictures and webs in the upper esophagus, the same considerations apply as for strictures in the lower esophagus. However, when dilating an upper esophageal stricture, the use of the short rigid esophagoscope is beneficial, since visualization through the short scope is superior to that through the standard scope.

REPEATED DILATION

Some patients require repetitive dilation for benign peptic esophageal strictures. This includes patients who for various reasons are not suitable candidates for an antireflux procedure and are managed in a conservative fashion. Other patients who have undergone an antireflux procedure for peptic stricture may require several postoperative dilations to maintain the caliber of the esophageal lumen during the postoperative healing phase. Patients with a benign postoperative anastomotic stricture following esophageal resection may similarly require periodic dilation. For all of these patients, dilation is easily performed on an outpatient basis using Maloney's dilators in an indirect fashion. Topical anesthesia is applied in the form of a gargle with 4 percent lidocaine solution. I like to coat the bougie with lidocaine lubricant, which may enhance the topical anesthesia, especially if more than one bougie is to be passed. Some patients may require administration of intravenous diazepam prior to the procedure, but most do not.

When periodic dilation is being performed for a previously diagnosed benign condition, it is important to recognize the possibility of malignant degeneration and obtain periodic radiologic and endoscopic assessment of the esophagus. Biopsies of a persistent strictured area should be obtained at intervals, and an esophageal brush should be passed through the lesion to obtain material for cytologic evaluation, as this often detects a malignancy more accurately than a random biopsy.

INTRAOPERATIVE DILATION

Prior to performing an antireflux procedure for peptic stricture, it is desirable to dilate the strictured area up to size 46 to 50 bougie. On occasion, this cannot be accomplished preoperatively. In such a situation, intraoperative dilation is utilized. Having mobilized the distal esophagus through a left thoracotomy, the surgeon's left hand is used to encircle the strictured area of the esophagus while the right hand reaches over the drapes to advance a previously positioned Maloney's bougie. The surgeon thus has good control over the amount of force being placed on the esophagus as he pushes down with the bougie with the one hand while stabilizing the esophagus in the other. An alternative technique is to mobilize the proximal stomach, make a small gastrotomy, and use Haeger's cervical dilators in a retrograde fashion to gradually dilate the strictured area. The gastrotomy is then closed prior to performing the antireflux procedure.

In summary, a wide variety of instruments and techniques are required to safely dilate the differing types and degrees of esophageal stricture.

SUGGESTED READING

Belsey RHR. Corrosive strictures of the esophagus. In: DeMeester TR, Skinner DB, eds. Esophageal disorders: pathophysiology and therapy. New York: Raven Press, 1985: 261.

Benedict EB. Peptic stenosis of the esophagus—a study of 233 patients treated with bougienage, surgery or both. Am J Dig Dis 1966; 11:761–770.

Cooper JD, Choinere L, Ilves R, Miller L. A simplified method for diagnostic esophageal pH monitoring for assessment of gastroesophageal reflux. Ann Thorac Surg 1983; 36:596–603.

Lilly JO, McCaffrey TD. Esophageal stricture dilatation: a new method adapted to the fiberoptic esophagoscope. Am J Dig Dis 1971; 16:1137–1140.

* Editor's Note: We have found it helpful to use the C-arm and fluoroscopy to check placement of the guidewire and observe the passage of the dilators.

I MOTOR DISORDERS

CRICOPHARYNGEAL DYSFUNCTION AND MYOTOMY

ANDRÉ DURANCEAU, M.D., F.R.C.S., F.A.C.S.
RAYMOND TAILLEFER, M.D.

Cricopharyngeal dysfunction results from a variety of causes. Neurologic disorders usually exhibit an assortment of functional abnormalities that may occur individually or in combination. Total absence of voluntary swallowing, poor initiation of swallowing, poor lingual control, and hesitancy are responsible for the deglutition problems. Weak pharyngeal propulsion with a poor relaxation response of the upper sphincter is seen in primary and secondary muscle disease. Idiopathic dysfunction of the upper sphincter with delayed opening or absence of opening or premature contraction is a frequent cause of oropharyngeal dysphagia. The pharynx in this situation retains its force. It is still unclear whether these abnormalities result in pharyngoesophageal diverticulum formation. In gastroesophageal reflux, pharyngoesophageal dysphagia is a frequent symptom, with possible physiologic abnormalities at the upper sphincter level. Neck surgery and radiotherapy may similarly alter upper esophageal sphincter function and laryngeal excursion.

APPROACH IN EVALUATION

Even today the most reliable approach to the patient with oropharyngeal dysphagia remains a thorough subjective evaluation of the symptoms with routine use of a detailed cineesophagogram or videoesophagogram to delineate the anatomic and functional alterations. The importance of these dynamic radiologic studies is emphasized by the fact that abnormal function is sometimes evident on only one or two frames of the evaluation. All phases of swallowing may reveal signs of dysfunction. Manometric evaluation of the whole esophagus is then completed. Absence of lower esophageal sphincter pressure with reflux complications may occur as cricopharyngeal dysfunction. Manometric abnormalities of the upper esophageal sphincter are usually seen with pressure, relaxation, or coordination values. This may be difficult to document because of the radial asymmetry of the sphincter coupled with the upward excursion of the larynx during swallowing. These technical limitations lead to underestimation of the true abnormalities present. The development and use of a long sleeve assembly should permit more accurate pressure recordings with less variation. Radionuclide pharyngoesophageal transit studies are performed to evaluate the effects of cricopharyngeal dysfunction or pharyngeal emptying. They add quantitative data to the functional abnormalities recorded by radiology and manometry. Their use should help to obtain more objective documentation of results before and after any therapy on the upper sphincter. Our final step in the evaluation of oropharyngeal dysphagia is endoscopy. Direct laryngoscopy and use of the short, rigid esophagoscope provide detailed evaluation of the pharyngoesophageal junction and rule out any endoluminal lesion. Evaluation of the distal esophagus and cardia is as important and may be completed later with the fiberoptic endoscope if therapy on the upper sphincter needs to be completed initially.

APPROACH TO TREATMENT

The management of cricopharyngeal dysfunction with medication alone brings unsatisfying results except in situations in which associated disorders are to be controlled: anticholinesterase medication in myasthenia gravis, thyroid and antithyroid medication in the metabolic myopathy of hypothyroidism and hyperthyroidism, and steroids in polymyositis and dermatomyositis. Although the use of medication like oxazepam, nitroglycerin, and calcium-channel blockers has been shown to be beneficial for a portion of patients with primary or secondary disorders affecting the esophageal body and the distal sphincter, their effects on the proximal sphincter area are still undocumented. Oropharyngeal symptoms resulting from reflux disease should be treated by managing the reflux problem. Dilatation of the upper esophageal sphincter can be easily performed using mercury-weighted bougies, but sustained relief cannot be expected from such a procedure unless a fibrotic component is present with the cricopharyngeal dysfunction. Pneumatic or hydrostatic dilatation of the upper sphincter area in the management of these disorders remains to be assessed. Dilatation should not be attempted if a diverticulum is present.

The best indications for cricopharyngeal myotomy are the presence of severe symptoms showing a correlation with pharyngeal and upper esophageal sphincter abnormalities on cineradiology and manometric recordings. Delayed hypopharyngeal clearance on radionuclide studies suggests upper esophageal sphincter dysfunction. The absence of voluntary deglutition and the absence of normal tongue movements represent contraindications to the myotomy, since the whole buccopharyngeal phase of deglutition remains nonexistent even if the upper sphincter is myotomized. Once an objective diagnosis is established there is no advantage in delaying the procedure, since other therapeutic means are lacking. Preoperative management should concentrate on appropriate tracheobronchial toilet, since aspiration is common in these patients. If pulmonary infection is present, aggressive antibiotic treatment must be initiated and the myotomy carried out as soon as the infectious process is under control: such a process will not improve in a patient who continues to aspirate.

TECHNIQUE

The technique for cricopharyngeal myotomy in cricopharyngeal dysfunction without diverticulum formation consists of raising a large rectangular muscular flap covering the distal pharynx, the cricopharyngeal muscle, and the proximal esophagus (Fig. 1). The patient is placed in a supine position with a small pillow under the shoulders. The head is hyperextended and turned to the right. The cricoid cartilage is located and marked at the level of attachment of the cricopharyngeus muscle. The incision is started above the sternal notch and extended toward the ear lobe, following the anterior border of the sternomastoid muscle. Division of the platysma is carried out next, and the superficial branch of the cervical cutaneous nerve is protected when it is in the upper third of the field. If it is in midfield it may have to be sacrificed; prior to the operation the patient is always informed that dysesthesia or anesthesia in the submandibular area may result. When the sternomastoid muscle is dissected free, the omohyoid muscle and the prethyroid muscles are exposed. The plane between these muscles and the thyroid gland is developed and the muscles cut along the axis of the incision. The carotid and the jugular veins are retracted laterally and the thyroid gland medially. When present, the thyroid vein is divided. The deep cervical fascia is open in the line of the incision, the inferior thyroid artery individualized, ligated, and cut laterally near the limits of the carotid sheath. This allows free access to the retropharyngeal space, and the pharyngoesophageal junction is freed by section of all cellular tissue. A No. 36 mercury bougie is used as an intraesophageal stent during the myotomy: it is large enough to ensure proper support during the myotomy, but not bulky enough to neutralize anterior retraction with simultaneous rotation toward the surgeon by the assistant. Excellent exposure is usually obtained, and the area to be myotomized is marked with a low-intensity cautery. After the cricoid cartilage is located, the myotomy is performed using a No. 15 blade. It extends for 5 to 6 cm, covering the distal pharynx, the cricopharyngeal area, and the muscularis of the cervical esophagus. The incision is started contralateral to the posterior midline, and meticulous hemostasis is completed. The muscularis of the cervical esophagus is cut first, and the myotomy extended toward the pharynx. The mucosa is denuded along the incision, and the pharyngeal submucosal plexus is easily identified by its large bluish vessels. The muscularis is then dissected free from the mucosa on the whole posterior aspect of the pharyngoesophageal junction, and the muscle is cut transversely at the proximal and distal limits of the myotomy. The resulting flap can be removed for histologic examination or fixed to retrothyroid tissue. The mercury bougie is then removed from the esophageal lumen and replaced by a Levin tube directed visually toward the stomach. A double 1/4-inch Penrose drain is introduced by a distal counterincision and placed behind the myotomized area and in the mediastinum at the thoracic inlet. The platysma is then closed and the skin reapproximated by a continuous subcuticular suture.

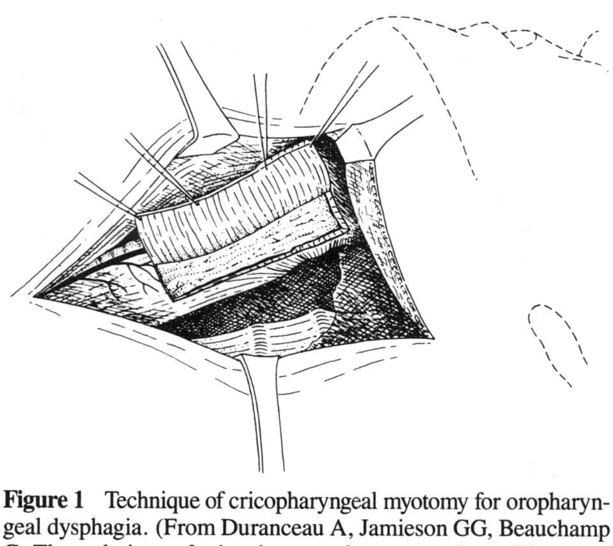

Figure 1 Technique of cricopharyngeal myotomy for oropharyngeal dysphagia. (From Duranceau A, Jamieson GG, Beauchamp G. The technique of cricopharyngeal myotomy. Surg Clin North Am 1983; 63:833-839.)

Postoperative care aims at preventing tracheobronchial aspiration and clearing pulmonary secretions. The gastric tube should keep the stomach empty of all secretions until normal peristalsis has returned. The rationale behind its use is that with the removal of the upper sphincter the last barrier against reflux is gone, and in addition blind introduction of this tube in an emergent postoperative situation will be avoided. Usually a liquid diet is allowed the next day. The two Penrose drains are removed on the second postoperative day if no undue drainage is observed after 24 hours of liquid intake. The patient is usually discharged on the third day with a soft diet.

RESULTS

Cricopharyngeal myotomy is presently the most useful treatment in the management of oropharyngeal dysphagia. A weaker upper sphincter and a shorter high-pressure zone result in diminished resistance to transit. In patients with dysfunction of neurologic origin, satisfactory to excellent results are obtained in more than 50 percent of patients. In muscular disorders, 75 percent of the patients who underwent operation will show sustained relief of the dysphagia. More than 85 percent of those with idiopathic dysfunction of the upper esophageal sphincter without diverticulum formation should show excellent results from the operation. Morbidity may include bleeding, infection, mucosal tear or perforation and fistula formation, recurrent laryngeal nerve palsy, and mediastinitis. Mortality is influenced by patient category. It can be as high as 10 percent for patients with dysfunction of neurologic origin and usually results from persistent aspiration or cardiopulmonary complications.

SUGGESTED READING

Bonavena L, Khan NA, De Meester TR. Pharyngoesophageal dysfunction: the role of cricopharyngeal myotomy. Arch Surg 1985; 120:541–549.

Duranceau A, Lafontaine ER, Taillefer R, Jamieson GG. Oropharyngeal dysphagia and operations on the upper esophageal sphincter. In: Nyhus LL, ed. Surgery annual. New York: Appleton-Century-Crofts, 1987:317.

Dodds WJ, Hogan WJ, Lydon SB, et al. Quantitation of pharyngeal motor function in normal human subjects. J Appl Physiol 1975; 39:692–696.

Payne WS, King RM. Pharyngoesophageal (Zenker's) diverticulum. Surg Clin North Am 1983; 63:815–824.

Winans CS. The pharyngoesophageal closure mechanism: A manometric study. Gastroenterology 1972; 63:768–777.

ACHALASIA

F. HENRY ELLIS Jr., M.D., Ph.D.

There is controversy regarding the choice of treatment of esophageal achalasia, a condition of unknown cause characterized by high resting pressure of the lower esophageal sphincter (LES), which fails to relax with swallowing, and simultaneous low-amplitude deglutitory contractions in the body of the esophagus. The controversy concerns whether forceful dilation or esophagomyotomy is the preferable primary form of therapy and whether an antireflux procedure should be added to esophagomyotomy. I believe that a short esophagomyotomy, limited for the most part to the distal esophagus and not accompanied by an antireflux procedure, is the preferred primary form of therapy and should be performed early in the course of the disease. Good results can be expected in a high percentage of patients after this procedure with few complications.

THERAPEUTIC ALTERNATIVES

Drug Therapy

In the past, drug therapy had little place in the management of patients with esophageal achalasia. Currently some reports suggest that nitrites and calcium-channel blockers, such as nifedipine (Procardia), may be useful in relaxing the LES. However, the proper role of these agents in the symptomatic management of patients with achalasia has yet to be defined.

Dilation

Simple bougienage has long been known to provide only temporary relief of dysphagia for patients with symptomatic esophageal achalasia. To be successful, esophageal dilation must be of the forceful type, employing a pneumatic, hydrostatic, or mechanical dilator. A review of the literature on forceful dilation over the past 15 years disclosed that an overall improvement rate of 70 to 80 percent can be expected. For this type of result to be achieved, patients often require repeated dilations. Of 431 patients reported on by the Mayo Clinic, 18 percent required repeated dilations to achieve good or excellent results. An esophageal leak developed in 19 patients, ten of whom required an operation, and two postoperative deaths occurred, so the technique is not without risk.

Esophagomyotomy and Fundoplication

The addition of fundoplication to esophagomyotomy was prompted by the reported high incidence of reflux esophagitis after esophagomyotomy; it ranged from 15 to 25 percent in some series. After analyzing the techniques employed by those who reported a high incidence of reflux, I am impressed by two factors: either the approach was abdominal rather than thoracic or the incision was carried far down onto the stomach. Clinical and experimental evidence shows that a long incision, i.e., carried 2 cm or more onto the stomach, can be expected to result in a high incidence of reflux esophagitis, whereas a short incision is not. A potential hazard of combining an antireflux procedure, particularly a total wrap, such as a Nissen fundoplication, with esophagomyotomy is esophageal obstruction postoperatively because of the absence of normal esophageal peristalsis in this disease. A lesser wrap, such as that provided by a Belsey or Hill procedure, is less likely to cause obstruction.

SHORT ESOPHAGOMYOTOMY

A correct diagnosis is essential, and in the early stages of the disease before esophageal dilatation has occurred, differentiation between esophageal stricture and carcinoma of the cardia may be difficult. In such cases, preoperative endoscopy is necessary. A definitive diagnosis requires esophageal manometry, the results of which disclose the characteristic motility abnormalities referred to earlier. In more advanced stages of the disease, when marked esophageal dilatation is accompanied by a long history of dysphagia, the diagnosis may be clear-cut, and endoscopy and manometry may be omitted.

Esophagomyotomy by the technique to be described is indicated in any symptomatic patient with esophageal achalasia if the patient's general condition permits. If operation is undertaken early in the course of the disease, no special preparation is required preoperatively. Only on rare occasions may some patients require preoperative respiratory therapy to relieve complications caused by aspiration or need nutritional improvement, i.e., hyperalimentation, if advanced malnutrition is present. The night before operation, only clear liquids are permitted by mouth, and the esophagus is completely lavaged both the night before and the day of operation to minimize the danger of aspiration during induction of anesthesia.

Techniques of Esophagomyotomy

The preferred approach for esophagomyotomy is a left thoracotomy, as it provides the most direct access to the distal esophagus. An incision through the bed of the nonresected left eighth rib has proved satisfactory. The mediastinal pleura is opened and the esophagus mobilized and encircled with a Penrose drain, preserving the vagus nerves. The esophagus is gently elevated, and the esophagogastric junction is delivered a short distance into the chest without dividing any of the hiatal attachments. With the esophagus under tension and compressed by the supporting fingers of the surgeon's left hand, the myotomy is begun on the left anterolateral surface and deepened through the circular muscle of the lower end of the esophagus down to the mucosa. The incision is extended distally across the esophagogastric junction just far enough to ensure complete division of the distal esophageal musculature. External identification of the esophagogastric junction may be facilitated by noting the increased vascularity of the gastric mucosa, evidenced by small vascular channels traversing it. The incision is carried onto the stomach for less than 1 cm. The proximal extent of the incision includes some of the distal dilated thick-walled portion, the total length varying between 5 and 7 cm. After the myotomy is completed, the muscle wall is dissected laterally from the mucosa so that half or more of the circumference is freed, permitting it to pout freely through the incision. The esophagus is then returned to its bed and the mediastinal pleura closed. The thoracic incision is closed in layers, and an intercostal catheter is left in place for postoperative drainage. Oral fluids are permitted the night of operation if desired, and a normal diet is resumed as soon as possible. The intercostal catheter is removed the day after operation, and the patient is usually ready for discharge in 5 or 6 days.

A rare complication after a short esophagomyotomy is an inadequate myotomy that does not sufficiently lower LES pressure, thus resulting in continued dysphagia. Incomplete mobilization of the muscle from the underlying mucosa may lead to healing of the myotomy with recurrent dysphagia. Both these complications require reoperation. A myotomy that extends too far onto the stomach predisposes the patient to gastroesophageal reflux with symptoms of heartburn making medical management necessary. If the myotomy is ineffective or if a stricture develops, more radical maneuvers are required. An antireflux procedure, such as the Belsey procedure, may control reflux. In the presence of a stricture, more radical surgery, such as resection and interposition, or resection with antrectomy and Roux-en-Y gastrojejunostomy may be required. An undetected mucosal injury may result in an esophageal leak with left empyema, a complication that necessitates closed or even open pleural drainage.

RESULTS OF OPERATION

A recent review of the reported results of large series of patients undergoing esophagomyotomy without an antireflux procedure revealed an overall improvement rate of approximately 90 percent. The only prospective randomized study comparing forceful dilation with esophagomyotomy disclosed an improvement rate of 60 percent after dilation compared with an improvement rate of 100 percent after esophagomyotomy.

Between January 1970 and January 1987, 151 esophagomyotomies were performed at the Lahey Clinic for achalasia with no deaths. Approximately one quarter of these patients had been treated on one occasion or more by forceful dilation, and 15 percent had had previous operations in the area of the esophagogastric junction. Analysis of the results in 113 of these patients revealed that 91 percent of patients were improved; the improvement rate was significantly better for patients having primary operation than for those having reoperation. Of the nine patients who had poor results, four had symptomatic gastroesophageal reflux that was controlled medically. None required reoperation. Other poor outcomes were in patients with an inadequate myotomy or in those operated on late when the disease was far advanced and after development of megaesophagus.

SUGGESTED READING

Ellis FH Jr, Olsen AM. Achalasia of the esophagus. Philadelphia: WB Saunders, 1969.

Ellis FH Jr, Crozier RE, Watkins E Jr. Operation for esophageal achalasia: results of esophagomyotomy without an antireflux operation. J Thorac Cardiovasc Surg 1984; 88:344–351.

Ellis FH Jr, Kiser JC, Schlegel JF, et al. Esophagomyotomy for esophageal achalasia: experimental, clinical, and manometric aspects. Ann Surg 1967; 166:640–656.

Murray GF, Battaglini JW, Keagy BA, Starek PJK, Wilcox BR. Selective application of fundoplication in achalasia. Ann Thorac Surg 1984; 37:185–188.

Okike N, Payne WS, Neufeld DM, et al. Esophagomyotomy versus forceful dilation for achalasia of the esophagus: results in 899 patients. Ann Thorac Surg 1979; 28:119–125.

SCLERODERMA AND DIFFUSE SPASM

ROBERT D. HENDERSON, M.B., F.R.C.S.(C), F.A.C.S.

In approximately 65 percent of patients with scleroderma and Raynaud's disease there is a loss of lower esophageal motor function. While this can occur in other collagen diseases it is much less frequent. With loss of motor power, high pressure zone (HPZ) tone is reduced or obliterated, lower esophageal motor waves are simultaneous and of low amplitude, with normal peristalsis occurring only in the proximal esophagus and cricopharyngeus. Patients with an adynamic esophagus are often asymptomatic and can swallow normally, using gravity for food descent. Once reflux develops there is a tendency toward ulceration and early development of strictures. This rapid deterioration is probably related to night reflux and lack of gravitational or propulsive clearance of the refluxed bolus. The problem of reflux may be further aggravated by poor gastric emptying.

INVESTIGATION

Investigation of these patients should include a careful history, manometric confirmation of an adynamic esophagus, pH studies, radiology, and endoscopy. Patients with symptomatic reflux and scleroderma are both a medical and surgical challenge. Medical management is standard for reflux and includes diet, bed elevation, antacids, H_2 blockers, and cholinergics. Failure of medical management is considered to have occurred with persistence of major symptoms or continuance of severe ulceration and stricture. Severe strictures are not uncommon, and patients continue to have severe dysphagia unless these can be dilated to 60 F. The combination of stricture and adynamic esophagus magnifies the dysphagia problems.

SURGICAL MANAGEMENT

Surgical management should be offered only to patients with a stable disease process and preferably those with the CREST variety of scleroderma. Surgery is aimed at effective reflux control. If reflux is prevented, if the esophagus is dilated to 60 F, and if the operative procedure does not produce overcompetence, then normal swallowing can be restored. In patients with severe esophageal shortening I use a transthoracic approach; however, when shortening is not severe by clinical estimation, I use a transabdominal incision with a modified short total fundoplication gastroplasty.

The details of the operation are described in the chapter *Recurrent Hiatal Hernia*. A gastroplasty tube is cut over a 60 F bougie. Posterior crural sutures are placed, to be tied later for loose crural approximation. The fundus is rotated clockwise around the gastroplasty tube and sutured through the suture line and to the distal 1.5 cm of esophagus and gastroplasty tube to produce a stable 6.5-cm intra-abdominal segment (5-cm gastroplasty and 1.5-cm esophagus). The completion fundoplication is approximated by one suture to give a completion length of less than 0.5 cm. Supporting sutures are placed to stabilize the fundoplication. Posterior crural sutures are now tied.

This operation is anatomically stable, requires only 1.5 cm of esophageal length, and is effective in reflux control but avoids overcompetence.

Of the 20 patients in whom this approach was used, 11 were followed up for five years and 9 were followed up for 1 to 5 years; 16 (80 percent) are asymptomatic, 3 (15 percent) are much improved, and 1 (5 percent) has moderate dysphagia. Considering the magnitude of the problem these results are most acceptable.

DIFFUSE ESOPHAGEAL SPASM

The diagnosis and management of diffuse esophageal spasm (DES) form one of the more controversial aspects of esophageal disease. Classic DES is easily diagnosed; however, less typical cases are problematic and require clear difinition.

History is not diagnostic; however, both pain and dysphagia are present in all patients. The most characteristic aspect of their pain complex is spontaneous pain, unrelated to eating, which occurs in 44 percent of patients. Occasionally dysphagia is profound and associated with rapid weight loss.

Manometric studies classically show a normal HPZ and severe high-amplitude disordered motor activity in the distal two-thirds of esophagus. Variations in the manometric pattern include low-amplitude, multipeaked, prolonged duration motor spasticity. Endoscopy is of value mostly in assessing reflux and excluding malignancy.

In my experience, radiology will show the diagnostic features of severe motorspasm and thickened esophageal wall in 47 percent of patients. Inaccurate radiologic assessment is a common problem.

MEDICAL MANAGEMENT

Medical management has variable success; however, some patients respond well to long-acting nitrates or calcium blockers. Although dilatation is usually ineffective, I have seen a few patients with dramatic improvement following passage of a 60 F Maloney bouge. Bag dilatation is also described.

SURGICAL MANAGEMENT

Surgery is reserved for failed medical management and persistent severe symptoms. The exact surgical approach is controversial. A review of seven major publications indicated 148 patients, six different methods of management, only two series with more than 15 patients, and no 5-year follow-up.

Myotomy length is controversial. The following have

been advocated: lower myotomy (aortic arch to stomach), lower myotomy with preservation of HPZ, total thoracic myotomy, and total myotomy with preservation of HPZ.

Anatomic and radiologic studies have shown that smooth muscle extends to the apex of the chest, with 85 percent immediately above the arch, 65 percent in the mid-upper esophagus, and 18 percent at the apex of the chest. Since this is a disease of smooth muscle, it makes sense to myotomize to the apex of the chest. Manometric and radiologic studies have shown that these methods are inaccurate in determining the proximal level of motor spasm. With use of total thoracic myotomy the incidence of residual motor spastic pain is very low.

Preservation of the HPZ is controversial. There are only two reports, and one of these indicated that two of seven patients required revision HPZ myotomy because of overcompetence. I have had five patients referred who had had proximal myotomy with preservation of HPZ. In each instance, overcompetence was a major problem. HPZ preservation should be more extensively investigated and reported on before this approach is considered a method of surgically managing DES.

The addition of hernia repair is also controversial. In my experience, reflux is a problem even with partial fundoplication, and reported series without hernia repair have had a significant incidence of reflux. The difficulty with hernia repair is devising a method that produces competence and avoids dysphagia.

My surgical approach uses a left thoracotomy. The esophagogastric junction is mobilized circumferentially up to the inferior pulmonary vein. Esophagus is mobilized along its mediastinal and pleural surfaces, preserving aortic blood supply, to the level of the aortic arch. A pleural window is opened above the arch to the apex of chest. The myotomy extends from the apex of chest through the HPZ.

Reflux control is obtained by means of a short total fundoplication. Esophagus is sutured to gastric fundus over a distance of 3.5 cm to create an intra-abdominal segment. The fundus is wrapped medially and laterally, fixed to the esophagus, and the completion fundoplication is maintained at less than 0.5 cm. In this method the intra-abdominal esophagus and completion fundoplication length are sutured separately. Reducing the fundoplication length allows tailored competence, which is effective in reflux control and avoids dysphagia.

Thirty-four patients have been treated by total thoracic esophageal myotomy and modified short total fundoplication. The first 17 had gastroplasty, and the second 17 a short fundoplication only. Follow-up ranges from 5 to 10½ years (average 7½ years). Of the 34 patients, 30 (88.2 percent) are asymptomatic; 2 (5.9 percent) have mild residual symptoms; 1 (2.9 percent) has moderate symptoms; and 1 (2.9 percent) has required revision surgery. Results are considered excellent in 94 percent. Each of the two patients with significant persistent symptoms had a gastroplasty, and each had dysphagia; however, one had had extensive previous surgery.

This is the first available 5-year follow-up of extended myotomy for DES and does demonstrate that effective results can be achieved by combining total thoracic esophageal myotomy with a short completion fundoplication.

SUGGESTED READING

Henderson RD, Pearson FG. Surgical management of esophageal scleroderma. J Thorac Cardiovasc Surg 1973; 66:686–692.

Henderson RD, Ryder D, Marryatt G. Extended esophageal myotomy and short total fundoplication hernia repair in diffuse esophageal spasm: Five-year review in 34 patients. Ann Thorac Surg 1987; 43:25–31.

Leonardi HK, Shea JA, Crozier RE, Ellis FH. Diffuse spasm of the esophagus: Clinical, manometric, and surgical considerations. J Thorac Cardiovasc Surg 1977; 74:736–743.

McGiffin D, Lomas C, Gardner M, McKeering L, Robinson D. Long esophageal myotomy for diffuse spasm of the oesophagus. Aust NZ J Surg 1982; 52:193–197.

Russell ML, Friesen D, Henderson RD, Hanna WM. Ultrastructure of the esophagus in scleroderma. Arthritis Rheum 1982; 25:1117–1123.

I ESOPHAGEAL DIVERTICULUM

CERVICAL AND THORACIC ESOPHAGEAL DIVERTICULUM

W. SPENCER PAYNE, M.D.
PETER C. PAIROLERO, M.D.
VICTOR F. TRASTEK, M.D.

Esophageal diverticulum occurs as the consequence of either extrinsic esophageal inflammatory reaction (traction diverticulum) or increased intraluminal pressure (pulsion diverticulum). Three anatomic locations are frequently implicated: (1) pharyngoesophageal (Zenker's), as a consequence of incoordination of the cricopharyngeus, leading to a pulsion pharyngeal mucosal sac; (2) midesophageal, as a consequence of healing granulomatous lymph nodal disease at the carinal level (traction diverticulum); and (3) epiphrenic, as a consequence of either specific functional disturbance of esophageal motility or organic distal esophageal stenosis, leading to pulsion diverticulum. All are capable of producing progressive symptoms, but only Zenker's diverticulum routinely requires surgical treatment. Midesophageal traction diverticulum is rarely symptomatic and rarely requires surgical management. Epiphrenic pulsion diverticulum is often totally asymptomatic, but 1 in 20 patients has significant disability from esophageal obstruction, retention, and regurgitation, and only these are candidates for surgical intervention.

Pharyngoesophageal diverticulum is safely and effectively managed by a one-stage left transcervical diverticulectomy. In recent years, cricopharyngeal myotomy has been added to diverticulectomy as a rational adjunct to diverticulectomy. Cricopharyngeal myotomy alone for a small symptomatic diverticulum is usually performed because diverticulectomy is not practicable, and symptomatic relief is universal. More recently, some have suggested myotomy alone for Zenker's diverticulum of all sizes, although others have championed myotomy with diverticulopexy. Although there may be some validity to these alternate approaches, limited published follow-up data on small numbers of patients fail to provide convincing evidence of progress. Failed myotomy, with or without diverticulopexy, is best managed by diverticulectomy. European throat specialists have developed a transoral endoscopic technique for laser or diathermic division of the spur and common wall between the diverticulum and cervical esophagus. This requires repeated endoscopic sessions, often with general anesthesia. Impressive morbidity, occasional development of cancer in the retained sac, and duration of repetitive treatment lessen enthusiasm for this approach.

The experience at the Mayo Clinic with 888 patients who underwent Zenker's diverticulectomy (age, 28 years to >90 years) indicated a 1.2 percent mortality, 1.8 percent leak rate, and 3.1 percent unilateral vocal cord paralysis. Morbidity and mortality were seen almost exclusively in patients who underwent reoperation after various unsuccessful procedures for diverticula. Long-term follow-up at 5 to 14 years after diverticulectomy showed that 93 percent of results were highly satisfactory and only 4 percent were unsatisfactory. Vocal cord paralysis, when seen, was almost always transient and thought to be the result of traction injury at operation. With appropriate Penrose drainage of the retropharyngeal space at operation, cervical leakage was rarely a serious complication. Spontaneous healing of leak, with parenteral alimentation and antibiotics, should be anticipated in most cases by 10 to 20 days.

Duration of hospitalization after the usual uncomplicated operation is 4 or 5 days, by which time the patient can return to full activities and diet. An esophagogram is usually obtained the morning after operation and, if this is satisfactory, oral diet is begun and rapidly advanced to general diet. Drains are removed once a solid diet is established and prior to dismissal from the hospital. This routine is followed whether the operation is diverticulectomy alone, with myotomy, or when myotomy alone is used. Occasionally patients with Zenker's diverticulum have acute instrumental or foreign body perforation. This complication should be managed as an emergency, and diverticulectomy is the most reliable treatment. Neglected diverticulum, with malnutrition and pulmonary complications of respiratory aspiration, has been uncommon in recent decades, but when seen, it is best managed by an immediate one-stage procedure. In this way, aspiration is terminated, and oral diet is quickly resumed. Cancer in a diverticulum is an uncommon complication that is seen mainly in neglected large sacs. When the neoplasm is well confined to the sac, diverticulectomy is often curative, but lymph nodal metastasis and direct extension to neighboring structures have a grave prognosis.

Traction diverticulum of the midesophagus is rarely a serious clinical problem. It is seen often as an incidental finding on upper gastrointestinal roentgenograms, but it is rarely appreciated at endoscopy. Its incidence appears parallel to that of specific granulomatous disease, especially tuberculosis or histoplasmosis. The chief complication is fistulization either with the tracheobronchial tree or, less commonly, with major or minor intrathoracic arteries or veins. Patients with the former have the classic "swallow-cough" symptom complex, with or without expectoration of identifiable ingested food or liquids. Expectoration of a broncholith with hemoptysis is not uncommon. Recurrent pneumonia, atelectasis, and even sepsis may be presenting features. Roentgenography, especially tomography, often defines significant mediastinal calcification from old granulomatous disease. Fistulas may elude routine contrast radiography of the esophagus, and a prone position may enhance fistula demonstration in some patients. Marker dyes or air infused into the esophagus during bronchoscopy may be required to demonstrate the site of some fistulas. Occasionally the contents of granulomatous mediastinal nodes are discharged into the esophagus, causing an intense inflammatory reaction locally, or alternatively, they may compress the esophagus and cause extrinsic narrowing.

When sizable vessels are eroded by ancient calcific granulomatous disease, bright red blood may be vomited, and at times, massive hematemesis is the prominent feature and can be life threatening. Location of the precise site or cause of bleeding may not be immediately apparent on endoscopy if bleeding is massive. Indeed, in some individuals it is even difficult to ascribe the source for such hemorrhage to the esophagus. Thoracic aortography with selective intercostal angiography should be considered.

When traction diverticulum becomes symptomatic, surgical management is indicated. Most of the length of the esophagus, and especially the pericarinal area, is accessible through a right thoracotomy, although other specifically defined problems may dictate a left-sided approach. Surgical treatment can usually be undertaken without fear of complication from specific organisms because inciting organisms have generally been eliminated by the time complications occur. Local excision of the traction diverticulum is effected conservatively, along with debridement of local mediastinal ancient granulomatous nodal disease and calcium. A layer closure of the esophageal defect over an indwelling 40 F to 50 F catheter prevents esophageal narrowing. Fistulization with the respiratory tract or blood vessels requires similar excision and closure. Occasionally it may be necessary to carry out concomitant pulmonary resection if portions of affected lung have been irreparably damaged. Recurrence or breakdown of repairs is minimized by interposition of viable pedicles of pleura, pericardium, or skeletal muscle. The integrity of esophageal closure is threatened if there is concomitant esophageal obstruction at, or distal to, the repair. Ease of passage of a 50 F bougie assures the absence of organic stenosis, but motility studies of the esophagus are required to define functional disorders. As a general rule, oral diet should not be resumed after such esophageal repairs for at least 7 to 10 days and then only when a contrast esophagogram reveals a normally patent esophagus without leak or obstruction.

Epiphrenic or pulsion diverticulum of the thoracic esophagus most commonly occurs in the distal 10 cm of the thoracic esophagus. A solitary diverticulum protruding into the right side of the chest is most frequent, but multiple bilateral sacs are not uncommon. They can be present without symptoms; in fact, most of those detected radiographically are modest in size, asymptomatic, and do not tend to progress in size or become symptomatic. Surgical intervention is indicated only when these sacs are rapidly enlarging or when clinical symptoms are present. Esophageal obstruction, retention, and regurgitation of fresh bland foodstuff and saliva are usual symptoms, and these symptoms are indistinguishable from the commonly associated esophageal motor disorders (achalasia and diffuse spasm) or the less frequently encountered organic distal esophageal stenoses. Current assessment should include complete evaluation of esophageal status prior to operation. This should include roentgenography, endoscopy, manometry, and acid pH reflux testing. Treatment is by left transthoracic esophageal diverticulectomy, with appropriate myotomy for associated motility disturbance. Some patients have an associated anatomic esophageal hiatal hernia and, occasionally, associated reflux complications. Almost all esophageal stenoses can be dilated to 50 F size, and an appropriate nonobstructive antireflux procedure with hiatal hernia repair can be effected. It is essential that all esophageal obstructive conditions be eliminated at operation because the incidence of leak or recurrent diverticulum is greatly increased in the presence of residual obstruction. Postoperatively the esophagus is kept at rest; a nasogastric tube is used for at least 7 to 10 days before study of the esophagus with water-soluble contrast medium. In the absence of definable obstruction or contrast extravasation, oral diet can be resumed. Confined leakage in the absence of sepsis is managed conservatively with antibiotics, hyperalimentation, and an additional 10 days of taking nothing by mouth before restudy. Leakage should be rare after these precautions. Sepsis from free leakage is extremely uncommon, but it may necessitate esophageal defunctionalization and subsequent delayed esophageal reconstruction.

Some authors recently suggested ignoring the presence of the diverticulum and concentrating on myotomy and relief of organic obstruction. Unfortunately this does not provide predictable relief of symptoms. Additionally, some patients present with symptomatic epiphrenic diverticulum alone, without definable motility or organic obstruction or reflux problems, and they require diverticulectomy for relief of symptoms. Symptomatic epiphrenic diverticulum of the thoracic esophagus is an uncommon and complex problem, and its treatment should not be entered lightly.

Stapling devices are widely used in thoracic surgery today, and their use is particularly applicable for diverticulectomy of the esophagus, whether in the neck or chest. It is important to define the neck of a pulsion diverticulum at the point where the mucosa protrudes through the esophageal musculature. The presence of an indwelling catheter within the lumen of the esophagus prevents stealing lumen as traction is applied to the sac at the time of diverticular neck transection and closure. If possible, and especially in Zenker's diverticulum, the mucosal neck should be amputated and closed at right angles to the long axis of the esophagus to minimize the risk of long stenosis. Muscularis should be approximated to bury the mucosal suture line, to minimize risk of leak. Thoracic esophageal myotomy should not be placed where it exposes a diverticulectomy site. Muscularis can be closed over the Zenker's diverticulectomy site after vertical myotomy by carrying out transverse extramucosal approximation of muscularis.

SUGGESTED READING

Debas HT, Payne WS, Cameron AJ. Physiopathology of lower esophageal diverticulum and its implications for treatment. Surg Gynecol Obstet 1980; 151:593–600.

Dukes RJ, Strimlan CV, Dines DE, et al. Esophageal involvement with mediastinal granuloma. JAMA 1976; 236:2313–2315.

Huang B-S, Payne WS, Cameron AJ. Surgical management for recurrent pharyngoesophageal (Zenker's) diverticulum. Ann Thorac Surg 1984; 37:189–191.

Payne WS, Reynolds RR. Surgical treatment of pharyngoesophageal diverticulum (Zenker's diverticulum). Surg Rounds 1982; 5:18–24.

Welsh GF, Payne WS. The present status of one-stage pharyngo-esophageal diverticulectomy. Surg Clin North Am 1973; 53:953–958.

I ESOPHAGEAL HEMORRHAGE

ENDOSCOPIC SCLEROTHERAPY IN ESOPHAGEAL VARICES

JAMES M. RICHTER, M.D., M.A.
ROBERT H. SCHAPIRO, M.D.

Injection sclerosis of esophageal varices was initially developed using general anesthesia and rigid endoscopic techniques. Although bleeding could be controlled acutely, the hemorrhage tended to recur and the technique fell into disfavor. Recognition of the limitations of portosystemic surgical shunt therapy and the development of flexible fiberoptic endoscopic instruments led to reevaluation of sclerotherapy for bleeding esophageal varices. Controlled clinical studies demonstrate that endoscopic injection sclerosis of varices can both stop acute bleeding and, when used repetitively, prevent future bleeding. There is also some evidence that injection sclerosis increases patient longevity, but it is less firmly established.

Patients presenting with hematemesis or melena and a history of chronic liver disease should undergo diagnostic esophagogastroduodenoscopy to identify the source of their bleeding. Generally, diagnostic endoscopy should be performed after circulatory resuscitation has been accomplished and the patient is stable. Endoscopy should be performed earlier in patients who are bleeding briskly or in those patients whom it may not be possible to stabilize promptly. In the actively bleeding patient, intravenous vasopressin is given to temporarily stop or slow the bleeding. If a skilled endoscopist is not available promptly, a balloon tube such as the Sengstaken-Blakemore or Linton-Nachlas tube can be used to stop the bleeding. If there is uncertainty about the security of the airway during the course of circulatory resuscitation or endoscopy, an endotracheal tube should be placed. Virtually all patients who require balloon tamponade should have endotracheal tubes.

Prior to the diagnostic endoscopy, the stomach is lavaged free of blood. If the bleeding is brisk or large volumes of blood and clot are present in the stomach, an Ewald tube should be used. With the patient in the left lateral position and the airway secure, the patient's pharynx is topically anesthetized with topical lidocaine and small amounts of diazepam (usually 2.5 mg) and meperidine (usually 30 to 50 mg) are given intravenously. Patients who are at risk for endocarditis should be given prophylactic systemic antibiotics. A standard endoscope is introduced orally into the esophagus and is advanced under direct vision into the stomach, where as much fluid as can quickly and conveniently be removed is aspirated through the suction channel. No attempt is made to remove large blood clots. The stomach and duodenum are inspected for the presence of gastritis or peptic ulcers, which are common coincident findings with esophageal varices. The endoscope is then withdrawn and retroflexed to inspect the gastroesophageal junction for the presence of gastric varices and gastroesophageal mucosal tears. If the dependent pool of blood in the stomach rises above the gastroesophageal junction, more fluid must be aspirated. If this cannot be done conveniently, the head and shoulders of the patient should be elevated sufficiently so that the top of the pool falls below the gastroesophageal junction to prevent the spontaneous reflux of blood into the esophagus.

The endoscope is then retracted into the distal esophagus, with the tip of the instrument generally 5 to 8 cm above the gastroesophageal junction. Fresh blood and clot are aspirated. The distal esophagus is inspected for the presence of varices and active bleeding. Even in the presence of serious upper gastrointestinal bleeding from esophageal varices, the specific bleeding varix is identified in less than one-third of cases. If a bleeding varix can be identified, either via active hemorrhage or by a sentinel clot, injection sclerosis begins with that varix. If a specific bleeding varix is not identified, treatment usually begins with the largest varix in the dependent position, provided that no other source of hemorrhage has been identified.

The optimal choice of sclerosant is uncertain. We have experience with 5 percent ethanolamine oleate, 5 percent sodium morrhuate, and 1 percent sodium tetradecyl sulfate. Each of these solutions appears to be equally effective. We have found no advantage to including antibiotics or thrombin in these mixtures, but have not tested them systematically. Currently we are adding a small amount of methylene blue to the sclerosant to use the pigment as a marker for injection sites. To control acute bleeding, injections are normally made by intravariceal puncture approximately 2 cm above the gastroesophageal junction. Three to four milliliters of sclerosant are injected intravariceally under direct vision, and the needle is left in place for 30 to 60 seconds and then withdrawn. If bleeding from the puncture site is observed, the needle is reinserted and another 1 ml of sclerosant is injected. The needle is then held in place for another minute. The tip of the endoscope is then held against the injection site until bleeding stops. We do no use an endoscope fitted with a balloon for tamponade. Injections are made in the other principal varices, moving from those that are most dependent to those that are most superior in the esophagus as viewed through the endoscope. Varices are not usually injected more than

5 cm above the gastroesophageal junction. We generally do four to six injections using 18 to 24 ml of sclerosant during the first course of therapy. As a rule, gastric or duodenal varices are not injected. Often gastric varices can be controlled by injection of the esophageal varices above them with retrograde propagation of clot. Under desperate circumstances, gastric varices may be injected from the retroflexed position.

A steady flow of air often is required to keep the esophagus open during sclerotherapy. This gas tends to collect in the patient's stomach, creating uncomfortable distention. It may be necessary to advance the endoscope into the stomach periodically and aspirate the air.

After the sclerotherapy, the patient is given nothing by mouth for at least 2 hours or until he or she is alert and oriented. A nasogastric tube is not replaced for patients who are stable, and they may take a liquid diet. Patients frequently experience some substernal discomfort for 1 to 3 days after each procedure. We treat this with a small amount of codeine, which can be given by mouth or by injection. Substernal pain that lasts longer than 72 hours may be associated with the development of a post-injection ulcer. When ulceration, a common occurrence, is observed, no further sclerosant is injected in the area of the ulcer. Late strictures are dilated in the conventional fashion using Maloney dilators after ascertaining that the possible ulcers have healed.

After the initial control of hemorrhage, attention turns to the prevention of rebleeding. The natural history studies of variceal bleeding following sclerotherapy show that the greatest risk for rebleeding is within the first 3 weeks after initial bleeding. We normally recommend that a second course of injection sclerotherapy be performed 3 to 5 days after the initial procedure. This is performed in a fashion similar to that of the initial injection sclerosis. The distal esophagus is carefully inspected for evidence of ulceration and thrombosis of previous varices. It may be difficult to visually determine whether or not a varix is thrombosed. We find that palpation with the injector apparatus while the needle is retracted is helpful. Large varices that do not appear to be thrombosed may be injected with 2 to 4 ml of sclerosant. In patients who have not bled again, smaller varices are purposefully injected submucosally to cause thrombosis while minimizing the risk of precipitating hemorrhage during the procedure. Multiple 1- to 2-ml injections are given totaling 15 to 20 ml of sclerosant. The procedure is repeated again between 7 to 10 days and 21 to 28 days after the initial bleed. The follow-up injections are often carried out on an outpatient basis. Subsequent injections are scheduled monthly until all varices are obliterated, depending upon the continued clinical status of the patient.

SUGGESTED READING

Cello JP, Grendell JH, Crass RA, et al. Endoscopic sclerotherapy versus portacaval shunt in patients with severe cirrhosis and acute variceal hemorrhage: long term follow-up. N Engl J Med 1987; 316:11–15.

Gryska PV, Hedberg SE. Injection thrombosclerosis of esophageal varices. Surg Gynecol Obstet 1985; 161:438–444.

Waren WD, Galambos JT, Riepe ST, et al. Distal splenorenal shunt versus endoscopic sclerotherapy for long term management of variceal bleeding: preliminary report of a prospective randomized trial. Ann Surg 1986; 203:454–462.

MALLORY-WEISS SYNDROME

KEITH S. NAUNHEIM, M.D.
ARTHUR E. BAUE, M.D.

In 1929 Mallory and Weiss described 15 patients with upper gastrointestinal hemorrhage resulting from mucosal tears across the gastroesophageal junction. Each patient was a heavy drinker and had recently had a bout of retching or emesis prior to the onset of bleeding. The authors postulated that the disorder was caused by explosive vomiting against a closed cardia producing high intraluminal pressures with resultant luminal dilatation and tearing of the mucosa. Two of the original 15 patients described were operated upon, both unsuccessfully. The first successful operative repair was performed in 1955 by Whiting and Barron, and since then many successive reports have been published.

Although Mallory-Weiss tears were initially felt to occur infrequently, the widespread use of fiberoptic endoscopy has shown that this disorder accounts for up to 15 percent of upper gastrointestinal bleeding episodes. This disorder has been strongly associated with significant alcohol ingestion, but it has also been reported to occur after emesis due to chemotherapy, migraine headaches, motion sickness, pregnancy, and ipecac ingestion and during cardiopulmonary resuscitation. The diagnosis must be seriously considered in any case of acute upper gastrointestinal bleeding with a history of antecedent vomiting, whether brief or prolonged. A high index of suspicion is essential in considering the diagnosis.

In the early reports the diagnosis was made intraoperatively or at autopsy. Soon thereafter attempts at preoperative diagnosis included barium swallows and, somewhat later, angiography. Unfortunately, barium contrast studies of the upper gastrointestinal tract do not demonstrate the lesion and in many cases are actually misleading. Over three-fourths of these patients will have a second potentially hemorrhagic lesion identified on barium contrast study or on endoscopy. Although these incidental lesions (varices, ulcer, or gastritis) may incite the vomiting, they are unrelated to the immediate hemorrhagic episode and could be misinterpreted as the cause of bleeding, leading to inappropriate treatment.

Angiography has also been used to localize the site of bleeding prior to operative intervention. Although specific, it is diagnostic only in cases with vigorous active bleeding, and its invasive nature makes it a less than ideal diagnostic test.

During the last two decades, flexible fiberoptic endoscopy has evolved as the principal diagnostic tool in Mallory-Weiss syndrome. After evacuation of clots from and lavage of the stomach, the endoscope is advanced through the esophagus, stomach, and duodenum. Because of the frequent presence of a second and usually more obvious pathologic lesion, the endoscopist must consistently make a thorough inspection of the gastroesophageal mucosal zone lest a tear go undetected and the hemorrhage be blamed on an incidental ulcer or gastritis. The diagnostic findings are one or more linear tears in the mucosa immediately above or below or across the gastroesophageal junction. Often fresh adherent clot or a small bleeding artery can be visualized at the base of these tears.

Nonoperative medical therapy is successful in more than 80 percent of Mallory-Weiss tears. Prior to endoscopy, virtually all patients will have undergone nasal or peroral gastric intubation with a large-bore catheter (i.e., 36 F Ewald tube). Lavage with saline is performed to evacuate clots, not only to facilitate full endoscopic visualization but also as medical management for upper gastrointestinal hemorrhage. In a small minority of patients, however, the bleeding will continue despite these measures. When this occurs we proceed to operative intervention in all but the most fragile patients. Further nonoperative attempts can be utilized in this small subset of patients in whom general anesthesia alone might prove lethal. This group is comprised mostly of elderly cirrhotic patients with a marked coagulopathy or other operative contraindications (i.e., recent stroke or infarction). In these patients, angiography with selective catheterization and Gelfoam embolization of the left gastric artery can be lifesaving. This is contraindicated in patients having had prior gastric surgery in whom the collateral arterial blood supply might be compromised, thereby leading to gastric infarction.

Although utilization of the Sengstaken-Blakemore tube has also been advocated in this disorder, we do not agree with its use because of the frequency of rebleeding and the potential for further gastroesophageal damage.

The operative approach is simple and straightforward. We use prophylactic antibiotics (1 g cephalothin intramuscularly) 1 hour before operation and for two doses at 6-hour intervals after operation. A laparotomy is performed through an upper midline incision. No dissection is required to expose the anterior surface of the stomach, which should be closely inspected. In many cases this will reveal a faint subserosal hemorrhage just at the level of the cardia, a pathognomonic feature of Mallory-Weiss tears. The stomach is opened in the middle third through a longitudinal gastrotomy, and all intraluminal clots are evacuated. Two Deaver retractors can be placed within the gastric lumen at the cephalad extent of the gastrotomy. Upward traction on these instruments will expose the gastroesophageal junction. Additional exposure may be gained from mild upward traction on the nasogastric tube, which can bring the gastroesophageal junction into even better view. There is but a single tear in the majority of these cases; however, multiple tears do occur, and the entire area should be carefully inspected. Any arterial bleeding point should be individually ligated, and then the mucosa and submucosa should be reapproximated with an absorbable 4–0 suture in running fashion. One last inspection for further bleeding points is carried out, and once this is accomplished, the stomach can be closed with a single layer of interrupted 3–0 silk sutures. The peritoneal cavity is liberally irrigated with saline, and the abdomen is closed in the standard fashion. Nasogastric sump suction is continued until gastric motility returns (evidenced by decreasing amounts of nasogastric return and by the passage of flatus). When this occurs the nasogastric tube can be removed and the patient rapidly advanced to a regular diet. The incidence of rebleeding should be near zero if all mucosal tears are visualized and properly repaired. The single greatest danger in the treatment of this disorder is failure to identify the primary lesion. When this occurs, the treatment or procedure may be inappropriate (i.e., gastrectomy) and followed by resumption of bleeding. In the Mallory-Weiss syndrome, recognition of the problem is nine-tenths of the solution.

SUGGESTED READING

Baue AE. Bleeding from lacerations of the cardia: a Mallory-Weiss syndrome. JAMA 1963; 184:325–328.

Bubrick MP, Lundeen JW, Onstad GR, Hitchcock CR. Mallory-Weiss syndrome: analysis of 59 cases. Surgery 1980; 88:400–416.

Mallory GK, Weiss S. Hemorrhages from lacerations of the cardiac orifice of the stomach due to vomiting. Am J Med Sci 1929; 178:506.

Sugawa C, Benishek D, Walt AJ. Mallory-Weiss syndrome: a study of 224 patients. Am J Surg 1983; 145:30–33.

Todd GJ, Zikria BA. Mallory-Weiss syndrome. A changing clinical picture. Ann Surg 1977; 186:146–148.

BARRETT'S ESOPHAGUS

BARRETT'S ESOPHAGUS

DOUGLAS J. MATHISEN, M.D.

Barrett's esophagus is lined with columnar mucosa. Compelling evidence suggests that Barrett's esophagus is a consequence of gastroesophageal reflux in most cases. A small but as yet undefined percent of patients have a congenital origin for this abnormal esophageal mucosa. It is predominantly a disorder of Caucasians and occurs in approximately 10 to 20 percent of patients who are found to have endoscopic evidence of esophagitis. What factors predispose patients to the development of Barrett's esophagus is unknown, although hypotheses have been proposed regarding the composition of refluxed material as responsible. The diagnosis of Barrett's esophagus is made by endoscopy and biopsy, which show a variety of columnar epithelia located in the tubular esophagus with squamous mucosa above it.

Barrett's esophagus and its management can be divided into three categories: (1) symptomatic reflux esophagitis, (2) complications of reflux esophagitis, and (3) adenocarcinoma arising within a Barrett's esophagus.

REFLUX ESOPHAGITIS

When patients with symptomatic reflux esophagitis have been documented to have Barrett's mucosa, proper management should include routine measures used to diminish reflux and institution of antacid and histamine H_2 blockers to manage the level of acid. I believe that endoscopic surveillance in these patients is important, despite claims to the contrary. The exact level of the squamocolumnar junction can thereby be measured, information gained as to its progression or regression while the patient is on treatment, and histologic changes of dysplasia or frank carcinoma in situ can be identified. Surgical intervention in this group of patients in the form of antireflux surgery should be considered for intractable symptoms of reflux, cephalad progression of the squamocolumnar junction, and progressively severe dysplastic changes of the mucosa. Following successful antireflux surgery, these patients still need to be followed carefully by means of endoscopy to see if regression of Barrett's mucosa occurs, to observe the histologic changes in the mucosa, to identify the possible development of cancer, and to monitor those in whom antireflux surgery has not been effective in controlling reflux. The choice of antireflux procedure is left to the discretion of each surgeon.

COMPLICATIONS OF REFLUX

Barrett's esophagus is frequently associated with significant esophageal bleeding, the development of severe esophageal ulceration, and a significant incidence of stricture formation. When these symptoms develop, aggressive medical management is clearly indicated, and there is some evidence that the use of antacids and H_2 antagonists together is more effective in managing the symptoms. Failure to control these complications should lead to early surgical intervention. Massive upper gastrointestinal bleeding, although uncommon, may limit the surgical options and therefore it should be treated vigorously. Large penetrating esophageal ulcers may be difficult to control medically and must always be evaluated for the presence of cancer. Some success has been achieved with aggressive medical treatment, including antacids and H_2 receptors. Failure of standard medical regimens, however, may lead to surgical intervention. Ulcers that are deeply penetrating or are found at surgery to show signs of perforation should be managed by resection and reconstruction. The use of short-segment colon or jejunum may be preferable to standard esophagogastrectomy because of the likelihood of recurrent severe reflux in this group of patients. Simple antireflux procedures in these patients may predispose them to future bleeding or perforation of the esophageal ulcer; therefore each patient must be given careful consideration as to appropriate surgical treatment. Strictures typically develop at the squamocolumnar junction, but may occur at any level in Barrett's mucosa. Initial management with dilation and aggressive medical treatment is warranted, especially in high-risk patients. Failure to control the stricture medically should lead to early surgical intervention. If shortening of the esophagus has occurred secondary to stricture, a gastroplasty plus a standard antireflux procedure is necessary. We have used the Collis-Belsey type procedure and have occasionally found the need for colon or jejunal interposition in this group of patients. These patients also require careful postsurgical follow-up for the development of cancer.

ADENOCARCINOMA IN BARRETT'S ESOPHAGUS

Dysplasia is a common finding in patients with Barrett's esophagus and may be identified in 68 to 100 percent of cases. Therefore, patients who are found to have dysplasia without carcinoma are presumably at high risk for the development of subsequent adenocarcinoma. Progression to severe dysplasia is an ominous finding. The prevalence of adenocarcinoma in patients with Barrett's esophagus is variously reported at between 10 and 20 percent. The exact incidence is unknown, but it appears that patients with Barrett's mucosa are 30 to 40 times more likely to develop adenocarcinoma than the population at large. The presence of carcinoma in situ or invasive carcinoma is an indication for surgical intervention. Long-term survival and even cure are possible, contrary to previously held opinions. Surgical resection should include the entire segment of esophagus containing Barrett's mucosa, since tumors may frequently be multifocal and retained Barrett's mucosa, of course, may be at risk of developing cancer in the future. The role of chemotherapy and radiation therapy in this group of patients is similar to that for all patients who have adenocarcinoma of the esophagus.

SUGGESTED READING

Cameron AJ, Ott BJ, Payne WS. The incidence of adenocarcinoma in columnar-lined (Barrett's) esophagus. N Engl J Med 1985; 313:857–859.

Naef AP, Savary M, Ozzello L. Columnar-lined lower esophagus: an acquired lesion with malignant predisposition: report of 140 cases of Barrett's esophagus with 12 adenocarcinoma. J Thorac Cardiovasc Surg 1975; 70:826–835.

Sarr MG, Hamilton SR, Marrone GC, Cameron JL. Barrett's esophagus: its prevalence and association with adenocarcinoma in patients with symptoms of gastroesophageal reflux. Am J Surg 1985; 149:187–193.

Skinner DB, Walther BC, Riddell RH, et al. Barrett's esophagus: comparison of benign and malignant cases. Ann Surg 1983; 198:554–566.

ESOPHAGEAL PERFORATION

SPONTANEOUS AND IATROGENIC ESOPHAGEAL PERFORATION

HERMES C. GRILLO, M.D.

Esophageal perforation is still not diagnosed promptly enough in many cases. Mortality rises steeply when there is delay in diagnosis. Although contained perforations, best defined as such some time after the incident, may be managed conservatively, especially after limited instrumental perforations, aggressive surgical therapy of esophageal perforation is usually the approach of choice.

TYPES OF PERFORATION

Iatrogenic perforation continues to be most common (Table 1). Next is "spontaneous" or effort perforation. Perforation caused by a foreign body is more common in children. Perforations may also result from external trauma, chemical burns, adjacent sepsis, or neoplasm.

Iatrogenic Perforation

Perforations occur after esophagoscopy and bougienage with and through flexible instruments as well as with rigid instruments. The cricopharyngeal region is most at risk; the lower end of the esophagus is the other likely spot. Stenosis and other lesions increase the hazards. Biopsy of lesions may also lead to perforation. A particularly severe injury may be caused by forceful dilation of achalasia. Forceful dilation of achalasia carries an incidence of perforation four times higher than the incidence of mediastinal leakage following esophagomyotomy. Other instruments intended either for the esophagus or the trachea have been known to cause perforation, including endotracheal tubes, nasogastric tubes, suction catheters, esophageal stethoscopes, and resuscitation tubes. Surgical procedures adjacent to the esophagus may also lead to erosion, devascularization, or septic perforation.

Spontaneous Perforation

This is generally the result of a postemetic tear of the lower esophagus. If the tear is partial, a Mallory-Weiss syndrome occurs, with bleeding into the esophageal lumen. If the tear rends the full thickness of esophageal wall,

TABLE 1 Causes and Locations of Esophageal Perforations*

Causes	*Location*			
	Cervical	*Thoracic*	*Abdominal*	*No. (%)*
Iatrogenic perforation				
esophagoscopy	6	2	—	8(9)
dilatation	2	19	1	22(26)
Blakemore or Linton tubes	—	9	—	9(11)
endotracheal tubes	7	—	—	7(8)
paraesophageal surgery	—	5	5	10(12)
Levin or Celestin tubes	—	2	—	2(2)
"Spontaneous" perforation	—	11	—	11(13)
Foreign body	5	4	—	9(11)
External trauma	4	3	—	7(8)
Total	24	55	6	85(100%)

* From Michel L, Grillo HC, Malt RA. Operative and nonoperative management of esophageal perforations. Ann Surg 1981; 194:58.

the Boerhaave syndrome results. Bleeding is rare in the latter. Rarely, submucosal hemorrhage occurs in the esophagus; this has been called esophageal apoplexy. The resulting hematoma may obstruct the esophagus. On rare occasion the mucosa may then rupture, and hematemesis follows.

Foreign Bodies

Foreign bodies may cause perforation directly or it may be due to erosion and ulceration. Traumatic extraction of the foreign body may lead to a tear in an already weakened wall.

External Trauma

The esophagus may be ruptured by closed trauma to the neck, the thorax, or the abdomen. Cervical injuries may result from a direct blow to the neck such as that from a steering wheel or dashboard. Usually the airway is simultaneously ruptured. Crushing chest injury may cause a tear of the esophagus in conjunction with a tear of the trachea. Penetrating wounds of the thoracic esophagus are rare because of the small size of the organ, the depth of its location, and the vital structures around it.

Chemical injury by corrosives may produce necrosis or inflammatory changes with later injury druing dilation.

CLINICAL PRESENTATION

Cervical Perforation

Subcutaneous emphysema is the most common manifestation, followed by pneumomediastinum, hydrothorax, and then dyspnea, pneumothorax, and a picture resembling shock. The last is uncommon after cervical perforation. Essentially all patients have cervical pain.

Thoracic Perforation

Mackler's diagnostic triad for spontaneous perforation of the thoracic esophagus consists of vomiting, pain in the thorax, and subcutaneous emphysema. This triad is seen in a minority of patients. Almost all patients with thoracic perforation suffer from pain early. Hydrothorax appears most frequently, followed by dyspnea and then shock. Pneumomediastinum, pneumothorax, and subcutaneous emphysema follow, in that order of frequency. Signs and symptoms following instrumental perforation of the thoracic esophagus are essentially the same as those seen after spontaneous perforation, although onset after the latter is usually more immediate and severe. With a free esophageal perforation into the thoracic cavity, progression is rapid, and the patient may be in shock within 24 hours. The picture of cervical perforation is more gradual and resembles that of progressive sepsis.

In *cervical perforation*, x-ray films show dissection of air in the neck tissues and widening (on lateral view) of the space between the airway and vertebrae. In *intrathoracic* perforations pneumothorax was seen in 26 percent of patients, pneumomediastinum in 41 percent and pleural effusion in 59 percent.

Spontaneous perforation may manifest initially with epigastric pain and thus be misdiagnosed as perforated ulcer or pancreatitis. The physician must keep the entity very much in mind in order to make a prompt diagnosis. If pain follows instrumentation, the diagnosis should be suspected immediately. Radiologic examination of the neck and chest should be done at once. Esophagograms should be performed preferably using water-soluble contrast medium. If there is any question or if the definition is inadequate, then barium may be used quite safely. If there is a suspicion of possible esophageal injury in conjunction with blunt injury to the trachea, barium should be used, since water-soluble material that might enter the airway would be too irritating. Endoscopy using methylene blue in the esophagus may be used.

TREATMENT

Cervical Perforation

The approach is through the classic avascular plane anterior to the sternocleidomastoid muscle, the carotid artery, and the internal jugular vein. This may be done either through a transverse collar incision or through an incision anterior to the sternocleidomastoid muscle. The middle thyroid vein and sometimes the omohyoid and inferior thyroid artery may be divided. Care must be taken not to injure the recurrent laryngeal nerve. If the perforation is accessible, it is closed (Table 2). Whether the perforation is sutured or not, an adequate soft suction drain must be placed. A rigid drain might cause vascular erosion. I prefer also to place gastrostomy and jejunostomy tubes. The stomach is drained to prevent reflux. The J-tube provides effective alimentation during healing. Antibiotic coverage is used initially. In late perforations when there is a retropharyngeal abscess, a similar approach is used, but no effort is made to suture the esophagus. In the latter case the time required for healing and closure of the perforation may be longer.

Thoracic Perforation

This is usually an urgent indication for operation, following fluid resuscitation. Although a chest tube may control massive hydropneumothorax for a brief time, an operative approach to the perforation should be made. Exceptions are patients who might have a small contained perforation with little evidence of systemic response or who have already shown stability for a time after perforation before being examined. Mortality figures clearly indicate that delay may be disastrous (see Table 2).

Through a thoracotomy, the pleural space is thoroughly cleansed and the area of perforation debrided. Usually the mucosa is in quite good condition, whereas the muscular wall may show considerable inflammatory change. The mucosa is repaired with interrupted 4–0 inverting silk

TABLE 2 Treatment of 72 Cases of Esophageal Perforations*

Type of Treatment	*Number of Patients*	*Mortality Rate*	
		Number	*Percent*
Cervical perforations			
nonoperative treatment	11	2	18
drainage	4	—	—
suture repair	6	—	—
Thoracic perforations			
nonoperative treatment	8	1	12.5
drainage	7	3	43
suture repair	10	2	20
suture and pleural flap	9	1	11
esophagectomy	8	1	12.5
exclusion-diversion	3	1	33
Abdominal perforations			
drainage	1	—	0
suture repair	4	1	25
Thal gastroplasty	1	—	0
Total	72	12	16.6

* From Michel L, Grillo HC, Malt RA. Operative and nonoperative management of esophageal perforations. Ann Surg 1981; 194:57.

sutures with the knots inside. The muscularis is closed with a layer of interrupted mattress sutures. I believe that it is always worthwhile to buttress the closure, even in a fresh perforation. The incidence of releakage from esophageal closure after perforation remains much too high and increases markedly with the time after perforation at which the repair was done.

I believe that repair should also be done after delayed perforation, even if it is 72 hours or longer after the event. In this case, thorough decortication of the lung is necessary so that it will expand to fill the pleural space postoperatively. Since the esophageal wall is much indurated by this time, a second-layer closure will probably not be wholly satisfactory or will be impossible. On the other hand, the mucosa may often be closed. In these cases buttressing is mandatory. A variety of tissue has been used, including pedicled intercostal muscle, a tongue of diaphragm, thickened pleura, pericardial fat pad, infolded gastric wall, and omentum. Pleura can only be used after *delayed* perforation, when it has already thickened markedly. A good method that does not require entering the abdomen is the pedicled intercostal muscle flap. In all of these techniques the buttressing flap should be sutured meticulously around the perforation as if it were an anastomotic layer. A few tacking sutures are not adequate. Chest tubes are then placed, the lung fully expanded, and chest closed. Gastrostomy and jejunostomy are performed for the reasons given.

Esophageal exclusion or diversion is rarely, if ever, necessary. Thus in a difficult case of early reperforation (seen 3 weeks after the original injury) with esophagopleurocutaneous fistula, treatment was by reoperation, mobilization and closure of the esophagus, and intercostal muscle flap buttress further supported by an omental pedicle flap. Total diversion above and below may present great difficulties in later esophageal reconstruction. Esophagectomy has a place in the treatment of esophageal perforation in a rare case such as perforation following biopsy of a carcinoma of the esophagus when the patient is otherwise an operative candidate.

In any patient with esophageal perforation, distal obstruction must be corrected if closure is to be successful. Thus, for example, if there is a perforation above an achalasia, a myotomy must be done. If there is pyloric obstruction, it must be relieved.

SUGGESTED READING

Bradham RR, Bridgeman AR, Scott SM, Betts RH. Spontaneous esophageal perforation. Management of the "intermediate" phase. Ann Thorac Surg 1967; 3:6.

Grillo HC. Esophageal perforation. Surg Rounds 1983; (Feb) 50–72.

Michel L, Malt RA, Grillo HC. Operative and non-operative management of esophageal perforations. Ann Surg 1981; 194:57–63.

Michel L, Malt RA, Grillo HC. Esophageal perforation. Ann Thorac Surg 1982; 33:203–210.

Skinner DB, Little AG, DeMeester TR. Management of esophageal perforation. Am J Surg 1980; 139:760–764.

ESOPHAGEAL INFECTION

MONILIASIS

MARK B. ORRINGER, M.D.

Candida albicans is a fungus that is a normal commensal inhabitant of the mouth, oropharynx, and lower gastrointestinal tract. In the setting of altered immunologic competence, this fungus may become a pathogen that typically has one of three clinical presentations. (1) It most commonly causes an acute, superficial, generally self-limited infection of oral and vaginal mucous membranes in infants, diabetics, denture wearers, and pregnant or physiologically normal women. (2) It may occur as a systemic infection of the bloodstream or viscera, most often gastrointestinal, respiratory, or renal, in patients with indwelling intravenous catheters; intravenous drug abusers; patients whose immunologic competence is altered by chronic disease, immunosuppressive therapy, or steroids; and in those receiving broad-spectrum antibiotics that can alter normal gastrointestinal flora. (3) Mucocutaneous candidiasis is the least common form of the infection, generally beginning in infancy or childhood, involving the skin, nails, and mucous membranes, and typically associated with a cell-mediated immunodeficiency and often failure of various endocrine glands. *Candida* esophagitis, therefore, typically occurs in patients with underlying malignant disease, those receiving immunosuppressive therapy, those with diabetes or primary immunodeficiencies, patients receiving prolonged broad-spectrum antibiotic therapy, those with endocrine abnormalities, severe cachexia, or protracted postoperative courses, and the elderly.

The diagnosis of *Candida* esophagitis is frequently unsuspected and therefore missed. Typically, in acute monilial esophagitis with oropharyngeal involvement, the patient complains of difficult or painful swallowing, symptoms easily attributable to the use of a nasogastric tube, which is common particularly in postoperative patients.

When *Candida* esophagitis is suspected, barium esophagography may confirm the diagnosis by demonstrating impaired motility; the cobblestone pattern of luminal nodularity due to mucosal ulceration and submucosal edema; or in advanced cases, a shaggy mucosal pattern due to mucosal ulceration, submucosal edema, and pseudomembrane formation. In the early stages of the disease, however, the patient's pain on swallowing may prevent him from distending the thoracic esophagus with a bolus of barium, giving the erroneous impression of either a deceptively normal esophagus or esophageal spasm.

Esophagoscopy is the mainstay of diagnosis of *Candida* esophagitis, which initially is seen endoscopically as characteristic raised, white plaque-like lesions. The mucosa is erythematous and nonulcerated. Direct brushings of the lesions for wet-mount microscopic examination and culture are far superior to esophageal biopsy in establishing the diagnosis. As the disease progresses and mucosal ulceration occurs, an overlying whitish, cheesy exudate, or pseudomembrane, is found. If the patient survives long enough from the underlying disease process, the inflammatory reaction may extend through the wall of the esophagus with invasion of the mucosal, submucosal, and muscle layers by the fungus. Healing of such extensive panmural esophagitis may result in a chronic stricture, an unusual but definite complication of monilial esophagitis. Strictures due to monilial esophagitis are seldom seen because (1) most patients with this condition are terminally ill and do not survive long enough to develop esophageal fibrosis, and (2) in the vast majority of cases, monilial esophagitis is a superficial disease confined primarily to the mucosa.

Candida may invade the thoracic esophagus either diffusely or segmentally, in which case there is a predilection for involvement of the distal and middle thirds. Curiously, however, the rare monilial esophageal stricture most often occurs in the upper and middle thirds of the thoracic esophagus. One likely explanation for this phenomenon is the fact that esophageal submucosal glands predominate in the upper half of the thoracic esophagus. Inflammation of these glands from infection, stasis, or distal obstruction can produce dilatation and the typical intramural outpouchings of these glands on barium swallow examination — "intramural esophageal pseudodiverticulosis." Inflammation of the tissues surrounding these dilated glands—peridiverticulitis — may result in stricture formation. That *C. albicans* has been cultured from the esophagus in half of the reported cases of intramural esophageal pseudodiverticulosis suggests a causal relationship.

Acute monilial esophagitis is the variety of monilial esophageal involvement that is most commonly encountered in debilitated, postoperative, or immunosuppressed patients, and it can progress, if unchecked, to panmural esophagitis, sepsis, and death. A high index of suspicion must therefore be maintained in the patient population most susceptible to this condition. The infection is usually controlled if it is diagnosed promptly and treated with oral nystatin (Mycostatin), 400,000 to 600,000 units of the suspension four times a day. Since postinflammatory mural fibrosis, typically involving the upper half of the thoracic esophagus, can subsequently occur, patients recovering from severe acute monilial esophagitis must be followed up with several barium swallow examinations during the first year to assure prompt recognition of a developing stricture and institution of dilation therapy.

Nystatin therapy is appropriate for mild cases of *Candida* esophagitis associated with reversible predisposing causes. In patients who fail to respond to nystatin, either parenteral miconazole or oral ketoconazole, 200 mg daily for at least 2 weeks, is indicated. This latter drug enhances the fungicidal properties of polymorphonuclear leukocytes and is therefore not effective in neutropenic patients. In neutropenic patients or those desperately ill with advanced *Candida* esophagitis, the drug of choice is amphotericin B (0.3 to 1 mg per kilogram per day). Additional data are emerging to suggest that prophylaxis against esophageal infection by *Candida* with either nystatin or ketoconazole is beneficial in immunocompromised patients, for example, seriously ill postsurgical patients receiving broad-spectrum antibiotics and post-transplantation patients.

A chronic esophageal infection with stricture formation may occur in mucocutaneous candidiasis, in which an intense mural inflammation results as a response to a relatively superficial esophageal mucosal infection. In these patients the narrowing seen on the barium esophagogram and endoscopy may be secondary to edema, inflammation, or spasm from the chronic infection and may respond to nystatin therapy without the need for dilation therapy. However, once a high-grade fibrotic stricture from *Candida* esophagitis is established, antifungal agents are of little value, and long-term esophageal dilation therapy is required. If comfortable swallowing is not achieved even with bougienage, the occasional patient with a monilial esophageal stricture will require esophageal replacement or bypass. My preferred surgical approach in this rare situation is transhiatal esophagectomy without thoracotomy and esophageal replacement with stomach anastomosed to the cervical esophagus. The stomach is relatively impervious to infection by *Candida*.

The use of immunosuppressants in organ transplantation, chemotherapeutics in oncology, and potent broad-spectrum antibiotics is clearly responsible for the increased incidence of monilial esophagitis encountered today. Physicians, and particularly surgeons, must have a high index of suspicion for this condition in immunocompromised patients and act aggressively in diagnosing and treating *Candida* esophagitis if life-threatening systemic infection and late esophageal stenosis are to be averted.

SUGGESTED READING

Gundry SR, Borkon AM, McIntosh CL, Morrow AG. Candida esophagitis following cardiac operation and short-term antibiotic prophylaxis. J Thorac Cardiovasc Surg 1980; 80:661–668.

Orringer MB, Sloan H. Monilial esophagitis: an increasingly frequent cause of esophageal stenosis? Ann Thorac Surg 1978; 26:364–374.

Scott BB, Jenkins D. Gastrointestinal candidiasis. Gut 1982; 23:137–139.

THE DIAPHRAGM

DIAPHRAGMATIC INJURY

ASHBY C. MONCURE, M.D.

Injury to the diaphragm in the setting of trauma may be a consequence of either penetrating or blunt trauma, usually of the lower chest and upper abdomen. The location of the injury to the diaphragm is quite variable. In that associated injuries to other anotomic structures are quite common, the presentation of the diaphragmatic injury is often obscured by the strident presentation of the other injuries. Common among these are injuries to ribs, spleen, long bones, cranium and contents, liver, colon, small bowel, pancreas, stomach, urinary bladder, kidney, heart, and major vessels.

ACUTE INJURY

Diagnosis

Diaphragmatic injury may be difficult to diagnose and is frequently an unsuspected finding at emergency exploration for penetrating trauma. Symptoms directly related to this injury involve the effects of encroachment and entrapment within the affected hemithorax by the herniated viscera. Hence dyspnea is the major symptom, along with pain related to the injured thorax or abdominal wall. In many patients, however, a history is not obtainable because of coma or immediate endotracheal intubation. Physical findings are those related to thoracic or abdominal injury, those related to other injured structures, and those specific to the diaphragmatic injury (dullness and diminished breath sounds over the affected hemithorax). However, of course, if massive herniation of the abdominal contents into the chest has not yet occurred, symptoms and signs specific to the diaphragmatic injury may not be present.

A major problem in diagnosis is the frequency with which the initial chest roentgenogram is either normal or has no specific findings; this occurs more frequently in blunt injury. Apparent elevation or irregularity of the diaphragm or extraneous shadows above the diaphragm suggest the diagnosis. In the stable patient, passage of a nasogastric tube and the use of a contrast (meglucamine diatrizoate or Gastrografin) study of the stomach may lead to a diagnosis. The use of ultrasonic examination or computed tomographic scan with visceral contrast may also be helpful in making a diagnosis. It should also be noted that herniation of abdominal viscera through a diaphragmatic rent may occur over a number of hours, and a chest film taken at an interval from admission may clearly demonstrate the diagnosis, even though the initial chest film may have appeared normal.

A high index of suspicion for the presence of diaphragmatic injury is necessary to avoid a delay in diagnosis. In that this lesion does not spontaneously heal, all diaphragmatic rents should be surgically repaired.

Management

The operative approach is largely determined by the condition of the patient and the suspected injuries. If hemodynamic instability is present, immediate initial anterolateral thoracotomy or median sternotomy may be necessary to control intrathoracic bleeding and relieve pericardial tamponade, after endotracheal intubation. Subsequent laparotomy or caudad extension of the midline incision made for sternotomy can thereafter be undertaken to deal with associated injuries, to include as well the repair of the diaphragm. Suspected injuries to thoracic organs also dictate thoracotomy or median sternotomy, and if need be, subsequent laparotomy for other injuries, during which diaphragmatic repair can be accomplished through either body cavity. Suspected intra-abdominal or retroperitoneal injuries dictate emergency laparotomy, and repair of the diaphragm through this route can also be accomplished.

In the hemodynamically stable patient, after the diagnosis has been made of acute diaphragmatic rupture, the patient may be approached on a semiurgent basis, recognizing that rapid respiratory deterioration or herniated visceral strangulation and perforation may occur fairly promptly. In these patients, the abdominal approach should be utilized because of the frequency of associated occult intra-abdominal injuries.

Most diaphragmatic rents may be closed with simple sutures of nonabsorbable material. In those instances in which the diaphragm is torn at its periphery, if there is lack of available lateral diaphragm for repair, the diaphragm may be advanced up several interspaces by placing horizontal mattress sutures through the edge of the torn diaphragm and then through the intercostal muscles on either side of the rib; thereafter the sutures are tied down external to the rib. Occasionally, it may be necessary to use prosthetic material, such as Marlex mesh, to bridge a gap in available tissue.

CHRONIC INJURY

The chronic presentation of diaphragmatic rupture represents the effect of entrapment of stomach, colon, or small bowel within the thorax, or the effect of longstanding collapse, from encroachment, on the affected lung. Early satiety, postprandial distress, productive sputum, and dyspnea are the presenting symptoms. A chest film with subsequent contrast examination of the gastrointestinal tract usually secures the diagnosis. The appropriate approach is usually thoracotomy, in order to allow separation of the adhesions that have developed between the trapped viscera and lung, with subsequent repair of the diaphragmatic defect through this route, as outlined previously.

SUGGESTED READING

Hood RM. Traumatic diaphragmatic hernia (collective review). Ann Thorac Surg 1971; 12:311–324.

Kirsh MM, Sloan H. Blunt chest trauma, general principles of management. Boston: Little, Brown, 1977.

Symbas PN, Vlasis SE, Hatcher C. Blunt and penetrating diaphragmatic injuries with or without herniation of organs into the chest. Ann Thorac Surg 1986; 42:158–162.

Wiencek RG, Wilson RF, Steiger Z. Acute injuries of the diaphragm: an analysis of 165 cases. J Thorac Cardiovasc Surg 1986; 92:989–993.

MORGAGNI HERNIA

MARK B. ORRINGER, M.D.

Herniation of intra-abdominal viscera into the pleural cavity through the anterior part of the diaphragm behind the xiphoid process was described by Morgagni in 1761. This diaphragmatic opening has since become known as the foramen of Morgagni, and a protrusion of intra-abdominal contents through it is referred to as a diaphragmatic hernia through the foramen of Morgagni.

Morgagni hernias are rare in both adults and children, constituting about 3 percent of diaphragmatic hernias reported in large series. This low reported incidence may be due to the fact that many patients with this condition are asymptomatic, and the condition goes undiagnosed. Foramen of Morgagni hernias protrude most often into the right side of the chest (90 percent), occasionally bilaterally (7 percent), and rarely on the left side (2 percent). Midline presentation and extension of the hernias into the pericardium have also been reported.

DEVELOPMENTAL ANATOMY

The foramina of Morgagni are small triangular areas of the diaphragm on either side of the inferior end of the sternum. If during embryologic development the retrosternal portion of the septum transversum does not form or the sternum and ribs fail to fuse, or both occur, a foramen of Morgagni hernia may result on either the right or left side. Thus a hernia may result from incomplete development of the diaphragm or from failure of the diaphragm to attach anteriorly. Since the pericardium reinforces the left side of the diaphragm, right-sided Morgagni hernias are most common. When anterior muscular reinforcement of the septum transversum does not occur, as is the case in 95 percent of patients, a hernia with a membranous sac forms. While it has been argued by some that these hernias are acquired, resulting from trauma, exertion, obesity, and the like, an embryologic origin is suggested by the consistent attachment of the hernia sac to the round ligament of the liver, its occurrence in children, its typical location in the right retrosternal area, and the frequency of associated malrotation of the colon.

PATHOLOGY

Foramen of Morgagni hernias are direct hernias that invariably have a membranous sac (95 percent). The sac most often contains omentum and transverse colon. Rarely the stomach and liver may be herniated. In infants the sac often contains the liver. With longstanding hernias the stomach may enter the sac, and sudden obstruction often ensues. Other organs in the hernia sac, such as cecum, terminal ileum, and ascending colon, are rare.

PRESENTATION

Morgagni hernias tend to be large and to contain abdominal viscera, but they are usually asymptomatic and discovered incidentally on routine chest roentgenography. The large bowel and omentum in most of these hernias are apparently less susceptible to strangulation and obstruction than small bowel or stomach. Symptoms, if present, are predominantly gastrointestinal or cardiorespiratory. The patient may experience epigastric pain and fullness aggravated by lifting or bending forward, bloating, cramping, nausea, occasional vomiting, or diarrhea. Recurrent partial large-bowel obstruction may occur, but complete large-bowel obstruction requiring emergency decompression is rare. Alternatively the patient may experience dyspnea, cough, or recurrent pulmonary infections from pressure on intrathoracic viscera by the hernia. Physical examination is seldom helpful, though occasionally intrathoracic bowel sounds will be heard.

DIAGNOSIS

Roentgenographic studies are the mainstay of diagnosing foramen of Morgagni hernias. Posteroanterior and lateral chest roentgenograms and the barium enema study suggest or establish the diagnosis in more than two-thirds of patients. Seldom is an upper gastrointestinal series or pneumoperitoneum needed. The PA chest roentgenogram characteristically shows a rounded shadow in the right cardiophrenic angle. On the lateral view this shadow is seen anteriorly, closely applied to the diaphragm and anterior chest wall. Loops of bowel in the sac give an intestinal bowel gas pattern, but more often, with omentum or transverse colon, the retrosternal shadow appears opaque and homogeneous. The barium enema study filmed in the upright position shows elevation of the midportion of the transverse colon, which is anchored retrosternally and cannot descend with the rest of the colon. If the diagnosis is not established with a barium enema study or upper gastrointestinal tract study, the differential diagnosis of the undiagnosed intrapleural mass includes pericardial cyst, mesothelioma, mediastinal lipoma, diaphragmatic tumor, thymoma, anterior chest wall tumor, and bronchogenic carcinoma. Computed tomography (CT) of the chest differentiates a cystic mass or solid chest wall tumor from a soft tissue mass. It is also usually effective in differentiating a primary pulmonary process from one within the mediastinum. Irrespective of the CT findings, however, exploration is generally indicated to establish a tissue diagnosis.

OPERATIVE APPROACH

Foramen of Morgagni hernias should be repaired whenever the diagnosis is made because of the danger of incarceration or strangulation of the abdominal contents herniated through the narrow diaphragmatic defect. When the diagnosis cannot be made preoperatively, surgery is still indicated to treat the other conditions in the differential diagnosis.

These hernias may be repaired through either a transthoracic or a transabdominal approach. When the diagnosis is known preoperatively the abdominal approach is preferred as it allows (1) treatment of associated gastrointestinal tract anomalies, (2) easier reduction of the herniated viscera by pulling them down rather than pushing them from above, and (3) repair of a bilateral hernia, which is not possible with a unilateral thoracic approach. An upper midline abdominal incision is usually used. An exploratory thoracotomy is performed when the diagnosis is not known preoperatively.

Irrespective of the approach, the repair is the same. The herniated viscera are returned to the abdomen, the peritoneal sac is excised, and the diaphragmatic defect is closed. Usually simple overlap of the adjacent diaphragmatic margins with interrupted nonabsorbable suture is adequate. Alternatively, in infants, mattress sutures can be placed between the edge of the diaphragmatic defect and the retrosternal periosteum. With large defects the anterior margin of the defect may be sutured to the posterior rectus sheath and anterior thoracic wall. The round and falciform ligaments may be used to strengthen the repair. Huge defects may necessitate insertion of a prosthetic patch. A chest tube is placed retrosternally in the large remaining space between the sternum and the intrathoracic viscera and is kept in place for several days. The operative mortality for repair of foramen of Morgagni hernias is low, and long-term results are excellent.

SUGGESTED READING

Orringer MB, Kirsh MM, Sloan H. Congenital and traumatic diaphragmatic hernias exclusive of the hiatus. In: Ravitch MM, ed. Current problems in surgery. Chicago: Year Book, 1975:3.

Thomas GG, Clitherow NR. Herniation through the foramen of Morgagni in children. Br J Surg 1977; 64:215–217.

Thomas TV. Subcostosternal diaphragmatic hernia. J Thorac Cardiovasc Surg 1972; 63:278–283.

EVENTRATION AND PLICATION

HAROLD C. URSCHEL Jr., M.D., LL.D.(Hon), D.Sc.(Hon)
JOHN DISIERE, M.D.
WROTEN M. McQUIRTER Jr., M.D.

Eventration of the diaphragm was first recognized and described by Jean Louis Petit in 1724 during autopsy studies; it was named by Beclard in 1829. Eventration is an abnormally high or elevated position of one leaf of the intact diaphragm as a result of paralysis, aplasia, or atrophy of varying degrees of the muscle fibers.

Classification of eventration includes (1) congenital (nonparalytic), which may be complete, partial, or bilateral, and (2) acquired (paralytic) or secondary to phrenic nerve injury, which can be unilateral or bilateral.

Diaphragmatic eventration is a rare clinical finding occurring in between .001 percent and .003 percent of new births. The majority of the eventrations are located on the left side and are most frequently found in males. The congenital (nonparalytic) form of eventration is due to a developmental defect resulting in an inadequate growth of muscle in the diaphragm. This leaves the diaphragm consisting primarily of fibrous tissue, with little or complete absence of skeletal muscle. Congenital eventration is often partial, since portions of the developing diaphragm may have normal myoblastic ingrowth. The acquired form is most often complete, since the entire nerve and, therefore, the entire motor supply, are usually damaged. In both the congenital and acquired types, the peripheral portion of the diaphragm usually contains normal musculature. In the acquired form the paralyzed diaphragm histologically resembles that of the congenital form, because of disuse atrophy. In either case the diaphragm is very thin and atonic and therefore is easily stretched and displaced upward by the abdominal contents. The acquired form (paralytic) is due to damage to the phrenic nerve or its origin from C3, C4, and C5 nerve roots. This may result from birth or other trauma, surgical sectioning, tumor ingrowth, or various infections.

The most common presenting symptoms in infants are those of acute respiratory insufficiency, especially noted after feeding. The diagnosis can usually be made by examination of posteroanterior and lateral chest roentgenograms, fluoroscopy, or CT scanning with oral contrast material (to differentiate eventration from congenital diaphragmatic hernia). In the adult the diagnosis is usually serendipitous, being made on routine chest x-ray examination, at thoracotomy for unrelated conditions, or at autopsy. Diagnostic pneumoperitoneography has been used to make the diagnosis. Radioscopic liver scans show the location of the dome of the diaphragm. Ultrasonography may be used to differentiate between diaphragmatic hernia, basilar lung masses, and partial eventrations by revealing the presence of the thin intact diaphragm.

In the adult, congenital eventrations often remain asymptomatic. They occasionally become symptomatic late in life, especially if obesity or acquired cardiopulmonary problems add to the burden of an already compromised lung. Symptoms may include dyspnea upon exertion, shortness of breath following a meal, severe dyspepsia, and bloating. With large, complete eventrations occasionally other gastrointestinal symptoms are present, such as intermittent bowel obstruction, dyspepsia, and inability to belch or an increase in incidence of belching and heartburn, which occur as the result of displacement of abdominal viscera.

In the adult, acquired (paralytic) eventration as the result of a mediastinal or cord tumor or infection must be ruled out and bronchoscopy and CME studies may be indicated. Cine-esophagography and upper gastrointestinal and barium enema examinations may also be of value to rule out gastrointestinal disease. All patients should undergo respiratory function studies to determine if the respiratory problem is restrictive. In addition, older patients should have ventilation-perfusion scans to determine the contribution of the eventration and the probability of improvement with surgical correction.

INDICATIONS FOR SURGERY

The decision for surgical repair is not based on the differentiation between congenital and acquired disease but rather on symptoms alone, except when phrenic nerve paralysis is due to incurable disease.

In the newborn who is suffering severe respiratory distress, surgical intervention may be the lifesaving factor. Infants who cannot be weaned from the respirator after adequate trial (5 to 10 days) should have surgical correction of the eventrated diaphragm. The neonate should be carefully screened for accompanying malformations such as patent ductus arteriosus or ventricular septal defect.

Symptomatic adults should also undergo surgical correction of the diaphragm along with cardioesophageal reconstruction to prevent gastroesophageal reflux, which often occurs as a result of change in cardioesophageal angulation.

OPERATIVE PROCEDURE

The transthoracic approach to the diaphragm is preferred except when bilateral eventrations are being repaired or in infants in whom the abdominal approach allows correction through one incision. Unless there is severe bilateral compression of the lungs, we prefer utilizing two separate thoracotomies several weeks apart. The goal is to return the diaphragm to a position of midexpiration, by eliminating all excess diaphragmatic material by plication, excision, or a combination of the two.

Through a sixth or seventh interspace posterolateral incision, the excess diaphragm is elevated, taking care to exclude underlying spleen, bowel, and abdominal contents. The excess is sutured at its base with large, nonabsorbable mattress sutures and folded over the remaining diaphragm. The edge is sutured at the site of its origin along the muscular diaphragmatic margin, leaving three layers of plicated diaphragm. Opening the diaphragm to explore the upper abdomen, excising the thinned-out portion, and closing by imbricating one layer over the other may be employed if abdominal viscera cannot be excluded from the underside. This method requires postoperative gastric decompression for resulting ileus. In the adult, a Colles-Belsey esophageal diaphragmatic repair is added to prevent reflux esophagitis with the new position of the diaphragm. If needed, additional support may be added using a prosthetic material such as a combination of two layers of Marlex mesh with a thin Silastic sheet. The procedure produces excellent results with low mortality and morbidity.

SUGGESTED READING

Beclard E. Cited by J. Cruveilhier in Atlas d'anatomie pathologique. Vol.I Book 17, Plate V; Paris: 1829:2.

Bisgard JD. Congenital eventration of the diaphragm. J Thorac Surg 1947; 16:484–491.

McNamara JJ, Paulson DL, Urschel HC Jr, Razzuk MA. Eventration of the diaphragm. Surgery 1968; 64:1013–1021.

Shah-Mirany J, Schmitz CL, Watson RR. Eventration of the diaphragm: physiologic and surgical significance. Arch Surg 1968; 96:844–850.

Symbas PN, Hatcher CR Jr., Waldo W. Diaphragmatic eventration in infancy and childhood. Ann Thorac Surg 1977; 24:113–117.

Taruer RD, Godwin JD, Putnam CE. Symposium on nonpulmonary aspects in chest radiology, the diaphragm. Radiol Clin North Am 1984; 22:615–631.

DIAPHRAGM PACING

WILLIAM W. L. GLENN, M.D.
JOHN A. ELEFTERIADES, M.D.

DEFINITION

Electrical stimulation of the phrenic nerve(s) by a programmed train of electrical stimuli of increasing intensity to effect a smooth contraction of the diaphragm muscle resulting in physiologic negative pressure inspiration is termed diaphragm pacing.

INDICATIONS FOR DIAPHRAGM PACING

Indications for diaphragm pacing in the treatment of chronic ventilatory insufficiency (CVI) are complete paralysis of respiration due to transection of the upper cervical cord, imperfect respiratory center control, and certain disorders of the peripheral components of the respiratory system. For pacing to be optimally effective, the phrenic nerves, diaphragms, chest wall, and lungs should be normal, but pacing may be recommended in the presence of organic disease that mildly or moderately compromises the function of these structures. In cases in which diaphragm pacing alone will not provide adequate ventilation it may be useful as an adjunct to mechanical forms of ventilatory assistance.

FUNCTIONAL INTEGRITY OF VENTILATORY SYSTEM FOR DIAPHRAGM PACING

Phrenic nerve function (viability of the phrenic nerve and the conduction time, as determined by transcutaneous [cervical] stimulation or direct stimulation of the nerve) is normal or near normal; diaphragm pacing probably will be inadequate if phrenic nerve function is impaired. The absence of a viable phrenic nerve renders pacing of the diaphragm impossible.

Respiratory center function is normal; there may be central alveolar hypoventilation (Ondine's curse), in which case the ventilatory response is blunted or absent to either normocapnic hypoxia or hypercapnic hyperoxia.

Lung function is normal or near normal as revealed by routine function tests, including ventilation and perfusion lung scans. In patients with chronic ventilatory insufficiency but with normal lungs, voluntary hyperventilation will result in normal arterial blood gas levels. Diaphragm pacing is not effective as a method of increasing ventilation in the presence of *severe* restrictive or obstructive lung disease.

Diaphragm function studies in the nonparalyzed patient demonstrate a minimum downward movement of 5 cm during inspiration and transdiaphragmatic pressures in the range of normal. In the paralyzed patient in whom the lower motor neurons of the phrenic nerves are viable the diaphragm contracts briskly in response to phrenic nerve stimulation.

Chest wall configuration that results in serious compromise of pulmonary function due to chest wall deformity may not benefit from diaphragm pacing.

TECHNIQUE OF IMPLANTING THE RADIOFREQUENCY DIAPHRAGM PACEMAKER

The operative procedure is simple, but surgical technique must be meticulous to avoid injury to the phrenic nerve. The operation consists of fixing firmly in place a monopolar platinum neural electrode behind (nonencircling) the phrenic nerve in the thorax by way of the second interspace anteriorly. (A cervical approach to the phrenic nerve may be used, but is less favored because of the possibility of missing some of the phrenic nerve components.) If bilateral pacing is indicated a phrenic nerve electrode is placed behind each nerve, the two units being implanted at separate operations 2 weeks apart. The electrode on the nerve is attached to the cathode terminal of a radio receiver implanted subcutaneously. The anode terminal of the receiver is attached to a metal plate implanted in a separate pocket in the subcutaneous tissue. A pulse train of radiowave impulses is generated in a transmitter located externally and transmitted to the subcutaneous receiver via an antenna inductively coupled to it, there converted to electrical pulses and transmitted by the electrode to the nerve. The electronic parameters that affect the rate, depth, and duration of inspiration are adjusted by manual controls on the externally located transmitter. Pacemaker function is tested in the operating room prior to closure of the chest. The schedule of pacing of the diaphragm is started 12 to 14 days postoperatively.

PACING SCHEDULE

The pacing schedule varies according to need and the efficiency of the pacing.

Part-Time

Ventilatory support. The respiratory rate in older children and adults is set at 10 to 14 inspirations per minute and the electrical frequency (pulse interval [PI]) at 25 to 20 Hz (40 to 50 msec PI). The current level is set to provide just maximal descent of the hemidiaphragm that corresponds to maximal tidal volume. Where only part-time support is prescribed, pacing is done for 10 to 12 hours during sleep to prevent hypoventilation or apnea. Longer periods of pacing at these electrical parameters are to be avoided.

Full-Time

Ventilatory support, preferably using simultaneous bilateral diaphragm pacing for 24 hours, requires conditioning of diaphragm muscle by stimulation with low frequency and a slow respiratory rate over a period of 4 to 6 months. Starting with both sides together for 15 minutes per hour at a rate of 10 respirations per minute and a frequency of 10 Hz (100 msec PI), the pacing parameters are gradually modified over the next 4 to 5 months until full-time pacing is achieved. At this point the respiratory rate will be 6 to 8 per minute and the frequency 7 to 8 Hz (130 to 140 msec PI). The ideal monitor of adequacy of ventilation during pacing is the level of the P_{et} CO_2. It should be measured at least every hour during conditioning and should range between 30 and 40 mm Hg. Alternate-side or alternate-breath pacing with stimulation at a higher frequency and faster rates has occasionally been used. An alarm is required that can be activated by the patient or is activated automatically in the event of ventilatory failure.

COMPLICATIONS

Accentuation of upper airway obstruction is the most common physiologic complication of pacing, and failure of the radio receiver is the most common complication involving the pacemaker apparatus. Both are easily corrected, the first by placement of a permanent tracheostomy and the second by replacement of the faulty component. Nerve injury from the nerve electrode cuff has not been a significant problem in cases in which the electrode has been monopolar and the application has been in the thorax. A serious complication, though a rare one, is wound infection involving the pacemaker components. This usually requires removal of all implanted components. Compression of the phrenic nerve by scar tissue or malposition of the neural electrode undoubtedly occurs in some cases, but this has usually been difficult to document. The complication is more likely to be seen in children, in whom growth is a factor, and particularly if an encircling electrode is used.

RESULTS

Approximately 600 patients in many different centers have been given diaphragm pacemakers. In the 81 patients in the Yale series, diaphragm pacing has been carried on for more than 17 years. Results are classified as follows: (1) success, meaning the ventilatory goal was achieved by pacing, albeit the ventilatory deficit was not always corrected. (Thirty-eight patients [47 percent] are so classified. Pacing was used for an average of 76 months, and in 36 of them, diaphragm pacing was the sole method of full-time or part-time ventilatory support.) (2) partial success, meaning there was significant benefit from pacing but another method of ventilatory support was also required. (Thirty-seven patients [46 per cent] are in this category.) Pacing was for an average of 66 months, and all but six required additional ventilatory support.) (3) failure, meaning ventilatory support was needed, but pacing proved ineffective or it worsened ventilation. (This was the case in five patients [6 percent] in whom pacing was utilized for a mean of 6 months but was then abandoned as being inadequate for their needs.) (4) pacing was never employed, meaning the potential for successful pacing existed, but spontaneous ventilation returned before a pacing schedule could be established. (This was the case with one patient.)

In some patients there was an adverse outcome directly or indirectly related to pacing. By related to pacing we mean to the appropriateness of the indications for pacing, to the operative technique, to the pacing regimen, to the patient's compliance with the pacing schedule, to physician or family support, to the integrity of the pacing equipment and to nonventilatory systemic disorders. These problems, which occurred in the early stages of the development of the technique of diaphragm pacing, would, for the most part, now be considered avoidable.

COMMENT

Effective long-term ventilatory support through diaphragm pacing has been demonstrated in a number of centers. The success of diaphragm pacing in the treatment of chronic ventilatory insufficiency depends on observance of several caveats: precise indications for instituting diaphragm pacing based on careful preoperative evaluation of the ventilatory needs and the structural integrity of the respiratory system; meticulous surgical technique during implanting of the stimulator; adherence to a prescribed pacing schedule and, when full-time pacing is indicated, to a program for conditioning the diaphragm muscle to improve its strength and endurance. In addition, a thorough understanding of the underlying disorder causing the chronic ventilatory insufficiency, its natural history, and the improvement in ventilation to be expected from diaphragm pacing, either alone or in conjunction with other aids to chronic ventilatory insufficiency, must be appreciated by all concerned. Finally, owing to the chronic nature of the disorder and the dependent state of the patients, it must be realized that the optimum result from long-term ventilatory assistance can be achieved only through dedicated professional care and unflagging family support to enable the patient to achieve the highest quality of life possible.

SUGGESTED READING

Glenn WWL, Phelps ML. Diaphragm pacing by electrical stimulation of the phrenic nerve. Neurosurgery 1985; 17:974–984.

Glenn WWL, Phelps ML, Elefteriades JA, Dentz B, Hogan JF. Twenty years of experience in phrenic nerve stimulation to pace the diaphragm. PACE 1986; 9:780–784.

Glenn WWL, Sairenji H. Diaphragm pacing in the treatment of chronic ventilatory insufficiency. In: Roussos CS, Macklem PT, eds. The thorax. New York: Marcel Dekker 1985:1407.

Ilbawi MN, Idriss FS, Hunt CE, Brouillette RT, DeLeon SY. Diaphragmatic pacing in infants; techniques and results. Ann Thorac Surg 1985; 40:323–329.

Schechter DC. Application of electrotherapy to non-cardiac thoracic disorders. Bull NY Acad Med 1970; 46:932–951.

SURGICAL TECHNIQUES

STAPLERS

FELICIEN M. STEICHEN, M.D.

PULMONARY SURGERY

Stapling instruments and techniques are useful in closure of the bronchus and pulmonary vessels in pneumonectomy and lobectomy; transpericardial closure in the right or left main bronchus for bronchopleural fistula after pneumonectomy; sealing of pulmonary parenchyma in wedge excisions; resection of emphysematous bullae; completion of interlobar fissures; modified, atypical and multiple segmentectomies; transsegmental and translobar resections.

Bronchial closure with staples in pneumonectomy and lobectomy offers the advantages of technical simplicity, saving of time, minimal if any contamination, efficient use of operating room resources, and immediate airtight sealing. While staple techniques have not eliminated bronchopleural fistulas, their use has led to a reduction of this dreaded complication to the level of 2 to 4.5 percent in most series, with the higher incidence usually related to pneumonectomy. For lobar bronchial closures I use the linear TA-30-3.5 instrument and the TA-30-4.8, or occasionally for very large main bronchi, the TA-55-4.8 instrument. The TA-30 stapler loaded with the special vascular (3mm) staples is used to achieve closure of the pulmonary artery and both pulmonary veins in pneumonectomy, the lobar vein in lobectomy, as well as the inferior pulmonary artery in lower lobectomy. For right upper and middle lobectomy, left upper lobectomy, and lingulectomy the segmental arterial branches are handled by manual ligation and transection. The small-sized vascular staples find their ideal application and usefulness in the intrapericardial closure of pulmonary vessels and left atrial wall. Similarly, in open heart surgery, the atrial appendage can be closed with the TA-30 vascular stapler. In my initial experience with 31 pneumonectomies and 91 lobectomies I have never found a malfunction of the staples used to close major pulmonary vessels. This series has now expanded to some 300 pulmonary resections, and the safety and reliability of vascular staples has remained the same, provided all safety recommendations are respected—as they should be in all uses of stapling instruments. Lastly, the linear TA-55, TA-90, and GIA instruments can be used for a variety of pulmonary parenchymal resections. Staples placed after the pulmonary tissue has been compressed and immobilized between the jaws of a linear stapler have completely eliminated the leakage of air and blood, especially in segmentectomy. Staples in pulmonary parenchyma are nontraumatic, preserve the blood supply, and maintain a safe, airtight hemostatic closure even as the pulmonary parenchyma is reinflated.

Staples greatly facilitate previously tedious technical steps, such as completing fissures in a lobectomy, extending the margins of resection from a lobectomy into the adjoining segment of another lobe without the need for a bilobectomy, and creating an airtight and watertight closure at the base of a large emphysematous bulla. For the various segmental resections the corresponding artery and bronchus are dissected and closed. The veins are included in the parenchymal staple line, and the segment is resected, resulting in a dry, airtight line of section—a far cry from the classic finger fracture technique. Resection across anatomic boundaries is possible without compromise of the remaining lobe. Staples have allowed the development of lung tissue—sparing metastatic node resections. Lung biopsies, especially in the patient with an opportunistic infection due to a diminished immune response, are facilitated by speed of technical execution, absence of trauma to the remaining lung and of pleural contamination, reduction of operating room exposure, anesthesia time, and elimination of accidental needle sticks to members of the operating team.

In conclusion, stapling instruments used in the various operations on the lung have led to a reduction in bronchopleural fistula rate to a level of 2 to 4 percent. Staples have added technical ease to the closure and transection of major pulmonary vessels and have made possible a whole variety of parenchymal pulmonary procedures with minimal morbidity, e.g., postoperative bleeding, air leaks, or sepsis.

ESOPHAGEAL SURGERY

The TA-55 instrument is ideally suited for closure of the neck of Zenker's and epinephric diverticula as well as the occasional midesophageal traction diverticulum. When indicated, the Collis-Nissen procedure can be accomplished with the GIA and end-to-end anastomosing (EEA) instruments; the transverse colon interposition operation can be achieved with the GIA, EEA, and TA instruments. In the various reconstructive operations after excision of a major portion or all of the esophagus for malignant disease or for irremediable caustic strictures, the various stapling instruments have found one of their most remarkable applications.

I have observed no complications related to the use of the instruments in the excision of various diverticula, the creation of a Collis-Nissen procedure, and in colon interposition in benign reflux strictures. In the early phase of stapling in surgery of the esophagus, complications essentially due to anastomotic leaks and bleeding occurred at a rate of 9 percent. In a series of 33 patients, most undergoing operation for esophageal substitution, two of three such patients died (6 percent) after complicated hospital courses in which the suture leak played a role but was not the major cause of death. More recently, especially with the added use of the EEA instrument for circular anastomosis, anastomotic leaks, often not apparent clinically, are observed at a rate of 3 to 5 percent and anastomotic strictures and occasional bleeding at a rate of 0.5 to 1 percent. Mortality due to the use of staplers has been reduced to an absolute minimum, i.e., it has been nearly eliminated.

Another attractive use of stapling instruments is for ligation of varices, either with the transgastric use of the EEA instrument placed into the lower esophagus to achieve transection and reanastomosis of the esophagus or with the GIA instrument *without the blade* and the placement of four linear rows of staples just beyond the esophagogastric junction on the posterior and anterior walls of the stomach. I do additionally perform ligation of the coronary vein and all of the collateral venous circulation in the lesser omentum and the gastropancreactic fold, as well as ligation of the splenic artery at the level of the tail of the pancreas, if this artery is more than 0.9 mm in diameter.

The various stapling instruments have had a profound influence on the technical operative aspects of thoracic surgery. Instruments that I have used with success are described in Table 1. In pulmonary operations their usage did not require basic changes in technical concepts, e.g., mucosa-to-mucosa closure of the bronchus. Furthermore, possible technical mishaps can be observed and corrected immediately, at the time of the primary operative procedure. In esophageal surgery the stapling instruments have more slowly established their worth by the demonstration that anastomoses formed with the EEA instrument are reliable and safe. Furthermore, the use of the instruments has led to the development of a large variety of substitute organs for the esophagus and the esophagogastric junction.

TABLE 1 Mechanical Sutures in Thoracic Surgery

Operation	*Staple Procedure*	*Instruments*	*Morbidity**	*Mortality**
Pneumonectomy	Closure bronchus Closure vessels	Linear TA-30,55-4.8 Linear TA-30 - V	B-P Fistula None	None
Lobectomy	Closure bronchus Closure veins and lower lobe arteries Completion fissure	Linear TA-30-3.5 Linear TA-30 - V Linear TA-55,90-3.5 GIA linear mode	B-P Fistula Early: 3.3% Late: 0% Air leak 1.1%	Early: 2.4% Late: 0%
Parenchymal resection of lung	Cuneiform, wedge, tangential excision(s) for biopsy, metastases	Linear TA-55-3.5/4.8 GIA linear mode	Air leak 2.3% Bleeding 4.6%	None
	Resection emphysematous blebs and bullae	Linear TA-90,55-3.5	None	None
	Modified,atypical,multiple segmentectomy	Linear TA-90-4.8 GIA linear mode	Early: Air leak 9% Bleeding 9%	None
	Transsegmental, translobar resection	Linear TA-90-4.8	Late: Air leak 0% Bleeding 0%	None
Excision, diverticulum Myotomy, esophagus	Closure neck of diverticulum	Linear TA-55-4.8	None	None
Collis-Nissen procedure	Tube gastroplasty in continuity with GE junction	GIA linear mode EEA gastric buttonhole	None	None
Transverse colon interposition	Transection-closure at limits colon segment Colocolostomy Esophagocolostomy Gastric closure Cologastrostomy	GIA linear and anastom. modes Linear TA-55-3.5/4.8 EEA circular anastom. LDS	None	None

TABLE 1 (Cont'd.) Mechanical Sutures in Thoracic Surgery

Operation	*Staple Procedure*	*Instruments*	*Morbidity**	*Mortality**
Thoracic esophagectomy or Palliative bypass, esophagocoloplasty	Transection-closure, rt. or lt. colon segment Ileocolostomy or colo-colostomy Esophagocolostomy Gastric closure Cologastrostomy Finney pyloroplasty	GIA linear and anastom. modes Linear TA-55-3.5/4.8 LDS EEA circular anastom.	Leak 3% Bleeding 3% Stenosis 1.5%	3%
Laryngopharyngoeso-phagectomy, reverse, greater curvature gastroduodenal tube	Transection-closure Duodenum Creation reverse gastric tube Billroth gastroduodenost.	GIA linear mode LDS EEA circular anastom. Manual anastomosis	Neck fistula 25% (healed)	None
Thoracic esophagectomy, reverse greater curvature tube Pyloromyotomy	Splenectomy Creation reverse gastric tube; gastric closure; esophagogastrost. (tube)	LDS GIA linear mode Linear TA-55-4.8 (EEA circular anastom.)	Leak 3% Stenosis 2%	3%
Esophagogastrectomy Isoperistaltic greater curvature tube Pyloroplasty	Creation isoperistaltic tube Esophagogastrost.(tube)	LDS GIA linear mode EEA semi-circul. (pyloroplasty) EEA circular anastom.	Leak 0% Stenosis 2%	None
Palliative bypass, thoracic esophagus Isoperistaltic greater curvature tube with antral continuity	Creation isoperistaltic tube Esophagogastrost.(tube)	LDS GIA linear mode EEA gastric buttonhole EEA circular anastom.	Leak 0%	None
Palliative bypass, G-E junction Esophagogastrostomy	Side-to-side anastomosis, lower esophagus to gastric fundus	GIA anastomotic mode TA-55-4.8 linear	None	None
Control bleeding, esophageal varices Ligation splenic artery and coronary vein and collateral	Esophagoesophagostomy High gastric wall stapling	EEA circular anastom. Linear Ta-55-4.8 SGIA linear mode (GIA without blade)	Leak 10%	10%

* Morbidity and mortality relate to the use of staplers only.
From Steichen FH, Ravitch MM. Contemporary stapling instruments and basic mechanical suture techniques. Surg Clin N Am 1984; 64(3):425–440.

SUGGESTED READING

Ravitch MM, Steichen FM. Surgical stapling techniques. Clin North Am. 1984; 64(3):425–440.

Ravitch MM, Steichen FM. Principles and practice of surgical stapling. Chicago: Year Book, 1987.

Steichen FM, Ravitch MM. Stapling in surgery. Chicago: Year Book, 1984.

LASER TECHNIQUES IN PULMONARY PROBLEMS

RICHARD B. McELVEIN, M.D.
GEORGE L. ZORN Jr., M.D.

A laser is a beam of coherent light of a specific wavelength. In thoracic surgery it is applied to tissue in the tracheobronchial tree with various reactions, depending on the type of laser used, the tissue treated, and the power density of the laser.

Two types of lasers are used. The carbon dioxide laser operates in the 10.6 μ range and has the advantages of good absorption, minimal scatter, and shallow penetration. It is absorbed in tissue containing water and operates independent of tissue color. A carbon dioxide laser cannot be transmitted through flexible fibers, and this necessitates a rigid system of articulated arms and mirrors.

The second type of laser is the neodymium-yttrium

aluminum garnet laser (Nd-YAG), which operates in the 1.06 μ range, has deeper penetration, and can be passed through flexible fibers. It has more scatter than a carbon dioxide laser, and the immediate tissue changes of laser impact are less evident, making it difficult to determine the depth of penetration.

We use lasers for the removal of a symptomatic obstruction of the tracheobronchial tree, either benign or malignant. Lasers do not cure cancer, but they do provide an improved airway. The use of a laser is compatible with previous or subsequent chemotherapy or radiation therapy.

We prefer the laser to other techniques such as morcellation of tissue with biopsy forceps extraction and cryotherapy because of the prompt response, control of bleeding and secretions, and probably longer survival rate.

We feel that there is no overwhelming advantage of one laser over the other, and we currently use both devices; the CO_2 laser for its cutting effect, and the Nd-YAG laser for vaporization. The shallow depth of penetration of a carbon dioxide laser reduces the risk of airway perforation, whereas the Nd-YAG laser is more effective for removing larger tumor volume.

Anesthetic management is very important. General anesthesia is initiated with an intravenous short-acting barbiturate and maintained with intravenous sedatives and muscle relaxants. Inhalation anesthetics are not applicable. A Dumon-type bronchoscope is passed, and ventilation is performed with a Sanders device attached to the side arm of the rigid bronchoscope. Ventilation is initiated with 100 percent oxygen. An electrocardiograph and a peripheral oximeter are used for monitoring. Compressed air is used to ventilate the patient while the laser is in use. This avoids the possibility of fire or explosion. If the oxygen saturation drops below 90 percent while using air ventilation, we stop using the laser and return to oxygen ventilation until saturation is improved.

Our choice for tracheal lesions is to pass the instrument distal to the obstruction if possible and work in a retrograde fashion. Obstruction of a main stem or lobar bronchus mandates working from proximal to distal while the opposite lung is used for ventilation, taking care to keep it clear of secretions, debris, and blood.

A flexible bronchoscope is passed through the rigid instrument for close inspection of the extent of the lesion both proximally and distally. The carbon dioxide laser is attached to the rigid bronchoscope after previous calibration. A joystick control with a helium-neon guidelight identifies the site of impact. If the lesion has a narrow base, we cut across the base and remove the obstructing lesion with forceps. If the base is broad, the surface of the lesion is treated, and charred material is aspirated with a straight suction tip.

We use the Nd-YAG laser in one of two ways. The fiber is passed through the flexible bronchoscope, which then is inserted through the rigid instrument to the level of the lesion and treatment carried out. The second method is to pass the laser fiber through the rigid bronchoscope with the Dumon attachments and use a Wolfe-Street telescope for close inspection of the lesion. By manipulation of the rigid instrument, the laser fiber, and the telescope, it is possible to align the Nd-YAG beam parallel to the axis of the bronchus for safe application. The use of a biopsy forcep with or without the telescope permits extraction of bulky portions of tumor that have been treated.

One alternative, which we rarely employ, is to pass the flexible bronchoscope through a large-bore endotracheal tube, maintaining ventilation with the side arm of the endotracheal tube connector. We find this unsatisfactory because of the difficulty in aspirating viscid or voluminous secretions.

We have learned that it is not necessary and may even be hazardous to unduly persist in eliminating all obstructions at one sitting. When charring of tissues and secretions distort the appreciation of the anatomy, the procedure is terminated. Retreatment is carried out in 48 to 72 hours.

Complications have been few. We have had four perioperative deaths in 221 cases—two from extremely vascular tumors that could not be controlled with the laser and two in the immediate postprocedure period. We have not had any instances of penetration of the tracheobronchial tree, probably because of our reliance on the carbon dioxide laser if we are in doubt as to the geometry of the tracheobronchial tree.

Only those patients with exophytic disease of the trachea and main stem bronchi should be treated. Patients who have extrinsic compression of the airway are not helped by laser treatment. Failures of laser treatment have occurred when it has been used to deal with extrinsic airway compression and in patients whose distal lung parenchyma will not re-expand despite removal of bronchial obstruction.

The preoperative evaluation of a patient includes standard chest x-ray films. CT scanning is of limited value because transverse cuts do not give an accurate picture of the extent of the disease. Digital chest radiography is available in our institution and has been helpful. Flow volume loops before and after surgery are a measure of the response to treatment and are useful in following a patient.

As we have gained experience with the laser, we have come to appreciate it as an instrument to be used with finesse and not brute power. We feel that this concept has prevented us from many of the poor outcomes reported by others.

In patients with benign lesions and particularly those with tracheal stenosis, we have observed that if there is a true exophytic lesion or web, it can be treated admirably by making radical cuts without circumferential removal of the lesion. The latter technique leaves a bare area that heals with a cicatrix, and a recurrence will result. If there is destruction of cartilaginous segments of the trachea and extrinsic compression or distortion, these patients are not candidates for laser treatment, but they should be treated with the standard methods of reconstruction.

Our results in 221 patients have been generally good. All 47 patients with benign lesions have had restoration of a normal lumen. Five of 10 patients with tracheal stenosis required subsequent reconstruction.

Of 174 patients with malignant disease, 91 have died, with an average life span of 5 months. Eighty-three are alive, with an average life span of 12 months.

SUGGESTED READING

Brutinel WM, McDougall JC, Cortese DA. Bronchoscopic therapy with neodymium-yttrium-aluminum-garnet laser during intravenous anesthesia. Chest 1983; 84:518–521.

Cortese DA, Kinsey JH. Hematoporphyrin derivative phototherapy in the treatment of bronchogenic carcinoma. Chest 1984; 86:8–13.

McElvein RB, Zorn GL. Indications, results and complications of bronchoscopic carbon dioxide laser therapy. Ann Surg 1984; 199:522–525.

Personne C, Colchen A, Leroy M, Vourc'h G, Toty L. Indication and techniques for endoscopic laser resections in bronchology. J Thorac Cardiovasc Surg 1986; 91:710–715.

Wolfe WG, Sabiston DC. Management of benign and malignant lesions of the trachea and bronchi with the neodymium-yttrium-aluminum-garnet laser. J Thorac Cardiovasc Surg 1986; 91:40–45.

LASER TECHNIQUES IN ESOPHAGEAL PROBLEMS

RICHARD B. McELVEIN, M.D.
GEORGE L. ZORN Jr., M.D.

We have used both the carbon dioxide and Nd-YAG laser for removing obstructing malignancies in the esophagus. The carbon dioxide laser has been used for very high lesions as part of our rigid bronchoscopic set-up. Other lesions have been treated using a flexible esophagoscope and the Nd-YAG with the patient under topical anesthesia.

We prefer the use of the laser to dilatation and placement of esophageal stents because we have found that the morbidity and mortality are lower and the results are better.

Laser treatment of carcinoma of the esophagus can be successful if there is an exophytic component of the disease, the involved segment is less than about 6 cm in length, and there is a normal gastrointestinal tract distally. Extrinsic compression of the esophagus does not respond to laser therapy, since a normal esophageal wall must be destroyed to obtain an adequate lumen.

Identification of the lumen may be difficult. The passage of a nasogastric tube or wire as a guide will help to identify the lumen. Care must be exercised not to impact the tubes in the esophagus, because combustion may occur. As in the tracheobronchial tree, several laser treatments may be necessary to provide an adequate lumen.

The Nd-YAG laser has a constant air flow through the fiber to keep the tip clear of debris, and this may result in gastric distention. This is readily controlled with the suction channel of the esophagoscope.

Our indication for using the Nd-YAG laser is the presence of symptomatic severe malignant obstruction of the esophagus. The laser can be used in conjunction with radiation therapy and chemotherapy given prior to, during, or subsequent to laser treatment. As a prelude to radiation therapy, laser treatment results in a patent esophagus much more rapidly, allowing patients to resume ingestion of food and fluid. We do not recommend the laser for patients who do not have symptomatic severe obstruction of the esophagus, since other modalities are available and more appropriate.

The complications of laser esophagoscopy include perforation and, infrequently, bleeding. Treatment in sequential sessions reduces the risk of perforation. Adequate visualization of the lesion and the lumen is necessary at all times.

The preoperative evaluation includes chest x-ray films and barium contrast studies.

Our experience to date has been limited, consisting of eight patients, all of whom have had restoration of their lumina and resumption of oral intake.

To date, we have had no experience with the use of hepatoporphyrin derivatives for treatment of carcinoma of the esophagus. We are aware of the work of others who have used these derivatives to sensitize tissue, and the laser is used to activate these compounds. One must not confuse the use of a laser and hepatoporphyrin derivatives with the use of the laser alone. In the case of the hepatoporphyrin derivatives, the laser is used to activate them to produce singlet oxygen with tissue destruction rather than for direct ablation of tissue.

SUGGESTED READING

McCaughan JS, Williams TE, Bethel BH. Palliation of esophageal malignancy with photodynamic therapy. Ann Thorac Surg 1985; 40:113–120.

Pietrafitta JJ, Dwyer RM. Endoscopic laser therapy of malignant esophageal obstruction. Arch Surg 1986; 121:395–400.

Tody L, Personne C, Colchen A, Vourc'h G. Bronchoscopic management of tracheal lesions using the neodymium yttrium aluminum garnet laser. Thorax 1981; 36:175–178.

I INCISIONS

MEDIAN STERNOTOMY

JOEL D. COOPER, M.D., F.R.C.S., F.A.C.S.(C)

Median sternotomy, widely used for cardiac surgery, has more limited, but nonetheless important application in general thoracic surgery. It has long been the incision of choice for mediastinal tumors. We increasingly favor it for resection of lesions in the distal trachea and for carinal resection. For patients with chronic postpneumonectomy bronchial stump fistula, especially right bronchial stump fistula, median sternotomy offers excellent exposure for division and closure of the proximal main bronchus through a clean uncontaminated field.

With experience, a variety of pulmonary procedures can be satisfactorily performed through the median sternotomy incision. It is particularly applicable when dealing with bilateral lesions such as multiple pulmonary metastases. On several occasions I have used the median sternotomy approach for patients with synchronous bilateral primary pulmonary carcinomas. Through the sternotomy approach, both sides can be assessed, and mediastinal lymph nodes can be staged to determine the most appropriate operation for the lesions. After such exploration and staging, one or both lesions may be resected. If both lesions require major resection, it may be preferable to perform one resection through the median sternotomy and defer the contralateral resection until a subsequent thoracotomy.

Several reports have advocated use of median sternotomy for young patients with a history of bilateral spontaneous pneumothoraces. However, I feel that staged transaxillary thoracotomies are a preferable approach in this situation, thus avoiding the more major incision and the more prominent scar associated with the median sternotomy. On the other hand, my experience with resection of emphysematous bullae has convinced me that the median sternotomy approach is generally the incision of choice for such persons. In patients undergoing resection for bullous disease, bilateral bullae are frequently present. Carrying out staged bilateral thoracotomies in such a patient is a major risk, and furthermore, complications from overexpansion or rupture of contralateral bullae may complicate the postoperative course if a thoracotomy is utilized to deal with one side only. With the sternotomy approach, both sides can be assessed completely, and when appropriate, bilateral plication or resection of bullae can be carried out. This offers the patient the maximum possible improvement with morbidity that is significantly less than that associated with lateral thoracotomy. The type of limited resection usually required for bullous disease poses no particular problem through the sternotomy approach, especially when the disease is concentrated in the upper lobes.

For pulmonary surgery via median sternotomy, anesthesia is generally administered using a double-lumen, Robert Shaw tube. This gives the ability to collapse either lung, greatly facilitating the exposure. The pulmonary ligament should be initially divided, which allows upward retraction of the lung into the field. Collapse of the lung permits careful palpation of the lung during search for multiple metastases and facilitates dissection of pulmonary vessels and bronchi during performance of lobectomy or pneumonectomy.

Left lower lobectomy may be technically difficult through the median sternotomy approach, as retraction of the heart is usually required, and this may be poorly tolerated in some patients. All other lobectomies, and either pneumonectomy, can generally be accomplished without undue difficulty, especially as the operator gains experience with this approach. A large pack placed behind the hilum of the lung to elevate the lung greatly improves the exposure.

In performance of right upper lobectomy through a median sternotomy approach, branches of the pulmonary artery to the right upper lobe are taken sequentially from above downward. Thus the recurrent branch of the pulmonary artery, to the anterior segment, is taken from in front, rather than through the major fissure as would normally be done via right thoracotomy. Because the median sternotomy approach is associated with less morbidity than a thoracotomy, it has been suggested that the sternotomy approach is the one of choice for elderly patients undergoing pulmonary resection. I have not adopted this approach, as I prefer the familiarity of the thoracotomy approach in case a difficult dissection should be encountered. Furthermore, with modern postoperative analgesia, especially with the use of postoperative catheter epidural analgesia, the morbidity associated with post-thoracotomy pain can be considerably lessened.

It is apparent to all who care for patients following

thoracic procedures that the discomfort and postoperative disability following median sternotomy is far less than that following lateral thoracotomy. Nonetheless this truism has been difficult to verify by objective measurement. We compared the effect of sternotomy with that of thoracotomy on postoperative pulmonary function in two groups of patients undergoing procedures not associated with pulmonary resection. Specifically the sternotomy group consisted of patients undergoing first-time, routine coronary artery bypass surgery, while the thoracotomy group consisted of patients undergoing transthoracic hiatal hernia repair. We utilized two simple measurements of lung mechanics, vital capacity and peak airway flow. Postoperative changes in vital capacity reflect the restriction imposed by the incisional pain. Peak flow correlates with the ability to produce an adequate cough, and reductions in the peak respiratory flow rate correlate best with the incidence of postoperative respiratory complications. Our study documented greater than 50 percent loss of both vital capacity and peak airway flow in both groups of patients on the second postoperative day, with no significant differences between the two groups. Subsequent measurements, however, demonstrated that patients undergoing sternotomy showed more rapid recovery with statistically significant differences, in favor of sternotomy, on days 4 and 7 after operation. One week following operation, peak airway flow had returned to 80 percent of the preoperative value for the sternotomy group of patients compared with 64 percent for patients having thoracotomy. At 1 week the vital capacity for the sternotomy group was 71 percent of the preoperative value compared with 58 percent for those undergoing thoracotomy. Even these measured differences, however, do not, in my opinion, reflect the lesser postoperative morbidity associated with sternotomy.

In spite of the superior postoperative pulmonary function afforded by the sternotomy approach, I generally choose a sternotomy incision primarily in situations in which the anatomic exposure afforded by this approach is superior to that from lateral thoracotomy. For pulmonary procedures, as noted previously, the chief indication is the desire to have access to both pleural spaces simultaneously. We have been concerned that the use of the sternotomy approach for pulmonary resection might give rise to contamination and subsequent infection of the sternotomy wound. Fortunately this has not been a significant problem, though there is little doubt that the consequences of an infected sternotomy are greater than that of an infected thoracotomy wound. Following unilateral or bilateral pulmonary resection through the sternotomy approach, we have generally placed the chest tubes directly into the pleural spaces rather than through the mediastinum.

Under certain circumstances, when one is operating on the upper mediastinum in the presence of a contaminated field, an upper partial sternotomy may be of some advantage. Such an incision is carried down from the sternal notch to the second or third intercostal space with lateral division of one side of the sternum into the right or left intercostal space allowing the upper divided sternum to be adequately spread. We have utilized this as the incision of choice when dealing with tracheoinnominate artery fistula. In this situation a contaminated tracheostomy wound is incorporated into the sternotomy incision, and hence the possibilities for sternotomy infection are great. If the lower half of the sternum is left intact, little if any postoperative respiratory morbidity results from infection and dehiscence of the upper, divided, portion of the sternum. This same approach may be utilized for emergency procedures related to trauma of the great vessels, especially when proximal control of the innominate or subclavian arteries is required.

Median sternotomy is utilized far less than lateral thoracotomy for general thoracic procedures. Nonetheless it would behoove the general thoracic surgeon to familiarize himself with thoracic anatomy via this exposure, as at times it does provide superior access and increased flexibility in dealing with diseases of the mediastinum, trachea, and lungs.

SUGGESTED READING

Cooper JD, Nelems JM, Pearson FG. Extended indications for median sternotomy in patients requiring pulmonary resection. Ann Thorac Surg 1978; 26:413–420.

Lima O, Ramos L, Dibiasi P, Judice L, Cooper JD. Median sternotomy for bilateral resection of emphysematous bullae. J Thorac Cardiovasc Surg 1981; 82:892–897.

Urschel HC, Razzuk M. Median sternotomy as a standard approach for pulmonary resection. Ann Thorac Surg 1986; 41:130–134.

FRENCH INCISION

RICHARD F. HEITMILLER, M.D.
DOUGLAS J. MATHISEN, M.D.

The anterolateral or French incision combines the advantages of a cosmetic muscle-sparing incision with good exposure. We have found the anterolateral incision to be a useful alternative incision.

TECHNIQUE

The patient is positioned on his or her side, angled at 45 degrees. This provides optimal exposure anteriorly, but still allows extension of the incision posterolaterally if necessary. An incision is made that extends from the inframammary crease to a point two finger breadths below the scapular tip. Subcutaneous skin flaps are then elevated to expose a greater length of the latissimus dorsi muscle to allow its mobilization. The medial edge of the latissimus dorsi muscle and its undersurface are then dissected. This dissection stays close to the muscle so as not to injure the neurovascular bundle of the serratus anterior muscle. The neurovascular bundle of the serratus runs longitudinally 2 to 3 cm posterior to the edge of the latissimus dorsi. The ribs are counted by external palpation to determine the level at which to enter the chest. The serratus anterior muscle is split along the line of its fibers over the anticipated interspace to enter the chest. This division of the serratus should stop 1 to 2 cm short of the neurovascular bundle to avoid injuring it. The serratus muscle can then easily be elevated off the chest wall, allowing exposure of the desired rib much farther posteriorly. If limited exposure is anticipated or if the patient is young with pliable ribs, the chest can be entered through an intercostal space and the rib spared. An extra long extension on the electrocautery is useful to gain access posteriorly. In some circumstances, in order to provide exposure and prevent rib fracture, a rib segment is removed and the chest entered through the periosteal bed. Two medium "square-holed" chest spreaders oriented at right angles are used for exposure. One retracts the ribs whereas the other retracts the soft tissue medially and the mobilized latissimus dorsi edge laterally, resulting in a square or rectangular window through which to operate. If additional exposure is required, it is easy to convert this to a standard posterolateral incision by extending the skin incision posteriorly, dividing the latissimus, and dividing the serratus at a lower level to preserve as much function as possible.

The chest is drained with one or two chest tubes brought through separate stab incisions placed low enough to enter the chest below the mobilized wound edges. If a segment of rib has been excised, the intercostal muscle edges are reapproximated with interrupted 0 silk stitches, and the serratus muscle is closed with running 0-Dexon reinforced with interrupted 0-Dexon stitches as needed. Subcutaneous tissue is reapproximated, and a subcuticular skin stitch is usually employed. If no rib is excised, then figure-of-eight pericostal stitches with No. 2 Vicryl are used.

ADVANTAGES

The principal advantages of this incision lie in its location and its anatomy. Because this incision lies entirely within the bra line, it is one of the most cosmetically appealing incisions. Moreover, the serratus anterior is divided in such a way as to maintain its neurovascular supply. Because it is a muscle-sparing incision, there is more rapid recovery, less functional impairment, and possibly less incisional pain. The incision can easily be extended posterolaterally to afford greater exposure in the event that this is necessary, which is difficult to do in other muscle-sparing incisions.

DISADVANTAGES

Hazards involved with this incision include choosing an incorrect interspace, long thoracic nerve injury, wound seroma, and limited exposure. Rib counting is most commonly performed by external palpation, counting up from the twelfth rib. In some patients this can be difficult, leading to some uncertainty about the specific interspace. Injury to the long thoracic nerve leads to a winged scapula and some disability. This can be avoided by limiting the incision in the serratus and avoiding excessive traction on the muscle. The edges of the incision are undermined in order to maximize thoracotomy exposure; this creates a potential space that can result in a seroma or hematoma. If the chest tubes are allowed to transgress this space, the risk of infection is markedly increased. A final disadvantage is the somewhat limited exposure from this incision. It is an anterior-based incision, and therefore exposure of the posterior hilus as well as the posterior gutter can be difficult. Lesions that are known preoperatively to involve these areas should be approached through a different incision.

The French incision combines a cosmetic muscle-sparing incision with reasonably good exposure. It can be used to perform a wide range of pulmonary resections. As a reasonably cosmetic incision, it is well suited for approaches to benign disease. In approaching more extensive pulmonary resections in which there is extensive chest wall involvement, posterior hilar involvement, or posterior mediastinal involvement, a standard posterolateral thoracotomy incision should be employed.

LATERAL THORACOTOMY: TECHNIQUE, INDICATIONS, AND COMPLICATIONS

WILLIAM H. WARREN, M.D.

The ideal thoracic incision should provide optimal exposure, cause minimal postoperative functional deficit, and be cosmetically acceptable to the patient. Much of the early postoperative morbidity can be related directly to the incision. The standard posterolateral thoracotomy causes moderate to severe postoperative pain. This promotes retention of secretions and atelectasis, sometimes leading to pneumonia and respiratory failure. The standard posterolateral thoracotomy may occasionally result in chronic shoulder disability due to limitation of motion.

A more limited incision that spares the latissimus dorsi and the muscles of the shoulder is associated with less postoperative pain and, as a result, fewer postoperative complications. This incision provides adequate exposure, and it is more cosmetic than the standard posterolateral thoracotomy.

OPERATIVE TECHNIQUE

The patient is placed in the lateral decubitus position, and the arm on the side of the incision is placed in an orthopaedic airplane splint. The back is perpendicular to the operating table. The shoulder may be abducted and flexed to a maximum of 90 degrees. The hips are stabilized with sandbags and tape after an axillary roll is placed under the contralateral axilla. This position provides optimal exposure of the axilla and lateral chest wall.

The limits of the surgical field are the elbow, the midline anteriorly, the iliac crest, and the spine posteriorly. A folded sterile towel is draped around the upper arm to provide optimal exposure of the axilla.

The incision is based on the appropriate interspace, which may be counted from the ribs below. The fourth interspace is optimal if a difficult hilar or upper lobe dissection is anticipated. The fifth interspace is chosen for middle lobe or lower lobe dissection. The choice of interspace may vary according to the configuration of the chest and the procedure.

In the female the skin incision can be modified to lie in the inframammary fold, carefully avoiding dissection into breast tissue. The breast may be elevated if further anterior exposure is necessary. The posterior limit of the incision is the anterior border of the latissimus dorsi. Behind this point lies the long thoracic nerve, and injury to it should be avoided. The intercostobrachial nerve may be visualized as it courses from the chest wall and also should be spared. The incision is carried down through the fibers of the serratus anterior to expose the ribs and intercostal muscles. The appropriate interspace having been identified previously, the intercostal muscles and the pleura are divided. It is not necessary to resect a rib. A lateral retractor elevates the belly of the serratus anterior posteriorly to avoid injury to the long thoracic nerve, and division of the intercostal muscles is extended posteriorly behind the axilla. Likewise, the intercostal muscles are divided anteriorly, care being taken not to injure the underlying lung. A surgeon's head light greatly facilitates the exposure, and the surgeon has equally good exposure standing on either side of the operating table. Collapse of the lung, using "one-lung anesthesia," is generally needed.

INDICATIONS

In my practice the lateral thoracotomy has become the incision of choice for standard and complicated pulmonary resections, including wedge resection, segmentectomy, lobectomy, and pneumonectomy. The exposure is adequate for bronchoplasty procedures and sleeve resections except in unusual circumstances. The posterolateral thoracotomy may be preferable if the tumor is bulky or in those cases in which a difficult hilar dissection is anticipated. The lateral thoracotomy does not provide adequate exposure of resection of a Pancoast tumor or other tumors with gross invasion of the posterior chest wall. Lateral and anterior chest wall resections can usually be managed through this incision without a counterincision.

Caution should be used in performing a lateral thoracotomy in the patient with previous mastectomy, especially if the incision was transverse and extending into the axilla or if the patient had postoperative radiotherapy to the axilla or chest wall. However, a lateral thoracotomy has been performed in several carefully selected such patients without wound healing problems.

The lateral thoracotomy should not be used in a patient who previously has had thoracotomy for pulmonary resection. Other absolute contraindications are open skin ulcers, suppurative infections in the axilla, and previous breast implant surgery. This incision is not adequate for exposure of a posterior mediastinal tumor with extension into the vertebral canal.

COMPLICATIONS

Several complications specific to this exposure may occur. Traction injury to the brachial plexus and neurovascular injuries at the elbow occur if the shoulder is extended beyond 90 degrees and if there is inadequate padding at the elbow (which rests within the airplane splint). A winged scapula may arise either from division of the long thoracic nerve or from excessive posterior retraction by an overenthusiastic assistant. If the injury is from traction it is usually reversible. If the intercostobrachial nerve is severed the patient may complain of an annoying numbness in the medial aspect of the upper arm and axilla. Post-thoracotomy pain has been a late complication with this exposure, but it occurs less frequently than with the more extensive dissection of posterolateral thoracotomy. The pain postoperatively is typically anterior in the inframammary area and seldom as debilitating as after posterolateral thoracotomy.

In conclusion, this incision gives adequate exposure for most pulmonary resections while causing less postoperative morbidity than the standard posterolateral thoracotomy.

SUGGESTED READING

Alley RD. Thoracic surgical incisions and post operative drainage. In: Cooper P, ed. The craft of surgery. Vol 1. Boston: Little, Brown, 1971.

Lees William M. Thoracic incisions. In: Shields TW, ed. General thoracic surgery. Philadelphia: Lea & Febiger, 1983.

Foster ED, Dobell ARC. Thoracic incisions. In: Ellis FH Jr, ed. Practice of surgery. New York: Harper & Row, 1985.

CARDIAC SURGERY | PRE- AND POSTOPERATIVE CARE

CARDIOPULMONARY BYPASS IN THE ADULT

JOE R. UTLEY, M.D.

The safety of cardiopulmonary bypass depends on precise management before, during, and after the procedure. We will present the steps in our routine procedures as well as the protocols related to managing specific abnormalities such as cerebrovascular disease or renal failure.

PREOPERATIVE EVALUATION

History. The patient's cardiovascular history may alter the technique of cardiopulmonary bypass. Previous stroke or transient ischemia require cerebrovascular evaluation and use of the brain protection protocol (to be described). Previous surgery may influence the site and techniques of incision and cannulation for perfusion or balloon pumping. Hypertension, diabetes, chronic lung disease, and peripheral vascular disease all may influence the conduct of cardiopulmonary bypass and must be noted preoperatively.

Preoperative medications may also influence the procedure. Hypertensive patients on medication may require vasodilators on bypass. Patients on diuretic therapy without adequate potassium supplementation may require aggressive replacement therapy. Diabetics, in addition to requiring closer glucose level monitoring, may require more frequent potassium determinations during cardiopulmonary bypass.

CONFIGURATION AND SET-UP OF HEART-LUNG MACHINE

The configuration of the heart-lung machine is designed to allow maximum safety and maximum flexibility of the system. The equipment we use is as follows:

Bentley BMR-1900 venous reservoir with Safe-T-Net Screen
Bentley BOSCM-50 hollow-fiber membrane oxygenator
Bentley BCR-3500 cardiotomy reservoir
Bentley AF-1040 arterial filter
Bentley tubing, except for pump-head tubing
Pump-head tubing: Tygon (S-50-HL) and (S-50-HL)
Sarns 7400 modular heart-lung machine
Haemonetics cell saver

The purge line from the venous reservoir bag can remove massive amounts from the venous reservoir if necessary. The purge line from the oxygenator to the cardiotomy reservoir is used in priming the system. This line has a one-way valve to prevent retrograde flow to the oxygenator from a pressurized cardiotomy reservoir.

A Sarns air bubble detector is placed around the line from the venous reservoir bag to the arterial pump head. It is capable of sensing small amounts of air and has back-up battery power. When it senses air, pump heads stop automatically.

The arterial filter is purged to the cardiotomy reservoir at all times. The cardiotomy reservoir is always open to air to prevent pressurization. The needle vent, pulmonary artery vent, and pump suction tubing are on separate roller pumps.

All positive pressure connections have either a bonding agent with nylon ties or Bentley locknuts. The negative pressure side of the pump head has a bonding agent and nylon ties at the pump head only. There is no tie or locknut at the venous reservoir outlet to allow quick changing of a ruptured reservoir bag. With this system, air is less likely to be pumped to the patient from an empty oxygenator because of the collapsable venous reservoir.

Cannulation. Routine arterial cannulation for cardiopulmonary bypass is of the ascending aorta below the innominate artery. Two concentric adventitial purse-string sutures without pledgets are used. The Sarns 6.5-mm high-flow aortic arch cannula is inserted through a stab incision that is gently dilated with a myocardial dilator. Correct placement of the arterial cannula is confirmed by vigorous blood flow from the cannula, transmitted pulsations to the line pressure monitor, and low line pressure during bypass. If the ascending aorta is very small, short, atherosclerotic, very calcified or is the site of dissection, alternative sites are used. Femoral arterial cannulation is used if the femoral and iliac arteries are not diseased. Other sites that may be used if the aorta has severe generalized atherosclerosis or is the site of dissection are the distal transverse arch or the right axillary artery.

For routine venous cannulation for coronary bypass procedures and aortic valve replacement, the single venous cannula (Sarns two-staged reinforced 40 F by 32 F) is placed through the right atrial appendage with the tip in the inferior vena cava. For mitral valve replacement or procedures opening the right side of the heart, bicaval cannulation with number 7 or number 9 Polystan venous cannulas are used.

The cardioplegia cannula (DLP, Inc, 12 ga) is placed in the ascending aorta. This cannula is used for cardioplegia delivery, for venting of the left ventricle after aortic clamping, and for air evacuation from the ascending aorta as the clamp is removed and after bypass is discontinued. Excessive negative pressure in this vent site is prevented by the VRV-200-B vacuum relief valve (Delta Medical Industries) in the vent line.

The pulmonary artery vent is an Argyle No. 14 F cannula placed through a single purse-string suture in the pulmonary artery. The pulmonary artery vent aspirates blood retrograde through the pulmonary circulation and recycles blood from the left atrium, left ventricle, and ascending aorta. After aortic clamping and cardioplegia delivery, the aortic and pulmonary artery vents provide complete left ventricular decompression. If the mitral valve is competent, ventricular distention may occur during cardioplegia delivery or after aortic clamp removal, before cardiac rhythm is restored. If distention is detected by palpation of the ventricle during cardioplegia, cardioplegia is stopped, and the ventricle is vented through the cardioplegia cannula; cardioplegia is then resumed. If distention is detected by palpation after removal of the aortic clamp and before stable cardiac rhythm is restored, the ventricle is compressed to empty it into the aorta.

TECHNIQUE DURING CARDIOPULMONARY BYPASS

Temperature. Temperature is monitored in the nasopharynx, rectum, pulmonary artery (Swan-Ganz catheter), and arterial and venous lines of the heart-lung machine. Nasopharyngeal and rectal temperatures drop to 34 to 36° C before cardiopulmonary bypass. The water bath is set at 20° C. The patient and water bath temperature will equilibrate at 27 to 28° C. If the bypass will be longer than 1 hour, the temperature is maintained at 28° C. With redo operations we may begin cardiopulmonary bypass before the heart is completely dissected. The temperature is maintained at 32° C until dissection is complete and then lowered to 28° C to avoid ventricular fibrillation before cardioplegia.

When aortic insufficiency is present, our goal is to maintain cardiac rhythm until aortic clamping in order to avoid ventricular distention. With procedures requiring less than 30 minutes of aortic clamping or less than 1 hour of cardiopulmonary bypass, the temperature is kept at 32° C to shorten rewarming.

Temperature is diminished if lower flow is anticipated. The temperature is lowered to 20° C or less before dropping flow to 1.0 L per minute per square meter or less. Diminished flow produces a drier operative field, diminishes noncoronary collateral flow, and avoids warming of the heart and cardioplegia washout. Diminished temperature and flow also help to deal with inadequate venous return, and lower temperatures are important when one anticipates difficult anatomic situations that may require arrest of the circulation. Hypothermia is used in patients with cerebrovascular disease or an atherosclerotic aorta in whom lowering of perfusion pressure or carotid artery clamping is anticipated.

The temperature of the water bath is raised to 40° C shortly before the aortic clamp is removed. The water bath is kept 10° C above venous blood temperature. Cardiopulmonary bypass is continued until rectal temperature reaches 35.0° C or venous blood reaches 37.5° C. Nasopharyngeal temperature may then be 39° C. Continuing bypass until these temperatures are reached has the advantage of less temperature drift when bypass is terminated, better cardiac performance, and improved coagulation.

Deep hypothermia and circulatory arrest are used in adult patients who require pulmonary artery endarterectomy, repair of complex aneurysms of the thoracic aorta, or other difficult technical problems. When circulatory arrest is anticipated, the water bath temperature is lowered to 10° C. Perfusion at low temperatures continues until the nasopharyngeal and rectal temperatures reach 16° C; the patient's head is packed in ice.

Before circulatory arrest, the aorta is clamped. Cardioplegia is infused if the myocardial temperature is above 15° C. Blood drains through the venous line to the oxygenator. When venous drainage has stopped, the venous line is clamped to avoid air entry.

Every 20 minutes reperfusion is instituted for 5 to 10 minutes if possible. Cardiopulmonary bypass is begun after all cardiotomy incisions have been closed. The water bath temperature is started at 10° C above the patient's venous blood temperature. The water bath temperature is progressively increased until the rectal temperature is 35.5° C or the venous blood is 37.5° C.

Contraindications to hypothermia include hepatic disease, sickle cell trait, and severe hyperlipidemia; microemboli from crystals of fat may occur at low temperatures with hyperlipidemia.

Flows. We determine flow primarily from patient temperature: flow of 2.4 L per minute per square meter at 37° C, 1.8 L per minute per square meter at 28° C, and 1.0 L per minute per square meter at 20° C. The resulting systemic pressure may influence flow in aged patients and those with cerebrovascular disease or atherosclerotic aortas. Patients who are less than 50 years old are perfused at a minimum pressure of 50 mm Hg and those above 50 years old are perfused at a minimum pressure (mm Hg) equal to their age (years). Also, flows may be increased to achieve a higher perfusion pressure in patients with cerebrovascular disease or atherosclerotic aortas.

Pressure. We maintain pressure according to the above criteria by increasing flow. If flow rates of 2.4 L per minute per square meter do not achieve the desired pressure, we use phenylephrine hydrochloride (Neo-Synephrine) boluses (1.0 mg). Pressure is lowered by decreasing flow when there is excessive noncoronary collateral flow, wet anastomoses, or a wet operative field.

Venous Saturation. The Bentley saturation meter measures venous saturation, which is maintained at higher than 55 percent by increasing flow. Venous saturation is usually 45 to 50 percent when beginning bypass and typically rises to 68 or 70 percent within 4 minutes. Venous saturation usually stabilizes near 60 percent at 28° C and flow of 1.4 to 1.6 L per minute per square meter. With rewarming, saturation rises to 75 percent with increased flow, but may drop to 55 percent as the patient's temperature rises. If venous saturation drops below 55 percent during bypass, we increase flow or lower the water bath temperature to 38° C.

Filters. The Bentley AF-1040 heparin-bonded arterial filter is used as an air-removal system as well as a filter. Heparin bonding of this 40-μ filter makes debubbling more efficient. The Bentley BCR-3500 cardiotomy reservoir with a 20-μ filter can handle very high flow rates.

Wet Coronary Anastamoses. To deal with wet coronary anastomoses requires a combination of reduced flow rates (down to 0.8 to 1.0 L per minute per square meter) and sodium nitroprusside to keep systemic pressures at 40 mm Hg or less during the anastamoses. Rarely does the venous saturation fall below 50 percent during this time. The patient's temperature may be decreased with reduction of flow, particularly if the brain protection protocol is used.

Brain Protection. Patients with a history of stroke, transient ischemic attack, carotid bruit, or noninvasive and angiographic evidence of cerebrovascular disease are given pharmacologic and physiologic brain protection. Pharmacologic protection includes phenytoin (Dilantin), 300 mg given preoperatively. Mannitol, 12.5 g, is given prior to bypass, and pentothal sodium is given at institution of cardiopulmonary bypass. Oxygen delivery is enhanced in these patients by maintaining mean pressure above 80 mm Hg and hematocrit above 25 percent.

Diabetes. Serum glucose level is checked every 30 minutes during bypass. With the ectothermic blood gas scheme, blood glucose is rarely over 150 mg per deciliter. A blood glucose level higher than 250 mg per deciliter is treated with 20 U of regular insulin in the oxygenator.

Serum Potassium. Serum potassium is determined every 30 minutes during bypass. Low serum potassium levels are treated only after rewarming; potassium usually falls with cooling and rises with warming. Boluses of potassium chloride (10 to 15 mEq) are given for potassium levels less than 4.0 mEq per liter during bypass. Serum potassium higher than 5.5 mEq per liter is treated with 50 ml of 50 percent glucose and 20 U of regular insulin. Furosemide (Lasix), 20 mg, is also given. Bypass is not terminated until the potassium level is less than 5.5 mEq per liter.

Hematocrit. Blood is used infrequently during bypass. We give blood when the hematocrit is less than 17 percent with a urine output greater than 100 ml per hour or when the hematocrit is less than 20 percent and the urine output is less than 100 ml per hour. Blood is given to keep the hematocrit above 25 percent with the brain protection protocol. Higher hematocrit values and viscosity are helpful when terminating bypass in patients with very poor ventricular function (ejection fractions less than 30 percent).

Blood Gases. We employ the ectothermic blood gas scheme not corrected for temperature. Regardless of the patient's temperature, blood gas determinations from a closed syringe are performed at 37° C. When the ectothermic scheme is used, patients warm and cool more quickly. We have observed less base deficit after hypothermia. Ventricular fibrillation is less likely to occur with cooling employing the ectothermic blood gas scheme.

Prime Solution. We employ the following priming components:

2 L Travenol Plasma Lyte A
12.5 g mannitol
1 g cefazolin
10,000 U heparin
25 g albumin — Total 2,160 ml

Heparin. The initial dose of heparin is 4 mg per kilogram and is injected by the surgeon into the right atrium. Activated clotting time is determined before instituting bypass to assure adequate anticoagulation. Activated clotting time is monitored every 30 minutes and is kept higher than 480 seconds by additional doses of heparin.

Air Lock. Air lock occurs infrequently during cardiac surgery in adults. With single venous cannulation, air can enter through transmural needle holes. If air lock occurs, our procedure is to turn off the pulmonary artery vent, translocate blood volume to the patient to increase venous pressure, and manipulate the venous line to move air to the venous reservoir. If the volume of air is great and cannot be resolved by these methods, it is necessary to stop the pump, clamp the venous line at the heart and at the oxygenator, disconnect the venous line from the venous cannula, and fill the venous line with saline at the operative field.

Hypotension. Hypotension is common at the beginning of cardiopulmonary bypass and is usually caused by hemodilution (low viscosity), narcotic anesthesia or pentothal sodium. If the hematocrit is less than 20 percent, blood is given; with a hematocrit higher than 20 percent, boluses of phenylephrine hydrochloride (Neo-synephrine 0.1 to 0.5 mg) are used. This initial hypotension usually resolves after 30 minutes of bypass.

Hypertension. Most patients receive low dose narcotic anesthesia and require treatment of hypertension during bypass. Treatment of hypertension may include giving more anesthesia (diazepam or fentanyl).

Isoflurane may be used in patients with good ventricular function. Boluses of sodium nitroprusside may be used during bypass; hydralazine (Apresoline), 10 mg, may be used during bypass, but may contribute to low vascular resistance after bypass.

Line Pressure. Line pressures above 300 mm Hg cause cavitation at the tip of the arterial line. With our technique, line pressure is 120 to 140 mm Hg when cold with low flow and 180 to 240 mm Hg when warming with high flows. High line pressure indicates a kinked arterial line or dissection of the aorta.

Renal Failure. Patients with preoperative serum

creatine levels higher than 1.8 mg per deciliter are given low dose dopamine during bypass; mannitol, 12.5 g is given before bypass. Furosemide, 10- to 40-mg boluses, is given to maintain urine output above 2 ml per kilogram per hour. If renal artery stenosis is proved or suspected, mean pressure is kept above 80 mm Hg.

Pulsatile Perfusion. In our experience the advantages of pulsatile perfusion are higher urine output, more rapid warming and cooling, and better renal and cerebral protection. Pulsatile perfusion is not easily achieved with a membrane oxygenator. We do not employ pulsatile perfusion if there is aortic dissection or aneurysm. With the Sarns pulsatile pump, we set the rate at 90 beats per minute and set the pulse width and duration to achieve maximum pulse pressure; the pump head is never allowed to completely stop, in order to avoid stagnation in the oxygenator.

Terminating Bypass. Bypass is terminated when the rectal temperature reaches 35° C or venous blood reaches 37.5° C. Before terminating bypass, an aortic needle vent must be functioning well, excessive blood must not be returned by cardiotomy suction, and cardiac rhythm must be stable. The pump is slowed until the appropriate filling pressures and cardiac performance are reached. The pump is kept on a slow setting to return the aortic needle vent flow until the vent is removed.

SUGGESTED READING

Taylor KM, ed. Cardiopulmonary bypass, principles and management. London: Chapman & Hall, 1966.

Utley JR, ed. Pathophysiology and techniques of cardiopulmonary bypass. Vol. 1. Baltimore: Williams & Wilkins, 1982.

Utley JR, ed. Pathophysiology and techniques of cardiopulmonary bypass. Vol. 2. Baltimore: Williams & Wilkins, 1983.

Utley JR, Stephens BD. Prevention of major perioperative neurologic dysfunction—a personal perspective. Perfusion. Vol. 1. 1986:135.

MYOCARDIAL PROTECTION

LELAND G. SIWEK, M.D.
WILLARD M. DAGGETT Jr., M.D.

The major objectives of cardioplegia are to produce a still heart and a relatively bloodless field and to protect the myocardium in order to ensure adequate function after the period of ischemic arrest. Hypothermia during ischemic arrest is clearly protective by reducing the metabolic demands of the heart, but even with deep hypothermia, demands are not reduced to zero. The goal of our system of myocardial protection is not only to reduce the metabolic demands of the myocardium to a minimal level but also to promote sufficient oxidative metabolism during cardioplegic arrest to meet these demands, thus preventing myocardial injury and depletion of high energy phosphate stores. In clinical practice, we use cold oxygenated dilute blood cardioplegia.

The problem of oxygen delivery to the arrested myocardium was first addressed by oxygenating asanguineous cardioplegic solutions. Oxygen solubility in water is enhanced by hypothermia, and all of the oxygen carried in solution is available for delivery. Although blood might seem attractive for cardioplegia because of its oxygen-carrying capacity, the leftward shift of the oxygen-hemoglobin dissociation curve with hypothermia severely impairs the ability of hemoglobin to deliver oxygen at low temperatures. At 10° C, oxygenated crystalloid cardioplegia is capable of releasing all of its oxygen, and this exceeds the oxygen-delivering capacity of oxygenated blood or oxygenated blood cardioplegia. The efficacy of cold oxygenated crystalloid cardioplegia was established in our laboratory by Bodenhammer and colleagues in an experimental study in dogs with 4 hours of aortic cross-clamping and infusion of cardioplegic solution every 20 minutes. The cardioplegic solution was bubbled with either room air or 100 percent oxygen. The recovery of ventricular function in the animals receiving aerated cardioplegia was uniformly poor, whereas most of the hearts receiving oxygenated cardioplegia had good functional recovery (Fig. 1). Consistent with this observation was the finding of significantly better adenosine triphosphate levels and myocardial ultrastructure in the oxygenated hearts. In addition, the oxygen consumption of these hearts was calculated over the entire 4-hour cross-clamping period. Several studies have indicated that at 10° C, the basal oxygen requirement of the arrested myocardium is 0.13 ml O_2 per minute per 100 grams left ventricle (LV). The hearts that received oxygenated cardioplegia had an oxygen consumption of 0.13 ml O_2 per minute per 100 grams LV, suggesting that this technique did indeed meet the basal myocardial oxygen requirements.

Although the oxygen dissolved in solution in cold oxygenated crystalloid cardioplegia appears adequate to meet the metabolic demands of the hypothermic myocardium, there are other reasons for the addition of a small amount of blood to the solution. One advantage of adding blood to the cardioplegic solution is related to the rheologic effect of erythrocytes. As early as the 1940s, Zweifach, studying the frog mesentery, found little or no circulation in the true capillaries with the use of crystalloid perfusates, but the addition of small quantities of red blood cells or even of carbon particles resulted in perfusion of the entire capillary bed. In experiments in our laboratory on 24-hour preservation of isolated perfused hearts, Saudeau and colleagues found that perfusion with crystalloid solution resulted in a progressive rise in coronary vascular resistance. Only the addition of a small number of red blood cells (hematocrit 2 to 5 ml per deciliter) prevented

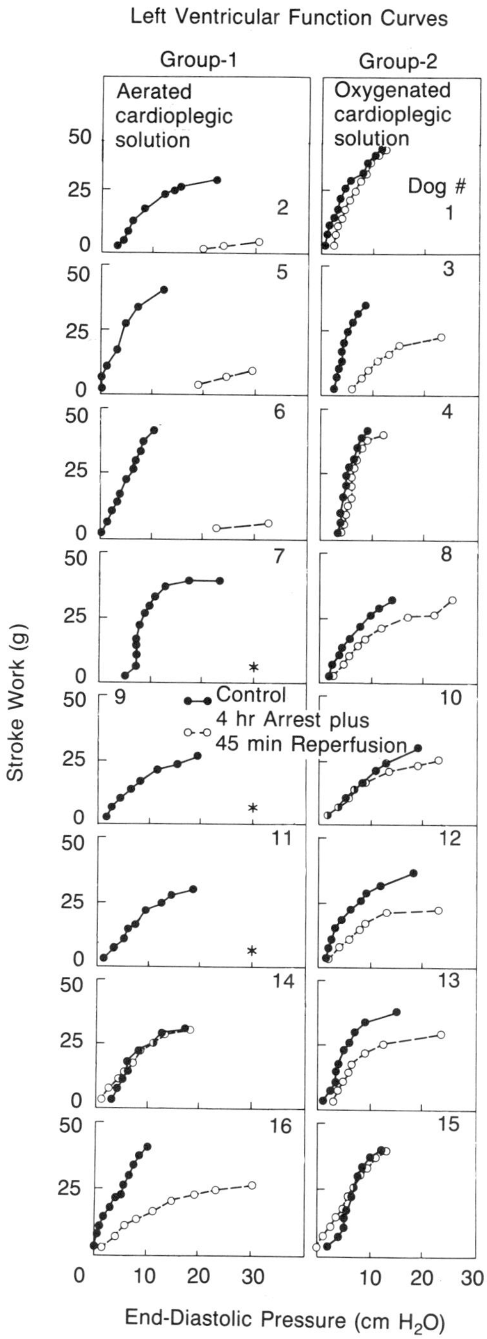

Figure 1 The comparison of ventricular function curves in eight canine hearts before (control) and after 4 hours of aortic cross-clamping and cardiac arrest with subsequent reperfusion. In the eight hearts studied in Group 1 (function curves shown on the left), ventricular function was markedly depressed in most hearts following 4 hours of protection with cardioplegic solution aerated with room air. In contrast, in the eight Group 2 hearts that were subjected to arrest with oxygenated cardioplegic solution, ventricular function curves following reperfusion show better preservation of myocardial function. (From Bodenhammer RM, DeBoer LWV, Geffin GA, O'Keefe DD, Fallon JT, Aretz TH, Haas GS, Daggett WM. Enhanced myocardial protection during ischemic arrest. Oxygenation of a crystalloid cardioplegic solution. J Thorac Cardiovasc Surg 1983; 85:769–780.)

this increased coronary vascular resistance, reduced myocardial edema, and increased oxygen consumption. In recent studies, we found that only blood-containing cardioplegic solutions were capable of maintaining perfusion of the entire canine posterior papillary muscle throughout a 5-hour cross-clamping period. We believe, therefore, that there is a rheologic basis for adding red blood cells to cardioplegic solutions that is unrelated to their hemoglobin content. If crystalloid perfusates cause capillary closure in the microcirculation, then dissolved oxygen must diffuse over greater distances to reach the mitochondria. Red blood cell-containing perfusates, by opening the capillary bed, shorten the diffusion distance for oxygen delivery to the cell, the oxygen being physically dissolved in the water fraction of the solution.

In addition to the rheologic effects of red blood cells, there are several other possible benefits of adding them to the cardioplegic solution. Red blood cells increase buffering capacity and provide a reliable source of calcium to prevent the calcium paradox. Our dilute blood cardioplegia contains approximately 0.1 mM ionized calcium. Red blood cells are also a rich source of catalase, an effective scavenger of oxygen-free radicals.

A small amount of calcium in cardioplegic solution is desirable to prevent the calcium paradox, which occurs upon readmission of calcium after a period of calcium-free perfusion. Calcium in higher concentrations, however, may actually increase oxygen consumption and deplete high energy phosphate stores. Recent studies in our laboratory have shown that in the isolated isovolumic rat heart, infusion of a cardioplegic solution containing a high calcium concentration is associated with ventricular contraction and depletion of high energy phosphates as well as with diminished functional recovery. The addition of magnesium to the cardioplegic solution greatly diminishes the calcium-induced ventricular contracture, preserves myocardial energy stores, and enhances function recovery.

In December of 1982, based on the principles described earlier, we began using oxygenated dilute blood cardioplegia in our clinical experience by the method to be described. The components per liter of our crystalloid cardioplegic solution are given in Table 1.

The system for delivery of the cardioplegia is illustrated in Figure 2. Two thousand milliliters of precooled cardioplegic solution are placed in a Bentley BCR-3500 cardiotomy reservoir. The solution is oxygenated by bub-

TABLE 1 Crystalloid Cardioplegic Solution Components

Component	*Part/L*
Potassium	25 mEq
Sodium	109 mEq
Chloride	108 mEq
Magnesium	32 mEq
Sulfate	32 mEq
Bicarbonate	27 mEq
Mannitol	10 g
Dextrose	5 g
Nitroglycerin	0.5 mg

bling oxygen through it. A 16-gauge, 8-inch long intravenous catheter (Deseret Intracath) is introduced via one of the ports on top of the reservoir and is inside the filter and defoamer built into the reservoir. The solution drawn out from the bottom of the reservoir will have passed through the filter and defoamer after being bubbled with oxygen. A mixture of 98 percent oxygen and 2 percent carbon dioxide is delivered through the catheter at the rate of 10 L per minute. The solution is continuously circulated by a separate roller pump at 600 ml per minute, both to rapidly oxygenate the solution and to cool it to 4° C by passing it through a stainless steel coil immersed in an ice bath. Once the patient is placed on cardiopulmonary bypass, 500 ml of hemodiluted pump blood are shunted from a filter in the arterial perfusion line into the cardioplegia reservoir to make dilute blood cardioplegia (final hematocrit is 3 to 6 ml per deciliter). In practice, we have found this oxygenation and cooling system to reliably provide maximal oxygenation of the cardioplegic solution (Po_2 > 700 mm Hg and dissolved O_2 content > 3 ml per deciliter), even when multiple doses of cardioplegia require refilling the reservoir with new solution and pump blood. We have changed from 100 percent oxygen to the 98 percent oxygen per 2 percent carbon dioxide mixture because bubbling with 100 percent oxygen removes carbon dioxide from bicarbonate-containing solutions and results in a highly alkaline pH (pH = 8.5 and Pco_2 < 8 mm Hg at 37° C), whereas the addition of 2 percent carbon dioxide to the gas results in a more physiologic pH (pH = 7.44 and Pco_2 = 35 mm Hg at 37° C).

Once the patient is prepped and draped, cardioplegia delivery tubing is passed from the surgical field to the perfusionist. This is double-lumen recirculating tubing with a stopcock at the end. Except during the actual infusion of cardioplegia, the cooled, oxygenated solution recirculates through this tubing, thus preventing a "dead space" of warm cardioplegic solution between the pump and the operative field. For coronary bypass procedures, we perform the proximal aortovenous anastomoses prior to initiating cardiopulmonary bypass. The advantage of this technique is that as each distal coronary anastomosis is performed, all subsequent doses of cardioplegia delivered into the aortic root automatically recruit all vein graft distal anastomoses in the delivery of cardioplegia. This is a matter of individual preference, and this cardioplegia system can be adapted to any surgical technique. Our prior experience with myocardial temperature mapping would suggest, however, that delivery of cardioplegia down vein grafts may help to achieve more uniform and complete myocardial cooling.

Once the patient is placed on cardiopulmonary bypass and while the temperature is being cooled, usually to 25° C, two catheters are placed in the ascending aorta, one for infusion of cardioplegia and the other for measurement of aortic root pressure during cardioplegia infusion. A single mattress suture is placed in the aorta and

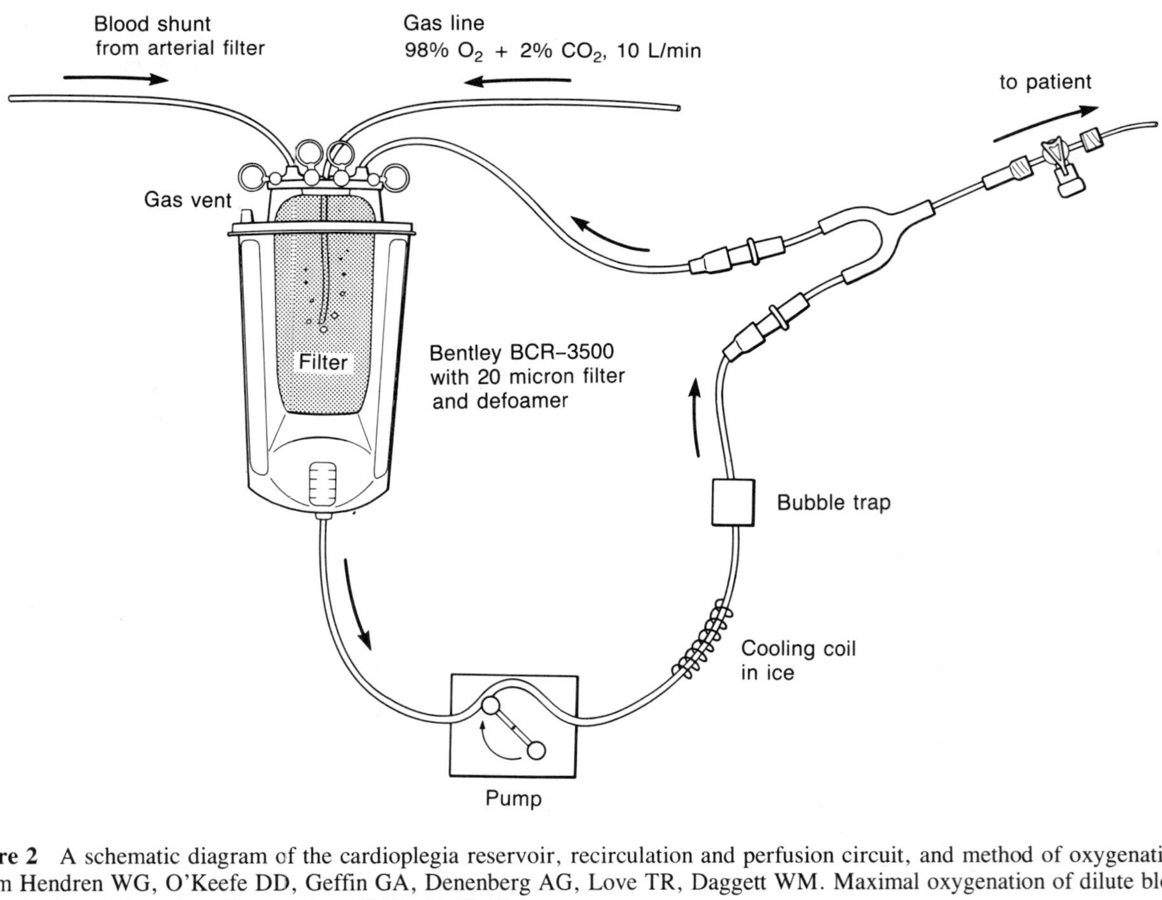

Figure 2 A schematic diagram of the cardioplegia reservoir, recirculation and perfusion circuit, and method of oxygenation. (From Hendren WG, O'Keefe DD, Geffin GA, Denenberg AG, Love TR, Daggett WM. Maximal oxygenation of dilute blood cardioplegic solution. Ann Thorac Surg 1987; 44:48–52.)

two 6-inch angiocatheters, one 14-gauge and the other 16-gauge, are inserted and tied to a tourniquet that tightens the suture around the catheters. Sterile pressure monitoring tubing is connected to the 16-gauge catheter and passed off the field to the anesthesiologist for monitoring of aortic root pressure. The 14-gauge catheter is connected to the stopcock on the cardioplegia infusion tubing. When the aorta is cross-clamped, the aortic root pressure is displayed on the monitoring screen to be viewed by both the surgeon and the perfusionist. The stopcock is turned open to the aortic root cannula, and cardioplegic solution is delivered by the perfusionist, who clamps the return line of the recirculating tubing and controls the infusion rate via the roller pump that has been recirculating the cardioplegia. The rate of administration is adjusted to produce an aortic root pressure between 80 and 100 mm Hg. In this way, we can assure that the rate of cardioplegia delivery is adequate to provide sufficient pressure at the coronary ostia to deliver the cardioplegia effectively. Although the aortic root pressure can be judged by palpation, we have found it more reliable to directly measure the pressure. This also enables the perfusionist to adjust the infusion rate or to detect insufficient aortic root pressure (as with aortic valve incompetence secondary to distortion) while the surgeon is occupied with other tasks.

It is important not to manipulate the heart during the infusion of cardioplegia, as this may cause aortic valve incompetence. As mentioned earlier, the routine monitoring of aortic root pressure may help to detect this. The loss of cardioplegia caused by a minimally incompetent valve often can be overcome by increasing the rate of infusion to achieve an adequate root pressure and also by delivering a larger volume. If mild aortic insufficiency is anticipated, we often place a 12-gauge rather than a 14-gauge infusion catheter to facilitate higher infusion rates. At times manipulation of the aortic annulus, particularly with a finger pressing on the noncoronary sinus of the aortic valve, may help to limit the amount of aortic insufficiency. In the presence of more severe aortic incompetence, one must generally infuse the cardioplegia directly into the coronary ostia.

The initial dose of cardioplegia is generally approximately 1.0 to 1.5 L, although larger volumes may be given in very ischemic or very hypertrophied hearts. For coronary bypass operations, the sequence of distal anastomoses is determined by the severity and distribution of obstructive lesions. Those regions that we feel are least likely to be well perfused (and thus cooled) via the native circulation, especially areas supplied by occluded arteries, are grafted early so that vein grafts will provide cardioplegia delivery and cooling to that segment of the myocardium. Our previous experience with temperature mapping during coronary bypass operations has helped to plan this aspect of the operation. We give additional doses of cardioplegia after every distal anastomosis, even though this may be at intervals of only 10 or 12 minutes. After the initial dose, subsequent doses of cardioplegia are generally 300 to 500 ml per dose. Once again, aortic root pressure is monitored during infusion of each dose of cardioplegia. For noncoronary bypass operations, even with extended cross-clamping times, cardioplegic solution is reinfused at intervals of 20 to 30 minutes at times that are convenient in terms of the conduct of the operation.

In addition to cardioplegia delivery, we feel that supplemental topical cooling contributes to myocardial protection by minimizing rewarming of the heart between infusions of cardioplegia. Sterile tubing is passed off the field and connected to a bottle of iced Ringer's lactate solution that is dripped into the pericardial sac, the rate being controlled on the surgical field. A laparotomy pad soaked in iced solution is placed behind the heart to minimize rewarming from the mediastinum, and a gauze sponge soaked in iced saline is placed over the exposed surfaces of the heart to prevent rewarming by operating room lights. When particularly long aortic cross-clamping times are anticipated, we employ more profound systemic hypothermia to 20 to 22° C to further decrease myocardial rewarming.

Approximately 10 minutes prior to anticipated removal of the aortic cross-clamp, systemic rewarming is begun. Once the aortic clamp is removed, it may take several minutes of reperfusion for electrical and mechanical activity to return. Our experience has shown greater than 70 percent spontaneous resumption of cardiac rhythm, and of those patients with sinus rhythm prior to operation, 93 percent had sinus rhythm at the end of the operation. Return of myocardial function has been excellent, even after prolonged aortic cross-clamping.

SUGGESTED READING

Daggett WM, Randolph JD, Jacobs M, O'Keefe DD, Geffin GA, Swinski LA, Boggs BR, Austen WG. The superiority of cold oxygenated dilute blood cardioplegia. Ann Thorac Surg 1987; 43:397–402.

Geffin GA, Love TR, Hendren WG, Torchiana DF, Titus JS, Redonnett BE, O'Keefe DD, Daggett WM. The effects of calcium and magnesium in hyperkalemic cardioplegic solutions on myocardial preservation. J Thorac Cardiovasc Surg (in press).

Heitmiller RF, DeBoer LWV, Geffin GA, Toal KW, Fallon JT, Drop LT, Teplick RS, O'Keefe DD, Daggett WM. Comparison of myocardial recovery following hypothermic arrest with oxygenated crystalloid and blood cardioplegia: the role of calcium. Circulation 1985; 72(Suppl II):241–252.

Saudeau J, Shaffer B, Daggett WM, Austen WG, Erdman AJ. Role of procaine and washed red cells in the isolated dog heart perfused at 5° C. J Thorac Cardiovasc Surg 1982; 84:886–896.

Torchiana DF, Love TR, Hendren WG, Geffin GA, Titus JS, Redonnett BE, O'Keefe DD, Daggett WM. Calcium-induced ventricular contraction during cardioplegic arrest. J Thorac Cardiovasc Surg 1987; 94:606–613.

VanderSalm TJ, Okike ON, Cutler BS, Paraskos JA, Ferulo J, Daggett WM. Improved myocardial preservation by improved distribution of cardioplegic solutions. J Thorac Cardiovasc Surg 1982; 83:767–771.

Zweifach BW. The distribution of blood perfusates in capillary circulation. Am J Physiol 1940; 130:512–520.

PULMONARY CIRCULATION: PHARMACOLOGIC MANAGEMENT

MICHAEL N. D'AMBRA, M.D.
JEAN-PAUL BELLER, M.D.

Pharmacologic management of the pulmonary circulation is, for practical purposes, limited to lowering impedance to forward blood flow across the lungs. If the lungs existed in isolation, treatment of pulmonary vascular hyper-resistance states would be relatively straight forward. Unfortunately, however, all the pulmonary vasodilating agents have the potential to cause life-threatening systemic hypotension.

We will detail a number of therapeutic approaches to the acute pulmonary hyper-resistance states that occur in cardiac surgical patients:

1. in response to the reversal of heparin by the administration of protamine,
2. after mitral valve replacement in patients with pulmonary hypertension,
3. with massive pulmonary embolism, following emergency embolectomy, and
4. after cardiac transplantation.

All four groups share, as their principal pathophysiologic derangement, an acute rise in pulmonary vascular resistance—high enough so that compensatory right ventricular (RV) reserve is exhausted. The right ventricle distends. The central venous and right atrial pressures rise. Simultaneously, the left atrium and left ventricle become relatively hypovolemic, resulting in diminished left ventricular stroke volume. Systemic hypotension develops rapidly (Fig. 1).

This pathophysiology (an overloaded right-sided circulation combined with a hypovolemic, hypotensive systemic circulation) is further complicated by changes in coronary perfusion to the right ventricle. RV dilation results in massively increased RV free-wall tension (RV myocardial oxygen consumption increases). The high wall tension can also deprive the RV free wall of the usually large systolic component of coronary blood flow.

THERAPEUTIC GOALS

Therapeutic intervention must meet seemingly conflicting requirements. It must simultaneously:

1. lower pulmonary vascular resistance,
2. assure adequate RV coronary perfusion pressure by raising systemic arterial pressure,
3. reduce preload of the distended right ventricle,
4. raise ventricular stroke volume in both chambers, and
5. reduce the radius of curvature of the RV free wall, thus decreasing myocardial oxygen consumption while enhancing coronary perfusion.

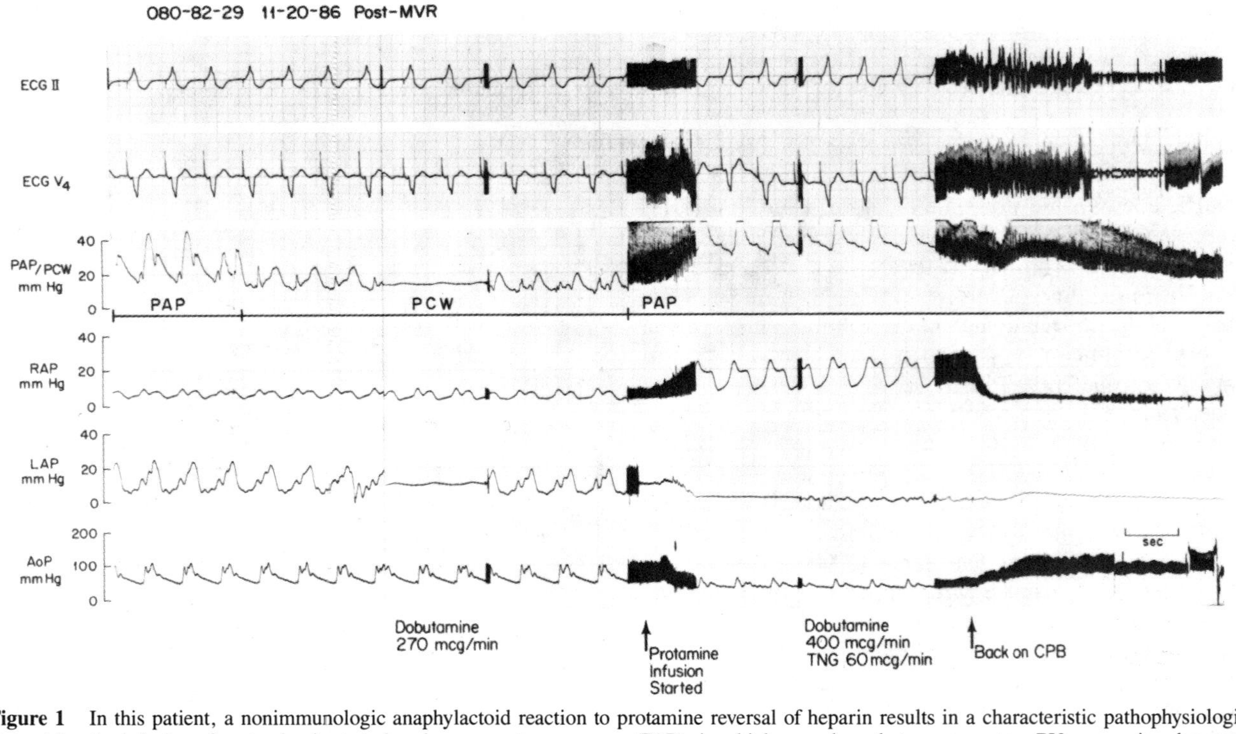

Figure 1 In this patient, a nonimmunologic anaphylactoid reaction to protamine reversal of heparin results in a characteristic pathophysiologic state. After the infusion of protamine is started, pulmonary artery pressure (PAP) rises high enough so that compensatory RV reserve is exhausted. The right ventricle distends, and the right atrial pressure (RAP) tracing shows evidence of tricuspid regurgitation. At the same time, the systemic circulation becomes relatively hypovolemic (low left ventricular filling pressure, LAP). Systemic hypotension aortic pressure (AoP) develops rapidly. This pathophysiology can also be seen after mitral valve replacement in patients with pulmonary hypertension, in those with massive pulmonary embolism, and after cardiac transplantation. ECG = electrocardiogram; PCW = pulmonary capillary wedge pressure; TNG = trinitroglycerin; and CPB = cardiopulmonary bypass.

THERAPEUTIC STRATEGY

Protamine Reaction

Pulmonary vasoconstriction associated with reversal of heparin by protamine is a nonimmunologic, anaphylactoid reaction. Systemic hypotension is usually due to inability to transfer blood across the lungs rather than to systemic vasodilation. The mediators involved are complement fractions C3a and C5a and thromboxane B2. Bronchospasm is usually the first manifestation of the reaction. Pulmonary vasoconstriction follows and is usually transient, often lasting no more than several minutes. Thus the clinical problem is to support the circulation during this short period. We have used left-sided (left atrial or aortic root) injections of calcium chloride to raise systemic pressure and right-sided infusions of epinephrine or isoproterenol (0.05 to 1.0 μg per minute) to dilate the pulmonary vasculature. If hypotension is profound or persistent, we reheparinize and reinstitute cardiopulmonary bypass for 5 to 30 minutes.

Factors predisposing to this reaction have not been identified. Although previous exposure to protamine-insulin preparations, diabetes mellitus, central venous or rapid bolus injection of protamine, preexisting pulmonary hypertension, and valvular heart disease have all been suspected, none has been consistently demonstrated. Since the response is nonallergic in origin, *it is safe* to administer protamine following an anaphylactoid reaction. We do this at a rate of 2 mg per minute by infusion.

On the other hand, *systemic hypotension* associated with protamine may be based on true allergy. With a true allergic protamine reaction, neither pulmonary hyper-resistance nor bronchospasm is likely, but histamine liberation does occur. The skin is flushed and pulmonary artery, central venous, and left atrial (or pulmonary capillary wedge [PCW]) pressures are generally very low. Pretreatment with corticosteroids (methylprednisolone 2 to 15 mg per kilogram intravenously), along with histamine (H_1 and H_2) receptor blockade with cimetidine (5 mg per kilogram intravenously) and chlorpheniramine (0.15 mg per kilogram intravenously), can moderate the response to subsequent protamine administration. Rarely, it is necessary to omit protamine reversal of heparin.

Mitral Valve Replacement and Pulmonary Embolism

Refractory pulmonary hyper-resistance can be seen in patients after mitral valve replacement or pulmonary embolectomy. Myocardial depression from bypass (and/or ischemic arrest) combines with increased RV afterload from the pulmonary hyper-resistance reaction to result in profound right-sided heart failure.

Separating right from left circulations regarding both hemodynamic monitoring and drug infusion sites allows for a logical solution to the simultaneous requirement for extremely potent pulmonary vasodilation and systemic vasoconstriction.

We accomplish this separation of the right and left circulations by adding a left atrial catheter prior to separation from bypass. The left atrial catheter is used for drug infusion to the systemic circulation, whereas the central venous and/or pulmonary artery catheters target the pulmonary circulation.

A left atrial catheter can be placed via a pursestring suture in the right superior pulmonary vein. In extremely unstable patients, two left atrial catheters are placed, one for continuous monitoring and intermittent drug injection (protamine, calcium) and one for continuous drug infusion (Fig. 2).

Allowing even short periods of low cardiac output and RV distress makes recovery extremely difficult. It is important, therefore, to plan for a sequence of therapeutic

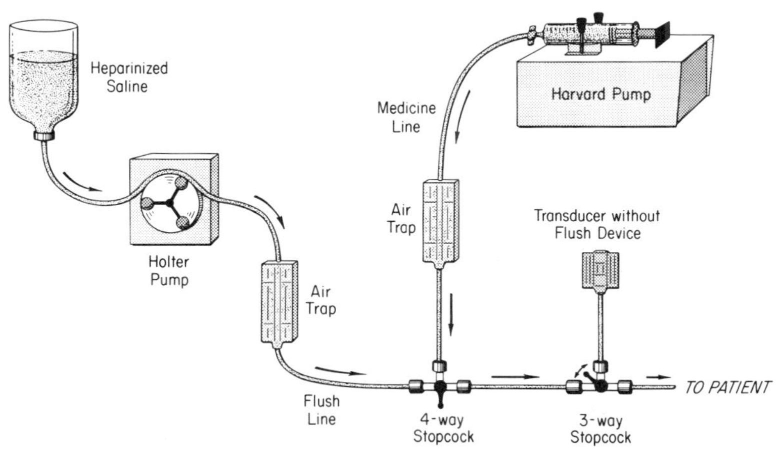

Figure 2 Schematic of left atrial line setup. The left atrial catheter can be used for drug infusion to the systemic circulation and for monitoring left ventricular filling pressure. Continuous infusion of heparinized flush solution with or without medication infusion is accommodated by the tubing arrangement shown. Left atrial pressure is obtained by briefly turning the threeway stopcock counterclockwise (causing a brief interruption in the flow of flush and/or medication). Air traps prevent entrainment of bubbles into the patient. Do not use transducers with automatic built-in flush devices.

escalations (following the therapeutic goals outlined above), with continuous monitoring of the effects of each step on right and left circulations. The following is such a sequence:

1. Generously correct any base deficit with bicarbonate *before* termination of cardiopulmonary bypass. Acidosis contributes significantly to pulmonary resistance and decreases the effectiveness of catecholamines. Also, these patients may have bronchoconstriction, which is generally at its worst in the first few minutes after cardiopulmonary bypass is terminated. Administering extra bicarbonate in anticipation of a brief period of elevated P_{CO_2} is wise.
2. Inject a 5 mg per kilogram calcium chloride bolus into the left atrium.
3. Establish an ideal pattern of ventilation: large tidal volume (15 to 20 ml per kilogram) delivered at rapid inspiratory flow rates without positive end-expiratory pressure and with a long expiratory time. Such a pattern is delivered best with two-handed manual ventilation. We have found that the mechanical ventilator capable of best mimicking this pattern is the Emerson Model 3PV. No anesthesia ventilators can provide such a ventilatory pattern.
4. Administer an epinephrine bolus (dose 4 to 10 μg) on the right side.
5. Give dopamine, 5 μg per kilogram per minute in a right-sided infusion. Give H_1 and H_2 blockers, and methylprednisolone 1 g intravenously (methylprednisolone administration may produce transient systemic vasodilatation; administer slowly).
6. If systemic blood pressure is acceptable: nitroglycerin 0.25 to 1.5 μg per kilogram (right-sided infusion). If systemic blood pressure is low: norepinephrine 0.01 to 0.3 μg per kilogram per minute via left atrial catheter, THEN, nitroglycerin 0.25 to 1.5 μg per kilogram (right-sided infusion).
7. If the patient does not stabilize, escalate to the sequence in Figure 3.

Prostaglandin E_1 (PGE_1 [Prostin VR]) is a stable metabolite of arachidonic acid that occurs naturally in humans and causes an increase in intracellular cyclic-adenosine monophosphate via a specific PGE_1 cell membrane receptor. It is almost completely metabolized in the first pass through a normal pulmonary circulation. Most patients with severe pulmonary compromise preoperatively seem to lose the capacity to metabolize this agent—hence the need for high doses of norepinephrine to compensate for systemic vasodilatation. PGE_1 has the desirable effects of specifically dilating coronary, renal, and cutaneous circulations in addition to its pulmonary effects. The in vitro inhibition of platelet aggregation by PGE_1 has not been reflected in clinically significant bleeding in cardiac surgical patients.

There are other potent pulmonary vasodilators that can be substituted for PGE_1 in the above therapeutic sequence (step 7). These include:

1. Amrinone lactate (Inocor), 0.75 mg per kilogram over 15 minutes, followed by 5μg per kilogram per minute as a right-sided infusion. Amrinone is a phosphodiesterase inhibitor. Because of this, it may act synergistically with PGE_1 and other agents that stimulate the production of cyclic adenosine monophosphate. Amrinone's adverse effects on platelet function and production, make it less applicable in some patients.
2. Phentolamine mesylate (Regitine), 0.1 to 0.2 mg per kilogram over 5 minutes followed by an infusion of 5 to 10 μg per kilogram per minute. This agent is an alpha-receptor blocker, and a drawback to its use is the volume loading that may be required. Glucose intolerance can develop during prolonged infusions, and an offset time of 4 to 6 hours prolongs weaning.
3. Aminophylline, a 2 to 4 mg per kilogram bolus directly into the pulmonary artery, followed by an infusion (5 μg per kilogram per minute). This agent should be avoided if tachycardia or arrhythmias are a problem. There also seems to be a tachyphylaxis to its pulmonary vasodilating effects in some patients.
4. Isoproterenol, 0.01 to 0.05 μg per kilogram per minute, as a right-sided infusion. This is a classic therapy for pulmonary hypertension and right-sided heart failure. Tachycardia and/or arrhythmias can be problematic.
5. Nitroprusside 0.5 to 3 μg per kilogram per minute.

If pharmacologic measures are not adequate, mechanical assist devices such as intrapulmonary artery balloon counterpulsation, extracorporeal membrane oxygenation, or right-sided ventricular assist should be considered.

Other Considerations

Arterial Pressure Monitoring Errors. Gradients between central and radial arterial pressures occur often in these patients. In this situation, the femoral artery or intra-aortic balloon pump central lumen should be utilized for systemic arterial blood pressure monitoring.

Weaning Patients from PGE_1. PGE_1 has been used for up to 10 days in adults with pulmonary hypertension and right-sided heart failure with good outcome. It is a potent dilator of pulmonary, coronary, renal, and cutaneous circulations, and there is a possibility of a rebound vasoconstriction if it is withdrawn rapidly. The manufacturer recommends weaning in decrements of 3 nanograms per kilogram per minute every 3 hours.

Care should be taken not to start weaning PGE_1 prematurely. It is best to have 24 to 48 hours of hemodynamic stability prior to starting the PGE_1 wean. However, in approximately 40 percent of patients it is possible to wean the norepinephrine before PGE_1, and this should be attempted in the first 24 hours. In those patients who require norepinephrine with the PGE_1, a simultaneous weaning of both drugs is our routine approach.

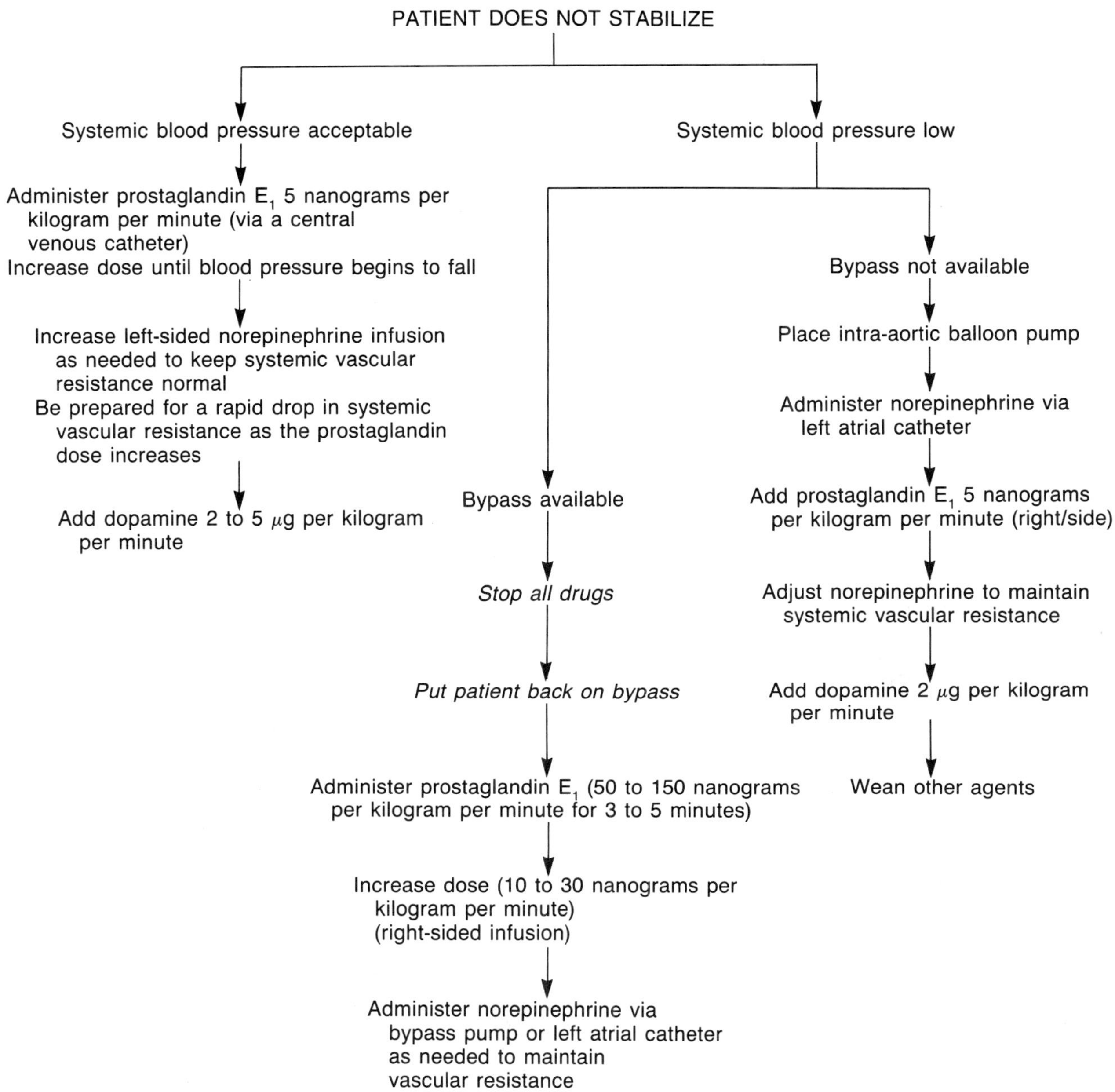

Figure 3 Procedure to be followed if patient does not stabilize following therapeutic escalations 1 to 6.

Cardiac Transplantation and Left Ventricular Assist Devices

Acute pulmonary hyper-resistance after cardiac transplantation or placement of left ventricular assist devices can be treated with dopamine (up to 5 μg per kilogram per minute) and isoproterenol (0.01 to 0.05 μg per kilogram per minute) initially. Nitroglycerin and sodium nitroprusside can be helpful in mild to moderately severe situations. For severe hyper-resistance, and in some centers as a first-line therapy, PGE_1 via a central venous cannula is utilized. PGE_1 is started at 30 nanograms per kilogram per minute and then increased until the systemic blood pressure just begins to fall (upper limit is usually in the range of 150 nanograms per kilogram per minute). PGE_1 is normally metabolized 99 percent on first pass by the pulmonary endothelium, and these patients rarely require alpha-adrenergic support of the systemic vascular resistance.

SUGGESTED READING

Bellamy RF, Lowensohn HS. Effect of systole on coronary pressure-flow relations in the right ventricle of the dog. Am J Physiol 1980; 238:H481–486.

D'Ambra MN, LaRaia PJ, Philbin DM, Watkins WD, Hilgenberg AD, Buckley MJ. Prostaglandin E_1 (PGE_1): a new therapy for refractory right heart failure and pulmonary hypertension after mitral valve

replacement. J Thorac Cardiovasc Surg 1985; 89:567–572.
Farrar DJ, Hill JD, Gray LA, et al. Heterotopic prosthetic ventricles as a bridge to cardiac transplantation: a multicenter study in 29 patients. N Engl J Med 1988; 318:333–340.
Jett GK, Siwek LG, Picone AL, Applebaum RE, Jones M. Pulmonary artery balloon counterpulsation for right ventricular failure. An experimental evaluation. J Thorac Cardiovasc Surg 1983; 86:364–372.
Morel DR, Zapol WM, Thomas SJ, Kitain EM, Robinson DR, Moss J, Chenoweth DE, Lowenstein E. C5a and thromboxane associated with pulmonary vaso- and broncho-constriction during protamine reversal of heparin. Anesthesiology 1987; 66:597-604.
Schaer GL, Fink MP, Parrillo JE. Norepinephrine alone versus norepinephrine plus low-dose dopamine: enhanced renal blood flow with combination pressor therapy. Crit Care Med 1985; 13:492–496.
Wilmshurst PT, Al Hasani SF, Semple MJ, Hamblin AS, Kioy PG, Lucas GF, Savidge GF, Webb-Peploe MM. The effects of amrinone on platelet count, survival and function in patients with congestive cardiac failure. Br J Clin Pharmacol 1984; 17:317–324.

BLOOD CONSERVATION

ROBERT L. THURER, M.D.

Transfusions of banked blood to patients having cardiac surgery increase the potential for complications related to blood administration (most importantly non-A, non-B hepatitis) and waste the limited blood resource. The increasing number of operations done on acutely ill and unstable patients has made it more difficult to eliminate blood transfusions. However, it should be possible to perform the majority of elective operations and a substantial portion of urgent and emergent procedures without the need for homologous blood or blood products. When needed, banked blood should be used sparingly. Therapy with components such as fresh frozen plasma, platelets, and cryoprecipitate is rarely indicated and frequently misused. This chapter reviews the blood conservation methods the author uses to avoid unnecessary transfusions.

GENERAL PRINCIPLES

First, limiting blood loss during surgery, catheterization, and diagnostic testing is extremely important in reducing transfusion requirements. Blood conservation techniques should not have to be used to make up for unnecessary blood loss during any phase of the patient's illness. For a blood conservation program to be successful, all physicians dealing with a patient must be committed to avoiding iatrogenic anemia. Laboratory tests should be limited and samples should be as small as possible. When blood is drawn from indwelling lines, the amount taken to clear the line should be reinfused rather than discarded. Meticulous hemostasis is mandatory for both catheterization and surgery.

Second, many transfusions may be avoided if physicians recognize that patients with satisfactory cardiovascular function can tolerate anemia. If normovolemia is assured by monitoring adequate intracardiac filling pressures, confirming appropriate levels of cardiac output by thermodilution determinations or clinical parameters, and observing satisfactory tissue perfusion, patients will recover satisfactorily with a reduced red cell mass. It is safe for patients to recover and be discharged with hematocrit and readings in the mid-20s. We usually accept hematocrit levels as low as 25 ml per deciliter; in selected cases, lower values may also be accepted. Banked blood transfusion should be given only for clinical indications such as hemodynamic instability, myocardial ischemia, or exercise intolerance rather than in automatic response to a "transfusion trigger." Standing transfusion orders frequently lead to the inappropriate transfusion of banked blood to patients whose only "problem" is a low hematocrit determination. However, because the normal response to anemia is an increase in cardiac output (mostly through an increased stroke volume rather than heart rate), patients with limited compensatory ability should be carefully monitored (with pulmonary artery thermodilution catheters) and their transfusion requirements determined by individual hemodynamic evaluation.

Finally, the risks associated with the transfusion of blood components, such as platelets and plasma, are similar to those associated with the transfusion of red cells. These risks are multiplied by the transfusion of products from multiple donors. In most cases, hemostatic defects related to platelet dysfunction and factor deficiencies in cardiac surgical patients do not cause excessive bleeding and resolve without transfusion of platelets or plasma. Their routine administration is inappropriate. Component therapy should be reserved for patients with ongoing bleeding, satisfactory surgical hemostasis, and specific, correctable deficiencies such as aspirin-induced platelet dysfunction. Desmopressin acetate has been shown to decrease bleeding after complex cardiac operations. In some instances, we give 0.3 μg per kilogram of body weight over 15 minutes after the postbypass protamine infusion is completed to patients who require prolonged bypass, reoperations, or those with increased bleeding. We do not use antifibrinolysins, factor concentrates, or cryoprecipitate.

PREOPERATIVE AUTOLOGOUS DONATION

We recommend preoperative autologous blood donation for all cardiac surgical patients except those with aortic stenosis or anemia. Typically, we collect three to four units of packed cells and separately frozen plasma over a 4-week period (weekly donations). Hematocrits are checked prior to each donation and the donation deferred if the hematocrit determination is less than 35 ml per deciliter. The patient is given ferrous sulfate (330 mg by mouth three times a day) or other iron supplementation, and the last blood donation is scheduled at least 72 hours before operation. Although this technique has been safe and effective for patients of all ages having congenital, valvular, and coronary operations, the patient's clinical status is reviewed before each donation, and blood is not taken if symptoms have worsened. Coronary patients and their anginal symptoms receive special attention. Isovolemic infusions of saline are given to reduce the rapidity of intravascular volume change.

The collected blood and plasma are available for transfusion to the donor-recipient during or after surgery. If the donor meets the criteria for volunteer donation, unused products are given to other patients. Of course, the transfusion of this autologous blood is not associated with the transmission of infectious diseases or febrile reactions. However, these donations can be inconvenient and delaying. Clerical complexity may complicate and frustrate the process. The surgeon and blood bank or transfusion service should work together to avoid these problems.

INTRAOPERATIVE BLOOD CONSERVATION

During surgery, we conserve blood by hemodilution, salvage of "discard" suction and oxygenator contents, the liberal use of the cardiotomy suction, and, of course, efforts to limit surgical blood loss. Hemodilution is effected by removing one or two units of whole blood before bypass. The amount of blood withdrawn is determined by the patient's hematocrit reading and weight, which are used to anticipate the hematocrit after dilution by the crystalloid prime on bypass. We adjust our blood removal to ensure a hematocrit of 20 to 22 ml per deciliter during bypass. The removed blood is stored at room temperature and reinfused after bypass. This technique allows a portion of the patient's blood to avoid extracorporeal circulation and to become a source of "fresh whole blood" after bypass. Blood is transfused during bypass only if the hematocrit falls below 18 ml per deciliter and cannot be raised by hemoconcentration. Although it is not routinely part of the bypass circuit, a Bentley hemoconcentrator is added if the oxygenator volume is excessive.

Before heparinization and after reversal, suctioned blood can be collected and reinfused. With this technique a minimal amount of blood is salvaged during routine operations. However, during complex procedures, reoperations, or when excessive bleeding occurs, we collect the "discard" suction in a Sorenson bag and anticoagulate it with a drip of heparinized saline (50,000 U in 500 ml) delivered through a T connector at the entrance to the bag. The collected product is washed with a Cobe 2991 Blood Cell Processor before infusion. We prefer this method to the more commonly used Haemonetics or Shiley cell washers because a single machine can be used to support several simultaneous procedures. Also, software costs are substantially less. However, this method is slower than the others, and the washed product is usually not available until 15 minutes after collection.

While the patient is heparinized, the cardiotomy suction is used to return salvaged blood to the pump circuit. At the conclusion of bypass, as much of the circuit contents as possible are infused through the arterial perfuser. After the cannulas are removed, the remaining contents of the bypass circuit are drained into a Sorenson bag, washed in the Cobe Blood Cell Processor, and the resulting washed packed cells are transfused. Alternatively, the blood salvaged from the circuit can be infused directly, packed by centrifugation, or washed in another device. "On-line" cell washing does not offer a significant enough advantage over these methods to justify its greater cost and complexity.

Surgical blood loss may be minimized by careful technique, early closure of the leg incisions used for vein harvest, and careful anticoagulation and reversal using activated clotting time. As discussed earlier, the routine use of blood components to improve the coagulation status is never sanctioned. Desmopressin acetate may be given selectively after heparin reversal.

POSTOPERATIVE SALVAGE OF SHED BLOOD

Because blood drained from the chest and mediastinal cavities after open heart surgery is defibrinogenated and sterile, it can be reinfused without washing. We collect this blood with the Pleur-Evac ATS system and return it to the patient within 4 hours of the start of collection. Typically, the shed blood is infused when 250 ml have been salvaged. If blood loss is ongoing, an additional collection bag is placed. If not, routine chest drainage is instituted. Other methods for infusion of shed blood include the Sorenson system and continuous methods using cardiotomy reservoirs. Intermittent methods are more simple and easy to use. On-line techniques do not offer any substantial advantage in handling the relatively small volumes involved. If blood loss is rapid, reoperation is undertaken promptly. Even for the bleeding patient, component therapy is unwise unless significant coagulopathy is documented. Surgical hemostasis should be ensured before postoperative bleeding is attributed to defects in the hemostatic mechanism.

SUGGESTED READING

Cosgrove DM, Thurer RL, Lytle BW, Gill GC, Peter M, Loop FD. Blood conservation during myocardial revascularization. Ann Thorac Surg 1979; 28:184–189.

Kruskall MS, Glazer EE, Leonard SS, Willson SC, Pacini DG, Donovan LM, Ransil BJ. Utilization and effectiveness of a hospital autologous preoperative blood donor program. Transfusion 1986; 26:335–340.

Salzman EW, Weinstein MJ, Weintraub RM, Ware JA, Thurer RL, Robertson L, Donovan A, Gaffney T, Bertele V, Troll J, Smith M, Chute L. Treatment with desmopressin acetate to reduce blood loss after cardiac surgery. A double-blind randomized trial. N Engl J Med 1986; 314:1402–1406.

Thurer RL, Hauer JM. Autotransfusion and blood conservation. Curr Probl Surg 1982; 19:97–156.

ANESTHESIA FOR CARDIAC SURGERY

ROBERT C. SCHNEIDER, M.D.

This chapter concentrates on the anesthetic management of patients undergoing surgical correction of the major acquired cardiac lesions. It does not discuss management of patients with congenital heart disease or special problems, such as patients with pericardial disease, implanted pacemakers, or the care of patients with cardiac lesions for noncardiac surgery.

PREOPERATIVE EVALUATION

The usual preoperative cardiac evaluation must be supplemented by additional information on respiratory, renal, endocrine, and hematologic dysfunction.

Respiratory

Patients with severe obstructive or bronchospastic disease are at significant risk for postbypass bronchospasm. This may embarrass the circulation by decreasing systemic venous return and increasing pulmonary vascular resistance, impairing right ventricular function with resulting inadequate cardiac output. Overdistended lungs may so compress the heart as to preclude chest closure. We administer steroids (prednisone 20 to 40 mg) the night before and the morning of surgery, and methylprednisolone up to 1 g through the operation, and into the postoperative period to help control this problem. We avoid agonist bronchodilators before surgery because increased heart rate may precipitate ischemia in patients with coronary artery disease or congestive failure in patients with significant stenotic valvular lesions.

Renal

Patients with severe renal dysfunction are at increased risk for postoperative renal failure. Hydration, high bypass flow rates, pulsatile bypass, and perioperative dopamine (3 to 5 μg per kilogram per minute) to maintain renal perfusion may help prevent this.

Endocrine

Patients with diet or oral drug-controlled diabetes mellitus frequently require intra- and postoperative insulin. Patients using neutral protamine Hagedorn insulin may be at increased risk for protamine reactions and are started on steroids the night before operation. Thyroid replacements are continued up to operation. Patients on long-term steroid therapy receive hydrocortisone 100 mg the night before and again intraoperatively in their first intravenous solution, with the dose tapered in the postoperative period.

Hematologic

Bleeding disorders need to be evaluated preoperatively to allow proper therapy following cardiopulmonary bypass. Aspirin, clofibrate, and fish oils are stopped at least 1 week (one platelet lifespan) prior to elective surgery to minimize the need for platelet transfusion. Other shorter-acting antiplatelet drugs (e.g., nonsteroidal anti-inflammatory drugs, dipyridamole, chlorpromazine, and diazepam) are stopped several days before operation. Patients on warfarin anticoagulation should be switched to a heparin infusion several days preoperatively to allow recovery of the prothrombin time. Patients on long-term high-dose nitroglycerin infusion may develop methemeglobinemia. The methemeglobin level can be determined preoperatively and, if elevated, treated with methylene blue.

Cardiac

The cardiac evaluation should determine the severity of symptoms, adequacy of cardiac compensation, and the effect of drug therapy. Preoperative stress testing with thallium imaging and two-dimensional echocardiography may supplement the electrocardiogram. A critical appraisal of catheterization results is essential: e.g., a low pulmonary capillary wedge pressure with an elevated left ventricular end-diastolic pressure usually indicates reduced left ventricular compliance, whereas elevation of both pressures is indicative of ventricular failure. Coronary angiographic lesions should be assessed physiologically: e.g., coexisting left anterior descending artery and circumflex artery stenoses do not carry the same significance as a left main coronary stenosis of equal degree, since two events are required to shut off blood flow to the same amount of muscle in the former instance but only a single event in the latter. However, total occlusion of a dominant right coronary artery with stenosis of a collateralizing left anterior descending artery can have the same physiologic significance as an equivalent left main coronary stenosis.

Medications to control ischemia, failure, and rhythm are given with preoperative medications. Beta-blockers, up to the equivalent of 120 mg propranolol per dose and calcium-channel blockers are continued at full dosage. Above 120 mg of propranolol per dose there may be an increased need for post bypass inotropic support. Patients who are receiving more than 90 mg per dose of diltiazem appear to require an elevated serum ionized calcium level for optimal ventricular function after bypass, and occasional patients on nifedipine appear to have persistent systemic vasodilation. Our experience with verapamil is small, but it has not caused noticeable problems. Nitrates at full dose have not caused hypotension if patients are kept recumbent after premedication. The angiotensin-converting inhibitors, captopril and enalapril, are continued to control hypertension or failure. However, they may interact with anesthetic induction agents and during bypass may produce troublesome vasodilation. Digitalis preparations are continued in patients in atrial fibrillation to control heart rate or in patients with congestive failure to prevent acute decompensation. If digitalis has been inadvertently discontinued and if it is needed to control heart rate, a supplemental dose is given the night before surgery to allow peak effect before the patient is brought to the operating room. Diuretics are continued only in those patients with difficult to control congestive failure.

Our standard premedication consists of morphine 0.1 to 0.15 mg per kilogram with scopolamine 0.3 to 0.4 mg intramuscularly about one-half hour before the patient is taken to the operating room. This is reduced in patients with borderline ventricular function to prevent oversedation. Fit patients also receive lorazepam 1 to 2 mg orally the night before and again the morning of operation to improve sedation.

MONITORING

All but patients with simple lesions, e.g., atrial septal defect, receive one or two 12- or 14-gauge intravenous catheters, an 18-gauge arterial catheter, and a thermodilution pulmonary artery catheter. Large-bore intravenous catheters are placed to assure free flow. If large forearm veins are not available, we employ a modified Seldinger's technique to cannulate an internal jugular vein. Patients undergoing first-time cardiac surgery receive one intravenous catheter, whereas patients undergoing cardiac reoperation or major aortic surgery receive two to allow rapid volume replacement and administration of blood coagulation products. The radial artery is our first choice for monitoring blood pressure. If this is not suitable or if the patient is on significant doses of pressor drugs, we cannulate a femoral artery. We avoid the axillary artery because hemorrhage into the neurovascular sheath can lead to troublesome compression of the axillary vein with congestion and edema. We use 18-gauge arterial catheters to facilitate withdrawal of blood before cardiopulmonary bypass when appropriate. This provides "fresh" autologous blood after bypass and can reduce homologous blood use. Pulmonary artery catheters are usually placed via the right internal jugular vein. This allows easy passage of the catheter and keeps the introducer out of the surgical field but accessible for intraoperative manipulation. In patients with carotid artery disease, the jugular vein on the more diseased side is chosen to assure the best carotid artery flow in the event that the carotid is inadvertently punctured. I routinely use a "venous infusion port" pulmonary artery catheter because of ease of placement and separate central venous pressure measurement and drug infusion lumina. Ventricular and atrioventricular pacing catheters are used when bradycardia or complete heart block may embarrass cardiac function, such as in patients with regurgitant valvular lesions or congestive heart failure. Pacing capability makes management of these problems routine. We monitor electrocardiogram leads II and V4 to V5. However, these may be changed if abnormalities are seen more easily in other leads. Precordial lead configuration frequently changes with opening the sternum, effectively moving the sensing electrode to more apical or lateral positions on the heart. The new configuration usually looks similar to V5 to V6 on the preoperative electrocardiogram. Temporarily bringing the sternum together should return the precordial electrocardiogram to its original configuration.

Urine output is monitored in all patients. Free flow of urine must be assured before initiating cardiopulmonary bypass, since obstruction to bladder emptying could result in serious distention and rupture. Patients with diabetes mellitus are maintained with 0 to 1^+ glycosuria.

We routinely monitor nasal and rectal temperatures using the pulmonary artery thermistor temperature as a check of absolute values. Nasal temperature reflects blood flow to the head, whereas rectal temperature reflects heat content of the body mass. All temperatures fall at the same rate during the prebypass period. With the initiation of bypass, nasal temperature falls slightly more slowly than pulmonary artery but much faster than rectal temperature. A slowly falling nasal temperature may indicate inadequate blood flow to the head. The presence of adequate blood flow in the arch vessels must be assured. Likewise, during rewarming, the nasal temperature should rise slightly more slowly than pulmonary artery but faster than rectal temperature. Warming should continue until the rectal temperature reaches at least 32 °C to minimize the chance of dangerous cooling after bypass.

ANESTHESIA—GENERAL COMMENTS

Anesthetics for cardiac patients are usually a combination of narcotic, inhalation agent, intravenous sedative, and muscle relaxant. Because of their limited effect on myocardial function and compatibility with other anesthetic drugs *narcotics* form the base of most cardiac anesthetics. Fentanyl (50 to 100 μg per kilogram) and sufentanil (10 to 20 μg per kilogram) have become the most popular narcotics because of their safety and ease of administration. Morphine (1 to 2 mg per kilogram) produces a slower and often smoother induction in patients with compromised cardiac function. It has less effect on heart rate and produces greater vasodilation than fentanyl, properties that make it attractive in patients with regurgitant valvular lesions. Hydromorphone (0.20 to 0.25 mg per kilogram) has similar characteristics to morphine without the vasodilation or histamine release. It is my drug of choice in very frail patients.

Narcotics may provide adequate control of the hemodynamic response to surgical stimulation in frail patients; however, supplementation is usually required. I prefer volatile *inhalation anesthetics* when possible, as they smooth out the prebypass course and are usually well tolerated, even by patients with compromised ventricular function. Three volatile anesthetics are available today. Halothane provides controllable myocardial depression, little peripheral vasodilation, and a negative chronotropic effect. It is, therefore, an ideal drug in patients with ischemic heart disease or a hyperdynamic response to surgical stimulation. Isoflurane produces little myocardial depression, significant vasodilation, and an increase in heart rate. It is useful in patients with regurgitant valvular lesions but frequently produces ischemia in patients with coronary disease. The effects of enflurane lie between those of these two agents, making it a more suitable general agent than isoflurane. All the volatile inhalation anesthetics are bronchodilators. This is a beneficial side effect in patients with obstructive or bronchospastic disease. I rarely use nitrous oxide, as it usually does not correct hemodynamic changes and by decreasing inspired oxygen to 50 percent or less, it reduces dissolved oxygen, a factor that may be important in patients with significant coronary disease.

Intravenous sedatives complement the inhalation anesthetics by reducing the response to stimulation. Droperidol (in 0.625- to 1.25-mg increments) rapidly lowers increases in blood pressure through a mild alpha-blocking action. In usual doses (up to 10 mg) it is practically devoid of myocardial effects. Thiopental (in 12.5- to 50-mg increments) likewise will lower blood pressure, but this effect is preceded by a transient rise caused by a shortlived vasoconstriction; myocardial depression may be significant in patients with borderline ventricular function. The benzodiazepines, lorazepam (1 to 2 mg) and midazolam (0.5 to 2 mg) can be used to sedate anxious patients prior to placement of invasive monitoring catheters. Careful observation is essential as some patients are very sensitive to intravenous benzodiazepines, especially with midazolam. They are also useful during rewarming on bypass to reinforce sedative blood levels and minimize chances of recall. I usually give 1 to 2 mg of lorazepam or 2 to 5 mg of midazolam for this purpose.

Muscle relaxants are usually chosen on the basis of their hemodynamic side effects. Vecuronium (0.1 mg per kilogram) is devoid of hemodynamic effects and is an ideal agent in the unstable patient. Metocurine (0.3 mg per kilogram) also has few hemodynamic effects. Onset is slower than that of vecuronium, and some patients have a fall in blood pressure from histamine release. Pancuronium (0.1 mg per kilogram) usually produces a transient increase in heart rate and may result in nodal rhythm. Gallamine (usually in a 10-mg bolus) also raises heart rate but in a more dose-dependent manner than pancuronium. When given as a large bolus, it may also precipitate nodal rhythm. Both metocurine and gallamine are eliminated only by renal excretion and should be avoided in patients with significantly impaired renal function. Both are also iodide salts and probably should be avoided in patients with previous reactions to iodine. Succinylcholine remains the most rapid-acting muscle relaxant. However, when it is used with fentanyl or sufentanil, and especially in patients on beta-blockers, significant bradycardia to the point of sinus arrest may occur.

Before bypass, *vasopressors, vasodilators* and *inotropic drugs* are used as indicated by the patient's condition. Transient vasodilation produced by anesthetic induction or other drugs (e.g., heparin) usually results in a fall in both systemic and pulmonary artery pressures. If needed, such changes are best treated with a short-acting vasopressor (e.g., phenylephrine, usually 10 to 40 μg per minute, but at a higher rate if required). Inotropic drugs increase myocardial oxygen consumption and may precipitate acute ischemia. Persistent systemic or pulmonary vasoconstriction is best treated with a controlled infusion of nitroprusside. Particular care must be used in starting nitroprusside in the treatment of elevated pulmonary vascular resistance to avoid systemic hypotension and right ventricular hypoperfusion; I start with 4 to 6 μg per minute and increase slowly as tolerated. Preinduction initiation of inotropic drugs is useful in patients with myocardial failure when anesthesia results in removal of endogenous catecholamine stimulation.

Patients with severe chronic obstructive lung disease or a history of bronchospasm are usually given histamine-blocking drugs (chlorpheniramine, 0.1 mg per kilogram, and cimetidine, 4 mg per kilogram) and steroids as discussed earlier. Narcotics and muscle relaxants that release histamine are avoided. Inhaled volatile anesthetics are administered before and during cardiopulmonary bypass for their bronchodilating effect. If bronchospasm does occur, treatment progresses from endotracheal aerosol bronchodilators (e.g., albuterol), to intravenous aminophylline (5 to 9 mg per kilogram loading dose followed by 0.5 to 0.9 mg per kilogram per minute infusion) or low-dose epinephrine (0.5 μg per minute) infusion, to prostaglandin E_1 infusion (1 to 4 μg per minute). Prostaglandin E_1 does not produce the tachycardia and arrhythmias common with aminophylline and epinephrine and may be used early in the course of treatment when bronchospasm is a particular concern.

ANESTHESIA—SPECIFIC LESIONS

Anesthesia for patients with *coronary artery disease* must maintain adequate myocardial perfusion and control myocardial oxygen consumption. To maximize coronary blood flow, control of heart rate (i.e., coronary perfusion time) is the single most important factor. I try to keep the heart rate in the 50s to 60s or at least in the range of the patient's resting heart rate. Systemic blood pressure should be kept in the normal range. Filling pressures should be kept as low as possible consistent with adequate blood volume and cardiac output. Continuation of beta-blockers, calcium-channel blockers, and nitrates will smooth the patient's prebypass course. Fentanyl or sufentanil, together with vecuronium, produces a smooth, rapid induction. Small doses of gallamine can be used to treat excessive bradycardia. If marked bradycardia occurs in response to laryngoscopy and intubation, then treatment is indicated, since a similar response may occur with sternotomy. A degree of vasodilation is common with induction and is usually self-limited. If it becomes troublesome, I prefer to treat it by placing the patient in the Trendelenburg position or by administering a vasopressor rather than with stimulation. Patients may respond to stimulation with increased heart rate and blood pressure, thus becoming ischemic.

A slow rise in heart rate with operation is common and usually of no significance. However, if necessary, small intravenous doses of a beta-blocker (e.g., propranolol, 0.2 to 0.5 mg, or metoprolol, 0.5 to 1.0 mg per dose) usually control the rate. Patients not on beta-blockers prior to operation are more prone to tachycardia, which may be more difficult to treat. Halothane may successfully decrease heart rate in this situation.

Systemic hypertension in the presence of adequate anesthetic depth can be treated with an inhalation anesthetic or a vasodilator. I prefer to start with inhalation anesthesia. If the patient has a very bad ventricle or is already on an inhalation anesthetic, I administer low doses of droperidol or start an infusion of nitroprusside (10 to 15 μg per minute). Nitroprusside produces balanced arterial and venous dilation. Therefore, an increased rate of volume infusion is frequently required.

Treatment of elevations of pulmonary artery and pulmonary capillary wedge pressures depends on the other hemodynamic and electrocardiographic conditions. Concurrent elevations of systemic and pulmonary pressures occur with stimulation and can be treated by deepening anesthesia, intravenous droperidol, or nitroprusside infusion in the absence or presence of ischemic electrocardiographic changes. Elevations of pulmonary artery and pulmonary capillary wedge pressures with little change or decrease in systemic arterial pressure usually indicates ischemia. These are best treated with an intravenous nitroglycerin bolus (starting with 10 μg and increasing as tolerated) or infusion (starting with 20 μg per minute and increasing as previously mentioned). Ischemic electrocardiographic changes in the absence of elevations of pulmonary capillary wedge pressure are best treated with a beta-blocker to slow heart rate and/or nitroglycerin. In the latter two circumstances, nitroprusside may worsen the ischemia.

Most patients can be separated from cardiopulmonary bypass with no drug support or with calcium chloride (1 to 2 g in divided doses of 3 to 5 mg per kilogram each). Patients with ventricular hypertrophy secondary to long-standing hypertension may require a brief period of blood pressure support with norepinephrine infusion to reperfuse the myocardium. It is uncommon to require long-term support. When cardiac output is inadequate, low-dose norepinephrine (0.33 to 2.0 μg per minute) alone or with dopamine or epinephrine may improve ventricular function.

Anesthesia for patients with *valvular heart disease* should preserve or enhance compensation to the valvular lesion. *Aortic stenosis* imposes a demand for increased strength of left ventricular contraction. Because of decreased ventricular compliance, atrial contraction may deliver up to 40 percent of ventricular filling. Changes in blood pressure are largely caused by changes in contractility. They tend to occur quite rapidly providing a saw-toothed blood pressure profile prior to anesthesia. Tachycardia is often poorly tolerated, resulting in significant elevations in pulmonary artery and capillary wedge pressures.

Aortic stenosis is the most dangerous lesion faced by the cardiac anesthesiologist because cardiac arrest does not respond to conventional management. Therefore, induction agents that depress contractility or change rhythm should be avoided. A slow induction with fentanyl or sufentanil and vecuronium usually maintains a slow heart rate, adequate blood pressure, and normal rhythm. Pancuronium should be avoided because of its propensity for causing nodal rhythm. An inhalation anesthetic can frequently be added before the skin incision is made and varied in concentration throughout the prebypass period to control the response to surgical stimulation. Vasodilators should be used with extreme caution and only with adequate monitoring because unexpected hypotension may result in ischemia and cardiac arrest.

After a short period of blood pressure support to reperfuse the heart after bypass, these patients usually become hyperdynamic and hypertensive. They respond well to a combination of beta blockade and vasodilation, e.g., labetalol or a combination of propranolol and nitroprusside.

Aortic insufficiency imposes a requirement for increased ventricular stroke volume, the absolute amount depending on the forward stroke volume and the regurgitant fraction. Myocardial hypertrophy reduces ventricular compliance, with significant ventricular filling occurring during atrial systole. These patients characteristically show gradual changes in blood pressure in the preinduction period and with induction of anesthesia, since decreases in systemic vascular resistance usually increase forward stroke volume. Increases in heart rate are well tolerated as there is no impediment to ejection. Bradycardia is frequently tolerated as well, and if pulmonary artery pressure is monitored, it need not be treated as long as cardiac output is maintained and pulmonary artery pressure remains acceptable.

Anesthesia may be induced with any of the previously-mentioned narcotics. Induction with morphine is smooth, with a slight lowering of blood pressure and increase in stroke volume. However, even 2 mg per kilogram is frequently inadequate to control the response to surgical stimulation. The sole use or addition of fentanyl or sufentanil is usually required. Not uncommonly increased ventricular performance with reduction of systemic vascular resistance maintains a high blood pressure, and the addition of an inhalation anesthetic to depress ventricular function is necessary. Unwanted bradycardia may be treated with small doses of gallamine or atropine or managed more simply with a pacing Swan-Ganz catheter. Muscle relaxation is achieved with vecuronium or a combination of pancuronium and metocurine. Large doses of pancuronium are avoided to minimize the chance of nodal rhythm. Reductions in stroke volume with increasing systemic vascular resistance respond well to nitroprusside infusion, or in patients with poor ventricular function, to a combination of nitroprusside and dobutamine (3 to 5 μg per kilogram) or dopamine (2 to 5 μg per kilogram).

Following cardiopulmonary bypass inotropic support is frequently required, since the presence of a competent aortic valve results in less ventricular wall stretch than before bypass. Dopamine, dobutamine, and low-dose epinephrine (0.33 to 1 μg per minute) alone or in combination with nitroprusside are all effective in increasing stroke volume.

In isolated aortic valve disease, the presence of a competent mitral valve preserves the pulmonary circulation despite far advanced aortic valve disease. Thus, pulmonary artery pressure is only mildly elevated and hemodynamic management is directed toward the systemic circulation and the left ventricle. In patients with mitral valve disease, the pulmonary circulation and right ventricle are involved early in the course of the disease and frequently constitute the greatest concern to the anesthesiologist. In this situation, airway or surgical stimulation results in elevations of pulmonary vascular resistance and, frequently, in varying degrees of right ventricular failure.

This may progress to inadequate left ventricular filling and systemic hypotension. Volume infusion in this situation may precipitate profound right ventricular failure and cardiovascular collapse. During management of anesthesia and hemodynamic support, these factors must be kept constantly in mind.

The majority of patients with *mitral stenosis* develop left atrial dilation and early atrial fibrillation. This group also develops progressive pulmonary vascular changes, pulmonary hypertension, pulmonary valvular insufficiency, and right ventricular distention; some patients develop tricuspid valvular insufficiency. A small group develops a thickened, small left atrium, and these patients tend to remain in sinus rhythm for a prolonged period. This group also tends to maintain a relatively normal pulmonary vasculature for a longer period of time.

Patients with mitral stenosis have impaired ability to compensate for changes in peripheral vascular tone with induction of anesthesia. Two clues to the sensitivity to induction are cardiac output (or stroke volume) and heart rate. Patients with a low cardiac output are usually very sensitive to narcotic and sedative drugs. They respond rapidly to small doses of induction agents. I prefer to start these patients with morphine or hydromorphone. Patients with a more normal cardiac output may require fentanyl or sufentanil. Patients with an elevated resting heart rate usually depend on endogenous catecholamine stimulation for hemodynamic stability and respond with systemic hypotension to induction of anesthesia. These patients are best managed with a slow induction with morphine or hydromorphone, using mild stimulation (e.g., placement of an oral airway, removal of covers, and placement of a urinary drainage catheter) to maintain hemodynamic stability. In both groups of patients, induction should proceed slowly but result in a good dose of induction drugs. Inadequate anesthetic depth may allow excessive response to intubation and surgical stimulation, with elevation of pulmonary vascular resistance and possible right ventricular failure. Continued response to surgical stimulation is best managed with the addition of an inhalation anesthetic. I prefer enflurane in low doses, as it produces mild pulmonary vascular dilation, and heart rate usually falls slightly. Muscle relaxation is produced with vecuronium, a combination of pancuronium and metocurine, or a succinylcholine infusion. Large doses of pancuronium and gallamine are avoided because they produce elevations of heart rate and may produce nodal rhythm in those patients in sinus rhythm. The response to intermittent increased surgical stimulation can be blunted with small doses of narcotic, droperidol or both just before the stimulus.

Following cardiopulmonary bypass these patients frequently require inotropic support. Dopamine, dobutamine, amrinone, and isoproterenol may all be used with good effect. Often a combination of inotropic drugs with or without a vasodilator avoids the complications of increasing doses of a single drug. I often start with dopamine because of its beneficial renal effects. Patients with significant elevations of pulmonary vascular resistance may exhibit pulmonary vascular constriction even at low doses. In this situation, the pure beta drugs are more useful. The relative inotropic and chronotropic effects of any drug vary from patient to patient and with each patient over time. However, isoproterenol, although the most potent of the beta drugs, is the most likely to cause tachyarrhythmias and should be used in the lowest effective dose. Persistent elevations of pulmonary vascular resistance and right ventricular failure can be managed with the addition of nitroprusside, phentolamine (up to 100 μg per kilogram loading dose in small increments, followed by an infusion of 1 to 5 μg per kilogram per minute), or prostaglandin E_1 (1 to 4 μg per minute). This is discussed in *Pulmonary Circulation: Pharmacologic Management.*

Patients with *mitral insufficiency* react to stimulation in much the same way as patients with aortic insufficiency. However, increases in systemic vascular resistance result in pulmonary vascular engorgement with elevation of pulmonary artery and pulmonary capillary wedge pressures, and left atrial enlargement frequently results in atrial fibrillation. Anesthetic management is similar to that for aortic insufficiency.

Patients with *dilated cardiomyopathy* usually present two problems to the anesthesiologist: congestive heart failure and arrhythmias. These patients usually present for operative management of their arrhythmia. Monitoring should include a pulmonary artery catheter, possibly with pacing capability to help maintain their tachycardia. Anesthesia should preserve cardiac contractility. Morphine alone or with small doses of ketamine (up to 1 mg per kilogram) are usually sufficient. Muscle relaxation with pancuronium or gallamine will maintain heart rate. Small doses of droperidol or a low-dose infusion of nitroprusside may increase stroke volume. A level of anesthesia that retains some responsiveness to stimulation is usually optimal. Patients with *hypertrophic cardiomyopathy* also present two problems: aortic outflow tract obstruction and arrhythmias. In this group of patients, maintenance of adequate blood volume and depression of myocardial contractility combine to minimize the outflow obstruction. Monitoring pulmonary wedge pressure assists in optimal fluid management. Induction should avoid excitement. Diazepam (0.3 to 0.5 mg per kilogram) with halothane or fentanyl followed by halothane should both be satisfactory. The level of anesthesia should prevent response to stimulation. Decreases in blood pressure should be treated with pure alpha drugs (e.g., phenylephrine starting with 10 μg per minute and increasing as needed to an effective dose) to avoid stimulating outflow tract contraction. Intravenous beta-blockade is also helpful in controlling obstruction and frequently is very effective in treating arrhythmias.

Patients with *constrictive pericarditis* or *pericardial tamponade* depend on high blood volume, elevated endogenous catecholamine levels, and high negative intrathoracic pressures (the "thoracic pump") for adequate ventricular filling and contractility. Stroke volume is limited by the external pressure on the ventricles and therefore cannot compensate for decreases in heart rate. Induction of anesthesia is often stormy, especially with tamponade. Hemodynamically significant pericardial effusions should be drained with local anesthesia prior to induction to improve hemodynamic stability. Light levels of anesthesia should be used to maintain responsiveness to stimulation until the pericardium is opened. Ketamine (0.25 to 1.0 mg per kilogram) is often satisfactory. Narcotics can be added as tolerated. Pancuronium or gallamine muscle relaxation will maintain heart rate. Patients with tamponade usually respond subsequent to opening the pericardium with marked hemodynamic improvement and require deepening of the anesthetic. Patients with constrictive pericarditis usually have marked hemodynamic lability during the pericardial dissection and must be managed on a minute-to-minute basis. They usually show progressive improvement as increasing amounts of ventricle are freed from the pericardium.

SUGGESTED READING

Kaplan JA, ed. Cardiac anesthesia. 2nd ed. New York: Grune & Stratton, 1987.

Lowenstein E, Koski EG. Anesthesia for cardiac surgery. In: Cheng TO, ed. The international textbook of cardiology. New York: Pergamon Press, 1986.

Ream AK, Fogdall RP, eds. Acute cardiovascular management. Anesthesia and intensive care. Philadelphia: JB Lippincott, 1982.

Reves JG, Hall KD, eds. Common problems in cardiac anesthesia. Chicago: Year Book, 1987.

Thomas SJ, ed. Manual of cardiac anesthesia. New York: Churchill Livingstone, 1984.

ARRHYTHMIAS FOLLOWING OPEN HEART SURGERY: ROLE OF CARDIAC PACING AND RECORDING

ALBERT L. WALDO, M.D.

It is well recognized that disturbances of cardiac rhythm and conduction are quite common in the postoperative period following open heart surgery. Fortunately, such disturbances are usually transient and are amenable to treatment when therapy is necessary. To this end, routine placement of temporary epicardial wire electrodes on the atria and ventricles at the time of open heart surgery for potential use in the diagnosis and treatment of disorders of rhythm and conduction in the postoperative period is highly recommended. These electrodes can be easily placed on the epicardium of the atria and ventricles at the time of operation and then can be brought out through the anterior chest wall for subsequent use. They have proved to be invaluable in the management of disorders of rhythm and conduction after open heart surgery using techniques that are reliable, rapid, easy to implement, and safe.

DIAGNOSTIC AND THERAPEUTIC USE OF TEMPORARY ELECTRODES

Temporary atrial wire electrodes can be used diagnostically in two ways: (1) to record atrial electrograms, i.e., electrical activity recorded directly from the atria; and (2) to pace the heart to assist in the diagnosis of an arrhythmia. The ability to record atrial electrograms, particularly simultaneously with a body surface electrocardiogram, provides a clear record of atrial activity and is particularly valuable in the diagnosis of arrhythmias in which either the nature of atrial activation or the relationship of atrial activation to ventricular activation is unclear in the standard electrocardiogram alone. Atrial pacing may be required to diagnose a narrow QRS complex tachycardia with a regular RR interval and a 1:1 atrioventricular relationship at a rate of 150 beats per minute, and it may also be used to assess atrioventricular conduction. Furthermore, these temporary epicardial atrial wire electrodes can be used effectively in the pacing treatment of virtually all abnormalities of rhythm and conduction that may occur in the postoperative period with the exception of atrial fibrillation, type II (very rapid) atrial flutter, sinus tachycardia, and ventricular fibrillation. Thus, atrial pacing may be used to suppress premature atrial or ventricular beats, to interrupt many tachyarrhythmias (atrial flutter, ectopic atrial tachycardia, atrioventricular nodal re-entrant tachycardia, atrioventricular reciprocating tachycardia involving an atrioventricular bypass pathway, some ventricular tachycardias, and sinus node re-entrant tachycardia), to increase heart rate as treatment of bradycardia from any cause, and to override or suppress undesirable rhythms with continuous rapid atrial pacing.

Temporary ventricular epicardial wire electrodes are also of great value. Although they are infrequently used diagnostically, they are of considerable use therapeutically, particularly in the treatment of bradyarrhythmias associated with atrioventricular block of any kind and for the treatment of tachyarrhythmias such as accelerated atrioventricular junctional tachycardia or recurrent ventricular tachycardia. And, with the advent of surgical therapies to treat ventricular tachyarrhythmias, they now have been used to perform postoperative programmed ventricular stimulation studies.

Number and Placement of Electrodes

It is recommended that at least one pair of temporary wire electrodes be placed on the right atrium, preferably high in the right atrium, and at least one and, better still, a pair, be placed on the right ventricle at the time of open heart surgery. In patients who have undergone surgical ablation of an atrioventricular bypass pathway (for the Wolff-Parkinson-White syndrome and associated arrhythmias), placement of four pairs of electrodes is recommended, one each on the right atrium, right ventricle, left atrium, and left ventricle for use in the postoperative period to test the efficacy of the surgical treatment with programmed electrophysiologic testing. In addition, placement of three pairs of electrodes is recommended (one on the right atrium, one on the right ventricle, and one on the left ventricle) in patients who have undergone surgical treatment of ventricular tachycardia to test the efficacy of the treatment postoperatively with programmed electrophysiologic testing. And finally, for patients undergoing placement of an automatic implantable cardioverter-defibrillator, similar placement of pairs of epicardial wire electrodes on the right atrium and both ventricles is recommended to permit programmed electrophysiologic testing of the device in the postoperative period. With the advent of the marriage of the antitachycardia pacemaker and the automatic implantable cardioverter-defibrillator, placement of temporary epicardial electrodes for postoperative use will be even more valuable.

TREATMENT OF POSTOPERATIVE BRADYCARDIA

Perhaps the most common and most useful application of epicardial wire electrodes is to provide an increased heart rate in the presence of temporary bradycardia, particularly in the period immediately following completion of the open heart surgery. Relative bradycardia is not uncommon, and simply pacing the atria at rates from 100 to 110 beats per minute provides a satisfactory rhythm, suppression of ventricular ectopic activity, and an adequate or improved cardiac output. In the presence of transient or even permanent complete heart block, ventricular pacing or atrioventricular sequential (DDD) pacing is quite simple to achieve and quite effective until spontaneous return of atrioventricular conduction occurs or a permanent pacing system is placed.

DIAGNOSIS AND TREATMENT OF SUPRAVENTRICULAR TACHYCARDIAS

Atrial Fibrillation and Atrial Flutter

These two rhythms are quite common in the postoperative period following open heart surgery and can often be diagnosed from an electrocardiogram alone. However, the recording of an atrial electrogram for diagnostic purposes is usually quite helpful, and, in fact, is sometimes necessary, as atrial flutter may not be detectable from the electrocardiogram and some forms of atrial fibrillation are relatively well organized, mimicking atrial flutter.

Bipolar atrial electrograms recorded from patients with atrial fibrillation are characterized by complexes having a myriad of shapes, polarities, and amplitudes as well as a broad range of rates and beat-to-beat cycle lengths. Thus, the diagnostic hallmark of atrial fibrillation based on recording of bipolar atrial electrograms is the characteristic beat-to-beat variability of these parameters. In contradistinction, the bipolar atrial electrograms during atrial flutter are characteristically of uniform morphology, polarity, and amplitude and have a remarkably constant beat-to-beat cycle length. Thus, the differentiation of atrial fibrillation from atrial flutter is quite easy to make using bipolar atrial electrogram recordings.

There are two types of atrial flutter. Both types are rapid, regular rhythms. Type I (classic) atrial flutter has a range of atrial rates from about 230 to 340 beats per minute and can always be interrupted with rapid atrial pacing. Type II atrial flutter has a range of atrial rates from about 340 or 350 to 430 beats per minute and cannot be influenced with rapid atrial pacing. Thus, when one makes a diagnosis of type II atrial flutter (a relatively uncommon rhythm following open heart surgery), it must be treated very much like atrial fibrillation.

Pacing Treatment of Type I Atrial Flutter

Rapid atrial pacing using the temporary atrial epicardial wire electrodes placed high in the right atrium is the treatment of choice for patients in whom type I atrial flutter develops following open heart surgery. To interrupt atrial flutter successfully with rapid atrial pacing, it is important to remember that one must pace at a sufficiently faster rate than the spontaneous rate, one must pace for a sufficient duration of time (generally at least 10 seconds or more), and one should use a large stimulus strength (at least 10 mA and sometimes more) to assure capture during the period of rapid pacing.

Currently, it is recommended that a ramp atrial pacing technique be used. In this technique, bipolar atrial pacing at a rate about 10 beats per minute faster than the spontaneous atrial rate is begun and electrocardiogram lead II is recorded continuously. When it is demonstrated that the atrial rate has increased to the pacing rate, the latter is gradually increased until the atrial complexes (flutter waves) in electrocardiogram lead II, which previously have been negative, become positive. The appearance of positive atrial flutter waves during atrial pacing is virtually always a marker that atrial flutter has been interrupted. When this occurs, the atrial pacing rate may be abruptly terminated or the pacing rate may be quickly slowed to a satisfactory rate (e.g., 100 to 110 beats per minute). Because the most successful rate for interruption of type I atrial flutter is approximately 120 to 130 percent (range 111 to 135 percent) of the spontaneous atrial rate, another technique is to initiate rapid atrial pacing at a rate within this percentage range and pace for 10 to 30 seconds or until the atrial complexes in the electrocardiogram lead II become positive. If pacing at the selected rate does not interrupt atrial flutter, the atrial pacing rate may be increased by increments of 5 to 10 beats per minute until successful interruption of atrial flutter is achieved.

Regardless of which atrial pacing technique is used, rapid atrial pacing will produce atrial fibrillation in some patients. Atrial fibrillation precipitated by rapid atrial pacing is almost always transient, lasting seconds to minutes before spontaneously converting to sinus rhythm. For those patients in whom atrial fibrillation persists, it is usually a more desirable rhythm than type I atrial flutter because atrial fibrillation is almost always associated with a slower ventricular response rate than that during atrial flutter. Also, in almost all instances, the ventricular response rate to atrial fibrillation can be quite easily controlled with digitalis, or, occasionally, with verapamil or a beta-blocker. Recently, we have noted that the administration of a type 1A antiarrhythmic drug (e.g., quinidine or procainamide) facilitates the interruption of atrial flutter with return to sinus rhythm.

For those patients in whom type I atrial flutter recurs despite interruption by rapid atrial pacing, continuous rapid atrial pacing at rates of 400 to 450 beats per minute to precipitate and sustain atrial fibrillation may be indicated. One would simply continuously pace the atria, controlling the ventricular response rate in a standard fashion to obtain a clinically satisfactory heart rate. Such pacing may be continued until one has achieved a therapeutic plasma level of a type 1A antiarrhythmic agent. Then, the rapid pacing may be discontinued, with the expectation that sinus rhythm will return promptly. Only infrequently is direct current (DC) cardioversion required to restore sinus rhythm following such treatment.

Paroxysmal Atrial Tachycardia

Fortunately, these rhythms, atrioventricular nodal reentrant tachycardia and atrioventricular reciprocating tachycardia involving an atrioventricular bypass pathway, are not very common following open heart surgery. Establishing the diagnosis may be quite helpful using atrial electrograms to identify atrial activity, since in these rhythms, the P wave is so often superimposed on the QRS complex of the electrocardiogram. In addition, pacing techniques to interrupt this rhythm help establish the diagnosis.

Paroxysmal atrial tachycardia probably is the simplest tachyarrhythmia to interrupt with atrial pacing, and after open heart surgery, atrial pacing is the treatment of choice. There are several acceptable methods of cardiac pacing to interrupt this arrhythmia. It can often be interrupted with an appropriately timed premature atrial beat, so that simple underdrive atrial pacing very frequently is effective. Since paroxysmal atrial tachycardia can always be interrupted with atrial pacing at a rate faster than the spontaneous rate, this simple and more predictable method of pacing therapy is recommended. For those patients in whom paroxysmal atrial tachycardia recurs despite its successful interruption by rapid atrial pacing, continuous rapid atrial pacing techniques, such as deliberate precipitation and maintenance of atrial fibrillation or pacing the atria at rates of 200 to 220 beats per minute and maintaining 2:1 atrioventricular conduction, may be required to suppress this arrhythmia and control the ventricular rate.

Ectopic (Nonparoxysmal) Atrial Tachycardia

In the postoperative period, this rhythm most often is a variant of atrial flutter and almost certainly results from re-entry in the atria. Its diagnosis may be established simply by recording the atrial electrogram simultaneously with the electrocardiogram when atrial activity in the electrocardiogram is not readily apparent. When present, ectopic atrial tachycardia is commonly associated with 2:1 atrioventricular conduction with the resulting ventricular rate being clinically acceptable. Thus therapy to interrupt this arrhythmia may not be required. When treatment is deemed advisable, atrial pacing will interrupt some forms of the rhythm and should always interrupt the form of the rhythm that is due to intra-atrial re-entry. The recommended pacing technique is similar to that described for type I atrial flutter.

Spontaneous Sinus and Atrioventricular Junctional Automatic Tachycardias

Generally, sinus and atrioventricular junctional automatic tachycardias in the postoperative period are transient and benign and do not require special attention apart from seeking the cause of the tachycardia. Both tachycardias are not readily amenable to therapy with standard atrial pacing techniques. Although they can be overdriven with rapid pacing, as soon as the external pacemaker is turned off or its rate is slowed to less than that of the spontaneous rate, the spontaneous automatic tachycardia again becomes apparent.

On occasion, in the presence of an atrioventricular junctional tachycardia, the absence of a P wave preceding the QRS complex results in a decreased cardiac output. Whenever it is desirable to provide an atrial contribution to cardiac output, this usually may be accomplished simply by pacing the atria at a rate just faster than the atrioventricular junctional rate. Occasionally, to accomplish this, it may be desirable to initiate atrioventricular sequential (DDD) pacing at a rate appropriately faster than the atrioventricular junctional rate. Whenever an automatic atrioventricular junctional tachycardia becomes life-threatening, generally because of marked hypotension and low cardiac output, ventricular paired pacing may be required and should be effective, particularly in children.

Ventricular Tachycardia

When the diagnosis of a wide QRS complex in the electrocardiogram is unclear, and if the patient's clinical status permits it, either recording or pacing through the bipolar atrial wire electrodes usually will enable the diagnosis to be established. A bipolar atrial electrogram may document atrioventricular dissociation. In the presence of a wide QRS complex tachycardia with a 1:1 atrioventricular relationship, if atrial pacing at a rate slightly faster than that of the tachycardia results in production of a fusion beat, a narrow QRS complex, or both, the diagnosis is established.

Either intravenous lidocaine therapy or DC cardioversion is generally the treatment of choice with ventricular tachycardia. However, this arrhythmia may be effectively treated by rapid ventricular or, occasionally, even rapid atrial pacing, with successful interruption of the tachycardia and resumption of sinus rhythm. As with rapid atrial pacing to interrupt type I atrial flutter, ventricular pacing to interrupt ventricular tachycardia must achieve a sufficiently rapid rate to interrupt the ventricular tachycardia. In addition, one must always be prepared to perform DC cardioversion or defibrillation promptly, because in a small percentage of patients, rapid ventricular pacing will produce a faster and hemodynamically intolerable ventricular tachyarrhythmia.

Supported in part by Grant RO1 HL38408 from the National Institutes of Health, National Heart, Lung, and Blood Institute, and a Research Initiative Award from the American Heart Association, Northeast Ohio Affiliate.

SUGGESTED READING

Pagé P, Arciniegas JG, Plumb VJ, Henthorn RW, Karp RB, Waldo AL. Value of epicardial programmed ventricular stimulation after surgery for ventricular tachyarrhythmias. J Am Coll Cardiol 1983; 2:1046–1052.

Waldo AL, MacLean WAH. The diagnosis and treatment of arrhythmias following open heart surgery. Emphasis on the use of epicardial wire electrodes. Mt. Kisco, NY: Futura, 1980.

Waldo AL, MacLean WAH, Cooper TB, Kouchoukos NT, Karp RB. Use of temporarily placed epicardial atrial wire electrodes for the diagnosis and treatment of cardiac arrhythmias following open heart surgery. J Thorac Surg 1978; 76:500–505.

Waldo AL, MacLean WAH, Karp RB, Kouchoukos NT, James TN. Continuous rapid atrial pacing to control recurrent or sustained supraventricular tachycardias following open heart surgery. Circulation 1976; 54:245–250.

Waldo AL, MacLean WAH, Karp RB, Kouchoukos NT, James TN. Entrainment and interruption of atrial flutter with atrial pacing. Studies in man following open heart surgery. Circulation 1977; 56:737–745.

MEDIASTINITIS AND THORACIC SPACE INFECTION

GUS J. VLAHAKES, M.D.
WILLARD M. DAGGETT Jr., M.D.
DOUGLAS J. MATHISEN, M.D.

In contemporary practice, mediastinitis following open heart procedures is not a frequent occurrence. When it occurs, however, it can still be a major source of morbidity and mortality. Our experience has been that early and aggressive management of the infection and of any recurrence, coupled with aggressive nutritional support, is essential to effect cure.

TREATMENT OF ACUTE INFECTION

In many cases, the diagnosis may be obvious, with fever, leukocytosis, and purulent sternal drainage; in some instances, however, a mediastinal pus collection may not spontaneously drain early in the course of the disease. The diagnosis must be suspected any time fever and leukocytosis occur without any other source. If wound tenderness and sternal instability are present, surgical exploration may be indicated, despite the absence of purulent drainage. A computed tomography (CT) scan is sometimes useful to identify a mediastinal collection or osteomyelitis. Once the diagnosis is made or strongly suspected, and blood has been drawn for cultures, broad-spectrum antibiotic coverage is promptly begun prior to operative intervention. This should include gram-negative and gram-positive coverage, including antibiotics effective against *Staphylococcus epidermidis*. It is our practice to use vancomycin and gentamicin until more specific bacteriologic identification and sensitivity determinations are made. If frank sternal drainage is present, initial antibiotic coverage is guided by Gram's stain analysis of the drainage.

Exploration is undertaken as soon as the diagnosis is made or strongly suspected and after administration of initial antibiotic doses. Operation should not be delayed; if septic shock is present, surgery should be done as soon as initial fluid and vasopressor resuscitation is completed. At operation, the mediastinum should be completely debrided of any necrotic tissue; fluid as well as tissue samples should be sent for bacteriologic analysis. Care should be taken to avoid damage to bypass grafts, if present, since anatomic landmarks may be difficult to find. Any temporary pacing wires or Teflon felt buttresses used at the original operation should be removed if at all possible. The presence of sternal osteomyelitis is an ominous sign. Any grossly infected portions of sternum must be debrided, as the presence of bone infection greatly increases the chances of recurrence. If an internal mammary graft or grafts were used, the sternum should be carefully inspected to ensure that adequate vascularity is still present; we debride all avascular sternal tissue. In all cases, we at least trim back the edges of each side of the sternum with an oscillating saw and submit the fragments for culture and pathologic analysis with staining for bacteria; this removes any potentially infected cut edges along with bone wax, if present. During debridement, it is important not to disturb planes that are not affected by infection, particularly in the left lateral pericardium or on the diaphragmatic surface of the heart. The majority of mediastinal collections of purulent material are in the immediate retrosternal area, and further mobilization of the heart is needed infrequently.

After complete debridement, the mediastinum is thoroughly irrigated with warm saline and hemostasis is secured; the use of antibiotic irrigation is optional, since any intraoperative irrigant does not produce sustained tissue levels of antibiotics. A single chest tube (No. 28 F) is inserted for drainage, and a No. 10 F pediatric feeding tube for irrigation is inserted through a stab wound near the upper end of the sternotomy incision; additional side holes are cut in the irrigation tube to promote better distribution of the irrigant. The sternum is then closed with multiple parasternal wires, using at least eight wires. In instances in which an entire half of the sternum has been removed or there are multiple transverse fractures, the costal cartilages are woven together with an additional sternal wire; this wire then serves as an anchoring point for the parasternal wires that close the chest. Since these tissues may be very soft, care must be taken not to overtighten the closure. The subcutaneous tissues are irrigated, and the linea alba and presternal tissues are approximated with interrupted absorbable monofilament sutures, such as No. 1 PDS. Skin edges are loosely approximated with interrupted nylon sutures; a type of delayed primary closure is achieved by placing strips of petrolatum-covered gauze (Adaptic) between each suture; these gauze strips are subsequently removed on the third postoperative day.

Broad-sprectrum antibiotic coverage is continued postoperatively until antibiotic sensitivities are obtained. Immediately following surgery, mediastinal irrigation is begun using 2.5 percent povidone-iodine (one-quarter strength Betadine) at a rate of 40 ml per hour, passing it through a warming coil if possible. Daily cultures of the mediastinal effluent are obtained, and irrigation is continued until culture results have been negative for 48 hours. Irrigation is then stopped, and on the following day, the chest tube is removed. Parenteral antibiotics are continued for at least 2 more weeks. The presence of sternal osteomyelitis may dictate longer treatment. Aggressive nutritional support is begun as early after surgery as possible, often supplementing oral intake with tube feedings, as required. Particularly if the remaining sternum is soft, or if closure was difficult, care should be taken to ensure that chest physiotherapy is not too vigorous. We usually minimize its use in this setting, unless specifically indicated.

After antibiotics are discontinued, patients are followed in the hospital for 2 or 3 days, to ensure that fever or leukocytosis does not reappear; patients are instructed to take their temperatures at home daily for at least 2 more weeks.

This regimen results in resolution of mediastinitis in approximately 75 percent to 80 percent of instances. An important factor in avoiding recurrence is early diagnosis and urgent, aggressive treatment, since sternal involvement predisposes to recurrence.

TREATMENT OF RECURRENCE

A recurrence usually means that there is a significant, residual anterior mediastinal cavity, residual sternal osteomyelitis, and/or impaired host defenses. In patients who have recurrences, treatment must be particularly aggressive, as they may be debilitated. As a first step, antibiotics are restarted, and the mediastinum is reexplored; infected portions of sternum and any other necrotic, infected tissue are removed. The irrigation and drainage system is reinserted, and irrigations are reinstituted to reduce the local bacterial count. Approximately 3 or 4 days later, an additional operation is carried out, and the mediastinal cavity is filled with vascularized tissue. Our preference is to use omentum, unless it is absent as a result of previous abdominal surgery, in which case rectus or pectoral muscle may be used. An upper midline abdominal incision is first made and an omental pedicle is mobilized, usually based on a single omental artery and vein. The omentum often must be mobilized off the transverse colon to achieve sufficient length; mobilization of the gastroepiploic artery off the stomach is rarely needed. The sternal incision is then reopened, and the anterior mediastinum is irrigated and debrided of any remaining necrotic tissue; material for cultures is obtained intraoperatively. The omentum is then laid into the mediastinum to fill the cavity. Care must be taken to avoid placing too much tissue into the mediastinum so that it does not become compressed when the sternum is reclosed. We use one or two Silastic Jackson-Pratt drains with bulb suction to drain the potential space behind the sternum and anterior to the omental pedicle. The chest is again closed, and antibiotic treatment and aggressive nutritional management are continued postoperatively. Antibiotics are continued for at least 2 to 3 weeks after surgery. In instances in which there has been extensive sternal osteomyelitis, antibiotic treatment may be requried for a longer period of time. In patients in whom the omentum is absent, we use rectus or pectoral muscle.

We have used this technique in eight cases of recurrent or chronic mediastinal infection following cardiac surgery. In six cases, recurrence came about after treatment by closed irrigation only, and in two cases, chronic, recurrent sinus tracts were present, related to infected Teflon felt at the site of aortotomy. In these two cases, not all of the felt could be removed, and the omentum obliterated the dead space and covered the exposed prosthetic material. In all eight cases, there were no recurrences, and patients are alive to date. In instances in which infections have been treated initially by closed irrigation only, recurrences requiring tissue obliteration of dead space may be predicted when infections are well established and the boundaries of an anterior mediastinal collection are not flexible enough to obliterate dead space. We have recently begun using follow-up CT scans to look for residual anterior mediastinal cavities that may require subsequent tissue obliteration; in one instance, omental transfer was performed based on the CT finding of a residual cavity overlying an aortotomy, before there were overt signs of recurrence.

SUGGESTED READING

Lee AB Jr, Schimert G, Shaktin S, Seigel JH. Total excision of the sternum and thoracic pedicle transposition of the greater omentum; useful stratagems in managing severe mediastinal infection following open heart surgery. Surgery 1976; 80:433–436.

Sarr MG, Gott VL, Townsend TR. Mediastinal infection after cardiac surgery. Ann Thorac Surg 1984; 38:415–423.

Schumaker HB Jr, Mandelbaum I. Continuous antibiotic irrigation in the treatment of infection. Arch Surg 1963; 86:384–387.

Seguin JR, Loisance DY. Omental transposition for closure of median sternotomy following severe mediastinal and vascular infection. Chest 1985; 88:684–686.

Thurer RJ, Bognolo D, Vargas A, Isch JH, Kaiser GA. The management of mediastinal infection following cardiac surgery. An experience utilizing continuous irrigation with povidone-iodine. J Thorac Cardiovasc Surg 1974; 68:962–968.

MALIGNANT PERICARDIAL EFFUSION

J. GORDON SCANNELL, M.D.

Malignant pericardial effusion is a serious complication but not necessarily a terminal manifestation of malignant disease. It may be the result of direct extension or mediastinal spread of intrathoracic malignancy, but equally common is a remote primary tumor, chiefly of the breast, the gastrointestinal tract (stomach and pancreas particularly), the ovary, and the prostate. It is also a troublesome complication of mediastinal lymphoma and Hodgkin's disease in which, in many instances, it is a late complication of radiation treatment.

The diagnosis of malignant pericardial effusion is the first step in its treatment. Increasing dyspnea, weakness, or substernal pressure may require urgent intervention, particularly when there are signs of tamponade. Records of increasing pulse rate, decreasing pulse pressure, and paradoxical pulse are useful monitors of progress. Conventional chest radiography and fluoroscopy have been replaced by ultrasonography and CT scanning. Other sophisticated imaging techniques may be useful. Ultrasonography and CT are helpful in the diagnosis, and in defining the extent and anatomy of the effusion, and in planning aspiration and drainage.

PERICARDIOCENTESIS

Pericardiocentesis by an infraxiphoid approach under local anesthesia is the time-honored method. Since aspiration is not without hazard, an operating room or cardiac catheterization laboratory environment is preferred, particularly for small effusions and when there is a thickened, inelastic pericardium. With the patient supine at a 30- to 45-degree angle and as much extension of the thoracolumbar spine as can be comfortably maintained, a short bevel No. 18 needle is introduced in the angle between the xiphoid and the costal margin on the left. The needle is directed beneath the costal margin and then upward toward the left clavicle. The thickened fibrous diaphragm can be appreciated, followed by entry into the pericardial sac. Aspiration at this stage should produce fluid, generally bloody. Once fluid has been obtained, the needle should be secured to prevent uncontrolled advance. The needle itself may be used as a precordial ECG lead, with due notice of any injury currents produced. Superficial laceration of the right ventricle is a major hazard, with dangerous bleeding from small superficial arteries into an already nondistensible, tense sac. The wall of the right ventricle is normally quite thin and vulnerable to an exploring needle. For this reason, flexible plastic catheters with needle stylets such as those used for intra-arterial puncture are preferred. As opposed to intracardiac blood, the bloody effusion of malignant disease does not clot. A drop or two on an available drape, paper towel, or filter paper produces a characteristic double contour.

The amount of fluid obtained by needle aspiration is variable and often disappointingly small. A favorable response should be immediately apparent with widening of the pulse pressure, increase in systolic pressure, and decrease in peripheral venous hypertension. Subjective relief is usually marked but may be deferred. For prolonged drainage, the introduction of a small catheter through an aspirating needle is so rarely productive that small plastic catheters introduced over guidewires in a modification of the Seldinger technique are preferred. These are placed under fluoroscopic control, a procedure best carried out in cardiac catheterization facilities with operators skilled in interventional radiologic techniques. Small 4- to 6-mm plastic catheters may be used to explore the pericardium and provide effective drainage for several days while adjuvant attack on the malignant process is begun.

The introduction of antitumor or sclerosing agents, e.g., tetracycline, has its advocates. Obliteration of the pericardial space is difficult to obtain by ordinary sclerosing agents, and a brisk pericardial reaction can be awkward if not disastrous. Penetration of sheets of tumor by surface agents is problematic but sometimes successful. Systemic chemotherapy or additional radiation, while pericardial drainage is maintained, is the most defensible rationale for therapy.

RECURRENT EFFUSION

A large number (probably a majority) of malignant pericardial effusions, can be managed, at least in the first instance, by pericardiocentesis and limited catheter drainage. If the fluid recurs, or signs of tamponade persist, pleuropericardial or abdominopericardial drainage may be necessary.

An infrapericardial approach with excision of the xiphoid is particularly useful in large effusions and thin individuals. A facile surgeon and a trusting patient can get by with local anesthesia and acceptable amounts of sedation.

My own preference has been limited left anterior thoracotomy under general anesthesia, carried to the lateral margin of the sternum with resection of the fifth or fourth costal cartilage. The incision may be extended intercostally beyond the anterior axillary line by splitting the serratus anterior in the direction of its fibers to provide a stable closure. The medial aspect of the left upper lobe is folded back, the phrenic nerve identified, and a generous window of pericardium resected or similarly folded. Gentle digital exploration of the pericardial sac is more readily carried out by this route than by the transxiphoid. Adequate pericardial biopsy is usually no problem, and a generous part of the pericardium is removed anterior to the phrenic nerve. The chest is closed with the customary tube drainage for as long as significant amounts of fluid are obtained.

The palliative results of pleuropericardial "windows" are surprisingly good, particularly if further adjuvant or radiation therapy is possible. The interesting paradox, of course, is that in a significant number of patients, radiation changes with contraction of a thickened pericardium are mistaken for recurrent malignant disease. In these instances, pericardiocentesis is hazardous; pleuropericardial drainage is remarkably effective if there has been no radiation damage to the myocardium.

SUGGESTED READING

Vignola P, Johnson RA, Scannell JG. Pericardial diseases. In: Johnson RA, Haber E, Austen WG, eds. The practice of cardiology. Boston: Little, Brown, 1980:664.

CONSTRICTIVE PERICARDITIS

FREDERICK O. BOWMAN Jr., M.D.

Constrictive pericarditis is a relatively uncommon but not rare entity. Over the past few decades, its etiology, understanding, and surgical management have undergone evolution. Concomitantly, the results of pericardiectomy for constrictive pericarditis have improved. Surgical mortality has declined. These improvements probably result from earlier recognition and from more extensive surgical removal of the constricting pathology. However, the patient with constrictive pericarditis frequently continues to present a challenge to surgical management.

ETIOLOGY

In past years, a high percentage of cases of constrictive pericarditis were either proved or deemed to be tuberculous in origin. Over the past 2 decades, other etiologies have replaced tuberculosis as the prime cause. Yet, in the areas in which it is endemic, tuberculosis continues to be a major etiologic factor. Although viral pericarditis is probably responsible for a large number of cases, therapeutic irradiation, metabolic and connective tissue disorders, and cardiac surgical procedures also account for many. In addition, trauma with resulting hemopericardium remains an occasional offender.

Therapeutic irradiation, most commonly for Hodgkin's disease or breast carcinoma, is an infrequent cause. The clinical picture may be quite subtle in its presentation but sometimes may be typical of constrictive pericarditis. Whereas pericardial disease is a consequence of irradiation of the mediastinum in 6 to 30 percent of cases, constrictive pericarditis is seen much less often. It usually requires years to develop and should be considered even many years after treatment when there is right-sided heart failure or elevated venous pressure.

Constrictive pericarditis has been increasingly reported as a late complication of open heart surgery. The incidence appears to be low, approximately 0.15 percent. Retained hematoma in the pericardial space, postpericardiotomy syndrome, low-grade infection, and irrigation with irritant solutions have been cited as etiologic factors. Although most blood is lysed and then absorbed from around the heart following surgery or trauma, perhaps a change in pericardial mesothelial fibrinolytic activity occurs in these instances, thereby leaving the hematoma to organize and fibrose. As for the postpericardiotomy syndrome, its incidence is high, but resulting constriction is uncommon.

A relatively high incidence of postoperative constriction has been reported after the use of povidone-iodine solution when it is used routinely to irrigate the pericardial cavity. Irrigation with Dakin's solution has also apparently yielded the same result. Therefore, irrigation of the pericardial cavity with irritant solutions should be avoided.

DIAGNOSIS

A high incidence of suspicion continues to be important in the diagnosis of constrictive pericarditis. The clinical picture develops slowly and subtely. Many patients continue to be treated for long periods for hepatic dysfunction, cardiomyopathy, or nutritional disorders. Evidence of right-sided heart failure, pericardial knock, and pericardial calcification with small cardiac silhouette are classic findings, and yet the classic picture is seldom seen. Typical findings at cardiac catherization of elevated venous pressures, rapid atrial X and Y descents, early ventricular diastolic dip and plateau, and equalization of mean right atrial, pulmonary wedge, and right and left ventricular end-diastolic pressure confirm the diagnosis. However, in the postcardiac surgical patient with other reasons for elevated pressures, such as valvular or myocardial damage, the diagnosis, both clinically and by cardiac catherization, may be extremely difficult. In recent years 2-D echocardiography and computed tomography have been of help in confirming the diagnosis by demonstrating the thickened pericardium. An example of this is when the diagnosis following therapeutic irradiation may be clouded by a degree of restrictive myocardial disease. In this instance, 2-D echocardiography and CT scanning may be extremely helpful.

INDICATIONS FOR SURGICAL THERAPY

At our institution, surgery is considered the primary treatment for constrictive pericarditis when the diagnosis is established and when there are no associated conditions that contraindicate major surgery. Pericardiectomy is the definitive treatment because constrictive pericarditis is a progressive lesion that tends to increasingly compromise cardiac function if treated nonoperatively. Perhaps an exception to this rule is the patient who has mixed valvular or myocardial disease and evidence suggesting only mild pericardial restriction. These patients may present difficult decisions as to timing of operative intervention.

SURGICAL TECHNIQUE

In this era of open heart surgery, some surgeons advocate cardiopulmonary bypass almost routinely, or pericardiectomy for constrictive pericarditis. Emptying the heart, thereby more clearly defining the plane of dissection and easing the management of cardiac perforation, if it should occur, is cited as an advantage of this technique. The obvious disadvantage appears to be an increased incidence of significant bleeding. Many surgeons reserve cardiopulmonary bypass for extremely difficult dissections or reoperations, or when there are concomitant cardiac lesions to be corrected. Most surgeons appear to prefer pericardiectomy with pump standby.

Routine monitoring of the patient is recommended, inserting an indwelling arterial line and a Swan-Ganz catheter to measure pulmonary wedge, pulmonary arterial, and right atrial pressures as well as to perform postoperative cardiac output determinations in the event of low-output syndrome.

The surgeon has a choice of three incisional approaches: median sternotomy, left anterior thoracotomy, or bilateral thoracotomy. The advantages of the median sternotomy are the ease of dissection and exposure of the right side of the heart, probably the best physiologic tolerance, and the least discomfort of the three. It is the incision of choice if one plans to use cardiopulmonary bypass. Its disadvantage lies in the relative difficulty of exposing the pericardium over the posterior left ventricle, left pulmonary veins, and left atrium.

Left anterior thoracotomy, through the fourth or fifth intercostal space, provides clear access to both left and right ventricles, including their diaphragmatic surfaces. Through it, minimal manipulation of the heart is required to achieve complete ventricular decortication. This incision can be readily extended across the sternum if further exposure on the right side is required.

Bilateral anterior thoracotomy offers the best exposure to the entire pericardial sac and its contents: both ventricles, both atria, both vena cavae, and left and right pulmonary veins. This incision, however, is the least well tolerated by the patient, both physiologically and symptomatically. A bilateral anterior thoracotomy, however, is especially useful in reoperation for inadequate prior pericardiectomy and for those occasional instances in which there is adjacent pleural disease that is constrictive and needs concomitant decortication.

Most commonly I use a median sternotomy for pericardiectomy, with pump standby in case dissection over the posterior left ventricle or left pulmonary veins cannot be satisfactorily completed without it. As noted in the preceding paragraph, however, bilateral anterior thoracotomy offers the greatest exposure and is used in isolated instances.

There continues to be some controversy and perhaps misunderstanding regarding the depth of pericardial resection. The classic four layers and planes are seldom readily seen. These four layers include the parietal and visceral pericardium and a layer of organized fibrin on each adjacent surface. Although it is not always necessary to remove the epicardium, this layer can be an important component of the constriction. Lack of removal may account for continued signs of constriction and a poor result; it should be removed if initial pericardiectomy does not immediately improve hemodynamic parameters. It should be noted that the epicardial layer may be especially constrictive in postirradiation cases.

Dissection of the pericardium should be planned so that the left ventricle is freed first. Acute right-sided heart failure may be seen if the right ventricle is released first. Via a median sternotomy, the dissection should start as far to the left as possible, thereby leaving most of the right ventricle protected until the left is decorticated. Incision is carried through the pericardium until the heart begins to bulge. It is wise to retain a flap of pericardium as one dissects, in case of inadvertent perforation or other tear. The old adage of using the flap to "reconstruct" the heart in case of excessive dilation and acute failure should rarely, if ever, be pertinent. If calcium spicules invade deeply into the myocardium, they should be circumscribed and left in place. Such small residues do not prevent the heart from expanding, and the danger of removing these islands is excessive. In the event of the involvement of the epicardium, the "waffle procedure," as described by Heimbecker, or a modification thereof, may be advisable. Removing the entire epicardium can result in coronary artery or myocardial laceration and excessive bleeding.

What should be the extent of the pericardial resection? Everyone agrees that it is necessary to completely free the anterolateral and diaphragmatic surfaces of both left and right ventricles. Some follow the advice of the late Emile Holman and recommend freeing of both atria, vena cavae, and pulmonary veins. Decortication of the atria and veins may be hazardous because of their thin walls, and it must be carried out with care. This author prefers as complete decortication of all structures as can be feasibly performed but would not hesitate to leave portions of the atria and veins unroofed if dissection became too difficult. There is no proof that decortication of more than the ventricles is necessary. One should expect that in every case, adequate pericardiectomy has been performed when both ventricles are freed and the filling pressures have decreased to normal levels.

RESULTS

The operation is usually well tolerated. However, the surgeon must be especially aware of postoperative low-output syndrome. The sicker the patient is preoperatively, the more likely it is that there will be a low cardiac output postoperatively. This, in some part, appears due to myocardial atrophy. Preoperative digitalization is advised for those patients who are not already digitalized. The use of early inotropic support, frequently beginning in the operating room, is indicated instead of relying on volume support alone. Occasional prompt insertion of the intra-aortic balloon pump may be lifesaving. Postoperative support with inotropes or the intra-aortic balloon pump may be required for several days. Other than this low-output problem, postoperative care does not differ from that following the usual thoracic operation.

Although the results from pericardiectomy for constrictive pericarditis have improved in recent years, the procedure is not without risk. Mortality rates in several recent series range from 4 to 14 percent. In a careful analysis of 81 patients, Seifert and associates found that the right ventricular end-diastolic pressure was the only significant predictor of in-hospital death. In patients with right ventricular end-diastolic pressure of 30 mm Hg, hospital mortality was 30 percent. This compared with 5 percent for those with a right ventricular end-diastolic pressure of 16 mm Hg and 10 percent for those with a reading of 20 mm Hg. McCaughan and co-workers, reviewing 231 patients, found the operative risk to be related to preoperative disability: 1 percent for New York Heart Association Class I or II, 10 percent for Class III, and 46 percent for Class IV patients.

Long-term results vary with the etiology of the condition and the successful outcome of the original surgery but not necessarily with the preoperative classification or the occurrence of postoperative low cardiac output. Many extremely ill patients can be returned to Class I and Class II status. Choice of incision is dictated by the patient's particular problems, and as complete pericardiectomy as possible is recommended.

SUGGESTED READING

Heimbecker RO, Smith D, Shimizu S, Kestle J. Surgical technique for the management of constrictive epicarditis complicating constrictive pericarditis (the waffle procedure). Ann Thorac Surg 1983; 36:605–606.

McCaughan BC, Schaff HV. Piehler JM. Danielson GK. Orszulak TA, Puga FJ, Pluth JR, Connolly DC, McGoon DC. Early and late results of pericardiectomy for constrictive pericarditis. J Thorac Cardiovasc Surg 1985; 89:340–350.

Miller JI, Mansour KA, Hatcher CR Jr. Pericardiectomy: Current indications, concepts, and results in a university center. Ann Thorac Surg 1982; 34:40–45.

Ribeiro P, Sapsford R, Evans T, Parcharidis G, Oakley C. Constrictive pericarditis as a complication of coronary artery bypass surgery. Br Heart J 1984; 51:205–210.

Seifert FC, Miller DC, Oesterle SN, Oyer PE, Stinson EB, Shumway NE. Surgical treatment of constrictive pericarditis: analysis of outcome and diagnostic error. Circulation 1985; 72 (Suppl II):II-264–273.

PULMONARY EMBOLISM

PULMONARY EMBOLISM

PETER VAN TRIGT, M.D.
WALTER G. WOLFE, M.D.

Pulmonary embolism continues to produce considerable morbidity and mortality in spite of a better understanding of its pathogenesis, presentation, and prophylaxis. It has been estimated that pulmonary emboli are responsible for 3 to 5 percent of in-hospital deaths, approaching 250,000 patients per year in the United States. Furthermore, over one-half million people sustain nonfatal pulmonary emboli each year. A high index of suspicion is extremely important if the outcome of this condition is to be successful, for the physician must consider pulmonary embolism early on as a clinical possibility so that appropriate diagnostic studies can be performed to confirm the diagnosis prior to beginning therapy. Delay in initiation of therapy often is responsible for the mortality associated with this disease.

The patient with a pulmonary embolus presents with nonspecific symptoms and signs associated with a wide range of cardiopulmonary disorders. Only one-third have evidence of venous thrombosis. The emboli originate from the iliofemoral venous system in approximately two-thirds of the patients and from the calf veins in the remaining one-third. Pulmonary emboli can also originate from thrombi in the right atrium, from septic thrombi in the pelvis, and from tumor emboli associated with hypernephroma. Pulmonary angiography remains the definitive study for diagnosis of pulmonary embolism. Although a normal six-view ventilation-perfusion ($V/\dot{Q}$) scan is sufficient to exclude the diagnosis, patients with low or intermediate probability interpretations of the $V/\dot{Q}$ scan should be studied with angiography if clinical suspicion is great. The high probability scan is usually adequate to establish the diagnosis, although if there is increased risk for systemic anticoagulation, an arteriogram should be obtained.

MEDICAL THERAPY

Approximately 90 percent of patients with pulmonary emboli are effectively managed with intravenous heparin once the diagnosis has been objectively established. Continuous intravenous infusion is preferable following a loading dose of 7,500 to 10,000 U. The activated partial thromboplastin time is maintained to stay at approximately two times control. The usual dose requirement is 800 to 1,000 U per hour to achieve the desired effect. Intravenous heparin given for 7 to 10 days is quite effective in the vast majority of patients with pulmonary emboli, as the heparin prevents clot propagation and allows for endogenous fibrinolysis. Symptomatic improvement occurs within days, and repeat perfusion scans usually demonstrate resolution of the thrombi after a course of intravenous heparin. Platelet count must be carefully monitored while the patient receives heparin, and at the first indication of a falling count, heparin therapy should be converted to sodium warfarin (Coumadin). Heparin-induced platelet aggregation and arterial small vessel thrombosis are rare but serious complications of hospitalized patients receiving heparin. Warfarin is started after the patient is asymptomatic, and once the prothrombin ratio reaches 1.7, heparin is discontinued and the patient is maintained on warfarin for 3 to 6 months.

The role of thrombolytic therapy for pulmonary thromboembolism has gained support as a result of the National Institutes of Health sponsored clinical trials of thrombolytic agents in acute pulmonary embolism. These studies indicated that the rate of resolution of embolic material can be greatly accelerated by streptokinase or urokinase, with normalization of hemodynamic disturbances and reperfusion of the lung. The best results are achieved when streptokinase or urokinase is used within 72 hours of the onset of pulmonary emboli. After 7 days no significant difference was found between heparin and streptokinase in restoration of blood flow to the lungs.

It is evident that the use of thrombolytic therapy achieves more rapid stabilization of the patient and more improved clinical results than is achieved with heparin in those patients who present with substantial, recent embolic occlusions (more than 30 percent of the pulmonary vasculature obstructed). In this group of patients, significant problems associated with arterial oxygenation and right ventricular dysfunction are usually present, and mechanical ventilation and inotropic support are commonly required in the early course. Familiarity with the use of streptokinase has increased recently with its application to acute coronary thrombosis, and we prefer its use to urokinase because of increased availability, greater temperature stability, and lower cost. The initiation of thrombolytic therapy with streptokinase, after objective documentation of the diagnosis, begins with a loading dose of 250,000 U administered intravenously over a 30-minute period. A maintenance dose of 100,000 U per hour is administered as a continuous pump infusion for 24 hours. During streptokinase therapy herparin is not used, but on completion of the lytic therapy heparin should be started at a continuous infusion when the activated partial thromboplastin time returns to two times control. Monitoring of systemic fibrinolysis during streptokinase therapy is necessary; for this purpose maintaining the thrombin clotting time at twice control is sufficient. A small number of patients may require higher doses of streptokinase to overcome high titers of antibodies that may be present in response to an occult streptococcal infection.

Contraindications to the use of streptokinase include an active site of gastrointestinal bleeding, recent surgery or trauma (within 10 days), or a recent stroke. Great care should be taken to minimize invasive monitoring during therapy in order to avoid bleeding from cutdown sites and around large-bore catheters. The single serious complication of thrombolytic therapy is bleeding, with a risk factor three times greater than that of heparin therapy. Because of the risk of bleeding complications, the use of streptokinase should be reserved for those patients sustaining *major* pulmonary emboli with significant pulmonary or cardiac decompensation, in order to achieve more rapid stabilization and provide the patient with a margin of safety in the immediate course. Dramatic effects can be seen within 12 hours following initiation of thrombolytic therapy.

SURGICAL MANAGEMENT

Surgical management of pulmonary embolism is considered for three specific conditions. Caval interruption is the procedure utilized for prevention of recurrent emboli from the inferior vena cava and lower extremities. Pulmonary embolectomy is performed for acute embolus associated with hypoxemia and hypotension that is not responsive to oxygen and inotropic support. Finally, pulmonary embolectomy also is considered for chronic pulmonary embolism associated with dyspnea, hypoxemia, and pulmonary hypertension caused by organized thrombus obstructing the main branches of the pulmonary artery.

Caval Interruption-Filtration

Vena caval ligation or partial interruption with a filter device can be associated with serious sequelae and may not completely prevent subsequent embolism. For these reasons, caval interruption should not be performed without objective documentation of deep venous disease involving the inferior vena cava or iliofemoral systems. Only rarely is chronic anticoagulation with warfarin not successful in controlling these patients' symptoms and risk of pulmonary emboli. Only those patients with well-documented recurrent episodes of pulmonary emboli while receiving adequate anticoagulation therapy or those with a strong contraindication to the use of anticoagulation should be considered candidates for such procedures. The Greenfield filter is preferable to open surgical ligation because of the severe, debilitating leg edema and venous stasis that result from ligation. The Greenfield filter is placed under fluoroscopy (preferably in the catheterization lab) through a right internal jugular venous approach under local anesthesia. The internal jugular vein is generally large and is opened transversely, with care being taken to avoid air embolism. Passage of the filter catheter–carrier assembly over a guidewire to the inferior vena cava avoids problems with navigation and the rare but troublesome eustachian valve overlying the caval-atrial junction. The filter is discharged at the level of the third lumbar vertebra, below the level of the renal veins. Potential problems associated with placement of the filter include discharging it in a tilted position and difficulty in passing the apparatus through a small jugular vein. Once released from the carrier, the filter should not be touched by the stylet or carrier, which can force the struts through the wall of the inferior vena cava. If placement occurs more superiorly than intended (at or above the level of the renal vein) little risk of renal impairment exists, as reported from prior experience with this situation. Long-term patency of the Greenfield filter is reported to be 95 percent, with an incidence of recurrent pulmonary embolism of less than 5 percent. Lower extremity edema and skin stasis ulceration are known complications but occur much less commonly than following surgical ligation. Long-term anticoagulation therapy is often combined with placement of a caval filter unless contraindicated by other clinical factors.

If caval ligation is undertaken, a right flank incision is usually performed in males, whereas in females a transabdominal route is used so that the ovarian veins may be ligated as well. The patient's legs should be elevated immediately after operation and elastic wraps should be applied to control leg swelling.

Pulmonary Embolectomy

Pulmonary embolectomy was first proposed by Trendelenburg in 1908 and was performed successfully for the first time by Kirschner in 1924. It was not until the advent of cardiopulmonary bypass that the mortality rate for removal of acute pulmonary emboli became acceptable. The first successful pulmonary embolectomy on cardiopulmonary bypass was performed by Bahnson and Sharp in 1961. Despite technological improvements, the mortality rate for acute pulmonary embolectomy has remained high, although with extreme variability in results among reporting centers. It is apparent that patient selection is one of the primary determinants of outcome. Usually patients with massive pulmonary emboli survive for a period of at least several hours, although a certain number experience sudden death. The majority of patients who survive the initial few hours following embolism respond to medical management. The difficulty lies in predicting which of the patients who survive long enough to have the diagnosis confirmed require embolectomy for survival. Once the diagnosis is made, patients who are unresponsive to medical therapy (oxygen, immediate heparinization or thrombolytic therapy, inotropic support), with refractory hypotension and hypoxemia, should be taken to the operating room for pulmonary embolectomy. A median sternotomy incision is employed, and cardiopulmonary bypass is instituted. The pulmonary artery is opened, and the emboli are removed under direct vision. Pulmonary parenchymal manual compression is used to force peripheral emboli into the central pulmonary artery where they can be removed, and the pulmonary arteries should be carefully irrigated of all debris. Caval interruption, which has been considered an integral aspect of the treatment of massive pulmonary emboli, should be used selectively. Most patients have not had adequate anticoagulation therapy at the time of embolectomy, and the usual clinical indications should be applied to placement of a caval filter or caval interruption.

Adequate oxygenation and hemodynamic improvement following embolectomy are usually dramatic, and the major cause of postoperative morbidity is cardiac complications. The mortality rate is still approximately 25 percent in this group of gravely ill patients.

CHRONIC PULMONARY EMBOLISM

Although the clinical course of most patients with pulmonary embolism is one of gradual resolution and reperfusion of the lung, a small but definite group of patients instead develop persistent, chronic obstruction of the pulmonary vasculature. This results in cor pulmonale and is classified as chronic pulmonary embolism. Patients present with dyspnea, cyanosis, and exercise intolerance associated with low arterial PO_2, pulmonary hypertension, and right ventricular hypertrophy. Usually more than half the major pulmonary arteries are occluded with organized thrombus. Evaluation includes pulmonary angiography with measurement of pulmonary artery pressures, measurement of arterial blood gases, and assessment of right ventricular function. Bronchial arteriography is needed to demonstrate patency of the distal pulmonary artery, and the ideal candidates have proximal main or lobar occlusion with a patent distal pulmonary artery filled via collaterals from the bronchial circulation, with hypoxemia but minimally impaired lung ventilatory function.

The surgical approach depends on the location of the majority of the thrombus. Extracorporeal circulation is preferable in most patients, as it provides a safer procedure. Median sternotomy is employed for access to the main pulmonary artery and its major branches. Anterior thoracotomy through the third intercostal space provides exposure to the main left or right pulmonary artery if only unilateral embolectomy is necessary. Proximal occlusion of the pulmonary artery can be performed during embolectomy to allow perfusion of the opposite lung. It is important to perform an extensive embolectomy, including the primary and secondary branches of the pulmonary artery, placing counterincisions in the distal vessel if necessary. Back bleeding from the pulmonary artery at the time of embolectomy is usually associated with a significantly improved clinical course postoperatively.

A series of 15 patients has been evaluated at Duke University Medical Center and selected for embolectomy as therapy for chronic pulmonary arterial obstruction. All patients had a history of chronic anticoagulation therapy with warfarin, and symptoms had been present for several years prior to evaluation for operation. Dyspnea on exertion was the most prevalent symptom (86 percent), followed by a history of previous thrombophlebitis (79 percent) and hemoptysis (50 percent). Following embolectomy, 83 percent improved their New York Heart Association functional status from Class IV to either Class I or Class II. Most patients were rehabilitated such that they either returned to work following recovery from operation or felt they were capable of resuming their previous occupations. There were two perioperative deaths in the series (13 percent mortality). One was due to hemorrhage in the reperfused lung after pulmonary arterial blood flow was reestablished, and the other patient died 3 days postoperatively as a result of persistent pulmonary hypertension and intractable right ventricular failure. Patients with severe pulmonary hypertension and resultant right ventricular failure are at significantly increased operative risk.

Pulmonary thromboembolism continues to be a difficult clinical problem as a major cause of morbidity and death. Once the clinical diagnosis of pulmonary embolism is considered, it must be objectively established or ruled out. Heparin anticoagulation with conversion to warfarin is still the treatment of choice in acute pulmonary emboli. In rare cases, caval interruption or filtration and/or pulmonary embolectomy may be necessary.

SUGGESTED READING

Greenfield LJ, Zocco J, Wilk J, Schroeder TM, Elkins RC. Clinical experience with the Kim-Ray Greenfield vena caval filter. Ann Surg 1977; 185:692–698.

Oldham HN Jr, Cox JL, Pass HI, Wechsler AS, Sabiston DC Jr. Effects of pulmonary embolism on regional myocardial blood flow. Surgery 1974; 76:160–169.

Parmley LF Jr, North RL, Oh BS. Hemodynamic alterations of acute pulmonary thromboembolism. Circ Res 1962; 11:450–465.

Sabiston DC Jr, Wolfe WG, Oldham HN Jr, Wechsler AS, Crawford FA, Jones KW, Jones RH. Surgical management of chronic pulmonary embolism. Ann Surg 1977; 185:699–712.

Wolfe WG, Sabiston DC Jr. Pulmonary embolism. In: Major problems in clinical surgery Vol. XXV. Philadelphia, WB Saunders, 1980.

TRANSPLANTATION, CIRCULATORY SUPPORT, AND CARDIAC PACING

CARDIAC TRANSPLANTATION

BRUCE A. REITZ, M.D.

Cardiac transplantation is among the most rapidly growing areas of cardiothoracic surgery. With the recent availability of improved immunosuppression using cyclosporine, many new cardiac transplant programs have been initiated, and an exponentially increasing number of patients are receiving cardiac transplants; it is estimated that over 1,500 patients will receive cardiac transplants in 1988.

Although there have been many improvements in our understanding of patient management, the principal factors contributing to a successful outcome in cardiac transplantation are the very careful attention to detail in the administration of immunosuppressive drugs and the detection and treatment of the side effects and complications of therapy. This chapter outlines our personal approach to the performance of cardiac transplantation, the control of immune suppression, and general aspects of patient management.

INDICATIONS FOR CARDIAC TRANSPLANTATION

Patients considered for cardiac transplantation must have end-stage disease that cannot be treated by standard medical or surgical alternatives. They are usually between 10 and 60 years of age, with no irreversible organ system failure, no active infection, medically compliant and motivated for recovery, and have insurance or other resources to pay for anticipated hospital and postoperative follow-up care. We consider insulin-dependent diabetes, a history of cancer, alcoholism, or drug abuse, or other serious systemic illnesses to be contraindications to transplantation. Patients younger than 10 or older than 60 have undergone transplantation successfully, but results in these age groups are uncertain, and transplantation in such patients should only be considered by experienced teams, and especially in the case of pediatric transplants, as an investigational procedure.

A high proportion of the patients receiving cardiac transplants at present require in-hospital intensive care because of low cardiac output syndromes prior to transplantation. Many patients now come to cardiac transplantation on inotropic drug support or with the intra-aortic balloon pump, and an increasing number have a mechanical ventricular support device. Although survival results in small numbers of such high risk patients have been equivalent to past experience with more favorable candidates, the best survival results occur in those patients falling well within the generally accepted guidelines presented above.

When a patient is accepted for cardiac transplantation, relevant information is obtained for matching with prospective donors. The patient's blood group, size and weight, and a very accurate and recent measurement of pulmonary vascular resistance are recorded. The patient's serology for cytomegalovirus, Toxoplasma, or herpes simplex exposure is verified, and tissue typing is done for later retrospective analysis. A survey of the patient's reaction against a panel of 50 random serum samples is performed to assess the presence of preformed antibody. Extensive preoperative teaching is given by transplant team members, particularly the nursing staff, who will be caring for the patient, and the team social worker, who can help with numerous details involved with family support. The patient's data are then entered on the national computer network United Network for Organ Sharing (UNOS) as well as with the local organ donor procurement group working with the transplant team. The length of wait for a donor organ depends primarily on the listing of the severity of the patient's medical condition; currently the longest waits are for those patients awaiting transplantation outside the hospital. Patients in the hospital in the most urgent category have an average wait of approximately 2 weeks, whereas patients outside the hospital in a stable condition may wait for 3 months or longer.

MANAGEMENT OF THE CARDIAC DONOR

The cardiac transplant team learns of potential donors from the organ procurement coordinator. The coordinator has basic information as to the donor's cause of death, associated injuries, age, size, and blood type, and details of the transplantation patient's condition and current management. The transplant surgeon must ensure that the potential heart is as near to normal as possible and of adequate size and function to adequately support the recipient's circulation. If the potential donor is not smaller than 20 percent of the body size of the recipient, and the recipient has a pulmonary vascular resistance of less than 6 Wood units, then standard procurement and orthotopic transplantation are usually acceptable for good cardiac function. When the donor's pulmonary vascular resistance is between 6 and 8 Wood units, the donor heart should be larger and a short ischemic time is required in order to safely perform orthotopic transplantation. If the recipient is especially ill and these criteria cannot be met, then consideration should be given to heterotopic cardiac transplantation in order to prevent the possibility of severe right-sided heart failure and early death.

It is important to emphasize continued close monitoring and care of the potential cardiac donor. Once brain death has been declared, adequate fluid resuscitation may be necessary, because donors are often allowed to become dehydrated in order to reduce cerebral swelling. Placement of a radial arterial line and central venous monitoring catheter is helpful in assessing fluid status. Furthermore, diabetes insipidus should be treated with vasopressin (Pitressin), hypothermia corrected with warming blankets, and inotropic drugs reduced to a minimum or discontinued after adequate fluid resuscitation. It is important to obtain blood, sputum, and urine cultures and then to start the donor on broad-spectrum antibiotics prior to harvesting the organ. Arrangements should be made to harvest the heart as expeditiously as possible, since the donor will inevitably deteriorate. Almost all qualified donors are appropriate for multiorgan donation, and this requires coordination with other transplant groups.

The donor procurement is carried out through a long midline incision with sequential dissection of the heart, liver, kidneys, or other organs to be removed. The quality of the heart should be carefully determined after initially opening the chest. All of the cardiac chambers are palpated to feel for valvular regurgitation, the coronary arteries are palpated for occult disease, and the heart is carefully inspected for areas of potential trauma and for regional contractility. After assurance that the heart is satisfactory, a call can be made to the transplant center to begin induction of anesthesia for the recipient.

Heart procurement begins with azygous vein ligation and division, vena caval inflow occlusion, the placement of an aortic cross-clamp when the systemic pressure falls below 30 mm Hg, and then the infusion of cold crystalloid cardioplegia solution into the proximal aortic root. The superior and inferior vena cavae are divided, allowing cardioplegia to vent from the right atrium, followed by division of the pulmonary veins and pulmonary artery. The heart is cooled topically while cardioplegia solution continues until 500 to 1,000 cc of solution has been administered. When this is completed, the aorta is finally divided, and the heart is wrapped sterilely with a protective gauze pad, stored in a sterile plastic bag with cold saline solution, and wrapped in several additional plastic bags before storage in a plastic container placed in a portable ice chest. The graft is then ready for transport back to the recipient operating room, with potential transport times of up to 3 hours and distances of up to 1,000 miles. The recipient team can judge the timing of the incision, depending upon the estimated time of arrival, and the need for dissection of adhesions as, for example, in patients who have had previous cardiac surgery. The donor heart should arrive in the recipient operating room at the time cardiopulmonary bypass is instituted and before the patient's heart is removed in preparation for transplantation.

RECIPIENT OPERATION

Cannulation for cardiopulmonary bypass in the recipient is performed in the high ascending aorta and in the vena cava by cannulating very low in the right atrium near the orifices of the two cavae. The heart is removed by transection just above the aortic and pulmonary valves and through the midportion of the right and left atria to remove the atrial appendages. A cautery is used to coagulate small bronchial-to-coronary vessels in the transected atria, and the pulmonary artery is digitally inspected for possible embolic material. The reimplantation is performed with 3–0 polypropylene suture beginning in the area of the left superior pulmonary vein and continuing down the left atrial free wall. When this has been brought down to the lower edge of the interatrial septum, the second arm of the suture is brought around the top of the left atrium and down the interatrial septum to complete the left atrial anastomosis. The donor right atrium is then opened with an incision from the inferior vena cava, obliquely toward the right atrial appendage. This is made big enough to match the recipient's right atrial cuff. The interatrial septum of the donor heart is inspected for a patent foramen ovale, and then the right atrial suture line is performed with 3–0 polypropylene material. When this is completed, the pulmonary artery is anastomosed with running 4–0 polypropylene suture. The caval tapes can be removed, air aspirated from the pulmonary artery, and volume gradually given to wash air through the lungs, the left atrium and left ventricle, and out the open aorta. The final aortic anastomosis is performed with 4–0 polypropylene suture, and then the aortic cross-clamp is removed.

Resuscitation of the heart may require as little as 20 minutes prior to obtaining good cardiac function and being able to separate from bypass. However, some hearts, especially those with ischemic times approaching 4 hours, may require up to 1 hour or even 90 minutes of additional resuscitation on cardiopulmonary bypass before they are ready to assume adequate function. It is especially important to follow a careful plan to remove air from the left side of the heart, since a good deal of air is trapped in the pulmonary veins after transection of the left atrium.

The chest is closed in routine fashion, except that we open the right pleural space widely as a mechanism for decompression of the very large pericardial space in case a pericardial effusion forms within the first 2 weeks following transplantation. Atrial pacing wires are placed on the donor right atrium and brought out through the skin for temporary pacing of the donor heart, should this be required. Isoproterenol, at 0.01 μg per kilogram, is started to maintain the heart rate at between 100 and 110 beats per minute. The patient is returned to the intensive care unit, where reverse isolation is used for the initial 3 days following transplantation. Since many of the recipients may have been taking sodium warfarin (Coumadin) to prevent pulmonary embolism, the prothrombin time may be elevated at the time of the transplant operation, and extra care may be required for hemostasis. Intravenous administration of vitamin K and fresh frozen plasma to partially correct the coagulation defect may be required.

On return to the intensive care unit, the patient is managed similarly to other patients who have had routine cardiac surgery. They awaken from anesthesia and are extubated when gas exchange and ventilatory mechanics are appropriate. The patient is allowed out of bed as soon as possible and begins a program of walking and light exercise, as tolerated. Early postoperative rehabilitation is often remarkable given the severe nature of the patient's preoperative condition. The patient is taught the medications and procedures and is moved from intensive care to an intermediate care monitoring ward in most cases within 5 days following transplant surgery.

IMMUNOSUPPRESSION

Since the availability of cyclosporine, virtually all patients have received initial treatment with this medication as the primary immunosuppressive drug. Our standard immunosuppressive protocol is given in Table 1. Cyclosporine administration is adjusted by maintaining the serum creatinine level below 2 mg per deciliter, and by cyclosporine serum levels measured by high-pressure liquid chromatography to be between 100 to 200 ng per milliliter in the first 3 months following transplantation. Cyclosporine is slowly tapered with a target value of 4 to 6 mg per kilogram at 6 months, maintaining levels between 75 to 150 ng per milliliter at that time. Patients are discharged from the hospital on prednisone at 30 mg per day. Steroids are tapered following the first 3 postoperative months to a maintenance dose of 0.2 mg per kilogram by 6 months.

Alternative strategies are used in patients who have associated medical conditions that may suggest complications with the proposed protocol or who develop such complications on therapy. If nephrotoxicity or poor renal function is apparent, cyclosporine is decreased to the lowest tolerable level, and azathioprine is instituted at 2 mg per kilogram per day and adjusted to keep the white blood cell count to less than 5,000 per cubic millimeter. Other patients with side effects of steroid therapy, including the onset of diabetes mellitus or severe osteoporosis, are switched from a prednisone protocol to one that uses cyclosporine and azathioprine. Azathioprine is instituted at 2 mg per kilogram and maintained for 2 weeks, followed by the reduction in prednisone dosage over the next 4 to 6 weeks down to zero.

Rejection is diagnosed by frequent endomyocardial biopsy based upon the Billingham criteria, with presence of an interstitial infiltrate indicating mild rejection and increased infiltrate with myocytic necrosis indicating moderate rejection. Treatment by augmented immunosuppression is given for patients with moderate rejection. Biopsies are obtained every 7 to 10 days for the first 6 weeks and then reduced to monthly intervals for the next 3 months. Thereafter, the biopsies are decreased to every 3 months or as dictated by rejection episodes.

Patients are frequently discharged from the hospital as early as 14 days following the transplant procedure. The mean hospital stay in our patients has been 21 days, and they are then followed with biweekly outpatient visits at which blood work can be monitored, including cyclosporine and serum creatinine levels and white blood cell count, and chest x-ray films and outpatient endomyocardial biopsy performed as indicated. We do not use any other specific type of immunologic monitoring to assess rejection at the present time.

Standard treatment for early (less than 3 months) rejection consists of intravenous administration of methylprednisolone, 1 g every day for 3 days. Oral prednisone is then increased to 100 mg and tapered over a 2-week period back to the maintenance level. Rejection episodes occurring 3 months or later after transplant are usually controlled by increasing the oral prednisone as indicated and tapering over 3 weeks back to maintenance level. Recurrent rejection episodes that are refractory to steroid therapy require additional agents, and we favor horse antithymocyte globulin (ATG) as the initial agent. This is given as indicated in Figure 1. When horse ATG is ineffective in reversing rejection, then either OKT_3 (murine monoclonal antibody) or rabbit antithymocyte globulin may be effective as rescue therapy. Patients with more than three rejection episodes in the first 6 months can also be considered for a triple drug protocol, combining maintenance cyclosporine with low-dose prednisone and azathioprine.

COMPLICATIONS

Infection is the major complication in immunosuppressed cardiac transplant recipients. In our patients it has occurred with a frequency of 0.05 episodes per patient month with pulmonary, cutaneous, urinary tract, and other

TABLE 1 Immunosuppressive Protocol

	Solu-Medrol (IV)	*Prednisone (Oral)*	*Cyclosporine (Oral)*	*Azathioprine (Oral)*
Preoperatively	—	—	10 mg/kg	—
Intraoperatively	500 mg	—	—	—
Perioperatively	125 mg q8h × 3 doses	1 mg/kg tapered to 30 mg/day by 2 weeks	10 mg/kg	2 mg/kg
Long-term	—	0.2 mg/kg	5 mg/kg	1–2 mg/kg

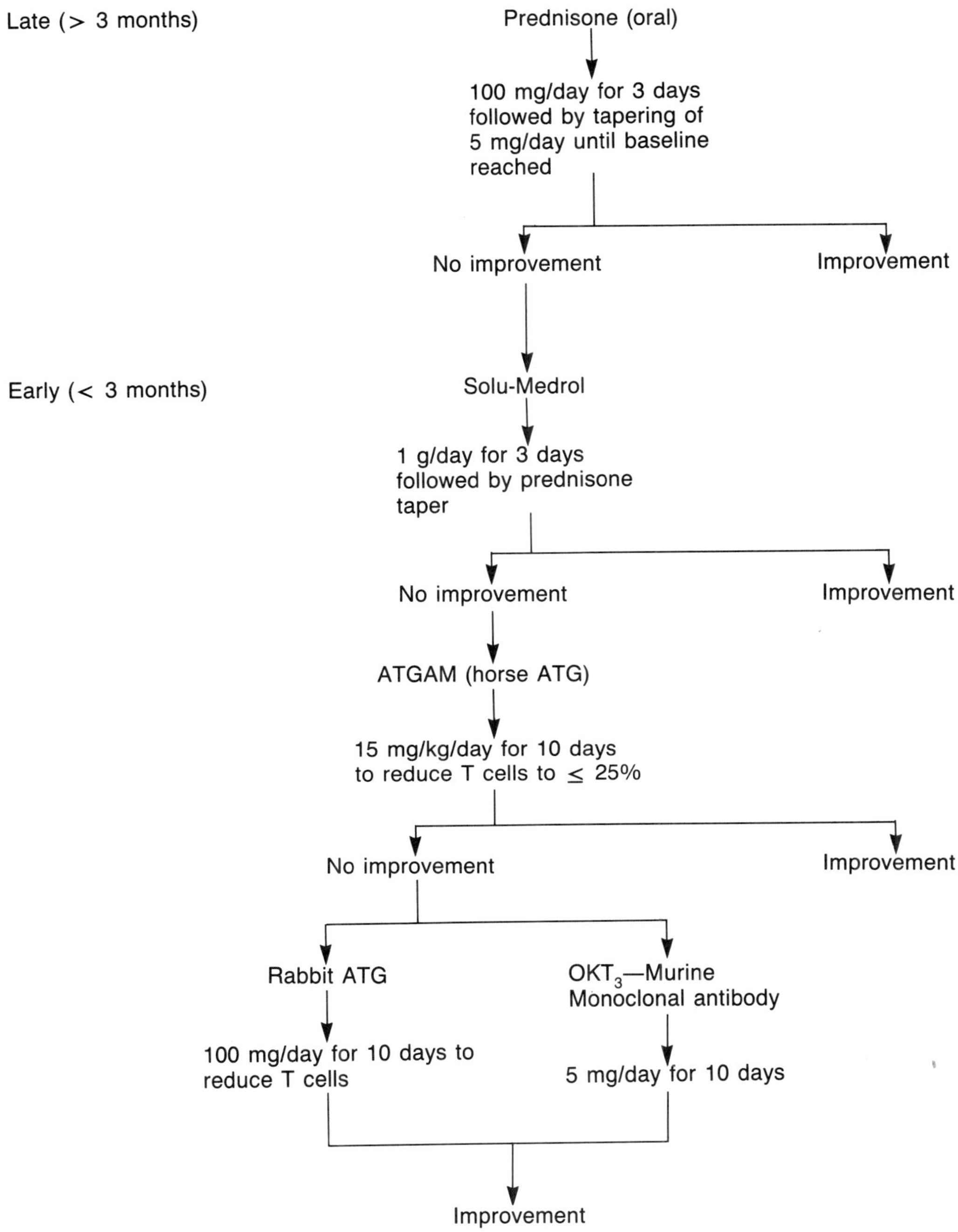

Figure 1 Treatment of transplant rejection.

associated infections as well as septicemia being encountered. These have included a wide spectrum of bacterial, viral, fungal, and protozoal infections. In order to reduce the incidence of cytomegalovirus (CMV), we avoid the use of CMV-positive blood products in patients who had previously had negative CMV titers.

A major complication of immunosuppression is nephrotoxicity associated with cyclosporine. This has been encountered in half of our patients and is manifested by a rising creatinine level or high blood pressure requiring treatment with at least one medication. In 10 percent of our patients, this has required reduction in the cyclosporine dose and the addition of azathioprine. Lymphoproliferative disorders have been encountered in 3 percent of patients within the first year following cardiac transplant; they are treated initially by reduction in immunosuppressive therapy. Additional chemotherapy or radiation therapy may be required, depending upon the site and severity of the lymphoma.

Intensive efforts are made at early patient rehabilitation. Patients are encouraged to return to a full and active lifestyle as early as can be tolerated. Despite the need for daily medication and frequent medical follow-up visits, more than 90 percent of patients return to an active lifestyle.

RESULTS

With the indications and treatment plans for cardiac transplantation that have been outlined, we have obtained a consistent 1-year patient survival of 87 percent, and 2-year patient survival of 83 percent. These results are similar to those of other transplant programs and suggest an anticipated 5-year survival of approximately 60 percent. The major late complication continues to be the development of graft coronary artery disease (30 percent of patients at 5 years), which is still poorly understood and controlled. Because of uniformly elevated serum lipid levels in patients receiving these immunosuppressive agents and the development of coronary artery disease, patients are instructed to stay on low-lipid diets, to engage in daily physical activity, and to maintain ideal body weight and as near normal blood pressure as possible.

Future efforts to improve cardiac transplantation as therapy must include improved immunosuppressive protocols, methods to prevent graft atherosclerosis, and efforts at markedly increasing the number of donor hearts available for transplantation.

SUGGESTED READING

Baumgartner WA, Reitz BA, Oyer PE, et al. Cardiac homotransplantation. In: Ravitch M, ed. Current problems in surgery. XVI, No. 9, Chicago: Year Book, 1979.

Billingham ME. Diagnosis of cardiac rejection by endomyocardial biopsy. Heart Trans 1982; 1:25.

Goldman MH, Barnhart G, Mohanakumar T, et al. Cyclosporine in cardiac transplantation. Surg Clin North Am 1985; 65:637–659.

Kaye M, Elcombe SA, O'Fallon WM. The international heart transplantation registry—the 1984 report. Heart Trans 1985; 4:290–292.

Lower RR, Shumway NE. Studies on orthotopic transplantation of the canine heart. Surg Forum 1960; 11:18–20.

HEART-LUNG TRANSPLANTATION

JOHN C. BALDWIN, M.D.

The treatment of patients with end-stage pulmonary vascular disease and related cardiac failure has long been a difficult and frustrating clinical problem. The successful reintroduction of combined heart and lung transplantation in 1981 ushered in an era of rapid development, focusing on donor selection criteria, heart-lung graft preservation methods, recipient selection criteria, and surgical technique. Heart-lung transplantation now offers a good prospect for survival and effective rehabilitation in properly selected patients with a variety of cardiopulmonary syndromes, including primary pulmonary hypertension, congenital heart disease with Eisenmenger's physiology, fibrotic and emphysematous lung disease with associated cor pulmonale, and cystic fibrosis.

SELECTION OF RECIPIENTS AND DONORS

The entire spectrum of pathophysiologic entities associated with end-stage pulmonary vascular disease and associated heart failure is characterized by unresponsiveness to medical therapy. This fact was a major impetus for the introduction of clinical combined heart and lung transplantation. There is a large population of patients with end-stage pulmonary vascular and parenchymal disease with associated right-sided heart failure who could be considered potential candidates for combined heart and lung transplantation. In addition, patients with congenital heart disease and Eisenmenger's physiology have received heart-lung transplants, and patients with ischemic or valvular disease with resultant fixed pulmonary hypertension could theoretically be considered. However, in the early stage of development of this technique, stringent selection criteria are applied within a limited number of disease categories.

Because of the continuing shortage of donor organs and the relatively favorable experience with younger recipients in heart transplantation, we currently limit heart-lung transplantation to patients who are less than 45 years of age. Patients should have severe symptoms, placing them in the New York Heart Association Class III or IV. Life expectancy may be difficult to estimate in many such patients, but clinical judgment should indicate a life expectancy measured in months. There should be agreement by medical and surgical consultants that all other modes of conventional medical and surgical therapy have been exhausted. Contraindications include the presence of other systemic diseases, which would, in and of themselves, be life-threatening. Renal dysfunction should be judged reversible and limited to the prerenal azotemia that is commonly seen among patients with heart failure. Passive congestion is present in all recipients, but severe liver dysfunction, characterized by a total bilirubin level in excess of 2.5 mg per deciliter, is a significant risk factor and a relative contraindication. Insulin-dependent diabetes mellitus is a contraindication because of the expected exacerbation by postoperative steroid therapy. The presence of an established systemic infection is also a contraindication. The risk of major postoperative bleeding is substantially increased in the setting of previous thoracic surgery, and this must be considered a relative contraindication at the present time. The degree of preoperative cyanosis does not correlate with postoperative bleeding, nor is it a notable risk factor.

The importance of preoperative psychologic assessment cannot be exaggerated; the patient's ability to cooperate with postoperative respiratory therapy and to comply with an immunosuppressive medical regimen is of paramount importance.

The rate-limiting factor in clinical heart-lung transplantation today is the continuing shortage of suitable donor organs. The problem is particularly acute in the case of heart-lung donors because of the propensity for neurogenic pulmonary edema, atelectasis, pneumonia, and other pulmonary complications in brain-dead, ventilated patients. Our current criteria stipulate that appropriate heart-lung donors are selected from those patients who have been declared brain dead and who are less than 35 years of age. There should be no history of preexisting cardiopulmonary disease, no evidence of established infection, and no chest trauma of sufficient severity to be likely to have caused myocardial or pulmonary contusion. As in the case of cardiac donors, there should be no sustained requirement for high-dose pressor support. In the case of heart-lung donors, aggressive fluid replacement should be avoided, and this consideration does dictate that alpha-pressor agents be used to manipulate peripheral vascular resistance for maintenance of adequate arterial pressure. Arterial Po_2 should be greater than 100 mm Hg on 30 percent inspired oxygen, and peak inspiratory airway pressure should be less than 30 cm H_2O. There should be no radiologic pulmonary abnormalities. In all cases of heart-lung transplantation performed in our program, the kidneys have been harvested. Frequently, the liver has also been harvested, and fluid considerations have not been a problem in this regard.

DONOR-RECIPIENT MATCHING

When a suitable heart-lung donor becomes available, initial matching should be according to ABO blood group compatibility. Within this constraint, matching of donor and recipient is carried out according to thoracic size and shape, as assessed by chest x-ray film. In general, the donor should be no more than 20 percent smaller in body mass than the proposed recipient. However, in the case of heart-lung transplantation, it is particularly important to ascertain an appropriate thoracic size match between donor and recipient. Significant difficulties with implantation of grafts have been encountered when donors have been matched with relatively small recipients, and inappropriately small grafts may predispose the recipient to persistent air spaces and pleural fluid collections. An ideal size match is one in which the donor thoracic dimensions are slightly smaller than those of the proposed recipient, to facilitate graft implantation and to allow for full lung expansion.

OPERATIVE TECHNIQUE

The donor operation is performed via median sternotomy. The heart is carefully inspected, as for cardiac transplantation, and the pleural spaces are entered for critical inspection of the lungs. Throughout the donor operation, manipulation and compression of the lungs are minimized. A complete anterior pericardiectomy is performed, removing both phrenic nerves and all thymic tissue. The azygous vein is ligated and divided. The ascending aorta and both venae cavae are encircled with umbilical tapes, and the trachea is exposed as high as possible, between the aorta and superior vena cava. For lung preservation, we currently employ a technique that includes aggressive vasodilation with prostaglandin E_1, beginning 15 minutes prior to aortic cross-clamping. The prostaglandin E_1 is administered via a central venous line and is commenced at a dose of 20 ng per kilogram per minute. We then titrate the dose gradually upward, usually to the range of 70 to 100 ng per kilogram per minute, depending on blood pressure tolerance; we usually accept a mean arterial pressure of 50 mm Hg or greater. The donor is then heparinized, the venae cavae are ligated, and the aorta is cross-clamped. The heart is arrested with crystalloid potassium cardioplegia and topical cooling. We then infuse cold, modified Collins' solution into the main pulmonary artery, and ventilation is continued with half-normal tidal volumes and room air. After placement of the aortic clamp, it is important to amputate the tip of the left atrial appendage to allow for egress of the pulmonary infusate and to incise the inferior vena cava to obviate the possibility of distention of the right side of the heart. After completion of the instillation of the cardioplegic and pulmonary cooling solutions, the venae cavae are completely divided, and the aorta is divided at the clamp. The pulmonary ligaments and posterior pleural reflections are divided using electrocautery, and the trachea is clamped at least five rings above the carina while the lungs are held inflated. The trachea is then divided above the clamp, so that the lungs are transported to the recipient operating room in the inflated condition. The graft is placed in a physiologic solution at 4° C.

In the recipient operation, emphasis should be placed on the safe and hemostatic removal of the recipient organs. Avoidance of injury to the phrenic nerves, the vagus nerves, and the recurrent laryngeal nerve and avoidance of bleeding in the posterior mediastinum are the essential features.

The operation is performed via median sternotomy. Prior to heparinization, incisions are made in both pleural spaces, and adhesions in these areas are divided using electrocautery. The pericardium is then opened, and cannulation is carried out in routine fashion as for cardiac transplantation, except that the cannulation of the ascending aorta should be as high as possible, near the innominate artery, and the aortic cannula should be brought out toward the top of the incision, to facilitate performance of the tracheal anastomosis.

After establishment of cardiopulmonary bypass, the venae cavae are snared, and the aorta is cross-clamped. Systemic cooling to 28° C is carried out. The heart is removed, dividing the aorta and pulmonary artery at the immediate supravalvular level and excising the heart at the midtrial level.

A left phrenic nerve pedicle of pericardium is then created, excising the pericardium anteriorly so as to leave a 3 cm border anterior to the phrenic nerve. The pericardium is incised posteriorly from the level of the pulmonary artery to the diaphragm to establish the pedicle. A vertical incision is then made in the oblique sinus of the left atrium, and the left-sided pulmonary veins are dissected, reflecting them into the left pleural space. The left pulmonary ligament is then divided. The left pulmonary artery is divided, and the left main bronchus is stapled and divided.

On the right side, a pericardial pedicle for the phrenic nerve is established in the same fashion. An incision in the left atrium is made from the lateral approach, as for mitral valve replacement. This allows for reflection of the right pulmonary veins into the right pleural space. After division of the pulmonary ligament, the pulmonary artery is divided, and the bronchus is stapled and divided, as done for the left side.

The pulmonary arterial remnant is removed, leaving a button (approximately 2 cm in diameter) in the area of the ductus diverticulum, thus avoiding injury to the recurrent laryngeal nerve. Clamps are then placed on the two stapled bronchi, and downward traction facilitates dissection of the bronchial tree proximally. During this phase of the operation, very careful attention must be given to hemostasis in the bronchial circulation. Application of metal clips to each vessel is usually sufficient; it is important to maintain a perfusion pressure of at lest 60 mm Hg during this phase in order to mimic the postoperative arterial pressure and thus unmask any potential bleeding points. This dissection is carried out up to the carina, and the trachea is divided at this level. It is exceedingly important to minimize more proximal dissection of the trachea and its blood supply.

The graft is then brought into the field, and the clamp is removed from the donor trachea. The donor trachea is divided one or two rings above the carina, and the tracheobronchial tree is carefully irrigated with normal saline and suctioned. The graft is then lowered into the wound, and the right lung is placed under the phrenic pericardial pedicle and the right atrial remnant. The left lung is placed under the left phrenic pericardial pedicle. It is important to avoid twisting of the pulmonary hilus at this juncture. The tracheal anastomosis is performed using an end-to-end running 3–0 polypropylene technique. No reinforcement or buttressing of this anastomosis is performed. After completion of the tracheal anastomosis, topical cooling of both lungs is instituted, and a third cooling line is placed in the tip of the left atrial appendage to enhance endomyocardial cooling and to exclude air from the left side of the graft.

The donor right atrium is then opened from the inferior vena cava up toward the base of the right atrial appendage, avoiding the area of the sinoatrial node. The right atrial anastomosis is then performed, beginning posteriorly in the area of the recipient atrial septum, which has become the posterior edge of the recipient right atrium. This anastomosis is carried out with a continuous running 3–0 polypropylene suture technique. Systemic cooling is employed to a level of 28° C during the operation, and rewarming is ordinarily begun during the performance of the right atrial anastomosis. The aortic anastomosis is then performed, using a running 4–0 polypropylene technique. Ordinarily, the use of the left atrial catheter, placed immediately after the tracheal anastomosis, eliminates the need for elaborate maneuvers for evacuation of air.

The heart is gradually resuscitated, and the lungs are ventilated with 40 percent inspired oxygen and 5 cm H_2O of positive end expiratory pressure. Approximately 30 minutes after removal of the aortic cross-clamp, the patient ordinarily can be weaned from cardiopulmonary bypass on low-dose isoproterenol support. Temporary epicardial pacing wires are left in place on the donor right atrium and right ventricle.

IMMUNOSUPPRESSION

Current immunosuppression for heart-lung transplantation is based on the fungal metabolite cyclosporine. Preoperatively, patients are given a single dose of cyclosporine, 10 to 15 mg per kilogram body weight orally. This dosage may be adjusted downward in cases of hepatic or renal failure. Patients are given an intravenous bolus of 500 mg methylprednisolone at the discontinuation of cardiopulmonary bypass, and intravenous methylprednisolone is continued for the first 24 hours after operation. Thereafter, steroids are withheld for 3 weeks in an effort to enhance early tracheal healing; three doses of intramuscular rabbit antithymocyte globulin are given immediately after surgery. Oral cyclosporine therapy is continued postoperatively, maintaining a cyclosporine level (radioimmunoassay) of 200 to 250 ng per milliliter during the first month. Thereafter, cyclosporine dosage is adjusted downward, to achieve levels of 100 to 150 ng per milliliter. Azathioprine is begun immediately postoperatively in a dose of 1 to 2 mg per kilogram per day, depending on white blood cell count. Azathioprine is continued indefinitely. Oral corticosteroids (prednisone 0.1 mg per kilogram per day, orally) are begun 3 weeks postoperatively.

COMPLICATIONS

The complications of combined heart and lung transplantation are, in large part, similar to those seen in cardiac transplantation. Therefore, infection and rejection are recognized as major causes of morbidity and mortality, and constant vigilance for these problems is required during the early postoperative phase. In addition, problems of accelerated graft atherosclerosis and immunosuppression-related phenomena such as renal failure, hypertension, hepatic dysfunction, and malignancy must be considered.

There are several special considerations in the case of heart-lung transplant recipients. With regard to postoperative pulmonary complications and management, it must be remembered that the lungs have suffered significant ischemic injury and that they are devoid of lymphatic drainage. Therefore, it is imperative to observe strict fluid restriction during the first week postoperatively. The so-called "reimplantation response" has been seen in many patients with heart-lung transplantation, although its frequency appears to be less with recently improved techniques for lung preservation. This remains a diagnosis of exclusion, and possibilities of infection or rejection must be continually eliminated.

MANAGEMENT OF REJECTION

Rejection has been significantly less common among heart-lung recipients than among heart recipients, and the basis for this finding is unclear; it is distinctly unusual for cardiac rejection to occur during this time. There is a statistically significant difference in this regard, such that heart-lung recipients have significantly less heart rejection than do heart recipients. Although serial endomyocardial biopsies remain the gold standard for diagnosis of cardiac rejection, the possibility of asynchronous pulmonary rejection must be considered in the setting of fever and the appearance of diffuse pulmonary infiltrates on chest x-ray films. Lung rejection can be exceedingly difficult to diagnose, and it remains a clinical diagnosis based on the assiduous exclusion of infectious causes for any radiologic abnormalities. When the picture is particularly unclear, it may be necessary to perform open lung biopsy to distinguish viral or other infections from rejection; endobronchial biopsy and transbronchial biopsy specimens are usually inadequate for establishing the diagnosis of pulmonary rejection. Even with an open lung biopsy, the matter may remain controversial.

When lung rejection is diagnosed, it is treated with pulse steroids in a manner similar to treatment of cardiac rejection. We utilize methylprednisolone 1 g intravenously daily for 3 consecutive days.

RESULTS

To date, we have performed 38 heart-lung transplantations in 37 patients. Nineteen of the operations were for congenital heart disease with Eisenmenger's physiology, and 18 were for primary pulmonary hypertension. Eighteen of these patients are currently living, at intervals of 1 month to 5 years after transplant. There were 11 hospital deaths, the majority related to postoperative bleeding and subsequent multisystem failure. This fact underscores the role of previous surgery as a significant risk factor and the importance of meticulous attention to hemostasis in the bronchial circulation. Five of the eight patients in the late mortality group developed obliterative bronchiolitis, which is likely to be a manifestation of chronic lung rejection. In patients who have experienced lesser degrees of long-term pulmonary deterioration, our recent experience with augmentation of immunosuppression through the addition of azathioprine to the previous cyclosporine and steroid regimen strongly suggests that the problem of chronic lung rejection can be arrested. It is hoped that the use of a three-drug regimen from the time of transplantation will eliminate this complication in most patients.

Among surviving patients, rehabilitation results have been excellent, with normal catherization and pulmonary function testing and with return to full, productive activity. Recent results have been particularly encouraging, and it is anticipated that, with improved understanding of proper recipient selection, donor surgical and lung preservation techniques, recipient surgical technique, and immunosuppressive regimens, early and late mortality rates will continue to decline. The recent introduction of successful distant procurement of heart-lung grafts should provide for greater clinical activity and resultant improvement in clinical technique.

SUGGESTED READING

Baldwin JC, Shumway NE. Cardiac and cardiopulmonary homotransplants. In: Sabiston DC, ed. The Davis Christopher textbook of surgery–the biological basis for modern surgical practice. 13th ed. Philadelphia: WB Saunders, 1985.

Baldwin JC, Stinson EB, Oyer PE, Jamieson SW, Shumway NE. The technique of cardiac transplantation. In: Hurst JW, ed. The heart. 6th ed. New York: McGraw-Hill, 1985.

Jamieson SW, Baldwin JC, Reitz BA, Stinson EB, Oyer PE, Hunt SA, Billingham ME, Theodore J, Modry D, Bieber CP, Shumway NE. Combined heart and lung transplantation. Lancet 1983; 1:1130–1132.

Jamieson SW, Stinson EB, Oyer PE, Baldwin JC, Shumway NE. Operative technique for heart-lung transplantation. J Thorac Cardiovasc Surg 1984; 87:930–935.

McGregor CGA, Baldwin JC, Jamieson SW, Yousem SM, Burke CM, Oyer PE, Stinson EB, Shumway NE. Isolated pulmonary rejection after combined heart-lung transplantation. J Thorac Cardiovasc Surg 1985; 90:623–625.

HOMOGRAFT MATERIAL IN CARDIAC SURGERY

JAMES L. MONRO, M.B., B.S., F.R.C.S.

The homograft materials discussed in this chapter are the antibiotic-sterilized unstented aortic valve and dura mater. Both are suitable for the correction of acquired and congenital defects. These materials have very low antigenicity; therefore graft rejection has not been a problem, and no special drugs or precautions are necessary.

The difficulties of obtaining homograft material vary in different countries. Despite the increasing number of transplantation programs, the availability and use of aortic homografts and dura mater have been very limited in the United States. Although the law has made the collection of this homograft material easier in the United Kingdom, because of the increased technical difficulty of inserting aortic homografts, relatively few surgeons use these valves.

HOMOGRAFT PREPARATION

Aortic Valve

Hearts are removed at routine post-mortem examination and refrigerated until the aortic root containing the aortic valve and ascending aorta are dissected, preferably as soon as possible but certainly within 72 hours of death. The anterior leaflet of the mitral valve is preserved and the internal aortic diameter measured. The valve is then sterilized and preserved in an antibiotic-nutrient medium, which is prepared by mixing 33.5 ml of antibiotic solution and 66.5 ml of nutrient medium (Table 1). The valve is kept in this solution at room temperature for 24 hours, and after sending small pieces of aortic wall for culture, it is stored in the same solution at 4° C for up to 8 weeks. Valve function will not be as good if stored for longer than this, and the sooner it is used the better.

Dura Mater

The dura mater, which is also collected at routine post-mortem examination, is put in the same antibiotic solution for 48 hours and then stored in 98 percent glycerol. It can be used up to 40 weeks later.

AORTIC VALVE REPLACEMENT

Ross and Barratt-Boyes independently started to use orthotopic aortic valve homografts in 1962 in an attempt to avoid the thromboembolic problems associated with prosthetic valves. Some of the early valves inserted by Barratt-Boyes were "fresh" in that they were taken under sterile conditions post mortem and used for aortic valve replacement within a short time.

However, because of the logistical problems associated with this mode of collection, valves were sterilized in beta-propiolactone. This, however, led to a disappointingly high failure rate, and by 1968 antibiotic sterilization had been introduced in an attempt to reachieve the "fresh" valve. The results with these antibiotic-sterilized valves were much better, but recently Yacoub has returned to using some "fresh" valves obtained from recipient hearts at the time of cardiac transplantation, and it will be interesting to see how the long-term performance will compare.

At present most units using homografts for aortic valve replacements have their own rather limited valve banks. However, preservation in liquid nitrogen as soon as the valve has been sterilized may increase the availability of valves. Careful valve selection reduces the number of suitable valves available still further, although small fenestrations in the cusps are frequently found and are not necessarily a contraindication to use. It is clear that the younger the donor and the shorter the time from death of donor to dissection and from sterilization to use of the valve, the better the quality of the valve. Furthermore, many valves that were inserted in the past did not fall within these parameters, and therefore past reported figures for valve failure may be worse than valve failure rates that should be achieved with currently implanted valves. Therefore one should only advocate aortic valve replacement with a homograft if a "perfect" valve is available. The technique of free-hand aortic valve replacement with a homograft is more difficult and time-consuming than with a prosthetic or bioprosthetic valve, which has an attractive man-made suture ring. For homograft insertion, a two-layered technique is used, and some apprenticeship is recommended in learning the technique. When homograft insertion was introduced in the early 1960s, many surgeons, attracted by the absence of thromboembolic problems, started to use these valves without a proper appreciation of the technical difficulties of the operation; therefore some very poor results were obtained.

Patient selection is also important if the best results are to be obtained. The apparent advantages of a free aortic homograft over a bioprosthetic valve would be a longer failure-free interval and a slightly lower risk of thromboembolic complications. However, the following factors mitigate against the use of a homograft:

1. Because the insertion of a homograft takes considerably longer than the insertion of a bioprosthetic valve, if a more lengthy procedure is contemplated e.g., the insertion of other valves or coronary artery bypass grafting, in the interests of myocardial preservation, a homograft probably is best avoided.
2. If the aortic root is dilated, tailoring can be used to narrow the root so that a homograft will fit. However, although Barratt-Boyes has not found this to be associated with an increase in late failure rate, it is not recommended. Certainly the presence of a Marfan root, sinus of Valsalva aneurysm, or other causes of an enlarged ascending aorta are contraindications. It is probably better not to use a homograft if the aortic ring (once the valve has been excised) is larger than 2.4 cm in diameter, and this will of course exclude a larger number of patients.
3. Hypertension has been shown to have a deleterious long-term effect on homografts (and no doubt on bio-

TABLE 1 Composition of Antibiotic Nutrient Medium*

Antibiotic Mixture Constituents	*Amount (mg)*	*Quantity (ml)*
Nystatin	83.3	10.0
Methicillin	1,000	1.4
Erythromycin	600	12.0
Gentamicin	400	10.0
Streptomycin	20	0.1
	Total	33.5
Nutrient Mixture Constituents		*Quantity (ml)*
Sterile distilled water		77.0
Medium 199 (bicarbonate-free)†		10.0
Preheated inactivated calf serum no. 1		8.0
Sodium bicarbonate (4.4%)		5.0
	Total	100.0

* Antibiotic nutrient medium = 33.5 ml antibiotic mixture + 66.5 ml nutrient mixture.
† Wellcome Tissue Culture Medium 199.

prosthetic valves), and therefore unless there are very strong indications for a tissue valve and the hypertension can be controlled, this is a contraindication.

Factors supporting the use of free aortic homografts are as follows:

1. Most cardiac surgeons put patients receiving bioprosthetic valves on anticoagulation therapy for 2 to 3 months postoperatively. However, it is not usual to give any anticoagulants after unstented homograft aortic valve replacement, and in some patients, e.g., those with gastric problems, this could be an indication for using a homograft.
2. In patients with active endocarditis of the aortic valve in whom replacement is required, the absence of prosthetic material (apart from sutures) makes homograft replacement particularly attractive, and the recurrence rate of endocarditis after homograft replacement is impressively low. The incidence of infective endocarditis after routine homograft aortic valve replacement is in the range of 1 percent, again lower than with other valves.
3. If there is a particularly small aortic root, e.g., less than 21 mm in diameter, and this is quite often the case in older women with aortic stenosis, the homograft is particularly suitable, since there is virtually no gradient across these homograft valves even in the smaller sizes in such patients. This also makes the homograft attractive in children; there is also a markedly decreased incidence of valve cusp calcification when compared with the use of porcine valves in young patients.

RESULTS WITH AORTIC HOMOGRAFT VALVE REPLACEMENT

Despite the increased technical difficulty of aortic valve replacement with a homograft, the early mortality (30 day) rate at about 3 percent is no higher than for aortic valve replacement with other valves. (Between 1973 and 1984, 200 patients underwent aortic valve replacement in Southampton, resulting in six early deaths). However, those patients having homografts are to some extent selected and may be slightly lower risk patients.

The long-term survival of patients having aortic valve replacement with a homograft is better than the survival rate of those with bioprosthetic or mechanical valves, 10-year survivals being in the region of 85 percent, 75 percent, and 70 percent, respectively. As already mentioned, patients receiving homografts may have been selected, but certainly the incidence of thromboembolic episodes in such patients is almost nil, and because they do not need anticoagulants, hemorrhage is not a problem.

The only significant problem with both homografts and bioprosthetic valves is valve failure. Valve failure can be defined as when the function of a valve is so poor as to require replacement or cause the death of a patient. As homografts are inserted free-hand, some minor distortion or deformity of the valve may occur that can cause an early diastolic murmur, audible from the time of operation. Many of these valves continue to function for years with trivial aortic regurgitation and cannot be considered to have failed. The late development of an early diastolic murmur may indicate moderate or severe valve failure, and valve replacement is likely to be necessary sooner or later. However, at 10 years about 15 percent of homografts will have failed, and this is usually due to cusp rupture. Endocarditis and calcific stenosis of the valve are rare. Valve failure seems to occur somewhat earlier with porcine valves, and it remains to be seen what proportion of tissue valves will still be functioning adequately at 15 and 20 years. However, even if as seems likely the failure rate approaches 50 percent at 20 years, patients will have been able to enjoy freedom from thromboembolic and anticoagulant-related problems. Moreover, when these valves fail there is usually sufficient time for valve replacement, which carries little more risk than the initial procedure, although of course the patient is older.

AORTIC ROOT REPLACEMENT

The antibiotic-sterilized aortic homograft is particularly suitable for complete replacement of the aortic root in both adults and children. In children with small aortic valve rings with or without tunnel subaortic stenosis, it provides a good alternative to root-widening procedures such as the Kono procedure. This is discussed in a separate chapter. It is particularly suitable in adults when infection is or has been present, since they would otherwise require a Dacron ascending aortic replacement. This is also discussed in a separate chapter.

However, the aortic wall of the homograft calcifies with time, and this may give rise to technical problems if the valve itself fails.

MITRAL VALVE REPLACEMENT

Stent-mounted aortic valves have been used for mitral valve replacement in the past, but there was a tendency for the commissure of the homograft to tear away from the stent, and they are not recommended in the mitral position.

AORTIC VALVE HOMOGRAFTS FOR THE TREATMENT OF CONGENITAL HEART DISEASE

Whole Homograft Conduits

Homograft conduits were first used in the late 1960s for the repair of pulmonary atresia (Ross, 1966), truncus arteriosus (McGoon, 1967), and tricuspid atresia (Fontan, 1968). In the repair of pulmonary atresia and truncus arteriosus, the homograft fills the gap between the top of the right ventricle and the pulmonary artery, lying almost in the position of the normal pulmonary artery. The anterior leaflet of the mitral valve comes down anteriorly to close the ventriculotomy, so that the homograft valve ring is not distorted. Occasionally it may be necessary to insert a patch of material such as pericardium in order to prevent distortion, and of course the coronary arteries of the homograft must be tied off.

By contrast, if a tube graft containing a porcine valve is used, it is usually sutured lower down on the right ventricle, and a loop of Dacron is taken laterally to reach the pulmonary artery. This can be pressed on by the sternum and is not as direct as the superiorly placed homograft.

Some of the homografts used in the early trials were freeze-dried, and this led to the calcification of a significant number, which had to be replaced. This, together with the difficulty many people had in obtaining homografts, led to the widespread use of porcine valves in Dacron tubes when they became available. However, these conduits have had considerable problems with valve stenosis and peel in the Dacron tube. Furthermore, relatively small sizes have to be inserted in infants requiring repair of truncus arteriosus, and therefore replacement is required later on. In contrast with the antibiotic-sterilized homograft, relatively larger sizes can be inserted initially and they last longer, although it remains to be seen whether patients operated on in infancy are able to reach adult size with the same homograft. The author's first patient operated on for truncus arteriosus in 1974 received a 1.7-cm homograft at the age of 7 weeks and is still quite well 12 years later with the same homograft, across which the gradient is 25 mm Hg.

When a conduit is used for the Fontan procedure and its variants, the homograft has been shown to be superior to the Dacron tube containing porcine valve conduits. Better flow characteristics where the flow is slower presumably make the homograft superior.

In the author's personal series of 67 patients who received homograft conduits between 1974 and 1986 (Table 2), there were 12 early and three late deaths. Of the 52 survivors, only one patient has required homograft replacement at 7 years following a Fontan procedure for tricuspid atresia. This patient, who was 21 at the time of operation and who had also had a baby, developed stenosis and calcification of the valve cusps; the homograft valve had been placed between the right atrium and outlet chamber. She has had successful reoperation. It would seem wise to use a valved conduit between the right atrium and outlet chamber if possible, since the outlet chamber can generate a systolic pressure that will be of less value without a valve. More Fontan procedures are being performed with direct anastomosis between right atrium and right pulmonary artery, obviating the need for a valve; however, when a valved conduit is used, the homograft appears to be the conduit of choice.

Unicusp Homograft Outflow Patches

If a whole aortic valve homograft is opened by cutting it open opposite the noncoronary cusp, those parts of the homograft wall bearing the right and left cusps can be removed to leave a diamond-shaped patch containing the noncoronary cusp and anterior leaflet of the mitral valve. This "unicusp" patch can be used to patch the outflow tract in the correction of the tetralogy of Fallot and so reduce the amount of pulmonary regurgitation that will otherwise inevitably occur. Although older patients tolerate pulmonary regurgitation well, at least initially, it may not be so well tolerated in infants. About 80 percent of patients with the tetralogy of Fallot undergoing correction in infancy require an outflow patch. If pulmonary regurgitation can be minimized in the all-important early postoperative phase, these infants will have an improved cardiac output. The author has used 43 unicusp patches in the correction of infants and young children with tetralogy of Fallot (Table 3). Sometimes a small enough homograft was not available, and then material such as pericardium or dura mater was used.

Although the cusp of the unicusp patch continues to function for many years, because the pulmonary valve ring grows but the homograft does not, central regurgitation almost inevitably occurs. Therefore late regurgitation can be a problem, as in other types of patches.

The homograft unicusp patch is good material to work with and much easier to use than Dacron. So far no late problems, such as aneurysm formation, have been encountered.

DURA MATER

After storage in glycerol, dura mater requires a brief soak and washing in saline to attain its normal soft texture. It is strong, water-tight and easy to suture to. It is cheap and plentiful in areas where the law allows and can be used in most positions where a patch is required. However, it is not recommended for closing ventricular septal defects.

TABLE 2 Homograft Conduits Inserted Between July 1974 and July 1986

Condition being Treated	*Number*	*Early Death*	*Late Death*	*Mean Age*
Truncus arteriosus	14	3	—	5.4 months
Tricuspid atresia (Fontan)	14	4	—	9.1 years
Pulmonary atresia + ventricular septal defect	14	1	1	6.3 years
Univentricular heart (Fontan)	9	2	1	12.0 years
Miscellaneous	16	2	1	9.1 years
Total	67	12	3	7.1 years

TABLE 3 Transannular Patching in 116 Consecutive Patients Undergoing Correction of Tetralogy of Fallot July 1974–July 1986

Type of Patch	*Infants (Less Than 1 Year)*	*Patients (Over 1 Year)*	*Total*
Unicusp Homograft	26	17	43
Homologous dura mater	5	16	21
Autologous pericardium	9	14	23
No patch	9	20	29
Total (% patched)	49 (82%)	67 (70%)	116 (75%)
Early deaths	2 (4%)	4 (6%)	

Dura mater is suitable for right ventricular outflow tract patches and is stronger than pericardium. Unlike the unicusp homograft patch, it of course results in pulmonary regurgitation. It is suitable for patching the aorta, either in the supra-aortic position or in the repair of coarctations. Dura mater has been used on more than 100 occasions in Southampton since 1979 and has been extremely satisfactory. No late problems have been encountered.

SUGGESTED READING

Barratt-Boyes BG. Homograft aortic valve replacement in aortic incompetence and stenosis. Thorax 1964; 19:131–150.
Osinowo O, Monro JL, Ross JK. The use of glycerol-preserved homologous dura mater grafts in cardiac surgery: the Southampton experience. Ann Thorac Surg 1985; 39:367–370.
Penta A, Qureshi S, Radley-Smith R, Yacoub MH. Patient status ten or more years after 'fresh' homograft replacement of the aortic valve. Circulation 1984; 70(Suppl I)1:182–186.
Ross DN. Homograft replacement of the aortic valve. Lancet 1962; ii:487.
Virdi IS. Monro JL, Ross JK. Eleven year experience of aortic valve replacement with antibiotic sterilized homograft valves in Southampton. Thorac Cardiovasc Surg 1986; 34:277–282.

THE ARTIFICIAL HEART: A BRIDGE TO CARDIAC TRANSPLANTATION

J. DONALD HILL, M.D.

The artificial heart has not evolved to the point of being a permanent replacement device for patients suffering from acute or chronic end-stage myocardial dysfunction. Although the permanently implanted pneumatic artificial heart has had limited success in extending a few lives and in generating invaluable scientific data, it has not provided a substantial quality or extension of life.

In contrast, excellent results are being achieved using heterotopic artificial hearts and there have been moderately good results using orthotopic artificial hearts for limited periods of time as a bridge to cardiac transplantation. This application provides an opportunity for a small population of patients to live extended, productive lives. It also generates valuable clinical experience with devices that may eventually become permanent prosthetic hearts.

THE DEVICES

Prosthetic hearts can be broadly classified into orthotopic and heterotopic prosthetic ventricles. Orthotopic prosthetic ventricles are placed in the mediastinum in the position of the natural heart after it is removed. Heterotopic prosthetic ventricles are positioned below or adjacent to the natural heart, which is not removed; the device is attached to the patient through short, wide diameter cannulas.

The most widely used orthotopic prosthetic heart is the Symbion Jarvik 7. Other orthotopic hearts include the Penn State heart, the Berlin heart, and the Unger heart.

The Thoratec prosthetic ventricle (Pierce-Donachy Design) is the most widely used heterotopic device. It can be used for univentricular (right or left side of the heart) or biventricular support; typically the prosthetic ventricles are positioned outside the body, on the anterior abdominal wall. Other clinical heterotopic pumps include the Novacor, Thermedics, Nimbus, and Abiomed systems.

INDICATIONS

A successful bridge to cardiac transplant requires the completion of a number of steps. These steps include the selection of an appropriate patient with irreversible heart failure but with no known contraindications to transplantation, implantation of heterotopic or orthotopic prosthetic ventricles for the period of time needed to locate a suitable donor heart, successful transplantation, recovery, and discharge.

There are three clinical indications for which a bridge to transplantation is being used: (1) in elective transplantation candidates who deteriorate before a suitable donor heart can be located, (2) for cardiogenic shock following acute myocardial infarction in a patient appropriate for cardiac transplantation, and (3) for acute cardiomyopathy in a patient appropriate for cardiac transplantation. Before prosthetic ventricle implantation can be considered, all conventional means of therapy should be attempted, including inotropic agents, afterload reduction, and intra-aortic balloon counterpulsation. If these adjuncts are unsuccessful, it is a mistake to persist with conventional therapies and to allow multiorgan failure to develop when prosthetic ventricles are available to maintain the patient. The decision to implant pumps is made when medical judgment determines that the patient will die within minutes to hours.

The use of prosthetic ventricles or ventricular assist devices for nontransplant applications is discussed in a separate chapter.

CONTRAINDICATIONS

Appreciating when not to implant a prosthetic device is crucial and often more difficult. The first rule is never choose a patient who already has any contraindication to transplantation, including primary or secondary organ dysfunction, cachexia, malnutrition, and/or infection. Prosthetic devices sustain life, they do not resurrect it. The critical clinical judgment in these situations is to determine if organ dysfunction is permanent or is only transiently depressed because of low cardiac output. Rule two is to use caution in choosing a patient for whom you are likely to have a difficult time locating a suitable donor heart. This includes presensitized patients or patients who have a large body size. Although devices have been used successfully for 3 months, there is probably an unknown but absolute time limit beyond which devices lead to morbidity, which could be a contraindication to transplantation. Rule three is if contraindications (including infection or emboli) develop during the implant period, do not proceed to transplantation unless they are sufficiently resolved to allow the transplant to be performed with good expectations of a successful outcome.

OPERATIVE PROCEDURES

Both heterotopic and orthotopic pumps can, if properly implanted, provide sufficient systemic oxygen delivery capacity for most patients.

Orthotopic Approach

The Jarvik blood pump, which comes in two sizes, is the only orthotopic prosthetic heart implanted frequently enough to evaluate this approach. The native heart is always removed by incising along both atrioventricular grooves, the intra-atrial septum, and just above the aortic and pulmonary valves. Separate cuffs are anastomosed to the atria and the pulmonary and aortic roots. The separate right and left ventricles are then joined to the cuffs by quick connects. A major operative concern is not to have any kinking or angulation that would reduce venous filling and substantially reduce cardiac output. Bleeding at any of the cuff anastomoses can also be a serious problem because once the pumps are attached, access to these suture lines becomes difficult, particularly at the posterior edges.

Heterotopic Approach

Heterotopic pumps offer several alternative implantation approaches. We are most familiar with the Thoratec pump, with which there is now a large clinical experience.

The native heart is not removed. There are at least three anatomic options available for placing cannulas for pump filling from the left side. If the eventual plan is to provide the patient with a cardiac transplant, the left ventricular apex is a good choice because it provides good pump filling (not affected by patient position), leaves no areas of blood stasis in the native heart, and keeps the cannula from interfering with chest closure. The cannula should be inserted under direct vision so that any thrombus in or near the apex can be removed. The disadvantages include (1) the cannula exit site on the abdominal wall is often located more laterally than one would like for easy nursing care and patient independence, (2) the surgical procedure requires extracorporeal circulation, and (3) it may be difficult to control any apical bleeding problems.

The direct left atrial appendage approach offers simplicity of insertion and removal. It provides good blood flow and pump filling but sometimes can be affected by patient position. A disadvantage is that if the left ventricle is not ejecting or is ejecting intermittently, stasis thrombosis can occur in the ventricular chamber.

The third approach is through the roof of the left atrium just adjacent to the right superior pulmonary vein, which is exposed by reflecting the right atrium along Sundergard's groove at the intra-atrial septum. This insertion is also simple and can be done without a heart-lung bypass procedure. The risk is that there can be stasis in the right superior pulmonary vein and variations in blood flow related to patient position.

Considering all of these advantages and disadvantages in a bridge to transplantation, we prefer the left ventricular apex as the best inflow cannulation approach because it ensures steady pump filling, decompresses the left ventricle, avoids stasis, aids in complete chest closure, and affords good patient mobility postoperatively. Return blood flow to the body in each approach involves the use of a woven Dacron graft anastomosed to the ascending aorta. We prefer to preclot this graft with cryoprecipitate followed by thrombin on the exterior of the graft. This produces perfect graft hemostasis.

For right heterotopic pump implantation, the pump inflow cannula is normally inserted through the right atrial appendage, which is removed at the time of transplantation. Sometimes moving the site of insertion inferiorly but still close to the atrioventricular groove positions the tip of the cannula more in the center of the right atrium and gives a more consistent flow rate. Return of right-sided heart blood flow to the body also involves use of a woven

Dacron graft that is anastomosed to the main pulmonary artery.

The blood-carrying conduits are brought out and secured separately through short vertical incisions in the epigastric area inferior to the wound. Chest tubes are often brought out laterally through the fifth or sixth intercostal space to avoid further incisions inferiorly and to increase available space for chest closure. The chest is not closed until complete hemostasis is accomplished. If coagulation parameters are abnormal, clotting factors are replaced by the appropriate use of fresh frozen plasma, cryoprecipitate, or platelets. It is our policy to close both the sternum and the soft tissues at the conclusion of the operation. We feel this substantially minimizes the risk of infection, decreases bleeding, allows the patient to be extubated, and facilitates postoperative nursing.

POSTOPERATIVE MANAGEMENT

Postoperative management is greatly simplified by the assurance of a normal cardiac output. All inotropic drugs are discontinued. Some patients with heterotopic pumps, particularly those who were in cardiogenic shock, may have intermittent cardiac arrhythmias such as ventricular tachycardia and ventricular fibrillation. We prefer that the patient be maintained in sinus rhythm. However, if the patient is going in and out of ventricular tachycardia and ventricular fibrillation, we would prefer to leave him or her in fibrillation rather than run the risk of thromboembolism resulting from alternating rhythms. Some patients have required low doses of epinephrine or norepinephrine to elevate systemic vascular resistance. The etiology of the low systemic vascular resistance is unclear but it is not related to sepsis.

Prophylactic antibiotics are used for 5 days and then discontinued. Careful watch is kept for signs of infection, and if infection is present, the source is specifically and appropriately treated. In long-term patients there may be superficial skin necrosis for approximately 2 mm around the cannula sites; this has not been a major problem. At the time of transplantation and removal of the device, the involved skin and subcutaneous tissues are removed.

The incidence of thromboembolism in patients having unilateral or bilateral Thoratec heterotopic pumps has been extraordinarily low. In many of these patients little or no anticoagulation therapy was used. However, we feel that in a patient with four valves and two pumping chambers, it is prudent to use some level of anticoagulation. After 24 to 36 hours, when coagulation parameters have returned to normal, continuous intravenous heparin infusion is begun at a rate of 600 to 1,000 U per hour, with a target activated clotting time of 1.5 times that of normal. For longer term support, warfarin (Coumadin) can be used, with the prothrombin time maintained at a range of from 16 to 18 seconds.

Patients are extubated as soon as feasible. They are encouraged to get out of bed; ambulation and even limited bedside exercises are possible.

RESULTS

Bridge to transplantation became a clinical entity in 1984 amid much controversy over medical and ethical issues. There was an obvious risk of infection and the potential for wasting good donor hearts. However, the results of bridge to transplantation have been excellent, with post-transplant survival in the Thoratec series equal to the current results of conventional cardiac transplantation.

For the heterotopic approach, using the Thoratec unilateral or bilateral system, of 57 patients implanted, 46 (81 percent) remained transplant candidates. Of the 11 patients who did not receive transplants, preexisting multiorgan involvement that was not reversible was the prevailing reason. Of the 46 patients who received transplants, 38 patients (83 percent) have survived to date.

The results in orthotopic transplantation using the Jarvik heart in 81 patients have been less successful than those with the Thoratec heterotopic system. Fifty-eight (72 percent) of the patients with implants maintained their clinical eligibility to receive transplants. Post-transplant survival rates using the Jarvik heart were 31 patients (53 percent) in the first 58 patients. The reason for these differences between heterotopic and orthotopic implant results is not entirely clear. Results with the orthotopic Jarvik heart have been adversely affected by mediastinal infection.

From the outset of this therapy, there has been an exciting medical controversy regarding the merits of the heterotopic versus the orthotopic systems. We advocated the heterotopic system for the bridge to a cardiac transplantation procedure for a number of reasons. First, the native heart does not have to be removed and therefore one is afforded time to evaluate the irreversibility of its condition. If the native heart recovers, the heterotopic pumps can be removed. Secondly, the magnitude of the heterotopic surgical procedure is much less than that of the orthotopic operation and can sometimes be done without a heart-lung bypass procedure. Third, the patient's size and the pump fit are seldom considerations with heterotopic pumps because they do not reside inside the chest.

Early in the development of this procedure, the orthotopic approach seemed to offer a measure of protection from infection by having the device inside the chest. However, experience has shown that this is not the case, and indeed, recent results indicate that the mediastinal position of large avascular prosthetic ventricles has led to significant mediastinal infection of up to 35 percent in some series. The relatively fixed boundaries of the mediastinum (sternum, vertebrae, and mediastinal pleura) do not collapse around the pump, and large areas of stasis and fluid collection develop in the mediastinum. In contrast, there has not been major infection at the percutaneous cannula sites for the heterotopic approach, as was originally expected.

TRANSPLANTATION

Once the device has been implanted, there is a temptation to relax and allow the patient's secondary organ function to recover before proceeding to transplantation. We have resisted this approach and immediately seek a donor heart so that the patient can undergo cardiac transplantation as soon as possible. Even if renal function is a problem, at present we prefer to perform the transplant early and deal with renal failure in the post-transplant period rather than risk the development of contraindications during the bridge period that would exclude the possibility of going forward with transplantation. However, with the increasing evidence of long safe bridge periods with the heterotopic system, we may modify this policy in the future.

IMMUNOSUPPRESSION FOLLOWING TRANSPLANTATION

Following transplantation, our immunosuppressive therapy consists of relatively low-dose methylprednisolone (1 to 2 mg per kilogram per day), cyclosporine, 10 mg per kilogram per day in two divided doses, and antilymphocyte globulin (Minnesota), 15 mg per kilogram per day (for 14 days). We feel that the lower dose of steroids reduces the incidence of wound complications in the immediate postsurgical state.

SUGGESTED READING

DeVries WC, Anderson JL, Joyce LD, et al. Clinical use of the total artificial heart. N Engl J Med 1984; 310:273–278.

Farrar DJ, Hill JD, Gray LA, et al. Heterotopic prosthetic ventricles as a bridge to cardiac transplantation. A multicenter study in twenty-nine patients. N Engl J Med 1988; 318:333–340.

Farrar DJ, Lawson JH, Avery GJ II, et al. Mechanical circulatory support in the treatment of heart failure: bridge to transplantation. In: Andrade JD, ed. Artificial organs. New York: VCH Publisher, 1987:159.

Hill JD, Farrar DJ, Hershon JJ, et al. Bridge to cardiac transplantation: successful use of prosthetic biventricular support in a patient awaiting a donor heart. ASAIO Trans 1986; 32:233–237.

Hill JD, Farrar DJ, Hershon JJ, et al. Use of a prosthetic ventricle as a bridge to cardiac transplantation for postinfarction cardiogenic shock. N Engl J Med 1986; 314:626–628.

SUPPORT OF THE FAILING HEART: LEFT HEART ASSISTANCE

JAMES A. MAGOVERN, M.D.
WILLIAM S. PIERCE, M.D.

During the past 10 years, the use of left ventricular assistance has moved from the experimental laboratory to clinical practice. In this chapter we review indications for left ventricular support, describe several available systems, discuss operative techniques, and briefly summarize results.

INDICATIONS

Postcardiotomy Cardiogenic Shock

If following a cardiac operation a patient cannot be weaned from cardiopulmonary bypass because of left ventricular failure, he or she may be a candidate for temporary ventricular assistance. The following criteria have helped us to define when to implement ventricular assistance:

1. A technically satisfactory cardiac operation has been done and the underlying cardiac pathology has been adequately repaired.
2. Volume infusion, pharmacologic support, and counterpulsation with an intra-aortic balloon pump have failed to adequately improve left ventricular function.
3. Left atrial pressure is greater than 25 mm Hg.
4. Systolic arterial blood pressure is less than 90 mm Hg.
5. Cardiac index is less than 1.8 L per minute per square meter.

Generally, patients older than 70 years are not candidates for left ventricular assistance, since the extent of their recovery rarely enables them to be discharged from the hospital. However, individual exceptions can be made if the patient is otherwise vigorous.

Bridge to Cardiac Transplantation

Patients who have already been accepted as heart transplant candidates, but who then suffer progressive left ventricular deterioration, are also candidates for insertion of a temporary left ventricular assist device. In this situation, hemodynamic criteria for insertion of an assist device are similar to those for patients with postcardiotomy cardiogenic shock. Many of these patients can be supported with a left venticular assist device if there is no elevation of the pulmonary vascular resistance, but some require biventricular support. For this latter group, there are two possible approaches: the use of biventricular assist devices or the use of a total artificial heart. It has not been determined which alternative is more desirable.

SYSTEMS AND TECHNIQUES

Pneumatic Devices

The Pierce-Donachy pump, developed at The Pennsylvania State University, consists of a smooth blood sac enclosed in a rigid case. Pulses of compressed carbon dioxide from an external source activate a flexible diaphragm, which then empties the blood sac. This system has supported a patient for as long as 21 days and therefore can be used for postcardiotomy cardiogenic shock and for bridge to heart transplantation. When it is used in patients with postcardiotomy cardiogenic shock, blood is removed from the left atrium via a No. 51 F cannula and returned to the ascending aorta through a 14-mm composite Dacron-polyurethane cannula. We have found that left atrial cannulation is superior to left ventricular cannulation because there is less bleeding from the cannulation site and less trauma to the already damaged left ventricle. In bridge to transplant procedures, when recovery of left ventricular function is not anticipated, the left ventricular apex is cannulated, so that the atria are spared for the subsequent transplantation procedure. The cannulas are brought out through the skin in the subcostal area, and the pump is positioned on the anterior abdominal wall. An assist pump flow of 4 to 6 L per minute is usually maintained, but the flow rate can only equal that of the natural right ventricle. Currently, this system is manufactured and marketed by the Thoratec Corporation, but its clinical use is restricted by the Federal Drug Administration.

Centrifugal and Roller Pumps

Satisfactory results with partial left-sided heart bypass from the left atrium to the ascending aorta have been reported by several groups using centrifugal or roller pumps. In essence, these methods are a continuation of partial cardiopulmonary bypass using equipment that is used in the operating room. A cannula placed through the superior pulmonary vein or directly into the left atrium diverts blood into a pump. Blood is returned to the patient through a cannula in the ascending aorta. The use of roller pumps has been described by several authors; recently, the use of a centrifugal (Biomedicus) system has also become popular.

Choice of System

The Pierce-Donachy ventricular assist device can provide flow of up to 8 L per minute, causes no significant hemolysis or fibrinolysis, and requires no systemic anticoagulation except, possibly, low molecular weight dextran. In addition, it can provide circulatory support for several weeks. Its primary disadvantage is its relative lack of availability. Several centers have permission from the Federal Drug Administration to use this system, but at present the system is not available to the entire cardiac surgical community.

The major advantage of the centrifugal and roller pump systems is availability; components are present in most centers that perform cardiac surgery. Because continuous flow is achieved with these pumps, smaller inflow and outflow cannulas can be employed. Cost is also less than with the Pierce-Donachy system, since no special equipment needs to be purchased. The major disadvantages are as follows:

1. Flow is nonpulsatile and is limited to a maximum of 4 to 5 L per minute, which in some cases is not sufficient to support the patient and can result in multisystem failure.
2. With roller pump systems, blood trauma occurs, resulting in hemolysis, fibrinolysis, and thrombocytopenia, especially when support is continued for more than 48 hours. Blood trauma is much less severe with the centrifugal pumps, but mild thrombocytopenia and fibrinolysis do occur.
3. One must constantly balance the need for heparin anticoagulation and the risks of thromboembolism and hemorrhage. With the centrifugal systems, heparin is given to keep the activated clotting time greater than 140 seconds, although thrombi still form in the pump head. Embolism has not been a problem, but the pump head should be changed every 24 hours. Roller pump systems require more heparin, and accordingly, bleeding has been a greater problem.
4. These systems are not suitable for long-term circulatory support if the surgeon is unable to wean the patient from the device within 5 to 7 days, and therefore they are not well suited for bridge procedures.

During the past several years, clinical application of the centrifugal pump system has been far greater than that of the roller pump systems because of less blood trauma, fewer bleeding complications, and reduced incidence of tubing cracks and air emboli.

RESULTS

Postcardiotomy Cardiogenic Shock

Since 1980, we have inserted the Pierce-Donachy left ventricular assist device in 16 patients who could not be weaned from cardiopulmonary bypass. Sixty-two percent were weaned from the device, and 44 percent were discharged from the hospital. Long-term follow-up has shown good functional recovery and minimal cardiac disability. Using roller pump systems, between 46 percent and 67 percent of patients have been weaned from the device and 33 percent to 35 percent have been discharged from the hospital. Similar results have been achieved using centrifugal pumps.

Bridge to Transplant

As of September 1986, a total of 14 patients have been supported at several institutions with a Pierce-Donachy system and have then undergone transplantation. Results have been excellent: 13 of the 14 patients are alive at present, and no major device-related complications have been reported. Patients have also been supported with centrifugal pumps before successful transplant procedures, but exact numbers and results have not been published.

Duration of Support

In postcardiotomy cardiogenic shock applications, we have used the Pierce-Donachy system for a mean of 4.8 days (range 1 hour to 25 days). However, this figure includes some patients who died early in the postoperative period. The mean duration of left ventricular assistance for those patients who were weaned from the device and subsequently discharged from the hospital was 7.4 days (range 4 to 12 days). Thus, recovery of ventricular function often can take as long as 1 week. In bridge to transplant procedures, we have used this device for as long as 21 days before successful cardiac transplantation.

Complications of Left Ventricular Assistance

We have had no device failures and no device-related thromboembolic complications. Postoperative hemorrhage is common in postcardiotomy patients, because these patients often have a coagulopathy caused by prolonged cardiopulmonary bypass before the device is inserted. This can usually be reversed with appropriate blood component therapy. We have not experienced infectious complications directly attributable to the device, but sepsis and multiple organ system failure develop in some patients who do not recover myocardial function.

Some degree of right ventricular failure is common and should be anticipated and treated promptly with volume loading, inotropic agents, and pulmonary vasodilators. A minority of patients require biventricular assistance. Arterial hypoxemia, secondary to right-to-left shunting across a patent foramen ovale, can occur if right atrial pressure exceeds left atrial pressure. This problem can be avoided by closure of the foramen ovale prior to initiating left ventricular assistance.

Temporary left ventricular assistance for postcardiotomy cardiogenic shock has become a well-established therapeutic technique. In the past, patients who could not be weaned from cardiopulmonary bypass would die in the operating room. Using the devices currently available, nearly one-half of these patients can be expected to recover good myocardial function and be discharged from the hospital. The long-term prognosis for these patients is also good.

Temporary use of a left ventricular assist device as a bridge to heart transplantation is a new application and appears to have been quite successful. However, before this can be considered an established therapeutic technique, prognosis after transplantation for bridge patients must be shown to be as good as it is for more stable patients who receive transplants electively.

In the future it is possible that left ventricular support might be helpful for patients with postmyocardial infarction cardiogenic shock. The early clinical results in this area have been disappointing, but largely because such support has been used in only the most desperately ill patients. With increased experience, improved technology, and better patient selection, left ventricular assistance may play an important role in improving the outlook for this group of patients.

SUGGESTED READING

Gaines WE, Pierce WS, Donachy JH, Rosenberg G, Landis DL, Richenbacher WE, Waldhausen JA. The Pennsylvania State University paracorporeal ventricular assist pump: optimal methods of use. World J Surg 1985; 9:47–53.

Hill JD, Farrar DJ, Hershon JJ, Compton PG, Avery GJ, Levin BS, Brent BN. Use of a prosthetic ventricle as a bridge to cardiac transplantation for post infarction cardiogenic shock. N Engl J Med 1986; 314:626–628.

Magovern GJ, Park SB, Maher TD. Use of a centrifugal pump without anticoagulants for postoperative left ventricular assist. World J Surg 1985; 9:25–36.

Pae WE, Pierce WS, Pennock JL, Campbell DB, Waldhausen JA. Long-term results of ventricular assist pumping in postcardiotomy cardiogenic shock. J Thorac Cardiovasc Surg 1987; 93:434–441.

Pennock JL, Pierce WS, Wisman CB, Bull A, Waldhausen JA. Survival and complications following ventricular assist pumping for cardiogenic shock. Ann Surg 1983; 198:469–478.

INTRA-AORTIC BALLOON CIRCULATORY SUPPORT

MORTIMER J. BUCKLEY, M.D.

The development of intra-aortic balloon assist at the Massachusetts General Hospital was initiated in our laboratory in 1966 in conjunction with the Avco Everett Research Laboratories. Our research was based upon the experimental work reported by Moulopoulos and Kolff and our experience with blood pumping in the form of counterpulsation from the groin vessels. Experimental studies indicated that the effectiveness of counterpulsation was related to the stroke volume of the balloon and the resulting augmented pressure response during diastole in the aortic root. These investigations showed that the stroke volume of the intra-aortic balloon was the most critical factor in determining predictable augmentation. Further evaluation in the laboratory demonstrated that the response of the ventricle in the shock state was dependent upon unloading of the ventricle (e.g., the rapid decrease in aortic root pressure with the deflation of the balloon) and upon diastolic augmentation resulting in increased coronary blood flow. Experiments carried out by Powell and Daggett demonstrated the independence of these functions in improving ventricular function. Clinical application of intra-aortic balloon assist was initiated in 1967 by Kantrowitz and in 1968 by our group.

HISTORICAL BACKGROUND

The patients selected in our early experience for intra-aortic balloon pumping were those in established cardiogenic shock subsequent to acute myocardial infarction. The following criteria were utilized: patients under 60 years of age with an acute myocardial infarction within the past 10 days and with severe hemodynamic compromise as evidenced by low urine output (less than 20 ml per hour) and a mean arterial blood pressure below 70 mm Hg. The patients were always treated first with established clinical approaches for the shock patient, e.g., the use of pressor agents, volume, heparin, and in most cases, anti-ischemic agents. In our initial experience patients did not receive intra-aortic balloon pumping unless they had been in established cardiogenic shock for at least 6 hours and were deteriorating. With this selection of patients, our rate of success, i.e., being able to wean the patient from the balloon and to discharge him or her alive from the hospital, was 16 percent. We learned, however, that these patients with whom we had success were the ones who had had the earlier balloon intervention and who had areas of myocardium with reversible ischemia. At the same time that these studies were being carried out, the Myocardial Infarction Research Unit (MIRU) centers developed criteria for the categorization of patients with compromised cardiac function after acute myocardial infarction. The most severe of these categories, Class IV cardiogenic shock, was characterized by a cardiac index of less than 2 L per minute per square meter of body surface, an elevated filling pressure of the left ventricle of greater than 17 mm Hg, and a mean aortic pressure of less than 70 mm Hg. These criteria were then applied to patients with acute myocardial infarction, and earlier intervention with intra-aortic ballooning was initiated. Patients who met the criteria of Class IV cardiogenic shock and who failed to improve after 1 hour of appropriate medical therapy were selected for intra-aortic balloon pumping. Patients who improved rapidly with this intervention were evaluated later as to the need for cardiac surgery. Those patients, however, who could not be weaned from an intra-aortic balloon pump within 24 hours, i.e., who could not improve their cardiac indexes above 2 L per minute per square meter of body surface and reduce their left ventricular filling pressures below 15 mm Hg independent of balloon assist were classified as balloon-dependent. These patients were then considered for urgent surgical intervention. Evaluation of these patients showed that coronary bypass grafting could achieve a survival rate of approximately 50 percent when applied early after the development of acute hemodynamic deterioration and application of intra-aortic balloon pump assist. The survival in patients with acute ventricular septal defect or mitral regurgitation secondary to acute myocardial infarction was somewhat higher.

Given the experience of increased survival with this severely ill group of patients, balloon assist was then applied to two other groups of patients—those who had failed to wean from cardiopulmonary bypass after technically successful cardiac surgery and those with medically refractory acute myocardial ischemia.

Patients who failed to wean from bypass after 1 hour of prolonged attempts of partial bypass and high-dose pressor support were selected for balloon intervention. The early results with these patients was an approximately 28 percent hospital survival rate. By applying the balloon earlier in the patient's course, e.g., well within the first failure to wean and before prolonged efforts with high-dose pressors, the survival rate improved to a level of approximately 70 percent. Success was found to be much more likely if there was evidence of reasonable left ventricular function before the surgical procedure and if evidence of reversal of ischemia developed during the operation.

The other area of application of balloon assist was for patients with medically refractory acute ischemia. The first group of patients within this category were those who developed angina, S-T segment elevation, and hemodynamic compromise within 10 days after an acute myocardial infarction in spite of medical therapy. These patients were treated with intra-aortic balloon assist, and appropriate medical therapy was continued. After cardiac catheterization and coronary angiography, surgery was carried out utilizing coronary bypass and other reconstructive techniques, as needed. The survival rate in these patients in the early experience was over 80 percent. The second group in which intra-aortic balloon assist was utilized was patients who developed medically refractory ischemia but who did not have recent myocardial infarctions. The balloon was used to control the ischemia, and then, after angiographic studies were completed, surgery was carried out as indicated. These patients were operated on in the mid-1970s with a mortality rate of less than 3 percent and an impressively low perioperative myocardial infarction rate of less than 2 percent. From these experiences, an aggressive approach to the utilization of intra-aortic balloon pumping has developed.

PRESENT INDICATIONS

At the present time *postmyocardial infarction cardiogenic shock* is considered a strong indication for the use of the intra-aortic balloon pump. Patients with a recent acute myocardial infarction who require increasing pressor support in the form of alpha-constrictive agents like norepinephrine and, in many circumstances, those requiring increasing doses of mixed agents such as epinephrine and dopamine, should be considered for intra-aortic balloon pumping. The insertion of the balloon has been facilitated in recent times by the development of percutaneous techniques. The placement of the balloon should be carried out in patients who have reasonable peripheral circulation, i.e., palpable femoral pulses, before their severely compromised hemodynamic state, and ventricles that were compensated without the need of digitalis and diuretics before the recent acute myocardial infarction or myocardial ischemia. The age of the patient is relative, but we have generally not used the balloon in patients over the age of 80 years. The ideal response to the balloon is an improvement in the hemodynamic situation with a reduction of pulmonary capillary wedge pressure below 15 mm Hg and a secondary rise in the cardiac index above 2.5 L per minute per square meter. Prompt cardiac catheterization and coronary angiographic study should be carried out. In order for coronary bypass surgery to be recommended, the coronary angiogram must show vessels that can be revascularized in the area of acute ischemia. These patients should be operated on urgently, and they have an expected survival rate of over 60 percent. Patients who fail to improve hemodynamically or who have a severely damaged ventricular myocardium as evidenced by lack of vessels perfused by collaterals in the area of ischemia should not be operated on. Survival in this latter group is extremely low.

Patients may also benefit from surgical intervention if mechanical lesions are present, such as *mitral regurgitation* or *ventricular septal defect* secondary to an acute myocardial infarction. The initiation of intra-aortic balloon pumping in these patients usually results in a reduction in the left atrial pressure when mitral regurgitation is present and improvement in left ventricular function, with variable effect on the left-to-right shunt in patients with ruptured intraventricular septum. Experience has shown that prolonged pumping is not therapeutic for these problems but should be used as a technique to make safe evaluation in the catheterization laboratory possible. In general, corrective surgery for the mechanical lesion should be carried out at the earliest possible time. The combination of balloon assist, early surgery, and improved techniques, particularly those described by Daggett for patients with ventricular septal defects, has resulted in an increase in the survival of these patients to at least 70 percent.

Ventricular irritability can often be a major complication of acute myocardial infarction, and when it leads to hemodynamic instability, intra-aortic balloon assist may be of value. Certainly, ventricular fibrillation or a very rapid ventricular tachycardia cannot be followed effectively by a balloon pump, but frequent episodes of ventricular tachycardia and life-threatening forms of multifocal ventricular irritability may be improved during intra-aortic balloon pumping. In patients who respond to the intervention with a marked reduction in irritability and improvement of ventricular function, we have found a better than 70 percent survival with acute surgery that might be required to correct reduced myocardial blood flow from severe coronary disease or, occasionally, to resect an acute aneurysm. However, patients who do not improve with intra-aortic balloon pumping have an extremely low survival rate, even when we have attempted to apply techniques of electrophysiology and arrhythmia localization. Thus, intra-aortic balloon pumping may serve not only to temporarily control arrhythmias in some patients but also to delineate those patients at high surgical risk.

The need for intra-aortic balloon counterpulsation in patients with *pump failure subsequent to cardiopulmonary bypass* has been greatly reduced with the use of effective myocardial protection during cardiopulmonary bypass procedures. Our present criteria for the use of such intervention are as follows. Patients who had reasonable ventricular function prior to surgery and who do not have significant aortic regurgitation should be identified and new ischemic changes in the electrocardiogram should be looked for. When cessation of total bypass is attempted after a reasonable period of myocardial perfusion and cardiac function deteriorates despite the use of inotropic agents, then intra-aortic balloon assist should be considered. The balloon may be inserted via the femoral artery by the percutaneous technique, by the open surgical technique, or, in circumstances in which there is severe peripheral vascular disease, by direct insertion into the ascending aorta. The latter technique is rarely used. Weaning from bypass is carried out as usual, now with appropriate diastolic augmentation and systolic unloading. In patients whom this technique fails to wean from bypass, partial circulatory bypass may be used with external units for appropriate pumping, or in some younger patients under consideration for cardiac transplantation, total artificial heart units may be implanted.

The management of *acute myocardial ischemia*, either with recent myocardial infarction or in association with severe unstable angina, may be greatly facilitated by the initiation of intra-aortic balloon pumping. Many patients with extensive coronary artery disease cannot tolerate the agents necessary to produce ventricular unloading or coronary dilation or both. The normotensive patient with an elevated wedge pressure and active ischemia may have a reduction in coronary blood flow with high-dose intravenous nitroglycerin. The reduction in aortic root diastolic pressure may result in a negative inotropic response in the patient because of a reduction in coronary blood flow. Similarly, the patient who is hypertensive and has extensive three-vessel coronary disease may not tolerate the degree of systolic unloading required to reduce the ventricular wall tension and oxygen consumption to control his or her ischemia. The use of an intra-aortic balloon pump facilitates appropriate medical therapy in these patients. The normotensive patient has a reduction in the peak left ventricular pressure as well as a marked augmentation of the diastolic pressure. The reduction in peak left ventricular pressure results in a marked decrease in left ventricular wall tension and reduction of oxygen demand. The elevation of diastolic pressure results in a rise in coronary blood flow to the myocardium. In addition, this mechanically increased diastolic pressure allows more aggressive use of alpha-blocking agents and vasodilators, especially in the hypertensive patient. Thus, the ideal intervention for therapy of acute myocardial ischemia, i.e., reduced left ventricular wall tension and increased coronary blood flow, can be more safely achieved during intra-aortic balloon pumping. Early efforts with intra-aortic balloon pumping brought up the question of whether this therapy would result in a rapid increase in coronary blood flow, development of coronary collaterals, and, potentially, a re-establishment of normal flow to ischemic areas. Our experience with intra-aortic balloon pumping indicated that this does not occur even during prolonged assist; thus, balloon pumping is used mainly to control the ischemic state and to allow appropriate evaluation of the heart, usually including coronary angiography. At the present time, these patients with medically refractory unstable angina ideally are operated on within 24 hours after intra-aortic balloon placement. Recent experience has shown that some properly selected patients may benefit by the utilization of coronary balloon angioplasty instead of coronary bypass; this usually requires that the patient have single- or double-vessel disease with high-grade proximal lesions. Intra-aortic balloon assist greatly improves the state of these patients by reducing their ischemia and allowing them a safer period of transient occlusion during the time of angioplasty. This may be especially true in those who have acute myocardial infarction with or without ongoing pain. Attempts to reperfuse the myocardium beyond thrombosed vessels have become more successful with the use of streptokinase or thromboplastin-activating factor (t-PA). Many of these patients have compromised hemodynamics, and intra-aortic balloon assist not only may provide some reversal of the ischemia to the surrounding myocardium but also may allow a more aggressive approach in the catheterization laboratory. Patients who evidence new ischemia with or without hemodynamic compromise during or immediately following elective or emergency balloon angioplasty can be greatly helped by intra-aortic balloon pumping. In some circumstances, enough stabilization is obtained so that further intervention is not necessary. In others, the patient is stabilized enough so that appropriate transfer to an operating room can be carried out and surgery can be achieved in a more controlled state.

TECHNIQUES OF INSERTION

Direct Insertion

In 1968, when intra-aortic balloon pumping was initiated, a surgical incision was required in the femoral area, with exposure of the common femoral artery. The technique for direct insertion is as follows. The area of the femoral artery is delineated on the side with the strongest palpable pulse. If the patient is in shock and no pulse can be felt, then any historical indication of a better side is used. The patient is prepped from the umbilicus to the midthigh on that side, and careful draping of a large field is carried out to protect the multiple instruments and catheters that will be used. A direct incision is made over the palpable femoral artery extending at least 3 cm above the inguinal ligament and 5 cm below. The incision must be longer if the patient has considerable fat in the area. The local anesthetic used can be infiltrated generously into the area or a regional block carried out if appropriate. Once the incision has been made, it is carried down through the fat, and the inguinal ligament is identified over the femoral artery and vein. The femoral sheath is entered and the femoral artery isolated. If the origin of the profunda femoris branch from the common femoral artery is high, then the inguinal ligament should be incised so that a total length of 3 cm of femoral artery can be placed between appropriate tourniquets. Careful palpation of the vessel must be carried out because this is a frequent site of plaque, and eccentric plaque is commonly present in patients with coronary artery disease. An appropriate soft segment is isolated, and the patient is heparinized with 50 mg of heparin. Once the artery is isolated between tourniquets, it is opened longitudinally for approximately 12 to 15 mm. If a wire-guided catheter is to be used, the wire can be inserted up through the tourniquet to enhance appropriate placement of the intra-aortic balloon pump. In cases in which fluoroscopy is not used to guide the catheter into place, a guidewire is extremely important. An estimate of how far the catheter should be inserted can be made by approximating how far it would have to go to reach the level of the distal aortic arch, which in most patients corresponds to the angle of Louis. The catheter is then marked with a tie at the level of the groin incision so that further insertion will warn the physician that he or she may be approaching the arch. The catheter is then inserted over the guide wire, with the proximal tourniquet being loosened enough to allow it to advance. The tourniquet is then tightened again around the catheter proximal to the femoral arteriotomy to reduce bleeding in the groin. When the catheter has been advanced to the position selected, a prepared 10-mm graft previously placed around the balloon catheter is anastomosed to the femoral arteriotomy. Once the graft is in place, it is ligated around the catheter shaft, and the tourniquet is removed from the femoral artery above. Any further bleeding is controlled with added ligatures or sutures, as necessary. The wound is irrigated copiously and closed in layers. The catheter should be sutured to the skin to prevent its movement. In the subsequent care of the patient, flexion at the level of the hip should be avoided if possible. The large size of these earlier balloon pumps and stiff catheters resulted in a vascular complication rate of approximately 4 percent. Failure to insert the balloon occurred in as many as 10 percent of the patients because of local disease of the vessel, tortuosity of the pelvic vessels, and poor flow around the catheter after insertion of the balloon.

The balloon is removed by first obtaining distal control of the femoral artery. Ligatures are removed from around the graft and the deflated balloon is withdrawn, allowing a small amount of blood to escape to flush out any clot that may have been present on the shaft of the balloon. A side-biting clamp is then placed on the graft, and it is trimmed to size and oversewn, thus leaving a small patch arterioplasty to prevent narrowing of the femoral artery. In our experience, the incidence of significant infection at the groin site has been less than 1 percent.

Percutaneous Insertion

Percutaneous balloon insertion has grown to be the most common technique utilized for the placement of an intra-aortic balloon pump. The technique requires the palpation of the femoral artery or its localization with a small-gauge exploring needle. Once the femoral artery has been identified and the needle inserted, a short guide wire can be inserted through the needle. Over this guide wire a small obturator is passed first; this initiates the hole in the femoral artery. A larger obturator that has a sheath over it is then inserted. The sheath has been designed to be of a diameter that will allow insertion of a tightly rolled intra-aortic balloon pump. Once the sheath has been placed into the iliac system, the short guide wire is removed and the intra-aortic balloon pump is inserted over a longer guide wire. The guide wire is advanced appropriately to the level of the subclavian artery, and the balloon is advanced up to this point. A secondary plug on the shaft of the balloon catheter is then advanced to seal any further bleeding from around the sheath. Once this has been done, the balloon is unfurled and primed and appropriate pumping can be initiated.

A modification of this technique may be used in certain circumstances. When the femoral artery cannot be palpated either because of shock or because the patient is on cardiopulmonary bypass, it may be exposed surgically. A soft spot is selected on the anterior surface of the common femoral artery, and a pursestring suture at least 1 cm in its long diameter is placed in this area; the technique of balloon insertion is carried out similarly to that described for the percutaneous technique. The advantage of this procedure is that a graft is avoided and that an elaborate surgical procedure may not be necessary at the time of the balloon removal. It also allows a catheter to be inserted directly through the femoral artery wall, and when it is properly positioned, the sheath through which it was inserted can be totally withdrawn and hemostasis obtained with a pursestring suture coming down around the catheter shaft alone. This reduces the volume and diameter of material left in the femoral artery to the catheter itself, which may be advantageous in patients with small femoral arteries.

The development of percutaneous techniques has greatly facilitated the use of intra-aortic balloon pumping. In addition, newer balloons have been designed with much smaller catheters and thinner balloon walls, allowing insertion into vessels that were previously unapproachable. This has resulted in increased ease of insertion of the balloon. At the present time, a balloon may be inserted in the catheterization lab within 10 minutes of the decision to do so. This time is even shorter if the patient already has a femoral arterial line in place. Thus, effective pumping for the acutely ischemic patient can be achieved within 15 minutes. The complication rate, as measured by vascular trauma or severe reduction in femoral artery flow resulting from insertion of a balloon, has been reduced from 11 percent in our first 100 patients to less than 5 percent. The balloon can be removed after effective pumping without an additional surgical procedure in over 98 percent of the patients. Approximately 2 percent of the patients require exploration of their femoral arteries and evacuation of clot and occasionally reconstruction of the vessel. The incidence of balloon-related deaths is less than 0.5 percent.

In our experience with 2,725 patients who have undergone intra-aortic balloon pumping, the change in insertion technique has produced the following results. All intra-aortic balloons placed from our first insertion on November 1986 up until February 1980 were implanted with direct surgical technique (1,208 cases). Since that time, 1,075 intra-aortic balloons have been inserted percutaneously, 90 percent of which have been placed in the cardiac catheterization unit. Surgical insertions have been carried out since that time in 442 patients. The majority of these balloons were placed surgically only after attempts at percutaneous techniques had failed; or, in over 200 patients they were placed in the operating room during cardiopulmonary bypass. Recently, however, even in the operating room, we have used the percutaneous techniques, since it is much less traumatic to the vessel and balloon removal is easier postoperatively.

BALLOON MANAGEMENT

Initiation of balloon assist depends on the proper placement of the balloon as previously described, and either a satisfactory electrocardiogram or arterial pressure wave needs to be utilized for the timing of the balloon. Two elements must be achieved: inflation of the balloon must be accomplished as early in diastole as possible, and deflation of the balloon must occur before ventricular ejection. In some circumstances, deflation timing may be sought that will reduce the pressure in the aortic root even more just prior to ejection. The most common technique for timing is the utilization of an appropriate R wave taken either from standard leads of the electrocardiogram or from precordial skin electrodes. In patients who have temporary pacemakers, such as those in the early postoperative period, the pacemaker signal may also be used as a timing signal source for the balloon pump. One of these timing impulses is used by the computer system of the balloon pump to project the appropriate times of inflation and deflation. The variations in electrical and mechanical function that occur in patients can be compensated for by the appropriate adjustment of the inflation and deflation controls in the console. Since consoles vary, the operator should consult the operating manual of the individual system to be used for proper selection of these timing points. Basically, however, the timing that is sought is one that produces slightly early closure of the aortic valve and reduction in aortic root pressure just prior to ventricular ejection. Generally, this reduction should not be below 50 mm Hg. While the patient is on the intra-aortic balloon, he or she should be protected from the possibility of thrombus formation on the balloon or catheter and potential embolization from these sites. The patient who has not undergone recent major surgery should be heparinized with a prolongation of the activated clotting time to at least twice the patient's control time. Patients who have undergone recent surgery, particularly extensive heart surgery, may be subject to bleeding at this level of heparinization and may be managed with low molecular weight dextran, generally at a dose of 20 ml per hour. Care must be taken regarding allergic reaction to this material. Careful monitoring of the peripheral circulation must be carried out, either by direct palpation of pulses distal to the balloon device, or, when appropriate, by Doppler monitoring of flow in the involved leg. The desired effect of balloon assist is marked augmentation of diastolic pressure and a secondary improvement of myocardial function, as evidenced by improvement of ischemic changes in the electrocardiogram, reduction in left atrial or pulmonary capillary wedge pressure, and a secondary improvement in cardiac output. Increased urinary output may be associated with this.

Weaning from balloon assist is critical. Just as ventricular function was utilized to determine if the patient required the assist device, a further evaluation of that function is necessary to determine if balloon assist is no longer needed. The condition of the left ventricle prior to the initiation of circulatory assist is critical in determining what level of function should be sought after balloon assist is discontinued. The easiest patients to manage are those who have required intervention for acute myocardial ischemia without myocardial infarction; thus, the patient who had a balloon inserted because of severe unstable angina and who has had successful multiple coronary bypass grafts and a low filling pressure coming off cardiopulmonary bypass can be weaned rapidly from the balloon in the operating room or shortly following operation. Our general practice is to allow this type of patient to stabilize in the intensive care unit and then initiate weaning from the balloon a few hours after the operation, with planned removal of the device within 24 to 48 hours. Since most of the balloons have been put in percutaneously, the major determinant of safe removal in most of these patients is restoration of normal coagulation factors. Thus, we wait until the patient's postoperative chest tube bleeding has diminished and remove the balloon when the appropriate coagulation studies are normal the next day. External compression over the balloon removal site is carried out for at least 1 hour, and close observation of the site is important for the next 12 hours. In patients with compromised cardiac function prior to surgery or who have developed compromised cardiac function during surgery, the following criteria are used for weaning. Twenty-four hours after surgery, when the patient has stabilized in the intensive care unit, discontinuation of the balloon assist is considered if the patient is off all pressor agents and has a left atrial filling pressure below 20. Adjustments in the accepted filling pressures must be made according to the presence or absence of a mitral prosthesis and the level of ventricular function previously determined. The balloon is weaned from a level of assist with each ventricular systole to a level of assist with every other ventricular systole. If, after 1 hour at this setting, the patient has not shown a rise in filling pressure of the left atrium or a greater than 10 percent decrease in the cardiac index, then the device is left in this mode. When the patient has shown stability for 2 hours at this setting, the assist may be reduced to one in every four systoles. If again deterioration has not occurred and the patient has remained stable in this mode of assist for 2 hours or more, further weaning may be carried out safely and balloon removal achieved. Patients who show marked deterioration when assist weaning has been initiated at 24 hours should not be weaned again for another 24 hours, and the previously described process should be initiated again. Some patients with poor ventricular function may have to be gradually weaned despite some deterioration in the cardiac index and rise in left ventricular filling pressures. This is especially true if prolonged balloon assist, i.e., for 1 week or more, has been carried out and severe ventricular dysfunction with infarction or previous scar is present.

Our experience now with intra-aortic balloon pumping involves over 2,750 patients. We feel that the use of this device allows us the most predictable intervention in the management of acute myocardial ischemia. There is a measurable reduction in peak ventricular pressure and, thus, a reduction in left ventricular wall tension. In addition, there is a predictable elevation in aortic root diastolic pressure and a potential secondary increase in coronary blood flow. These two changes are ideal in the management of coronary artery disease. They complement ongoing medical therapy for ischemia, allow safe catheterization study of the patient, and where indicated allow safer surgical intervention for coronary artery disease and its complications. In addition, intra-aortic balloon pumping may be beneficial in allowing an appropriate period of reduced ventricular work subsequent to cardiopulmonary bypass and restoration of acceptable ventricular function in the postoperative period.

SUGGESTED READING

Buckley MJ. Surgery for acute myocardial infarction: evolution and current status. In: Moran JM, Michaelis LL, eds. Surgery for the complications of myocardial infarction. Orlando: Grune & Stratton, 1980:247.

Buckley MJ, Craver JM, Gold HK, Mundth ED, Daggett WM, Austen WG. Intra-aortic balloon pump assist for cardiogenic shock after cardiopulmonary bypass. Circulation 1973; 48(Suppl III):90–94.

Buckley MJ, Leinbach RC, Kastor JA, Laird JD, Kantrowitz AR, Madras PN, Sanders CA, Austen WG. Hemodynamic evaluation of intra-aortic balloon pumping in man. Circulation 1970; 41(Suppl II):130.

Buckley MJ, Mundth ED, Daggett WM, Gold HK, Leinbach RC, Austen WG. Surgical treatment of ventricular septal defects and mitral regurgitation complicating acute myocardial infarction. Ann Thorac Surg 1973; 16:598–609.

Dunkman WB, Leinbach RC, Buckley MJ, Mundth ED, Kantrowitz AR, Austen WG, Sanders CA. Clinical and hemodynamic results of intra-aortic balloon pumping and surgery for cardiogenic shock. Circulation 1972; 46:465–477.

Kantrowitz A, Tjonneland S, Freed PS, Phillips SJ, Butner AN, Sherman JL Jr. Initial clinical experience with intra-aortic balloon pumping in cardiogenic shock. JAMA 1968; 203:113-118.

Laird JD, Madras PN, Jones RT, Kantrowitz AR, Kothari ML, Buckley MJ, Austen WG. Theoretical and experimental analysis of the intra-aortic balloon pump. Trans Am Soc Artif Intern Organs 1968; 14:338–343.

Martin RS, Moncure AC, Buckley MJ, Austen WG, Akins CW, Leinbach RC. Complications of percutaneous intra-aortic balloon insertion. J Thorac Cardiovasc Surg 1983; 85:186-190.

CARDIAC PACING

J. WARREN HARTHORNE, M.D.

On October 9, 1958, Dr. Ake Senning implanted the world's first epicardial pacemaker in Arne Larsson, an electronics engineer suffering from complete heart block caused by prior myocarditis. Both surgeon and patient are alive and active today. The concept of electrical treatment of cardiac rhythm disturbances dates back to the 19th century. Albert Hyman described an "artificial cardiac pacemaker" for temporary use in 1932. C. Walton Lillehei, during the early days of cardiac surgery, was among the first to describe methods of temporary postoperative pacing. Today's modern dual-chamber cardiac pacemaker, although seemingly elaborate in circuit complexity, shares the same basic goal of preventing symptomatic bradyarrhythmias.

BASIC CONSTITUENTS OF A PACEMAKER SYSTEM

A cardiac pacemaker, whether temporary or permanent, should be thought of as a *system* composed of a power supply, housing, leads, and an electronic circuit.

Power Supply. Temporary pacemakers are never line powered because of the possible hazards of current leakage into the myocardium. Most are powered by a 9-V alkaline battery. Care must be taken to ensure a supply of fresh batteries, and a regular maintenance schedule of battery testing and replacement is mandatory. All implantable pacemakers are powered by lithium batteries of varying design. A detailed description of cell types and electrochemistry is not pertinent here, beyond noting that one cannot specify pacemaker longevity simply by knowing the energy source. Wide variations of usable energy capacity, coupled with programmable variations of electronic current settings, rate of stimulation, and differences in lead design, create a complex interplay of factors that determine individual pacemaker performance. In general, small, cosmetically attractive pacemaker generators have decreased battery size and capacity, whereas larger units offer greater longevity although in a bulkier device.

Housing. Although it is not often thought of as a discrete subunit of a pacemaker system, the can that encloses the power supply and electronic circuit constitutes a critical element in reliability of the device. Most implantable devices are triply sealed, with the power supply and circuitry independently enclosed within hermetically sealed containers, and the final assembly also hermetically sealed within yet another enclosure. Defects of welding techniques as well as flaws of electronic "feed-through" design* have created premature failures in some devices.

Lead. The lead acts as the conductor of the stimulating energy to the myocardium. The electrode is that portion of the lead that is in actual contact with the myocardium. The insulation of the lead may be of silicone rubber or of various forms of polyurethane; the latter ensures ease of handling and tougher resiliency.

Electronic Circuit. The predominant purpose of all pacemaker devices is to stimulate the heart; this is accomplished by the *output* circuit (or amplifier). This circuit modifies the energy available in the power supply so that the pacing stimulus has duration (pulse width) and amplitude (measured in volts or milliamperes). The frequency of stimulation is determined by the *timing* circuit, which, like many modern wrist watches, consists of a crystal oscillator. Depending on the nature of the pacemaker device and the lead orientation, the output stimulus may be applied to the atrium or to the ventricle or to both chambers in sequence (Fig. 1). In the last instance, two output and

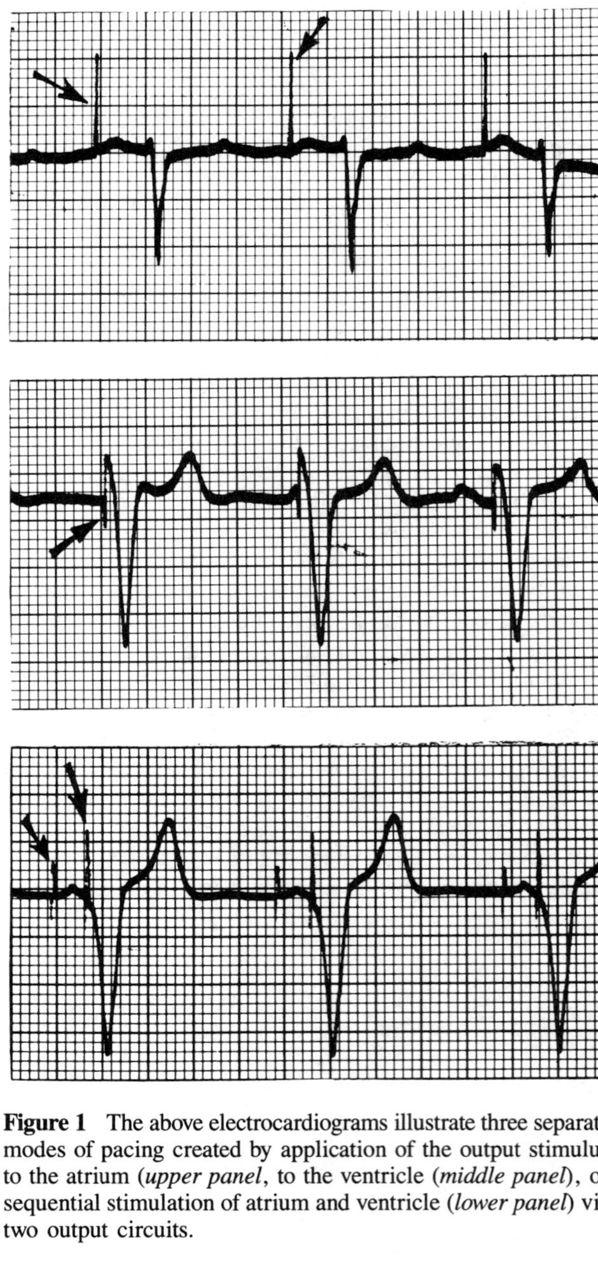

Figure 1 The above electrocardiograms illustrate three separate modes of pacing created by application of the output stimulus to the atrium (*upper panel*, to the ventricle (*middle panel*), or sequential stimulation of atrium and ventricle (*lower panel*) via two output circuits.

* Feedthrough is a conductor surrounded by an insulator that allows passage of electricity between circuit components separated by a nonconductive partition.

timing circuits are required for sequential stimulation. Finally, to avert competition with native rhythms, a *sensing* circuit (or amplifier) is interposed between the output circuit and the appropriate cardiac chamber. The pacing lead offers the "efferent" pathway by which the output stimulus reaches the heart. It serves a second role as an "afferent" limb by which the sensing amplilfier of the pulse generator detects native intracavitary P waves or QRS complexes.

The increasing complexity of modern-day cardiac pacing systems has mandated the use of a descriptive code for the various modes of pacing (Table 1). Conventional VVI pacemaker devices remain in common use, often modified by a biologic sensor that modulates pacing rate in response to various measures of physical exercise (venous temperature, respiratory rate, Q-T interval, body vibrations). Dual-chamber systems employ output, sensing, and timing circuits for both atrial and ventricular channels with separate timing for the atrioventricular delay.

INDICATIONS FOR PACING

Clinical evidence of symptomatic bradyarrhythmia predominates as the leading indication for temporary or permanent cardiac pacing. Transient bradycardia following cardiopulmonary bypass with or without ventricular ectopy often responds to single-chamber atrial pacing (AOO or AAI) or to dual-chamber (DVI) stimulation without having to resort to implantation of a permanent device. Concerns over inappropriate use of permanent pacing systems have been voiced at local, state, and national levels and have been the subject of congressional review. Physicians who prescribe or implant pacing devices must familiarize themselves with existing Medicare implant guidelines (Table 2). Preadmission, preprocedure approval of all pacemaker procedures (except those performed as emergencies within 24 hours of hospital admission or those performed as outpatient procedures) is now required by Medicare through the regional Peer Review Organization (PRO). In general, the guidelines are reasonable, although accurate, graphic documentation in the patient's hospital record is essential, since the records of all Medicare age pacemaker patients are now reviewed before payment to the hospital is approved.

TECHNIQUE OF PACEMAKER INSERTION

A detailed description of all of the technical aspects of pacemaker implantation is not appropriate. The pacing leads in the past were inserted via cutdown on the cephalic or external jugular vein, but this technique has been almost completely displaced by the subclavian puncture technique. Epicardial pacing is confined to temporary postoperative pacing, infants, or those patients in whom a mechanical prosthesis in the tricuspid position precludes transvenous passage of a pacing lead into the right ventricle. The technique of dual lead insertion via a single subclavian puncture is our preferred method and is shown in Figure 2. J-shaped leads are positioned in the right atrial appendage when this structure is present. For those patients who have undergone prior surgical resection of the appendage, an active fixation lead containing an extendible fixation screw is employed. Tined ventricular leads are positioned in the right ventricular apex, with the tips snared in the trabeculations to minimize subsequent displacement. Results vary according to individual operator experience and patient population. In a busy center (over 50 implants per year), fewer than 1 percent of ventricular leads should require subsequent repositioning as a result of displacement. The atrial lead position is less reliable, and somewhere between 5 to 10 percent of atrial leads can be expected to show partial or complete failure to perform as intended during the early weeks following insertion. This is often a time-related phenomenon and tends to diminish with continued observation as the lead tip becomes more firmly fixed to the atrial endocardium.

TABLE 1 International Pacemaker Code *

Code Position	*I*	*II*	*III*	*IV*	*V*
Designation**	Chamber(s) paced	Chamber(s) sensed	Pacemaker response	Programmable options	Tachyarrhythmia options
Letters used	0 = No pacing V = Ventricle A = Atrium D = Dual (i.e., A and V)	0 = None V = Ventricle A = Atrium D = Dual (i.e., A and V)	0 = None I = Inhibited T = Triggered D = Dual (i.e., I and T)	0 = None P = Simple programmable (rate output) M = Multiprogrammable C = Communicating; i.e., telemetry R = Responsive rate pacing	B = Bursts N = Normal rate competition S = Scanning E = External

* The five position pacemaker code. At present, it is conventional to utilize the first four positions routinely, with the fifth position being specified only when antitachycardia pacing functions are available.
**Manufacturer's designation only: S = single chamber

TABLE 2 Medicare Indications for Cardiac Pacemakers (Medicare Carriers Manual, Transmittal #1094, May 1985)

Group I Single-Chamber Pacemakers		*Group II Dual-Chamber Pacemakers*	
Covered	Not Covered	Covered	Not Covered
A. Conditions under which implantation of a cardiac pacemaker is generally considered acceptable or necessary provided the condition is chronic or recurrent and not due to transient causes, such as acute myocardial infarction, electrolyte or drug imbalance.	B. Additional claims development may be required; conditions that although used by some physicians as bases for permanent pacing are considered unsupported by adequate evidence of benefit and therefore should not be considered appropriate uses for single-chamber pacers in the absence of foregoing indications.	A. Conditions under which implantation of a dual-chamber cardiac pacemaker is considered acceptable or necessary in the general medical community unless conditions 1 and 2 under Group II B are present.	B. Whenever the following conditions that represent overriding contraindications are present, dual-chamber pacemakers are *not* covered.
1. Acquired complete heart block 2. Congenital complete heart block with severe bradycardia or symptoms due to slow rates. 3. Type II second-degree heart block. 4. Type I second-degree heart block with significant symptoms of hemodynamic instability due to the heart block. 5. Sinus bradycardia (heart rate below 50/min) with major symptoms (e.g., syncope, seizures, confusion, congestive heart failure). Must correlate association of symptoms with bradycardia. 6. Sinus bradycardia of 50–59/min with dizziness or confusion clearly due to the bradycardia. 7. Sinus bradycardia that is the consequence of necessary drug therapy for which there is no alternative and when the bradycardia clearly causes symptoms (i.e., seizures, syncope, congestive heart failure).	1. Syncope of undetermined cause. 2. Sinus bradycardia without significant symptoms. 3. Sinoatrial block or arrest without significant symptoms. 4. Prolonged R–R' intervals in atrial fibrillation without third-degree heart block or with other causes of transient ventricular pause. 5. Bradycardia during sleep.	1. Patients in whom single-chamber ventricular pacing at the time of insertion elicits a definite drop in blood pressure, retrograde conduction, or discomfort. 2. Patients in whom pacemaker syndrome due to atrial or ventricular asynchrony and significant symptoms has already been experienced with a pacemaker that is being replaced.	1. Ineffective atrial contractions such as chronic atrial fibrillation, flutter, or giant left atrium. 2. Frequent or persistent supraventricular tachycardias except when the pacemaker is used for the control of the tachycardia. 3. A clinical condition in which pacing takes place only intermittently and briefly and is not associated with a reasonable likelihood that the pacing need will become prolonged, such as in the occasional patient with hypersensitive carotid sinus syndrome with syncope due to bradycardia that is unresponsive to medical measures.

INTRAOPERATIVE LEAD TESTING

The physician performing the implant attempts to work the ventricular lead tip into the trabeculations of the right ventricular apex. A properly positioned lead will "hold" its tip position when slight traction is created on the body of the lead. Measurement of the stimulation threshold and the intracavitary QRS amplitude is essential to ensure subsequent acceptable lead performance. A ventricular lead that is properly impacted against healthy endocardium will display elevation of the S-T segment on the endocardial electrogram with a QRS amplitude in excess of 6 mV. Although such recordings may be accomplished by a conventional, properly grounded ECG machine or oscilloscope, a commercial pacemaker systems analyzer offers a more accurate determination of parameters. A stimulation threshold of below 1 V and 1 mA is expected with present-day ventricular leads when testing at a pulse duration of 0.5 msec. For atrial leads, a 'P" wave amplitude of 2.0 mV or greater and a threshold comparable to that of the ventricular lead are anticipated. When comparable figures are not obtained, repositioning of the lead(s) in another location or switching to a different lead design (such as active fixation) is appropriate, since high stimulation thresholds and low intracavitary signals almost invariably lead to subsequent unacceptable pacemaker performance postoperatively. Representative lead positions are illustrated in Figure 3.

TABLE 2 Medicare Indications for Cardiac Pacemakers (Medicare Carriers Manual, Transmittal #1094, May 1985) (Continued)

Group I Single-Chamber Pacemakers		*Group II Dual-Chamber Pacemakers*	
Covered	Not Covered	Covered	Not Covered
8. Sinus node dysfunction with or without tachycardias when accompanied by significant symptoms. 9. Sinus bradycardia plus potentially life-threatening ventricular tachyarrhythmias. 10. Bradyarrhythmias associated with supraventricular tachycardia when the bradycardia is associated with significant symptoms. 11. The occasional patient with hypersensitive carotid sinus syndrome with syncope due to bradycardia. 12. Bifascicular or trifascicular block accompanied by syncope, which is attributed to transient complete heart block. 13. Prophylactic pacer following acute myocardial infarction associated with complete heart block plus bundle branch block. 14. "Overdrive" pacing for refractory ventricular tachycardia. 15. Type I second-degree heart block with a prolonged QRS complex.	6. Right bundle branch block and left axis deviation and other forms of fascicular or bundle branch block without syncope or other symptoms of intermittent atrioventricular block. 7. Asymptomatic second-degree heart block of type I unless the QRS complexes are prolonged or electrophysiologic studies have demonstrated that the block is at or beyond the level of the bundle of His.	3. Patients in whom even a relatively small increase in cardiac efficiency will importantly improve the quality of life, e.g., in patients with congestive heart failure that is refractory to medical treatment. 4. Patients in whom the pacemaker syndrome can be anticipated, such as young active individuals.	4. Prophylactic pacemaker use following recovery from acute myocardial infarction associated with temporary complete and/or type II second-degree atrioventricular block in association with bundle block.

PACEMAKER FOLLOW-UP

As with most forms of medical care, the physician's responsibility does not end with the implantation of a cardiac pacemaker. Not only does the patient require periodic assessment of general medical and cardiovascular problems and regulation of medications, but the pacemaker device, itself, must be subjected to careful scrutiny. With most patients, this overall care is provided through a blend of direct physician-patient contact at 3- to 6-month intervals coupled with intervening telephone monitoring of pacemaker performance according to a schedule established by Medicare. In brief, this latter schedule acknowledges the need for high-risk and low-risk device follow-up schedules, and the choice is left up to the prescribing physician based on individual device and patient considerations. The majority of present-day, lithium-powered pacemaker devices offer dependable performance for 5 to 10 years with differences based upon battery capacity, frequency and mode of stimulation, and pacer output settings.

The risk of the pacemaker implant procedure should be close to zero as far as operative death is concerned. Infection following a primary implant procedure should be well less than 1 percent; infections, when they occur, are most commonly the result of mechanical erosions or of reoperations for revision of lead position. Technical flaws in the pacemaker system design, are, fortunately, extremely rare despite articles in the news media to the contrary.

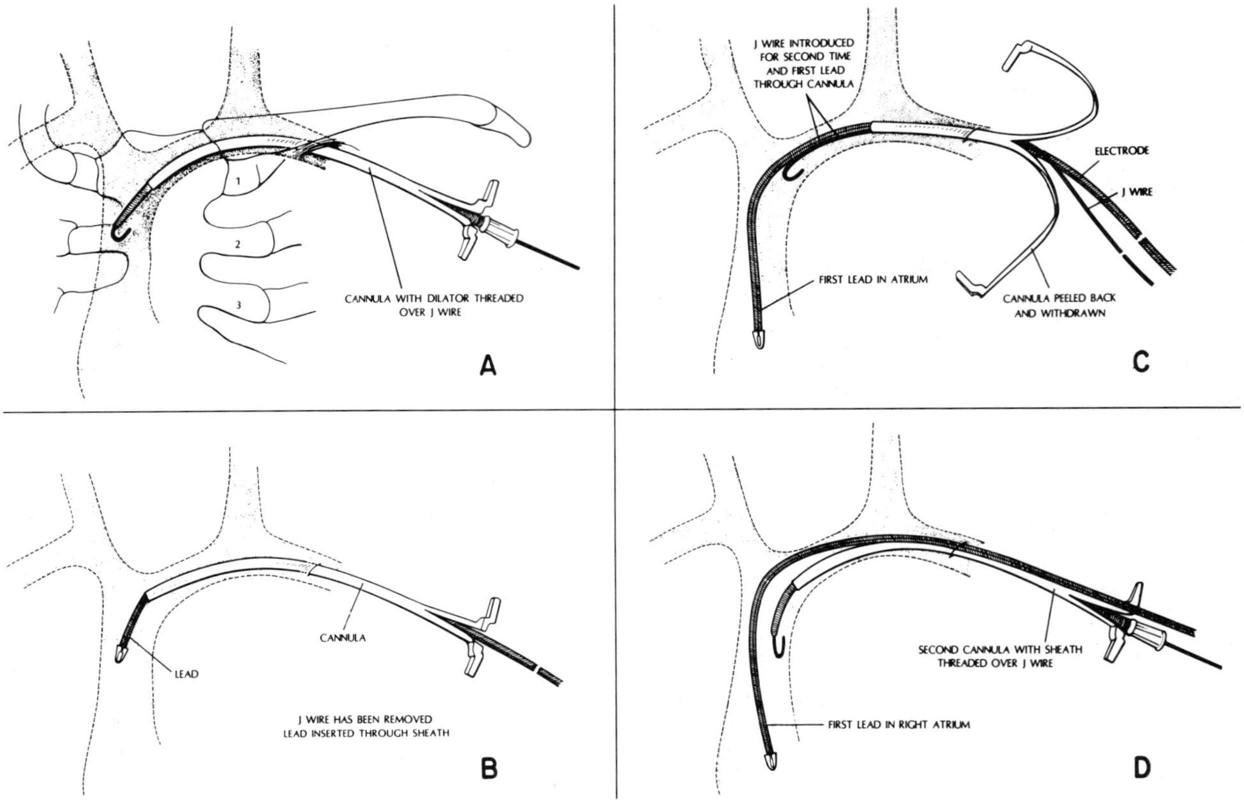

Figure 2 The consecutive steps that are followed to insert two pacing leads via the subclavian approach with a single puncture are illustrated. In *A*, after successfully puncturing the subclavian vein, a curved wire guide and overriding introducer sheath are advanced to the level of the right atrium (confirmed by fluoroscopy). In *B*, the obturator and wire guide have been removed and replaced with a pacing lead. In *C*, the introducer sheath is "peeled away" after reinserting another introducer wire alongside the pacing lead. In *D*, a second introducer is advanced over the wire guide, and the steps illustrated in *B* and *C* are repeated. Note that it is essential to position the patient in the Trendelenburg position throughout this maneuver to minimize ingress of air, and that the introducer sheath should be occluded by manual compression until the lead is inserted. Similarly, it is appropriate to clamp the guidewire to the sterile drapes to minimize dislodgement out of or into the venous system.

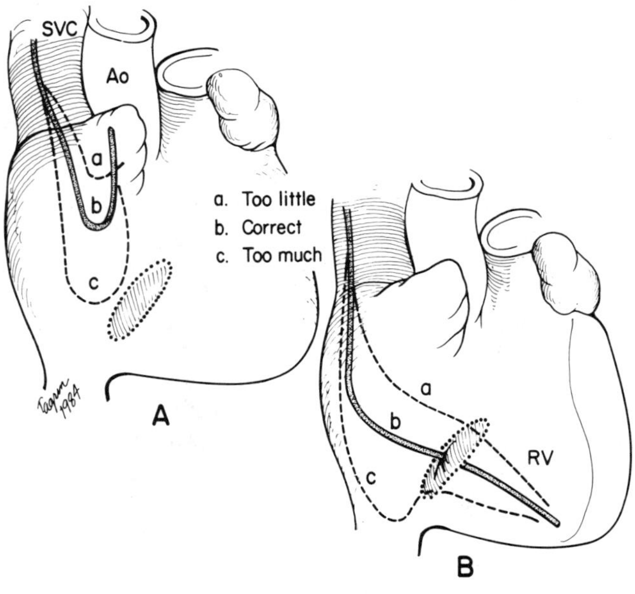

Figure 3 Fluoroscopic image of atrial and ventricular leads during normal respiration when properly positioned. (From Harthorne JW. Cardiac pacing. In: Cheng TS, ed. International textbook of cardiology. New York: Pergamon Press, 1986:387.)

SELECTION OF PACEMAKER DEVICE

As noted in Table 2, Medicare guidelines are now fairly precise as to what type of device is considered suitable for the individual patient. Nonetheless, those responsible for the patient's welfare must prescribe what best suits the patient's individual needs from the standpoint of cardiovascular physiology. Conventional, single-chamber pacemakers are best suited for those patients who have chronic atrial fibrillation and slow ventricular rates. When exercise bradycardia (chronotropic incompetence) is also documented, one of the newer, sensor-based pacemakers that raises ventricular paced rates in response to activity, Q-T interval, or respiratory rate offers improved exercise capacity. It must be recognized that ventriculoatrial conduction following paced ventricular beats may occur and negate the advantages of such adaptive rate devices. When the atria remain in normal sinus rhythm, coupled with the presence of complete heart block or sinus node dysfunction, the advantages of atrial transport to cardiac function in the active patient favor the selection of a dual-chamber pacemaker device (or less frequently an atrial pacemaker). Each patient must be considered individually and the choice of device made with a clear recognition of the ultimate goal of pacing relative to the patient's age and lifestyle.

SUGGESTED READING

Barold SS, ed. Modern cardiac pacing. Mt. Kisco, NY: Futura Publishing, 1985.

Furman S, Hurzeler P, DeCaprio V. Cardiac pacing and pacemakers. III. Sensing the cardiac electrogram. Am Heart J 1977; 93:794–801.

Harthorne JW, McDermott J, Poulin FK. Cardiac pacing. In: Johnson RA et al, eds. The practice of cardiology. Boston: Little, Brown, 1980.

TUMORS

CARDIAC TUMORS

GRADY L. HALLMAN, M.D.
R. CRAIG KUYKENDALL, M.D.

Primary neoplasms of the heart are rare, and autopsy series report incidences ranging from 0.001 percent to 0.28 percent. Approximately 70 percent of such tumors are benign, and in adults nearly one-half are myxomas. The other 30 percent of primary cardiac neoplasms are malignant. These malignant tumors are usually highly aggressive, and death may occur within one year of diagnosis. In children and infants, the most common cardiac neoplasm is the rhabdomyoma.

The clinical presentation of benign tumors varies, depending upon size and location, and ranges from asymptomatic to severe incapacitation. Most commonly signs are related to obstruction of blood flow through valves or cardiac chambers. For example, a myxoma in the left atrium may mimic mitral stenosis because of obstruction of the mitral valve. Prolapse of a tumor through a valve orifice may produce annular dilatation and result in valvar regurgitation, usually in addition to partial obstruction. Fragments of the tumor may produce emboli. The conduction system may be disturbed, and life-threatening arrhythmias may be present.

The gold standard for diagnosis of cardiac tumors is cardiac catheterization and angiocardiography. Two-dimensional echocardiography may be sufficient, especially with intracavitary lesions such as myxomas.

BENIGN CARDIAC TUMORS

Myxoma

Myxoma is the most common cardiac tumor, and approximately 75 percent occur in the left atrium. Operation is indicated after the lesion is demonstrated by appropriate studies. If the lesion is pedunculated and on the left side of the heart, operation should not be delayed and may be necessary on an urgent basis, particularly if embolization has occurred.

Surgical Technique

The heart is exposed through a median sternotomy. Manipulation of the heart during cannulation is kept to a minimum in order to prevent intraoperative fragmentation and embolization. Total cardiopulmonary bypass is instituted, using a single arterial and double caval cannulas for left atrial lesions. The aorta is cross-clamped, and cold cardioplegic solution is infused into the aortic root to obtain diastolic arrest. If the myxoma is in the left atrium, the first incision is made into the left atrium posterior to the interatrial groove. The cavity is gently explored to confirm the diagnosis and locate the tumor's site of origin, which usually is the fossa ovalis. A second incision is made in the lateral right atrial wall, and the right atrium and right ventricle are explored. When the tumor arises at the fossa ovalis, the entire atrial septum is excised, working from the right side and perhaps guided by an instrument or finger in the left atrium. Care must be taken not to fragment the tumor. The septum and tumor then can be removed en bloc through the right atrium. Routine wide excision of tumor and septum should prevent local recurrence. If the tumor arises from a site other than the fossa ovalis, it should be removed with a full-thickness of atrial wall if possible, or a wide resection of endocardium should be performed in continuity with the base of the tumor.

After the specimen is removed, the mitral valve and left ventricle are explored for mitral valve damage, residual tumor fragments, or multicentric tumors. Rarely, the mitral valve or annulus has been damaged to the extent that valve replacement or annuloplasty is required. The cardiac chambers are irrigated with saline solution to remove any tumor fragments. The atrial septal defect is then closed with a Dacron patch. Atrial incisions are closed, air is evacuated from the heart, and the operation is completed.

Right atrial myxomas are approached in a slightly different way, but the goals are the same. Venous cannulation for cardiopulmonary bypass is accomplished by placing one cannula directly into the superior vena cava and the second into the inferior vena cava via a common femoral vein or perhaps directly into the supradiaphragmatic inferior vena cava. An incision is made into the lateral aspect of the right atrium, and the tumor is excised widely as described earlier, removing the atrial septum if the tumor is attached to it. The left atrium can be explored through the excised septum or via an incision posterior to the interatrial groove. If the tricuspid annulus is dilated sufficiently, annuloplasty may be required. The atrial septal defect is repaired with a Dacron patch, and all atriotomies are closed.

Myxomas of either the left or right ventricle are extremely rare. They should be approached through the corresponding atrium and atrioventricular valve (AV). Excision should include tumor and adjacent tissue at its base. Full-thickness excision usually is not necessary because local recurrence after excision of ventricular myxomas has not been reported.

We have had no deaths and no tumor recurrences in our experience with this approach. Arrhythmias, particularly supraventricular, are common during the early postoperative period, but most patients have converted to sinus rhythm by the time of discharged from the hospital.

Rhabdomyomas

Cardiac rhabdomyomas are the most common cardiac neoplasms in infants and children. They occur in the ventricles and may be multicentric. Approximately half of these patients have tuberous sclerosis and a short life span.

Indications for operation vary with the clinical situation. For instance, infants with tuberous sclerosis who are asymptomatic and have multicentric tumors should not have surgery. On the other hand, otherwise healthy infants who are symptomatic and have a single tumor obstructing flow through a ventricular cavity with resultant heart failure should undergo excisional therapy.

Surgical Technique

Operation is accomplished using cardiopulmonary bypass and moderate hypothermia. The tumor location is usually known preoperatively, and the approach is tailored appropriately. If possible, the tumor is approached via an atriotomy, working through an atrioventricular valve, although a ventriculotomy may be required. All gross tumor including the base is excised. If the tumor involves valve structures or impinges on conduction pathways, palliative resection is indicated. Rhabdomyomas do not have significant growth potential, and some have spontaneously regressed. Resulting defects in the septum or ventricular free wall are closed primarily or patched with Dacron or pericardium.

Other Benign Tumors

The clinical presentation and operative approach to benign primary cardiac tumors other than myxomas or rhabdomyomas depend on their size and location and on the effect they may have on cardiac rhythm.

In adults, the diagnosis and location of a tumor are usually made by echocardiogram or cardiac catheterization during the work-up of a symptomatic patient. Thus, diagnosis of the tumor is indication enough for excision to relieve the patient of disabling symptoms. Moreover, all patients with a diagnosis of cardiac neoplasm require exploration to make a histologic diagnosis and rule out malignancy. Specific complications caused by the tumor need to be addressed. For instance, tumor-induced valve dysfunction may require valve replacement or annuloplasty, irritative foci may necessitate cryoablation in addition to tumor excision to eradicate arrhythmogenic foci, and intracavity tumors require excision to allow unimpeded flow of blood.

Surgical Technique

Operation is performed through a median sternotomy. After the heart is inspected, cardiopulmonary bypass is instituted and cardioplegic solution injected. Epicardial tumors are excised, and the resultant defect closed primarily. Endocardial tumors are removed through an appropriate atriotomy working across the AV valve. If this is technically not feasible, then a ventriculotomy is made, the tumor excised, and the ventricle is closed. Since these tumors are benign, careful judgment must be used in deciding on extent of excision, because the tumor may involve critical cardiac structures such as valves or conduction pathways. It may be wiser to debulk such tumors, leaving behind gross disease, rather than to attempt total excision if radical surgery might prejudice recovery.

Special Considerations in Infants

Infants with small tumors may present with refractory ventricular tachyarrhythmias that may lead to sudden cardiac arrest or death. Fourteen such infants recently have been treated successfully at the Texas Heart Institute. Eleven had hamartomas, sometimes called Purkinje cell tumors. Only rarely can a tumor mass be seen preoperatively by the usual diagnostic modalities such as echocardiogram or catheterization, but electrophysiologic studies pinpoint the location of an ectopic focus. Operative exploration of these infants is the treatment of choice because most do not respond to currently used antiarrhythmic agents.

Surgical Technique

The gross appearance of most of these tumors is subtle. Operative mapping confirms preoperative electrophysiologic studies and indicates which area to excise. Care is taken to maintain normothermia during mapping of arrhythomogenic foci because they are sensitive to body temperature changes. Chronotropic anesthetic agents also are avoided for similar reasons. After the heart is exposed through a median sternotomy, epicardial mapping is performed in the beating heart. A removable clip-on lead that acts as a bipolar reference electrode is placed near the apex of the beating heart. Sensing probes are passed over the epicardium until the point of earliest excitation is identified. Operative mapping has confirmed preoperative electrophysiologic mapping in all cases. Once the focus is identified, the patient is cannulated and placed on cardiopulmonary bypass using standard techniques. Cardioplegia is used to arrest the heart. If an obvious tumor is seen, simple excision is adequate, since malignancy or recurrence has not been encountered. Often the findings are subtle, consisting of flat, gray areas; some have appeared completely normal. The suspected area is excised or is biopsied and cryoablated. Results so far have been excellent, and tachycardia has not recurred in any patient.

Antiarrhythmic drugs have not been required following surgery.

MALIGNANT CARDIAC TUMORS

Most primary malignant tumors are sarcomas, most commonly angiosarcomas arising in the right atrium. These are extremely aggressive, and few patients survive beyond one year. They locally invade the heart and surrounding mediastinal structures, and almost 80 percent have metastasized at the time of diagnosis. Clincial manifestations vary widely and include chest pain, heart failure, conduction abnormalities, obstruction of blood flow, and hemopericardium. All patients with malignant cardiac neoplasms require exploration to assess potential for resection or debulking or both. Resection requires judgment and is rarely for cure. Palliative resections are the rule and must be tailored to meet individual circumstances. Our experience has included valve replacement, resection or debulking of tumor, and cardiac repair. Hemopericardium progressing to tamponade requires emergency exploration and pericardectomy. Postoperative radiation and chemotherapy may provide satisfactory palliation.

SUGGESTED READING

Kabbani S, Cooley DA. Atrial myxoma: surgical considerations. J Thorac Cardiovasc Surg 1973; 65:731–737.

Kirklin JW, Barratt-Boyes BG. Cardiac tumors. In: Kirklin JW, Barratt-Boyes BG, eds. Cardiac surgery: morphology, diagnostic criteria, natural history, techniques, results and indications. New York: John Wiley & Sons, 1986.

McAllister HA, Fenoglio JJ. Tumors of the cardiovascular system. In: Subcommittee on Oncology of the National Research Council's Committee on Pathology, ed. Atlas of tumor pathology. Fascide 15, series 2. Washington, DC: Armed Forces Institute of Pathology, 1978.

Ott DA, Garson A, Cooley DA, Smith RT, Moak J. Cryoablative techniques in the treatment of cardiac tachyarrhythmias. Ann Thorac Surg 1987; 43:138–143.

Reece IJ, Cooley DA, Frazier OH, Hailman GL, Powers PL, Montero CG. Cardiac tumors: Clinical spectrum and prognosis of lesions other than classical benign myxoma in 20 patients. J Thorac Cardiovasc Surg 1984; 88:439–446.

TRAUMA

CARDIAC AND THORACIC AORTIC TRAUMA

ALAN D. HILGENBERG, M.D.

The attraction of high-speed vehicle travel, alcohol, drugs, and weapons to some elements of our society leads to injuries that often involve the cardiovascular system. Although cardiac and thoracic aortic injuries may be immediately fatal, emergency management in the field and rapid transportation to the hospital allow some of these patients to reach emergency departments alive. Motor vehicle accidents are responsible for most of the blunt trauma to the heart and aorta, and these patients typically have additional injuries involving the head, abdomen, and skeleton. Penetrating thoracic wounds are now more often the result of handguns than knives; the amount of visceral damage is great and the mortality rate is high.

BLUNT TRAUMA

Cardiac contusion is not a well-defined clinical entity because the diagnosis is not always easily made, the findings are typically transient, the condition is usually well tolerated, and pre-existing cardiac disease may confuse the picture. It is probably common after major blunt chest trauma and varies in seriousness from minor injuries with only electrocardiographic changes or arrhythmias to more serious damage resulting in depressed cardiac output. Chest pain and tachycardia are common. Electrocardiographic changes consisting of S-T segment and T wave abnormalities, conduction disturbances, and arrhythmias occur in about 80 percent of patients with cardiac contusions. Two-dimensional echocardiography and radionuclide angiography are promising diagnostic studies in patients with significant cardiac contusions. Abnormalities noted include those of segmental ventricular wall motion and depressed ejection fraction of either the right or left ventricle. Management involves monitoring and treatment of arrhythmias, and in patients with hemodynamic instability, monitoring and treatment of pulmonary artery and wedge pressures and cardiac output. The prognosis is related to the degree of ventricular dysfunction and to the severity of the associated extracardiac injuries. The mortality rate for patients with cardiac contusions is about 10 percent, although the deaths are usually due to noncardiac causes.

Coronary artery occlusion from blunt trauma occurs infrequently, but it is possible to separate these patients from those with cardiac contusion. These patients present with electrocardiographic evidence of acute myocardial infarction immediately following chest trauma. Once they are stabilized, they should undergo coronary angiography and assessment of ventricular function. Their monitoring and treatment is identical to that of patients with nontraumatic acute myocardial infarction. As yet no direct surgical intervention has been reported, but urgent coronary artery bypass might be considered if the traumatic occlusion is located proximally in a large coronary artery and the diagnosis is established within 1 to 2 hours of the injury. Postinfarction complications such as ventricular aneurysm or ventricular septal defect may require surgical correction, and late coronary artery bypass grafting may be necessary if angina occurs. Repair of these sequelae is usually successful, and operative mortality is low.

Intracardiac defects include valvular injuries, ventricular septal defects, and ventricular aneurysms, and all are rare occurrences after blunt trauma. Aortic, mitral, and tricuspid injuries are noted in descending order of frequency. All lesions present as valvular insufficiency. Traumatic aortic insufficiency is typically diagnosed weeks or months after injury, and it is due to avulsion of the valve attachment to the aorta at a commissure or to leaflet rupture. Most patients require elective surgical treatment, since the lesion is usually progressive. Surgery is indicated if the patient is symptomatic or if left ventricular function is deteriorating. Aortic valve replacement is recommended, since attempts at valve repair have had a high failure rate. Elective valve replacement can be done with a low mortality and excellent prognosis. The very rare mitral and tricuspid valve injuries present as valvular insufficiency caused by papillary muscle disruption, ruptured chordae tendinae, or a leaflet tear. The indication for operative intervention is the development of symptoms of congestive heart failure that are unresponsive to medical management. Valve repair or replacement is necessary depending upon the exact site of injury, and if done electively, it should be associated with a low operative risk.

Blunt trauma can result in a ventricular septal defect (1) directly from the forces of injury; (2) from delayed rupture of a severely contused septum; and (3) from traumatic coronary artery occlusion, septal infarction, and then rupture. Most patients with a traumatic ventricular septal defect complain of dyspnea and have signs of a loud systolic murmur and congestive heart failure from the left-to-right shunt. Studies should include right-sided heart catheterization, left ventriculography, and coronary arteriography. Medical management should be tried initially. Surgery is required with continuing symptoms and the presence of a 2:1 or larger shunt. If urgent repair is necessary soon after the injury, the defect is exposed through the most severely damaged area of ventricular myocardium and closed with a prosthetic patch. If the patient can be treated medically for several weeks, then elective repair can be done with minimal risk.

A true ventricular aneurysm can develop after blunt trauma from a severely contused segment of myocardium or from an infarcted area secondary to traumatic coronary artery occlusion. Symptoms and radiologic findings usually occur weeks or months after the injury. Once the diagnosis is established by catheterization, elective aneurysm repair is usually recommended regardless of the severity of symptoms, since complications in untreated patients are common. The operative risk is low since the patients are usually young and do not have diffuse coronary artery disease.

Rupture of the heart after blunt trauma is compatible with short-term survival if the cardiac injury is small (particularly if located in one of the atria) and the pericardium is intact. These patients uniformly present with cardiac tamponade and often have cyanosis of the upper half of the body. Pericardiocentesis may be diagnostic and may provide temporary hemodynamic improvement. When this injury is suspected, urgent thoracotomy offers the only hope of survival. If the patient's hemodynamics deteriorate, an emergency room left anterior thoracotomy can provide adequate exposure. However, the ideal situation is to transport the patient to the operating room for a median sternotomy. The sites of injury in the reported cases in order of frequency are right atrium (50 percent), left atrium (24 percent), right ventricle (17 percent), and left ventricle (9 percent). Direct suture repair without cardiopulmonary bypass is usually possible.

Traumatic rupture of the aorta requires urgent diagnosis and therapy for survival of the minority of patients with this injury who reach a hospital alive. The history of an accident involving sudden deceleration and the finding on a chest x-ray film of mediastinal widening and obscuring of the aortic knob contour strongly suggest an aortic injury. We find the computed tomographic scan unable to consistently make the diagnosis of an aortic false aneurysm or to reliably exclude it. Therefore we proceed directly with an aortogram to demonstrate the presence of the injury and to pinpoint its location. Ninety-five percent of the clinical injuries are located in the upper descending aorta just distal to the left subclavian artery. The remaining 5 percent occur in the ascending aorta, the aortic arch, the distal thoracic aorta, or in multiple sites. Once the diagnosis is established, in most cases treatment involves emergency surgical repair. For the usual injury in the upper descending aorta, exposure is via a left thoracotomy, and the aorta is repaired by insertion of a short tubular Dacron graft. If the injury appears straightforward, we use simple cross-clamping and control of the proximal blood pressure by pharmacologic means and try to keep the occlusion time less than 30 minutes. If distal perfusion is to be used, a 9-mm Gott shunt is placed between the proximal aortic arch and the distal thoracic aorta. In our experience survival following surgical repair occurs in approximately 75 percent of the patients, and paraplegia occurs in less than 5 percent. If the false aneurysm is located in the ascending aorta, the operation includes median sternotomy, cardiopulmonary bypass, and insertion of a Dacron graft. For aortic arch injuries, which usually involve avulsion of an arch branch, operation involves median sternotomy, placement of a Dacron bypass graft from the ascending aorta to the innominate artery or other involved arch branch, and oversewing of the aorta at the origin of the false aneurysm. Shunts have not been used, but electroencephalographic monitoring is desirable in order to detect the rare patient who requires shunting.

Under highly selected circumstances, initial medical management with beta-blocking drugs and antihypertensive agents may be appropriate. These circumstances include concomitant severe head injuries, burns, respiratory failure, and sepsis. Once these conditions have been appropriately treated, aortic repair can be carried out.

PENETRATING TRAUMA

Penetrating wounds to the heart and intrapericardial great vessels can present as cardiac arrest, hemorrhagic shock, or cardiac tamponade.

Cardiac arrest in the presence of a precordial wound requires emergency room thoracotomy if the patient's arrest occurred immediately prior to or shortly after arrival in the emergency room. Treatment involves intubation and ventilation, blood volume expansion, immediate left anterior thoracotomy with digital control of the myocardial injury, rapid suturing of the cardiac wound, manual compression of the heart, and treatment of the underlying rhythm. Survival in approximately one-third of such patients has been reported.

Hemorrhagic shock occurs when a cardiac wound communicates freely with the mediastinum or pleural space through a sizable defect in the pericardium. These patients usually have a gunshot wound and require rapid blood volume administration that may include autotransfusion and prompt thoracotomy with digital and suture control of the cardiac injury. If an emergency room thoracotomy is required, a left anterolateral incision with possible extension across the sternum is most suitable. If the patient can be taken to the operating room, a median sternotomy provides excellent exposure for most injuries. Cardiopulmonary bypass is needed only rarely. Survival of approximately 50 percent of these patients is reported.

Cardiac tamponade should be diagnosed by rapid clinical evaluation. The key signs are hypotension, distended neck veins, elevated central venous pressure, and at times cyanosis of the upper body. Pericardiocentesis may result in temporary hemodynamic improvement in some patients, but it should not be overly relied on as a diagnostic maneuver, since both false-positive and false-negative results may occur. When the diagnosis of tamponade is strongly suspected, we recommend prompt thoracotomy with repair of the cardiac wound. If the hemodynamics deteriorate and do not respond to pericardiocentesis, emergency room left anterior thoracotomy is necessary. If the patient is sufficiently stable to be transported to the operating room, either a median sternotomy or a left anterior thoracotomy can be used, depending on the site of the entrance wound. The right ventricle is the most frequently involved chamber, followed by the left ventricle, atria, and intrapericardial great vessels. Digital control and direct suture repair are usually possible, and cardiopulmonary bypass is rarely necessary. Survival of approximately 90 percent of these patients is reported. We rarely use the limited subxiphoid exploration for suspected cases of tamponade.

Late sequelae of penetrating cardiac wounds are noted in approximately 25 percent of patients who survive initial treatment. The common lesions consist of left-to-right shunts, valvular insufficiency, and ventricular aneurysms. Ventricular septal defects are the most common shunts found, and they are suspected when a systolic murmur is heard in the period of recovery after repair of a penetrating cardiac wound. Asymptomatic patients who have less than 2:1 shunts and normal right-sided heart pressures can be observed. Surgical closure employing cardiopulmonary bypass is required in patients with symptoms of congestive heart failure and shunts greater than 2:1. Communications between the ascending aorta and a right-sided heart chamber such as the right atrium, right ventricle, or pulmonary artery virtually all result in severe symptoms of heart failure, and they all require operative correction. Employing cardiopulmonary bypass, the defect is approached through the ascending aorta with a secondary opening of the right-sided heart chamber if required; the defect is closed either with a prosthetic patch or with direct sutures, depending upon its size. Connections between a coronary artery and a cardiac chamber are rare, but they typically result in progressive enlargement of the fistulous communication with eventual evidence of myocardial ischemia and heart failure. For this reason, the communication should be repaired when discovered, usually by opening the affected right-sided heart chamber and closing the fistula directly with sutures. Valvular insufficiency requires surgical correction if the patient becomes symptomatic and has significant hemodynamic impairment noted on catheterization. Post-traumatic ventricular pseudoaneurysms should be repaired when discovered, since the incidence of complications is high in unoperated patients.

SUGGESTED READING

Akins CW, Buckley MJ, Daggett WM, et al. Acute traumatic disruption of the thoracic aorta: a 10-year experience. Ann Thorac Surg 1981; 31:305–309.

Harley DP, Mena I, Narahara K, et al. Traumatic myocardial dysfunction. J Thorac Cardiovasc Surg 1984; 87:386–393.

Hilgenberg AD, Austen WG. Trauma to the heart and great vessels. In: Haber E, Austen WG, eds. The practice of cardiology. 2nd ed. Boston: Little, Brown, 1988.

Leavitt BJ, Meyer JA, Morton JR, et al. Survival following nonpenetrating traumatic rupture of cardiac chambers. Ann Thorac Surg 1987; 44:532–535.

Tavares S, Hankins JR, Moulton AL, et al. Management of penetrating cardiac injuries: the role of emergency room thoracotomy. Ann Thorac Surg 1984; 38:183–187.

THORACIC AORTA

REPLACEMENT OF THE THORACIC AORTA

E. STANLEY CRAWFORD, M.D.

The diseases or conditions of the aorta for which graft replacement or bypass is employed are trauma, aortitis, infection, coarctation, aortic manifestations of Marfan's syndrome, tumor, medial degenerative aneurysm, aortic dissection, and dissecting aortic aneurysm. The pathologic concepts of disease and the application of grafting techniques employed for its treatment vary with the disease, its location, and extent. These are discussed accordingly except for dissection, which is considered in the chapter *Acute and Chronic Aortic Dissection.*

TRAUMA

Acute Trauma

The author's personal experience in the treatment of acute aortic injury is so small (six patients) that it would not be included here if one observation had not been made. Two patients had severe associated cerebral and skeletal injuries. Quality survival was not expected in either case. Moreover, these and other associated injuries were considered to pose prohibitive risks for operation for laceration and dilatation of the distal aortic arch in one, and laceration, dilatation, and partial upper descending thoracic aortic obstruction in the other. The aortic injury in both cases was treated medically, i.e., as in uncomplicated type III aortic dissection with frequent monitoring of aortic size. Both patients totally recovered, and the injured segment of aorta was successfully replaced at 18 months in one and 24 months in the other because of increase in size.

This anecdotal observation may seem insignificant, but when taken in context with the relatively large number of similar cases reported, its impact on treatment of this potentially lethal injury could be highly significant. Currently, surgeons are under pressure to routinely repair the injury. The results of medical treatment with careful monitoring and tight blood pressure control in selected cases offer a viable option to surgical treatment in the critically injured patient with stable aortic injury.

Chronic Trauma

Traumatic lesions of the aorta tend to remain stable and not rupture after a period of 2 weeks, when they are considered to enter the chronic stage. Subsequently, the injured segment gradually dilates, and its wall becomes calcified in many instances. These calcified lesions are relatively rare, and free rupture into the pleural cavity is not common. These characteristics suggest that when calcified, these lesions are benign, rarely cause trouble, and may be treated conservatively.

This author has employed graft replacement in 34 patients with chronic traumatic aneurysms of the thoracic aorta. The location of the aneurysms was arch in four, upper descending thoracic aorta in 29, and upper abdominal aorta in one. The interval between injury and operation varied from 10 weeks to 37 years. Complications requiring operation included rupture, airway obstruction, compression of other adjacent structures, and erosion into lung, bronchus, and chest wall. All of the author's patients survived operation without significant complications; consequently, elective operation is recommended regardless of size of the aneurysm after a year of recovery from associated injury. Mandatory operation is indicated for appearance of symptoms or sudden increase in size. These patients are usually young, and operation poses little risk. Prophylactic surgery at this age is well tolerated.

AORTITIS

The two common forms of aortitis are Takayasu's and granulomatous or giant cell arteritis. Both are autoimmune diseases, and the systemic manifestations in the active stages of both respond well to steroid therapy. Medical treatment does not cure or relieve either aneurysm or occlusion. In fact, both lesions may arise in the patient while he or she is on steroid therapy.

Takayasu's Aortitis

This disease occurs in both males and females but is most common in females less than 30 years of age. The disease affects the aorta and its major branches. Accurate diagnosis is made only by total aortography visualizing the aorta and its branches. Two-thirds of the lesions are occlusive in nature and one-third are aneurysms. Both types of lesions occur in the same patient. The former produce myocardial infarction, stroke disease, renovascular hypertension, symptoms of aortic obstruction, and aortic dissection. The most common causes of death are aortic dissection and rupture of fusiform aneurysms, either of the aorta or aortic branches.

Aneurysms and dissection may be located in the ascending aorta, ascending aorta and arch, descending thoracic aorta, abdominal aorta, or both descending thoracic and abdominal aortas. Most patients with aneurysms have associated branch vessel obstruction or aneurysm. The aneurysmal disease is treated by graft replacement therapy regardless of stage of disease, and this is usually done in association with branch vessel bypass. Operation is successful in the acute stage using current techniques in contrast to old reports of frequent failure. Failure reported attributable to the acute nature of the disease probably resulted from older techniques.

Granulomatous Aortitis

This disease is the third most common cause of aneurysms after medial degeneration and dissection and occurs in the upper age groups, i.e., over 55 years. Most patients are women over 65 years of age. Although aneurysmal disease may involve any aortic segment, it most commonly involves the thoracic segment and tends to be diffuse in nature, involving the entire thoracic aorta or even the entire aorta. Death occurs from rupture caused by spontaneous aortic laceration (simple bursting) or dissection. Treatment consists of graft replacement, frequently in stages. Steroid therapy relieves systemic manifestations, improves appetite, and may be helpful in preparation of the patient for operation. But surgery should not be delayed if symptoms suggest early rupture, or for more than 7 days in any case.

INFECTION

Mycotic aneurysms occur from bacteremia following instrumentation or distant infections. Bacteria identified from blood or aneurysm culture include *Staphylococcus, Streptococcus, Salmonella*, pneumococci, *Haemophilus influenzae, Bacteroides, Escherichia coli*, and others. The common sites of these aneurysms are the ascending aorta, aortic arch, descending thoracic aorta, and the abdominal aorta in the region of visceral artery origins. Appropriate medical therapy does not prevent rupture. The author recommends immediate submission of preoperative blood cultures and/or material aspirated from the aneurysm by needle before surgery for culture and institution of intravenous broad-spectrum antibiotic therapy. Graft replacement is performed within 24 hours or immediately if there are signs of leakage or rupture. Excised material is submitted for additional cultures. The aortic graft is inserted directly into the débrided aneurysmal cavity. The aneurysmal wall is left open. Intensive intravenous antibiotic therapy is continued for 1 month, and then appropriate oral antibiotics are continued for the rest of the patient's life. This form of therapy has proved effective in 22 patients, 19 of whom have been long-term survivors (>1 year).

Local excision of aneurysm, proximal and distal aortic ligation, and extra-anatomic bypass were not considered in these cases because of the frequency of involvement of aortic segments from which major branches arise, e.g., visceral and brachiocephalic arteries. Moreover, this has not been a satisfactory procedure in treatment of patients with descending thoracic aortic graft infection because of late rupture of false aneurysms of the proximal sutured aortic stump.

Thoracic Aortic Graft Infections

Most graft infections occur following operations on the ascending aorta and arch and result from chest wall wound complications. The infection is usually associated with ruptured false aneurysm located at suture lines. Manifestations include large mediastinal blood collections and intermittent aortocutaneous bleeding. Bacteriologic and antibiotic management of this complication is similar to what has been described for mycotic aneurysm. Surgery is performed by first establishing profound hypothermia and circulatory arrest using femoral vein–femoral artery partial cardiopulmonary bypass. The midsternal wound is then opened, the hematoma evacuated, and the false aneurysm closed by simple suture or, in rare cases, by insertion of an extension of the previously inserted graft or new graft. The area of aortic reconstruction is débrided, cleaned, and covered by viable tissue, muscle flaps mobilized from either the chest wall or omentum. The chest wall is completely closed after inserting tubes for drainage and for local irrigation with antibiotic solution. Eight of the author's nine patients treated by this technique are still alive. One death occurred from a coagulopathy developing at the time of operation.

Bacterial endocarditis including infection of a valve-conduit site may also occur. This type of infection may develop early from bacteremia caused by distant infection, i.e., urinary tract and pulmonary complications, or from infected intravascular catheters. These infections are usually cured by antibiotics and removal or successful treatment of the source. Late infections from bacteremia are also observed. The causes of such bacteremias include the well-known distant sources: dental, urogenital, skin, and others. About 50 percent of these may be successfully treated medically. Operation consisting of valve-conduit or valve replacement is indicated for valve complications. Simple false aneurysms may be treated as above.

Excision of graft and extra-anatomic bypass was performed in two patients who developed infected grafts of the descending thoracic aorta. Despite long-term antibiotic therapy, these patients died at 2 and 3 years, respectively, from rupture of false aneurysms of the aortic stump, even though they were free of infection. Local excision and insertion of new grafts covered with omentum, combined with long-term antibiotics, would now be the procedures of choice for treatment of infected grafts in the descending thoracic aorta.

AORTIC COARCTATION

Late results, 6 months to 2 years, following dilation treatment of coarctation of the aorta have revealed a high incidence of complications, including aneurysms and recurrent obstruction. These findings clearly indicate that surgical treatment by end-to-end anastomosis, patch graft techniques, or graft replacement is the preferred method of treatment of this condition. Because of space limitations, the treatment of the ordinary case will not be discussed.

As Maude Abbott showed many years ago, the aorta in these patients is frequently abnormal, being affected by medial degenerative disease. Aneurysms sometimes occur in association with coarctation or appear later after repair. These lesions may be located in the aortic root or transverse aortic arch, above and below the coarctation. They occur proximal, distal, or both proximal and distal to hemodynamically insignificant coarctation in older patients (pseudocoarctation). These lesions are susceptible to dissection, laceration, and rupture, complications that accounted for 25 percent of the deaths in Abbott's series. Appropriate treatment of coarctation requires total thoracic visualization of the aorta before treatment and careful annual monitoring by appropriate methods after operation and graft replacement of the aneurysms. This author has successfully treated 12 patients with these unusual aneurysms by graft replacement.

AORTIC MANIFESTATIONS OF MARFAN'S SYNDROME

In the natural course of the disease, half of patients with Marfan's syndrome die by the age of 32. The majority of deaths are caused by complications of the cardiovascular system, principally rupture of fusiform aneurysm or aortic dissection. Although fusiform aneurysm may involve any and all segments of the aorta, the most common segment is the ascending aorta and transverse aortic arch. Operation consisting of composite valve graft is now successful in over 95 percent of these cases and should be employed in all patients with complications and electively in others when the diameter of the annular segment is twice that of the uninvolved distal aorta (5 to 6 cm). More distant aneurysms including dissection should be replaced if they are a similar size.

These patients should be closely monitored because multiple aortic segments or even the entire aorta may require replacement in the course of the disease. This author has performed multiple operations including total aortic replacement in 125 patients. Actuarial survival at 15 years is 50 percent, which suggests that surgical treatment of these complications as they appear may double the life expectancy of these patients.

PRIMARY AORTIC TUMORS

Primary aortic tumors are extremely rare. Clinical manifestations include symptoms of aortic obstruction and branch vessel embolic obstruction. Treatment consists of wide local excision and graft replacement for the primary lesion and embolectomy for distal embolization. These tumors are malignant and permanent cure has not been reported, but treatment as described significantly extends life and preserves extremities as well as vital organs.

MEDIAL DEGENERATIVE DISEASE

Most aneurysms of the thoracic aorta are due to medial degenerative disease of unknown etiology. Atherosclerosis may be superimposed on the disease but is rarely the primary cause. Although aneurysms may be localized to a segment, diffuse or multiple segmental involvement including the entire aorta is frequent. Rupture occurs within 5 years in over 90 percent of patients. Operation is recommended when the diameter of the aneurysm is twice that of uninvolved proximal and distal segments and may be performed in stages for diffuse disease or when multiple segments are involved.

TECHNIQUES

The technical aspects of replacement of various aortic segments have been presented in detail by other authors. This section deals only with generalities of current preference of this author. The total experience, including results of operation for aneurysm according to aortic segment for nondissection regardless of factors such as previous operation, infection, and associated diseases, is shown in Table 1.

Ascending Aorta and Arch

Ascending and arch operations are combined since the aneurysm replaced in these cases frequently involves both segments; and although treatment may vary, results are similar regardless of extent. Excision including most of the ascending aorta is performed in most cases to prevent recurrence. Separate valve and graft technique is employed in patients with diseased valves and normal sinus segments. Composite valve grafts are employed when sinus segments are involved. St. Jude valve and valve-conduits are preferred. Porosity of grafts is reduced by albuminization. Coronary arteries are reattached by modified Cabrol's technique using separate 10 mm albuminized Dacron grafts. Brachiocephalic vessels are reattached to the graft by suturing the island of aorta from which they arise to an opening made in the graft. Associated aneurysms of brachiocephalic vessels may be replaced by smaller grafts attached to aortic graft. The aneurysmal wall is excised. Inclusion technique is rarely employed, as in the past.

Cardiopulmonary bypass is required in these patients. Profound hypothermia and circulatory arrest are employed to prevent hemorrhage and to protect the central nervous system, as indicated previously in the treatment of large aneurysms and in those that may be entered during exposure. The technique is also employed during replacement of distal ascending aorta and arch lesions. The author finds that brain temperatures of 21° C allow safe arrest

TABLE 1 Results of Aortic Replacement for Nondissecting Disease

Segment	*Period of Treatment*	*Number of Operations*	*30-Day Survival*
Ascending aorta and aortic arch	12/20/77–6/2/87	325	302 (93%)
Descending thoracic aorta	12/12/56–6/2/87	355	326 (92%)
Thoracoabdominal aorta	6/20/60–6/2/87	753	688 (91%)
Total		1,433	1,316 (92%)

for periods exceeding 1 hour. Peripheral temperature measurements are unreliable in these cases. The electroencephalogram becomes isoelectric at brain temperatures of 21 to 22° C. Patients are monitored with a 12-lead electroencephalograph and are cooled an additional 2 to 5° C (rectal temperature) after brain activity ceases. The arch segment of graft is inserted first, and rewarming is started while the proximal graft is being inserted. The patient is rewarmed to 38° C (rectal). The water bath temperature is maintained at 42° C, and the temperature of the blood returning to the patient is not allowed to exceed 39°C.

Myocardial protection is achieved by hypothermia and intermittent direct coronary artery perfusion with cold hyperkalemic blood solution. Five to 8 L of the latter solution may be used and excess water removed by a Hemofilter unit (Bentley HF-700).

Descending Thoracic Aorta

Operation is performed using double-lumen endotracheal tubes to allow collapse of the left lung. This permits greater exposure and prevents retraction injury to the lungs. The aorta is separated proximally from the left pulmonary artery and clamped proximally either proximal or distal to the subclavian artery and distally beyond the aneurysm. The aneurysm is opened longitudinally and blood recovered for autotransfusion. Bleeding intercostal arteries are transfixed with suture. The graft is inserted by inclusion technique using continuous suture of proximal and distal anastomoses. Air is removed from the graft by flushing and needle aspiration to avoid cerebral embolization.

Thoracoabdominal Aortic Replacement

Anesthesia management is similar to that described previously. Operation is performed through a posterolateral incision that is extended across the costal arch down to the pubis as a midline incision. The descending thoracic aorta is exposed as previously described. The abdominal segment is exposed retroperitoneally by incising the peritoneum in the left gutter and mobilizing the left colon, kidney, spleen, and body and tail of the pancreas upward and to the right. The thoracic aorta is clamped proximally, and the aorta or iliac arteries are clamped distally. The aneurysm is opened and the graft inserted by inclusion technique. Visceral vessels and routes of spinal cord blood supply, D8–12 and L1–2, are reattached to the graft by suturing their origins to openings made in the graft.

Hemodynamic Control and Organ Protection

Cardiac function and proximal blood pressure may be controlled using pharmacologic agents or pump bypass or both. These are monitored by peripheral blood pressure and balloon catheters floated into the pulmonary artery. Equally good results may be achieved by either method and are dependent upon the skill of the anesthesiologist. Distal protection, i.e., renal function and spinal cord, is debatable. Pump bypass both with and without SEP monitoring or hypothermia has not been protective in the author's experience (Tables 2 and 3).

SPECIAL TECHNIQUES

Diffuse aneurysms involving the ascending aorta, arch, and more distal segments require special therapeutic strategies. Survival is best when such extensive aneurysms are replaced in stages, the ascending aorta and arch in one stage and the descending thoracic aorta or thoracoabdominal aorta in another. The order of operation is based on symptoms, size of aneurysm, and cardiac complications. Large symptomatic distant aneurysms are replaced first and then ascending and transverse arch aneurysms are replaced 6 weeks or 2 months later. The order of operation is reversed in patients with large proximal aneurysms associated with aortic insufficiency or coronary artery occlusive disease. Rarely, both segments are removed at one operation through a thoracoabdominal incision using profound hypothermia and circulatory arrest obtained by partial femoral vein–femoral artery cardiopulmonary bypass in the lateral position. This procedure is employed selectively because of the increased incidence of complications and mortality and because aortic root reconstruction cannot be accomplished with this exposure.

The technique of profound hypothermia and circulatory arrest using femoro-femoral partial cardiopulmonary bypass prevents exsanguination and provides a dry field without the need for aortic isolation and clamping. This

TABLE 2 Results with Pump Bypass Including Somatosensory Evoked Potential Monitoring

Extent	*Number of Cases*	*Survival*	*Par/Plg*
Descending thoracic	78	72 (92%)	2 (3%)
Thoracoabdominal	74	63 (85%)	20 (27%)
Total	152	135 (89%)	22 (14%)

TABLE 3 Results without Pump Bypass

Extent	*Number of Cases*	*Survival*	*Par/Plg*
Descending thoracic	277	254 (92%)	13 (5%)
Thoracoabdominal	679	625 (92%)	28 (9%)
Total	956	879 (92%)	41 (4%)

adjunct is useful in treatment of patients with descending thoracic and thoracoabdominal aortic aneurysms in the lateral position. Indications include patients in whom the proximal aorta cannot be isolated for clamping (such as those with huge aneurysms and those with inflammation and scarring), to avoid hemorrhage and exsanguination in patients with contained rupture or clamp lacerations of the aorta or pulmonary artery, and to avoid clamping of the distal aortic arch in patients with atherosclerotic disease of the arch and brachiocephalic vessels that may cause cerebral emboli.

SUGGESTED READING

Cabrol C, Pavie A, Mesnildrey P, Gondjvakhch I, Laughlin L, Bors V, Corcos T, Grondin P. Long-term results with total replacement of the ascending aorta and reimplantation of the coronary arteries. J Thorac Cardiovasc Surg 1986; 91:17–25.

Crawford ES, Crawford JL. Diseases of the aorta including an atlas of angiographic pathology and surgical technique. Baltimore: Williams & Wilkins, 1984.

Crawford ES, Crawford JL, Safi HJ, Coselli JS. Redo operations for recurrent aneurysmal disease of the ascending aorta and transverse aortic arch. Ann Thorac Surg 1985; 40:439–455.

Crawford ES, Stowe CL, Crawford JL, Titus JL, Weilbaecher DG. Aortic arch aneurysm: a sentinel of extensive aortic disease requiring subtotal and total aortic replacement. Ann Surg 1984; 199:742–752.

Gott VL, Pyeritz RE, Magovern GJ, Cameron DE, McKusick VA. Surgical treatment of aneurysms of the ascending aorta in the Marfan syndrome. Results of composite-graft repair in 50 patients. N Engl J Med 1986; 314:1070–1074.

Kouchoukos NT, Marshall WG Jr, Wedige-Stecher TA. Eleven-year experience with composite graft replacement of the ascending aorta and aortic valve. J Thorac Cardiovasc Surg 1986; 92:691–705.

ACUTE AND CHRONIC AORTIC DISSECTION

E. STANLEY CRAWFORD, M.D.

It is generally accepted that life expectancy from untreated aortic dissection is limited, with death occurring frequently during the acute stage from cardiac complications, rupture, arterial obstruction, and multiple organ failure, or during the chronic stage from residuals of these complications and from rupture of fusiform aneurysms that develop in the weakened dissected aortic wall. In fact, follow-up studies of large groups of patients collected from multiple institutions and from single population-based patients indicate that most patients died within 3 months and all were dead within 5 years from onset of disease when untreated. This dismal prognosis of the natural course of the disease may not be entirely correct, as evidenced by the number of patients seen with chronic untreated aortic dissection at all aortic levels. Despite these observations, the author shares the view that dissection is a serious, life-threatening disease because he has rarely participated in the care of a patient with acute aortic dissection involving the ascending aorta who survived without operation and has observed numerous patients with terminal complications of chronic dissection.

It appears that treatment, frequently consisting of surgery, even in the terminal stages of the disease, favorably alters its course. For example, early survival after surgery in the author's 453 patients with both acute and chronic dissection treated by multiple operations (median age of 60 years at first operation) was 85 percent, and long-term actuarial survival at 5 and 10 years was 50 percent and 30 percent, respectively. The effectiveness of surgical intervention was, however, dependent upon early diagnosis and timely application appropriate to the presence or incidence of likely complications. These considerations are determined by the location, extent, and duration of disease. Current therapy is discussed accordingly.

EARLY DIAGNOSIS

Computed tomographic (CT) scanning is the most accurate simple screening test for determining the presence and extent of dissection and outside aortic diameter. It is available to the general medical public to search for etiology of chest, back, and abdominal pain. Its early and frequent application permits diagnosis and more timely referral for surgical therapy. Magnetic resonance imaging, cineangiography, echocardiography, and digital subtraction angiography may be helpful but are inconvenient, impractical, or inadequate and should be reserved for special indications.

Aortography by experienced operators, visualizing the entire aorta and its branches, is equal to or better than CT scanning for diagnosis and gives more information regarding branch vessel involvement and aortic valvular insufficiency (AI). Patency of renal arteries is necessary in the anuric patient. The demonstration of a patent superior mesenteric artery is also advisable in the early acute stage because manifestations of early intestinal ischemia may be masked by other factors and by treatment, including narcotics and anesthesia. Injection of both true and false lumina with contrast agent may be necessary for this purpose.

It is recommended that nonsurgeons use prompt CT scanning for diagnosis and that surgeons add or use aortography to plan treatment and use CT scanning to screen patients later for progression of disease in unreplaced segments or to determine aortic diameter.

CLASSIFICATION OF LOCATION, EXTENT, AND DURATION

The DeBakey classification of location and extent of dissection is employed for this discussion. Type I usually begins at a tear in the proximal ascending aorta and extends distally to involve varying segments up to and including the entire aorta. In rare cases, the tear may be located either in the transverse aortic arch or the descending thoracic aorta and extend distally. In either case, the dissection extends retrograde for varying distances into arch and ascending aorta. The retrograde dissection may be limited to the tubular segment of ascending aorta, or it may extend more proximally and involve both tubular and sinus segments. In still other cases, the aortic commissures and coronary arteries may be involved. Complications of this form include rupture into the mediastinum, pericardium, and heart chamber, cardiac tamponade, myocardial infarction, and AI. Distal complications in type I include distal vessel obstruction and affected organ failure or gangrene in the acute form and chronic ischemia in the chronic form.

Type II dissection arises from a tear in the proximal ascending aorta but rarely extends beyond the innominate artery origin. Proximal extension into the aortic root with complications similar to those enumerated previously is common. This type is more often seen in patients with pre-existing fusiform aneurysms of the ascending aorta, as in patients with Marfan's syndrome.

Type III dissections arise from a tear located in the proximal descending thoracic aorta and extend for varying distances beyond the tear up to and including the entire remaining aorta. Complications include rupture and distal vessel obstruction.

The disease is labile, unpredictable, and frequently associated with complications of the dissecting process during its early stage (2 weeks), after which it becomes more stable and tends to heal (the chronic stage). Regardless, milder complications, for example, AI, may persist and progress, and the dissected aortic wall may gradually dilate into fusiform aneurysm, particularly at the site of origin, and produce the complications associated with other forms of aneurysmal disease.

TREATMENT

Because of the frequency of serious and fatal complications from ascending aortic involvement and the sudden and unpredictable manner in which they may occur, operation is recommended in all patients with acute types I and II dissection as soon as the diagnosis is made. Exceptions include the moribund, the elderly, and those with other limiting, associated nondissection disease.

Treatment of Acute Types I and II

Operation is directed to the ascending aorta regardless of the presence of distal aortic or aortic branch vessel occlusion. Appropriate early proximal operation usually decompresses the distal false lumen and restores distal circulation. When this result is not achieved, distal procedures are more safely performed at the same operation following repair of the ascending aorta.

Patients who enter the hospital with cardiac tamponade are admitted directly to the operating room. The pericardium is aspirated as femoral vein-femoral artery partial cardiopulmonary bypass is instituted under local anesthesia. The patient is then anesthetized, the mediastinum is explored, and appropriate surgery is performed after establishing total cardiopulmonary bypass. Patients without tamponade are admitted to the intensive care unit, fully monitored, and blood pressure reduced with appropriate medication, including narcotics. Total aortography is then performed, and the patient is admitted to the operating room, usually within 2 to 3 hours after admission.

Selection of operative techniques is based on principles dictated by personal experience in primary treatment of 62 patients with acute dissection of the ascending aorta and 120 patients treated for aneurysm, frequently dissecting in origin, occurring after previous ascending aorta or heart operations. Aortoplasty with or without patches is no longer employed because of the tendency of the disease to recur or progress and the tendency of the ascending aorta to dilate into large aneurysm in later stages. The preferred procedure is routine replacement with tubular graft, replacing the entire involved ascending aorta. Replacement is even extended into the arch when it is weakened by the dissection, particularly in patients in whom the tear occurs in the arch and in those with arch rupture. This frequently allows redirection of flow into the true lumen to decompress distal vessel origins and to prevent later fusiform dilation locally beyond the graft. Distal reconstruction is performed without clamps with the patient in the head-down position with the support of cardiopulmonary bypass, profound hypothermia, and circulatory arrest.

Techniques of Distal Reconstruction

Circulation is arrested after the electroencephalogram becomes isoelectric. The ascending aorta is opened and explored. The aorta is transected just proximal to the origin of the innominate artery in patients with types I and II dissections in whom the tear is located proximally and in whom the outer dissected wall has not been damaged distally. The distal dissected aortic wall proximal to the innominate artery in such cases is sandwiched between two strips of Teflon felt, one being placed inside the true lumen, using interrupted sutures placed on tension to stretch the aortic lumen to normal size in order to avoid narrowing. End-to-end anastomosis is then performed between this reconstructed aortic segment and an albuminized knitted Dacron graft. Arch extension requires excision of its lesser curvature. The segment of greater curvature containing the brachiocephalic vessels is preserved and its edges sandwiched between two strips of Teflon felt. The distal anastomosis is performed either between the beveled end of the graft and the reconstructed greater curvature of the aortic arch or to the upper end of descending thoracic aorta. The preserved island of greater curvature containing the origins of the brachiocephalic vessels is reattached to an opening made in the side of the graft.

After completing the distal anastomosis, cardiopulmonary bypass is slowly resumed to fill the aorta, brachiocephalic vessels, and graft with the patient in the head-down position to remove air. The graft is then clamped proximal to the innominate artery origin, full cardiopulmonary bypass is resumed, and rewarming is started. The proximal reconstruction is performed with the patient in the neutral position.

Techniques of Proximal Reconstruction

The currently employed method of proximal reconstruction is based on ascending aortic involvement. In some cases involvement is confined to the tubular segment, which is excised about 10 mm distal to the aortic commissures. The edge of residual proximal aorta is sandwiched between two strips of Teflon felt and attached to the proximal end of the distal graft by continuous suture. The heart and graft are filled in the head-down position to remove air. The clamps are removed, the cardiac apex aspirated, and the proximal graft is vented. The patient's head is elevated when cardiac output returns to normal.

In other cases in which there are undilated sinus segments, the retrograde dissection process may extend into the sinus segment and even dislodge the aortic commissures and produce AI or involve the origins of coronary arteries without producing obstruction or rupture of the outer wall. Proximal reconstruction may be performed in these cases by techniques just described. Resuspension of aortic commissures is made more certain using interrupted through-and-through pledgeted sutures at the level of commissural reattachment.

More commonly, the sinus segment of ascending aorta is either dilated from pre-existing medial degenerative disease or the outer wall of dissection is too thin to preserve or has ruptured or leaked, evident by active bleeding or the presence of epicardial hematoma. In any case, proximal reconstruction is best achieved by composite valve and graft replacement. The aortic valve is excised and the valve end of an albuminized St. Jude composite valve graft is sutured to the aortic annulus. The coronary arteries are reattached according to their involvement. When the coronary artery origins are not involved, they are first reattached by Dacron tubing. One end of a 10-mm albuminized Dacron tube is sutured around the origin of the left coronary artery, and after the composite valve graft has been attached to the annulus proximally and the other graft distally, the other end of the 10-mm Dacron tube is placed posteriorly and along the right side of the aortic graft and attached to the origin of the right coronary artery anteriorly. Coronary artery reattachment is completed by side-to-side anastomosis of this smaller graft to the aortic graft.

When the dissection involves the origins of the coronary arteries, these vessels are oversewn and the coronary circulation is restored by double or triple coronary artery vein bypass grafting extending between the aortic graft and distal coronary artery segments. In the settings described, both methods allow secure reattachment without tension and prevent intraoperative hemorrhage or obstruction and later false aneurysm formation.

Of the 62 patients with acute dissection treated by ascending and arch operation during the past 24 years using techniques available at the time of treatment, 47 (75 percent) survived. Seventeen (85 percent) of the 20 patients treated during the past 2 years employing the principles described were early survivors (30 days). The most important factors determining survival appeared to be earlier diagnosis, immediate operation, profound hypothermia and circulatory arrest permitting open operation, more extensive replacement, and the more recent methods of managing sinus segment involvement.

Treatment of Chronic Types I and II Dissection

The indications for proximal operation in patients with chronic types I and II dissection are dependent on previous treatment. Primary operation is indicated to replace fusiform aneurysms of the ascending aorta or both ascending aorta and arch, either to prevent or relieve complications, including AI, rupture into a heart chamber or externally, and compression of vital structures. Operation is indicated in those previously treated to remove aneurysms occurring proximal and distal to previous operations, false aneurysm at suture lines, AI, infection, aorto-heart chamber fistulas, and other indications listed previously.

In general, the principles of operative technique are similar to those described for patients with acute dissection. Differences in patients with chronic dissection include valve replacement for all patients with AI, and either separate valve and graft replacement in those patients with undilated sinuses, or a composite valve and graft in those with dilated sinus segments. The currently preferred method of coronary artery reattachment is use of Dacron grafts, as described. Vein grafts and internal mammary grafting are employed only in the presence of associated atherosclerotic obstruction; however, previously inserted coronary artery vein bypasses are reattached to the aortic grafts. Teflon felt baffling is rarely necessary, and sandwiching the dissected walls is impossible because of fibrous contraction of wall of true lumen and relative dilatation of false lumen. To avoid distal artery obstruction, the "septum" between true and false lumina is partially excised prior to anastomosis.

The objectives of the redo operation are similar to those described, but techniques may differ. Exposure frequently requires arrest of the circulation prior to chest entry. This is accomplished by femoral vein-femoral artery partial cardiopulmonary bypass and profound hypothermia. Old grafts are removed and replaced with longer grafts, including composite valve-grafts. False aneurysms are simply sutured in some, in others native and old malfunctioning prosthetic valves are replaced, and in still others good functioning prosthetic valves may be preserved by suturing the proximal graft directly to the aortic sewing ring and aorta. Coronary artery origin reattachment is performed by using Dacron grafts. Infections are treated by drainage, débridement, and simple closure of false aneurysms by direct suture. The ascending aorta and arch are covered and perigraft space filled with viable tissue, either muscle from the chest wall or omentum.

Survival in patients treated by graft replacement for chronic dissection of ascending aorta and arch with the full spectrum of complications outlined was 87 percent (118 out of 135). Survival varied with extent of replacement and previous ascending aortic operation. Thus, survival according to these variables was (1) *first operation*, ascending aorta, 94 percent (42 of 45), transverse arch, 100 percent (3 of 3), ascending aorta and transverse arch, 88 percent (25 of 29); *redo operation*, ascending aorta, 88 percent (20 of 23), transverse arch 100 percent (4 of 4), and ascending aorta and arch, 79 percent (24 of 31).

The most common indication for operation in the patient with chronic type I dissection treated initially for acute dissection was for aneurysm of the distal aorta. Chronic obstruction of distal branch vessel was second. These are discussed later.

Acute Type III Dissection

In the experience of the author, the prognosis and treatment of acute type III dissection has depended on its complications at the time of hospital admission. Nineteen patients were treated medically according to Wheat's protocol. One patient, who died, had stroke, paraplegia, renal failure, and poor lung function at the time of admission. Another patient had separate chronic dissection limited to the ascending aorta and acute dissection arising distal to the left subclavian artery. The ascending aortic aneurysm was replaced because a diagnosis of acute type I dissection was made. The distal acute dissection was treated medically, but the patient died 7 days after operation from rupture of the distal aorta. The other 17 patients (90 percent) who entered the hospital in good condition without complications were long-term survivors.

Graft replacement of long segments of the aorta, including descending thoracic or both descending thoracic and abdominal aortas, was performed as a lifesaving procedure in 48 patients who had had complications for some time before admission. These included dissection superimposed on pre-existing large degenerative aneurysms of the descending and thoracoabdominal aortas or enlarged false lumina in patients without pre-existing aneurysmal disease. Both of these groups of patients frequently had rupture. Other complications included obstruction of the aorta or its branches. Five of these patients had irreversible gangrene of the gastrointestinal tract. In addition to extensive replacement, some required partial cardiopulmonary bypass, profound hypothermia, and circulatory arrest in the lateral position to control circulation during operation in order to limit bleeding from rupture or for cerebral protection for arch clamping or reconstruction during operation. The survival rate in these 48 patients was 65 percent (30 of 48). The causes of death were gangrene of the gastrointestinal tract, uremia, sepsis, pulmonary failure, paraplegia, and old age.

Improvement in results may be attributable to early diagnosis and treatment, including medical, prophylactic graft replacement of degenerative aneurysms, and early operation for branch vessel obstruction consisting of proximal graft replacement at the site of the aortic tear and distal redirection of flow into the true lumen. This possibility is suggested by survival in 10 of 11 patients surgically treated during the past 2 years.

Chronic Type III Dissection

Although careful control of hypertension may prevent aneurysmal dilation of untreated dissected aortic segments, many patients developed this complication, including those whose blood pressure continued to be normal. Dilatation occurred in the previously dissected outer wall of the false lumen. Personal observations made in patients with rupture and in those followed without surgical therapy suggest that elective operation is indicated when the external diameter of the dissection is 6 cm or twice that of proximal or distal aorta. Death occurred in 76 percent of such nontreated patients followed for 2 years, with half of the deaths being caused by rupture.

Progression of old dissection in the chronic stage was not observed. New acute dissection was seen occasionally either in the undissected aortic circumference, the outer wall of the old dissection, or at a new aortic site not involved in the initial episode. The presence of new dissection was rarely suspected prior to operation performed for aortic dilatation, and symptoms were thought to be caused by rupture.

Although the initial dissection process may have involved all or mostly all of the aorta, the dilatation requiring operation varies in extent from the proximal descending thoracic aorta in type III to the entire aorta in type I. The ascending aorta and arch are replaced first in the latter cases, and then the remaining aorta is replaced at a second operation. When indications warrant, the order may be reversed.

Distal replacement is performed by inclusion technique. The aorta is clamped between the left common carotid artery and the left subclavian artery (which is also clamped) proximally and distally at appropriate levels. Proximal blood pressure is controlled either by left atriofemoral bypass or by nitroprusside or both, depending on the surgeon's choice. The false lumen is entered, and the inner wall of dissected true lumen is excised. An albuminized knitted graft is sutured proximally to previously inserted graft (type I), or to the aorta just distal to the subclavian artery proximal to the site of the tear (type III) and distally to undilated aorta from which the dissected septum is partially removed, or to the iliac arteries using a bifurcation extension graft. Visceral vessel origins and origins of D8 to L2 intercostal and lumbar arteries are reattached in patients with extensive aneurysms. Reconstruction is completed by suturing the old aortic wall tightly around the graft.

Survival in the author's 117 patients who required replacement of the descending thoracic aorta for chronic dissection was 106 (90 percent), with neurologic disturbances occurring in 6 (5 percent) patients. Survival in 131 patients who required replacement of the descending thoracic aorta and segments up to and including the entire abdominal aorta was 123 (94 percent), with 35 (26 percent) developing lower limb neurologic disturbances. Methods to prevent or reduce paraplegia employed by the author include hypothermia, temporary bypass with and without evoked potential monitoring, and vessel reattachment. These have not been successful. Renal failure, which occurs in 3 percent of patients (primarily in those with pre-existing impaired renal function), has not been prevented by bypass or direct renal artery perfusion with cold Ringer's lactate solution during the period of renal artery isolation from the aortic circulation.

SUGGESTED READING

Cabrol C, Pavie A, Mesnildrey P. Long-term results with replacement of the ascending aorta and reimplantation of the coronary arteries. J Thorac Cardiovasc Surg 1986; 91:17–25.

Crawford ES, Crawford JL, Safi HJ, Coselli JS. Redo operations for recurrent aneurysmal disease of the ascending aorta and transverse aortic arch. Ann Thorac Surg 1985; 40:439–455.

Crawford ES, Crawford JL, Safi HJ, Coselli JS, Hess KR, Brooks B, Norton HJ, Glaeser DH. Thoracoabdominal aortic aneurysms: preoperative and intraoperative factors determining immediate and long-term results of operations in 605 patients. J Vasc Surg 1986; 3:389–404.

Crawford ES, Snyder DM. Treatment of aneurysms of the aortic arch: a progress report. J Thorac Cardiovasc Surg 1983; 85:237–246.

DeBakey ME, McCollum CH, Crawford ES, Morris GC Jr, Howell JF, Noon GP, Lawrie GM. Dissection and dissecting aneurysms of the aorta: twenty-year follow-up of five hundred twenty-seven patients treated surgically. Surgery 1982; 92:1118–1134.

Wheat MW Jr, Palmer RF, Bartley TB, Seelman RC. Treatment of dissecting aneurysms of the aorta without surgery. J Thorac Cardiovasc Surg 1965; 50:364–373.

AORTIC ARCH REPLACEMENT

M. ARISAN ERGIN, M.D.
RANDALL B. GRIEPP, M.D., Ph.D.

Replacement of the aortic arch presents the cardiothoracic surgeon with a unique and demanding technical and tactical challenge. The fundamental logistical problem involves the preservation of the integrity of the central nervous system during the period in the procedure when the aortic arch must be excluded from the circulation for replacement. In the past, a number of cerebral perfusion techniques have been utilized, with unpredictable results. The complexity of these support techniques has contributed to the substantial morbidity and mortality traditionally associated with attempts at replacement of the aortic arch.

The most significant advance in the surgical management of lesions of the aorta requiring the replacement of the aortic arch has been the introduction of "profound hypothermia and circulatory arrest" as the methods of choice for central nervous system preservation during the exclusion of the aortic arch. This has greatly simplified a formidable surgical undertaking and has led to uniformly improved results.

INDICATIONS

Atherosclerotic aneurysms involving the aortic arch constitute the most frequent indication for its resection and replacement. Isolated saccular aneurysms of the arch are rare. Frequently the arch of the aorta is involved in an extension of aneurysmal dilation of varying portions of the ascending and descending aorta with fusiform dilation, requiring concomitant replacement of these segments together with the arch.

Individuals with previously repaired type A or type B dissections often have residual dissection in the aortic arch and go on to develop aneurysmal dilation. The condition of this group of patients represents the second most frequent indication for aortic arch replacement in our experience.

In about 10 to 15 percent of patients with acute dissections of the aorta, the initial intimal tear is located in the arch. These patients should be considered for partial or total replacement of the aortic arch during the acute stage in order to exclude the primary intimal tear.

Among the less frequent indications for replacement of the aortic arch are traumatic tears with subsequent development of false aneurysms, mycotic aneurysms, and aneurysms of the arch related to connective tissue disorders involving the aorta.

Most aneurysms of the aortic arch are detected as a result of findings on a routine chest x-ray film or during the course of a routine work-up for associated cardiovascular disease. Computed axial tomography, digital subtraction aortography, and magnetic resonance imaging delineate the vascular origin of the mediastinal widening seen on the plain films of the chest. Contrast angiography is the mainstay of definitive diagnosis and is invaluable in the preoperative evaluation. It is also the only certain means of localizing the intimal tear in the aortic arch in acute dissections.

In patients with symptoms of compression of surrounding structures, e.g., hoarseness or venous distention and pain, and in those with aneurysms of the arch measuring 9 cm or more, the risk of spontaneous rupture is substantial, and elective replacement of the aortic arch is indicated. Patients with evidence of leak or impending rupture and those with acute dissection of the aorta suspected of having the initial intimal tear in the arch should be considered for emergency replacement of the aortic arch.

There are relative contraindications to the replacement of the aortic arch in patients with advanced biologic age or in those with underlying systemic conditions that preclude a good functional result or a meaningful survival time.

SURGICAL CONSIDERATIONS

Because of the extent of their underlying cardiovascular disease, some patients with aneurysms of the aortic arch require concomitant replacement of various portions of the ascending and descending aortas and of the aortic valve in addition to resection of the aneurysm and the replacement of the aortic arch. A small number of saccular aneurysms of the arch may be amenable to resection with partial occlusion of the aortic arch and aortorrhaphy. Even in these cases, manipulation of the aneurysm may dislodge thrombus and result in distal embolization, with troublesome consequences, especially in the cerebral circulation. For this reason controlled resection and replacement of all arch aneurysms with the aid of cardiopulmonary bypass are the safest surgical methods available. The current method of choice for total prosthetic replacement of the aortic arch is profound hypothermia and circulatory arrest. In this method a combination of surface cooling and cardiopulmonary bypass is used to produce profound total body hypothermia. The aortic arch is then replaced during a single period of circulatory arrest. Cardiopulmonary bypass is then utilized for rewarming.

The anesthetic regimen consists of oxygen, halothane, and morphine sulfate. The electrocardiogram, arterial pressure, pulmonary artery pressure, and esophageal and rectal temperatures are continuously monitored. Arterial blood gases are checked periodically. Following the induction of anesthesia and endotracheal intubation, 250 mg of methylprednisolone is given intravenously and surface cooling is begun with a combination of ice packs and a cooling blanket. We believe that the initiation of hypothermia with surface cooling is essential, since a substantial amount of heat is removed from the body, particularly from the periphery. This considerably shortens the period of core cooling and, more importantly, prevents the shifting of heat from a poorly cooled periphery to central organs during the period of circulatory arrest. When the esophageal temperature reaches 30° C, the ice packs are removed, and the patient is positioned and prepped for a median sternotomy incision.

Operative Technique

A median sternotomy is performed with extension of the incision superiorly along the medial border of the sternocleidomastoid muscle. The left sternothyroid and sternohyoid muscles are transected, and the innominate vein is ligated and divided. Care is taken to preserve the recurrent laryngeal and phrenic nerves as the aortic arch and its three branches are exposed. The pericardium is opened, and following heparinization, cannulation of the superior and inferior vena cavae is carried out. Simultaneously the left common femoral artery is dissected out and used for cannulation for the arterial return. Cardiopulmonary bypass with cooling is begun at a flow rate of 2,500 to 3,000 ml per minute with a disposable bubble oxygenator and an auxiliary heat exchanger. During the period of core cooling, the patient's head is wrapped in towels and packed circumferentially with ice bags to prevent central nervous system warming during the circulatory arrest period.

In cases in which ascending aortic replacement is required, the ascending aorta is cross-clamped at this time, and cardioplegic solution is infused either into the ascending aorta or directly into the coronary orifices. Cardioplegia is supplemented with topical hypothermia during the period of myocardial ischemia for optimal myocardial protection. The proximal portion of the ascending aorta is then excised. The aortic valve is resuspended or replaced as necessary, and a preclotted and autoclaved low-porosity Dacron graft is sutured to the aorta immediately above the aortic valve and coronary ostia with a single continuous 4–0 monofilament suture. If the graft inclusion technique is not feasible, this suture line should be reinforced with a strip of Teflon felt on the outside. The completion of this phase of the operation usually coincides with the end of the core cooling, when the esophageal temperature drops to 12 to 15° C. At this point the flow rate in the bypass circuit is reduced to 100 ml per minute, and arch vessels are clamped individually, or alternately, the patient's head is placed in an extreme Trendelenburg's position to prevent air entrapment in the brachiocephalic vessels during the period of circulatory arrest.

The aneurysm is opened, and the inside of the aortic arch is inspected. Once the aorta, free of significant disease is reached, it is circumferentially incised to prepare for a direct end-to-end graft-to-aorta anastomosis or alternately for anastomosis with the graft inclusion technique. This end-to-end anastomosis is reinforced with an outside strip of Teflon felt, sandwiching the aorta between the graft and the Teflon felt.

Circulatory arrest makes possible the exploration of the arch from within and allows one to accomplish the distal anastomosis in a quiet, bloodless field. The superior portion of the aortic arch is then trimmed to leave a cuff of tissue approximately 5 mm wide around the orifices of three arch vessels. A strip of Teflon felt is tacked to this cuff anteriorly and posteriorly. An ellipse is cut from the top of the graft coming from the descending aorta, and the prepared cuff containing the orifices of the brachiocephalic vessels is anastomosed to this area with a running 4–0 monofilament suture. Alternately, if graft inclusion technique is used, the ellipse cut on top of the graft is anastomosed from inside the aortic arch to immediately around the orifices of the brachiocephalic vessels as a single anastomosis. The new aortic arch is then carefully aspirated and washed to remove any foreign material. The flow rate is increased to 500 ml per minute, and the free end of the graft is held vertically and allowed to fill with blood. The clamps are then removed from the arch branches, with the proximal end of the graft still open and freely bleeding. Meticulous attention to detail is mandatory during this part of the procedure in order to prevent air or particulate embolization into the cerebral circulation. Following restoration of the cerebral circulation, a clamp is placed across the graft just proximal to the anastomoses to the arch vessels. The perfusion rate is then increased to 2,500 ml per minute with full warming, and the warming blanket is activated. The proximal portion of the graft is trimmed and anastomosed with a continuous suture to the graft replacing the ascending aorta.

During rewarming, packed red blood cells are added to the pump, progressively raising the hematocrit to 30 to 35 ml per deciliter at the end of the period. Also during warming the anastomoses are carefully examined and any bleeding points are controlled with individual sutures. The operating table is placed in the Trendelenburg position, the ascending aortic graft is aspirated for air, and the clamp across the graft is removed, reestablishing myocardial perfusion. Within several minutes the heart is defibrillated and the perfusion rate is increased to 3,500 ml per minute with continued warming, and any bleeding points are controlled with individual sutures. If the graft inclusion technique was used, during the rewarming period all suture lines are checked and the remnants of the aneurysm are then closed around the graft for immediate hemostasis. Most residual oozing into the wrap stops after the coagulation mechanism is restored to normal. In some cases we have found it useful to create a communication between the wrap and the right atrium either directly or via a short piece of Goretex graft in order to decompress the wrap until all oozing stops. Once the patient's esophageal temperature reaches 37° C, four units of fresh frozen plasma are added to the pump, and shortly thereafter the bypass is discontinued. Protamine sulfate and 20 units of platelets are then infused within the next few minutes. After adequate clotting is observed, decannulation and routine closure are carried out.

Close observation of the coagulation mechanism with repeated determination of the coagulation profile is important for adequate component therapy in the immediate postoperative period. If proper attention is given to component therapy, coagulopathy is not a major problem.

RESULTS

The described standard method of profound hypothermia and circulatory arrest was used to replace the aortic arch in a series of 60 patients. Concomitant procedures included replacement of varying portions of the ascending and descending aorta, resuspension or replacement of the aortic valve, and coronary artery bypass grafting. Thirty-six patients underwent elective and 24 patients emergency arch replacement. The overall mortality for the entire group stands at 18.3 percent (8.3 percent for elective operations and 37.5 percent for emergency arch replacement).

There have been no deaths since 1982 among patients undergoing elective arch replacement. The mortality rate of emergency arch replacement still remains high; however, this is primarily due to the high number of ruptured aneurysms included in this group. In the last 10 patients undergoing emergency arch replacement, six had preoperative rupture of their aneurysms, and there were only two postoperative survivors in this subgroup. If one excludes the ruptures, the mortality rate of emergency arch replacement remains around 20 percent.

Similar results with excellent figures for elective procedures and respectable results for emergency procedures are reported by other groups utilizing profound hypothermia and circulatory arrest for replacement of the aortic arch. Long-term outlook for these patients depends on the underlying cardiovascular pathology and is not different from the prognosis following surgical treatment of ascending or descending aneurysms.

SUGGESTED READING

Crawford ES, Saleh SA. Transverse aortic arch aneurysm: improved results of treatment employing new modifications of aortic recon-

struction and hypothermic cerebral circulatory arrest. Ann Surg 1981; 194:180–188.
Crawford ES, Snyder DM. Treatment of aneurysms of the aortic arch. J Thorac Cardiovasc Surg 1983; 85:237–246.
Ergin MA, O'Connor J, Guinto R, et al. Experience with profound hypothermia and circulatory arrest in the treatment of aneurysms of the aortic arch: aortic arch replacement for acute dissections. J Thorac Cardiovasc Surg 1982; 84:649–655.
Griepp RB, Stinson EB, Hollingsworth JF, et al. Prosthetic replacement of the aortic arch. J Thorac Cardiovasc Surg 1975; 70:1051–1063.
Livesay JJ, Cooley DA, Reul GJ, et al. Resection of aortic arch aneurysms: a comparison of hypothermic techniques in 60 patients. Ann Thorac Surg 1983; 36:19–28.

VALVULAR HEART DISEASE

SURGICAL VALVOTOMY AND PERCUTANEOUS BALLOON VALVOTOMY FOR MITRAL STENOSIS

W. GERALD AUSTEN, M.D.
PETER C. BLOCK, M.D.

Tremendous progress has been made in the surgical treatment of mitral stenosis since the pioneering efforts of Harken in Boston, Bailey in Philadelphia, and Brock in London in the late 1940s with closed digital valvotomy. Although closed mitral valvotomy was certainly a significant success, it became clear in time that the amount of relief of stenosis by finger fracture alone was sometimes rather modest and so various knives, valvulotomes, and dilators were developed. With the advent of safe cardiopulmonary bypass, open mitral valvotomy in recent years has become the procedure of choice in most circumstances. The recent advent of interventional therapy in the cardiac catheterization laboratory has led to the development of a promising new technique of percutaneous mitral valvotomy with a dilating balloon.

INDICATIONS FOR INTERVENTION

The ideal case for mitral valvotomy is a patient with significant mitral stenosis and no or minimal mitral regurgitation and no or minimal valvular calcification. The risk of mitral valvotomy is quite low, and the results of intervention are good. With proper patient selection, the chances of requiring mitral valve replacement and the attendant complications are unlikely. Thus, patients with moderate symptoms from their mitral valve disease should usually be offered intervention. The calculated mitral valve area in patients appropriate for surgery usually is 1.2 cm^2 or less, occasionally up to 1.5 cm^2. Evidence of significant pulmonary hypertension due to mitral stenosis, even in patients with mild or no symptoms, should also usually be an indication for intervention. Although the best candidates for intervention are patients in the New York Heart Association Classes II and III, sicker patients in Class IV and beyond are also appropriate candidates. This includes patients with severe pulmonary hypertension and even pulmonary artery pressures higher than systemic. Patients with peripheral embolism should be considered for operative intervention if there is significant mitral stenosis, regardless of cardiac symptoms; relief of the stenosis and operative removal of the atrial appendage (as well as the removal of any atrial clot) are associated with a marked reduction in thromboembolism.

The primary contraindications to surgical intervention include other severe diseases such as end-stage renal disease, severe chronic lung disease, or incurable malignancy. With the recent advent of percutaneous balloon valvotomy, even some of these patients with limited survival related to noncardiac problems can be considered for palliative intervention.

TECHNIQUE AND RESULTS OF SURGERY

Open Mitral Valvotomy

In recent years open mitral valvotomy has become by far the most common approach for these patients and closed mitral valvotomy is a very rare operative procedure in the United States. We prefer open mitral valvotomy because of the increased control that the surgeon has with this technique. The considerable risk of serious hemorrhage and the complication of peripheral embolism associated with closed valvotomy without cardiopulmonary bypass are markedly lessened in the open operation with cardiopulmonary bypass. Further, there is no doubt that the surgeon can do a better job in terms of relief of stenosis and correction of any mitral regurgitation by the open technique.

Prior to instituting cardiopulmonary bypass, we usually palpate the tricuspid valve by inserting a finger through the right atrial appendage to determine if the valve is stenotic or regurgitant. Cardiopulmonary bypass is performed in the usual manner, with aortic cross-clamping and protection of the myocardium with 4° C cardioplegic solution and bathing the outside of the heart in 4° C Ringer's lactate solution. The systemic temperature is lowered to 25° C.

The left atrium is opened with a longitudinal incision posterior and parallel to the interatrial groove. Any atrial thrombus is removed. The mitral valve is then visualized, and a traction suture is placed in each mitral leaflet. The two traction sutures are pulled horizontally by right-angle clamps to put tension on the area of commissural fusion. The two commissures are then identified. A third right-angle clamp is then placed beneath the commissure to be cut. The clamp is opened slightly to further indicate the exact location of the commissure and to push the chordae to the side where they are attached, protecting them from the surgeon's knife. The commissure is carefully cut, incising 2 or so millimeters, then inserting the right-angle clamp further to protect the chordae tendineae, extending the incision another 2 or so millimeters and repeating this process until the commissure is completely open. The commissure should be incised up to approximately 1 or 2 mm from the annulus. The other commissure is opened in the same fashion. Both commissures curve anteriorly. Any debris that is loosened in carrying out the commissurotomy should be removed. On occasion, calcium deposits on the valve leaflet can be removed with a rongeur, which improves leaflet mobility. It is important at this point to evaluate the subvalvular structures. If the chordae tendineae are fused with resultant leaflet immobility, the chordal fusion should be released by a knife incision. The incision may need to extend into the middle of the fused papillary muscles to further improve leaflet mobility.

When the stenosis has been relieved, the mitral valve should be evaluated for any mitral regurgitation. This can be accomplished by a number of techniques, all of which try to mimic the normal distention of the left ventricle by passive filling with fluid. One method consists of inserting a No. 12 or 14 F catheter antegrade across the mitral valve into the left ventricle and injecting saline with a syringe while evaluating leaflet approximation and regurgitation; alternatively, this can be achieved by insertion of the catheter into the left ventricle via the ventricular apex. By whatever technique chosen, areas of mitral regurgitation may be identified and can usually be corrected by placement of strategically located sutures and/or, on occasion, the performance of a mitral annuloplasty. A full discussion of mitral valve reconstruction for the treatment of mitral regurgitation is found in the chapter entitled *Mitral Valve Reconstruction*.

The left atrial appendage should be removed from the circulation to minimize the chance of postoperative thromboembolism. This can be accomplished by oversewing the orifice of the left atrial appendage from the inside, being careful that the running suture is superficial and thus does not cause damage to the left circumflex coronary artery. Alternatively, we frequently suture ligate the base of the atrial appendage; this is accomplished with a pursestring suture placed on the outside of the base of the atrial appendage.

Prior to closure of the heart, a left ventricular vent (No. 24 F chest tube) is placed across the mitral valve into the left ventricle and is brought out through the left atriotomy. The left atrium is then closed. Great care is taken to ensure that all air is removed from the left side of the heart and aorta, and once this has been accomplished and with a large needle hole in the ascending aorta, the heart is defibrillated.

After cardiopulmonary bypass has been terminated and the patient is hemodynamically stable, simultaneous left atrial and left ventricular pressure measurements are performed to determine the function of the mitral valve and whether there is any residual mitral stenosis or regurgitation. In very rare circumstances, reinstitution of cardiopulmonary bypass for further surgery on the mitral valve or, more likely, mitral valve replacement is required.

Results of Open Mitral Valvotomy. The results of open mitral valvotomy have improved over the years with advancements in preoperative and postoperative care, protection of the myocardium with better cardioplegic techniques, and improved methods of mitral valvotomy. Operative mortality and results depend on the preoperative state of the patient. Mortality ranges from less than 1 percent for patients in New York Heart Association Class II to approximately 5 to 10 percent for patients in New York Heart Association Class IV. Overall operative mortality is approximately 1 percent. The complication of embolism at the time of surgery is almost nonexistent. The recurrence rate following open mitral valvotomy is significantly lower than that reported for closed mitral valvotomy. This is due to many factors. Patients selected for open mitral valvotomy do not have significant mitral regurgitation or valvular calcification, and open valvotomy achieves excellent relief of stenosis without significant regurgitation. If this is not accomplished, the patient usually has a mitral valve replacement at the time of the initial operation. In any event, reoperation because of functional deterioration of the mitral valve in patients who have previously undergone open mitral valvotomy is in the range of 15 percent at 10 years. The incidence of peripheral emboli following open mitral valvotomy is low, in the range of 2 or 3 percent over a 10-year follow-up period. The 5- and 10-year survival statistics of patients who have undergone open mitral valvotomy are approximately 94 percent and 87 percent, respectively.

Closed Surgical Mitral Valvotomy

Closed surgical mitral valvotomy can be carried out with or without cardiopulmonary bypass. Closed mitral valvotomy without cardiopulmonary bypass was the surgical method of choice for treating patients with mitral stenosis from the time of the initial successes with this treatment in 1947 until the late 1960s and early 1970s. It is now a technique employed almost exclusively in parts of the world where cardiopulmonary bypass is not available or sufficiently safe. We employ it only in very rare circumstances, such as in a pregnant woman with severe mitral stenosis and uncontrolled congestive heart failure. The procedure should be performed in a room where open heart surgery can be carried out and with "pump standby." The operation is usually done through a left posterolateral thoracotomy. The atrial appendage is carefully examined to be certain that there is no clot present. The surgeon's finger is inserted into the atrium through a pursestring in the left atrial appendage. The function of the mitral valve can be well evaluated, since the heart is working in a reasonably normal fashion while the surgeon's finger is examining the size of the mitral orifice and estimating the amount of mitral regurgitation by the force and size of any regurgitant jet. The carotid arteries are occluded manually by the anesthetist for brief periods of approximately 20 to 40 seconds; this is done whenever there is a significant risk of embolization, such as when the surgeon enters the left atrium and when the mitral valve is split. The mitral valve was originally opened by exerting digital pressure on each of the fused commissures to gradually separate the leaflets without tearing them or the chordae tendineae. A number of modifications of this initial technique resulted in the mid 1950s in the Tubbs' transventricular dilator technique.

The use of the transventricular dilator requires little change from the finger fracture approach. The left posterolateral thoracotomy is extended anteriorly to achieve exposure of the left ventricle. The surgeon's finger is inserted through the atrial appendage, and the mitral valve is palpated. A pursestring suture is placed at the tip of the left ventricle in an avascular area. The closed transventricular dilator is inserted into the left ventricle and is guided through the mitral orifice with the surgeon's finger in the left atrium. The transventricular dilator should be moved back and forth to be certain that no chordae are caught in the dilator mechanism. In addition, the tip of the dilator should be pressed against the surgeon's finger in the left atrium to be sure that, when the dilator is opened, it remains through the valve and does not pop back into the left ventricle; if this occurs, the open dilator may tear the chordae tendineae or papillary muscles. The dilator, with its two heads pressing against the two leaflets, supplies its own counterpressure and achieves a considerably increased force to separate the fused commissures. Although there is disagreement as to the appropriate orientation of the dilator in relation to the valve commissures, we prefer to have the dilator blades open at right angles to the commissures and against the valve leaflets. Depending on the estimate of the patient's valve size by the surgeon's finger, we initially set the dilator to an opening of between 2.5 and 3.5 cm. After each dilation, the dilator is moved back into the ventricle and the valve function is examined with the surgeon's left atrial finger both in terms of residual stenosis and of regurgitation. The dilator diameter is increased by increments of 0.5 cm as long as no significant regurgitation has occurred and as long as the surgeon feels that residual stenosis can still be relieved. We have, on occasion, found it of help to dilate the mitral valve with the left atrial finger while the transventricular dilator is across the valve and expanded. When adequate mitral valve function has been achieved, the transventricular dilator is removed and the left ventricular pursestring suture is tied. When the procedure on the mitral valve has been completed and a stable hemodynamic state has been achieved, the mitral valve is once again evaluated by the surgeon's left atrial finger and, in addition, we usually perform simultaneous measurement of left atrial and left ventricular pressures.

If an adequate result is not achieved by the closed technique or if there is evidence of clot in the left atrium, the closed procedure may be converted to an open operation. For patients operated on via a left thoracotomy, this is accomplished by the insertion of one venous line through the left common femoral vein into the inferior vena cava, a second venous line through the right ventricular outflow tract into the main pulmonary artery with a tourniquet around the main pulmonary artery, and the insertion of the arterial line into the left common femoral artery.

For the past 15 years we have, on occasion, performed closed mitral valvotomy with cardiopulmonary bypass employing the Tubbs' transventricular dilator. We have employed this procedure in some patients who have pure mitral stenosis with essentially no mitral regurgitation and no mitral valve calcification and who by catheterization and echocardiography do not appear to have significant subvalvular involvement. This technique has the added safety and hemodynamic stability of cardiopulmonary bypass combined with the simplicity of a closed technique using the transventricular dilator. Further, if an open approach is required, it can be accomplished immediately. A median sternotomy incision is employed and standard cardiopulmonary bypass is achieved. Since we want to be able to evaluate the function of the mitral valve intermittently following the transventricular dilations, we take the systemic temperature to approximately 30° C and do not cross-clamp the aorta. A large pursestring suture is placed in the left atrial wall immediately anterior to the right pulmonary veins. The surgeon's left index finger is inserted through this pursestring for evaluation of the mitral valve. An additional pursestring is placed in an avascular area at the tip of the left ventricle. The Tubbs' transventricular dilator is inserted through the tip of the left ventricle and guided through the mitral valve to the tip of the surgeon's finger in the left atrium. The dilation of the mitral valve is accomplished in a manner similar to that described previously. Because the patient is on cardiopulmonary bypass, the procedure can be done in a much more relaxed fashion and the dilation can be accomplished in a more deliberate way. Between each dilation, the function of the mitral valve can be estimated by the surgeon's finger in the left atrium. When an adequate mitral valve opening has been achieved, the transventricular dilator is removed and the left ventricular pursestring suture is tied down. The heart is then positioned in as normal a location as possible, and a stable hemodynamic state with reasonably normal left ventricular systolic pressure is achieved; an additional evaluation of the function of the mitral valve is then performed by the surgeon's finger in the left atrium. Once the patient is off cardiopulmonary bypass with a normal temperature, simultaneous left atrial and left ventricular pressure measurements are done to further assess the function of the mitral valve.

Results of Closed Surgical Mitral Valvotomy. Operative mortality for closed mitral valvotomy with or without cardiopulmonary bypass is comparable to that of open mitral valvotomy, in the range of 1 percent.

In the closed valvotomy without bypass, the primary problems at the time of surgery include a relatively high incidence of peripheral thromboemboli from atrial clot (or mitral valvular particulate matter), problems with tearing of the left atrial wall and resultant hemorrhage, inadequate relief of mitral stenosis, and creation of mitral regurgitation. The late results have been less satisfactory with closed mitral valvotomy without bypass than with open mitral valvotomy. At 10 years after the initial surgery, approximately 20 percent of the patients have died and approximately 30 percent have required reoperation because of mitral valve dysfunction. The use of the transventricular dilator has resulted in better relief of the stenosis, but there appears to be a higher incidence of regurgitation following this technique.

The use of cardiopulmonary bypass decreases the incidence of some of the previously mentioned complications with the closed technique such as inadequate handling of left atrial thrombus and problems with tearing of the left atrial wall and resultant hemorrhage. Although our results with this technique have been better than the results in patients who have undergone closed mitral valvotomy without cardiopulmonary bypass, the recurrence rate is still somewhat higher than in open mitral valvotomy.

PERCUTANEOUS BALLOON VALVOTOMY

Percutaneous mitral valvotomy using dilating balloon catheters has been recently developed as a therapeutic alternative to surgery for patients with mitral stenosis. The appeal of percutaneous mitral valvotomy is that it is done in the catheterization laboratory, percutaneously, without general anesthesia. Patients usually leave the hospital within 24 hours after the procedure.

Patient Selection. The best results of percutaneous mitral valvotomy are in mitral stenosis patients with minimally or noncalcified mitral valves without severe subvalvular fibrosis. Previous mitral valvotomy, severe pulmonary hypertension, mild mitral regurgitation (1+/4+), and left ventricular dysfunction are not contraindications. Patients with severe pulmonary hypertension should be monitored carefully to avoid hypovolemia, hypotension, and right-sided heart failure. Patients who are not good candidates for mitral valve surgery because of associated noncardiac diseases such as pulmonary or renal disease may also be candidates for percutaneous mitral valvotomy.

Technique of Percutaneous Mitral Valvotomy. Using the standard transseptal puncture technique performed from the right femoral vein, a Mullin's sheath (USCI, Billerica, MA) is placed in the left atrium. Heparinization is achieved with 100 U per kilogram given intravenously. A floating No. 5 F balloon-tipped catheter (Arrow, Inc., Reading, PA) is passed through the sheath antegrade across the mitral valve. The mitral valve gradient is recorded, and the floating balloon catheter is then advanced out the aortic valve. A 0.038 inch diameter transfer wire guide is advanced through the catheter to the descending aorta. The catheter and Mullin's sheath are removed, leaving the wire guide behind (Fig. 1). A 5- or 6- mm dilating balloon catheter is advanced over the wire to the atrial septum, and the atrial puncture is dilated to allow passage of larger dilating balloon catheters. A second wire guide is then placed parallel to the first by using a double-lumen catheter (Mansfield Scientific, Mansfield, MA). Then two dilating balloon catheters (usually 20-mm diameter) are advanced antegrade, one over each wire guide, and both balloons are positioned

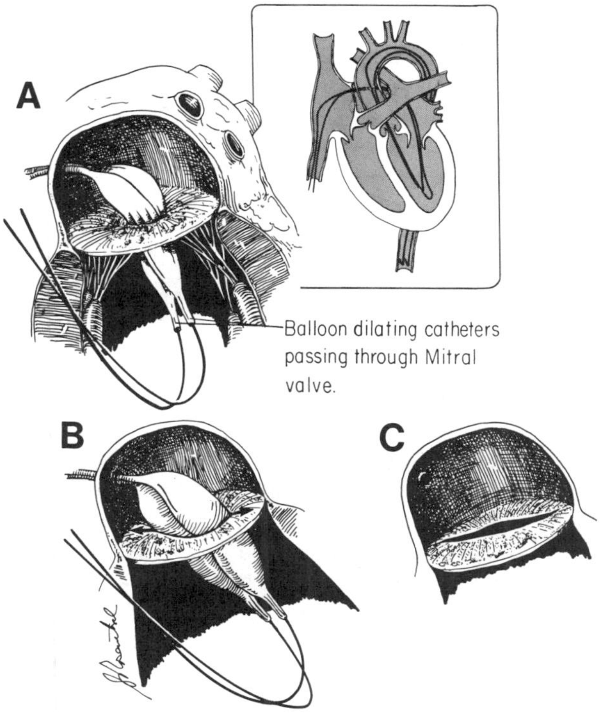

Figure 1 Diagram of percutaneous mitral valvotomy. Two transfer wire guides are placed from the femoral vein through the right atrium, across the atrial septum, left atrium, across the mitral valve, and the left ventricle to the aorta (insert). *A*, two dilating balloon catheters (deflated) are advanced over the wire guides and positioned across the stenotic mitral valve. *B*, the balloons are inflated simultaneously, splitting the fused commissures. *C*, the dilating catheters and wire guides are removed; the mitral orifice is enlarged.

across the stenotic mitral valve. Two or three full simultaneous balloon inflations within the valve orifice are usually adequate to open the valve. Frequently a "waist" is seen on the initial inflation because of the fused mitral commissures.

The best results of percutaneous mitral valvotomy are achieved with simultaneous inflation of two balloons (20 and 20 mm; 25 and 15 mm) so as to lower left atrial pressure to less than 14 mm Hg (assuming that left ventricular diastolic pressure is normal). Percutaneous mitral valvotomy should *not* be considered satisfactory unless the left atrial pressure is reduced to this level.

The dilating balloon catheters are removed. Simultaneous left ventricular and left atrial pressures are again recorded to evaluate the final mitral gradient. Left ventriculography should be performed to evaluate mitral regurgitation as the final step.

Results of Percutaneous Mitral Valvotomy. The initial results of percutaneous mitral valvotomy in our first 75 patients are shown in Table 1. Overall, mitral valve area increased from 0.8 $\pm$ 0.1 to 1.7 $\pm$ 0.2 cm^2 ($p<0.0001$). Mitral valve gradient fell from 19 $\pm$ 1 mm Hg to 7 $\pm$ 1 mm Hg ($p<0.0001$).

Multiple stepwise regression analyses of the factors that predicted the best results of percutaneous mitral valvotomy identified the following characteristics: minimal

TABLE 1 Results of Percutaneous Mitral Valvotomy (75 Patients)

	Before Percutaneous Mitral Valvotomy	*After Percutaneous Mitral Valvotomy*
Valve area	0.8 ± 0.1 cm^2	1.7 ± 0.2*
Mitral gradient	1.9 ± 1 mm Hg	7 ± 1*
Cardiac output	3.8 ± 2.4 L/min	4.6 ± 0.2
Mean pulmonary artery pressure	41 ± 2 mm Hg	27 ± 2*
Pulmonary resistance	338 ± 45 dynes/sec/cm^{-5}	260 ± 33*

* = $p<0.0001$.

valve calcification; mobile mitral valve; minimal subvalvular fibrosis; and minimal valve thickening. Patients with these characteristics had the most optimal results: valve area increased from 0.9 ± 0.1 cm^2 to 2.0 ± 0.1 cm^2.

Complications of Percutaneous Mitral Valvotomy. Complications include the production of mitral regurgitation, thromboembolic events, and problems related to transseptal catheterization such as tamponade or the creation of a left-to-right shunt through the atrial septum. In our series of the first 75 patients, one patient (1.3 percent) died at emergency surgery of right-sided heart failure caused by severe pulmonary hypertension. One additional patient died of an acute myocardial infarction due to atherosclerotic coronary artery occlusion 24 hours after a successful percutaneous mitral valvotomy. Two patients had emboli (2.7 percent), and two had heart block at the time of balloon inflation (one required a permanent pacemaker). One patient developed mitral regurgitation but did not require surgery. Left-to-right shunting occurred immediately in six patients but had disappeared 24 hours later.

Long-Term Follow-Up of Percutaneous Mitral Valvotomy. Clinically, 75 percent of patients improved their New York Heart Association Class by one or two steps at initial follow-up. No improvement was seen in 25 percent. Cardiac catheterization studies show that if patients have an initial good result and have little subvalvular or valvular thickening or calcification before percutaneous mitral valvotomy, restenosis does *not* occur by 1-year follow-up examination. Patients with subvalvular disease and thickened, calcified valves have a higher chance of restenosis. Longer term follow-up studies are needed to evaluate the results of percutaneous mitral valvotomy and to determine its ultimate role in therapy. It is hoped that if an adequate valvotomy is accomplished, long-term clinical improvement may be similar to that achieved with closed surgical valvotomy.

SUGGESTED READING

Block PC, Palacios IF, Jacobs ML, Fallon JT. Mechanism of percutaneous mitral valvotomy. Am J Cardiol 1987; 59:178–179.

Commerford PJ, Hastie T, Beck W. Closed mitral valvotomy: actuarial analysis of results in 654 patients over 12 years and analysis of preoperative predictors of long-term survival. Ann Thorac Surg 1982; 33:473–479.

Gross RI, Cunningham JN Jr, Snively SL, Cantinella FP, Nathan IM, Adams PX, Spencer FC. Longterm results of open radical mitral commissurotomy: ten year follow-up study of 202 patients. Am J Cardiol 1981; 47:821–825.

Kirklin JW, Barratt-Boyes BG. Mitral valve disease with or without tricuspid valve disease. In: Cardiac surgery. New York: John Wiley & Sons, 1986:323.

Palacios I, Block PC, Brandi S,Blanco P, Casal H, Pulido JI, Munoz S, D'Empaire G, Ortega MA, Jacobs M, Vlahakes G. Percutaneous balloon valvotomy for patients with severe mitral stenosis. Circulation 1987; 75:778–784.

MITRAL VALVE RECONSTRUCTION

AUBREY C. GALLOWAY, M.D.
STEPHEN B. COLVIN, M.D.
FRANK C. SPENCER, M.D.

At New York University (NYU) 225 patients with mitral insufficiency have been operated on with the Carpentier techniques of mitral valve reconstruction since 1979. A detailed analysis with a 99 percent complete follow-up has been completed for the first 148 patients. Operative mortality was 1.2 percent for isolated mitral valve reconstruction, 4 percent in the overall series. The mitral insufficiency resulted from degenerative disease prolapse, or ruptured chordae in 43 percent of patients; rheumatic fever in 30 percent, ischemic heart disease 11 percent, endocarditis 10 percent, and congenital heart disease in 3 percent.

Before operation 19 percent of patients were New York Heart Association Class IV, 59 percent Class III, and 20 percent Class I or II.

RECONSTRUCTION VERSUS REPLACEMENT

Reconstruction seems possible in at least 90 to 95 percent of patients with mitral insufficiency. Relative contraindications are principally advanced left ventricular dysfunction, presence of acute endocarditis, or severe cardiomyopathy. Reconstruction is a more complex procedure than prosthetic valve replacement; therefore it is not undertaken when other diseases indicate that a shorter and simpler operation is preferable. Mitral reconstruction is strongly preferred to replacement whenever possible because of the freedom from the well-known complications of prosthetic valves. Serious thromboembolism is virtually unknown after the first few months following reconstruction. Chronic anticoagulant therapy is not routinely needed, and endocarditis is rare.

Currently the principal uncertainty is the durability of reconstruction, which has been the main problem with different forms of mitral reconstruction intermittently tried for over 3 decades. The Carpentier techniques, however, were the first to emphasize the multiple anatomic causes of mitral insufficiency, with specific techniques for each abnormality found; these abnormalities are asymmetric annular dilatation, leaflet prolapse, chordal rupture, leaflet perforation, and restricted motion of the valve apparatus. Durability in the New York University series has been very good; actuarial analysis found that 90 percent of patients have remained free from late valve replacement 5 years following operation; in patients with prolapse or ruptured chordae, only one late valve replacement has been necessary.

TIMING OF OPERATION

Prompt operation is recommended for virtually all symptomatic patients. It is also recommended for asymptomatic patients with angiographic demonstration of severe mitral insufficiency with progressive cardiac enlargement and a fall in ejection fraction with exercise. Thus early operation is recommended to prevent the insidious evolution of irreversible ventricular injury in minimally symptomatic patients.

OPERATIVE TECHNIQUE

A median sternotomy incision is used. Standard cardiopulmonary bypass with membrane or bubble oxygenator and roller pump is used. The perfusion rate is approximately 2 to 3 L per square meter per minute, with moderate hemodilution and a temperature near 30° C. The Carpentier sternal retractor (Fig. 1) is essential for providing adequate exposure and a still operative field because operative decisions are principally made from visual inspection of the different valvular abnormalities found. A safe form of cardioplegia is essential, as periods of ischemia for 1, 2, or more hours may be required, especially if associated procedures are performed. The NYU cardioplegia technique uses a cold blood potassium method in combination with topical hypothermia, maintaining a myocardial temperature well below 15 °C, confirmed by periodic thermistor measurement of regional myocardial temperatures.

An incision is made in the left atrium posterior to the interatrial groove, carrying the incision to the left beneath the superior cava above and the inferior cava below. A proper adjustment of the blades of the Carpentier retractor is essential, positioning the tips of the blades so traction is applied to the atrial wall 2 cm from the mitral annulus.

Mitral Valve Inspection

A detailed inspection is done to detect abnormalities of the annulus, leaflets, chordae, or papillary muscles. Jet lesions help to identify the defective leaflet. Reconstruction may be performed with confidence as long as the aortic leaflet is satisfactory; it has been satisfactorily completed in virtually every patient in whom it was undertaken. *Annular dilatation* is principally an asymmetric enlargement of the annulus of the mural leaflet. The annulus of the aortic leaflet is not involved, as it is part of the basic fibrous skeleton of the heart. This anatomic fact is the basis for uniform applicability of annuloplasty. Disease of the valve leaflets, such as fibrosis, calcification, prolapse, or ruptured chordae can be determined by precise inspection while lifting different chordae with a nerve hook. *Elongation of chordae* is best evaluated by using chordae near the commissures as a reference point, for these are seldom elongated. Significant elongation of chordae exists when the leaflet tissue can be elevated more than a centimeter above the normal plane of the annulus.

Techniques of Repair for Mitral Insufficiency from Different Causes

Repair of Mitral Insufficiency from Prolapse or Ruptured Chordae

Mural Leaflet Disease. A flail mural leaflet from either chordal elongation or rupture is treated by excision. Extensive disease in the mural leaflet does not preclude reconstruction, for at least 60 to 70 percent of the leaflet can be safely resected as a quadrangular excision, leaving some intact leaflet tissue near each commissure. The resulting defect may be as much as 4 to 5 cm wide (Fig. 2A). A radical excision of diseased leaflet tissue is performed, making little effort to minimize the extent of resection. Wide resection may be done for multiple ruptured chordae or for intrinsic leaflet disease. Following the quadrangular excision, the annulus of the excised segment is plicated with a figure-of-eight suture of 2–0 Tevdek, carefully inserting the suture so that the plicated annulus approximates the margins of the residual leaflet tissue without tension (Fig. 2B). This is a key point. Occasionally with a large defect following quadrangular excision, two separate annuloplasty sutures have been used. The margins of the leaflet tissue are then sutured with figure-of-eight 4–0 or 5–0 Prolene sutures (Figs. 2C and 2D). Usually three or four are required. Saline is injected into the ventricular cavity through a bulb syringe to elevate and approximate the mitral valve leaflets, demonstrating the degree to which the insufficiency has been corrected. This intermittent injection of saline during performance of reconstruction is a valuable technique. At this time the

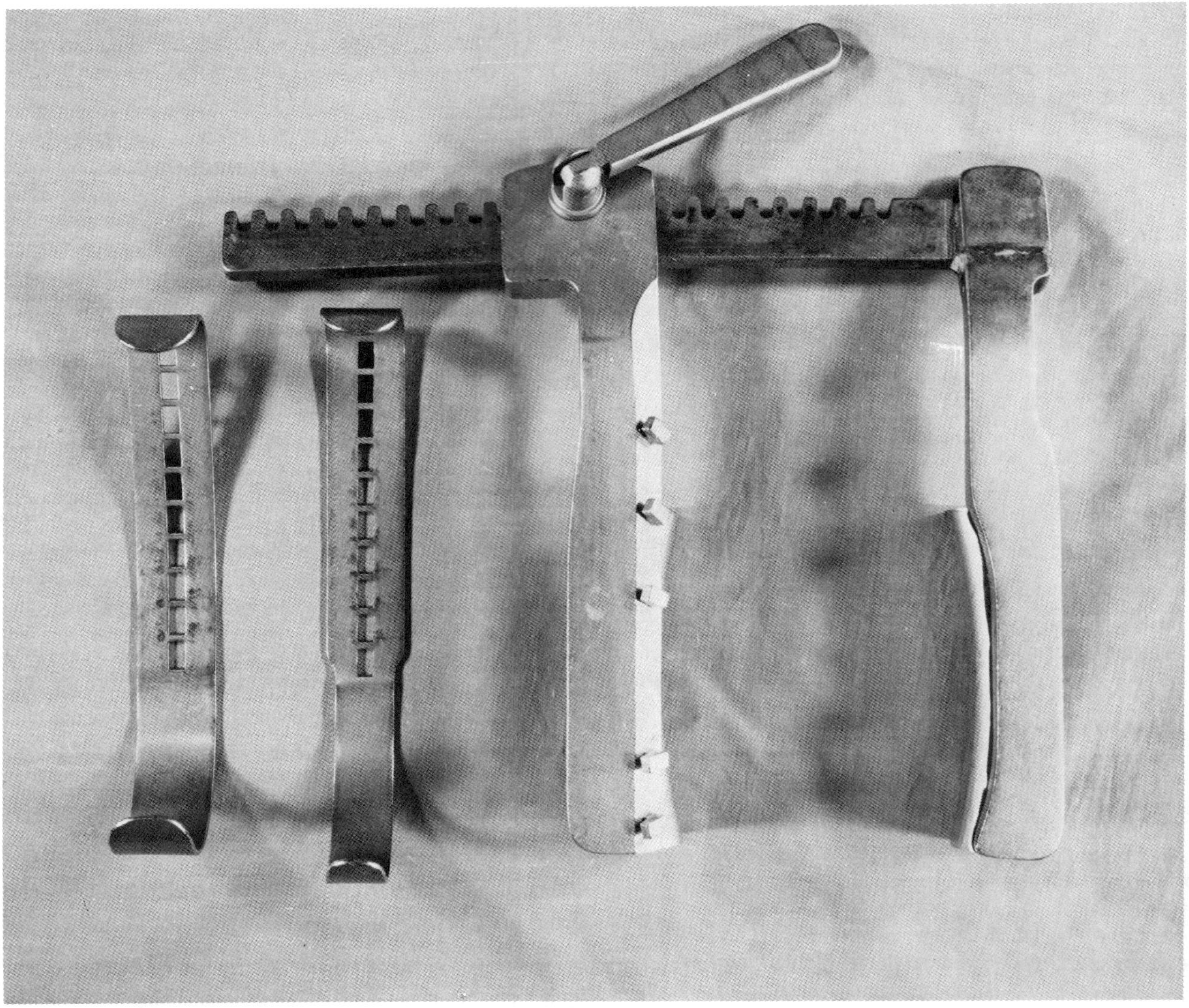

Figure 1 The Carpentier sternal retractor with atrial traction blades.

amount of insufficiency remaining from the annular dilatation can be estimated.

Calcification. Extensive calcification of the annulus of the mural leaflet has not been found to be a contraindication as long as the aortic leaflet is not severely diseased. Since plication of the mural leaflet annulus is a key part of the operative technique, sufficient calcium must be débrided from the annulus to permit plication without perforation of the ventricular wall. Cautious débridement of calcium has been successfully performed in 26 patients without injury.

Ruptured Chordae of Aortic Leaflet. Ruptured chordae of the aortic leaflet are usually treated by resuspension of the free margin of the leaflet to an intact secondary chorda. Transposition of chordae from a segment of mural leaflet, as described by Carpentier, was occasionally used.

Elongated Chordae. Elongated chordae are corrected by the Carpentier technique of making a 1-cm incision in the tip of the involved papillary muscle and implanting sufficient lengths of the elongated chordae into this muscular trough to restore the proper length.

Repair of Mitral Insufficiency from Rheumatic Valvular Disease

When mitral insufficiency is the dominant problem, excellent results can be obtained with reconstruction. However, when significant mitral stenosis is present, in combination with insufficiency, the least satisfactory results are obtained. Mitral stenosis is treated with an extensive commissurotomy that stops 3 or 4 mm from the annulus where the small commissural leaflets are located. Separation of fused chordae is extensively performed, often splitting the underlying papillary muscle for over a centimeter. The shortened fibrotic secondary chordae of the mural leaflet may be cautiously divided. The valve leaflets must be mobilized sufficiently to appose properly in systole and to open widely in diastole. Annular dilatation is usually minimal.

Repair of Mitral Insufficiency from Other Causes (Endocarditis; Coronary Artery Disease; Congenital)

Only limited experience has been obtained with these unusual forms of mitral insufficiency, but identification of the valvular abnormality producing the insufficiency has made reconstruction feasible in the majority of the patients operated on. Identification of the pathologic changes causing the insufficiency by careful inspection, combined with the bulb syringe test, is the basic approach. As long as the aortic leaflet of the mitral valve is satisfactory, reconstruction is achievable, for the mural leaflet can be radically excised, plicated, and an annuloplasty ring inserted, correcting insufficiency in the majority of patients.

The Annuloplasty Ring

Insertion of the annuloplasty ring is considered a key component of the operation for several reasons, although others with much less experience than Carpentier have minimized the importance of routine insertion of the ring (Fig. 3). The ring was inserted in 84 percent of the patients operated on, the usual exceptions being children or patients with a small mitral annulus. The insertion of the ring not only stabilizes the repair, removing tension from the suture lines in the mitral leaflets, but it also prevents dilation of the annulus in future years, which could occur if minimal insufficiency began from recurrent disease.

Selection of the proper sized annuloplasty ring is crucial, measuring the length of the annulus of the aortic leaflet between the two commissures. The fact that this portion of the mitral annulus does not dilate with mitral insufficiency is one of the key concepts that makes reconstruction possible. The usual size ring is between 28 and 34 mm. Initially sutures are placed in the annulus at each commissure, after which a ring of proper size can be chosen, noting where the "commissures" of the annuloplasty ring should be located. The degree of plication of the dilated and distorted mural leaflet annulus that must be done as the annuloplasty sutures are inserted can also be estimated.

Precise insertion of each annuloplasty suture is crucial. No. 2–0 Tevdek suture has usually been employed. The needle is inserted perpendicular to the annulus, located about a millimeter beyond the visible junction of the mitral leaflet tissue with the atrial wall (the "hinge" area).

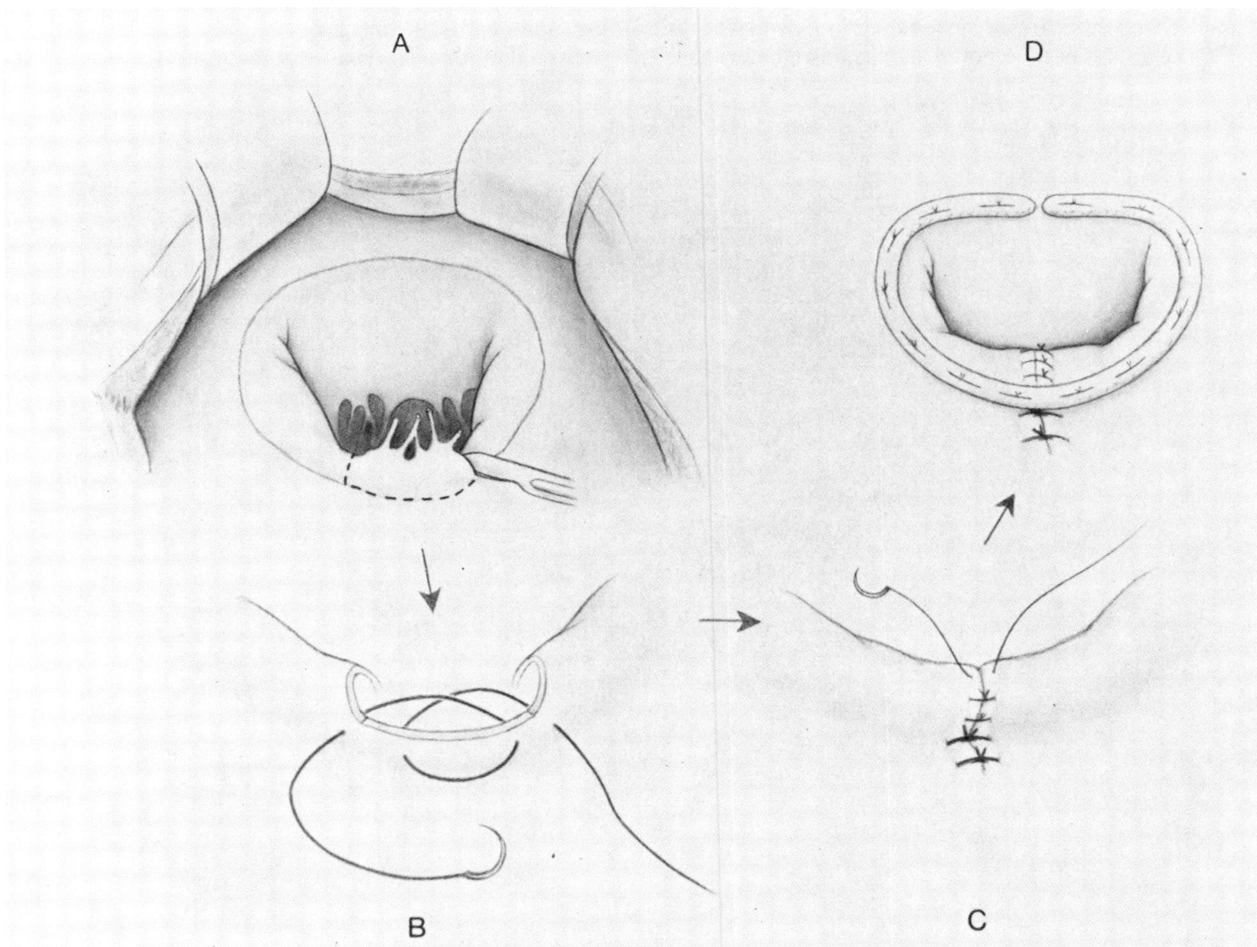

Figure 2 Repair of mitral insufficiency by resection of mural leaflet. *A*, quadrangular resection of mural leaflet. *B*, plication of the annulus of the excised segment. *C*, suture of the margins of the leaflet tissue. *D*, appearance after completion of the reconstruction.

The needle is advanced down through the annulus and curved to emerge again, encompassing 10 to 15 mm of tissue. A helpful mental image from plane geometry is to envision the annulus as a circle; the suture is placed as a tangent to the circle. Improper placement of the suture laterally may injure the circumflex coronary artery or conduction tissue, while improper placement medially may injure a leaflet chordae. Not securely placing the suture in the fibrous tissue of the annulus may lead to dehiscence of the annuloplasty ring. Eight or 10 annuloplasty sutures are customarily inserted, "gaining" appropriate amounts in the annulus of the mural leaflet and in the commissures, to plicate and correct the dilatation present. After the annuloplasty ring has been tied in position, the bulb syringe test is again performed to see if an additional suture is needed to correct any insufficiency near the mitral orifice.

Finally, the original figure-of-eight annuloplasty suture is covered with two or three 4–0 Prolene sutures in the atrial wall. The orifice of the left atrial appendage is oversewn with a continuous 3–0 or 4–0 Prolene suture to eliminate the appendage as a future source of embolism. Careful placement of the sutures just beneath the endothelium of the atrial appendage avoids injury to the circumflex coronary artery.

The left atrial incision is closed with continuous suture, after which fibrillation is induced, the aorta unclamped, and intracardiac air removed in a standard manner. Once air has been removed and the heart defibrillated, the perfusion rate and blood volume are adjusted to permit the left ventricle to eject blood at a systemic pressure above 80 mm Hg. The index finger is then inserted through the untied atrial suture line to palpate the functioning mitral valve. Usually no insufficiency is found. It has been noted that the visual appearance of the leaflets when distended with the bulb syringe test during operation corresponds well with the findings on palpation of the functioning mitral valve with the heart beating, which in turn corresponds well with intraoperative and postoperative 2-D and Doppler echocardiographic assessment.

The operative technique as described has proved a reliable one for repair and has been successfully completed in almost all patients operated on; we have virtually never abandoned repair for replacement because of unanticipated technical problems or had to return a patient to the operating room a few days after operation because of residual insufficiency. Certain key aspects of technique merit repetition for emphasis. A key component of the operation is the ability to resect liberally a wide segment of diseased mural leaflet and to safely suture the edges of the remaining mural leaflet segments together. Two features of the technique appear important to protect from disastrous dehiscence of the suture line in the mural leaflet. First, the figure-of-eight annuloplasty suture must be placed so that there is absolutely no tension on the edges of the remaining mural leaflet segment. Second, the annuloplasty ring further stabilizes the repair, for these sutures also protect

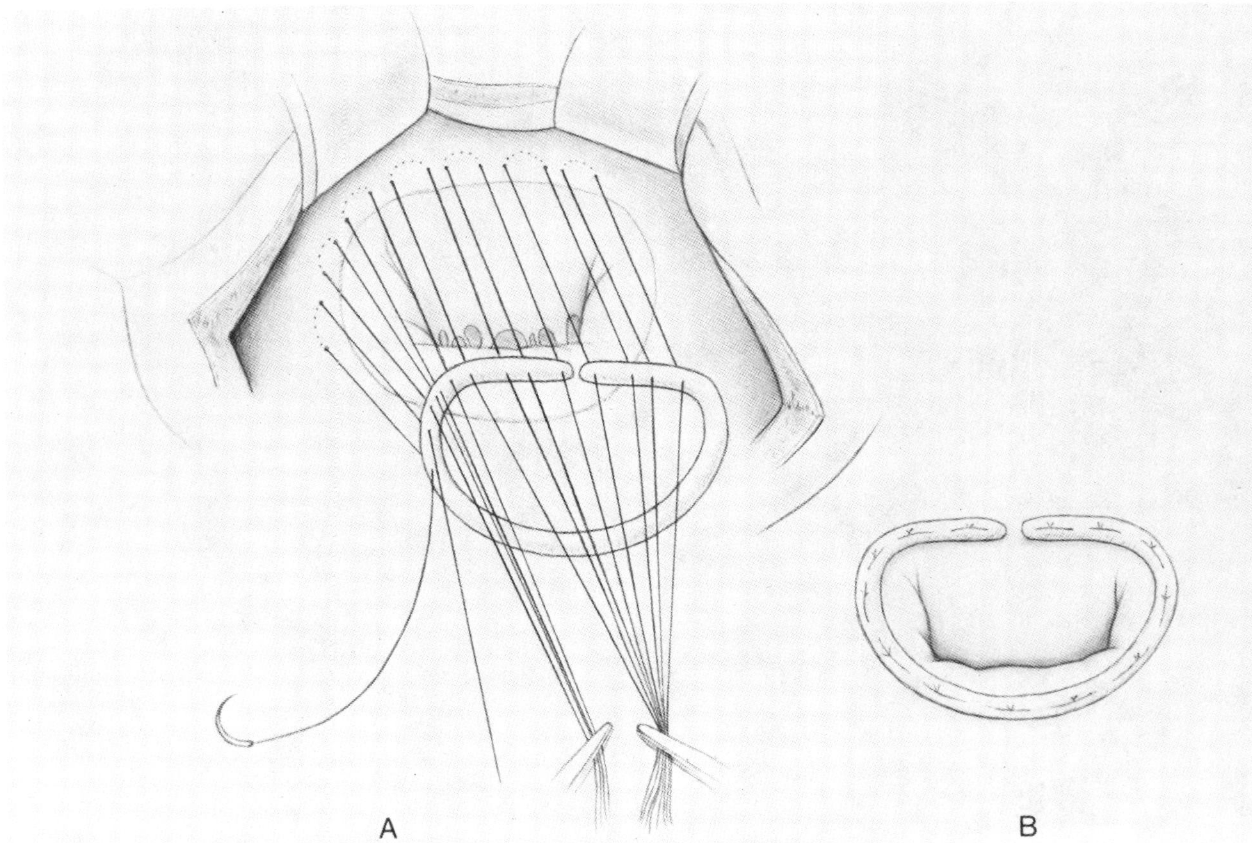

Figure 3 The Carpentier mitral annuloplasty ring. *A*, suture placement. *B*, appearance after sutures are tied into place.

from any tension on the mural leaflet suture line. The importance of a still, dry operative field that permits careful inspection of the valve in a detailed, unhurried manner is most important because key decisions on the type of reconstruction performed must be determined by inspection during the operation. In over 90 percent of the patients operated on, two or more techniques of reconstruction were used, usually segmental resection of a diseased mural leaflet (65 percent of patients) and insertion of an annuloplasty ring (84 percent of patients).

POSTOPERATIVE AND CONVALESCENT CARE

Postoperative care is usually uneventful, with the patient being discharged from the hospital 7 to 9 days following operation. 2-D Doppler echocardiography is routinely done before discharge to detect any residual mitral insufficiency. Anticoagulant therapy with warfarin and dipyridamole (Persantine) is started 2 days after operation and continued for at least 3 months when feasible, keeping the prothrombin time near 20 seconds. The main risk of significant thromboembolism is in the first 3 months following operation. Subsequently warfarin is stopped and aspirin added to the antiplatelet program, continuing both drugs for at least 1 year. After 3 months, thromboembolism is fortunately rare. Patients who have been in severe congestive heart failure with a large left atrium and permanent atrial fibrillation perhaps should continue warfarin indefinitely because of the hazards of thrombi developing in these large atria. One of the great advantages of reconstruction is that significant thromboembolism has been of negligible importance, especially in patients who remain in a sinus rhythm following the operation. Transient ischemic attacks have occurred in some patients for a few months, perhaps representing platelet emboli, but no neurologic defects have occurred, and such episodes have stopped after the first several months.

Standard antibiotic prophylaxis is used to protect from endocarditis. However, late endocarditis is less common after reconstruction than after valve replacement and has not been a significant problem in our series.

In the NYU series, the patient is seen annually for 2-D and Doppler echocardiography to detect any recurrent insufficiency. Cardiac catheterization has been performed only in a small percentage of patients, as this has virtually always confirmed the findings of echocardiography. To date, only one patient with degenerative disease has developed significant late insufficiency, although 10 to 15 percent of patients with rheumatic valve disease have developed some recurrent insufficiency.

The 7-year NYU experience with 250 mitral reconstruction operations has shown durable results after repair of mitral insufficiency from any cause, obtaining the best results in patients with degenerative prolapse or ruptured chordae. The late freedom from recurrent insufficiency, thromboembolism, anticoagulant related complications, and endocarditis has been most encouraging, making mitral reconstruction the procedure of choice for most patients with mitral valve insufficiency.

SUGGESTED READING

Carpentier A. Cardiac valve surgery—the "French correction." J Thorac Cardiovasc Surg 1983; 86:323–337.

Carpentier A, Chauvaud S, Fabiani JN, et al. Reconstructive surgery of mitral valve incompetence. Ten-year appraisal. J Thorac Cardiovasc Surg 1980; 79:338–348.

Spencer FC, Colvin SB, Culliford AT, Isom OW. Experiences with the Carpentier techniques of mitral valve reconstruction in 103 patients (1980–1985). J Thorac Cardiovasc Surg 1985; 90:341–350.

TRICUSPID VALVE REPAIR

CARLOS M. G. DURAN, M.D., Ph.D.

The surgical treatment of acquired tricuspid valve disease remains an elusive problem. Tricuspid pathology is often silent, it may follow the dictates of mitral disease, and diagnosis is often difficult to make; these factors make both the treatment and the postoperative evaluation difficult. As a result, there are wide differences in the surgical approaches to tricuspid valve disease, ranging from valve replacement to ignoring the lesions completely. Contemporary reparative techniques with low mortality and morbidity have encouraged a much more aggressive approach to tricuspid repair.

DIAGNOSIS OF ACQUIRED TRICUSPID VALVE DISEASE

There is a lack of precise clinical criteria to determine the presence and degree of tricuspid disease. The well-known clinical signs of disease are unmistakable; however, their absence does not exonerate the surgeon from suspecting and treating pathology. Indeed, some patients have required reoperation only to repair the previously ignored tricuspid valve disease, whereas in others, the ignored tricuspid insufficiency disappeared spontaneously when left-sided valve lesions were corrected. To add to the diagnostic difficulty, the intraoperative digital assessment of tricuspid disease may be very subjective; it is further complicated by changes in cardiac output during surgery and uncertainties about the future evolution of the disease.

The diagnostic issues that must be addressed are (1) whether or not the patient has tricuspid disease; (2) whether it is "organic," i.e., lesions at leaflet and/or commissural level, or "functional," i.e., annular dilatation without any other pathology; and (3) severity of the disease.

In all patients with valvular heart disease, the tricuspid valve should be evaluated preoperatively. Clinical signs should be taken as an unmistakable diagnosis of the disease; their absence, however, does not mean a study can be dispensed with. An echo-Doppler study should be performed, and if it is not conclusive, a right ventriculogram with a malleable pulmonary balloon catheter trapped in the inflow trabeculae should be carried out. With careful technique, there should not be any false-positive results.

The presence of an organic tricuspid lesion should be considered a priori in all rheumatic patients. Detection of insufficiency in the presence of a nondilated annulus, irregularity of the valvular plane, jet-like regurgitation, and hemodynamic gradients are signs of organic disease.

Finally, the degree of insufficiency should also be established preoperatively in order to decide whether to correct or surgically ignore the disease. It is generally accepted that functional tricuspid insufficiency is caused by annular dilatation secondary to right ventricular failure due to altered contractility or pressure load or both. Two factors must be responsible for the severity and reversibility of functional tricuspid insufficiency (TI): first, the degree of annular dilatation, and second, the capacity for systolic reduction of the dilated annulus. Both of these parameters of annular diameter and its percentage of shortening are easily measurable either in a right anterior oblique ventriculogram or in a high resolution 2-D echocardiogram. Those patients with a normal tricuspid valve have a small annular diameter and a large percentage of systolic annular shortening. Those with mild TI start systole with an enlarged annulus, but good shortening capacity reduces it to normal levels before the end. Those with severe TI start with a very enlarged annulus that never reaches normal levels because of impaired contractility. Whenever the end-systolic diameter is above what we have established as critical (angiographically above 27 mm), the regurgitation is pansystolic and therefore severe. Furthermore, those patients with severe regurgitation with a normal annular diameter have obvious organic tricuspid valve disease.

INDICATIONS FOR TRICUSPID SURGERY

All tricuspid regurgitation lesions do not require surgical treatment; those patients with functional TI and low pulmonary resistance can be expected to improve annular dilatation once the left-sided valve lesions have been surgically corrected. Therefore, our present recommendations regarding tricuspid annuloplasty in the setting of functional TI are as follows:

1. Mild TI, characterized by a palpable regurgitant jet in the right atrium that can be felt within 1 or 2 cm of the tricuspid valve, can be ignored if elevated pulmonary resistances are below 500 dynes per second per m^{-5} (normal is 250).
2. Moderate tricuspid regurgitation, with a regurgitant jet palpable in the right atrium at least 3 cm from the tricuspid valve, should be repaired even with low pulmonary resistance. Although tricuspid regurgitation should be expected to disappear spontaneously, we have no data on the time required for this to occur, and a better early postoperative course would be expected if the regurgitation were surgically corrected.
3. Patients with severe, functional tricuspid regurgitation and high pulmonary resistance or severely affected right ventricular function should undergo a repair procedure. Spontaneous disappearance of their regurgitation cannot be expected.

In principle, all "organic" tricuspid lesions should be managed surgically. If a transvalvular gradient is present and is ignored, the left-sided repair results in increased cardiac output, and any tricuspid gradient increases. It would be tempting to ignore these organic lesions with minimal gradients, mild-to-moderate regurgitation, and low pulmonary resistances. However, our experience has shown postoperative persistence of regurgitation. We therefore recommend repair of "organic" lesions when even mild stenosis and/or mild-to-moderate TI has been diagnosed. A conservative procedure is nearly always possible, although the surgical results are less satisfactory than in cases with pure functional regurgitation.

OPERATIVE TECHNIQUES

The surgical approach to all patients is through a midline sternotomy incision. Finger palpation of the right atrium is still performed because it is such a traditional, easy maneuver. A finger can be inserted through a purse-string suture in the right atrial appendage to feel the tricuspid apparatus and to grade the regurgitant jet. This approach may miss organic lesions, which always require visual confirmation.

Both cavae are independently cannulated with right-angled cannulas* to provide a large unobstructed operative field. Arterial return is through the ascending aorta. Moderate general hypothermia and topical hypothermia through a cold continuous drip into the pericardium are employed in all cases. All procedures on the left side are performed during a single, uninterrupted period of aortic cross-clamping; cold cardioplegia is used in all cases. Once the left-sided surgery is finished, the aorta is unclamped and rewarming is begun. All tricuspid surgery is conducted under nonischemic conditions; an oblique right atriotomy is performed, extending from the right atrial appendage toward the inferior vena cava. Two separate retractors are always used, but of different sizes according to the right atrial size. A "coronary suction" is placed in the coronary sinus to achieve a relatively dry field. The tricuspid valve is carefully explored using nerve hooks, particularly when an organic lesion is suspected.

Tricuspid Commissurotomy

All "organic" lesions include some degree of commissural fusion. It is essential to identify all three commissures and decide whether they require splitting. In most cases, the two septal commissures are incised, ignoring the anteroposterior commissure. Observation of a line of leaflet fusion is not sufficient; it is of paramount importance to identify the always present fusion of two of the

* Polystan A/S Walgerhoem, Denmark.

underlying commissural cords. Retraction of the corresponding leaflets with nerve hooks shows the often very thin, fused cords. The incision is started at the exact point of insertion of these cords and extended downward, separating the two cords, and then it is extended radially along the commissure without reaching the annulus. Casual incision of the commissure between any two commissural cords can result in an unsupported leaflet and secondary insufficiency; the importance of examining the supporting, subvalvular apparatus cannot be overstated.

In most cases some degree of cuspal thickening and consequent shrinkage are present, and therefore an annuloplasty has to be performed to compensate for the reduced amount of tissue available to the tricuspid orifice. The results cannot be expected to be as good as those obtained in "functional" insufficiency. Leaflet retraction has to be compensated for by a significant reduction in annular diameter, which either induces some stenosis or otherwise maintains some insufficiency. It is, however, our opinion that a commissurotomy followed by annuloplasty is far superior to present-day valve replacements, which carry a higher mortality and morbidity and residual gradients. Only approximately 5 percent of our patients with organic tricuspid disease have required valve replacement.

Tricuspid Annuloplasty

Tricuspid annuloplasty is probably the more universally accepted surgical technique, but also less accurately performed due to the lack of feedback attributed to the difficulty in evaluating its results. The technique proposed by Kay in 1965, which transforms the tricuspid into a bileaflet valve by plicating the posterior leaflet, has been practically abandoned. At present, two basic techniques are available: (1) the techniques of Cabrol and DeVega that use a semicircular double continuous suture along the tricuspid annulus to reduce it selectively, and (2) the techniques of Carpentier, Duran, and Puig Massana that incorporate a prosthetic ring that is sutured to the annulus. The double continuous suture technique is simpler, faster, and more economical. However, besides tendency of the suture to become detached from its anchoring points, the procedure carries the danger of being overdone. The surgeon often has a tendency to be more concerned with residual insufficiency than with stenosis, which in the case of the atrioventricular valves is of more physiologic importance. We favor the use of a prosthetic ring whose size is selected according to the tissue available and that is anchored by numerous stitches. Two types of rings are available: the Carpentier-Edwards rigid ring, shaped like the normal systolic tricuspid orifice, and the Duran-Hancock flexible ring. I prefer the latter ring because (1) total flexibility reduces tension at each suture and therefore decreases the chances of dehiscence, (2) it follows closely the continuous movements of the tricuspid annulus both in the horizontal and vertical planes, and (3) it is less stenotic, as it can increase its area in diastole by adopting a more circular shape. In systole, the atrioventricular muscle shapes the ring into a configuration similar to that of the Carpentier-Edwards ring. The Puig Massana-Shiley ring is flexible and can be reduced in circumference by pulling two strings placed inside the ring material; unfortunately, in order to maintain this capability, a continuous suture has to be used.

For the placement of the Duran-Hancock flexible ring, all sutures are passed through the base of the leaflets in a U-fashion and parallel to the direction of the annulus. Double armed 2–0 sutures are used throughout. At the septal leaflet area, it is important that the needle be seen crossing the leaflet substance into the ventricular cavity and back through the leaflet into the atrium to avoid damage to the conduction system. For the remaining perimeter, the stitches can be passed through the annulus which, in the tricuspid, is more of a theoretical structure and therefore should be passed very close to the base of the leaflet. The bites should be approximately 3 to 5 mm wide and a maximum of 1 cm apart. As with the mitral valve, at each commissure the stitches are wider and encompass both sides of the commissural area, so as to selectively plicate those areas. About 12 stitches are used in all. Sizing is done by choosing an obturator that fits the distance between the two stitches placed at the extremities of the septal leaflet before the septal commissures. The rings have three equidistant markers, 27, 29, 31, 33, or 35 mm apart. The number indicated in the obturator corresponds to the distance between any two markers of the corresponding ring. For instance, if the distance between the extremities of the septal leaflet is 33 mm, a 33 obturator will fit, and the selected 33-mm ring will have 33 mm between any two markers. All stitches are then passed through the ring, which has a marker line to avoid twisting it when handling. The sutures should be placed in the ring more closely than through the annulus to already achieve some annular reduction. They should be distributed evenly to avoid buckling of the flexible ring. This often happens early in one's experience and carries no harmful consequences, except that it further reduces the tricuspid orifice. When a rigid ring is used, this mistake cannot be seen because it will be the annulus and not the ring that compensates for the error.

The result of the annuloplasty is checked with the heart beating since the tricuspid procedure is performed under nonischemic conditions, and in the approximately 15 minutes that it takes to place the ring, the heart is rewarmed. Saline is injected with a thin cannula placed across the tricuspid orifice in order to visualize any regurgitation. It should be stressed that some degree of incompetence in the tricuspid valve is well tolerated and does not have the same consequences as in the mitral position. Once cardiopulmonary bypass has been terminated, the valve can be palpated by the surgeon's finger, and any residual jet may be graded. The anticoagulation policy for these patients is determined by the left-sided surgery.

RESULTS OF TRICUSPID SURGERY

This technique carries a low mortality and morbidity, although it can be expected that about one-third of patients, if restudied, will show residual gradients, and one-fifth will show some residual insufficiency. To date, 510 Duran flexible rings have been used in the tricuspid position. A review of our experience was conducted in

1980, covering the period June, 1974 to December, 1979. At the time of that review, 368 patients had undergone tricuspid surgery, either replacement (nine patients) or conservative treatment (359). Nine isolated commissurotomies and 350 annuloplasties were performed utilizing 306 Duran flexible rings, 31 Carpentier rings, and in 13 cases, a DeVega procedure. All patients had a full preoperative catheterization study. The overall hospital mortality was 8.4 percent. One hundred nineteen patients with a Duran flexible ring were restudied postoperatively with a full catheterization, including biventricular ventriculography; 64 patients had "organic" and 55 had "functional" tricuspid disease.

A residual gradient was found in 45 patients (38 percent); 32 were detected at rest and 13 only after volume loading. The average gradient was 2.8 plus or minus 1.6 mm Hg. The incidence of residual gradient was 44 percent among those patients with organic disease and 31 percent among patients with functional regurgitation. The incidence of postoperative gradients found with this technique compared favorably with that reported with other techniques (50 percent with the DeVega procedure and 48 percent with the Carpentier ring). Thirty percent of the patients restudied showed residual regurgitation, which again compared favorably with the 41 percent found with the DeVega procedure and 31 percent following Carpentier ring annuloplasty.

These data reflect the technical difficulty of achieving a perfect surgical result with the available surgical techniques of tricuspid annuloplasty and are a consequence of the underlying principle of these techniques. Competence must be achieved at the expense of an annular constriction down to the systolic area necessary for leaflet coaptation; this area may be necessarily much smaller than the normal diastolic orifice. A careful sizing could reduce these difficulties, but only partially. It has been stressed, however, that these are hemodynamic data that may have little bearing on clinical results, which in this group of patients were excellent, since postoperatively, 87 percent were in Functional Classes I and II.

SUGGESTED READING

Cabrol C. Annuloplastie valvulaire. Un nouveau procede. Nouv Presse Med 1972; 1:1366.

Carpentier A, Deloche A, Hanania G, et al. Surgical management of acquired tricuspid valve disease. J Thorac Cardiovasc Surg 1974; 67:53–65.

DeVega NG. La anuloplastia selectiva, regulable y permanente. Rev Esp Cardiol 1972; 25:555–560.

Duran CG, Ubago JLM. Clinical and hemodynamic performance of a totally flexible prosthetic ring for atrioventricular valve reconstruction. Ann Thorac Surg 1976; 22:458–463.

Duran CG, Pomar JL, Colman T, et al. Is tricuspid valve repair necessary? Thorac Cardiovasc Surg 1980; 80:849–860.

CHOOSING A HEART VALVE SUBSTITUTE

W. GERALD AUSTEN, M.D.

The development of heart valve substitutes that function satisfactorily for prolonged periods has dramatically changed the care of patients with valvular heart disease. In 1954, Hufnagel placed a caged-ball Hufnagel valve in the descending thoracic aorta of a patient with aortic regurgitation. The valve was designed for quick insertion without circulatory support. Although it did result in partial relief of the aortic regurgitation, the valve had many problems, including a high rate of thromboembolism, correction of only a portion of the aortic regurgitation, and excessive noise. When it became possible in the late 1950s to operate with cardiopulmonary bypass under direct vision on the valves of the heart, a number of investigators developed valve leaflets or whole valves made of Teflon, Dacron, silicone, and other similar materials. Although initial results with the valve substitutes were encouraging, late valve degeneration because of calcification and/or tearing of the leaflets was extremely common. It was clear that different designs and/or different materials would be required for long-term success. Returning to the caged-ball concept, Harken, in March of 1960, was the first to successfully replace an aortic valve with this type of prosthesis, and in September of 1960, Starr successfully replaced a mitral valve. Thus began the present era of valvular surgery.

Over the last 28 years, a great deal of progress has been made in the design and development of materials for mechanical valves and in the preparation and design of biologic tissue valves to achieve more normal flow characteristics, to decrease pressure gradients across the valves, to avoid thromboembolic complications, and to improve the durability of the valve substitutes. There have thus evolved a number of very good mechanical and tissue valve prostheses. The current popular valve substitutes function remarkably well, but each has specific shortcomings that must be taken into consideration when a patient is evaluated for valve replacement and when the type of valve substitute is recommended.

GENERAL INFORMATION REGARDING VARIOUS VALVE SUBSTITUTES

There are two broad categories of valve substitutes—mechanical valves and tissue valves. When evaluating the choice of a particular valve substitute, the primary areas to be considered should include valve function, the incidence of thromboembolism (including the need for anticoagulants), and the durability of the valve. Other points to be mentioned are prosthetic valve size relative to orifice size, ease of insertion, intensity of valve noise, and (in the case of homografts) ease of procurement.

The mechanical valves that we will consider here are the standard Starr-Edwards caged-ball valve (Models 1200 and 1260 aortic and Model 6120 mitral), the standard Björk-Shiley and the Medtronic-Hall tilting disk valves and the St. Jude Medical bileaflet valve. In the tissue valve category, we will consider the porcine Carpentier-Edwards and Hancock heterograft valves and the allograft (homograft) valve.

The *Starr-Edwards valve* is easy to insert but requires a somewhat generous space because of its large ball and cage. The transvalvular gradients are larger than comparable diameter tilting disk or bileaflet valves but are still usually very satisfactory except in the very small sizes, and thromboembolic rates are comparable to those with the tilting disk and bileaflet valves used today. As with the use of all mechanical valves, patients should be anticoagulated with warfarin, and there is thus a significant incidence (approximately 2 percent per patient year) of bleeding complications. Most patients are aware of some increase in valve noise, but it is rare for this to be a significant problem. An important plus for the Starr-Edwards valve is that there is long-term experience (up to 20 years) with this valve with excellent durability statistics.

The tilting disk valves with reasonable intervals of clinical observation that we have used include the Björk-Shiley valve and the Medtronic-Hall valve. These valves are easy to insert, and their valve noise intensity is similar to that of the Starr-Edwards valve. Anticoagulation is, of course, necessary. The *standard spherical disk Björk-Shiley valve* has been used extensively throughout the world. The convexo-concave Björk-Shiley valve has had serious durability problems and has been withdrawn from use. The Björk-Shiley monostrut valve is in use in Europe at present but is not yet available in the United States. The standard Björk-Shiley valve has very good hemodynamic characteristics, and the incidence of thromboembolic complications with its use has been similar to that for the Starr-Edwards valve. Valve thrombosis in the aortic and particularly the mitral positions has occurred in a small but important percentage of patients; this very serious complication has been noted significantly more frequently with the Björk-Shiley valve than with other mechanical valves. Further, a small percentage of patients with Björk-Shiley valves has experienced the catastrophic complication of strut fracture and disk escape. The bad publicity from strut failure, primarily with the convexo-concave Björk-Shiley valve, but also on rare occasions with the early model standard Björk-Shiley valve, has dampened our enthusiasm for this valve, and we have not used it for the last year or two. Indeed, the manufacturer terminated sales of the standard Björk-Shiley valve as of January 1, 1988.

The *Medtronic-Hall valve* is a newer tilting disk valve. The flow characteristics of this valve are slightly better than those of the standard Björk-Shiley valve in that the disk opens to a larger angle. The thromboembolism rate appears similar to that for the Björk-Shiley valve, and there still remains a small incidence of thrombotic occlusion with this valve, particularly when used in the mitral position. As already mentioned, the hemodynamics of the valve are very good, even when small sizes are employed. Thus far, the durability of the valve has been excellent.

The *St. Jude Medical bileaflet valve* has become extremely popular in recent years. It has now had considerable clinical trial and is clearly an excellent mechanical valve. It is easy to insert and designed so that there is central flow; the hemodynamics are excellent, and the pressure gradients across this valve are the least associated with any of the available prostheses. Although there was some initial hope that anticoagulation might not be required, this is not the case, and all patients with St. Jude Medical valves should be given anticoagulation therapy if possible. Thromboembolic complications (approximately 1.8 percent per patient year in aortic valves and approximately 3.2 percent per patient year in mitral valves) are similar to or less than those with the other popular mechanical prostheses, and the valve has thus far demonstrated excellent durability. Valve noise appears to be slightly less than with the Starr-Edwards and the tilting disk valves.

The porcine heterograft tissue valves (*Carpentier-Edwards and Hancock valves*) have now been used for prolonged periods. The valves are supported on a stent and are thus easily inserted. They have central flow. The hemodynamics of these valves are quite good in the average and large sizes and have been improved in the smaller sizes with better design. Still, the smaller porcine heterograft valves may have significant gradients if inserted in normal- or large-sized adults. The thromboembolic complications with these valves are low, and most patients can be treated without long-term warfarin anticoagulation. The incidence of thromboembolic complications in patients with Carpentier-Edwards or Hancock valves and without anticoagulation is less than in patients with mechanical valves and warfarin anticoagulation. There are some data to suggest that patients in atrial fibrillation may have significantly more embolic problems if they are not put on anticoagulation therapy, and therefore we administer anticoagulants to all our patients with a heterograft mitral valve replacement who are in atrial fibrillation. The valve sounds are similar in intensity to those of normal valves. The primary problem with the porcine heterograft valve is, of course, late failure—leaflet calcification or rupture or both. This rarely occurs in the first 4 or 5 years after insertion in adult patients. At 6 to 7 years, however, the valve failure rate in adults is approximately 5 to 10 percent, and by 10 years it is approximately 20 to 30 percent. Some studies suggest that mitral valves may fail at a somewhat greater rate than aortics. The failure rate in children is markedly increased with a significant increase in calcification, and young adults have more rapid valvular degeneration than older adults.

The *aortic homograft valve* has been used in the aortic position as a stented as well as an unstented valve substitute. In the mitral position, the valve has been used only with a stent. When a stent is used, the technical aspects of homograft valve replacement are simplified and identical to those for insertion of the other valves that we have discussed. When an unstented valve is placed in the aortic position, the technical considerations are considerably increased. The homograft valve has excellent flow characteristics with central flow. The unstented valve in the aortic position has excellent hemodynamics, and the stented valve has very good hemodynamics except possibly in the smaller sizes. The durability of the homograft valve appears to be very much related to the method of handling and preservation. All of the early techniques of chemical sterilization and/or irradiation resulted in unsatisfactory long-term durability. More recent techniques of preparing fresh valves in physiologic salt solution and antibiotics and storing them for up to a number of weeks at 4° C have resulted in improved durability but still a significant late valve failure rate. Very recent reports concerning aortic homograft valves preserved in a nutrient media employing cryopreservation techniques with temperatures as low as −196° C have indicated extraordinarily good durability results with minimal valve degeneration at 10 years. This recent encouraging information has stimulated a number of groups, including our own, to investigate the use of this valve substitute. The incidence of thromboembolic problems with the unstented aortic homograft valve is very low, almost zero, without use of anticoagulants. The incidence with stented valves is similar to the relatively low thromboembolic incidence found with the porcine heterograft valves. The valve sounds with the unstented homograft valve are essentially normal. It should be emphasized that procurement of homograft valves is a problem; there is not an abundant supply of normal aortic valves, and processing of the valve requires considerable effort and cost.

WHEN TO USE WHICH VALVE SUBSTITUTE

We feel that each patient who requires a valve replacement should be considered individually in terms of the particular valve that would be most suitable for that individual. On the one hand, the mechanical valves have the advantage of long-term durability, but they all require lifetime warfarin anticoagulation and carry an increased risk of thromboembolism, as well as a significant risk of hemorrhage secondary to anticoagulation. The tissue valves have the advantage of low thromboembolic rates without warfarin anticoagulation, but the significant incidence of valve degeneration is an important negative point.

We consider the overall health status and estimated life expectancy of the patient in making a recommendation regarding a mechanical versus a bioprosthetic valve. In general, in patients under approximately 65 to 70 years of age, we prefer to use a mechanical valve if there is no contraindication to anticoagulation. We prefer the St. Jude Medical valve in most circumstances if we are going to use a mechanical valve, and we particularly like it in patients with small aortic roots or small left ventricles because of the excellent hemodynamics and small transvalvular gradients, even in the smaller-sized valves. We use the Starr-Edwards prosthesis in a modest number of patients who are appropriate for a mechanical valve replacement and who have an appropriately large aortic root or left ventricle; the Starr valve has stood the test of time with excellent durability. Some members of our group like the Medtronic-Hall valve because of its excellent hemodynamics.

In patients older than approximately 65 to 70 years of age, we usually employ the Carpentier-Edwards heterograft tissue valve if the aortic root or the left ventricular cavity is large enough. We recommend this approach because of the patient's limited life expectancy and the increased bleeding problems from anticoagulation in these older patients. If the aortic root is so small that we are concerned about an excessive transvalvular gradient associated with a small Carpentier-Edwards valve, we enlarge the aortic root by incision across the annulus in the noncoronary sinus and insertion of a Dacron patch so that a larger sized heterograft valve can be employed. We also employ the Carpentier-Edwards porcine xenograft in younger adults who are not appropriate candidates for long-term anticoagulant treatment. In young adult women who require valve replacement and who wish to have children, we prefer a bioprosthetic valve replacement so that warfarin anticoagulation can be avoided. Usually there is sufficient time before valve degeneration may become a problem for childbearing to have occurred.

As mentioned earlier in this chapter, there is some evidence that patients with atrial fibrillation should have anticoagulation therapy to avoid an increased risk of systemic emboli; therefore, in such patients, there seems less reason for using a heterograft valve, since it does not avoid anticoagulation. Thus, we usually employ a mechanical valve prosthesis in mitral patients who have been in atrial fibrillation for an extended period of time. In general, we also avoid the use of a mitral bioprosthesis in patients with small, soft, left ventricles because we worry about myocardial perforation from the valve stent.

In patients requiring tricuspid valve replacement, our philosophy regarding the type of substitute is similar to that stated above. In patients under the age of approximately 65 to 70, or in patients requiring anticoagulants for other reasons, we usually employ the St. Jude Medical valve. We prefer this valve in the tricuspid position because of its low inertial resistance and excellent hemodynamic characteristics. In older patients not requiring anticoagulants, we usually implant a Carpentier-Edwards heterograft tissue valve.

SUGGESTED READING

Arom KV, Nicoloff DM, Kersten TE, Northrup WF, Lindsay WG. Six years of experience with the St. Jude Medical valvular prosthesis. Circulation 1985; 72 (Suppl II):153-163.

Beaudet RL, Poirier NL, Doyle D, Nakhle G, Gauvin C. The Medtronic-Hall cardiac valve: 7½ years' clinical experience. Ann Thorac Surg 1986; 42:644-650.

Bjork VO, Henze A. Ten years' experience with the Björk-Shiley tilting disc valve. J Thorac Cardiovasc Surg 1979; 78:331-342.

Kinsley RH, Antunes MJ, Colsen PR. St. Jude Medical valve replacement. An evaluation of valve performance. J Thorac Cardiovasc Surg 1986; 92:349-360.

Magilligan DJ Jr, Lewis JW Jr, Tilley B, Peterson E. The porcine bioprosthetic valve. Twelve years later. J Thorac Cardiovasc Surg 1985; 89:499-507.

Miller DC, Oyer PE, Stinson EB, Reitz BA, Jamieson SW, Baumgartner WA, Mitchell RS, Shumway NE. Ten to fifteen year reassessment of the performance characteristics of the Starr-Edwards Model 6120 mitral valve prosthesis. J Thorac Cardiovasc Surg 1983; 85:1-20.

Miller DC, Oyer PE, Mitchell RS, Stinson EB, Jamieson SW, Shumway NE, Baldwin JC. Performance characteristics of the Starr-Edwards Model 1260 aortic valve prosthesis beyond ten years. J Thorac Cardiovasc Surg 1984; 88:193-207.

O'Brien MF, Stafford EG, Gardner MAH, Pohlner PG, McGiffin DC. A comparison of aortic valve replacement with viable cryopreserved and fresh allograft valves, with a note on chromosomal studies. J Thorac Cardiovasc Surg 1987; 94:812-823.

MITRAL VALVE REPLACEMENT

ADNAN COBANOGLU, M.D.
ALBERT STARR, M.D.

It is now more than a quarter of a century since the first successful replacement of a mitral valve on September 21, 1960, at The Oregon Health Sciences University. The problems that were given particular attention at that time were (1) fixation of the device to the living heart tissue to provide a permanent implant without perivalvular leak and without eventual dislocation, and (2) efforts to diminish the occurrence of thrombosis. These goals and application of sound surgical technique during heart valve replacement are even more important today, as more operations are being performed on much higher risk patients.

No single technique in mitral valve replacement is uniformly applicable to all patients and disease processes. The nature of the underlying disease process, the age of the patient, the fragility of tissues, and the type of prosthesis used all affect the implantation techniques. The surgeon should have an open mind and be versatile enough to adapt to different individual circumstances. Some of the techniques that are described in this chapter not only are of historical value but also could be applied in special, unusual situations.

ETIOLOGY OF MITRAL VALVE DISEASE

The most common etiology of mitral valve disease is rheumatic fever. Nonrheumatic causes of mitral stenosis include congenital abnormalities of the valve, mitral annular calcification, endocarditis, and myxoma. Some of the nonrheumatic causes of mitral regurgitation include floppy valve syndrome, myxomatous degeneration, congenital abnormalities, ischemic papillary muscle dysfunction, endocarditis, and idiopathic chordal rupture.

INDICATIONS FOR SURGERY IN MITRAL STENOSIS

The most common presenting symptoms of mitral stenosis are exertional dyspnea and hemoptysis. After the onset of symptoms, the mean duration of life is 5 to 10 years. There is uniform agreement that when a symptomatic patient reaches New York Heart Association (NYHA) Functional Class III or IV, surgery is indicated. Occurrence of supraventricular tachycardia such as rapid atrial fibrillation indicates severe derangement of atrial myocardial geometry and may have a negative effect on long-term survival. Earlier surgery in this subset of patients with mitral stenosis may provide better long-term outcome.

In patients with mitral stenosis who develop pulmonary hypertension, intrinsic alterations in the pulmonary arterioles and parenchyma may lead to irreversible pulmonary vascular disease. Valve replacement is the only effective means of preventing irreversible pulmonary vascular changes. If right ventricular failure related to pulmonary hypertension has supervened, surgical intervention is definitely indicated.

In general, surgery can be deferred in patients with mild stenosis with a mitral valve area index of 1.0 cm^2 per square meter of body surface area (BSA) or greater, whereas it is recommended for moderate or severe stenosis in which the mitral valve orifice is reduced to less than 1.0 cm^2 per square meter of BSA.

INDICATIONS FOR SURGERY IN MITRAL REGURGITATION

The most common symptoms of mitral regurgitation are dyspnea and chronic weakness and fatigue secondary to low cardiac output.

The timing of operation in patients with mitral regurgitation is more controversial than that for mitral stenosis. It is uniformly agreed that the symptomatic patient in New York Heart Association Class III or IV who has documented mitral regurgitation should have surgery. The problem arises from the fact that asymptomatic or minimally symptomatic patients with mitral regurgitation may pass insidiously into a stage in which irreversible left ventricular dysfunction occurs, thus obviating maximum benefit from surgery. Thus, in the patient who is asymptomatic or only mildly symptomatic (New York Heart Association Class II), close follow-up with noninvasive tests such as the electrocardiogram, chest x-ray, echocardiogram, and radioisotope ventriculogram is of paramount importance to prevent progression to an irreversible cardiomyopathic state. Enlarging heart size and left ventricular dysfunction should be indications for cardiac catheterization and early surgery. The maximum benefit of surgery is obtained in patients with preoperative normal ejection fractions. In patients with normal resting hemodynamics and left ventricular contractility, these should also be evaluated during exercise.

SURGICAL APPROACHES TO MITRAL VALVE REPLACEMENT

Left Thoracotomy

The origin of the left-sided approach to the mitral valve goes back to the early days of closed mitral operations by Cutler and Levine, Henry Souttar, and subsequently Charles Bailey in Philadelphia. Although this approach is still preferred in centers that continue to do closed mitral commissurotomy, it is an uncommon approach for mitral replacement.

The chest is entered through a full left thoracotomy incision through the fifth intercostal space or through the bed of the resected sixth rib. In most cases direct aortic cannulation is carried out in the ascending aorta or the aortic arch; if not, the external iliac or femoral artery may be used. For venous return primarily the right ventricular outflow tract is cannulated, since cannulation of the right atrium is more difficult, especially after previous surgery. A large pursestring of 3–0 suture material is placed, and a No. 34–36 F catheter is introduced into the outflow tract through a transverse incision. During this maneuver the incision in the right ventricular outflow tract is controlled with the left index finger, and the cannula is introduced retrograde into the right ventricle. An alternative cannulation for venous return is through a pursestring in the main pulmonary artery and again by threading a large-bore catheter across the pulmonary valve into the right ventricle. Decannulation is done in a similar manner, with the left index finger in place controlling the bleeding, and the incision is closed with interrupted or continuous sutures. If the infundibulum is friable, cannulation can be difficult. With atrial traction sutures placed appropriately, good exposure of the mitral valve can be achieved (Fig. 1), although at times exposure is not ideal. It is difficult to assess the results of repair. This incision is particularly useful for closed commissurotomy with pump standby.

Right Thoracotomy

The first successful human mitral valve replacement in 1960 was done through the right side of the chest. Right anterolateral thoracotomy may be applied for exposure of the mitral valve in selective cases when isolated mitral valve surgery is contemplated. In our experience, a full thoracotomy has very rarely been necessary.

The patient's right arm can be kept overhead or at the side; we prefer the overhead position. The right side of the chest is entered through the fifth intercostal space. The incision involves at least 1 to 2 inches of the latissimus dorsi muscle for optimal exposure.

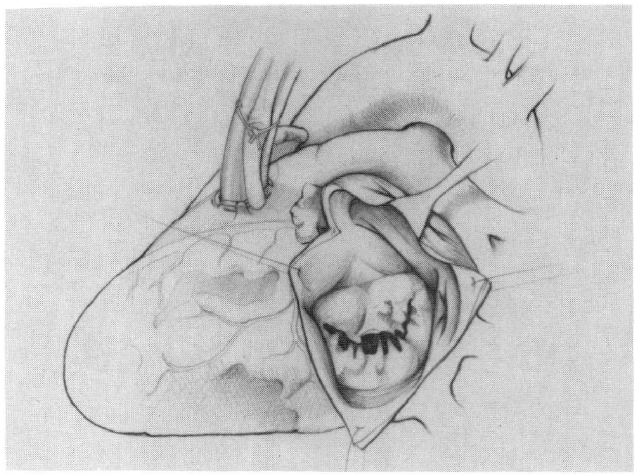

Figure 1 Exposure of the mitral valve through a left atriotomy (left thoracotomy).

Right anterolateral thoracotomy is particularly applicable in patients who have had previous cardiac operations. The mitral valve is approached relatively safely through the virgin right side of the chest with minimal dissection of the heart, avoiding extensive scar tissue and bleeding. The incision in the atrium is in the usual location, parallel to the interatrial groove. Evacuation of air is easy, since the left atrium is the highest chamber when the patient's right side is upward.

With this approach the exposure is limited, and surgery for associated coronary artery disease or aortic valve disease would be impossible.

Cannulation is carried out in the usual manner with two venous cannulas and an arterial cannula. The ascending aorta is preferred for aortic cannulation, and this can be done safely in almost every instance. Femoral cannulation is employed only as a second choice if a problem with aortic cannulation is encountered.

Median Sternotomy

The definitive approach to the heart in dealing with surgical problems was arrived at in the mid-1960s with the use of median sternotomy. This is the prevailing approach on most cardiac surgical services, as it is on ours; the surgeon has unimpeded access and total control of all cardiac chambers and great vessels. Arterial and venous cannulation, concomitant surgery (aortic valve replacement, coronary artery bypass), and evacuation of air are all carried out with ease. From the patient's standpoint, it is a much less painful incision than a left or right thoracotomy. Although median sternotomy is the most common approach to the mitral valve, one must realize that it is not a direct line approach, and certain maneuvers are necessary to facilitate exposure of the mitral valve. We have found aortic cross-clamping and the use of cardioplegia to achieve a completely relaxed heart to be necessary adjuncts to mitral surgery with this approach.

The incision starts at the suprasternal notch and extends about 1 to 2 inches below the xiphoid process. There is no reason to start high up in the neck; as a matter of fact, particularly in female patients, the incision could start an inch below the suprasternal notch. Following sternotomy and pericardial incision in the midline, the pericardium is tagged to wound stockinettes (Fig. 2). The aorta is controlled with a tape and the superior vena cava with a tape and tourniquet. Two venous cannulas are used. The superior vena cava is cannulated with a catheter through the right atrial appendage, and the inferior vena cava is cannulated low, close to the atriocaval junction. Thus, with the two venous catheters away from each other, after the left atrium is opened retraction provides wider exposure.

Arterial return from the pump oxygenator is via a No. 24–26 F cannula introduced into the high ascending aorta. A 12-gauge catheter with a Y-arm is introduced into the aortic root through a small pursestring suture for administration of cardioplegic solution and later for evacuation of air while the patient is coming off bypass (see Fig. 2).

The extracorporeal circuit consists of a roller pump system and a membrane oxygenator. After initiation of cardiopulmonary bypass, the inferior vena cava is controlled with a tape and tourniquet. While the patient is cooled down to 26° C, the interval between the inferior vena cava and the right inferior pulmonary vein is developed, and the pericardial reflection in this area is incised. The interatrial groove is developed so that the right atrium is rolled off the left atrium. A small pursestring of 4–0

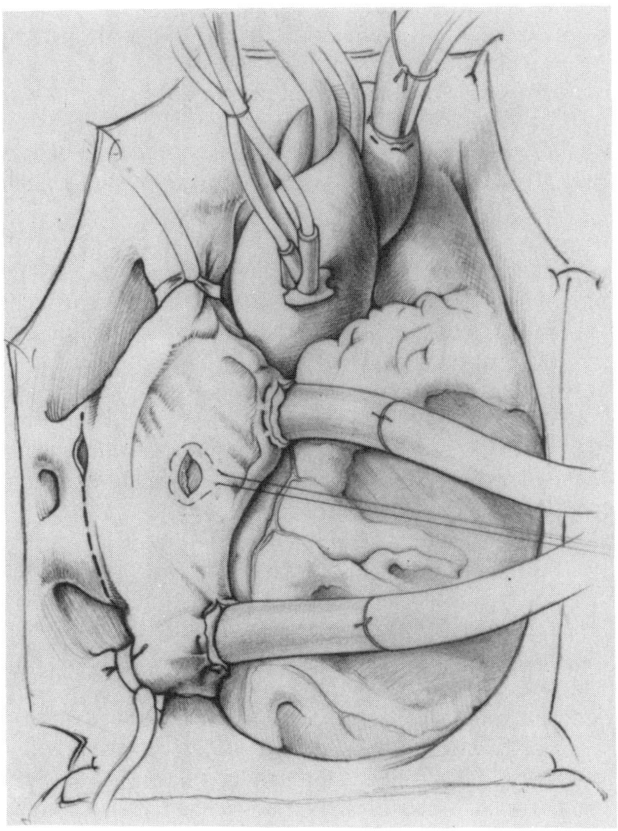

Figure 2 Exposure of the heart and cannulation through a median sternotomy.

polypropylene is placed on the right atrial free wall to drain the cardioplegic solution following its administration into the aortic root.

At 26° C body temperature or when cardiac fibrillation occurs, the ascending aorta is cross-clamped, the caval tapes are tightened, and cold potassium-blood cardioplegia is administered into the aortic root. This solution is recirculated and kept at 3 to 4° C. The interventricular septal temperature is continuously monitored and kept close to 10° C throughout the cross-clamping period with additional aliquots of cardioplegic solution. Topical cooling also is utilized by filling the pericardial well intermittently with an ice-cold balanced electrolyte solution. In cases of aortic insufficiency, the aorta is opened through a small transverse aortotomy and the cardioplegic solution is given via the individual coronary ostia with hand-held cannulas. The solution is drained from the right atrium through the previously placed pursestring suture. Retrograde coronary sinus perfusion has occasionally been applied in cases with concomitant severe coronary artery disease or in some reoperative cases with patent grafts (e.g., patent internal mammary artery graft).

Once satisfactory myocardial cooling is achieved, a longitudinal incision is made in the left atrium posterior and parallel to the interatrial groove (Fig. 3A). This incision is carried as far as necessary inferiorly underneath the inferior vena cava, and it enhances exposure of the mitral valve (Fig. 3B). We prefer two hand-held Army-Navy retractors for exposure of the valve, unless the left atrium is extremely large. When the left atrium is very large, a Cooley's left atrial retractor works very well. The Carpentier mitral retractor reduces the amount of assistance required but in our experience necessitates a wider opening of the sternal retractor. In our hands the two hand-held retractors have worked well. Cephalad and caudad retraction provides undistorted views of the subaortic curtain and the mitral valve (Fig. 3C). During this retraction, one should be careful not to let the tips of the retractors dig in and injure the interatrial septum.

The mitral valve is carefully inspected as to the nature of the disease process, the quality and mobility of the leaflets, involvement of the subvalvular structures (chordae, papillary muscles), amount of fusion, scarring, and calcification. Visualization of the valve is facilitated by engaging a cardiotomy sucker into the mitral orifice. Any thrombus or other loose material is removed. Once the decision to replace the valve is made, a backhand traction suture is placed into the middle of the anterior leaflet (Fig. 4A). Using a No. 15 knife blade on a long handle, the surgeon incises the anterior leaflet parallel to the free margin about 8 to 10 mm away from the annulus (Fig. 4B). This incision is carried around in both directions. The now mobile leaflet is grasped with an Allis clamp while a Metzenbaum scissors is used to separate the aortic leaflet at each commissure from the annulus. The papillary muscles are divided at their apex where there still is a whitish tinge to the muscle (Fig. 4C). During this maneuver care should be taken not to transect too low, i.e., resection of the papillary muscles themselves (particularly the posterior papillary muscle), which may weaken the ven-

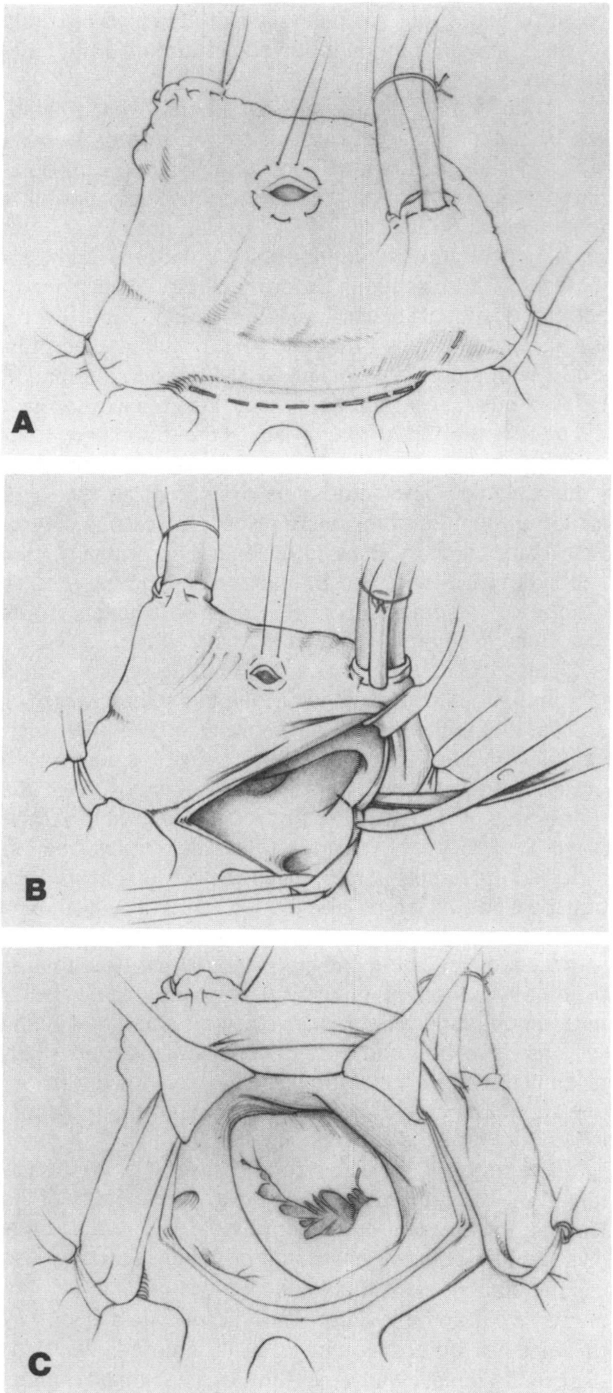

Figure 3 Transatrial exposure posterior to the interatrial groove. *A*, Location of atriotomy. *B*, Extension of atriotomy inferiorly underneath the inferior vena cava. *C*, Retraction of anterior lip of atriotomy incision with two hand-held retractors.

tricular wall and cause ventricular rupture. At this point a decision is made on the amount of posterior leaflet to be resected based on its pliability. Too vigorous a resection should be avoided in this area, and as much of the secondary and tertiary chordae as possible should be retained (see Fig. 4B). (At times, if the left ventricular function is poor, the entire posterior leaflet is left in.) One should be careful not to leave loose chordae, since they can interfere with the occluder mechanism of some mechanical prostheses. Too much resection in the posterior leaflet area weakens this already weak portion of the annulus further and may give way to atrioventricular separation. Also, one should leave enough of a rim for suture placement in this area in order to avoid deep bites with risk of injury to the circumflex coronary artery or the coronary sinuses. The same caution is taken in the area of the posteromedial commissure to avoid injury to the conduction system.

Once the valve is excised, the left atrium and the ventricle are flushed with cold solution, and all debris is removed. We prefer vertical everting mattress sutures for valve implantation (Fig. 5A). With everting vertical mattress sutures a three-dimensional fixation of the sewing ring is achieved, which we believe is important in order to diminish the problem of periprosthetic leak (Fig. 5B). Other techniques utilized (Fig. 6) are simple interrupted, figure-of-eight, horizontal mattress sutures with or without pledgets (pledgets on the atrial or ventricular side) or continuous suture technique. Porcine bioprostheses are best implanted with pledgeted horizontal mattress sutures with the pledgets on the ventricular side. Pledgets bolster the narrow sewing ring of these prostheses (Fig. 7).

The annulus is sized after placement of two sutures in areas corresponding to the anterolateral and posteromedial commissures. Downsizing is not necessary. The prosthesis should be a snug fit but should not be forced in with difficulty. With the Starr-Edwards Silastic ball prosthesis, the transparent valve sizer makes sizing easier, since one sees the annulus and adjacent tissues, gets a feel for pressure on the tissues, and can size the ventricle at the same time. The mechanical prosthesis of choice at our institution has been the Starr-Edwards Model 6120 Silastic ball valve. It is very easy to handle at the time of surgery. The lack of projections and the closed-cage design prevent the possibility of sutures becoming looped. The sewing ring is amply upholstered to avoid the problem of decubitus ulceration at the zone of contact with living tissue, also reducing the possibility of perivalvular leak. When sized appropriately to the size of the annulus and the left ventricular cavity, left ventricular outflow tract obstruction with this prosthesis is never a problem.

When valves of other design, e.g., bileaflet or tilting disk valves, are used, it is important to orient the valve in the particular position recommended to achieve optimal hemodynamic performance.

After placement of all sutures (2–0 braided Tevdek) into the annulus, the sutures are passed twice through the sewing ring of the Silastic ball valve, and then the valve is seated down and the sutures tied. The knots are directed toward the outside of the sewing ring during tying (Fig. 8A). We prefer to do mitral valve surgery without a left ventricular apical vent but use a No. 16 Foley catheter (in the case of bioprostheses, a No. 16 left atrioventricular vent), which is positioned through the valve in the left ventricular cavity and brought out through the atriotomy incision (Figs. 8A, 8B). The left atriotomy is closed with two sutures of 3–0 Prolene in a single layer with sutures

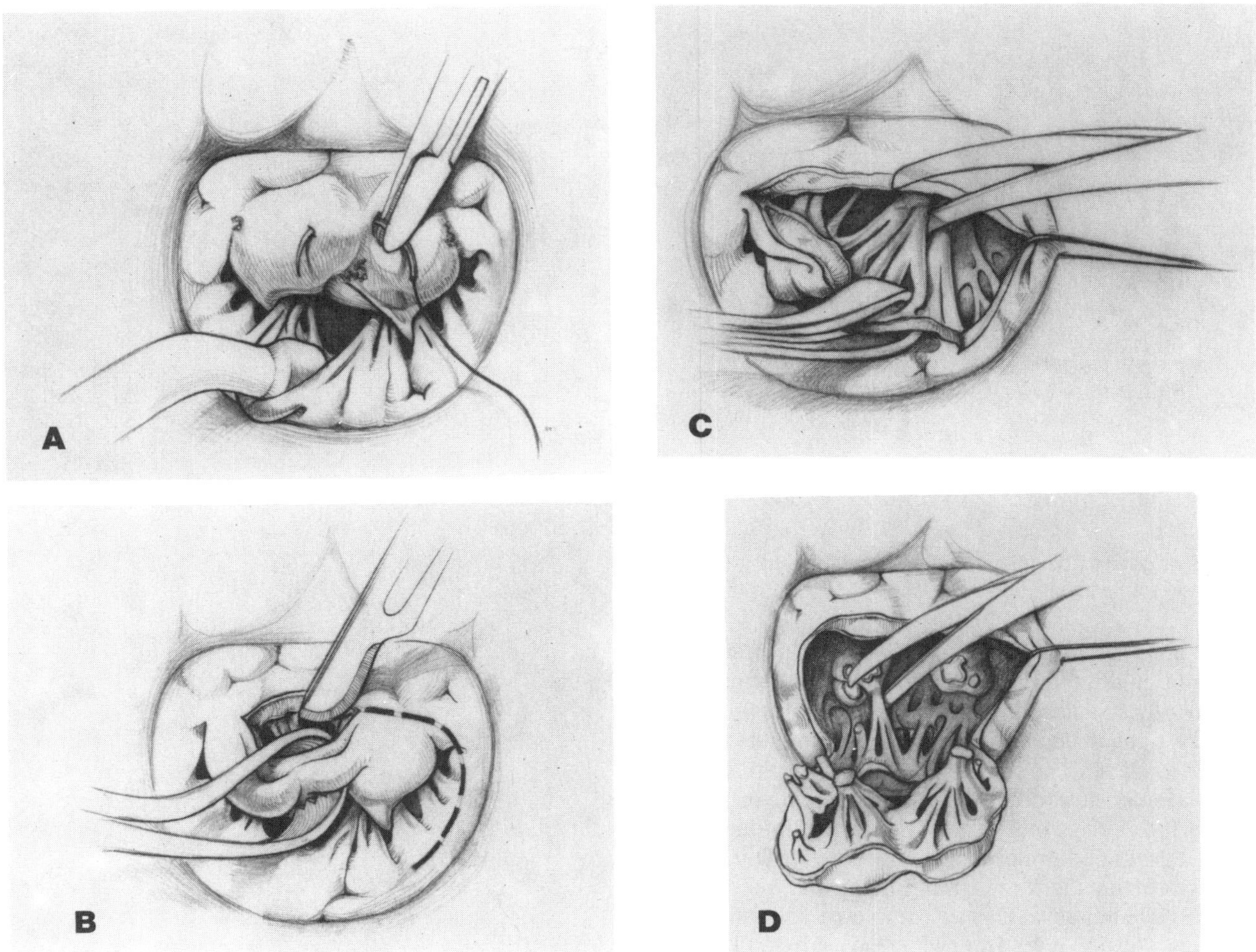

Figure 4 Excision of native mitral valve. *A*, Traction suture placed into anterior mitral leaflet. *B*, The anterior mitral leaflet is incised with a No. 15 knife blade. *C*, Division of papillary muscle at its apex. *D*, Retention of secondary and tertiary chordae in the posterior leaflet area.

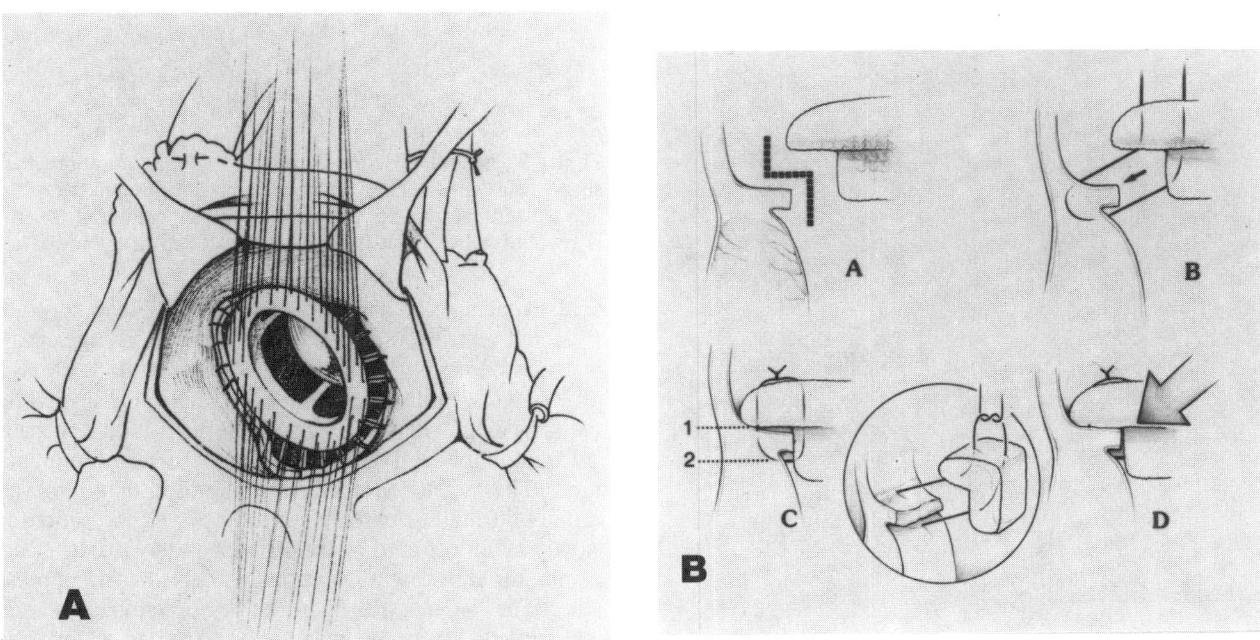

Figure 5 Mattress suture technique for valve implantation. *A*, Vertical everting mattress sutures for implantation of the Silastic ball valve. *B*, Three-dimensional fixation of a prosthesis with vertical everting mattress sutures.

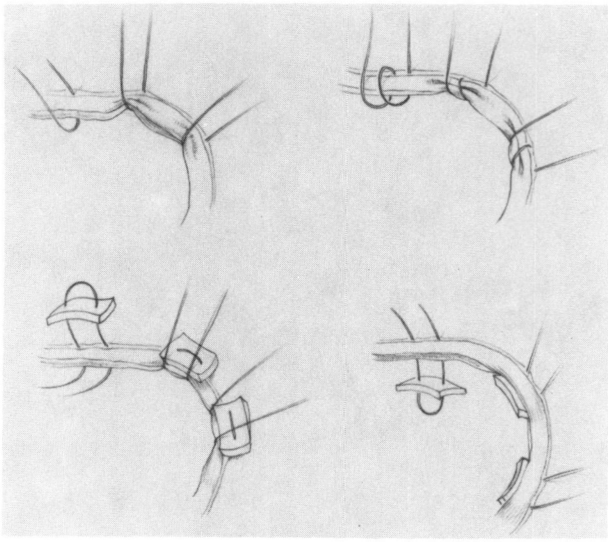

Figure 6 Various techniques of suture placement for mitral prosthesis implantation.

started at each end of the incision. Some of the fat in the atrioventricular groove is incorporated into this closure as a bolster. The Swan-Ganz catheter that at times lies close by in the right atrium is avoided by not taking suture bites that are too deep. The sutures are left untied until the last possible moment in order to allow for venting of the left side of the heart if necessary. The vent is brought out through the untied Prolene atriotomy sutures. During left atrial closure, patient rewarming is started.

With the left atrial closure completed, the ascending aortic cross-clamp is removed while the heart is still fibrillating. Air that may have entered the ascending aorta is evacuated through the side arm of the catheter used to administer cardioplegic solution into the aortic root. Air is evacuated from the left atrium through the untied atrial closure suture while the lungs are inflated by the anesthesiologist. The heart is lifted up gently, and the left

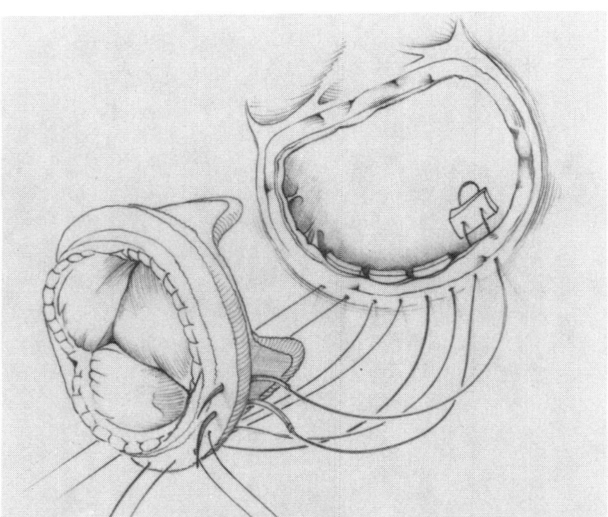

Figure 7 Implantation of porcine bioprosthesis with pledgeted horizontal mattress sutures (pledgets on the ventricular side).

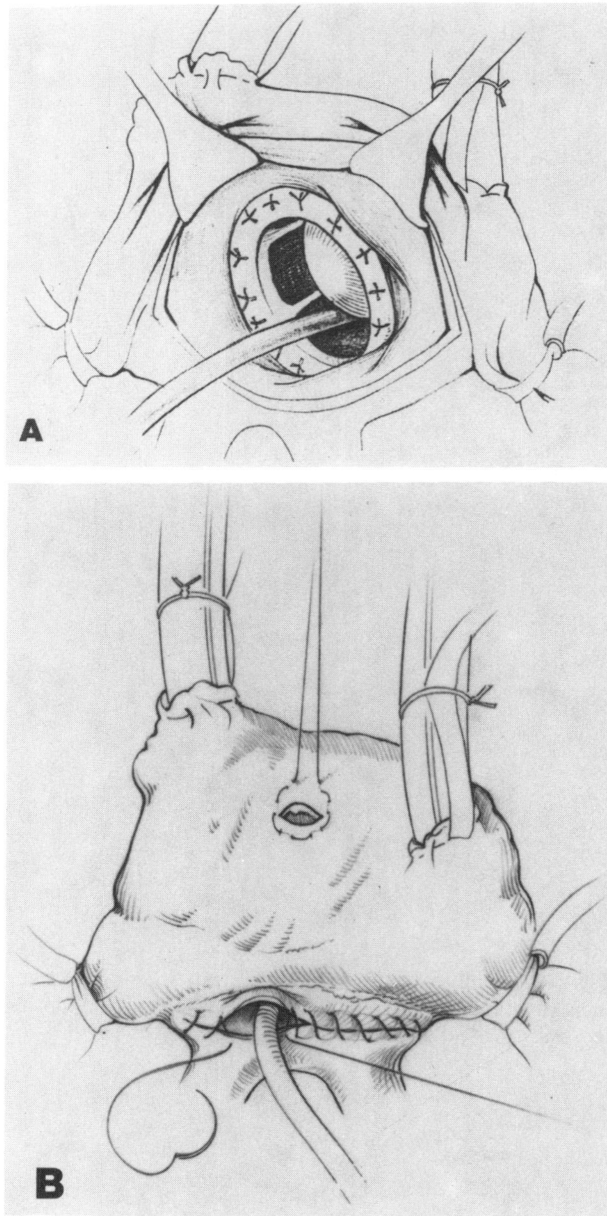

Figure 8 Seating of mitral prosthesis. *A*, The mitral prosthesis is seated, and a Foley catheter is placed through the valve into the left ventricular cavity. *B*, The Foley catheter (or vent) is brought out through the midportion of left atriotomy.

ventricular apex is aspirated with a needle and syringe. If the left ventricular apex does not lift up easily, the cavity is aspirated across the interventricular septum. After all air evacuation maneuvers have been carried out and while the ascending aorta is still vented, the heart is defibrillated. Adequate time is given for the heart to recover and gain vigor. The catheter across the mitral prosthesis is removed rapidly during one cardiac cycle. At 37° C, the patient is slowly taken off cardiopulmonary bypass, and the heart is monitored by direct inspection and also by filling pressures. The cannulas are removed while protamine is started and cannulation pursestring sutures are tied down. The aortic cannulation site is routinely reinforced with a second suture. After placement of two large chest tubes, closure of the sternotomy is routine with stainless steel wires for the sternum and absorbable running sutures for the presternal fascia, linea alba, and the subcutaneous fat. The skin is closed in a subcuticular manner.

Other Methods of Left Atriotomy

The Superior Approach. Incising the dome of the left atrium between the aorta and the superior vena cava was advocated and popularized by some in the mid-1950s. This approach gives broad exposure of the mitral valve, particularly when the left atrium is enlarged. The aorta collapses following cross-clamping and is retracted to the left and anteriorly, exposing the dome of the left atrium. One can injure the artery to the sinus node, particularly when it originates from the circumflex coronary system, with subsequent sinus node dysfunction and atrial arrhythmias.

Biatrial, Transseptal Approach. As described by Dubost, this approach is particularly applicable in cases of small left atria to enhance exposure of the mitral valve. An incision is started on the right superior pulmonary vein and continued perpendicularly toward the interatrial groove and on to the right atrium and interatrial septum (Fig. 9A).

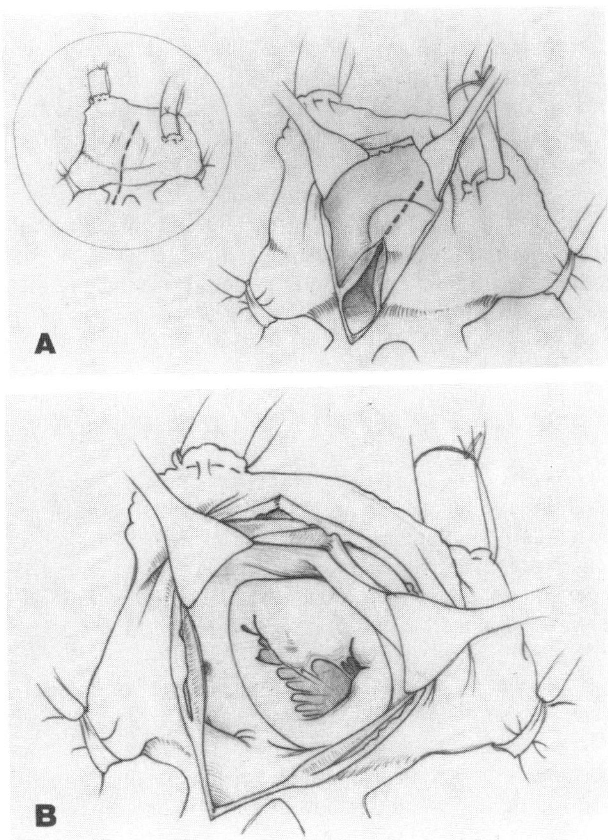

Figure 9 Transseptal approach to the mitral valve. *A*, Biatrial transseptal approach to the mitral valve; incision across interatrial septum at region of fossa ovalis. Inset: Incision starting on right superior pulmonary vein, extending onto right atrium. *B*, Excellent exposure of mitral valve (and tricuspid valve if necessary) through biatrial transseptal approach.

This approach provides excellent exposure of both the mitral and the tricuspid valves (Fig. 9B). It carries with it the risk of difficulty in closing both atria and in repairing the interatrial septum and the increased possibility of atrial arrhythmias.

A variation of the biatrial approach includes a longitudinal right atriotomy and longitudinal incision in the interatrial septum that is carried onto the dome of the left atrium in between the superior vena cava and the aorta. The right and left atria are opened up like a book page, and excellent exposure of both atrioventricular valves is accomplished. This is a cumbersome incision to close and carries with it the risk of injury to the sinus node artery and an increased incidence of atrial arrhythmias.

MITRAL VALVE REPLACEMENT UNDER UNUSUAL CIRCUMSTANCES

At times mitral valve replacement may become necessary following an attempted reparative procedure. Although the replacement techniques are similar, it becomes even more important to monitor myocardial temperatures and to have good myocardial protection with multidose cardioplegia. Additional core cooling may have to be undertaken in cases of rapid myocardial rewarming.

In patients with a markedly dilated annulus, it is not necessary to use a valve prosthesis as large as the annulus. The prosthesis will plicate the annulus against the sewing ring, and this is particularly easy to achieve with the Model 6120 Silastic ball valve with its amply upholstered sewing ring.

If concomitant aortic valve replacement is necessary, this is done following mitral replacement. In the cases of concomitant coronary revascularization, all distal anastomoses are done prior to mitral replacement. Multidose cardioplegia is utilized both through the aortic root and the vein grafts. Following mitral valve replacement, the proximal anastomoses are performed during rewarming of the patient.

Heavy calcification of the annulus is occasionally encountered. In most cases it is possible to squeeze the calcified area with a heavy forceps or a rongeur and make it pliable enough for suture placement. At times one has to place the suture around the calcified zone.

When mitral surgery is done as a reoperation it is not necessary to dissect the left ventricle completely free of adhesions. The left side of the heart and the apex are left alone. Thus the adherent pericardium in this area reinforces the back wall of the ventricle, and ventricular rupture or injury is avoided.

It is quite clear that there are different approaches and techniques employed when dealing with the diseased mitral valve. Any one of these methods will work well for the patient and for the cardiac surgeon as long as the choice is based on sound surgical principles and reproducible good results.

RESULTS WITH MITRAL VALVE REPLACEMENT

Utilizing one of the above techniques, the operative mortality for isolated mitral valve replacement is approximately 5 to 10 percent and is dependent on the preoperative functional class of the patient, the etiology of the valvular heart disease, and the degree of left ventricular dilation and dysfunction. Survival rates of 70 to 80 percent 6 years postoperatively can be expected.

SUGGESTED READING

Cobanoglu A, Grunkemeier GL, Aru GM, et al. Mitral replacement: clinical experience with a ball valve prosthesis—25 years later. Am Surg 1985; 202:376–383.

Cobanoglu A, Starr A. Starr-Edwards Silastic ball prosthesis: state of the art 25 years later in cardiac surgery. In: Crawford FA Jr, ed. State of the art reviews. Vol. 1, no. 2. Philadelphia: Hanley & Belfus, 1987

Dubost C, Guilmet D, Parades B, Pedeferri G. Nouvelle technique d'ouverture de l'oreillette gauche en chirurgie a coeur ouvert: l'aboard bi-auriculair transseptal. Presse Med 1966; 74:1607–1608.

Elkins RC, Bender HW, Brawley RK, et al. Technique for prosthetic replacement of the mitral valve. Surg Gynecol Obstet 1972; 134:485–488.

Meyer BW, Verska JJ, Lindesmith GG, et al. Open repair of mitral valve lesions: the superior approach. Ann Thorac Surg 1965; 1:453–457.

Starr A, Edwards ML. Mitral replacement: clinical experience with a ball valve prosthesis. Ann Surg 1961; 154:726–740.

PRESERVATION OF THE POSTERIOR CHORDAE TENDINAE IN MITRAL VALVE REPLACEMENT

TIRONE E. DAVID, M.D., F.R.C.S.(C), F.A.C.S.

The left ventricle is an anatomic and functional component of the mitral valve. The mitral valve, in turn, assists the left ventricle in maintaining its normal geometry and mechanics.

Experimentally, mitral valve replacement with complete excision of the native valve impairs left ventricular function. This impairment can be minimized by preserving the chordae tendinae during mitral valve replacement. It has been shown that the chordae tendinae of the anterior leaflet are more important than those of the posterior leaflet for left ventricular function. This is probably because the anterior leaflet and its chordae anchor the posterior and lateral walls of the left ventricle to the central fibrous body.

Clinically, successful mitral valve repair provides better results than mitral valve replacement. This is because mitral valve repair restores left ventricular geometry to a situation closer to normal and, consequently, results in better postoperative left ventricular function. The basic difference between mitral valve repair and mitral valve replacement is that the attachments between the mitral annulus and left ventricular wall are left intact in the former and they are severed in the latter. Thus, the chordae tendinae seem to be important determinants in the outcome of mitral valve surgery.

Mitral valve replacement with preservation of the chordae tendinae is an operation that mimics mitral valve repair. It has been shown that mitral valve replacement with preservation of the chordae tendinae provides better postoperative results than conventional mitral valve replacement in patients with chronic mitral regurgitation. This operation is particularly valuable in patients with chronic mitral regurgitation and impaired left ventricular function. Mitral valve replacement with complete excision of the native valve in these patients is sometimes followed by a stormy postoperative course, sometimes with minimal or no symptomatic improvement. Mitral valve replacement with preservation of chordae tendinae allows for a safer operation, and the majority of patients experience symptomatic improvement.

Patients with mitral stenosis who require mitral valve replacement usually have rigid, fibrotic, and frequently calcified valves. The rigidity of the mitral valve is such that it interferes with distention and contraction of the muscle fibers around the posterior and lateral walls of the left ventricle. Preoperative left ventricular wall motion is quite abnormal in patients with advanced mitral stenosis. Mitral valve replacement with complete excision of the native valve does not usually affect left ventricular function in these patients. Mitral valve replacement with preservation of the chordae tendinae in patients with advanced mitral stenosis is practically impossible, since the nature of the pathologic process is such that it would prevent the implantation of a prosthesis in the mitral orifice.

SURGICAL TECHNIQUE

As with any operation, good exposure is of the utmost importance. To accomplish that, each cava must be individually cannulated; the superior vena cava should be mobilized; and a generous incision extending from the superior to the inferior walls of the left atrium should be performed. A self-retaining mitral valve retractor helps to improve the exposure.

Every effort should be made to repair a diseased mitral valve. The surgeon should accept a mildly stenotic or mildly incompetent valve, since it is probably superior to any prosthetic valve. Nonetheless, valve replacement is usually required in more than one-half of all patients undergoing mitral valve surgery. This is either because of the advanced disease of the leaflets and chordae tendinae, as seen in patients with rheumatic heart disease, or because of disease of the papillary muscles and left ventricular wall, as seen in those with ischemic heart disease. The majority of patients with degenerative disorders of the leaflets and chordae tendinae have repairable mitral valves.

Mitral Stenosis

We believe that a patient with advanced mitral stenosis should have the valve completely excised before a prosthesis is implanted. Some surgeons advocate preservation of the posterior leaflet or parts of it as a measure to decrease the rare possibility of left ventricular rupture. This procedure does not have any effect on postoperative left ventricular function. The mitral annulus is usually small in patients with mitral stenosis, and it may be difficult to insert a prosthetic valve of adequate size when the posterior leaflet is preserved. It is our opinion that left ventricular wall rupture is caused by trauma during the excision of the mitral valve or the insertion of the prosthetic valve. A carefully planned and executed operation should prevent this dreaded complication of mitral valve replacement.

Mitral Regurgitation

All attachments between the mitral annulus and the left ventricle should be preserved during mitral valve replacement in patients with mitral regurgitation. However, this is not possible in all patients. Thus, in patients with rheumatic mitral regurgitation, parts of the anterior leaflet and at times some chordae tendinae may have to be excised in order to insert a prosthetic valve of adequate size that will function normally. We believe that the important ingredient in this operation is to preserve some leaflet tissue and its chordae tendinae so as to maintain continuity between the central fibrous body and both papillary muscles as well as between the posterior part of the mitral annulus and the papillary muscles. In most patients with rheumatic mitral regurgitation, a triangular excision of the anterior leaflet, as shown in Figure 1A, and preservation of most chordae tendinae are all that is required to allow the safe implantation of a 31- or 33-mm bioprosthesis or a somewhat smaller St. Jude valve. The edges of the anterior leaflet may have to be resuspended to keep the chordae tendinae taut. This can be accomplished by incorporating the edges of the anterior leaflet into the sutures used to secure the prosthetic valve in the mitral annulus, as illustrated in Figure 1A. The occasional patient with very fibrotic and retracted posterior leaflet and chordae tendinae may need two or three relaxing incisions to accommodate a larger mitral prosthesis (Fig. 1A). We prefer sutures with pledgets to secure prosthetic valves. The pledgets can be left either on the atrial or ventricular side. In patients with rheumatic valves, we usually place the sutures in such a way as to leave the pledget behind the leaflet (Fig. 1B).

No leaflet tissue has to be excised in patients with mitral regurgitation secondary to papillary muscle or left ventricular wall disorders. An incision is made along the midline of the anterior leaflet between the insertion of the chordae tendinae from the anterior and posterior papillary muscles. The two free edges created by this incision are then sutured to the mitral annulus using the same sutures to secure the mitral prosthesis (Fig. 1C). When some shortening of the posterior leaflet is desirable, the pledget should be left on the atrial side and the suture passed through the mitral annulus first and then through the leaflet at the desired point for shortening (Fig. 1D).

The anterior leaflet in patients with mitral regurgitation secondary to degenerative disorders is dealt with in the same way as in patients with ischemic heart disease. The posterior leaflet is often redundant and should be

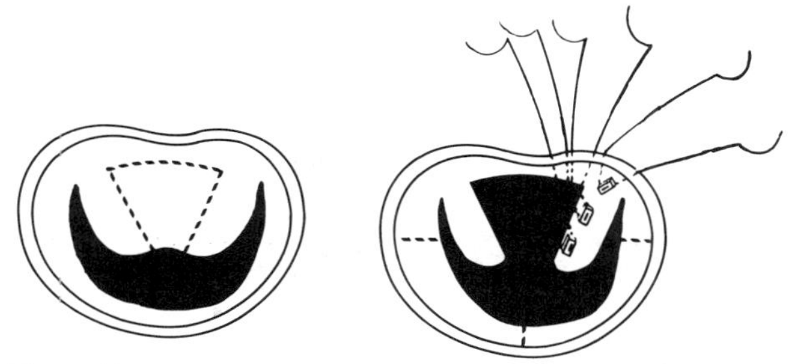

Figure 1A Rheumatic mitral regurgitation. The anterior leaflet is partially excised and its edges are resuspended to maintain the chordae tendinae taut.

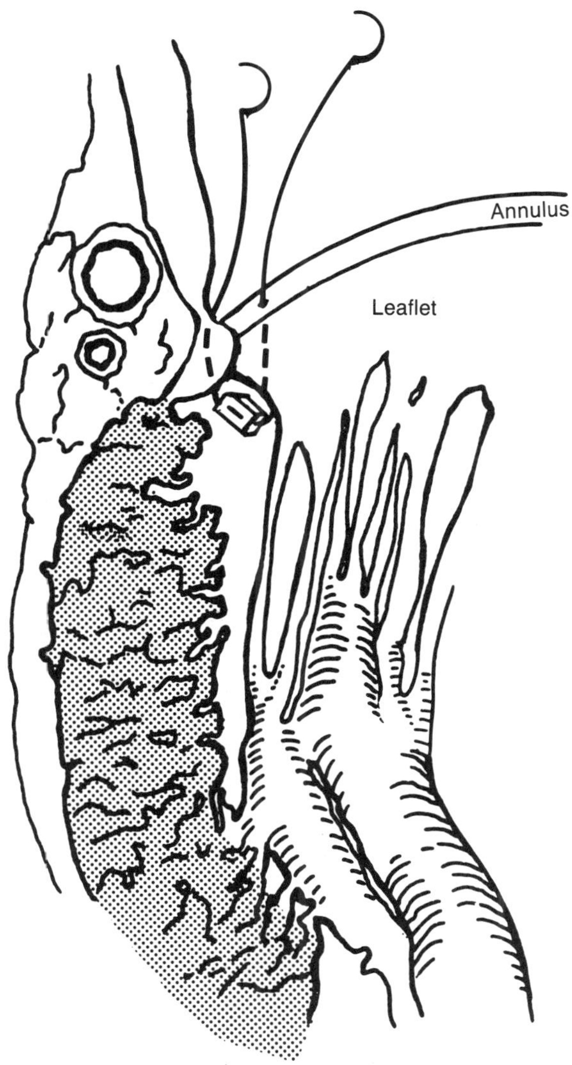

Figure 1B A method to secure the mitral prosthesis leaving the pledget behind the leaflets.

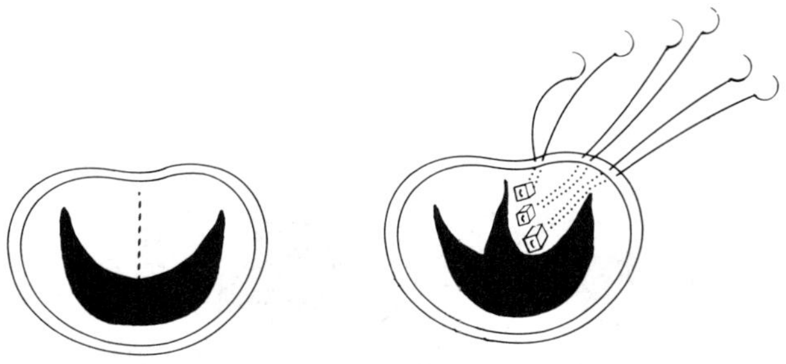

Figure 1C Mitral regurgitation with pliable leaflets. A simple incision in the center of the anterior leaflet suffices to allow the implantation of a mitral prosthesis.

shortened by incorporating parts of it in the sutures used to secure the mitral prosthesis (Fig. 1D).

Mitral Prosthesis

Certain mechanical valves should not be used when preservation of the chordae tendinae is desirable. Ball and disk valves that protrude into the left ventricular cavity during diastole may not function well in these patients. Mechanical bileaflet valves, such as the St. Jude Medical, have been used in a number of patients without apparent problems, as assessed by postoperative echocardiographic and Doppler studies. All commercially available bioprostheses can be implanted without adverse effect in their function.

CLINICAL RESULTS

The operative mortality and morbidity after mitral valve replacement for chronic mitral regurgitation are significantly decreased when the chordae tendinae are preserved. This method of mitral valve replacement also enhances long-term survival.

We replaced the mitral valves of 127 patients with mitral regurgitation during the past 7 years at the Toronto Western Hospital. The mitral regurgitation was secondary to myocardial infarction in 57 patients, and when operated on, 18 of these patients were in cardiogenic shock. See Table 1 for operative mortality and 5-year survival.

We believe that these differences are explained by the effect of the chordae tendinae in left ventricular function. We found that systolic left ventricular function after mitral valve replacement is significantly better in patients who

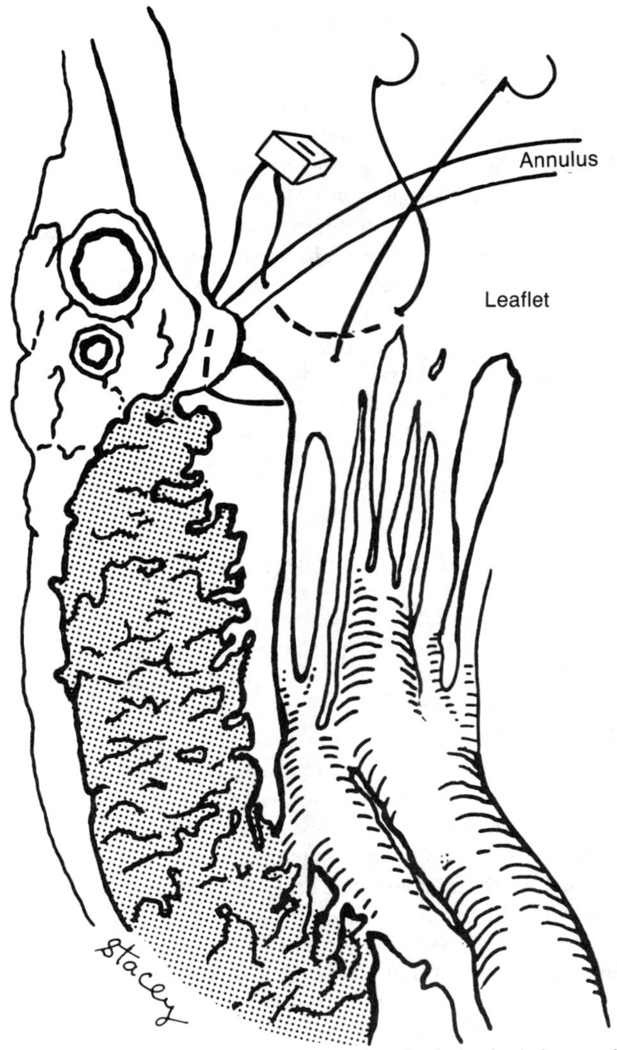

Figure 1D The suture used to secure the mitral prosthesis is passed in such a way as to shorten the leaflets to keep the chordae tendinae taut.

have had preservation of the chordae tendinae. Thus, left ventricular ejection fraction during exercise frequently increased when the chordae tendinae were preserved and frequently remained unchanged when the chordae tendinae were excised.

SUGGESTED READING

David TE. Mitral valve replacement with preservation of chordae ten-

TABLE 1 Mitral Valve Replacement: Operative Mortality and 5-Year Survival

	Operative Mortality		
	Hemodynamically stable	*Cardiogenic shock*	*Five-year actuarial survival*
Mitral valve replacement with preservation of chordae tendinae	0/68	1/12	87 ± 7%
Mitral valve replacement with excision of chordae tendinae	2/41	3/6	55 ± 4%

dinae: rationale and technical considerations. Ann Thorac Surg 1986; 41:680–682.
David TE, Burns RJ, Bacchus CM, Druck MN. Mitral valve replacement for mitral regurgitation with and without preservation of chordae tendinae. J Thorac Cardiovasc Surg 1984; 88:718–725.
David TE, Ho WC. The effect of preservation of chordae tendinae on mitral valve replacement for post-infarction mitral regurgitation. Circulation 1986; 74(1):116–120.
Hansen DE, Cahill PD, Derby GC, Miller DC. Relative contributions of the anterior and posterior mitral chordae tendinae to canine global left ventricular systolic function. J Thorac Cardiovasc Surg 1987;93:45–55.
Spence PA, Peniston CM, David TE, et al. Toward a better understanding of the etiology of left ventricular dysfunction after mitral valve replacement: an experimental study with possible clinical implications. Ann Thorac Surg 1986; 41:363–371.

ACUTE AND CHRONIC MITRAL REGURGITATION IN THE ISCHEMIC HEART

MARSHALL D. GOLDIN, M.D.
HASSAN NAJAFI, M.D.

Surgical repair of ischemia-induced mitral valve disease is associated with one of the highest mortality rates for treatment of acquired heart disease. The mortality for repair of acute mitral regurgitation (MR) following myocardial infarction ranges from 20 to 60 percent. Improvements in surgical technique and in pre- and postoperative care have contributed to gradually decreasing mortality rates. Long-term survival depends primarily on the amount of residual viable myocardium and its blood supply.

MR secondary to coronary insufficiency may be classified into two categories: (1) the acute process following a fresh infarction, often inferior, associated with papillary muscle rupture, and usually catastrophic in onset; and (2) the chronic type caused by multiple infarctions that lead to progressive cardiac decompensation. There may be intermittent mitral regurgitation due to acute episodes of ischemia; these exacerbations may resolve spontaneously and do not recur following revascularization.

Acute and chronic mitral regurgitation secondary to ischemic heart disease differ in various aspects. The pathophysiologic aspects and diagnostic features of each are summarized in Table 1.

ACUTE MITRAL REGURGITATION

Mortality secondary to acute MR diminishes in proportion to how well the acute process is tolerated; however, it is rarely possible to delay surgery for acute valvular disruption. Although intensive management and intra-aortic balloon pump support afford some degree of stability, it is essential to avoid delay in treatment in order to avoid compromising the function of vital organs. Prolonged periods of poor perfusion may result in extension of infarction and neurologic, renal, hepatic, or pulmonary failure.

For those patients with acute congestive heart failure who respond to intensive management, preoperative assessment includes cardiac catheterization and coronary angiography, with subsequent urgent operation. Patients in cardiogenic shock require intra-aortic balloon assist and emergent cardiac studies followed immediately by surgery. On occasion, profound cardiogenic shock may mandate emergency mitral valve replacement based on clinical examination and confirmation of the diagnosis by Swan-Ganz catheter. In general, however, it is preferable to obtain complete evaluation to determine the extent of underlying myocardial and coronary disease.

In most cases, preoperative management includes monitoring with a Swan-Ganz catheter, arterial line, Foley catheter, and often intra-aortic balloon pump. For those patients without preoperative intra-aortic balloon pump assist, with or without a radial arterial cannula, we prefer to include a transfemoral arterial line in the operative field to facilitate percutaneous introduction of the intra-aortic balloon pump catheter in the event that it is required perioperatively. In unstable patients, particularly those with hypoperfusion, it is preferable to avoid antibiotics that are potentially nephrotoxic.

SURGICAL STRATEGY IN ACUTE MITRAL REGURGITATION

Timing of Study and Surgery

Intensive medical therapy includes the administration of digoxin, diuretics, vasopressor and inotropic agents as needed, frequently insertion of an intra-aortic balloon pump, and, occasionally, transvenous pacing. As soon as stabilization has occurred, full cardiac studies must follow. Operation is essential if left-sided heart failure persists despite maximum therapy. Definition of left-sided heart failure includes the manifestations of low output with elevated left-sided filling pressures: a pulmonary capillary wedge pressure greater than 20 mm Hg, mean arterial pressure less than 60 mm Hg for over 1 hour in a previously normotensive patient, a cardiac index less than 1.4 L per minute per square meter of body surface, urine output of less than 20 ml per hour for 4 hours, and progressive acidosis. These patients are particularly vulnerable to cardiac arrest and demand expeditious evaluation followed promptly by surgery.

Mitral valve replacement is necessary in most patients. In a few selected patients, mitral valve reconstruction may be considered. Coronary bypass grafts should be included for significantly narrowed coronary arteries of adequate caliber that supply viable myocardium.

TABLE 1 Ischemic Mitral Regurgitation

Comparison	*Acute*	*Chronic*
Etiology	Papillary muscle rupture	Papillary muscle dysfunction/annular dilation
Frequency	Infrequent	Frequent
Location of myocardial infarction	Inferior	Multiple
Onset of congestive heart failure	Sudden	Gradual
Etiology of congestive heart failure	Mitral regurgitation ± left ventricular dysfunction	Left ventricular dysfunction ± mitral regurgitation
Onset of congestive heart failure following myocardial infarction	2–7 days	Weeks-months
Mortality	50% within 24 hours	Delayed
Diagnosis		
Echocardiography	Flail leaflet	Dilated left ventricle and annulus
Right heart catheterization	Giant V wave	Moderate V wave, elevated pulmonary capillary wedge pressure
Size of left atrium	Normal	Variable, often enlarged
Surgical intervention	Early, emergent	Semielective

Intra-Aortic Balloon Pump Assist

Balloon pumping may be used in the management of acute MR due to ischemic heart disease in three settings: (1) for preoperative stabilization of patients in shock who cannot be stabilized with pharmacologic support or those with ongoing ischemia prior to or following studies and prior to surgery; (2) intraoperatively to treat inadequate cardiac output and occasionally to assist patients who manifest marginal hemodynamics during weaning from cardiopulmonary bypass; (3) postoperatively to treat gradual deterioration of cardiac output; however, late insertion to reverse deterioration in this circumstance is generally associated with poor results.

Management of Cardiopulmonary Bypass and Myocardial Protection

Bicaval cannulation, perfusion via the ascending aorta, and systemic hypothermia to 26 to 28° C with a mean blood pressure of 60 to 80 mm Hg at a flow rate of 2 L per minute per square meter constitute our routine. Blood gases, electrolytes, blood glucose level, and urine output are monitored at intervals throughout the procedure and in acute patients, more frequently as indicated.

The aorta is cross-clamped gradually to ensure closure and to prevent intimal injury. We use intermittent multidose cardioplegia (4°C, 20 to 25 mEq potassium chloride), administered initially at a dose of 700 to 1,200 ml (depending on heart size), and supplemented at volumes of 200 to 300 ml every 15 to 30 minutes thereafter. Pressure in the ascending aorta during infusion is limited to approximately 100 mm Hg and is confirmed by palpation. We utilize iced slush for external cooling, including the right ventricle, with careful attention to avoid contact with the phrenic nerves. In patients with total coronary occlusions or poor collateral flow, cardioplegia infusion via completed bypass grafts supplements myocardial protection. In general, except in young patients with excellent left ventricular function and prognosis, we do not employ the internal mammary artery for coronary bypass in acutely ill patients.

Surgical Procedure

With awareness of greater tissue fragility in these patients, mitral valve replacement is performed in standard fashion. In patients requiring combined coronary revascularization and mitral valve replacement, all distal anastomoses must be completed prior to valve replacement. Manipulation of the empty heart can then proceed without the risk of posterior ventricular rupture secondary to torsion on the annulus or strut injury of the posterior wall. Although total revascularization is preferable, the duration of aortic cross-clamping is an important consideration. The three major vessels with viable myocardium should be the primary targets; additional branches should be considered on the basis of caliber, viable myocardium, collateral flow, and the total anticipated duration of aortic cross-clamping.

Approach. The size and configuration of the left atrium are the most important factors in selection of the incision for exposure of the mitral valve. If the superior portion of the left atrium that presents between the aorta and superior vena cava appears to be of sufficient size, as it may be in chronic MR, an anteroposterior incision will provide excellent exposure. Venting can be accomplished via this incision or via the right superior pulmonary vein. The presence of a short, immobile, or calcified aorta precludes this approach.

The standard approach with mobilization of the superior vena cava and inferior vena cava with dissection of the atrial groove is advantageous when the left atrium is small; this is often the case in acute MR. Avoid extension of the incision too far cephalad or behind the superior vena cava. Despite the above maneuvers, exposure may be somewhat limited in patients with small atria, even with the relaxation achieved with cardioplegic arrest. An alternative incision originating in the right superior pulmonary vein and extending obliquely into the right atrium and across the atrial septum to the fossa ovalis often provides satisfactory exposure. Another approach consists of separate incisions in both the right atrium and atrial septum; this exposure is generally satisfactory in the small heart with acute mitral regurgitation. In both of the latter approaches, it is preferable to place the inferior vena cava cannula as caudad as possible. Placement of a sump catheter in the most dependent portion of the left atrium provides a clear field. Utilizing the above approaches, it has not been necessary to divide the superior vena cava to obtain exposure of the mitral valve. In reoperative cases, mobilization of the entire heart facilitates exposure and minimizes the risk of traction on the annulus.

During total cardiopulmonary bypass with caval encirclement, it is often advantageous to allow cardioplegia draining from the coronary sinus to exit via a small (5-mm) stab wound in the lower aspect of the right atrium. Advantages include excellent myocardial preservation and avoidance of hyperkalemia and fluid overload; this may be particularly important in patients with acute MR if urine output was low prior to surgery.

In cases of anterior or posterior left ventricular aneurysm or a large akinetic area associated with MR of sufficient magnitude to require valve replacement, exposure via the left ventriculotomy affords remarkable access for removal of mural thrombi and mitral valve replacement.

Assessment of Mitral Valve. Upon entering the left atrium, determine the status of the mitral valve. For papillary muscle rupture, we believe that valve replacement is the operation of choice. If structural components of the valve are preserved, reconstruction should be considered except during emergency surgery, in which case mitral valve replacement is the most definitive and dependable procedure. As a rule, we avoid reconstruction if the patient is too ill or if the anatomy is questionable.

Selection of Mitral Valve Prosthesis. The most important considerations in selecting a prosthesis include the size of the left ventricular chamber, the anticipated longevity of the patient, and the risks of anticoagulation in that particular patient. Quite often, especially in patients with mitral valve disruption secondary to acute myocardial infarction, the left ventricle may be small and hence a low profile mechanical prosthesis should be selected, such as a St. Jude Medical valve or Medtronic-Hall prosthesis.

Since many of the patients in this group are also older and have limited longevity, the modest incidence of bioprosthetic valve failure should not be a significant factor against selection of this type of valve in cases in which the size of the ventricular cavity and the size of the annulus (29 mm or larger) permit such a prosthesis to be used. In younger patients with good left ventricular function, selection of a mechanical prosthesis such as the Starr-Edwards valve provides the greatest freedom from valve-related failure.

Evacuation of Air. Evacuation of air following mitral valve replacement requires meticulous attention to detail. With the patient in the Trendelenburg position, vigorous ventilation is performed by the anesthesiologist while venting is accomplished via one or more of the following routes: (a) left atrial vent, (b) aortic root cardioplegia catheter, and (c) incompletely closed left atrial suture line.

Construction of Proximal Anastomoses. Rewarming via cardiopulmonary bypass and a warming blanket is begun during closure of the left atrium. Maintenance of myocardial preservation requires continued application of iced slush to the heart until the aorta is unclamped. Gradual return of cardiac function, ventilation of the lungs, and gentle manipulation of the heart with or without the patient in the Trendelenburg position, rotation from side to side, and suction via the left atrium and left ventricle all assist in evacuation of intracardiac air. Continuation of ventricular venting during proximal anastomoses with side clamp exclusion of the ascending aorta prevents ejection of air during cardiac recovery. Prior to tying the last proximal anastomosis, coronary bulldog clamps are placed proximally on each saphenous vein graft prior to removal of the side clamp. Increasing cardiac ejection assists in further evacuation of any remaining air.

If the ascending aorta is calcified, fragile, or obviously atheromatous, the proximal anastomoses should be performed with the aorta still cross-clamped. When aortic access is limited, additional inflow may be obtained utilizing Y-graft anastomoses. Subsequent to recovery from cross-clamping, improved cardiac ejection and diuresis may occur prior to weaning from cardiopulmonary bypass. In such favorable circumstances, weaning from bypass may be accomplished without insertion of a Swan-Ganz catheter, balloon pump, or cardiotonic medications. Not infrequently, however, impaired cardiac activity associated with low cardiac output and marginal systemic perfusion pressure require meticulous attention to weaning while utilizing all measures to improve cardiac performance.

Weaning from Cardiopulmonary Bypass. Low cardiac output following combined repair for mitral regurgitation, particularly in the acute setting, requires a stepwise strategy designed to obtain graduated increments in perfusion with the least physiologic expense. Low-output syndrome may be defined as systolic blood pressure less than 90 mm Hg with a cardiac index less than 1.4 L per minute per square meter of body surface. Initial volume infusion during monitoring of pulmonary wedge pressure (up to an optimal level of 13 to 18 mm Hg) to maximize cardiac output and improve stability is followed by administration of a cardiotonic agent (dopamine 3 to 5 μg per kilogram per minute).

If the cardiotonic drug requirement increases without significant improvement in perfusion and cardiac output, intra-aortic balloon pump insertion must be considered.

Prior to insertion of this device, assessment of the systemic vascular resistance is essential. Elevated systemic vascular resistance (>1,600 dynes per second centimeter^{-5}) often responds favorably to dobutamine (3 to 5 μg per kilogram per minute), in addition to or instead of dopamine. Nitroprusside (1 to 3 μg per kilogram per minute) may also be used to reduce systemic vascular resistance. Rarely, systemic vascular resistance will be very low, requiring norepinephrine (2 to 4 μg per minute). Dexamethasone 10 to 12 mg intravenously and 4 to 6 mg every 8 hours for 24 to 48 hours may also be of benefit.

Often, low cardiac output related to atrioventricular dissociation, atrial asystole, or prolonged second-degree heart block responds favorably to sequential atrioventricular pacing (ideal A–V interval approximately 150 msec). Temporary electrodes are routinely placed medial to the junction of the superior vena cava and the right atrium for atrial pacing, and in the anterior aspect of the right ventricle for ventricular pacing. For sequential pacing, two electrodes are placed 1 cm apart in both the atrial and ventricular sites. In patients with recent onset atrial fibrillation, cardioversion (5 to 10 joules) is usually successful in converting atrial arrhythmias; this contrasts with patients with long-standing atrial arrhythmias, in whom sustained sinus rhythm may be difficult to achieve.

Rather than continued titration of medications, which also stress the myocardium, it is most logical to proceed with an intra-aortic balloon pump. Prior insertion of a femoral artery cannula facilitates introduction of the percutaneous device. Following institution of mechanical assist, stabilization or reduction of the dose of cardiotonic agents with improvement of cardiac output allows termination of cardiopulmonary bypass, reversal of heparin, and careful closure of the sternum.

Supplemental doses of digoxin and furosemide occasionally may be useful in the treatment of heart failure, supraventricular arrhythmias, and oliguria. Hyperkalemia that is unresponsive to diuresis may be treated with intravenous insulin 10 U and intravenous glucose 50 g.

SPECIAL CONSIDERATIONS IN CHRONIC MITRAL REGURGITATION

In patients with chronic mitral regurgitation secondary to chronic myocardial ischemia, the valvular regurgitation may be a result of annular dilation and/or ischemic papillary muscle dysfunction. These patients may present with varying degrees of angina and only occasionally require preoperative insertion of an intra-aortic balloon pump. In general, preoperative preparation may proceed in routine fashion.

The relative significance of valve dysfunction versus ventricular impairment must be evaluated when deciding whether mitral valve replacement will be necessary. Considerations include the degree of regurgitation, left atrial size, the amplitude of the V wave in the atrial pressure tracing, the response to medical management, and intraoperative evaluation. The advantages of combining coronary revascularization with mitral valve replacement are well recognized, with lower early mortality and better long-term results.

Important issues in regard to decision making in these patients include left ventricular function, the degree of mitral regurgitation and whether or not it is episodic, and the severity of angina, if present. In patients with angina, modest MR, and well-preserved left ventricular function without chronic congestive heart failure, coronary revascularization with or without mitral valve repair is the procedure of choice. Another subset of patients presents with recurrent exacerbations of mild or moderate MR associated with an acute episode of myocardial ischemia; in these patients, MR results from ischemic ventricular dysfunction rather than annular dilation or papillary muscle dysfunction, and coronary revascularization alone is also the procedure of choice.

In patients with moderately severe MR with good left ventricular function, the long-term prognosis is good. An aggressive approach toward restoration of mitral valve competence is warranted. In addition to revascularization, consideration should be given to mitral valve replacement or, when appropriate, mitral valve reconstruction. The final subset of patients includes those with severe MR and poor left ventricular function. These patients generally have chronic congestive heart failure, and their long-term prognosis is poor. Treatment is by revascularization and restoration of mitral competence; whether the latter is best achieved by mitral valve replacement (with or without preservation of the posterior leaflet) or by mitral valve reconstruction is not yet resolved.

ANTICOAGULATION

Anticoagulation with warfarin is generally begun on the second postoperative morning (following chest tube removal). In selected patients with long-standing mitral or tricuspid valve disease, meticulous monitoring of the prothrombin time is necessary, particularly if there is any hepatic dysfunction.

Long-term anticoagulation is maintained in all patients with mechanical prostheses, a previous history of emboli, and atrial thrombi. In those patients with bioprostheses, anticoagulation is preferable in the presence of atrial fibrillation, relatively low cardiac output, poor runoff following coronary artery bypass grafting, or when left ventricular thrombectomy or ventriculotomy has been performed.

MORBIDITY AND MORTALITY

Postoperative complications and mortality in patients with acute mitral regurgitation are related primarily to low cardiac output with or without associated infarction, whereas multiple organ failure accounts for most of the remaining mortality. In those patients with a postoperative low output state, the surgical mortality is 40 percent, with a 5-year survival rate of approximately 40 to 50 percent and only 16 percent for patients operated on who are in cardiogenic shock. Combined mitral valve replacement and coronary revascularization in patients with ischemic MR are associated with an operative mortality rate of 20 percent and an actuarial survival rate of 85 percent. Most late deaths occur secondary to arrhythmias, congestive heart failure, and recurrent infarction.

SUGGESTED READING

Buckley MJ, Mundth ED, Daggett WM, Gold HK, Leinbach RC, Austen WG. Surgical management of ventricular septal defects and mitral regurgitation complicating acute myocardial infarction. Ann Thorac Surg 1973; 16:598–609.

Christakis GT, Kormos RL, Weisel RD, Fremes SE, Tong CP, Herst JA, Schwartz L, Mickleborough LL, Scully HE, Goldman BS, Baird RJ. Morbidity and mortality in mitral valve surgery. Circulation 1985; 72 (Suppl II):120–128.

Minale C, Messmer BJ. Combination of mitral and coronary artery surgery. J Cardiovasc Surg 1986; 27:480–487.

Najafi H, Javid H, Hunter JA, Goldin MD, Serry C, Dye WS. Mitral insufficiency secondary to coronary heart disease. Ann Thorac Surg 1975; 20(5):529–537.

AORTIC VALVE REPLACEMENT

WILLIAM G. MARSHALL Jr., M.D., F.A.C.C.
NICHOLAS T. KOUCHOUKOS, M.D.

Aortic valve disease is the most common valvular disorder for which surgical treatment is indicated. Degenerative calcific aortic stenosis is the valvular lesion that most frequently requires valve replacement. Rheumatic aortic valve disease, which produces both stenosis and insufficiency, is encountered less frequently. Other conditions that may require aortic valve replacement include bacterial endocarditis, atherosclerotic ascending aortic aneurysm, ascending aortic dissection, annuloaortic ectasia, and various arteritides.

INDICATIONS FOR OPERATION

The three major symptoms of aortic stenosis are syncope, angina, and congestive heart failure. The presence of any of these is an indication for surgery, since survival is significantly shortened after the onset of symptoms if valve replacement is not performed. The presence of these symptoms is usually associated with a measured aortic valve gradient of greater than 50 mm Hg, or a calculated aortic valve area of less than 1.0 cm^2. The calculated aortic valve area is a useful indicator of significant aortic stenosis in patients with impaired left ventricular function, since cardiac output may be reduced and a significant pressure gradient may not be present between the left ventricle and aorta. Aortic valve replacement is also indicated in asymptomatic or minimally symptomatic patients if an aortic valve gradient of greater than 50 mm Hg or an aortic valve area of less than 1.0 cm^2 is present.

The indications for valve replacement in patients with aortic insufficiency are less precise, since the severity of the insufficiency is often difficult to quantitate, and the adverse effects of left ventricular volume overload (as opposed to the pressure overload of aortic stenosis) are more difficult to predict. Congestive heart failure New York Heart Association Class III—IV is considered an indication for valve replacement, since evidence of left ventricular dysfunction is usually present. The presence of Class IV symptoms is associated with increased operative risk and a lesser degree of functional improvement postoperatively. Because of the lack of functional improvement in a substantial number of Class IV as well as some Class III patients, valve replacement earlier in the course of the disease should be considered in less symptomatic patients who have echocardiographic evidence of left ventricular enlargement (left ventricular end-systolic dimension greater than 50 mm) and subnormal fractional shortening (less than 25 percent), and those who have roentgenographic evidence of left ventricular decompensation (cardiac to thoracic wall ratio greater than 0.55 on a standard chest roentgenogram, or a left ventricular ejection fraction of less than 40 percent).

Patients with moderate or severe aortic insufficiency as a result of annuloaortic ectasia, aortic dissection, or atherosclerotic aneurysm of the ascending aorta usually require replacement of the aortic valve in conjunction with resection and replacement of the ascending aorta. Valve replacement in patients with native or prosthetic valve endocarditis is ideally performed after a 2- to 4-week course of antibiotic therapy but may be required more urgently if significant cardiac failure or persisting bacteremia is present.

From 25 to 50 percent of patients with aortic valve disease have significant coexisting coronary artery disease. The exact etiology of the symptom of angina is difficult to determine when these disorders coexist. Since isolated valve replacement in this setting is associated with a higher incidence of persistent symptoms, late myocardial infarction, and death, combined aortic valve replacement and myocardial revascularization is recommended for virtually all patients in whom the two lesions coexist. Addition of coronary artery bypass grafting to aortic valve replacement is not associated with increased hospital mortality or perioperative myocardial infarction.

Patients with symptomatic coronary artery disease who undergo coronary artery bypass grafting and who have aortic valve disease (aortic valve gradient of greater than 50 mm Hg, aortic valve area of less than 1.0 cm^2, or moderate to severe aortic regurgitation) should have concomitant aortic valve replacement even in the absence of symptoms. Aortic valvular disease of this severity can be expected to progress, and a second operation to replace the aortic valve frequently is necessary. These secondary procedures are associated with increased risk. In addition moderate or severe aortic regurgitation may result in severe left ventricular distention after initiation of cardiopulmonary bypass or if ventricular fibrillation develops. If this occurs after release of the aortic clamp, it may be difficult to establish an effective rhythm and to discontinue cardiopulmonary bypass.

There are few contraindications to aortic valve replacement in patients with hemodynamically significant aortic stenosis. Removal of the outflow obstruction usually results in adequate left ventricular function, even in the presence of severe preoperative myocardial dysfunction, if intraoperative myocardial protection is adequate. Patients with associated right ventricular failure without organic mitral or tricuspid valvular disease, and those with critical valve areas (less than 1.0 cm^2) but with gradients less than 30 to 40 mm Hg, are at significantly higher risk for operation. Patients with aortic regurgitation and marked left ventricular dysfunction (ejection fraction of less than 25 to 30 percent) are also at higher risk. Currently methods to accurately identify patients with myocardial dysfunction who will not benefit from correction of the valvular lesion, are not available.

TECHNICAL CONSIDERATIONS

A median sternotomy incision is used, and the ascending aorta is cannulated just proximal to the innominate artery. A single two-stage venous cannula is placed through the right atrial appendage for venous return, and the left side of the heart is decompressed with a catheter placed through the right superior pulmonary vein and positioned in the left ventricle. A polyvinyl catheter for measurement of left atrial pressure is also placed through the right superior pulmonary vein. Cardiopulmonary bypass is established at an initial flow of 2.2 L per minute per square meter using a crystalloid priming solution. The myocardium is cooled to 25 to 27° C by stepwise reduction of the perfusate temperature to 15° C. The ascending aorta is then clamped. During the period of aortic clamping, systemic perfusion is maintained at 1.6 to 2.0 L per minute per square meter at 24 to 28° C. The pericardial cavity is continuously irrigated during this period with 1 to 2 L of 4° C Ringer's solution.

A transverse incision is made in the aorta just above the right coronary ostium. It is extended obliquely into the center of the noncoronary sinus. Hypothermic (4° C), hyperkalemic (30 mEq K+ per liter), oxygenated crystalloid cardioplegia is infused directly into the coronary ostia, using Silastic balloon-tipped catheters. Initially, 350 ml per square meter are infused during a 2- to 3-minute interval. If necessary, the infusion is continued until the myocardial temperature, measured with a thermistor probe in the anterior ventricular septum, reaches 10 to 12° C. Additional infusions are given when the myocardial temperature exceeds 18° C, if ventricular fibrillation occurs, or every 20 to 30 minutes. The left main coronary artery may be very short, and care must be taken not to infuse only the anterior descending or circumflex artery. This can result in severe ischemia of the anterior or lateral left ventricular wall. Preoperative coronary arteriography is helpful in identifying this anatomic finding.

A sponge is placed in the left ventricular cavity, and a small piece of umbilical tape is placed in the left coronary ostium to prevent embolization of calcium. Excision of the valve is begun at the commissure between the right and noncoronary cusps. The right coronary cusp is excised first. The left coronary cusp is excised next, followed by the noncoronary cusp. Use of a No. 15 scalpel blade allows the cusps to be excised at their junction with the annulus. If necessary, a rongeur is used to remove residual calcium from the annulus. Its removal is necessary to permit optimal placement of the sutures and firm seating of the prosthesis. The débridement must be done carefully in the left coronary sinus to prevent perforation. After the valve is excised, the packing is removed and the ventricular cavity is copiously irrigated with saline to remove all particulate matter. The size of the aortic annulus is determined, and the appropriate prosthesis is selected.

If coronary artery bypass grafting is required, the grafts are anastomosed to the coronary arteries at this time. Cardioplegic solution can then be infused directly into the vein grafts as well as the coronary ostia. This is advisable if the coronary artery disease is severe and diffuse, and if myocardial cooling is not optimal. The aortic prosthesis is then sewn in place.

If a bioprosthesis is used, pledgeted 2–0 Ticron horizontal mattress sutures are placed with the pledgets on the ventricular side of the annulus. This often permits insertion of a prosthesis that is one size larger than that used if the pledgets are placed on the aortic side of the annulus. This technique is particularly useful in the patient with a small aortic root. If a mechanical prosthesis is inserted, simple interrupted sutures of 2–0 Ticron are generally used. If the annulus is thin, friable, or large (larger than 25 mm), pledgeted horizontal mattress sutures are used with the pledgets placed on the aortic side of the annulus to prevent interference with the motion of the occluder. When an aortic allograph is used, a valve 2 to to 3 mm smaller in diameter than the measured diameter of the annulus is selected. It is thawed, trimmed, and inserted using two layers of continuous 4–0 polypropylene suture.

After insertion of the valve, the aorta is closed with a single layer of continuous 4–0 polypropylene suture. Before completing the closure, the heart is filled with blood to evacuate air. When the closure is completed, the aortic cross-clamp is removed and air is evacuated from the aorta with a needle vent attached to suction. If coronary bypass grafts have been placed, the anastomoses of the grafts to the aorta are now performed using a partially occluding clamp. After release of this clamp, residual air is evacuated from the ventricle and ascending aorta. The ventricular vent is removed, and the patient is weaned from cardiopulmonary bypass. Pairs of pacing wires are placed on the atrium and ventricle. Two mediastinal drainage tubes are inserted, and the wound is closed.

Patients with bioprostheses do not usually receive anticoagulant therapy but are given antiplatelet agents (aspirin, dipyridamole). Patients with mechanical prostheses are placed on warfarin sodium beginning on the second postoperative day.

RESULTS OF OPERATION

Operative mortality for elective isolated aortic valve replacement is less than 5 percent. Age at operation and the severity of preoperative left ventricular dysfunction are the primary determinants of risk. Operative and late mortality rates are generally higher among patients with aortic incompetence than in patients with aortic stenosis. This is related primarily to the presence of more severe preoperative left ventricular dysfunction preoperatively. The adequacy of intraoperative myocardial protection becomes an important determinant of risk during procedures that require prolonged periods of myocardial ischemia (greater than 90 minutes). Major complications following aortic valve replacement include perioperative myocardial infarction (1 to 3 percent), permanent or transient neurologic deficits (1 to 3 percent), and the development of complete heart block, (less than 1 percent).

Long-term survival is approximately 85 to 90 percent at 5 years. Factors that adversely affect survival include preoperative left ventricular dysfunction, advanced age, concomitant untreated coronary artery disease, and ventricular arrhythmias. Approximately 80 to 90 percent of patients achieve New York Heart Association Class I and II status postoperatively. Some studies have suggested that the type of prosthesis inserted may have an effect on long-term survival, but this is not clearly established. Late complications, including thromboembolism, prosthetic valve endocarditis, prosthetic valve malfunction, and bleeding secondary to anticoagulant therapy, each occur at a frequency of 1 to 2 percent per year and are related in some degree to the type of prosthesis implanted. To date, no prosthesis has been found to be completely free of complications or superior to any other one currently employed.

SUGGESTED READING

Barrett-Boyes BG, Roche AHG, Whitlock RML. Six year review of the results of free-load aortic valve replacement using an antibiotic sterilized homograft valve. Circulation 1977; 55:353–361.

Borkon AM, Soule L, Baughman KL, et al. Ten year analysis of the Bjork-Shiley standard aortic valve. Ann Thorac Surg 1987; 43:39–51.

Kouchoukos NT, Lell WA, Rogers WJ. Combined aortic valve replacement and myocardial revascularization—experience with a cold, cardioplegia technique. Ann Surg 1983; 197:721–727.

Richardson JV, Kouchoukos NT, Wright JO, Karp RB. Combined aortic valve replacement and myocardial revascularization: results in 220 patients. Circulation 1979; 59:75–81.

Ross J Jr. Afterload mismatch in aortic and mitral valve disease: implantation for surgical therapy. J Am Coll Cardiol 1985; 5:811–826.

AORTIC VALVE REPLACEMENT IN THE ADULT WITH SMALL AORTIC ANNULUS

LAWRENCE H. COHN, M.D.

Development of reliable replacement devices for the human aortic valve has been one of the most important therapeutic advances in this century. Aortic valve replacement with the bioprosthetic or prosthetic devices available at present is established as an adequate and safe method of dealing with the wide variety of pathologic lesions in the aortic root. In the adult, aortic valve replacement is by far the most common procedure, although calcific débridement of aortic leaflets and occasionally aortic commissurotomy are still techniques that may be utilized in some patients. Since there are a variety of excellent and durable prosthetic and bioprosthetic valves, it is now possible to use a particular valve taking into consideration the patient's clinical history and anatomic findings. In the vast majority of cases, such a satisfactory valve-patient match is obtainable.

In some adult patients with classic degenerative aortic valve disease or in adults in whom inadequate results were obtained after valvulotomy when they were children, the aortic annulus is so small that either no prosthesis or a prosthesis of suboptimal size can be inserted without special surgical techniques to enlarge the aortic root. Aortic valve replacement with a small aortic prosthesis may leave an unacceptable resting and exercise gradient in adult patients. The size of the aortic prosthesis therefore should be proportional to the size of the patient and consistent with the probable cardiac output because a minimal gradient across the prosthetic aortic valve is one of the objectives of valve replacement. This chapter details the therapeutic possibilities of aortic valve replacement using the appropriate size prosthesis in the small adult aortic root and the surgical options within that framework.

There are eight therapeutic alternatives for the surgical treatment of the patient with a small aortic annulus in whom the desired valve to be implanted may be too large or possess an unacceptably large resting and exercise gradient in a particular patient.

1. Change the prosthesis from the initially desired one to one with superior hemodynamics. In elderly patients in whom it has been shown that anticoagulation is a higher risk therapy and in whom a biologic valve would be desirable, the annulus may be too small for a bioprosthetic valve. In our clinic, 21-mm Modified Orifice Hancock and 21-mm Carpentier-Edwards porcine valves are used without hesitation in the elderly age group. The gradients in these valves have been acceptably low in smaller patients and in those in the elderly age group with a relatively low cardiac output, but an annular diameter of less than 21 mm usually would necessitate a change of valve selection to a mechanical valve. We have used the Ionescu-Shiley pericardial valve in the 19 mm range (actual diameter is 20 mm), a biologic valve hemodynamically superior to the porcine valve. The 19-mm Ionescu valve, however, has high rigid struts that may be a disadvantage in pa-

tients with extremely calcified and/or narrowed aortic roots above the aortic valve. Thus, in this situation we have turned to the 19-mm St. Jude bileaflet valve in the elderly patient, despite the fact that anticoagulation is required.

2. If there is an absolute contraindication to anticoagulation together with a small aortic root, and a St. Jude valve is unacceptable because of this reason, then a tissue valve, probably a 19-mm Ionescu valve, will be inserted. In order to close the ascending aorta, a second therapeutic option may be necessary—the placement of an oval Dacron or Goretex gusset in the ascending aorta beginning at the annulus and completely filling out the aortotomy with increased width without impinging on the high struts of the Ionescu or porcine valve.
3. In the event that the annulus is smaller than 19 mm in diameter, the aortic incision may be extended through the noncoronary cusp and into the anterior leaflet of the mitral valve. This operation, which has been named the Manouguian or Nicks procedure, allows for the upsizing of at least one valve size (2 mm). Valve annular sutures are placed at the apex of the incision in the mitral valve and then passed through the valve annulus. A patch gusset is usually needed to close the aorta.
4. In the event that procedure number 3 has not increased the size of the annulus sufficiently for the patient, an extension of this incision into the left atrium as well, suggested by Rittenhouse, may be a therapeutic alternative in rare instances. This involves the use of a double-patch technique to enlarge the roof of the left atrium and the anterior leaflet of the mitral valve as well as to promote fixation of the aortic prosthesis at the annular ring.
5. In endocarditis of the aortic valve and annulus, it often is required that a low profile valve prosthesis be inserted in a tilting position because of annular abscess or other infection in the periannular aortic root. This technique of tilting a low-profile prosthesis (either the St. Jude or the Björk-Shiley valve) allows the sutures to be placed in relatively noninfected tissue and still results in satisfactory valve mechanics and perfect hemodynamics. Placing the valve in the partial supra-annular position in one area of the aortic annulus while maintaining its normal position for at least half or two-thirds of normal aortic annular circumference allows for insertion of a larger aortic valve prosthesis. The surgical technique must avoid any entrapment of the valve leaflets or valve disk by subvalvar tissue, usually prevented by everted horizontal mattress sutures. This maneuver should allow for placement of a larger valve prosthesis than ordinarily would be possible by placing the valve in the straight annular position.
6. Total supra-annular supracoronary placement of the valve is a possible alternative but is a rare procedure for enlargement of the aortic root. It is usually done only in the presence of a small aortic root and endocarditis when there is not enough room to place a prosthesis at a tilted angle to achieve a satisfactory cardiac output in the large adult patient and when concomitant annular infections and abnormalities exist. The valve used should be a low profile valve, generally sutured to the wall of the aorta with pledgeted mattress sutures passed from outside to within. With the coronary ostia below the valve, coronary bypass grafts must be constructed from the ascending aorta above the valve to the distal left anterior descending and to the distal right coronary arteries.
7. Aortoventriculoplasty, or the Konno procedure for enlargement of the aortic root, is a more radical surgical operation that allows for considerable enlargement of the aortic annulus by at least two or three prosthetic sizes. Most patients who have need of this approach have had prior operations for congenital aortic stenosis. Most would have had a prior valvotomy or subaortic resection. In this procedure an incision is made vertically into the ascending aorta and is carried down into the right coronary sinus toward the junction of the aortic and pulmonary valves to the left of the right coronary orifice. A ventriculotomy is made in the right ventricle and then extended into and across the aortic annulus to join the incision in the aorta. A septotomy is made near the membranous septum so as not to sever the left and right bundle branches and to join and open the left ventricle as well. Once the incisions are made, the aortic valve is excised, and the ventricular septum is reconstructed with Dacron utilizing part of the septum for placement of aortic valve sutures. In these cases we recommend that a prosthetic valve rather than a bioprosthesis always be used for the obvious reason that the bioprosthesis, even though generally reliable in the aortic position, may require reoperation in 10 to 15 years. A St. Jude valve is our choice for this procedure. The septal patch then is carried up over onto the aorta and closed. A final second Dacron patch is used to close the right ventriculotomy up to the aortotomy.

   A considerably larger prosthesis may be inserted, leaving no left ventricular outflow obstruction. The disadvantages are that the procedure takes considerably longer, there may be damage to the right coronary artery or to one or both bundle branches, or complete heart block may be initiated during the procedure. Obviously, bleeding from the Dacron patches is a major risk. This procedure has been reserved for those with unusually small annuli and prior valvular operations. Further details about this approach may be found in the chapter *Options in the Treatment of Aortic and Subaortic Stenosis in Children: Role of Aortoventriculoplasty.*
8. Left ventricular apical-aortic conduit. This procedure has been used in pediatric patients and more recently in young adults with severe recalcitrant left ventricular outflow obstruction. It is a radical approach in which a valved conduit is placed in the left ventricular apex and brought out to the descending aorta. Less interest has been shown in this procedure recently because the Konno and other procedures mentioned previously have gained in popularity and familiarity. This technique uses a secondary approach to left ventricular outflow obstruction, leaving the hypoplastic aor-

tic root intact. It adequately reduces left ventricular aortic gradient and peak left ventricular pressure; however, the apical-aortic conduits usually contain a tissue valve and hence often require re-replacement via an abdominal or thoracic incision.

A considerable amount of judgment, knowledge of the patient's clinical history, (including reaction to anticoagulation), of annular anatomy, and of body surface area all must be taken into consideration before replacing the appropriate valve in the patient with a small aortic root. Clinical and anatomic considerations therefore dictate the therapeutic option to be employed in each patient.

SUGGESTED READING

Campbell DB, Waldhausen JA. The Konno procedure for enlargement of the aortic root. J Cardiac Surg 1986; 1:69–78.

Cohn LH. The long-term results of aortic valve replacement. Chest 1984; 85:387–396.

Cohn LH, Allred EN, DiSesa VJ, et al. Early and late risk of aortic valve replacement: a 12-year concomitant comparison of the porcine bioprosthetic and tilting disc prosthetic aortic valves. J Thorac Cardiovasc Surg 1984; 88:695–705.

Konno S, Imai Y, et al. A new method for prosthetic valve replacement in congenital aortic stenosis with hypoplasia of the aortic ring. J Thorac Cardiovasc Surg 1975; 70:909–917.

Manougian S, Weybold-Epting W. Patch enlargement of the aortic valve ring by extending the aortic incision into the anterior mitral leaflet. J Thorac Cardiovasc Surg 1979; 78:402–412.

COMPOSITE AORTIC VALVE AND AORTIC ROOT REPLACEMENT IN ANEURYSMAL DISEASE

CARY W. AKINS, M.D.

Aneurysms of the ascending aorta, particularly when they are associated with aortic valvular insufficiency, continue to provide a diagnostic dilemma for the physician and a technical challenge for the cardiovascular surgeon. While the exact risk of rupture of aneurysms of the ascending aorta is not as well defined as the risk of rupture of abdominal aortic aneurysms, surgery is frequently recommended when the ascending aorta approaches 7 cm in transverse diameter or is more than two times the size of the rest of the aorta, or if aortic valvular insufficiency causes significant symptoms, leads to ventricular enlargement, or is associated with a fall of greater than 0.10 in the left ventricular ejection fraction during exercise.

While the causes of ascending aortic aneurysms are wide ranging, from atherosclerosis to trauma to giant cell aortitis to infectious processes, the most common cause remains cystic medial necrosis. In this setting, the aortic valvular insufficiency is frequently not caused by the actual enlargement of the annulus of the aortic valve but by splaying of the commissural attachments due to the aortic widening; although the aortic valve leaflets may be normal, they will thus fail to coapt in diastole, resulting in central regurgitation. Thus the term annuloaortic ectasia may be something of a misnomer.

While our institution and many others had good early results with separate replacement of the aortic valve and grafting of the ascending aorta, leaving a cuff of ascending aortic tissue containing the coronary arteries between the two prostheses, significant bleeding from the proximal anastomosis was occasionally encountered. Later problems of recurrent aneurysm formation in the segment of retained aorta have led us to a more widespread use of composite replacement of the aortic valve and ascending aorta with reimplantation of the coronary arteries. It is my basic feeling that any time that aortic insufficiency is caused by disease of the aorta and not of the aortic valve itself, the patient is best treated by composite aortic valve and root replacement, in order to remove as much of the diseased aorta as possible. Although the operative mortality rate would be expected to be higher for what is a more involved surgical procedure, recent results have demonstrated that it is no different, and in fact may be lower, than for separate replacement of the aortic valve and ascending aorta.

PREOPERATIVE PREPARATION

Aortography remains the gold standard for evaluation of ascending aortic aneurysms. Although echocardiography, nuclear magnetic resonance scanning, CT, and digital subtraction angiography can demonstrate aneurysms of the aorta, we prefer detailed evaluation in two planes with aortography. This is particularly important in delineating the extent of distal aortic involvement. Separate coronary angiography is also performed in any patient who has angina pectoris as a symptom, ischemic changes on the electrocardiogram, or is over the age of 35. Whether or not a stenotic coronary artery is bypassed concurrently depends upon the patient's symptoms, the severity of the stenosis, and the amount of myocardium at risk.

OPERATIVE PROCEDURE

The operation is performed using standard cardiopulmonary bypass, usually, however, with cannulation of the left common femoral artery. Occasionally if the aneurysmal disease is strictly confined to the ascending aorta, the aortic arch can be cannulated for arterial return.

Prior to opening the pericardium, control of the aorta is obtained by passing a tape around the distal neck of the aneurysm just proximal to the innominate artery. The patient is then heparinized and the left common femoral artery and vein are cannulated. The pericardium is then opened, and a superior vena caval drainage cannula is inserted through the right atrium.

Because I prefer extra low porosity woven Dacron grafts, I have constructed the conduits myself, since until recently there have been no commercially available conduits with extra low porosity grafts. The size of the conduit is generally chosen by the size of the aorta where the distal anastomosis is to be performed, which is presumed to be closer to the size of the normal aorta and thus more appropriate to the size of the aortic annulus that will be found inside the aneurysm. I do not preclot or bake the grafts with plasma because I have had no important bleeding problems through the graft. The large majority of patients undergoing this operation have a mechanical valve placed in the graft. If the patient is elderly or cannot be anticoagulated, the composite graft is constructed with a Carpentier-Edwards porcine prosthesis. My mechanical valve of choice currently is the Medtronic-Hall tilting disk prosthesis. A mitral valve of the appropriate size is chosen, rather than an aortic prosthesis, because the sewing ring is better. The valve is turned upside down and sewn into the end of a Meadox Veri-Soft ultra low porosity Dacron graft using 2–0 Teflon-coated braided polyester sutures. A commercially prepared conduit is now available with the Medtronic-Hall valve and the same graft material.

If separate coronary grafting needs to be performed, segments of saphenous vein harvested from the leg are prepared at this time using the patient's own heparinized blood.

Cardiopulmonary bypass is instituted and the patient is cooled, usually to 22° C. If the aneurysm extends into the aortic arch or if an inspection of the aortic arch is required, then the temperature is lowered to 15 to 18° C. For the standard composite replacement that is confined to the ascending aorta, cooling is continued until the heart fibrillates, at which time the pump is immediately shut off to avoid distension of the ventricle from the associated aortic valve insufficiency. The aorta is then cross-clamped just proximal to the innominate artery using a soft rubber-jawed clamp, and a left ventricular vent is inserted. An incision is made into the aneurysm. The right and left main coronary arteries are individually cannulated and infused with cold, oxygenated, dilute blood potassium cardioplegia. Approximately every 15 to 20 minutes during the procedure additional infusion of cardioplegia solution is performed. The cavae are then occluded. The aneurysm itself is excised, as I do not favor operating inside it. Careful attention is paid to the dissection along the main pulmonary artery and the right pulmonary artery so as not to damage these structures. The left and right coronary arteries are isolated with islands of aortic tissue measuring approximately 1.5 cm in diameter. Special care must be used for the dissection of the inferior wall of the left coronary artery aortic island to avoid damaging the left main coronary artery itself. The aortic valve is then excised.

When the patient has significant obstructing lesions of the coronary arteries in addition to aneurysmal disease of the aorta and aortic insufficiency, separate grafting is performed utilizing reversed saphenous vein. The segments of vein are anastomosed distally to the coronary arteries as soon as the aneurysm has been opened and cardioplegia has been instilled into the main coronary artery ostia. Individual plastic cannulas are retained in the proximal end of the vein grafts, and when cardioplegia is inserted at intervals into the main coronary ostia, it is also inserted into the vein grafts to the obstructed coronary arteries. The proximal anastomoses are performed after the aortic grafting procedure has been completed but prior to the removal of the aortic cross-clamp.

If aortic arch replacement is required, it is performed after any distal coronary grafting but prior to anastomosis of the composite graft to the left ventricular outflow tract. A separate segment of identically sized aortic graft is anastomosed to the distal aorta either directly with 3–0 polypropylene or after the aortic layers of a dissection have been initially buttressed inside and outside with Teflon felt strips. When the valve-containing graft is in place with the coronary arteries reattached, the two aortic grafts can be joined with 4–0 or 3–0 polypropylene suture on a tapered needle.

Anastomosis of the conduit to the aortic outflow can be performed either with interrupted or continuous sutures. When utilizing pledgeted mattress sutures of 2–0 Teflon-coated braided polyester, the pledgets are left on the aortic side of the valve annulus if a tilting disk prosthesis is used, but they may be placed on the ventricular side of the aortic annulus if a porcine prosthesis is used. If Teflon pledgets are placed on the ventricular side of the annulus with a tilting disk prosthesis, the portion of the disk that opens into the ventricle can catch on the pledgets. Currently, however, I attach the conduit to the aortic outflow tract with three running sutures of 2–0 monofilament polypropylene, utilizing one suture for each cusp of the valve.

Once the conduit has been sewn to the left ventricular outflow tract, the island of aortic tissue holding the left main coronary artery is carefully prepared, and a hole is cut in the back of the conduit for the coronary anastomosis. Because the underside of the anastomosis of the left main coronary artery to the conduit is virtually impossible to reach once the grafting procedure has been accomplished, I perform the inferior portion of this anastomosis with multiple sutures of pledgeted 4–0 polypropylene suture, placing the pledgets on the aortic button that holds the left coronary artery. This is particularly useful in cystic medical necrosis or with acute dissections of the aorta involving the main coronary arteries. The upper portion can then be run with 4–0 suture. In a similar fashion, the right coronary artery is then anastomosed to the conduit after a hole has been cut in the anterior portion of the graft. Because this anastomosis is somewhat easier to reach in the event of bleeding after completion of the grafting procedure, two or three running 4–0 prolene sutures are frequently utilized.

Preparation for the distal anastomosis is then made. In any situation in which the aorta is particularly friable, especially with acute ascending aortic dissections, resection of the aorta is extended to an area just short of the innominate artery. The inner and outer layers of the aorta are reapproximated with 3–0 polypropylene suture buttressed inside and outside of the aorta with Teflon felt. Then the graft is trimmed and anastomosed to this edge with 2–0 prolene suture as rewarming is begun. Air is vented from the graft as the cross-clamp is released and as digital pressure is held on the right main coronary artery to avoid air embolism into the right coronary artery. Two atrial and two ventricular pacing wires are routinely placed on the heart, and a left atrial pressure catheter is placed through the hole in the left superior pulmonary vein that was used to vent the left ventricle. If there has been no associated coronary artery bypass grafting, the pericardium is routinely closed, leaving two catheters inside and one outside for drainage. All patients are placed on anticoagulation therapy for a minimum of 2 to 3 months when porcine prostheses are used and indefinitely when mechanical prostheses are used.

RESULTS OF SURGERY

During the past 6 years I have employed composite aortic valve and ascending aortic replacement in 27 patients; 13 were done emergently for acute ascending aortic dissections, five also required partial or total aortic arch replacement, and seven had associated coronary artery bypass grafting. Hospital mortality has been 7 percent, with the causes of death in the two patients being an anaphylactic reaction to medication in one patient and *Aspergillus* endocarditis in the other.

SUGGESTED READING

Akins CW, Buckley MJ, Austen WG, Daggett WM, Levine FH. Myocardial protection with hypothermia and potassium cardioplegia for the surgery of ascending aortic aneurysms. J Thorac Cardiovasc Surg 1980; 79:700–704.

Bental H, DeBono A. A technique for complete replacement of the ascending aorta. Thorax 1968; 23:338–339.

Grey DP, Ott DA, Cooley DA. Surgical treatment of aneurysm of the ascending aorta with aortic insufficiency. J Thorac Cardiovasc Surg 1983; 86:864–877.

Kouchoukos NT, Marshall WG, Wedige-Stecher TA. Eleven-year experience with composite graft replacement of the ascending aorta and aortic valve. J Thorac Cardiovasc Surg 1986; 92:691–705.

TRICUSPID VALVE REPLACEMENT

GUS J. VLAHAKES, M.D.
W. GERALD AUSTEN, M.D.

Tricuspid valve replacement is employed infrequently in the practice of cardiac surgery. When required, it is usually indicated because of concomitant left-sided disease and consequent severe functional tricuspid regurgitation, not amenable to valve reconstruction, or because of severe organic rheumatic tricuspid valve disease also not amenable to reconstructive surgery. An additional small group of patients who may ultimately require tricuspid valve replacement are those who have undergone prior tricuspid valve excision for the management of right-sided bacterial endocarditis. Rarely, blunt trauma results in severe tricuspid regurgitation, which may require tricuspid valve replacement.

DIAGNOSIS

The diagnosis of *tricuspid regurgitation* can be made in instances of moderate to severe tricuspid insufficiency solely on the basis of physical examination. Jugular venous pulses demonstrate prominent waves during systole followed by sharp descent during diastole. There may be a holosystolic murmur audible along the right sternal border that may increase with inspiration; however, physical findings associated with left-sided disease may make auscultatory findings difficult to differentiate. When venous pulsations are prominent, the liver edge may be enlarged and pulsatile on examination. In advanced cases of tricuspid regurgitation, there may be ascites and peripheral edema as well. The diagnosis is further suggested by findings of right atrial enlargement on chest x-ray and echocardiogram. Two-dimensional echocardiography with Doppler examination is very sensitive for determining the presence of tricuspid valve regurgitation and provides an approximation of its severity. At the time of a catheterization study of left-sided lesions, right-sided heart pressure studies and right-sided ventriculography should be carried out. The presence of regurgitant V waves in the right atrial pressure tracing strongly suggests the diagnosis, which can be confirmed subsequently by right ventriculography. The absence of V waves does not exclude the diagnosis. In instances in which tricuspid regurgitation occurs in the setting of mitral and/or aortic valve disease, final diagnostic confirmation and estimation of the severity of tricuspid regurgitation should be achieved at the time of left-sided valve surgery; digital exploration of the right atrium and tricuspid valve prior to institution of cardiopulmonary bypass permits a good estimation of the severity of tricuspid regurgitation. In rare instances in which this entity is being considered as a diagnosis by itself, right-sided heart pressure study and ventriculography should be included in the evaluation in addition to echocardiography and physical examination in order to confirm the diagnosis and help in the decision regarding operation.

Tricuspid stenosis may present more diagnostic difficulties and may be particularly difficult to diagnose because of the usual, concomitant left-sided disease. The diagnosis may be further obscured in patients who have long-standing atrial fibrillation. Tricuspid stenosis may produce nonpulsatile elevation in jugular venous pressure as well as hepatic enlargement without a pulsatile liver edge. A diastolic murmur may be present at the lower left sternal border and may increase in intensity during inspiration. This physical finding may be difficult to distinguish from aortic regurgitation. If the diagnosis of tricuspid stenosis is suspected, the tricuspid valve should be assessed by echocardiography. A gradient can usually be demonstrated by a Doppler examination, and the motion and thickness of the tricuspid valve leaflets and subvalvular apparatus should also be assessed. Confirmation of the diagnosis usually requires cardiac catheterization with simultaneous recording of right atrial and right ventricular pressures. Significant tricuspid stenosis may be diagnosed when the diastolic gradient is in the range of 4 to 5 mm Hg. This must be assessed in the light of the patient's overall cardiac output; if the patient is in a relatively low output state because of advanced, concomitant left-sided disease, then lesser gradients may also indicate significant tricuspid stenosis.

INDICATIONS FOR TRICUSPID VALVE REPLACEMENT

Tricuspid Valve Disease in the Setting of Multivalve Heart Disease

When rheumatic *tricuspid stenosis* is present as part of multivalve disease, operative intervention is often dictated by the left-sided lesions of the heart. In these instances, the degree of tricuspid stenosis should be determined by digital examination and also possibly by direct vision at the time of left-sided surgery. Even moderate tricuspid stenosis should be considered for either valvuloplasty or valve replacement, since replacement of left-sided valves may increase cardiac output and make the manifestations of tricuspid valve stenosis more severe.

The decision whether to perform tricuspid valvuloplasty versus valve replacement to correct tricuspid stenosis is controversial and involves decision-making processes similar to those used in patients with mitral valve disease. The degree of thickening and the mobility and pliability of the valve leaflets and subvalvular apparatus must all be considered in the decision. If satisfactory function of the tricuspid valve cannot be achieved by incising the commissures and valve reconstruction, tricuspid valve replacement should be carried out. How much tricuspid regurgitation can be safely left depends on the degree of pulmonary artery hypertension which, in turn, is dictated by the presence of any left-sided disease.

The decision regarding treatment of functional *tricuspid regurgitation* with concomitant left-sided disease may be difficult and is still somewhat controversial. In situations in which surgery is being performed for multivalve disease, it is important to evaluate and grade tricuspid regurgitation prior to instituting cardiopulmonary bypass; this can be done by digital exploration of the tricuspid valve. If it is anticipated that the treatment of left-sided valvular heart disease will result in significant improvement in pulmonary hypertension, and particularly if only mild to moderate tricuspid regurgitation is present, then consideration should be given to the possibility of only treating the left-sided disease. After cardiopulmonary bypass is terminated following left-sided replacement(s) or reconstruction, tricuspid regurgitation should again be graded by digital palpation. If tricuspid regurgitation is absent or mild, no further intervention is required. If there is still significant tricuspid regurgitation even with anticipated improvement in pulmonary hypertension, we proceed to reconstruct the tricuspid valve. This is outlined in a separate chapter entitled *Tricuspid Valve Repair.*

If significant functional tricuspid regurgitation is present because of pulmonary hypertension secondary to left-sided disease, we feel that the decision of whether to reconstruct or replace the tricuspid valve depends in part on the anticipated prognosis for the pulmonary hypertension. Particularly in patients in whom pulmonary hypertension is severe (near systemic) and in whom it is anticipated that there will be significant, residual pulmonary hypertension, consideration should be given to replacement of the tricuspid valve instead of reconstruction. It has been our experience that, in patients with this type of severe left-sided valvular heart disease, tricuspid valve reconstructions do not yield durable results, and replacement is preferred.

If significant tricuspid regurgitation results from primarily organic tricuspid valve disease, the decision to repair versus replace the tricuspid valve must take into consideration not only the degree and prognosis of pulmonary hypertension but also the quality of the tricuspid apparatus. In general, patients with significant organic tricuspid regurgitation in the setting of concomitant left-sided disease require tricuspid valve replacement.

Isolated Tricuspid Regurgitation

In patients who have undergone prior tricuspid valve excision for endocarditis or who have developed tricuspid regurgitation from trauma, the necessity for subsequent valve replacement is determined by symptoms and the presence of any manifestations of right-sided heart failure. In particular, hepatic congestion and its consequences should be considered as indications for replacement of a tricuspid valve in these instances. In the endocarditis patients, this must, of course, be balanced against the risk of reinfection, since many of these patients have acquired their tricuspid endocarditis from drug abuse.

Isolated Tricuspid Stenosis

Tricuspid stenosis as a single entity requiring tricuspid valve replacement is extremely rare. Surgical intervention, either as a valvuloplasty or valve replacement, is dictated by symptoms and physical findings. Moderate degrees of tricuspid stenosis may not produce symptoms at rest or with mild activity; however, patients in this category may have significant limitation of activity, as venous pressure will rise during exercise. Intervention is certainly indicated when more advanced stenosis is present with evidence of hepatic congestion, or in even more severe cases with ascites and peripheral edema. If possible, it is important to plan operative intervention before significant hepatic dysfunction develops, as this will increase the risk of surgery. In instances of moderate stenosis, consideration should be given to operative intervention if significant lifestyle and activity limitations are present. The decision of whether to perform valvuloplasty versus valve replacement is identical to that discussed earlier in patients with multivalve disease.

SURGICAL TECHNIQUES

Tricuspid valve replacement is performed through a right atriotomy with the patient on cardiopulmonary bypass. Whether the operation is being performed for tricuspid valve disease alone or as part of multivalve surgery, the tricuspid valve should be evaluated by digital palpation through an atrial cannulation site prior to the institution of bypass. An initial assessment of the degree of functional or organic disease should be made. In instances in which valve replacement is being considered because of severe regurgitation, particularly in association with left-sided valve surgery, it is important to grade the amount of regurgitation before bypass, as this will assist in the decision-making process as to whether or not tricuspid surgery is needed, and, if so, whether replacement or reconstruction is appropriate. Tricuspid valve replacement may be performed without aortic cross-clamping and with only mild to moderate degrees of hypothermia. When it is performed at the time of replacement of left-sided valves, we complete the left-sided procedures, evacuate air from the left side of the heart, and remove the aortic cross-clamp. The patient is rewarmed until the perfusate temperature reaches approximately 32° C, at which it is maintained. We utilize an oblique atriotomy in the right atrial free wall to visualize the tricuspid valve. It is helpful to determine from preoperative studies whether an intra-atrial communication exists, as this may present a risk for air entrapment in the left atrium and consequent air embolism. In addition, care is taken not to touch the area of the fossa ovalis in the event that probe patency is present through the atrial septum. The anterior and posterior leaflets of the valve are excised removing chordae but leaving an approximately 3-mm cuff of valve tissue for suturing. A little more cuff of the septal leaflet is left intact to be used for subsequent suturing to help avoid damage to the conduction system. Care is taken in the region around the coronary sinus to ensure that excessive traction is not applied in areas near the conduction system and that these areas are not touched with instruments. By performing tricuspid valve replacement with the heart beating, the electrocardiogram can be monitored for the appearance of conduction delay or heart block; suture placement can be modified accordingly if either of these manifestations of conduction system injury is observed. At the time of valve excision, the Swan-Ganz pulmonary artery catheter, if present, is withdrawn, and the end of the catheter is placed to the side of the operative field.

The choice of tricuspid valve prosthesis is dictated by the types of prostheses selected for the left side. In general, once a patient is committed to life-long anticoagulation because of left-sided mechanical prostheses, we place a mechanical prosthesis in the tricuspid position. Our preference is the St. Jude Medical valve because of its excellent flow characteristics and low transvalvular gradient. In patients receiving porcine heterograft valves for their left-sided valvular disease, we insert a porcine heterograft valve in the tricuspid position as well, if the right ventricular cavity is of sufficient size. In patients who do not have left-sided prostheses, we prefer to use a mechanical valve, usually a St. Jude Medical, up to the age of approximately 65 to 70, unless there is a contraindication to anticoagulation therapy. After the age of approximately 65 to 70, we usually use a porcine heterograft valve, unless the patient requires anticoagulation for other reasons.

For suturing of the valve, we prefer to use horizontal mattress sutures of 2–0 Ticron with Teflon pledgets. The Teflon pledgets are placed on the atrial side of the tricuspid annulus when we insert a mechanical prosthesis, and they may be placed on the atrial or the ventricular side when we insert a bioprosthesis. The sutures are placed through the annulus; extreme care is taken in the area of the conduction system to ensure that the stitches do not extend posteriorly beyond the tricuspid annulus. The sutures are then threaded through the prosthetic annulus and the prosthesis is seated. At this point, rewarming of the patient is instituted, and the sutures are tied into place. If a bioprosthesis has been selected, we replace the Swan-Ganz catheter across the prosthesis into the right ventricle. It may subsequently be flow-redirected across the pulmonic valve. If a mechanical prosthesis has been inserted, we use alternative means of postoperative monitoring, as will be described. The atriotomy is then closed. Prior to completion of the atriotomy closure, the caval tapes are removed to expel air from the right side of the heart, and the atriotomy closure is completed. Temporary ventricular pacing wires are placed in all cases, and in patients who are in sinus rhythm, atrial pacing wires are placed for pacing as well as for postoperative diagnostic purposes. Cardiopulmonary bypass is then discontinued. A finger is then reintroduced into the right atrium, and the functioning of the prosthesis is checked.

When mechanical prostheses are placed in the tricuspid position, transvenous pulmonary artery catheters cannot be placed. In these instances, we have monitored pulmonary artery pressure and determined cardiac output with special pulmonary artery catheters introduced into the pulmonary artery through a pursestring suture in the right ventricular outflow tract (American Edwards Laboratories, Irvine, CA; 5 F double-lumen thermodilution and pressure monitoring catheter, Model No. 792004). When used in conjunction with cold injections through a central venous catheter, the thermodilution transducer in the pulmonary artery provides a good estimate of cardiac output. We have also placed this catheter in the left atrium, and in conjunction with right-sided cold injections, it can be used to estimate cardiac output by the thermodilution technique. Alternatively, when this catheter is not available, we have placed Swan-Ganz catheters through pursestring sutures in the right ventricular outflow tract; these catheters often produce some bleeding when removed postoperatively, and this is not recommended in instances in which significant postoperative pulmonary hypertension is expected. Because the prosthesis is in direct continuity with venous return, it is essential that extreme precautions be taken with intravenous and central venous lines from the standpoint of maintenance of sterility.

In instances of reoperations, usually because of a degenerated tricuspid bioprosthesis or because of severe tricuspid regurgitation resulting from left-sided disease, reopening the sternum can be difficult, particularly if a hypertensive and distended right atrium is adherent to the posterior table of the sternum. The enlarged right atrium may be strongly suggested by the chest x-ray film or by preoperative echocardiography. This should always be suspected when the right atrial pressure exceeds approximately 18 mm Hg. In these instances, we have administered vasodilator agents, such as nitroglycerin or nitroprusside, to decrease right-sided filling pressures temporarily and thus make opening the sternum safer. In some instances, we have used initial femoral vein and femoral artery cannulation and partial bypass to decrease filling pressures and permit safer sternal opening.

Heart block may occur late following tricuspid valve replacement and, thus, careful attention should be paid to monitoring after surgery; this is particularly likely when both tricuspid and mitral valves have been replaced. If, at the usual time of discharge, patients in atrial fibrillation have unusually slow ventricular rates, or patients with sinus rhythm have prolonged P-R intervals, consideration should be given to an additional period of time in the hospital for monitoring to ensure that difficulty with the conduction system does not continue to evolve.

RESULTS

The morbidity and mortality rates of tricuspid valve replacement are usually dictated by other valve procedures performed on the left side of the heart. Thus, the risk of operative mortality following tricuspid valve replacement varies widely, ranging from very low to approximately 20 percent, depending on other associated cardiac surgery. When it is performed in conjunction with mitral valve replacement, the risk is approximately 5 to 8 percent, depending on the severity of the left-sided disease and associated pulmonary hypertension. When tricuspid valve replacement is performed in conjunction with mitral and aortic valve replacement, the risk may range from 10 to 20 percent, again depending on the severity of the left-sided disease and pulmonary hypertension. In patients undergoing tricuspid valve replacement alone, the risk of operative mortality is usually quite low, in the range of 0 to 5 percent.

SUGGESTED READING

Arneborn P, Bjork VO, Rodriguez L, Svanbom M. Two-stage replacement of the tricuspid valve in active endocarditis. Br Heart J 1977; 39:1276–1278.

Baughman KL, Kallman CH, Yurchak PM, Daggett WM, Buckley MJ. Predictors of survival after tricuspid valve surgery. Am J Cardiol 1984; 54:137–141.

Carpentier A, Deloche A, Hanania G, Forman J, Sellier PH, Piwnica A, Dubost CH. Surgical management of acquired tricuspid valve disease. J Thorac Cardiovasc Surg 1974; 67:53–65.

P'eterffy A, Bjork VO. Surgical treatment of Ebstein's anomaly. Scand J Thorac Cardiovasc Surg 1979; 13:1–7.

Singh AK, Christian FD, Williams DO, Georas CS, Riley RR, Nanian KB, Karlson KE. Follow-up assessment of the St. Jude Medical prosthetic valve in the tricuspid position: clinical and hemodynamic results. Ann Thorac Surg 1984; 37:324–327.

PROSTHETIC AND NATIVE VALVE ENDOCARDITIS

ADOLF W. KARCHMER, M.D.

Essential to designing effective treatment for infective endocarditis is an understanding of the causative organisms and their antimicrobial susceptibility, the pathologic consequences of infection, and the physiologic derangements that result from intracardiac complications of endocarditis. Important differences exist in the microbiology of native versus prosthetic valve endocarditis (Table 1). Native valve endocarditis (NVE) and prosthetic valve endocarditis (PVE) with onset more than a year after surgery are caused primarily by streptococci, enterococci, staphylococci (primarily *Staphylococcus aureus*) and fastidious gram-negative coccobacilli. In contrast, PVE during the year after cardiac surgery is predominantly due to *Staphylococcus epidermidis*, with additional cases caused by diphtheroids, fungi, and *S. aureus*. Notably, 80 percent of the *S. epidermidis* causing PVE during the year after surgery are resistant to methicillin and other beta-lactam antibiotics, including cephalosporins. Only 30 percent of *S. epidermidis* isolated from later onset cases are resistant to methicillin. Drug addict-associated NVE is commonly caused by *S. aureus* (especially if the tricuspid or pulmonic valve is involved) and streptococci (primarily involving valves on the left side); however, unique regional differences are noted in the organisms causing addict-associated infective endocarditis, such as *Pseudomonas aeruginosa* in Chicago and Detroit and methicillin resistant *S. aureus* in Detroit. Infection involving native valves is localized primarily to the leaflet. In contrast, infection extending beyond the valve into the annulus and perivalvular tissue is common with PVE on mechanical valves and porcine bioprosthetic valves during the year after implantation. As a result, dehiscence of the prosthesis with consequent regurgitation and myocardial abscess is often encountered. Occasionally, large vegetations partially obstruct the prosthetic orifice, a complication usually associated with infection of a mitral valve prosthesis. With

TABLE 1 Causes of Endocarditis at Massachusetts General Hospital

Organism	*Native Valve Endocarditis* 1975–1983*	*Prosthetic Valve Endocarditis† 1975–1982*	
		Onset Following Surgery	
		< 12 mo	*> 12 mo*
Streptococci (nonenterococcal)	89 (42)	1 (1)	11 (25)
Enterococci	15 (7)	2 (3)	4 (9)
Pneumococci	2 (1)	—	1 (2)
S. aureus	64 (30)	5 (7)	5 (12)
S. epidermidis	10 (5)	41 (57)	10 (23)
Gram-negative bacilli	6 (3)	3 (4)	1 (2)
Fastidious gram-negative coccobacilli‡	10 (5)	1 (1)	7 (16)
Diphtheroids	—	4 (6)	1 (2)
Fungi	3 (1)	4 (6)	1 (2)
Others and mixed	4 (2)	5 (7)	1 (2)
Culture-negative	8 (4)	6 (8)	2 (5)
Total	211	72	44

* From DiNubile MJ, Calderwood SB, Steinhaus DM, Karchmer AW. Cardiac conduction abnormalities complicating native valve active infective endocarditis. Am J Cardiol 1986; 58:1213.
† From Calderwood SB, Swinski LA, Karchmer AW, et al. Prosthetic valve endocarditis analysis of factors affecting outcome of therapy. J Thorac Cardiovasc Surg 1986; 92:776.
‡ Includes *Haemophilus* species, *Actinobacillus actinomycotemcomitans*, *Cardiobacterium*.

NVE and infected porcine bioprosthetic valves, leaflets may be damaged severely, resulting in valve incompetence. Hemodynamic deterioration as a consequence of valve dysfunction is a major cause of death in patients with infective endocarditis and is the cardinal derangement prompting surgical therapy. Electrocardiographic conduction abnormalities, particularly those which are new, persistent, and associated with aortic valve infection, suggest a myocardial abscess involving the conduction system and warrant placement of a demand pacemaker as well as surgery. Although some extracardiac complications of infective endocarditis are life-threatening, e.g., immune complex-mediated renal failure and intracranial mycotic aneurysm, therapy of these infrequent events is beyond the scope of this discussion. However, a thorough understanding of the microbiology, pathology, and intracardiac complications of endocarditis enables physicians to provide optimal care for most patients with this disease.

TREATMENT

Antibiotic therapy. The guiding principles of antibiotic therapy for endocarditis serve equally well for NVE and PVE. A bactericidal antibiotic or combinations of agents that are bactericidal are administered parenterally, in high doses for prolonged periods. When choosing between effective antimicrobial regimens, considerations to minimize toxicity must prevail. Once the etiology of infective endocarditis is known, there is no reason to delay antibiotic therapy. However, the decision to initiate therapy prior to the isolation of an agent must be weighed carefully. Premature administration of antibiotics can interfere with the all important effort to recover a causative organism from blood cultures. In turn, the inability to carefully evaluate the antimicrobial susceptibility of the organism may confound the effort to design optimal therapy. If the course of the infective endocarditis has been indolent, and clinical findings do not suggest hemodynamic impairment requiring urgent surgical intervention, blood cultures should be obtained and administration of antibiotic therapy delayed. If the initial cultures are negative, as often occurs when patients have received antibiotics recently, this delay provides an opportunity to repeat cultures or to use special culture techniques. The delay does not place patients at risk for complications of endocarditis that would have been prevented by immediate empiric therapy. However, if the infective endocarditis is acute or if the presence of valve dysfunction and congestive heart failure indicates a need for early valve replacement, four to six separate blood cultures should be obtained over an hour and empiric antibiotic therapy begun immediately thereafter.

The regimens recommended for treating infective endocarditis caused by a specific organism are based on the in vitro bactericidal activity of antibiotics against the organism and clinical experience (Table 2). Three regimens have been found to be effective in the treatment of NVE caused by penicillin-susceptible (minimum inhibitory concentration [MIC] ≤ 0.2 μg per milliliter) nonenterococcal streptococci, including *Streptococcus bovis*. Streptomycin is used in two of these regimens with a consequent risk, although small, of ototoxicity. Experience with the 2-week regimen is limited; it is not recommended for PVE, infection due to nutritionally deficient streptococci, and NVE associated with neurologic complications or hypotension. The combination of penicillin G and streptomycin for 2 weeks, followed by 2 additional weeks of parenteral penicillin, is recommended for PVE caused by penicillin susceptible streptococci. This regimen is also recommended for treatment of NVE and PVE caused by some of the relatively penicillin-resistant streptococci (MIC ≥ 0.2 μg per milliliter to ≤ 0.5 μg per

TABLE 2 Antimicrobial Therapy of Endocarditis in Adults

Organism		*Regimen of Choice*		*Alternate Regimen**	*Duration of Therapy (Weeks)* *NVE*	*PVE*
Streptococci: nonenterococcal penicillin-susceptible (MIC <0.2 μg/ml)	1.	Aqueous penicillin G 2 to 4 MU IV q4h	1.	Vancomycin† 7.5 mg/kg IV q6h or cephalothin 2 g IVq4h	4	4–6
	2.‡	Aqueous penicillin G as above for 4 weeks plus streptomycin† 500 mg IM q12h for the initial 2 weeks	2.‡	Cephalothin in the above doses plus streptomycin‡ 500 mg IM q12h for 2 weeks	4	4–6‡
	3.	Aqueous penicillin G and streptomycin† in the above-noted doses	3.	None	2	N/A
Relatively penicillin-resistant						
a. MIC ≥0.2 μg/ml to ≤0.5 μg/ml	1.	Use regimen #2 above	1.	Use regimen #2 above	4	6
b. MIC >0.5 μg/ml	1.	Treat as for enterococcal endocarditis	1.	Use alternate regimen for enterococcal or cephalothin plus streptomycin† in above doses	4	6
Enterococci	1.	Aqueous penicillin G 4 MU IV q4h plus gentamicin‡ 1 to 1.3 mg/kg IV q8h	1.	Vancomycin† 7.5 mg/kg IV q6h plus gentamicin† 1 to 1.3 mg/kg IV q8h	4–6	6
Staphylococci:						
S. aureus (methicillin-susceptible)	1.	Nafcillin or oxacillin 2.0 g IV q4h	1.	Cephalothin 2.0 g IV q4h or vancomycin† 7.5 mg/kg IV q6h	4–6	6
S. aureus (methicillin-resistant)	1.	Vancomycin† 7.5 mg/kg IV q6h	1.	None	4–6	6
S. epidermidis (methicillin-susceptible)	1.	Use regimen for methicillin-susceptible *S. aureus*	1.	Use regimen for methicillin-susceptible *S. aureus*	4–6	6
S. epidermidis (methicillin-resistant)*	1.‡	Vancomycin† 7.5 mg/kg IV q6h plus rifampin 300 mg orally q8h plus gentamicin† 1 to 1.3 mg/kg IV q8h for the initial 2 weeks	1.‡	Vancomycin† 7.5 mg/kg q6h plus other agents based on susceptibility studies	4–6	6
Diphtheroids:						
Gentamicin-susceptible (MIC ≤4 μg/ml)	1.	Aqueous penicillin G 4 MU IV q4h plus gentamicin† 1.3 to 1.5 mg/kg IV q8h	1.	Vancomycin† 7.5 mg/kg IV q6h	4–6	6
Gentamicin-resistant (MIC >4 μg/ml)	1.	Vancomycin† 7.5 mg/kg IV q6h	1.	Design based on susceptibility studies	4–6	6
Fastidious gram-negative cocco-bacilli§	1.	Ampicillin 2 to 2.5 g IV q4h	1.	Cefotaxime 2 g IV q4h	4–6	4–6
	2.‡	Ampicillin 2 to 2.5 g IV q4h plus streptomycin† 500 mg IM q12h	2.‡	Cefotaxime 2 g IV q4h plus streptomycin† 500 mg IM q12h	4–6	4–6
Pseudomonas aeruginosa	1.	Ticarcillin 3 g IV q3h plus tobramycin† 2.7 mg/kg IV q8h	1.	Synergistic bactericidal combination based on susceptibility studies	6–8	6–8
Fungi and yeast	1.	Amphotericin B 0.6 mg/kg to 1.0 mg/kg IV once daily (for *Candida* species add flucytosine† 35 to 40 mg/kg orally q6h)	1.	Design based on susceptibility studies		

* Alternate regimens are for use in patients who cannot tolerate the regimen of choice.
† Doses must be adjusted for decreased renal function.
‡ Preferred regimens for patients with PVE.
** If causing NVE, treat as NVE caused by methicillin-resistant *S. aureus*.
§ Includes *Haemophilus* species, *Actinobacillus actinomycetemcomitans*, *Cardiobacterium hominis*, and *Kingella kingii*.
Abbreviations: MU = million units, IM = intramuscularly, NA = not advised.

milliliter), whereas the regimen used for enterococcal endocarditis is preferred for the more resistant strains (MIC >0.5 μg per milliliter). Enterococcal endocarditis, regardless of valve type, is treated with a synergistic bactericidal combination of penicillin and gentamicin. Although streptomycin was the aminoglycoside combined with penicillin previously, high-level resistance to streptomycin that precludes synergy is found among 40 percent of enterococci. The frequency of high-level resistance makes the routine use of streptomycin for treating enterococcal endocarditis unacceptable.

Endocarditis due to *S. aureus* is treated with a penicillinase-resistant penicillin, cephalosporin, or vancomycin unless the strain is confirmed to be penicillin-susceptible (does *not* produce penicillinase), and then penicillin can be used. Vancomycin is the only agent recommended for treatment of infective endocarditis caused by methicillin-resistant *S. aureus*. Enhanced killing of methicillin-susceptible *S. aureus* can be achieved by combining gentamicin and nafcillin (synergy). Nevertheless, given the potential nephrotoxicity of gentamicin, I do not routinely initiate therapy for *S. aureus* endocarditis with this combination. However, if after 4 to 5 days of treatment a clinical response is not evident, if the organism is susceptible, I add either intravenous gentamicin (1.3 mg per kilogram body weight every 8 hours) or rifampin (300 mg orally every 8 hours). The addition of gentamicin is preferred when the risk of nephrotoxicity is not high.

Prosthetic valve endocarditis caused by *S. epidermidis* is treated with a combination of antimicrobials. These organisms are commonly resistant to all beta-lactam antibiotics; therefore, vancomycin serves as the primary antimicrobial and is combined with rifampin and gentamicin; the latter is limited to the initial 2 weeks of treatment. When PVE is caused by *S. epidermidis* strains documented to be methicillin-susceptible, beta-lactam antibiotics are recommended. The role of combination therapy for these cases is not established. Unless infection is acquired nosocomially, *S. epidermidis* that cause NVE are usually methicillin-susceptible. NVE caused by *S. epidermidis* can be treated with the regimens designated for endocarditis caused by *S. aureus* with comparable susceptibility to methicillin.

Optimal regimens for treating endocarditis caused by gram-negative organisms have not been established. Experience using the new very potent penicillins and cephalosporins is limited. For PVE caused by fastidious gram-negative coccobacilli, high cure rates have been achieved using ampicillin and streptomycin. Experience in drug addicts with endocarditis due to *P. aeruginosa* indicates a need for the synergistic combination of tobramycin (very high doses are used—8 mg per kilogram per day) and ticarcillin; in addition, surgery is often required to excise infected valves. Treatment for infective endocarditis caused by other gram-negative bacilli must be designed on the basis of in vitro susceptibility studies with consideration given to the very potent new beta-lactam antibiotics and to the role of combinations of antibiotics.

Patients with infective endocarditis must be monitored closely while receiving antibiotic therapy. During the initial 3 to 5 days of treatment, blood cultures should be obtained to document that the bacteremia has been suppressed. Thereafter, if early cultures are negative, repeat blood cultures are obtained only to assess complications or unexplained fever. Some bacteria are called tolerant because there is a 32-fold or higher difference in the MIC and the minimum bactericidal concentration (MBC) for cell wall–active antibiotics (penicillins, cephalosporins, vancomycin). However, only rarely does this phenomenon have clinical significance and require that a noncell wall–active antibiotic be added to the treatment. In monitoring therapy, the serum bactericidal titer (dilutions of the patient's serum that kill the infecting organism) is determined at the time of expected highest (peak) and lowest (trough) serum antibiotic concentrations. While high titers are preferred, they do not guarantee a successful outcome of infective endocarditis. Antibiotic therapy that effects killing of the causative organisms by at least a 1:8 dilution of the serum at peak and trough times is desirable. Nevertheless, when endocarditis is due to more resistant organisms, trough titers of 1:8 are often not achieved, and yet therapy is effective. Daily physical examinations and periodic laboratory testing should be focused on the early detection of complications of infective endocarditis and adverse reactions to antibiotics.

Surgical Treatment. Débriding infected paravalvular tissue, removing infected valves, and replacing dysfunctioning cardiac valves with prosthetic ones have become increasingly important in the management of patients with both NVE and PVE. In some patients antibiotic therapy alone cannot eradicate infection or remedy intracardiac complications. Among these patients, the survival rate of those undergoing surgery is higher than that of those treated medically. Furthermore, the risk of recrudescent infective endocarditis is low. Nevertheless, when deciding to operate, the risk of surgery must be considered: operative mortality, recurrence of original endocarditis, new onset PVE and associated mortality, the need for reoperation to correct valve dysfunction, and thromboembolic complications and bleeding from anticoagulation. Given these risks, there are few absolute indications for surgery in infective endocarditis; rather, many clinical and laboratory observations are relative indications and only when viewed together may they warrant surgery.

The clinical situations for which surgery should be considered during active infective endocarditis are listed in Table 3. Hemodynamic deterioration due to valve dysfunction, either regurgitation or stenosis, is the most common indication for surgery. When congestive heart failure is moderate to severe, surgery is required if mortality rates of 75 to 90 percent are to be avoided. Similarly, unresponsive infection and infection caused by organisms for which there is no adequate antimicrobial therapy, e.g., fungi and yeast, warrant surgery. Evidence of infection extending beyond the valve leaflet is increasingly accepted as an indication for surgery. Patients with PVE who have invasive disease (especially occurring within the year after valve implantation) or who have a relapse of endocarditis usually require surgery. Patients with NVE who relapse despite treatment with a recommended regimen are often cured

TABLE 3 Indications for Cardiac Surgery in Patients with Active Infective Endocarditis

Absolute Indications:

- Moderate to severe heart failure due to valve dysfunction
- Uncontrolled infection with persistent bacteremia
- No adequate antimicrobial therapy—fungal endocarditis

Relative Indications:

- Evidence of invasive and destructive infection: valve dysfunction; new and persistent conduction system disturbances; unexplained persistent fever for 9 days despite appropriate antibiotic therapy; abscess shown by echocardiography or cardiac catheterization
- Detected organisms: *S. aureus, S. epidermidis** antibiotic-resistant gram-negative bacilli
- Relapse of infective endocarditis after appropriate therapy*
- Recurrent systemic emboli

* For PVE.

with a more intensive course of antimicrobial therapy; surgery may be required if complications supervene or antibiotics remain ineffective. If there are no intracardiac complications, NVE caused by *S. epidermidis* can usually be cured with antibiotic therapy. In contrast, PVE due to *S. epidermidis*, especially that occurring in the year after valve surgery, is often an invasive infection and usually requires surgical intervention. There is great controversy regarding the role of surgery in treating *S. aureus* endocarditis. Surgery is rarely necessary when treating right-sided *S. aureus* endocarditis in drug addicts. However, when patients with left-sided NVE or PVE caused by *S. aureus* do not show a prompt and progressive response to antibiotic therapy, early surgical intervention may improve survival rates. The mortality rate of *S. aureus* endocarditis in nonaddicts is 25 to 40 percent; therefore the threshold to operate should be low. A similar approach should be used for patients with infective endocarditis due to relatively antibiotic-resistant gram-negative bacilli.

Recurrent arterial emboli are often noted among the indications for surgery; however, it has not been established that further emboli will be prevented by surgery. If, after arterial emboli vegetations remain according to echocardiography, the argument for surgery seems more cogent, although it is still not absolute. Vegetations on the aortic or mitral valve seen on echocardiography define a group of patients who are likely to have complicated courses, to require surgery, or to die. Nevertheless, a vegetation alone is not an indication for surgery but must be considered in the context of the entire clinical and laboratory evaluation of the patient. When other relative indications for surgery are present, the vegetation may strengthen the argument to proceed.

The benefits of surgery for patients with infective endocarditis depend on the timing of the procedure. Operative mortality is proportional to preoperative hemodynamic disability; thus, surgery should be performed before severe heart failure develops. Ideally patients with infective endocarditis receive 7 to 10 days of antibiotic therapy prior to surgery. However, if absolute indications for surgery are present, the procedure should not be delayed to allow additional antibiotic therapy. Prolonged antibiotic therapy prior to surgery has not been associated with a more favorable outcome in patients with either NVE or PVE. In fact, additional antibiotic therapy that delays surgery may result in a less favorable outcome.

When weighing indications for surgery for infective endocarditis, all aspects of the patient's medical history and condition must be considered. If time permits, evidence of extracardiac infection should be sought, and if found, eradicated. For example, a renal or splenic abscess should be drained or removed before valve replacement. The risk of recurrent endocarditis on prosthetic valves and the attendant mortality are very high in drug addicts who continue to abuse narcotics. In consideration of this, tricuspid and pulmonic valvulectomy (without valve replacement) have been used to treat addict-associated right-sided infective endocarditis that is unresponsive to antibiotics. The risk of recrudescent endocarditis on a prosthesis is not related to prosthesis type; therefore, valve selection is determined by the same technical and clinical considerations that guide selection during elective valve replacement.

The duration of antibiotic therapy after surgery is determined by the evidence that infection was present at the time of surgery. The combined preoperative and postoperative antibiotic treatment should provide at least a full recommended course. However, if the gross appearance of perivalvular tissues, the histopathology of the resected tissue, or the intraoperative cultures indicate continued active infection, a full course of antibiotics is administered after surgery. Prolonged courses of oral antibiotics after parenteral therapy are not generally used in patients with infective endocarditis. Only very rarely, when infection cannot be eradicated and surgery cannot be performed, is long-term suppressive oral antibiotic therapy used.

Anticoagulation Therapy. Although systemic emboli occur in 15 to 30 percent of patients with NVE, anticoagulant therapy is not used in an attempt to prevent these. On the other hand, if a clear indication for anticoagulation arises in a patient with NVE, it is not contraindicated. In contrast, among patients with PVE involving a prosthesis for which maintenance anticoagulant therapy is indicated, this therapy is continued cautiously (prothrombin time increased 1.5 times the control value). If a hemorrhagic complication occurs, the anticoagulation is reversed until the risk of further bleeding abates. Anticoagulant therapy is not initiated when the prosthesis that is infected would not otherwise merit it.

PROGNOSIS

The prognosis for patients with NVE or PVE for whom surgery is indicated is clearly improved by appropriately timed surgical intervention. Among NVE patients for whom valve replacement therapy is required, in-hospital mortality can be reduced from at least 50 percent to approximately 15 percent. For patients discharged from the hospital after surgical treatment of NVE, actuarial estimates indicate that 80 to 90 percent survive 12 months and 70 percent survive 5 years. Patients with PVE treated surgically experience a 25 percent mortality rate during hospitalization. Following discharge, the actuarial estimate of survival at 12 months is 80 to 85 percent and at 4 years 60 to 75 percent. Patients with surgical treatment of either NVE or PVE may experience late endocarditis-related complications, including relapse of endocarditis and prosthetic valve dysfunction due to periprosthetic leakage. These complications are more commonly seen in patients with invasive perivalvular infection or with positive cultures or Gram's stain of excised material; hence, these patients require very careful follow-up care.

While the prognosis for NVE and PVE has improved with the increased availability of potent antibiotics and the increased frequency of early surgical intervention, mortality and morbidity remain high. Consequently, when treating NVE and PVE, the portal of entry for the causative organism should always be sought and corrected. Dental health should be assessed and corrected routinely. Endocarditis due to *S. bovis* may be a clue to cryptic colonic polyps or carcinoma, and careful study of the colon is indicated in these patients. Similarly, any patients with prosthetic valves or prior NVE are at risk for recurrent endocarditis; they must be instructed to assiduously use antibiotic regimens as prophylaxis against infective endocarditis (American Heart Association Recommendations. Circulation 1984; 70:1123A).

SUGGESTED READING

Alsip SG, Blackstone EH, Kirklin JW, Cobbs CG. Indications for cardiac surgery in patients with active infective endocarditis. Am J Med 1985; 78(Suppl 6B):138–148.

Baumgartner WA, Miller DC, Reitz BA, et al. Surgical treatment of prosthetic valve endocarditis. Ann Thorac Surg 1983; 35:87–102.

D'Agostino RS, Miller DC, Stinson EB, et al. Valve replacement in patients with native valve endocarditis: what really determines operative outcome? Ann Thorac Surg 1985; 40:429–438.

Karchmer AW, Archer GL, Dismukes WE. Staphylococcus epidermidis causing prosthetic valve endocarditis: microbiologic and clinical observations as guides to therapy. Ann Intern Med 1983; 98:447–455.

Mills SA. Surgical management of infective endocarditis. Ann Surg 1982; 195:367–383.

Sande MA, Kaye D, Root RK, eds. Endocarditis: contemporary issues in infectious diseases. Vol. 2. New York: Churchill Livingstone, 1984.

IDIOPATHIC HYPERTROPHIC SUBAORTIC STENOSIS

CHARLES L. McINTOSH, M.D., Ph.D.

The continued use of the terminology idiopathic hypertrophic subaortic stenosis (IHSS) appears appropriate in the surgical literature, since the etiology of hypertrophy continues to be idiopathic and by operative criteria obstruction (subaortic stenosis) must be present. The current alternative term hypertrophic cardiomyopathy, with or without obstruction, is probably more suited to the spectrum of patients under medical management.

Dyspnea, shortness of breath, fatigue, chest pain, presyncope, and syncope are the symptoms usually associated with IHSS. These symptoms are thought to be caused by (1) decreased compliance, (2) obstruction of left ventricular outflow, (3) ischemia, (4) arrhythmias, or (5) a combination of these. Patients with IHSS are first treated maximally with beta-blockers, calcium-channel blockers, and diuretics, in various combinations. In addition, patients with coronary artery disease may require nitrates. Therapeutic management of problematic supraventricular and ventricular arrhythmias is based on preoperative Holter monitoring and, in some high-risk patients, on electrophysiologic study. The majority of patients having IHSS may be effectively treated medically, but for those who fail treatment or cannot tolerate their drugs, operation is recommended.

INDICATIONS AND CONTRAINDICATIONS FOR OPERATION

Absolute indications for operation include

1. Patients with demonstrated resting and provocable obstruction and persistent symptoms (New York Heart Association Functional Class III or IV) after maximum medical therapy.
2. Patients with sudden death followed by resuscitation without neurologic deficits who have significant (>50 mm Hg) resting or provocable obstruction.

Operation is indicated but with reservations about maximum relief of symptoms following medical therapy in

1. Patients with provocable obstruction only.
2. Patients in chronic atrial fibrillation.
3. Patients with severe coronary artery disease that may not be suitable for complete revascularization or possibly may demonstrate limited coronary flow reserve secondary to small vessel disease.

Absolute contraindications to operation in

1. Patients with dilated left ventricles and depressed ejection fractions according to radionuclide angiograms (<40 percent) and with small resting and/or provocable obstructions only, who have previously been shown to have hypercontractile left ventricles with normal (>45 percent) to supernormal ejection fractions.
2. Patients whose symptoms are secondary to supraventricular or ventricular arrhythmias.

PREOPERATIVE EVALUATION AND MANAGEMENT OF PATIENTS

History, physical examination, electrocardiogram, chest x-ray examination, exercise tolerance testing and M-mode and 2-D echocardiograms are obtained routinely. The echocardiograms are useful in determining operability based on septal thickness and morphology, degree of mitral systolic anterior motion, aortic root and left atrial dimensions, and level of systolic anterior motion contact below the aortic annulus.

Cardiac catheterization should be performed after all cardiac drugs have been discontinued for 24 to 72 hours in order to determine resting and provocable obstruction in addition to right- and left-sided hemodynamics. Provocation with Valsalva's maneuver, amyl nitrite, and isoproterenol simulates the effects on gradients of changing preload and afterload and increasing heart rate and cardiac output. Possible right ventricular outflow tract obstruction should also be ruled out. Spurious gradients may be obtained using a multiple side-hole catheter; therefore, an endhole pigtail catheter should be used. A left ventriculogram is performed to evaluate the presence and degree of mitral regurgitation and left ventricular contractility. The presence of mitral annular calcification should be noted on fluoroscopy in the event that a mitral valve replacement is anticipated. Coronary arteriograms are routinely performed.

Preoperatively, beta-blockers, calcium-channel blockers, and diuretics are tapered and then discontinued 24 hours prior to operation. If moderate to severe symptoms occur, the patient may be treated with lower doses of intravenous beta-blockers or calcium-channel blockers, which are continued up to the time of operation. In the presence of significant coronary artery disease, medical therapy with nitrates is continued. Unless this is contraindicated, patients should be off amiodarone 3 to 6 months prior to operation.

MONITORING AND ANESTHESIA

Monitoring includes an arterial line, Swan-Ganz catheter, electrocardiogram, and urinary output catheter. A pacing Swan-Ganz is used in patients with a history of or demonstrated complete heart block, Mobitz type II, sick sinus syndrome, or conduction abnormalities which, especially after a left ventricular myotomy and myectomy, may lead to heart block.

Following induction with thiopental sodium and relaxation with pancuronium, anesthesia is maintained with 100 percent oxygen ventilation and supplemented narcotics (fentanyl, sufentanil, or morphine sulfate). Hypotension is treated with volume replacement or an alpha agent. Supraventricular or ventricular arrhythmias are treated pharmacologically or electrically if the patient is hemodynamically unstable.

OPERATIVE THERAPY

Various approaches to relief of left ventricular outflow tract obstruction secondary to IHSS include left ventricular myotomy; left ventricular myotomy and myectomy (Morrow's procedure); mitral valve replacement; left ventricular myotomy and myectomy via the left ventricular apex approach; left ventricular myotomy and myectomy via the left atrium; and right ventricular myotomy and myectomy. It is desirable to approach the left ventricular outflow tract obstruction directly and not to compromise left ventricular function with the operation. Objectives of the operative therapy are (1) to maximally relieve resting and provocable obstruction; and (2) to do so with minimum mortality and morbidity.

Since 1982 operations performed in this clinic for treatment of obstruction include left ventricular myotomy and myectomy and mitral valve replacement based upon information obtained from the intraoperative echocardiogram. An Irex Echo instrument is currently used. The transducer is gas sterilized and vented for 16 to 18 hours prior to use. Once the pericardial sac is opened, long and short axis 2-D echocardiograms are obtained to determine septal thickness, distribution of septal hypertrophy (i.e., localized or homogeneous), and systolic anterior motion contact point on the septum. Table 1 summarizes our current criteria for choice of operation. The intraoperative echocardiogram is essential to tailoring the operative approach and to minimizing iatrogenic complications, such as creation of a ventricular septal defect and incomplete relief of obstruction. Figure 1 illustrates some of the variations of extent and distribution of septal hypertrophy seen in IHSS. Figure 1A, the "classic morphology," is seen in only 12 to 15 percent of patients.

Generally, the operative approach for both left ventricular myotomy and myectomy and mitral valve replacement is through a median sternotomy, although in the presence of an increased anteroposterior diameter, a normal sized left atrium, and marked septal and free wall-hypertrophy, the mitral valve replacement may be facilitated by a left posterolateral or right anterior thoracotomy. Either femoral artery or aortic arch cannulation is used. Venous drainage is by a single cannula (left ventricular myotomy and myectomy) or double cannulae (mitral valve replacement).

LEFT VENTRICULAR MYOTOMY AND MYECTOMY—AN OPERATIVE APPROACH

The left pleural space is opened widely, and the left ventricular vent is brought in at the middle to posterior axillary line and inserted into the left ventricular apex. The left ventricle can be vented via the superior pulmonary vein, but the apex vent is preferable for subsequent air removal when the left ventricular myotomy and myectomy is completed. Excellent venous drainage requires minimal left ventricular venting, thus facilitating the passage of instruments into the left ventricular cavity.

The previously described anoxic flaccid arrest at 30° C is no longer used, and myocardial preservation is accomplished using 26° C total body hypothermia, ice slush, and cold National Institutes of Health oxygenated alkalotic crystalloid cardioplegia. Cardioplegia administration is repeated every 20 minutes.

TABLE 1 Indications for Left Ventricular Myotomy and Myectomy Versus Mitral Valve Replacement

Indications for Left Ventricular Myotomy and Myectomy	*Indications for Mitral Valve Replacement*
Septal dimension ≥18 mm in region of resection	Septum <18 mm in thickness in area of resection
Previous inadequate left ventricular myotomy and myectomy	Atypical septal morphology (i.e., prominent basilar notch or unusual distribution of hypertrophy)
Note: The hypertrophy must be located within the "operative window," i.e., aortic annulus. The presence of 3 to 4+ mitral regurgitation in the absence of primary mitral valve disease *or* of severe pulmonary arterial hypertension is not a contraindication for left ventricular myotomy and myectomy	Previous "adequate" left ventricular myotomy and myectomy with persistent symptoms and demonstrated significant obstruction
	Mitral regurgitation secondary to primary mitral valve disease
	Note: Heavy mitral valve annular calcification may make mitral valve replacement difficult

Operative exposure is shown in Figure 2. The aorta is opened vertically to within 5 mm of the aortic annulus in the noncoronary sinus. Bimanual digital palpation of the septum allows the surgeon to translate the intraoperative echocardiogram to the operative findings. The exposure of the interventricular septum is accomplished by retraction of the right coronary leaflet anterior and to the patient's left, using a cloth-covered thin tubular retractor. Further fixation and exposure of the basilar portion of the interventricular septum are facilitated by external pressure over the septum using a stick sponge. Patients who have resting obstruction usually have a contact lesion from the systolic anterior motion of the anterior mitral valve leaflet, as evidenced by thickened endocardium (as shown). Patients with only provocable obstruction most often have no endocardial thickening. This contact point (as determined by the intraoperative echocardiogram) normally lies 2 to 3 cm below the aortic annulus and should be the point of maximal resection. The proximal portion of the left ventricular myotomy and myectomy need not begin directly beneath the right coronary leaflet, because (1) obstruction does not occur at this point, and (2) the septum is often thin in this region and support for the aortic annulus may depend on this part of the septum's being intact. Normally a resection starting 0.5 to 1.0 cm below the annulus and extending 4.0 cm toward the apex is effective in relieving the obstruction. If the contact point is lower on the septum, as seen in the presence of posterior mitral valve systolic anterior motion, the myotomy-myectomy should be extended toward the apex by the appropriate amount.

Figure 3, a longitudinal view of the operative field, shows the proper placement of the lighted 18-mm retractor to protect the mitral valve apparatus (A) and to provide a cutting surface for the vertical incisions (B). Care

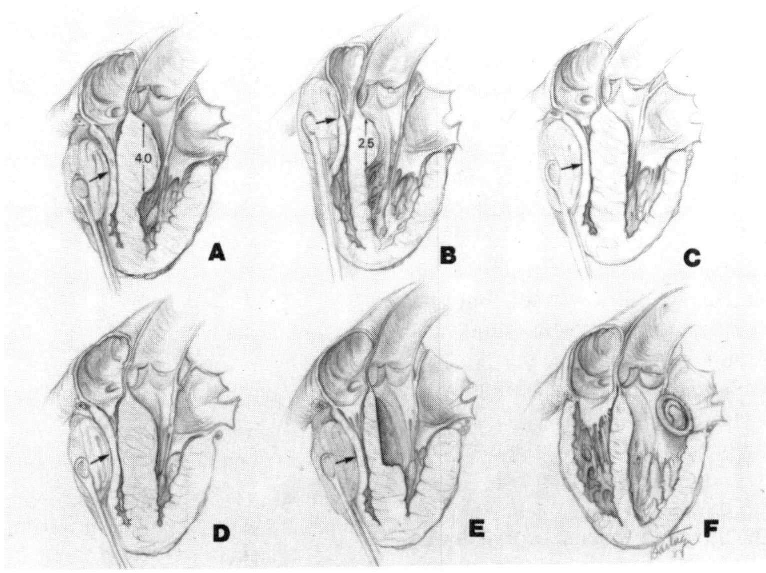

Figure 1 Variations of distribution and extent of septal hypertrophy seen in patients with IHSS. *A*, classic morphology: 4.0 cm basilar septal hypertrophy and normal distal septum; *B*, limited (2–2.5 cm) basilar septal hypertrophy and normal distal septum; *C*, diffuse or homogeneous hypertrophy of septum and normal left ventricular free wall; *D*, concentric septa and free wall hypertrophy; *E*, following left ventricular myotomy and myectomy of *D*; *F*, mitral valve replacement indicated by thin basilar hypertrophy of septum. From Morrow AG. Hypertrophic subaortic stenosis. Operative methods utilized to relieve left ventricular outflow obstruction. J Thorac Cardiovasc Surg 1978; 76(4):423–430.)

must be taken to assure that all chordae tendineae are behind the retractor to avoid damaging them. Retractors larger than 18 mm in width may provide greater protection of the mitral valve apparatus, but a larger retractor combined with anterior retraction of the right coronary leaflet may stretch the aortic annulus, producing iatrogenic aortic regurgitation.

The Morrow procedure, as shown in Figures 3 through 5, has been modified only slightly. The rule for the depth of septum resected is usually one-half of the septal thickness at the systolic anterior motion contact point.

The first vertical myotomy incision is made using a No. 10 knife blade, attached to an angled handle, starting 2 to 3 mm to the right of the midpoint of the right coronary leaflet and 0.5 to 1.0 cm below the aortic annulus. This incision, parallel to the axis of the retractor, is extended 4.0 cm toward the apex unless the basilar septal hypertrophy is of shorter length (see Fig. 1B). As the knife blade is withdrawn, the septum is incised against the lighted retractor. The hypertrophied muscle associated with IHSS often has a gritty consistency secondary to the interstitial fibrosis. The second vertical myotomy, as shown in Figure 4, is made counterclockwise 10 to 15 mm, depending upon the amount of interventricular septum exposed, and is made parallel to the first incision and extended 4.0 cm. There is a tendency to point the tip of the knife blade down toward the retractor rather than parallel to its axis, creating a shallow distal myotomy-myectomy. Digital palpation confirms the depth and length of the myotomy incisions. The transverse myotomy is made connecting the two vertical myotomies 0.5 to 1.0 cm below the aortic annulus using a No. 10 knife blade attached to a handle angled on the flat. This incision is again made parallel to the axis of the lighted retractor and extends 4.0 cm toward the apex.

In patients who have isolated basilar septal hypertrophy (see Figs. 1A and 1B), the resection is now complete and the muscle mass resected is shown in Figure 5A. The channel created is shown in Figure 5B. Additional muscle may be removed by a 45-degree longitudinal incision of the first vertical myotomy incision. It may be important to preserve the vertical depth and not to taper the myotomies severely in order to prevent the anterior leaflet from again contacting the newly created roof of the trough in a very narrowed left ventricular outflow tract. Additional thickened endocardium may be resected to further "relax" the left ventricular outflow tract, but care should be taken to avoid damage to the anterior mitral valve leaflet if scar is contiguous with the valve per se.

In patients who have homogeneous thickening of the interventricular septum (see Figs. 1C and 1D), the distal portion of resection may be facilitated by advancing the cloth-covered retractor into the proximal channel, retracting anteriorly and to the patient's left. This usually exposes the distal part of the attached specimen, which may then be divided with a scissors. Care must be taken to avoid the chordae tendineae when the distal resection is completed. If it is necessary to remove additional muscle, which is often the case, the roof of the trough is first digitally palpated to assess the thickness of the remaining muscle. If the trough tapers distally, it should be squared off with appropriate incisions. The completed longitudinal resection in a homogeneous hypertrophied interventricular septum is shown in Figure 1E. The muscle may then be removed by additional incisions or in small portions with a pituitary rongeur. Fragments of the distal resection are removed with a rongeur.

The coronary ostia are now blocked with either coronary perfusor tips or a Kitner's sponge, and the ventricle is lavaged with 2 L of cold saline to remove debris. The aortic valve leaflets are inspected to be certain they were not damaged during the procedure. The aortic incision is closed, and the absence of aortic regurgitation is confirmed when the aortic cross-clamp is removed by placing the left ventricular vent to gravity drainage. Patients with IHSS have "super hearts" that may begin to override the pump even at lower temperatures; therefore, thorough removal of air should be performed early to avoid air emboli. Temporary atrial and ventricular wires are used routinely, and when indicated, permanent wires are implanted. The thresholds of the ventricular wires may be somewhat higher than expected secondary to the interstitial fibrosis. In patients with demonstrated potential lethal ventricular arrhythmias, usually polymorphic, consideration should be given to the placement of defibrillator pads for potential use of an automatic internal cardiac defibrillator.

Following termination of cardiopulmonary bypass, a repeat intraoperative echocardiogram is performed. The adequacy of the channel, absence or presence of systolic

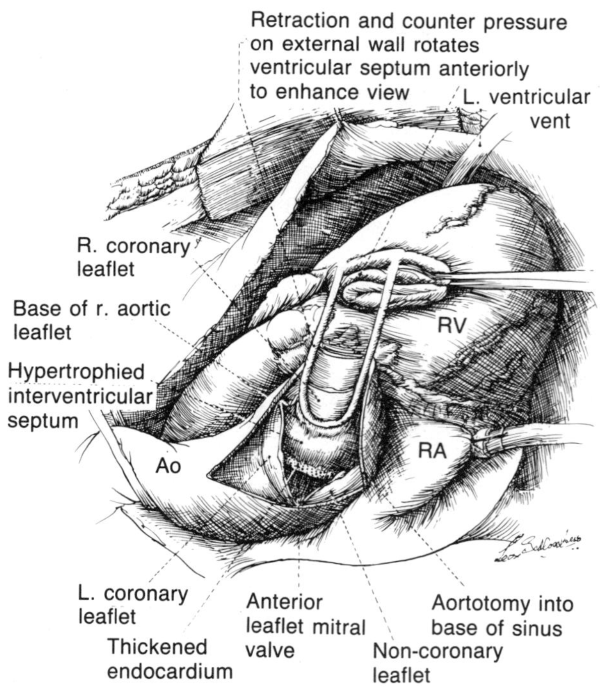

Figure 2 Operative approach through a median sternotomy. The septum is exposed through a vertical aortotomy, with retraction of the right coronary leaflet and external compression of the septum using a stick sponge. Note thickened endocardium representing point of obstruction by systolic anterior motion of the mitral valve leaflet. (From Morrow AG. Hypertrophic subaortic stenosis. Operative methods utilized to relieve left ventricular outflow obstruction. J Thorac Cardiovasc Surg 1978; 76(4):424.)

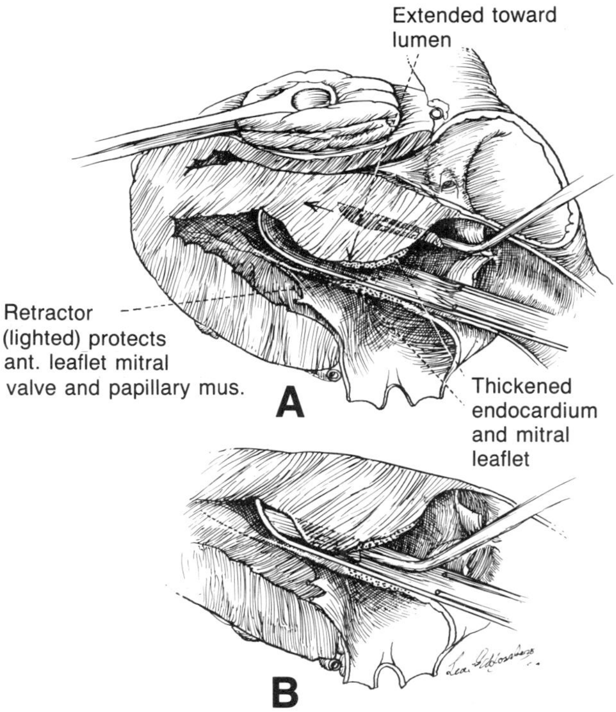

Figure 3 *A*, longitudinal view of operative field showing placement of the lighted retractor to protect the mitral valve apparatus and to provide a cutting surface for the vertical myotomy incisions. *B*, note that the scalpel blade is parallel to the lighted retractor to provide uniform depth of myotomy. (Redrawn from Morrow AG. Hypertrophic subaortic stenosis. Operative methods utilized to release left ventricular outflow obstruction. J Thorac Cardiovasc Surg 1978; 76(4):425.)

anterior motion, increase in left ventricular outflow tract area, and absence of a ventricular septal defect or damaged chordae tendineae producing a flail mitral valve leaflet are determined. If an inadequate channel has been created with persistent systolic anterior motion and obstruction, revision of the left ventricular myotomy and myectomy should be performed if sufficient septum remains at that time; if not, a mitral valve replacement can be performed.

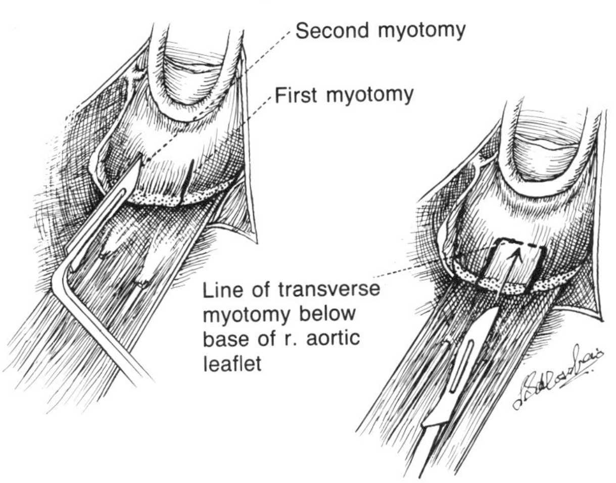

Figure 4 Positions of the vertical and horizontal myotomy incisions. Note resection starts 0.5 to 1.0 cm below right coronary annulus. (Redrawn from Morrow AG. Hypertrophic subaortic stenosis. Operative methods utilized to release left ventricular outflow obstruction. J Thorac Cardiovasc Surg 1978; 76(4): 427.)

If an iatrogenic ventricular septal defect has been created, it should be closed through a right atriotomy or a right ventriculotomy. A small ventricular septal defect may enlarge with increasing left ventricular pressures once the patient is off bypass. The location is usually just below the crista supraventricularis. The ventricular septal defect should be repaired as one would an ischemic defect, i.e., with a large Teflon patch secured to good tissue using pledget-reinforced sutures. Unfortunately, complete heart block may result from this complication and repair and should be treated with an atrioventricular sequential pacemaker in patients with previous normal sinus rhythm. If the ventricular septal defect is not initially detected or occurs late and if the Q_p:Q_s is less than 2:1 in a hemodynamically stable patient, the ventricular septal defect may be closed at a later date by direct suture technique once endocardial fibrosis has formed around the defect. The incidence of complete heart block should be lower in this instance.

MITRAL VALVE REPLACEMENT FOR OPERATIVE TREATMENT OF IHSS

Mitral valve replacement is performed according to standard operative technique. Myocardial preservation follows the regimen outlined for left ventricular myotomy and myectomy. Mitral valve replacement procedure should employ a low profile disc or bileaflet valve to avoid problems associated with a small left ventricular outflow tract. Spherical Björk-Shiley valves (usually 23 to 27 mm) or a Hancock bioprosthesis when anticoagulants are contraindicated has been routinely employed in this clinic. With the changing availability of Björk-Shiley valves, the St.

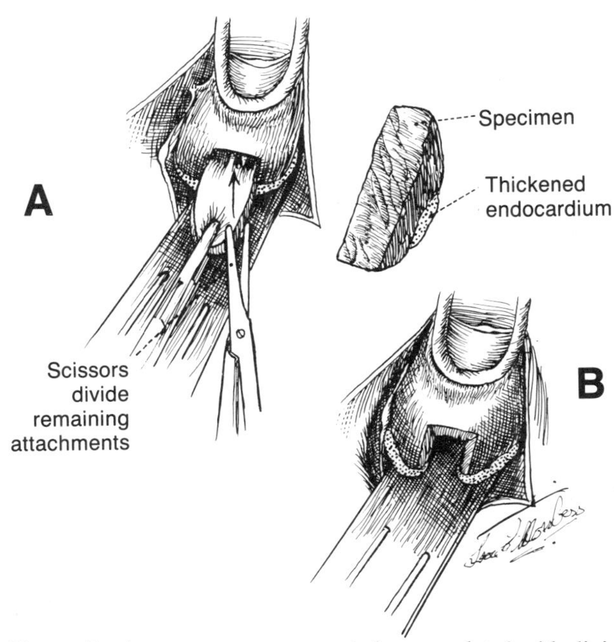

Figure 5 *A*, myotomy-myectomy being completed with division of muscle attachment with a scissors; *B*, completed myotomy-myectomy. Residual endocardial thickening is resected from septum. (Redrawn from Morrow AG. Hypertrophic subaortic stenosis. Operative methods utilized to release left ventricular outflow obstruction. J Thorac Cardiovasc Surg 1978; 76(4): 427.)

Jude Medical valve is an alternative. The recommended suture technique is pledget-reinforced horizontal mattress sutures, since the valve remnant and annulus are usually normal. The Björk-Shiley valve is usually positioned with the major orifice directed toward the left ventricular free wall. The Hancock bioprosthesis is positioned with the widest intrastrut distance beneath the left ventricular outflow tract. If the mitral valve is difficult to visualize through a median sternotomy, a transatrial septal approach may be beneficial. A routine intraoperative echocardiogram after mitral valve replacement is not performed.

POSTOPERATIVE MANAGEMENT

Management problems of these patients include supraventricular and ventricular arrhythmias and hypotension. Generally, if the patient has been identified preoperatively as having a significant supraventricular or ventricular arrhythmia that has responded to digoxin, beta-blockers, calcium-channel blockers, or type 1A antiarrhythmic drugs, these agents are employed in the immediate postoperative period to avoid hemodynamic compromise. A rapid ventricular response to atrial fibrillation or loss of the "A kick" may result in significant reduction in cardiac output and systemic blood pressure. If the patient is hemodynamically unstable, electrocardioversion should be performed promptly and the appropriate drug therapy given to maintain normal sinus rhythm. If atrial fibrillation recurs, appropriate drugs should be given to slow the ventricular response. Digoxin normally can be used safely in postoperative left ventricular myotomy and myectomy or mitral valve replacement patients for treatment of atrial fibrillation. Atrial flutter can often be converted to normal sinus rhythm using rapid atrial pacing and, therefore, the temporary atrioventricular wires are left in situ for 5 to 7 days postoperatively.

Treatment of ventricular tachycardia consists initially of intravenous lidocaine or procainamide followed by the appropriate oral agent. Treatment of short runs of ventricular tachycardia in IHSS patients remains controversial, but, as a rule, a 15-beat run will be treated. Isolated unifocal or multifocal premature ventricular contractions, couplets, and triplets are not treated.

Following left ventricular myotomy and myectomy, 70 percent of patients in this clinic have a left bundle branch block. If complete heart block occurs in the presence of normal sinus rhythm, treatment is with an atrioventricular sequential pacemaker, or, in the absence of an atrial mechanism, an activity-sensing device.

Hypotension may be treated with volume replacement if indicated and the appropriate inotropic agent. Generally, phenylephrine is used if the patient is still obstructed on provocation; otherwise, epinephrine or dopamine is utilized. The intraoperative postprocedure echocardiogram may prove helpful in determining the appropriate inotropic agent.

Patients with a mechanical prosthesis are anticoagulated with warfarin and the prothrombin time is maintained at two times that of controls. Paroxysmal or chronic atrial fibrillation usually requires anticoagulation.

TABLE 2 Sex and Age Distribution in Patients Operated on for IHSS, 1982–1987

	Left Ventricular Myotomy and Myectomy (N=108)	*Mitral Valve Replacement (N=48)*
Males	62	19
mean age (range)	43.8 (18–80 yr)	44.5 (29–63 yr)
Females	46	29
mean age (range)	48.1 (11–72 yr)	50.3 (16–78 yr)

RESULTS

Five hundred and forty patients have been operated on for IHSS at the National Heart, Lung, and Blood Institute. The majority of these patients (83 percent) have had IHSS alone and the remainder other associated cardiac lesions. Morrow performed the left ventricular myotomy and myectomy or Morrow procedure on 350 patients between 1960 and 1982. Operative mortality in his series was approximately 8 percent. Analyses of 120 patients operated on by him from 1960 to 1975 demonstrated good long-term symptomatic improvement, with 85 percent and 51 percent of patients in New York Heart Association Functional Class I or II at a mean of 5.2 and 10.2 years, respectively. Late deaths thought to be related to IHSS occurred in 11 (9 percent) at a mean of 5.2 years and 35 (29 percent) at a mean of 10.2 years, with a cumulative total of 62 (49 percent) deaths in this group over the entire follow-up period. Causes of death included congestive heart failure (ten), known arrhythmias (five), sudden (five), unknown (13), and repeat operation (two). Calculated annual mortality following operation for IHSS is 4 percent per year. Contrary to earlier predictions, very few patients progressed to a dilated cardiomyopathy.

Since 1982, 108 left ventricular myotomy and myectomy procedures and 48 mitral valve replacements have been performed in patients having symptoms and obstruction secondary to IHSS. Thirty-seven additional patients have undergone treatment for IHSS in combination with other cardiac lesions. Sex and age distributions are shown in Table 2. It is of interest that in spite of the advent of

TABLE 3 Complications Following Operative Treatment for IHSS

Left Ventricular Myotomy and Myectomy	(N=108)
Acquired ventricular septal defects (two repaired early, one late; all survived)	3
Cardiac arrest—resuscitation	1
Iatrogenic aortic insufficiency requiring valve replacement	2
Seroconverted to human immunodeficiency virus (+)	1
Compartment syndrome	1
Central embolus (air)	1
Complete heart block requiring pacemaker	2
Mitral Valve Replacement	(N=48)
Cardiac arrest—resuscitation	1
Paravalvular leak—reoperation	1
Central embolus (thrombus)	1
Descending thoracic aortic dissection	1

TABLE 4 Hemodynamic Summary Following Operation for IHSS (1982–1987)

	Preoperatively	*Left Ventricular Myotomy and Myectomy Postoperatively*	*Postoperatively Only*	*Preoperatively*	*Mitral Valve Replacement Postoperatively*	*Postoperatively Only*
PAW	(N=46) 14.6±1.2	(N=46) 12.1±0.9	NA	(N=23) 14.7±1.4	(N=23) 13.4±0.9	NA
LVEDP				(N=26) 17.5±1.2	(N=26) 10.9±0.7	NA
0-CP	(N=23) 16.8±1.9	(N=23) 15.0±1.2	NA			
+-CP	(N=33) 19.3±1.2	(N=33) 15.6±1.1	NA			
CI				(N=23) 2.6±0.1	(N=23) 2.7±0.1	NA
0-CP	(N=20) 2.6±0.2	(N=20) 2.3±0.1*	NA			
+-CP	(N=31) 2.7±0.1	(N=31) 2.8±0.1*	NA			
Gradients						
Rest	(N=58) 80.8±6.0	(N=58) 16.1±3.9	NA	(N=26) 68.2±9.1	(N=26) 3.8±1.0	NA
Valsalva	(N=36) 103.9±5.3	(N=36) 24.7±5.2	(N=26) 47.8±8.0	(N=17) 96.2±5.3	(N=17) 11.1±3.5	(N=15) 10.1±2.7
Amyl nitrite	(N=28) 94.4±4.4	(N=28) 30.6±4.8	(N=32) 49.6±6.9	(N=15) 95.1±6.1	(N=15) 17.4±4.4	(N=17) 20.7±5.2
Isoproterenol	(N=16) 118.3±7.7	(N=16) 37.2±6.45	(N=41) 63.1±6.5	(N=10) 121.0±8.8	(N=10) 28.2±6.7	(N=20) 21.6±4.1

Key: PAW=pulmonary arterial wedge pressure (mm Hg); LVEDP=left ventricular end-diastolic pressure (mm Hg); CI=cardiac index (liters/min/m^2), values report mean±standard error of the mean; NA=not applicable; 0-CP=no cardioplegia; +-CP=cardioplegia used.
*p=0.01 for cardiac index±cardioplegia.
All gradients measured peak to peak—mm Hg.

beta-blocking agents and calcium-channel blockers, the mean age at operation has not changed significantly (see Table 2) when compared with a mean of 44 (range 8 to 75 years) reported in 120 patients operated on from 1960 to 1975.

Current operative mortality (1982 to 1987), defined as in the hospital or less than or equal to 30 days after the procedure, is 2.7 percent (three patients) following left ventricular myotomy and myectomy and 6.3 percent (three patients) after mitral valve replacement during the same time period. Cause of death in the left ventricular myotomy and myectomy patients was low cardiac output in all three patients; two of these had had 30° C anoxic flaccid arrest. Following mitral valve replacement, low cardiac output (one patient), hepatic renal failure (one patient), and prosthetic malfunction (one patient) accounted for operative mortality. Four (3.8 percent) patients have died late after left ventricular myotomy and myectomy, three suddenly and one of congestive heart failure. Two patients (4.0 percent) have died suddenly following mitral valve replacement. Complications following treatment of IHSS are shown in Table 3.

Seventy-three patients have returned for postoperative follow-up after left ventricular myotomy and myectomy; 59 (80.1 percent) are New York Heart Association Functional Class I or II and 10 are Functional Class III. Following mitral valve replacement, 26 (72 percent) of 36 patients are Functional Class I or II, three remained Functional Class III, and five improved from Class IV to III.

Hemodynamic findings are summarized in Table 4. These data reveal that pulmonary arterial wedge pressure is not significantly increased in patients following mitral valve replacement, in spite of smaller sized valves (23, 25, and 27 mm Björk-Shiley) being used. Current myocardial preservation methods preserve the preoperative cardiac index, as shown in 31 left ventricular myotomy and myectomy patients receiving cardioplegia and ice slush, as did all the mitral valve replacement patients (N = 23), compared with 20 left ventricular myotomy and myectomy patients who had 30° C anoxic flaccid arrest (p= 0.01). Both left ventricular myotomy and myectomy and mitral valve replacement predictably relieve resting obstruction, but mitral valve replacement more predictably relieves provocable obstruction. Patients who have obstruction at rest greater than or equal to 100 mm Hg are not routinely provoked preoperatively, and the data shown as postoperative probably represent only the patients with severest obstruction preoperatively.

SUGGESTED READING

Braunwald E, Lambrew CT, Rockoff SD, Ross J Jr, Morrow AG. Idiopathic hypertrophic subaortic stenosis: 1. A description of the disease based upon an analysis of 64 patients. Circulation 1964; 30 (Suppl 4):IV-3-IV-119.

Cooley DA, Wukasch DC, Leachman RD. Mitral valve replacement for idiopathic hypertrophic subaortic stenosis: results in 27 patients. J Cardiovasc Surg 1976; 17:380–387.

Maron BJ, Bonow RO, Cannon RO III, Leon MB, Epstein SE. Hypertrophic cardiomyopathy: interrelations of clinical manifestations, pathophysiology, and therapy (Part I). N Engl J Med 1987; 316:780–789.

Maron BJ, Bonow RO, Cannon RO III, Leon MB, Epstein SE. Hypertrophic cardiomyopathy: interrelations of clinical manifestations, pathophysiology, and therapy (Part II). N Engl J Med 1987; 316:844–852.

Maron BJ, Merrill WH, Freier PA, Kent KM, Epstein SE, Morrow AG. Long-term clinical course and symptomatic status of patients after operation for hypertrophic subaortic stenosis. Circulation 1978; 57:1205–1213.

Morrow AG. Hypertrophic subaortic stenosis. Operative methods utilized to relieve left ventricular outflow obstruction. J Thorac Cardiovasc Surg 1978; 76:423–430.

APICOAORTIC CONDUITS

DENTON A. COOLEY, M.D.

A few patients with aortic stenosis cannot be managed successfully by conventional techniques. Included in this group are those with fibrous tunnel obstruction of the left ventricular flow tract, calcific aortic stenosis, hypoplasia of the aortic annulus, and tubular hypoplasia of the ascending aorta. Patients with significant recurrent aortic valvar stenosis, after prior attempts at aortic root repair or valvotomy, may also be considered for radical outflow tract reconstruction, especially if infection has contributed to the failure of the previous procedure.

At the Texas Heart Institute, we have treated a number of such patients with left ventricular outflow tract obstruction by using an apicoaortic conduit. Our initial review of nine such procedures in 1976 was among the first clinical reports, and it was expanded to include 27 patients in 1980. By September, 1986, 13 additional patients had been seen, making a total of 40 patients in the series to date. Of these, 22 were men and 18 were women. Ages at surgery ranged from 2 to 77 years (mean age, 29.5 years), and the average follow-up period is now 8.3 years.

Prior aortic valvotomy, annular enlargement, coronary artery bypass, or valve replacement had been performed in 22 of these patients; the indications for apicoaortic conduits in these patients were recurrent obstruction with impending heart failure or active hemolysis from a diminutive ventricular outlet. The 18 remaining patients had not undergone any previous procedures, but they were considered candidates for apicoaortic shunts because of either outflow obstruction or severe aortic calcification in conjunction with coronary artery disease.

OPERATIVE PROCEDURE

A median sternotomy is made, and cannulations of the venae cavae and ascending aorta are performed in the usual manner. Special partially occluding caval clamps are used to ensure capture of venous return. In most instances, total cardiopulmonary bypass with cold potassium cardioplegia is used to effect a diastolic cardiac arrest. The left atrium is vented via the right superior pulmonary vein. The ascending aorta is cross-clamped just proximal to the origin of the innominate artery, and a mixture of 500 ml of 5 percent dextrose and 0.45 percent sodium chloride with cardioplegic solution is infused into the aortic root. Topical hypothermia is induced with iced saline.

After the heart stops, the left ventricular outflow tract, aortic valve, and ascending aorta are examined to determine the feasibility of creating an apicoaortic shunt. We continue to favor the supraceliac abdominal aorta as the site of re-entry, and the median sternotomy can easily be extended into the upper abdomen. An aperture is coned from the left ventricular apex, a semirigid inlet prosthesis is inserted into the ventricular cavity, and the sewing ring is secured to the apex with mattress sutures and Teflon felt pledgets (Fig. 1). The valved Dacron conduit is anastomosed end-to-side to the supraceliac aorta after retracting the left lobe of the liver and dividing the right crus of the diaphragm. This approach avoids the left pleural cavity and free peritoneum; it ultimately positions the conduit superficially in the abdomen, where subsequent valve replacement can easily be done without the need for cardiopulmonary bypass, thoracotomy, or another median sternotomy. The two grafts are tailored to a gentle curve through the left hemidiaphragm and are anastomosed within the abdomen with continuous 4–0 or 3–0 braided polyester suture.

Before the ascending aortic cross-clamp is released, precautions are taken to evacuate any residual air from the composite conduit proximal and distal to the valve, the left ventricle, and the ascending aorta. Depending on the time required for performing the procedure, the entire operation may be accomplished during cold cardioplegic arrest. Intermittent coronary perfusion with release of the aortic clamp may also be used. In the presence of adequate cardiac hypothermia with pharmacologically induced cardioplegia, a period of circulatory arrest of more than 60 minutes is well tolerated.

After the cannulae have been removed, pressures are measured in the left ventricle, in the conduit proximal and distal to the valve, and in the ascending aorta. In most patients, we have temporarily occluded the ascending aorta to determine the effect on the systemic circulation. Generally, after a brief decrease in blood pressure of approximately 20 percent, the systemic pressure rises to a normal level, indicating that the conduit could, if necessary, conduct the entire left ventricular output.

POSTOPERATIVE CARE AND RESULTS

For most patients in whom the conduit contained a heterograft valve, no long-term anticoagulants have been used. There has been no known instance of thromboembolism in our patients despite the lack of anticoagulation therapy. In some patients, aspirin and dipyridamole were started on the third postoperative day. Sodium warfarin was continued in those patients who already had a mechanical prosthetic valve in the aortic or mitral annulus. In our last few patients, we have used Björk-Shiley convexo-concave valves in the conduit, and these patients have been anticoagulated with sodium warfarin. Antibiotic coverage has been used in all patients during the early postoperative period.

Among the 40 patients in our series, there have been six (15 percent) early deaths. Eight initial survivors have died an average of 2.5 years after their procedures; four of the deaths were unrelated to the conduits. Of the remaining four late deaths, two patients had infections of the conduit (at 1 and 4 years, respectively), and two had ruptures of left ventricular false aneurysms (at 2 and 5 years, respectively). Four patients have required a laparotomy for replacement of the porcine valve at 3, 4, and 8 (two patients) years after the initial procedure. In the sixth postoperative year, one patient needed correction of a fibrotic obstruction of the conduit that developed at the egress from the left ventricle; another patient developed a false aneurysm of the left ventricular apex that required surgical correction in the fifth postoperative year.

In both children and adults, the shunt relieves signs and symptoms of left ventricular outflow tract obstruction. Analyses of postoperative angiograms and pressure tracings show that the left ventricular aortic gradient has been corrected, ventricular function has been preserved or improved, and blood flow has been distributed normally through the coronary and systemic circulations. Hemolysis has been reversed. Follow-up, now approaching 11 years for many patients, demonstrates that the procedure is well tolerated and does not hinder normal growth or exercise in children and young adults. Although formal exercise testing has not been done routinely, none of the patients

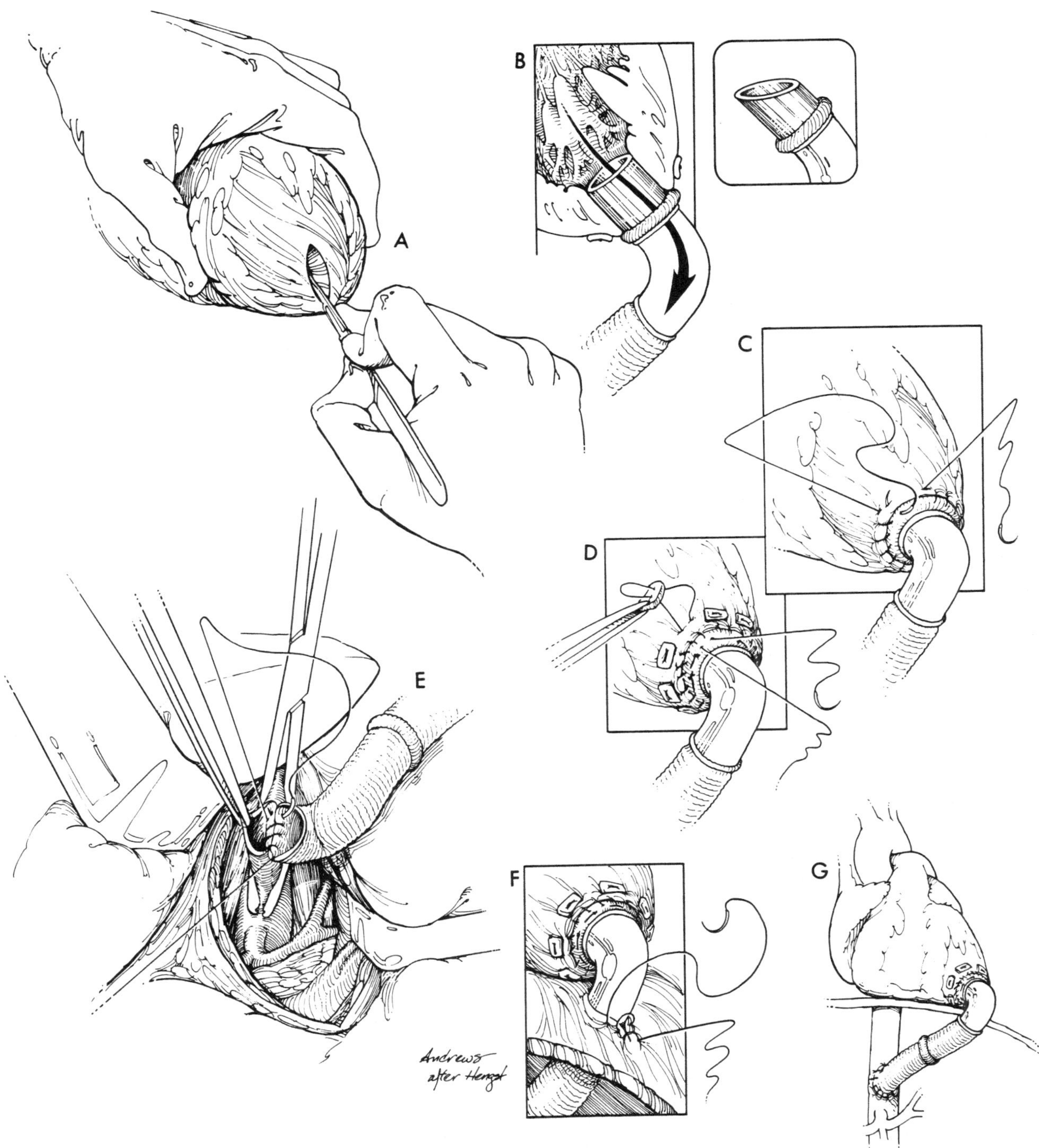

Figure 1 Technique for insertion of an apicoaortic conduit. (From Cooley DA. Techniques in cardiac surgery. Philadelphia: WB Saunders Co, 1984:194.)

have reported symptoms with exercise and none are restricted physically. Three older patients with significant angina and severely calcified aortas that precluded routine bypasses have had good results with vein grafts from the conduit to the involved coronary vessels.

Recognized late problems with these conduits include disruption of the conduits from the ventricular apices, infection, thromboembolism, and porcine valve failure. Only one of our patients, however, developed obstruction of the conduit at the insertion into the ventricle, and we have not had any recognized instances of thromboembolism, a significant difference from all other groups of our patients undergoing various types of valve replacement procedures. The late development of ventricular false aneurysms is disconcerting. Although two of our patients died suddenly of rupture of such false aneurysms without premonitory symptoms, our experience shows that successful repair may be possible if the problem is detected on time. The optimal follow-up of these patients by way of monitoring the potential development of apex-conduit disruption has yet to be defined, but may well include echocardiography, computed tomography, and, perhaps, occasional contrast ventriculography.

SUGGESTED READING

Carrell A. On the experimental surgery of the thoracic aorta and the heart. Ann Surg 1910; 52:83.

Cooley DA. Apico-aortic conduit. In: Techniques in cardiac surgery. 2nd ed. Philadelphia: WB Saunders, 1984:198.

Cooley DA, Norman JC, Mullins CE, Grace RR. Left ventricle to abdominal aorta conduit for relief of aortic stenosis. Cardiovasc Dis Bull Tex Heart Inst 1975; 2:376.

Sarnoff SJ, Donovan TJ, Case RB. The surgical relief of aortic stenosis by means of apical-aortic valvular anastomosis. Circulation 1955; 11:564–575.

Sweeney MS, Walker WE, Cooley DA, Reul GJ. Apicoaortic conduits for complex left ventricular outflow obstruction: 10-year experience. Ann Thorac Surg 1986; 42:609–611.

COMPLICATIONS OF AORTIC VALVE ENDOCARDITIS

DONALD ROSS, D.Sc., F.R.C.S.
PHILIP BELCHER, M.B., B.S. F.R.C.S.

The aortic valve continues to be the most commonly affected in both native and postprosthetic endocarditis. The chief surgically treatable complication of native endocarditis is valve regurgitation, and the onset of ventricular failure during treatment is the usual indication for surgical intervention. Recurrent peripheral embolism with echocardiographic demonstration of vegetations and uncontrolled infection are additional indications.

Native endocarditis may resolve with antibiotics, but it is usually treated by valve replacement. Not infrequently, a quiescent and localized destructive perforation of a cusp may be simply patched with autogenous pericardium and may provide an excellent long-term result (Fig. 1).

The regurgitant jet of blood and bacteria onto the mitral valve gives rise to jet lesions, which should always be suspected in aortic valve endocarditis. Again they can be closed, patched with pericardium, or plicated, depending on the progression of the lesion. The important thing is to be aware of the possibility of jet lesions, to look for them, and to deal with them if they are present.

Previously unsatisfactory results in our hands with postprosthetic or advanced native valve endocarditis have led to a more radical approach in these circumstances. This involves the complete removal of all infected tissue or promoting its free drainage into areas outside the circulation. In particular, bacterial endocarditis resulting in abscesses of the aortic root poses severe anatomic and therapeutic problems. Operations designed simply to replace the infected valve or prosthesis plus local debridement are likely to fail because of the persistence of residual infected material retained within the circulation. To exclude such material from the bloodstream and to debride the annulus effectively usually involves excision of the whole aortic root. Reconstruction of this area becomes mandatory, but we are reluctant to insert further prosthetic material. For this reason it has been our policy to replace it with an antibiotic-sterilized homograft. The coronary arteries attached to disks of aorta are reanastomosed to the homograft.

Root abscesses characteristically occur around the annulus, sometimes causing detachment of the aorta from the ventricle (Fig. 2). Others burrow posteriorly within the mitral valve leaflet to lie behind or to the left of the pulmonary artery. Standard methods of dealing with this complication have included curetting the cavities, treating with local antiseptics, and approximating the edges with buttressed sutures. Pericardium or Dacron cloth may also be used to cover the defects. Others have described the use of a composite valved Dacron graft to replace the aortic root in addition to coronary reimplantation. However, the insertion of a large amount of prosthetic material within the infected area is a source of concern. With any of these methods, recurrent prosthetic endocarditis is likely.

The National Heart Hospital, London, organizes and maintains an aortic homograft bank and has a 25-year experience of homograft aortic valve replacement. The incidence of endocarditis after homograft replacement of the aortic valve has been low (0.5 percent per patient year), and the mean survival time of the valves has been about 10 years. They are flexible, easy to handle, embolism is virtually unknown, and anticoagulation is consequently not required. Aortic homografts have been our first choice

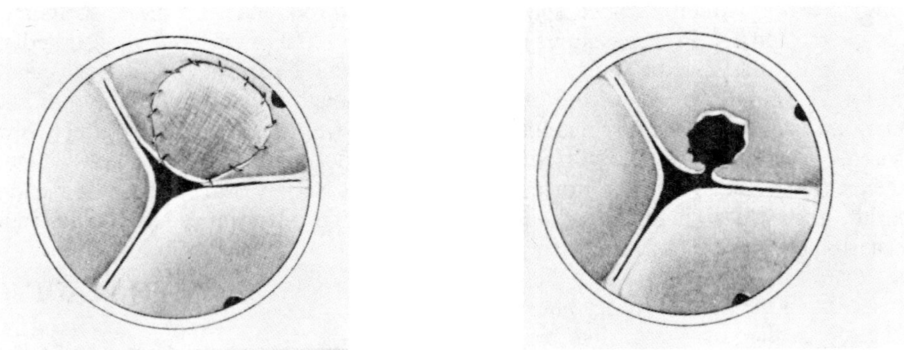

Figure 1 Patch of autogenous pericardium to repair a healed destructive lesion of endocarditis.

for valve replacement in this institution, particularly in young patients. Also because they are stored in antibiotics they are, in our view, particularly suitable for cases with infection. When inserted as a complete functional aortic root, not unexpectedly the valves are invariably competent.

The timing of operation in general depends on the patient's past history and hemodynamic state. When a number of previous operations have been performed, the indication is clear. The use of cross-sectional echocardiography has made possible the early detection of root abscesses before their more florid manifestations such as heart block become apparent. Because we consider abscesses to be relatively inaccessible to antibiotics, we prefer to operate whenever they are found or if the hemodynamic picture indicates that there is increasing detachment of a prosthesis.

The first homograft aortic root replacements were for hypoplastic or tunnel aortic stenosis over 14 years ago, but more recently we have looked upon the method as particularly applicable in prosthetic valve endocarditis.

The operation is performed under appropriate antibiotic coverage with standard anesthetic management. The heart is exposed by a median sternotomy incision; cardiopulmonary bypass is established with a single right atrial cannula, and the patient is cooled to 25° C. A vertical aortotomy is made and extended into the noncoronary sinus. Cardioplegia is infused via the coronary ostia. The aorta is transected about 1 cm above the commissures, and dissection proceeds between it and the common and right pulmonary arteries. The left coronary artery is in danger at this point and a curved metal probe is placed within it so it can be avoided and mobilized with safety. This coronary is fully mobilized with a button of aorta. The right coronary artery is dealt with similarly. The abscesses are opened fully while the valve annulus is excised. Any large tissue deficiencies may have to be made up with autogenous pericardium. Remnants of fibrous tissue are usually left on the ventricular septum for the subsequent attachment of sutures. The root excision is extended across the anterior leaflet of the mitral valve; this is inspected for jet lesions, and the excision skirts the upper margin of the membranous septum to avoid the conducting tissue (Fig. 3).

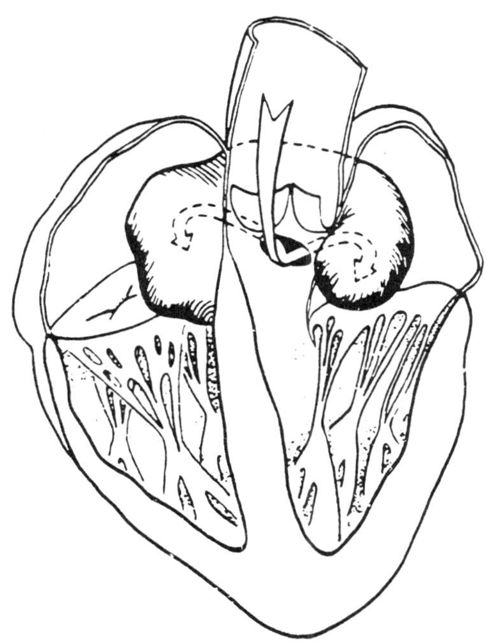

Figure 2 Root abscess arising below the aortic valve and encircling the valve root.

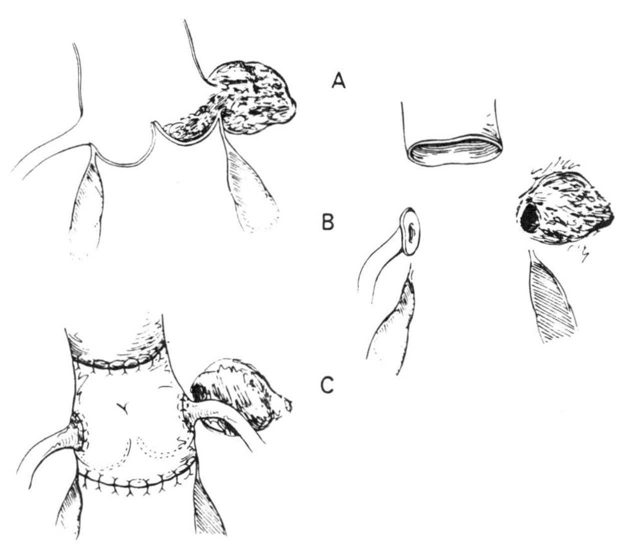

Figure 3 Steps in aortic root replacement: *A*, Periaortic root abscess communicating with infected valve. *B*, Infected root excised allowing abscess to drain freely outside the circulation. *C*, Completed root replacement.

A complete homograft root is then trimmed and inserted using multiple interrupted 4–0 Prolene sutures tied over a thin strip of Teflon felt that may be soaked in iodine and squeezed dry. The circumference of the proximal end of the homograft is divided into four quadrants taking about eight sutures in each. The well-mobilized left coronary artery is then anastomosed to the appropriate position on the homograft, after which the upper end of the homograft aorta is anastomosed to the transected ascending aorta. The aortic clamp is removed to assess the appropriate point of insertion of the right coronary because of the frequent variations in the position of that vessel.

Out of a total of 112 homograft root replacements, 58 have been for infective endocarditis, 31 (29 percent) with primary endocarditis and 27 (25 percent) with post-prosthetic endocarditis.

There were seven early deaths (22.6 percent) and five late deaths (16.1 percent) among the 31 patients operated on for primary endocarditis. Recurrent endocarditis was responsible for two deaths. One patient had Q-fever (*Coxiella burnetii*), and this was retrospectively diagnosed from culture of the removed prosthesis. Infection persisted but was successfully dealt with at reoperation by another homograft root and appropriate chemotherapy. Follow-up from 1 to 120 months has demonstrated a reinfection rate of less than 2 percent per patient year.

Although the early mortality has been high, we believe this represents the most effective means of curing aortic endocarditis with root abscess, particularly the post-prosthetic variety. Earlier diagnosis and radical root excision as a primary procedure should reduce the mortality.

SUGGESTED READING

Dhalla N, Radley-Smith R, Yacoub M. Early and long-term performance of aortic homograft root replacement. In: Bodnar E, Yacoub M, eds. Biologic bioprosthetic valves. Yorke Medical Books, 1986.

Donaldson RM, Ross DN. Homograft aortic root replacement for complicated prosthetic valve endocarditis. Circulation 1982; 70 (Suppl 1): 178–182.

Lau JKH, Robles A, Cherian A, Ross DN. Surgical treatment of prosthetic endocarditis. Aortic root replacement using a homograft. J Thorac Cardiovasc Surg 1984; 87:712–716.

Okita Y, Franciosi G, Matsuki O, Ross DN. Early and late results of aortic root replacement using antibiotic sterilized aortic homograft. Submitted for publication, 1987.

Somerville J, Ross DN. Homograft replacement of aortic root with reimplantation of coronary arteries. Br Heart J 1982; 47:473–482.

I CORONARY ARTERY DISEASE

CONDUIT OPTIONS FOR CORONARY ARTERY BYPASS SURGERY

BRUCE W. LYTLE, M.D.

The standard conduits used for coronary bypass grafting are the greater saphenous vein and the internal mammary artery (IMA). The saphenous vein is easy to procure, has favorable handling characteristics, is versatile, can be used for many grafting patterns, and is large enough so that it can provide an excess of blood flow for virtually any coronary artery. The disadvantage of using the saphenous vein is graft failure, which increases in frequency beyond 5 postoperative years, when vein graft atherosclerosis becomes prevalent. Compared with the saphenous vein, the IMA is a smaller vessel, more difficult to procure, not as versatile, and more technically demanding to use as a bypass graft. The advantage of IMA grafts is that they stay patent; even 10 years after surgery the patency rate of internal mammary artery grafts is over 90 percent. The goal of the surgeon must be to tailor an operation for myocardial revascularization to the patient, maximizing the advantages and disadvantages of the available conduits. The following is a personal approach.

For patients undergoing operation for primary isolated revascularization, I use the left IMA in virtually all cases, usually as a graft to the left anterior descending coronary artery. Our studies of long-term results after coronary bypass surgery have shown that patients who received left IMA grafts to the left anterior descending coronary artery (often in addition to vein grafts) had better 10-year survival and fewer reoperations than did patients who had vein grafts alone. Furthermore, the superior patency rate of IMA to left anterior descending coronary artery grafts has been established by postoperative angiographic studies involving thousands of grafts. The clinical and angiographic success of the operation is not a matter of opinion but of record. If a graft to the left anterior descending coronary artery is not required, or on the rare occasion when it is not a very important vessel, the left IMA is used to graft the circumflex system. In the past, concern has been expressed that IMA grafting might lead to perioperative complications, but experience has shown that single IMA grafting has not been associated with increased perioperative morbidity. Surgeons have also worried that IMA grafts might not provide enough flow to relieve ischemia and prevent infarction. Some judgment must be exercised in matching IMA grafts to recipient arteries. When the left IMA is small (less than half the diameter of the vessel to be grafted) or has insufficient flow to supply the needs of a large, critically obstructed left anterior descending coronary artery, I use the IMA to graft a secondary target, such as the diagonal or a circumflex branch, although that strategy is employed less that 10 percent of the time. With time, the IMA can increase in size to accommodate for more demand for flow, so concern about adequate IMA flow applies mostly to the perioperative period. The relative contraindications to use of the IMA are emergency operations to graft an acutely occluded vessel (such as sometimes occurs during attempted percutaneous transluminal coronary angioplasty), atherosclerosis of the IMA, a severe obstruction of the subclavian artery, or a dissection involving the IMA.

Whereas the position of the left IMA to the left anterior descending coronary artery graft as the preferred bypass operation is secure, the status of bilateral IMA grafting is evolving. Bilateral IMA grafting increases the complexity of coronary bypass grafting, and there is a slight increase in perioperative morbidity, manifested primarily as an increase in the prevalence of reoperations for bleeding. We have also noticed a trend (not statistically significant) toward an increase in wound complications. The long-term results of bilateral IMA grafting have been superb, with excellent late survival and symptom status, a very low rate of reoperation, and excellent patency of right and left IMA grafts to branches of the left coronary system. On the other hand, if reoperation is ever needed, it will be difficult for the patient with an IMA graft crossing beneath the sternum.

I currently use bilateral IMA grafts in approximately half of the operations I do for primary revascularization. I do not routinely use both IMA's for patients over 70 years of age, since advanced age appears to be a determinant of increased morbidity, or for patients at increased risk of needing future operation. Included in the latter group are patients with valvular dysfunction and those with single- or double-vessel disease who have major coronary vessels that are not in jeopardy at the time of initial surgery.

When matching the conduits to coronary arteries during bilateral mammary grafting, my first principle is to use the left IMA to the most important left-sided vessel. In most cases, this means that the left IMA is used to graft the left anterior descending coronary artery and the right IMA is crossed over (either in front of the aorta or through the transverse sinus) to graft the circumflex. This pattern usually provides the best graft to the left anterior descending artery system, permits sequential grafting to the artery and a diagonal, if needed, and protects the most important graft in the event that reoperation is required. Another scheme is to use the left IMA to the left anterior descending artery as an in situ graft and to use the right IMA as a free (aorto-to-coronary) graft to the circumflex system. This works well when the right IMA does not reach the circumflex as an in situ graft and also avoids grafting across the midline beneath the sternum. Long-term data regarding free IMA grafts are quite favorable, but only dozens rather than thousands of grafts have been studied; hence, we still do not have the same degree of confidence in them as we do in the in situ grafts. The right IMA can be used to graft the main right coronary artery in most cases and sometimes, but not always, it will reach to the posterior descending branch. However, the late patency rate of right IMA grafts to the right coronary artery is not quite as good as that of right IMA grafts to branches of the left coronary system. The left IMA will reach almost any circumflex branch as an in situ graft and can be used in conjunction with a right IMA graft to the left anterior descending coronary artery, although that pattern does expose the graft to potential injury if reoperation is ever needed.

If the superb late survival rate we have documented for our patients after bilateral IMA grafting is confirmed by a longer follow-up of the broad spectrum of patients who are now receiving this operation, bilateral IMA grafting will become the standard method of revascularization. At present, specific indications for this technique are young age (all patients under 50 years of age should receive bilateral IMA grafts), absence of a suitable saphenous vein, and severe ascending aortic atherosclerosis.

Sequential mammary artery grafting is also a technique in the process of evolution. The favorable long-term results documented for single and bilateral IMA grafting make it seem logical that sequential IMA grafts might represent an improvement over vein grafting, but as yet few data exist to support that view. Sequential IMA grafting is technically difficult, and the surgeon must be careful not to jeopardize an important IMA graft to a major coronary artery in order to graft a vessel of secondary importance. If coronary vessels are intramyocardial or buried in epicardial fat, the difficulties of sequential IMA grafting are magnified. Finally, although the IMA can sometimes provide adequate flow for multiple coronary vessels, that is not consistently predictable. Currently, I use sequential IMA grafts in less than 10 percent of patients, most often in the left anterior descending coronary artery diagonal system and occasionally in the circumflex system. I have never done more than two anastomoses per IMA.

I use the saphenous vein to graft vessels not grafted with the internal mammary artery. If the vein is of good quality, I prefer separate vein grafts to coronary vessels with an internal diameter of 1.5 mm or greater. I try to graft coronary vessels with an internal diameter of 1.25 mm or less as part of a sequential graft, with a larger coronary vessel as the most distal anastomosis on the vein. I do not use Y-type grafts because of their poor late patency rate.

Reoperations present special problems. Often, fewer conduits (particularly saphenous vein) are available; lesser saphenous veins may be useful in these situations. On the other hand, there are often fewer coronary vessels that need grafting. IMA grafts are particularly useful in reoperations, since an aortic anastomosis is not needed, and space on the aorta may be at a premium during reoperation. It is a common situation that the patient presenting for reoperation has had the myocardium supplied by one of the major coronary systems damaged by infarction, and if the remaining areas of viable myocardium can be revascularized with grafts that will stay patent, a third operation need not be a consideration. Bilateral IMA grafting fits this situation. Scarring of endothoracic fasciae sometimes makes it more difficult to obtain length for the IMA pedicle at reoperation. However, free IMA grafts can be employed. Thickening of the aortic adventitia at reoperation makes the aortic anastomosis of a free graft more difficult, but that problem can be solved by anastomosing the proximal IMA to the residual "button" of occluded vein grafts.

Caution must be exercised, however, in the use of IMA grafts in one reoperative situation in particular. It is the policy of many surgeons (including me), to remove stenotic (but not totally obstructed) atherosclerotic vein grafts at reoperation. When a stenotic vein graft supplying a totally obstructed native coronary system is removed, it should be replaced with another vein graft, not an IMA. The IMA may not be able to increase flow acutely enough to supply the entire coronary system, which has been devascularized by removal of the previous vein graft.

Lack of available conduits and the desire to extend the use of arterial grafts have led me to use the right gastroepiploic artery for grafting the right coronary artery on several occasions. The right gastroepiploic artery is freed from the stomach to the level of the pylorus, brought posterior to the stomach through a hole in the diaphragm, and anastomosed to the right coronary artery. Although a useful technique, this must still be considered experimental.

The use of conduits other than the IMA and lower extremity vein has been disappointing. Artificial grafts, human umbilical vein, homologous saphenous vein, bovine carotid artery, arm vein, and radial artery have all been used and in all cases the long-term results have been terrible. Fortunately, if one becomes familiar with the use of the internal mammary arteries, lower extremity vein (including sequential grafting techniques and lesser saphenous vein), and right gastroepiploic artery, other conduits are rarely needed.

SUGGESTED READING

Campeau L, Enjalbert M, Lesperance J, et al. Atherosclerosis and late closure of aortocoronary saphenous vein grafts: sequential angiographic studies at 2 weeks, 1 year, 5 to 7 years, and 10 to 12 years after surgery. Circulation 1983; 68(Suppl II):1–7.

Loop FD, Lytle BW, Cosgrove DM, et al. Influence of the internal mammary artery graft on 10-year survival and other cardiac events. N Engl J Med 1986; 314:1–6.

Lytle BW, Cosgrove DM, Loop FD, et al. Perioperative risk of bilateral internal mammary artery grafting: analysis of 500 cases from 1971–1984. Circulation 1986; 74(Suppl III):37–41.

Lytle BW, Loop FD, Cosgrove DM, et al. Long-term (5–12 years) serial studies of internal mammary artery and saphenous vein coronary bypass grafts. J Thorac Cardiovasc Surg 1985; 89:248–258.

Tector AJ, Schmahl TM. Techniques for multiple internal mammary artery bypass grafts. Ann Thorac Surg 1984; 38:281–286.

NONINVASIVE EVALUATION OF PATIENTS WITH CARDIAC DISEASE

CHARLES A. BOUCHER, M.D.

Almost any cardiac disorder can result in cardiac arrest and sudden death. With this severe end point always possible, each cardiology consultation must answer the following question: Is the patient stable enough to be reassured that adverse cardiac events are unlikely to occur in the near future, or is the patient at increased cardiac risk and to be considered for additional therapy? Sometimes this distinction can be made from the basic clinical examination, and at other times further testing is required. This chapter reviews the noninvasive approaches available to help the cardiologist answer this question. The strategy discussed is applied specifically to patients who are referred for elective, major, noncardiac surgery, but it can be generalized to any patient. For the purpose of this discussion, the primary focus is on coronary artery disease because of its high prevalence.

BASIC EVALUATION IN CORONARY ARTERY DISEASE

Central to the cardiac evaluation are the history, physical examination, electrocardiogram, and chest x-ray films. If there is no history of chest pain or previous myocardial infarction, a normal cardiac examination, a normal electrocardiogram, and a normal cardiac silhouette and pulmonary vasculature on the chest film, the likelihood of coronary artery disease is small. A cardiology consultation is seldom necessary in this setting. However, if some of these tests are abnormal, a cardiology consultation is appropriate, and additional laboratory tests are often needed to clarify the severity of the underlying disease. The number of preoperative tests needed depends on several variables that are often unrelated to the cardiac disease itself. First, a younger, working patient who is likely to undergo significant "stress," such as manual labor or frequent travel, tends to be evaluated more thoroughly than an older sedentary patient. Second, if the cardiac abnormality is chronic and the patient has already demonstrated an ability to tolerate it by virtue of previous surgery or some other previous cardiology evaluation, these laboratory tests may not be necessary. For example, the finding of left bundle branch block in a patient that has been present for 20 years is of little concern, whereas if it is of new onset, further investigation is called for. Third, if the surgery is emergent or the patient has other severe medical problems that preclude ease of testing, the tests may be deferred. For example, an 80-year-old blind patient with aphasia and chronic renal failure may not be an appropriate candidate for noninvasive cardiac testing to determine if severe coronary disease is present.

The major risk of coronary artery disease during major noncardiac surgery is the development of new ischemia leading to hemodynamic deterioration with congestive heart failure and severe arrhythmias. The presence of a previous infarction with congestive failure is also a risk but is not as devastating and difficult to control as the development of new ischemia, especially if it is severe. Because of the significant physical and emotional stress associated with major surgery, any underlying cardiac condition might be exacerbated and provoke cardiac decompensation. This may occur even if there is little or no evidence of it before surgery, and the patient is entirely stable at rest. One factor that may be different for peripheral vascular surgery is that these patients may be physically inactive because of claudication and therefore provide little history of exertional cardiac symptoms preoperatively. A factor that may be different for thoracic surgery is that the respiratory therapy needed for optimal postoperative management of these patients (e.g., chest physical therapy, bronchodilators) often exacerbates any underlying cardiac condition. Therefore, a clear understanding of the exact nature and severity of any heart disease is crucial for optimal perioperative management. If the cardiac disease is severe, either close monitoring with arterial and pulmonary artery catheters is warranted or a patient may be sent first for coronary angiography and cardiac surgery or coronary angioplasty if warranted.

With the widespread prevalence of coronary artery disease in older adults, who should be suspected of having coronary artery disease? Who should have further tests? Who should be considered for coronary angiography and myocardial revascularization? If a patient has a history of some exertional chest, midepigastric, shoulder, arm, or jaw discomfort or has an abnormal electrocardiogram or a history of a previous myocardial infarction, coronary artery disease is likely to be present.

Patients having obvious classic angina either on minimal exertion or at rest are candidates for coronary angiography even without additional noninvasive tests. In most cases, however, the assessment is not so clear and simple. Neither the severity of the symptoms nor the electrocardiogram is a useful marker of the severity of the disease. Patients with mild symptoms may have advanced disease, and patients with severe symptoms may have mild disease. The symptom itself often is not painful and may be dismissed by the patient as an ache or heartburn. In some cases, coronary artery disease may be entirely asymptomatic. Nearly half of patients with acute myocardial infarctions have no antecedent warning in terms of previous chest pain, and 30 percent of infarctions themselves go unrecognized clinically.

NONINVASIVE TESTING IN CORONARY ARTERY DISEASE

Because of the limited value of the clinical assessment, objective testing is justified to quantify the extent of coronary artery disease in patients in whom it is suspected. Quantifying the severity of disease rather than detecting the disease per se is the most common reason why the stress thallium test described below is ordered in our institution. Because coronary perfusion is often adequate at rest despite the presence of severe disease, this evaluation usually involves some kind of stress.

Traditionally, exercise electrocardiography has been used for this purpose, but because of the limited accuracy of the electrocardiogram alone, especially if the at-rest tracing is already abnormal or if the patient has hypertension, the procedure of choice in our institution is stress thallium myocardial perfusion imaging. The electrocardiogram is both less sensitive and less specific than the thallium image results. In this test, the patient is exercised to symptom-limited levels, preferably while off beta-blocker therapy, similar to the level of a conventional stress test. Then, a small amount of a short-lived radionuclide tracer, thallium-201 chloride (a radioactive analogue of potassium chloride), is injected intravenously at peak exercise time. This is rapidly extracted from the blood into the heart muscle in relation to myocardial perfusion. Images in multiple views are taken 5 minutes and 3 hours after injection. On the early images, defects in myocardial thallium uptake represent regions of reduced myocardial perfusion. On the late images, perfusion defects that fill in (redistribute) partially or completely represent ischemia or underperfused viable myocardium, whereas defects that persist represent regions of old infarction. In addition, if abnormally increased pulmonary activity of thallium is present in the early images, this suggests that the patient developed exercise-induced elevations in left ventricular filling pressures during exercise. This occurs because some of the thallium bolus accompanies edema fluid into the lungs, which occurs transiently when left ventricular filling pressures are elevated at peak exercise. Thallium lung uptake is therefore a noninvasive marker of lung fluid and pulmonary artery wedge pressure at peak exercise.

The combination of thallium redistribution (fill in) and increased pulmonary activity provides important functional information of the impact of coronary disease. These variables are most associated with adverse cardiac events in any patient and in patients after surgery. Such patients should be seriously considered for either special invasive monitoring during surgery or coronary angiography in advance of their surgery.

The decision to proceed to myocardial revascularization after the coronary angiogram is an extensive and controversial topic. With the relatively low morbidity and mortality of both coronary angioplasty and elective coronary bypass surgery, we consider myocardial revascularization in advance of elective noncardiac surgery in the following general situations:

1. The patient has angina that affects his or her lifestyle or has unstable angina despite adequate medical therapy. The patient is likely to undergo this procedure anyway in the near future.
2. The patient is stable but has laboratory data known to be associated with increased risk of future cardiac events, such as fall in blood pressure on a stress test, profound ischemic S-T segment changes at a low heart rate, multiple redistributing thallium segments, increased thallium lung uptake, or left main or severe three-vessel coronary disease.
3. The surgery is so stressful or the recovery so difficult that cardiac ischemic events are likely. Examples might be a right pneumonectomy or repair of a thoracoabdominal aortic aneurysm.

In many adult or older patients, there is limited or no ability to exercise, usually because of coexisting conditions (e.g., claudication, arthritis). In these patients, the diagnostic value of exercise testing is obviously limited. In such cases, we perform nonexercise stress testing using intravenous or oral dipyridamole instead of exercise. This approach is superior to inadequate exercise in demonstrating the severity of underlying coronary artery disease. The dipyridamole produces maximal coronary vasodilation, which accomplishes chemically what the exercise achieves during a physical stress test. Flow to the most normal zones is maximized, and this permits delineation of regions of reduced perfusion with a tracer such as thallium. The dipyridamole primarily affects myocardial blood supply and has a minimal affect on myocardial oxygen demand; therefore, it cannot be used as a conventional stress test without thallium. Redistribution of thallium occurs in a fashion similar to that with the exercise thallium test. When redistribution is present, it identifies patients with ischemic potential and increased cardiac risk.

Another widely applied noninvasive test is the radionuclide ventriculogram (also known as the gated blood pool scan or MUGA scan, which means MultiGated Acquisition). In this study, the red blood cells are labeled with technetium-99m, and images of right and ventricular motion are obtained in multiple views. This allows measurement of ejection fraction and regional wall motion, both of which are important, along with the thallium perfusion study, in understanding the impact of coronary disease (especially previous infarction) on the right and left ventricles.

Finally, some centers have been testing a new perfusion agent that uses technetium-99m instead of thallium-201, because of its better imaging properties. This agent is technetium hexamibi (hexakis 2-methoxy isobutyl isonitrile) or Cardiolite (formerly RP-30) and may provide superior imaging quality compared with that of thallium. It may be useful in distinguishing ischemic viable myocardium from infarcted nonviable myocardium in the setting of acute myocardial infarction.

The two major indications for proceeding to coronary angiography and consideration of myocardial revascularization are relief of severe angina and prevention of future cardiac events. The former is easy to assess clinically, but the latter is not. It depends on accurate risk stratification, which usually cannot be determined on clinical grounds. Prognosis is poorest in patients with the worst left ventricular function (lowest ejection fraction), but these patients are not usually candidates for myocardial revascularization. When left ventricular function is reasonable, the ability to unmask ischemia or left ventricular decompensation with exercise (increased lung uptake) by thallium scan identifies the high-risk patient. Because left ventricular function is an important variable in coronary disease, some have suggested that the left ventricular function response to exercise, as determined by radionuclide ventriculography (blood pool scanning), is also valuable in this regard. Although this is generally true, we prefer the thallium stress test for three reasons: other diseases of the left ventricle affect ventricular function, such as hypertension or primary cardiomyopathy, which may produce abnormalities similar to those seen with coronary disease; the modification in the bicycle stress test required to acquire the images is difficult for many older patients compared with the treadmill test used with thallium, and inadequate levels of exercise are more common; and radionuclide ventriculography is not suitable for nonexercise stress testing with dipyridamole.

CONGESTIVE HEART FAILURE

Patients with dyspnea, fatigue, or an abnormal chest x-ray examination should be evaluated to determine several issues. First, is the symptom or finding caused by cardiac or pulmonary disease? The best screening approach is to determine room air arterial blood gases, pulmonary function tests, including a diffusion capacity to assess the lungs, and a radionuclide ventriculogram or an echocardiogram to assess right and left ventricular function. The decision to order one or the other of the last two tests depends on the quality of the imaging and interpretation, which can vary from laboratory to laboratory. The cardiologist is usually very aware of which test in a given has been most accurate in assessing ventricular function. When the quality of both is good, the radionuclide ventriculogram is generally favored because of the difficulties that may be encountered in ultrasound imaging in visualizing parts of the heart through the rib cage (bone) and lung (air).

Causes of dyspnea may be right or left ventricular dysfunction, pulmonary vascular disease, coronary artery disease, pulmonary mechanical limitations (restrictive or obstructive), or disorders of the pulmonary interstitium with inadequate diffusion of oxygen and carbon dioxide. Poor conditioning and anxiety (hyperventilation) are other causes of dyspnea. If a combination of pulmonary and cardiac disease is evident or if the symptoms are discordant with the laboratory tests with the patient at rest, it may be appropriate to stress the patient by measuring right and left ventricular function by radionuclide ventriculography and pulmonary gas exchange analysis at rest and during exercise so that the precise mechanism of the limitation can be determined.

If the dyspnea is thought to be associated with the heart and the diagnosis of congestive heart failure is made preoperatively, its etiology is important and has implications for the management of the patient. Usually, it is coronary artery disease, and if so, it often represents an end stage of this disorder with ejection fractions below 30 percent. The overall long-term prognosis is poor. Sometimes angina presents as congestive heart failure. There are two mechanisms for this. (1) The pain or tightness may be perceived as a choking or smothering feeling and described as dyspnea. True exertional dyspnea may occur, since the ischemia occurring with stress may depress left ventricular function to the point where left ventricular filling pressures rise to the levels seen in heart failure. This should be suspected when the ejection fraction at rest is better preserved and should prompt serious consideration of coronary angiography and coronary bypass surgery to prevent further irreversible deterioration of left ventricular function. (2) If the heart failure is caused by a primary cardiomyopathy or a disorder of diastolic dysfunction such as severe hypertension and left ventricular hypertrophy, the prognosis is usually better. All patients with heart failure should have a noninvasive assessment of right and left ventricular function, and close hemodynamic monitoring is indicated at the time of surgery.

If the dyspnea symptoms are associated with a heart murmur, a two-dimensional echocardiogram with Doppler examination is useful to determine the presence and severity of associated valvular heart disease. Any valve lesion, when severe, can contribute substantially to adverse cardiac events during and following surgery, but the two most important situations to recognize are severe valvular aortic stenosis and a hypertrophic left ventricle with obstruction, both of which can lead to unpredictable swings in cardiac hemodynamics with minor shifts in circulatory volume and blood pressure. In valvular aortic stenosis, there is a fixed obstruction of the aortic valve. With a hypertrophic left ventricle, there is excessive hypertrophy that may be associated with impaired left ventricular ejection. In addition, patients with severe mitral disease are at risk for heart failure and atrial arrhythmias. The presence of these abnormalities should be evident by the combination of the initial cardiac evaluation and the echocardiogram. In the setting of an aortic stenosis murmur, one clinical clue to the presence of critical aortic stenosis is the second heart sound. When the second heart sound is single, the aortic stenosis is usually severe. When the second heart sound can be heard to split in the adult, the aortic stenosis is seldom critical and usually does not warrant further noninvasive evaluation.

ARRHYTHMIAS

Patients are frequently referred for evaluation simply because of the presence of an irregular pulse, symptoms of palpitations, or frequent premature ventricular or atrial contractions noted on the electrocardiogram. The appropriate work-up is similar to the above if associated chest pain or dyspnea is present. If there is no other evidence of heart disease, simple electrocardiographic monitoring during surgery is usually adequate. If there are symptoms of dizziness, lightheadedness, or syncope that according to history seem to be potentially cardiac-related, preoperative Holter monitoring is indicated. Evidence of a cardiac etiology is sudden unexplained onset or symptoms related to exertion. Evidence of a noncardiac etiology includes associated localized neurologic symptoms or postictal phenomena. Obviously, if an arrhythmia is unmasked, appropriate antiarrhythmic therapy should be instituted. Patients with bifascicular block with first-degree atrioventricular block and a bundle branch block are at potential risk for higher degrees of atrioventricular block and warrant preoperative insertion of a temporary transvenous ventricular pacemaker. Right bundle branch block and left anterior hemiblock alone with a normal P-R interval are not such indications. A pacemaker is also obviously indicated on a permanent basis if a patient has any evidence of symptomatic bradycardias with Stokes-Adams attacks (sudden loss of consciousness without warning or postictal phenomena). A 24-hour Holter electrocardiographic recording is helpful to ascertain whether the symptom is on a cardiac basis and should be repeated until the symptom in question is reproduced during the recording.

The most common arrhythmia, however, is atrial flutter or atrial fibrillation. Patients with premature atrial contractions often develop atrial fibrillation postoperatively, and they are usually prophylactically begun on digoxin. Normal hearts conduct this rhythm at a high rate (above 150 beats per minute) without developing angina or congestive heart failure. If angina or failure occurs, some disorder is present and should be clarified. Rapid atrial fibrillation is equivalent to a stress test. If the ventricular response rate is below 120 beats per minute without any therapy, there is intrinsic conduction system disease, and the patient may have severe sinus bradycardia upon conversion to sinus rhythm.

SUGGESTED READING

Beller GA, Gibson RS. Sensitivity, specificity and prognostic significance of noninvasive testing for occult or known coronary disease. Progr Cardiovasc Dis 1987; 29:241–270.

Boucher CA, Brewster DC, Darling RC, Okada RD, Strauss HW, Pohost GM. Determination of cardiac risk by dipyridamole-thallium imaging before peripheral vascular surgery. N Eng J Med 1985; 312:389–394.

Steinberg EP, Klag MJ, Bakal CW, Strauss HW, Boucher CA, Guiney TE. Exercise thallium scans: patterns of use and impact on management of patients with known or suspected coronary artery disease. Am J Cardiol 1987; 59:50–55.

Strauss HW, Boucher CA. Myocardial perfusion studies: lessons from a decade of clinical use. Radiology 1986; 160:577–584.

SELECTION OF PATIENTS FOR CORONARY ARTERY SURGERY

RONALD M. WEINTRAUB, M.D.

Twenty years of experience with over a million patients have given the cardiology community the data base for a more rational approach to patient selection for bypass surgery. The pendulum has swung through several cycles of enthusiasm and skepticism as a large number of retrospective reviews and several prospective, randomized studies have gained ascendence in the medical and lay communities. However, a cautionary note is appropriate in drawing general conclusions from the Veterans Administration Cooperative, CASS, European Cooperative, and National Cooperative Unstable Angina studies, because some of the populations studied were narrowly defined. Furthermore, surgical and technical advances such as cardioplegia and the use of internal mammary grafts have altered the studies in midstream. In the last 5 years, advances in invasive cardiology have changed the picture even further, modifying selection criteria for revascularization in general and actually increasing the number of patients studied. Finally, issues of cost containment and the threat of medical rationing are beginning to intrude on purely medical decision making.

GENERAL SELECTION CRITERIA

The decision to perform revascularization depends on the answers to three questions: (1) Will well-being be significantly and favorably affected over a reasonable period of time? (2) Is survival likely to be prolonged? and (3) What is the operative risk? The answers to these questions must be considered in the context of other patient characteristics.

Patient-Controlled Factors. Elective revascularization should not be offered to patients who are markedly obese or who refuse to stop smoking.

Age. In patients above the age of 70, urgent (nonelective) operation for myocardial ischemia carries a higher mortality than does elective operation. In our experience octogenarians appear to present special problems. Urgent operation carries with it a significantly higher mortality (approaching 20 percent), and the combination of diffuse coronary disease and severe left ventricular dysfunction carries a prohibitively high operative mortality.

Psychosocial Factors. In general cardiac surgeons should be selective with respect to such factors as dementia and the need for long-term nursing home care as exclusion criteria for surgery. Making decisions on an ad hoc basis, we should exclude those who cannot live reasonably independent lives, and those dependent patients without family or other strong social support systems.

Coexisting Disease. Prognosis for a coexisting disease may be a limiting factor in the selection of patients for coronary revascularization. A prognosis of more than 3 years would seem to be a reasonable discriminator for those who would benefit from cardiac operations. For example, chronic renal dialysis or renal transplantation ought not to be exclusionary if the overall prognosis exceeds 3 years. Patients with recently identified pulmonary, gastrointestinal, or renal malignancies may be appropriate candidates for revascularization, particularly as a first step toward definitive control of their malignancy. Although revascularization is generally contraindicated in advanced malignancy, certain patients with slow growing but incompletely controlled neoplasms such as lymphoma or breast and prostate carcinoma may be considered for operation. Again, the prognosis for the noncardiac illness should be the guide to selection for bypass. Note, however, that some patients with lymphomas or hematopoietic malignancies face a higher surgical risk because of hemorrhagic tendencies or host resistance factors. Finally, a history of previous tumor therapy, particularly irradiation of the chest wall, may modify or alter proposed coronary revascularization. When venous conduits are unavailable, internal mammary angiography may be required to demonstrate patency in these patients. Finally, previous lower limb amputations may affect a patient's operability not only with respect to availability of conduits but also because of limits in postoperative mobility.

Physiologic and Technical Factors As Modifiers. Although past studies have indicated that left ventricular dysfunction was an incremental risk factor in coronary bypass operations, more recent data have suggested that this may be less important. Nevertheless, we have found that very low cardiac outputs (cardiac index < 1.8), in conjunction with ejection fractions less than 0.20, have carried a high mortality. Similarly, severe pulmonary hypertension (above 55 mm Hg) has been associated with a high operative mortality. Diffuse coronary disease, particularly with intense coronary calcification, presents higher risks, as does extensive aortic calcification, particularly of the "eggshell type." Finally, although we have usually been able to find adequate conduits, even in reoperations, it is probably wise to obtain internal mammary angiograms if venous conduits are not available and the internal mammary artery is not seen on a left ventricular angiogram.

INDICATIONS FOR ELECTIVE CORONARY BYPASS OPERATION

Failure of medical management to provide symptomatic relief continues to be the primary indication for operation in chronic stable angina. This criterion tends to be somewhat flexible, depending on the age, general medical condition, lifestyle, and wishes of the particular patient. In addition, a general body of knowledge has evolved from retrospective and prospective studies that emphasizes the importance of anatomy in the selection of patients for revascularization. Furthermore, the importance of inducible ischemia is becoming increasingly more recognized not only in chronic stable angina but also in the postinfarction state. For instance, the very low medical mortality in patients with two vessel disease in the CASS study as compared with the higher mortality in anatomically similar patients in the European Cooperative study is associated with a low incidence of positive exercise tests in the former and a higher incidence in the latter. There is also a large body of data demonstrating that the presence of inducible ischemia in the early (3-week) postinfarction state is a discriminator for high risk with medical management. Such patients should be offered coronary revascularization surgery.

Patients selected for elective coronary bypass surgery should be those with severe or poorly controlled symptoms, patients with significant left main coronary artery stenosis, or patients with triple vessel obstructive disease, especially with left ventricular dysfunction and positive exercise tests, or patients with positive submaximal exercise tests within 3 weeks of myocardial infarction. Patients with two vessel or single vessel disease in which the proximal left anterior descending artery is stenotic and whose exercise test results are positive, or similarly patients with large territories subtended by compromised, dominant vessels should also receive careful consideration.

The category of silent myocardial ischemia or "failure of the early warning system" is receiving increased recognition. The management of these patients remains controversial, particularly since the natural history is not well documented, but it would appear prudent to revascularize those patients with documented ischemia in whom large territories of myocardium are at risk.

Elective revascularization is an area in considerable flux because of the increasingly aggressive role of angioplasty as a means for revascularization. The increasing skill of the cardiologist with invasive procedures, the political prospect of reducing the cost of revascularization, and the lack of any studies that might engender skepticism about angioplasty are markedly altering the population of patients being referred to cardiac surgeons. Angioplasty is generally being applied to patients with anatomically simpler disease, leaving the sicker, older patients with more diffuse disease to the cardiac surgeon. A rise in surgical mortality has already been documented. Federally sponsored clinical trials hold some hope for an objective evaluation of open versus closed revascularization, but these studies are just being formulated, and the results in terms of patient selection for the most appropriate therapy cannot be expected for at least 5 years.

Patients with congestive heart failure continue to challenge the cardiac surgeon. Our ability to differentiate between irreparably injured and scarred myocardium and myocardium that is capable of some improvement remains poor. In general, coronary bypass has not been helpful in patients who do not have demonstrable ischemia. Patients with intermittent acute ischemia that presents as "flash" pulmonary edema have greatly benefited from revascularization, but those with more chronic failure have not. The development of the dipyridamole thallium scan may be helpful in separating the different types of chronic injury. We have achieved some limited success in treating patients with ischemic cardiomyopathy by combining revascularization with new inotropes such as milrinone.

NONELECTIVE CORONARY BYPASS

Unstable angina may be defined as the new appearance of angina or the change in a previously stable pattern of angina culminating in angina at rest or with minimal activity and associated with transient electrocardiographic changes requiring an intensive care setting. Although there are sufficient data to suggest that such patients can often be stabilized and then revascularized at a time of election, many patients today who are already on triple therapy present in a more advanced stage of disease. We feel that *all* such patients should undergo catheterization before leaving the hospital, even if they become stable and do not require urgent intervention. A small percentage of patients who stabilize on medical therapy and who are found not to have threatening anatomic conditions may not require further treatment. However, the incidence of significant left main artery disease in this population is 12 to 15 percent, and two-thirds may have either left main artery disease or significant trivessel disease with large regions of myocardium at risk; surgical revascularization is advised for these patients. The remaining third, many with new-onset angina, have single or double vessel disease that may be appropriately treated with angioplasty. In a recent study of 100 consecutive catheterization days at Boston's Beth Israel Hospital, 127 patients underwent initial diagnostic catheterization for the evaluation of coronary disease. In this group 60 percent proceeded to revascularization, slightly over half of whom were treated by open operation. During this study, 61 percent of the angioplasty procedures and 65 percent of the open operative procedures were performed on an urgent basis. In this tertiary referral hospital virtually two-thirds of all revascularization procedures were performed on an urgent basis. Furthermore, the growing confidence and skill of our cardiology colleagues in applying angioplasty techniques to a wider population of patients with ischemia ensure that the patients who remain for open operation will be those who are sicker and anatomically more complex.

In a setting in which there is a shortage of operative time for patients requiring surgery urgently, the management of these patients waiting in-hospital bears some examination. In addition to the usual measures (beta-blockade, calcium-channel blockers, and nitrates), we have found that intravenous heparin is extremely useful. Interestingly, many patients, on discontinuation of heparin for one reason or another, have suffered recurrent ischemia. The administration of intravenous heparin also allows the discontinuation of aspirin. For those patients who have remained on aspirin or who have been placed on aspirin concomitant with a failed angioplasty, the administration of desmopressin may mitigate the antiplatelet effect of aspirin. Most useful, however, is the education of cardiologists in the avoidance of aspirin when possible and the substitution of heparin for any hospitalized patient who might be a candidate for open operation on the same hospital admission.

Finally, although the intra-aortic balloon pump is less frequently used in the perioperative treatment of patients with unstable angina, its application cannot only be lifesaving in patients with hemodynamic instability but also helpful when used for stabilization while trying to fit patients into tight operative schedules.

Postinfarction Angina. Operation on patients with postinfarction angina is undertaken to prevent threatened extension in the area of injury or new infarction in distant areas. As a general rule, operations should be avoided within the first 48 hours after infarction, the period of stunned myocardium. Continued instability, however, may force an earlier operation as the lesser of two evils. The size of the infarction injury, the amount of left ventricular dysfunction, and the temporal proximity to infarction influence operative risks, as has been pointed out by Hochberg. When intervention is mandated by continuing ischemia or hemodynamic instability in the face of extensive left ventricular injury, the intra-aortic balloon pump may be of great value. We also use counterpulsation liberally when enzymatic, angiographic, or radionuclide estimation of injury is moderate or greater.

Acute Events in the Catheterization Laboratory. With the growing application of angioplasty, acute arterial injury or abrupt postangioplasty closure are increasingly common facts of surgical life. When acute closure occurs and is associated with acute myocardial ischemia, a few basic principles should be followed. First, myocardial support should be instituted in the catheterization laboratory by either passage of a "bail-out" (multihole) catheter or, failing its passage, an intra-aortic balloon pump. The patient must then be operated on in as expeditious a manner as possible. Early aortic cross-clamping with administration of cardioplegia and the construction of distal anastomoses first may be the techniques of choice in those patients exhibiting continued ischemia. Using these principles, we have had only one surgical death in covering over 3,500 angioplasty patients.

SUGGESTED READING

Barbash G, Rabkin MT, Kane NM, Baim DT. Coronary angioplasty under the prospective payment system: the need for a severity-adjusted payment scheme. J Am Coll Cardiol 1986; 8:784–790.

European Coronary Surgery Study Group. Long-term results of prospective randomized study of coronary artery bypass surgery in stable angina pectoris. Lancet 1982; 2:1173–1180.

Gottlieb SO, Weisfeldt ML, Ouyang P, Mellits ED, Gerstenblith G. Silent ischemia as a marker for early unfavorable outcomes in patients with unstable angina. N Engl J Med 1986; 314:1214–1219.
Hochberg MS, Parsonnet V, Gielchinsky I, Hussain SM, Fisch DA. Timing of coronary revascularization after acute myocardial infarction. J Thorac Cardiovasc Surg 1984; 88:914–921.
Passamani E, Davis KB, Gillespie MJ, Killip T, and the CASS. Principal Investigators and Their Associates. A randomized trial of coronary artery bypass surgery. Survival of patients with a low ejection fraction. N Engl J Med 1985; 312:1665–1670.

INTRAOPERATIVE CORONARY ANGIOPLASTY

NOEL L. MILLS, M.D.

Surgeons who perform coronary artery bypass are now being presented with patients who have much more extensive, distal coronary artery disease. Regardless of the causes of this phenomenon, the end result is that the cardiac surgeon must be more inventive in his or her endeavor to effect a complete revascularization of the coronary arteries. Distal coronary atherosclerotic lesions that limit runoff may result in early failure of grafts or inhibit collateral circulation to other potentially perfused areas of the heart. In this situation, intraoperative balloon catheter dilation of a distal lesion becomes an important tool in the armamentarium of the cardiac surgeon in order to offer more complete myocardial revascularization. The technique was first introduced in 1978 but in general has been overshadowed by the tremendous interest in percutaneous coronary angioplasty.

Intraoperative coronary angioplasty is used to dilate lesions that are not able to be bypassed or lesions that are not feasible for a coronary endarterectomy. Intraoperative coronary angioplasty is always performed in conjunction with a bypass graft. The angioplasty is performed through the coronary arteriotomy used for the anastomosis. As opposed to percutaneous transluminal coronary angioplasty, operative angioplasty is performed under direct visualization with the aid of palpation of the lesion and measurement of catheter length from the arteriotomy to the area to be dilated. The success or failure of the dilation can immediately be ascertained with the use of calibrated probes, angioscopy, or both.

The development of newer, more refined catheter systems for use at the operating table in general has lagged far behind the development of the percutaneous coronary angioplasty catheter systems. The limitations of the various operative angioplasty devices have been carefully reported in previous communications. Fixed guidewire coaxial systems have been the standard for use at the operating table. The SCIMED catheter system with its smaller profile deflated balloon is preferred by this author and is the device used for the cases in this report. The balloon is located close to the catheter tip, and the system has centimeter markings for ease in measuring coronary arteriotomy to lesion distances. The system is essentially a balloon on a guidewire that enables balloon passage through smaller, tighter lesions. Catheter hang-up or plaque dislodgement or both are minimal with this device.

INDICATIONS AND PHYSIOLOGIC CONSIDERATIONS

The mechanisms by which coronary atherosclerotic lesions are opened by balloon dilation are (1) intimal fracture, (2) stretching of the media and adventitia, (3) plaque disruption, and (4) a longitudinal splitting of the plaque. After dilation, increased laminar flow across the area that was dilated in conjunction with "remodeling" allows stability of the lumen and increased perfusion of the myocardium. Previous studies have revealed that certain lesions are more amenable to angioplasty than others. For example, if the atherosclerotic disease is involved with circumferential calcification, the calcified "ring" may not be able to be broken by the dilating catheter in spite of high pressures. Dilations at bifurcations may produce undesirable results because of closure of one side of the bifurcation. Liquid cholesterol and debris in lesions may offer an increased chance of embolization into distal branches, and therefore operative angioplasty of such lesions should be avoided, especially in proximal disease.

Specific indications for operative angioplasty involve basically those lesions in which the distal coronary artery beyond the lesion is too small to accept a graft. In addition, in certain situations a lesion may be in an anatomic location that is inaccessible to normal, safe coronary bypass techniques and an operative angioplasty may be indicated. Calcification in itself is not a contraindication to either percutaneous transluminal coronary angioplasty or operative angioplasty. The most common arterial lesion to be dilated intraoperatively is located in the distal left anterior descending coronary artery near the apex of the heart. On occasion, tandem left anterior descending lesions may be managed by angioplasty. Specific contraindications for operative angioplasty are (1) anastomoses should not be dilated when they have been narrowed due to technical reasons, (2) an artery should not be dilated in order to enlarge it to enhance the technical ease of coronary artery bypass grafting, (3) dilation of proximal lesions that could embolize debris after release of the aortic cross-clamps should be avoided, and (4) in no situation should an operative dilation be performed that establishes significant competition with the bypass graft from the native circulation.

TECHNIQUE

Previous reports have carefully outlined the standard technique for performing operative angioplasty. Briefly, the epicardium, whenever possible, is opened over the lesion and the lesion is visualized and palpated. A coronary arteriotomy is performed proximal to the lesion, and a calibrated probe is used to measure the internal diameter of the coronary artery and the distance from the arteriotomy to the lesion itself. The operative angioplasty balloon size is chosen in relation to the size of the coronary artery. The balloon diameter should be equal to or slightly larger than that of the coronary artery in which the lesion resides. Using the previous linear measurement, the balloon system is then passed across the lesion, and the balloon is situated such that it straddles the lesion. Dilation is performed using a commercially available syringe-manometer with normal saline in the balloon. The hand-held device is used to inflate the balloon to 7 to 10 atm, and this pressure is held for 30 seconds. Three consecutive inflations and deflations are carried out, and the balloon is withdrawn. The appropriate-sized calibrated probe is carefully passed across the dilated lesion to record the enlarged diameter. A silver clip is placed adjacent to the lesion as a future angiographic reference point. The coronary anastomosis is then performed.

The procedure is considered successful if the lesion can be dilated to a calibrated probe size of the adjacent coronary artery. An unsuccessful operative angioplasty is one in which the lesion cannot be crossed or cannot be dilated once it is crossed with the balloon. Dilation is limited strictly to the area of the lesion and is not performed on normal-sized areas of the coronary artery. Early experience with this technique of dilation in normal-sized areas resulted in a high incidence of coronary artery thrombosis. Antiplatelet therapy is a standard part of the postoperative care after operative angioplasty.

CLINICAL MATERIAL AND RESULTS

The clinical experience with intraoperative coronary balloon angioplasty has been reported previously by our group with respect to the use of four different catheter systems. Those clinical data clearly document the success rate of operative angioplasty, patency rates, and problems associated with the technique. During the course of obtaining the data, it became clear that one system (SCIMED) had distinct advantages over others (Fig. 1). Failures at operation due to inability to cross lesions were improved upon significantly by use of a smaller balloon profile. The steerable angioplasty system for operative use was not found to be particularly advantageous because at operation the lesion is usually visualized and the catheter can be bent to accommodate the configuration of the coronary artery.

The data reported herein encompass a 2½ year period from July 1984, to January 1987. There were 67 patients whose ages ranged from 36 to 80 years. Nine patients were females. Four patients were undergoing reoperation coronary artery bypass, and one patient had a concomitant aortic valve replacement. One patient in the group

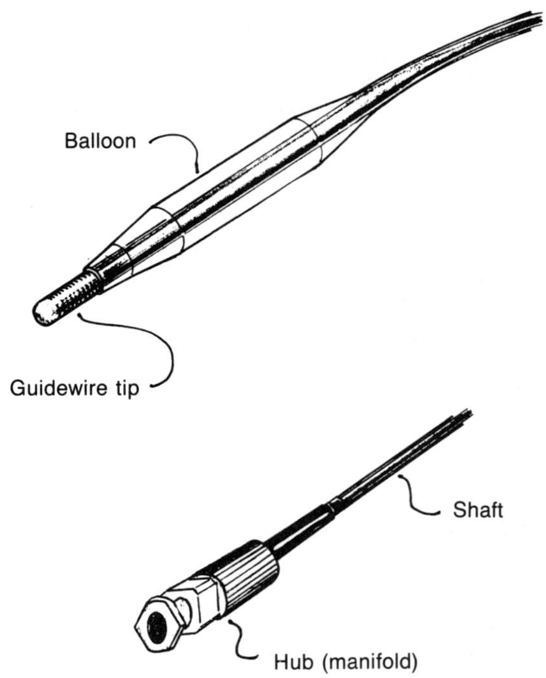

Figure 1 The low profile operative angioplasty device (SCIMED) has no catheter body. The system is basically a balloon over a malleable guidewire that allows an easier passage of the balloon across stenotic coronary artery lesions.

was undergoing an acute myocardial infarction at the time of operation. Two to seven coronary artery bypasses were performed in these patients, and three or more bypasses were performed in 63 of the 67 patients. Twenty-five patients in the group had such extensive coronary disease as to require endarterectomy on one or more coronary arteries. Two patients had angioplasty in more than one coronary artery. The left anterior descending artery was the vessel treated by angioplasty in 57 patients, the posterior descending artery in nine patients, the inferior ventricular branch of the right coronary artery in two patients, and the first marginal branch of the circumflex artery in one patient (Table 1).

There were two hospital deaths in the group. One 77-year-old male patient died in the intensive care unit within 2 weeks after operation of renal complications. The patient had pre-existing renal disease, had had a recent myocardial infarction, and had a successful angioplasty of the proximal posterior descending coronary artery at the time of operation. The angioplastied artery was patent throughout at post mortem. There was no evidence of perioperative myocardial infarction. The second patient, a 78-year-old male, expired 1 month postoperatively of a bleeding ulcer and respiratory failure after undergoing a ventricular aneurysm repair and sextuple coronary bypass. Angioplasty was performed on the distal left anterior descending artery at operation, and there was no evidence of vessel thrombosis or perioperative myocardial infarction. There were five operative failures (7.5 percent) due to inability to cross the lesion with the catheter device. There was one failure secondary to a rupture of a 2.5-mm balloon at 8 atm pressure; a distal endarterectomy was suc-

TABLE 1 Operative Angioplasty of 69 Coronary Arteries in 67 Patients

SCIMED Low Profile Catheter

Coronary Artery	*No.*	*Successful*	*Failure*
Left anterior descending	57	52	5
PD	9	8	1
Inferior Vent	2	2	0
CFfxMarg	1	1	0
Total	69	63	6

cessfully performed. The operation consisted of a sextuple coronary artery bypass with an endarterectomy of the distal right coronary system as well as angioplasty and endarterectomy of the left anterior descending artery. The patient had no clinical or chemical evidence of perioperative myocardial infarction. One month after operation, the patient had a normal exercise stress test. There were two late deaths in the series. One patient succumbed at 3 months postoperatively of noncardiac causes secondary to Dubin-Johnson syndrome. Postmortem examination of the angioplastied left anterior descending artery revealed a widely patent angioplastied vessel with no evidence of recurrent stenosis or thrombosis. A second patient died at 26 months postoperatively of carcinoma of the lung. Postmortem examination was not performed. Postoperative cardiac catheterization has been performed on 11 of the 69 patients. Nine of eleven of the angioplastied vessels (82 percent) were patent and stenosis-free. One patient had a distal left anterior descending artery occluded at the angioplasty site, and a second had a distal posterior descending artery occluded at the angioplasty site. Patency rate in this group is comparable to the 71 and 72 percent success rate in previous reported series.

CONCLUSIONS

Operative transluminal angioplasty of the coronary arteries has proved to be a safe technique that can afford increased runoff in vessels with distal coronary artery disease. The technique is best reserved for short, isolated distal lesions as opposed to extensive lesions of more than 1 cm in length; in these latter instances, endarterectomy is indicated. Acceptance of the technique has been hindered by poor design of early, prototypic intraoperative balloon catheters and the fact that later devices (e.g., SCIMED low-profile catheter system) have required cumbersome data collecting to meet clinical experimental standards for government approval. Re-stenosis after operative angioplasty is difficult to document because of the general well-being of postoperative coronary artery bypass patients and their reluctance to submit to the expense and hazard of repeat cardiac catheterization. Failures or unsuccessful operative angioplasties due to the inability to cross lesions with the angioplasty device have continued to decrease to a low of 7.5 percent with the use of an improved catheter system. Whether the re-stenosis rate of operative angioplasty mirrors that of percutaneous coronary angioplasty is unknown. Certainly, vessels subjected to operative angioplasty in general are smaller than those undergoing percutaneous transluminal coronary angioplasty. However, a precise balloon positioning under direct vision with operative angioplasty offers a distinct advantage with less chance of dissection or perforation. Postoperative follow-up has shown no detectable difference in groups of patients having operative angioplasty and those having standard coronary bypass procedures. It should be emphasized that coronary arteries that are amenable to bypass or endarterectomy should be treated accordingly, and operative angioplasty should be reserved for coronary artery lesions that are not amenable to standard coronary artery bypass operative techniques.

SUGGESTED READING

Jones EL, King SB. Intraoperative balloon-catheter dilatation in the treatment of coronary artery disease. Am Heart J 1984; 107:836–837.

Mills NL. Angioplasty. In: Jang CD, ed. New York: McGraw Hill 1986:337.

Mills NL, Doyle DP. Does operative transluminal angioplasty extend the limits of coronary artery bypass surgery? A preliminary report. Circulation 1982; 66 (Suppl I):1-26–29.

Mills NL, Doyle DP. Experience with operative angioplasty of the coronary arteries. Am Heart J 1984; 107:838–840.

Mills NL, Ochsner JL, Doyle DP, Kalchoff WP. Technique and results of operative transluminal angioplasty in 81 consecutive patients. J Thorac Cardiovasc Surg 1983; 86:689–696.

Mills NL, Solar RJ. In: Roberts AJ, Richard C, eds. Current surgery of the heart. Philadelphia: JB Lippincott, 1987:27.

Roberts AJ, Alexander JA, Knauf DG, et al. Clinical and angiographic experience with intraoperative transluminal balloon-catheter dilatation and coronary artery bypass surgery. J Cardiovasc Surg 1985; 26:207-211.

PERCUTANEOUS ANGIOPLASTY: THE ROLE OF THE CARDIAC SURGEON

DOUGLAS A. MURPHY, M.D.

Percutaneous transluminal coronary angioplasty has enjoyed tremendous growth in the United States over the last 6 years. At Emory University Hospital over 5,000 angioplasties were performed over this period of time, and 196 patients have required urgent coronary bypass surgery for angioplasty-related myocardial ischemia. This experience with acutely ischemic angioplasty patients has provided the foundation for a rational approach to this challenging patient group. Successful surgical support of an angioplasty service demands four areas of understanding and planning: surgical goals, patient selection, team organization, and technical considerations.

SURGICAL GOALS

The primary concern in the mind of the coronary surgeon confronted with the acutely ischemic angioplasty patient is to ensure the patient's survival by revascularization of the ischemic myocardium. Only if the survival of the patient appears secure can consideration be given to the revascularization of threatened but nonischemic segments of the myocardium. Similarly, it may be necessary to perform revascularization using saphenous veins if time and patient instability do not allow the safe use of the preferred internal mammary artery. These priority factors must be understood by both the cardiologist and the patient. In the medicolegal environment of the 1980s it is important for the surgeon to document in the medical record the factors that forced him or her to compromise the revascularization procedure in any way in the rescue of the ischemic angioplasty patient.

PATIENT SELECTION

The surgeon's role in selection of appropriate angioplasty patients is to anticipate potential difficulties in the event of angioplasty failure. Of primary concern is the extent of left ventricular dysfunction that follows closure of the instrumented artery. When the portion of myocardium in jeopardy exceeds 40 to 50 percent of the left ventricular mass, severe hemodynamic compromise can be anticipated with angioplasty misadventure. Clinically, we have seen such compromise with angioplasty of very proximal left anterior descending arterial lesions complicated by inadvertent left main artery dissection and with angioplasty of left anterior descending artery lesions when collaterals from this artery supply a previously occluded right or circumflex artery. Caution must also be exercised in the angioplasty of patients with a previous myocardial infarction in the distribution of another coronary artery. In this setting, if the sum of the previously damaged myocardium and the myocardium in jeopardy by the angioplasty exceeds 40 to 50 percent, severe hemodynamic compromise can complicate angioplasty. The potential risk of hemodynamic decompensation with angioplasty is increased when intra-aortic balloon pump insertion is not possible.

A second area of major concern for the surgeon is the recognition of factors that might delay an emergency bypass procedure. Factors that delay restoration of flow to the ischemic myocardium increase the extent of necrosis. In our experience causes of delay have included patient reluctance to go promptly to surgery, protracted efforts to reopen the artery in the angioplasty suite, previous median sternotomy, and absent or diseased saphenous veins.

Potential hemodynamic deterioration or conditions that may result in time delay do not contraindicate angioplasty, but the difficulty of surgical rescue and myocardial salvage is increased. This must be appreciated by both the cardiologist and the patient.

TEAM ORGANIZATION

Efficient and effective management of the failed angioplasty patient requires the cooperative effort of the cardiologist, the anesthesiologist, and the cardiac surgeon. Every institution must develop a plan for surgical rescue of ischemic angioplasty patients that incorporates the unique personnel and equipment characteristics of the facility. Smaller hospitals may require close coordination of angioplasty and operative schedules to ensure immediate availability of an operating room and personnel.

Criteria for emergency surgical intervention must be firmly established for each patient prior to the actual angioplasty procedure. Compromise of a major coronary artery with ongoing ischemia is the usual indication for surgical revascularization. Compromise of a small side branch or closure of an artery jeopardizing a small segment of myocardium may be better managed conservatively. Occasionally angioplasty may be deemed appropriate in patients who are not surgical candidates, and this decision should not be reversed if angioplasty fails.

Integral to the success of managing these patients when surgical intervention seems likely has been the early involvement in the angioplasty suite of a team of cardiac anesthesiologists. The presence of this team to manage the patients' respiratory and cardiovascular systems frees the cardiologist to concentrate on attempts to resolve the ischemic process and/or to insert an intra-aortic balloon pump. By initiating care in the angioplasty suite, the anesthesia team can provide hemodynamic stability and a coordinated transfer to the operating room.

The rationale for revascularization in these patients is the prevention or reduction of myocardial infarction. Since infarction is directly proportional to the duration and severity of the ischemia, the surgical rescue effort should be designed to reduce these two factors.

It is difficult to correlate salvage of myocardium with speed of surgical revascularization in our own experience because the patients with the most intense ischemia are routinely afforded the most expeditious surgery. Nonetheless, the greatest cause of postoperative transmural infarction after failed angioplasty has been delay in revascularization. The most common delay in our experience has been persistent attempts by the cardiologist to reopen the artery after the onset of ischemia. A policy regarding this situation must be established at each institution. Once the decision has been made to proceed to surgery, every effort should be made to revascularize the patient as quickly as possible.

If the intensity of the myocardial ischemia can be reduced, the risk of myocardial infarction will be less. If S-T segment elevation is absent on the electrocardiogram, the incidence of myocardial necrosis has been less than 10 percent in failed angioplasty patients in our hospital. Use of a catheter with multiple proximal and distal side holes to stent open the damaged artery has been quite effective in temporarily reversing ischemia until bypass surgery can be accomplished. Such a "bail-out" catheter may also allow delivery of potassium cardioplegia solution to the distal artery after aortic cross-clamping. When coronary flow through the damaged artery cannot be directly achieved, the intra-aortic balloon pump can be utilized to stabilize hemodynamics and reduce myocardial oxygen requirements. Criteria for the insertion of the intra-aortic balloon pump in ischemic angioplasty patients at our institution include hypotension, persistent S-T segment elevation, or an anticipated delay in surgical revascularization. Acute ischemia may complicate angioplasty several hours after the procedure is completed, and for this reason the surgical team must remain available for at least 24 hours after the procedure. The following policy for the management of patients with delayed ischemia has been effective in our hospital: If the angiographic appearance of the instrumented artery at the original procedure demonstrated evidence of dissection, then the patient is taken directly to surgery. If the initial angioplasty result was ideal, the patient is frequently returned to the angioplasty suite for an attempt at resolution of the ischemic process by catheter-related techniques.

SURGICAL TECHNIQUE

The basic techniques utilized in the failed emergency angioplasty patient are similar to those applied to the revascularization of any acutely ischemic coronary patient. There are, however, three unique situations that can occur in the setting of the failed angioplasty patient and that may require technical modifications. These situations include distal coronary embolization, rupture of the coronary artery, and distal coronary dissection.

Distal coronary embolization may occur with attempts to dilate lesions in diseased saphenous vein grafts. These grafts may contain atherosclerotic debris that may be dislodged into the native coronary artery beyond the distal anastomosis. The angiographic recognition of embolization is critical to proper therapy, and the localization of distal debris on angiography can be very helpful in proper placement of a new graft. Retrograde coronary perfusion of cardioplegia may also be useful in situations of multiple distal emboli.

Rupture of a coronary artery by an angioplasty balloon may present as free rupture with cardiac tamponade or as a large epicardial hematoma overlying the instrumented artery. Free rupture is managed by relief of tamponade, ligation of the artery at the rupture site, and distal revascularization. When the rupture is walled off by the adventitia, however, it is possible to manage the lesion by distal bypass in an area uninvolved by the hematoma. When the distal artery is large enough for such a bypass, it is possible to avoid ligation of the native artery. When the artery has to be opened in an area of hematoma, it is usually necessary to ligate the native artery proximal to the graft anastomosis.

Distal coronary dissection has been quite common in our experience and occurs when the dissection process extends beyond the point of anticipated anastomosis construction. Distal dissection is recognized when coronary arteriotomy reveals first a false lumen with a convex posterior wall and then a deeper true lumen. Revascularization is best afforded in this situation by construction of a routine anastomosis incorporating the walls of both the true and false lumina together. This technique, which can be facilitated by carefully placed stay sutures to align the walls, assures anastomosis of the bypass graft to the true lumen. Ligation of the dissected native coronary is not necessary.

Revascularization in these settings can be performed equally well with the saphenous vein or the internal mammary artery. Consideration must be given to the degree of stability of the patient if an internal mammary graft is to be used; the additional time needed to take down the graft must be factored in. With the use of the intra-aortic balloon pump and the "bail-out" catheter, many patients can be stabilized to permit the time to use an internal mammary artery graft; this decision must be considered on an individual basis.

RESULTS

Over the last 6 years, 196 out of 5,000 angioplasty patients at the Emory University Hospital required urgent coronary bypass surgery for angioplasty-related myocardial ischemia. The overall survival in this surgical group has been 98 percent. Patients with S-T segment elevations prior to urgent operation had myocardial enzyme level elevations postoperatively. Approximately 18 percent developed new Q waves in the postoperative electrocardiogram. Myocardial necrosis did not correlate with the time to revascularization, the number of diseased vessels, the artery being instrumented, the mechanism of ischemia, or the presence of collateral flow. These patients had a greater chance of requiring postoperative inotropic agents or antiarrhythmic drugs than did elective coronary bypass patients.

SUGGESTED READING

Jones EL, Murphy DA, Craver JM. Comparison of coronary artery bypass surgery and percutaneous transluminal coronary angioplasty including surgery for failed angioplasty. Am Heart J 1984; 107:830–835.

Murphy DA, Craver JM, Jones EL, et al. Surgical management of patients following unsuccessful percutaneous transluminal coronary angioplasty. J Thorac Cardiovasc Surg 1982; 84:342–348.

Murphy DA, Craver JM, Jones EL, Curling PE, Guyton RA, Gruentzig AR, Hatcher CR Jr. Surgical management of acute myocardial ischemia following PTCA. Role of the intraaortic balloon pump. J Thorac Cardiovasc Surg 1984; 87:332–339.

Murphy DA, Craver JM, Jones EL, King SB III, Curling PE, Douglas JS Jr. Hemodynamic deterioration following coronary angioplasty in the presence of previous left ventricular infarction. Am J Cardiol 1984; 54:448–450.

Murphy DA, Craver JM, King SB III. Distal coronary artery dissection following PTCA. Ann Thorac Surg 1984; 37:473–478.

THROMBOLYTIC THERAPY

JACQUES G. LOSMAN, M.D., F.A.C.C.

Twenty years ago the management of an acute myocardial infarction was described by C. K. Friedberg as: "reduce the work of the heart until the infarcted area is healed, alleviate pain or other discomfort, overcome shock and cardiac failure if present and cope with dangerous cardiac arrhythmias or any complication that may arise." No attempt to reestablish blood flow or save jeopardized myocardium was envisioned. Our improved understanding of the pathophysiology of acute infarction and of the correlation between coronary anatomy, thrombosis, and extent of necrosis has resulted in a more rational treatment that attempts to restore adequate blood flow before irreversible myocardial damage has occurred or within a period of delay brief enough to minimize the extent of myocardial necrosis. This has involved lysis of the coronary thrombus and mechanical correction of the causal stenosis by percutaneous transluminal coronary angioplasty (PTCA) or surgical revascularization (coronary artery bypass grafting).

PATHOPHYSIOLOGIC BASIS OF THROMBOLYTIC THERAPY

The rationale for the use of thrombolytic therapy in the early stages of an acute infarction is based on a body of experimental and clinical evidence: (1) the seminal role of a complete or near-complete epicardial coronary artery thrombosis, interrupting the blood flow to an area of the heart muscle, (2) the ability of lytic agents to dissolve a fresh thrombus, and (3) the assumption that early reperfusion abrogates or limits myocardial damage. Most often the thrombosis occurs in a preexisting atherosclerotic and narrowed segment of the artery. Platelet aggregation, spasm, and/or plaque hemorrhage may all play a role in the initial event leading to thrombus formation. Coronary angiography performed early in the course of acute myocardial infarctions has shown that complete occlusion is present in over 80 percent of transmural infarcts, although spontaneous recanalizations may occur later. The efficacy of thrombolytic agents is well established; streptokinase (STK), extracted from group C beta-hemolytic streptococci, in the presence of plasminogen, activates the latter, producing plasmin, a proteolytic enzyme. STK is antigenic and may trigger a severe anaphylactic reaction if used repeatedly.

Thrombolysis using tissue plasminogen activator (t-PA) is under investigation and has recently been approved for clinical use. This agent has a high specificity for fibrin and does not produce as much systemic fibrinolysis; although some systemic fibrinolysis occurs, most patients maintain approximately 60 percent of their control fibrinogen levels. All these fibrin lysing agents have been shown to dissolve clots effectively, particularly fresh ones. Newer fibrinolytic agents with higher specificity and greater efficacy are being produced and will soon be available for clinical trials.

INDICATIONS FOR THROMBOLYTIC THERAPY

Currently, thrombolytic therapy is indicated for the initial treatment of most acute myocardial infarctions. Exceptions to this may be the patient with a small inferior infarction that is stable and has become pain-free. In view of the importance of early therapy, some centers now provide emergency teams equipped with thrombolytic agents to initiate the treatment at home as soon as the patient is reached; the precise efficacy of this approach is not known, since coronary angiography is not available to demonstrate the occluded vessel prior to therapy.

Absolute contraindications to thrombolysis include active internal bleeding, a history of cerebrovascular accident, recent operation (within 2 weeks), trauma, prolonged resuscitation, and severe, uncontrolled hypertension or a patient over the age of 75. Relative contraindications include a history of cerebrovascular disease, gastrointestinal and genitourinary bleeding, hypertension, or any other factor that increases the risk of bleeding.

TECHNIQUES OF ADMINISTRATION OF THROMBOLYTIC AGENTS

Intracoronary Streptokinase. STK, the most widely used thrombolytic agent, has been given directly in the ostia of the occluded coronary or, employing selective catheterization, at the site of occlusion. The intracoronary dose of STK varies from 200,000 to 500,000 U, given over a short period of time. After routine preparation, heparin (3,000 U intravenously) and hydrocortisone (100 mg intravenously) are given, followed by the performance of selective coronary angiography (Seldinger's technique). The thrombosed vessel is catheterized, and the tip of the catheter is positioned close to the obstruction. Nitroglycerin, 200 μg to 300 μg, is injected, followed by a 20,000 U bolus of STK. The STK infusion is started at a rate of 4,000 U per minute for 20 minutes, then 2,000 U per minute for 45 minutes. Repeated injections of contrast medium are given to monitor the progress of recanalization. When successful, a continuous heparin infusion (1,000 U per hour) is started. If required, intravenous lidocaine and/or sublingual nifedipine is given to control arrhythmias.

The advantage of intracoronary delivery is that low doses are effective, the drug has relatively little systemic effect, and it yields a high rate of recanalization (70 to 75 percent). In addition, most studies on STK indicate that the intracoronary route is more efficacious than the intravenous route in dissolving the thrombus. However, intracoronary administration requires a cardiac catheterization procedure that is time-consuming, delays the initiation of thrombolysis, and is not available in all institutions or around the clock.

Intravenous Streptokinase. An increasingly popular technique consists of giving a high dose of STK intravenously, producing a generalized thrombolytic state that lyses the coronary thrombus in 50 to 60 percent of cases. This approach involves intravenous administration of a high dose during a 60-minute infusion. First, hydrocortisone (100 mg intravenously) and heparin (3,000 U intravenously) are given, followed by the STK infusion. The total dose varies from 1,250,000 to 2,500,000 U. Lidocaine and/or nifedipine is given to control arrhythmias. The major advantages of intravenous STK are its low cost and ease of use.

Intravenous t-PA. More recently, t-PA has become part of the clinical armamentarium. This agent successfully recanalizes 80 to 85 percent of thrombosed coronary arteries. Patients receive 100 mg of intravenous t-PA (10 percent of the dose as a bolus, 50 percent as an infusion during the first hour, and 20 percent during the second and third hours). Heparin is given before or after t-PA is started (a 5,000-U bolus followed by 1,000 U per hour infusion, keeping the partial thrombin time between 1.5 and 2.0 times that of control). Lidocaine and/or nifedipine is given to control arrhythmias.

RESULTS

The rates of recanalization for various thrombolytic agents are given in the preceding section. The thrombolytic state lasts 24 hours, and rethrombosis of the coronary artery is prevented by heparin given for a number of days or until the patient undergoes revascularization by PTCA or coronary artery bypass grafting, if indicated. The decision to revascularize by PTCA or by coronary artery bypass grafting is made by the same criteria used in any patient with coronary artery disease; in general, most patients who undergo successful thrombolytic therapy need at least PTCA of the lesion that was the source of the thrombosis. Without PTCA or coronary artery bypass grafting, rethrombosis will occur within the first week in 20 to 30 percent of patients in spite of anticoagulation.

By combining thrombolysis with PTCA, patency rates in excess of 90 percent have been reported. More commonly, however, the reocclusion rate following angioplasty in the setting of a recent, acute infarction ranges from 10 to 12 percent within the first few days following the procedure; this is in contrast to the 2 to 4 percent reocclusion rate seen following elective angioplasties in patients without recent infarctions. The reason for this difference in PTCA patency rates is unknown; it may be related to differences in the coronary artery lesion that has recently thrombosed (e.g., possible effects of recent plaque hemorrhage) or to the fact that the region of infarcting myocardium distal to a recanalized artery may have less myocardial blood flow and hence a slower flow through the coronary artery itself.

Thrombolysis may be complicated by hemorrhage, sometimes severe, such as gastrointestinal bleeding, but most of the time the bleeding is minor, consisting primarily of oozing at the arterial puncture sites, which can be controlled by application of local pressure. Severe hemorrhages require clotting factor replacement therapy with fresh frozen plasma and fibrinogen. When an emergency operation is indicated during the thrombolytic state, the procedure can be performed exercising great care for hemostasis and appropriate blood component therapy.

Effect of Thrombolysis on Myocardial Infarction Size

The usefulness of thrombolysis has been demonstrated by many experiments in which the timely reopening of an occluded coronary vessel significantly reduced the area of eventual myocardial necrosis. Although 20 minutes of severe ischemia at normothermia is known to be lethal to the cardiac myocyte, an acute myocardial infarction is a more complex event involving areas in different degrees of jeopardy. In the absence of recanalization, it progresses from reversible ischemic changes to irreversible injury and cellular death in 4 to 6 hours after the onset of severe ischemia. Ultimate infarction size depends on multiple factors, such as the extent of atherosclerosis of the other coronary arteries and the presence of collateral circulation, heart failure, cardiogenic shock, arrhythmias, or other pathologies. When recanalization is achieved, the residual infarct size depends on the degree and length of ischemia before reperfusion and the other factors that affect the acute infarction. Controversy has surrounded the concept that reperfusion results in a hemorrhagic infarction larger than the initial injury. In animal experiments, it has been shown that reperfusion after ischemia disrupted the microvascular endothelium, resulting in a hemorrhage into the ischemic area; however, in humans it appears that when a hemorrhagic infarct develops following reperfusion, the area involved is not greater than the area of necrosis at the center of the acute infarction.

Time is the major factor, and when thrombolysis is initiated less than 2 hours after the onset of ischemia (defined as at least 30 minutes of continuous severe typical chest pain unresponsive to sublingual administration of nitrates and/or nifedipine and accompanied by new S-T segment elevations with reciprocal changes), the prospect of reperfusion is excellent and myocardial damage may be minimal in terms of effects on left ventricular function. A series of patients with acute anterior infarctions who received thrombolysis within 2 hours of the onset of pain sustained minimal damage. Reperfusion within 2 to 4 hours still salvaged a significant amount of myocardium. Beyond 4 hours the results are less consistent and the benefits questionable. Early relief of pain, within 3.5 hours, correlated with a small infarct. It has been our experience that, following reperfusion and at the time of a coronary bypass operation, the area of myocardial infarction is nearly always small, sometimes absent on the epicardial surface of the heart.

Of course, it is difficult to accurately quantitate the amount of myocardium in jeopardy in the initial phase of an acute infarct and thus difficult to quantitate the amount of muscle that is saved. Nevertheless, large published series strongly suggest that early reperfusion by thrombolysis decreases acute myocardial infarct size significantly. Conversely, when coronary angiography is performed later, the presence of a patent artery is not necessarily a sign of success because the thrombolysis might have occurred after the damage was already done.

Effect of Thrombolysis on Patient Survival and Cardiac Function

A number of studies have shown that successful early reperfusion significantly reduces the early and late mortality following acute infarction if adequate measures are taken to prevent the high incidence of late reocclusion and reinfarction; the benefit of successful thrombolysis is not apparent at the end of the first year after the initial acute infarction unless the hemodynamic causal lesions are corrected.

Future improvement in the salvage of myocardium essentially depends on more expeditious application of thrombolysis. Still, too often critical time is wasted first between the onset of symptoms and the admission to an emergency room (because of insufficient public awareness about "heart attack") and second between admission, diagnosis, and initiation of therapy. Administration of thrombolytic agents by paramedics and a better education of the public, prompting a patient to seek medical attention at an early stage of chest pain, will both reduce the crucial time factor. The development of safer and more efficient thrombolytic agents and the early correction of coronary artery stenoses also will improve the outlook of patients with acute myocardial infarction.

During the acute phase, the role of the cardiothoracic surgeon remains limited to those patients who may require an emergency operation because of failed thrombolysis and life-threatening ischemia; this group includes patients with continuous severe ischemia in spite of pharmacologic and lytic therapy and intra-aortic balloon pump support, patients presenting with cardiogenic shock (refractory to catecholamine infusion and intra-aortic balloon pump support), and those with acute mitral valve regurgitation and cardiac rupture. When the lytic state is reversed, those patients with persistent high-grade stenoses that cannot be satisfactorily managed with angioplasty should undergo a revascularization procedure without delay to avoid the consequences of reocclusion. Today's management of all acute infarctions should combine early lytic therapy when possible, followed by emergency PTCA and early coronary artery bypass graft when indicated to minimize the loss of myocardium.

SUGGESTED READING

Erbel R, Pop T, Henrichs KJ, et al. Percutaneous transluminal coronary angioplasty after thrombolytic therapy: a prospective controlled randomized trial. J Am Coll Cardiol 1986; 8:485–495.

Losman JG, Finchum RN, Nagle D, et al. Myocardial surgical revascularization after streptokinase treatment for acute myocardial infarction. J Thorac Cardiovasc Surg 1985; 89:25–34.

Rovelli F, DeVita C, Feruglio GA, et al. GISSI trial: early results and late follow-up. J Am Coll Cardiol 1987; 10:33B–39B.

Simoons ML, Serruys PW, van den Brand M, et al. Early thrombolysis in acute myocardial infarction: limitation of infarct size and improved survival. J Am Coll Cardiol 1986; 7:717–728.

Tennant SN, Dixon J, Venable TC, et al. Intracoronary thrombolysis in patients with acute myocardial infarction: comparisons of the efficacy of urokinase with streptokinase. Circulation 1984; 69:756–760.

Topol EJ, Califf RM, Kereiakes DJ, George BS. Thrombolysis and angioplasty in myocardial infarction (TAMI) trial. J Am Coll Cardiol 1987; 10:65B–74B.

CORONARY REVASCULARIZATION: DISTAL ANASTOMOSES PRECEDING PROXIMAL ANASTOMOSES

FLOYD D. LOOP, M.D.

The protection offered by cold cardioplegia allows the surgeon to perform all anastomoses during one period of cross-clamping and obviates much of the discussion about whether to perform proximal before distal anastomoses or vice versa. Delivery of cardioplegia into potentially ischemic areas through the distal anastomosis, or from the aorta through the aortocoronary graft, permits cross-clamping of the aorta for 1 to 2 hours without perceptible myocardial damage, even in the face of diffuse coronary atherosclerosis. The advantage of first performing proximal vein graft anastomoses within a tangential clamp is that it theoretically provides cardioplegia delivery as soon as the distal anastomosis is completed and shortens the cross-clamping time. However, this method requires more manipulation of the aorta of the beating heart.

Performing distal anastomoses first followed by proximal anastomoses, all during one period of cross-clamping, began with reoperation patients and has continued with primary elective cases. One may perform each distal anastomosis followed by its respective proximal anastomosis and thus deliver cardioplegia through the aorta down the graft sequentially. The advantages of this technique are that it requires minimal cardiac or aortic manipulation, all anastomoses are performed under one aortic cross-clamp application, and cardioplegia delivery may be decided according to severity of ischemia or atherosclerotic narrowing. As the technique becomes familiar, it is easier to perform proximal anastomoses on the complete cross-clamped aorta rather than within the confines of a U-shaped vascular clamp, especially in reoperations, because the aorta requires no further mobilization.

CANNULATION AND VEIN PREPARATION

Cannulation has been simplified to an aortic perfusion line and a two-stage right atrial catheter that drains the inferior vena caval and right atrial blood. In patients with poor left ventricular function or those who require combined valve or aneurysmectomy procedures, some surgeons prefer bicaval cannulation and a left atrial or left atrioventricular vent passed through the right superior pulmonary vein. Under those circumstances, a tourniquet may be placed around the inferior vena caval cannula, but it is not necessary to do the same for the superior cava unless the right atrium is opened during the operation. If the common femoral artery and vein are used as cannulation sites, as in complicated reoperations or aortic surgery, the inferior vena cava may be cross-clamped to reduce the amount of warm blood reaching the septum and other subendocardium. For most cases, however, an aortic arterial perfusion line and a large venous drainage cannula in the right atrium suffice.

Since approximately 90 percent or more of patients receive an internal mammary artery graft, the mobilization of this arterial pedicle is the first step after entry. We procure the saphenous vein at the latest possible moment so that it is stored for the least amount of time. As the internal mammary artery dissection is completed, the leg incisions are made, and the vein is removed after cannulation. The protocol that we follow in vein removal includes gentle handling, low distention pressure (the end is not clamped), and ligation of side branches 1 to 2 mm from the vein wall. The vein is flushed with a dilute heparin solution (balanced pH), sprayed with a dilute papaverine solution (3 parts saline: 1 part papaverine), filled with the heparin solution, occluded on each end with small bulldog clamps and wrapped in gauze moistened with the same solution. The vein specimen is not stored in any medium.

Lesser saphenous veins have comparable patency to the greater saphenous system, but the cephalic or basilic arm veins generally have a lower patency. Homologous saphenous veins, umbilical veins, or polytetrafluoroethylene grafts are unacceptable and should not be used except in dire circumstances.

The Mayo Clinic experience indicates that adherence to a protocol of dipyridamole for 2 days preoperatively and the combination of aspirin and dipyridamole postoperatively significantly improve vein graft patency. This combination of antiplatelet agents sometimes produces gastric side effects and should not be used in patients with previous ulcer history or those with known bleeding tendencies. In these patients and in patients 70 years or older, we prefer low-dose aspirin alone, which amounts to one "baby" aspirin tablet or approximately 81 mg of aspirin per day; there is some evidence that this regimen also reduces intimal hyperplasia and may significantly enhance vein graft patency. If tolerated, these drugs should be prescribed for at least 1 year and perhaps indefinitely.

Unfortunately, there is no known preventive for vein graft atherosclerosis. Trauma during vein preparation may be an inciting factor. Patients should be advised to modify their diets to reduce serum cholesterol levels. This admonition may not be applicable to older patients, but it is sound advice for the typical patient with coronary atherosclerosis.

GRAFTING TECHNIQUES

As mentioned earlier, we accomplish all anastomoses under one period of cross-clamping, and this method includes performance of aortic vein graft anastomoses with the aorta fully cross-clamped. At this stage in the evolution of bypass grafting and in my practice, core cooling and cold blood cardioplegia are used for all cases, including coronary bypass combined with other procedures and surgery for acute ischemic syndromes. A continuous drip of cold saline into the pericardial cavity is not necessary and may be harmful to respiratory mechanics by causing temporary phrenic nerve dysfunction. This complication assumes even greater importance in the elderly, who may be more prone to cold injury.

Small vessel anastomoses, e.g., internal mammary artery grafts and side-to-side vein to coronary artery anastomoses, are constructed with interrupted siliconized 7–0 silk. End-to-side vein graft anastomoses are frequently performed with continuous 7–0 polypropylene. However, when the recipient artery is 1.0 to 1.5 mm, we revert to the interrupted 7–0 silk technique because, in our opinion, it enables the surgeon to perform the graft under the most direct vision and carries the least risk of anastomotic stricture.

If the lumen is small and the vessel diffusely atherosclerotic, an endarterectomy is frequently the best solution. One must be sure that all atherosclerotic remnants are removed, particularly from the distal segment that carries the arterial runoff. If the plaque is not feathered upon removal, the remnant should be retrieved, either by extending the arteriotomy or by making another arteriotomy over the remaining plaque and then bridging the two anastomoses in a sequential graft. A good endarterectomy frequently takes significantly more time than ordinary grafting; the plaque must be teased out gently and compulsively so that every remnant of the distal artherosclerotic process is removed. An inadequate endarterectomy results in myocardial infarction unless the vessel is already totally occluded. Even then, an inadequate endarterectomy may jeopardize the collaterals already in existence.

Sequential grafts are advantageous for three reasons: (1) arterial runoff may be improved by linking two or more coronary arterial vessels into one graft; (2) graft length may be conserved; and (3) in sequential vein grafting, fewer aortic anastomoses are required. Measurement between anastomoses is critical, and graft closure may compromise perfusion to a large area. For this reason, both sequential vein and arterial bypasses should probably be restricted to two arteries, usually within the same arterial system, and rarely more than three. The patency for sequential grafts is the same as that recorded for individual grafts with one coronary anastomosis.

Although graft length measurement to the aorta after completion of the distal anastomosis is generally easier to gauge than the opposite measurement, i.e., proximal first and distal last, length under both circumstances is crucial. For circumflex grafts, it is best to follow curvature of the pericardium around, over the pulmonary vein, to the aorta. Following this gentle curve results in satisfactory length. In anterior descending artery grafts, the vein must curve out over the pulmonary artery and down to the anterior descending artery in a loop rather than straight across. Veins tend to retract, and retraction may tent the distal anastomosis. Right coronary artery vein grafts are placed either between the right atrial appendage and the right ventricle over the margin of the heart, or angled more inferiorly around the right atrium. Some surgeons use a methylene blue stripe on the vein to avoid twisting. Vein grafts that do not follow the intended course or show obvious length problems must be redone.

The trend toward arterial grafting is based on recent evidence that an internal mammary artery graft to the anterior descending coronary artery, either alone or combined with vein grafts, significantly improves 10-year survival compared with the use of vein grafts only; it also significantly reduces the incidence of late myocardial infarction, hospitalization for cardiac events, and reoperation. Based on this information, use of the internal mammary artery has expanded to sequential, bilateral, and free (aortocoronary) arterial grafting. Preliminary evidence indicates that bilateral internal mammary artery grafting leads to an even higher intermediate term survival than single internal mammary artery grafting. Whether this observation will be confirmed by later analysis is unknown.

In most patients, the anterior descending coronary artery is the most important of the three major coronary vessels. Occlusion of the anterior descending results in a greater incidence of death than closure of any other vessel. Also, an anterior descending arterial lesion affects prognosis more than a lesion in all other coronary arteries combined, except for the left main coronary artery. Therefore, the left internal mammary artery should be used for anterior descending artery grafting whenever indicated and technically feasible.

Patency of sequential arterial grafts is essentially the same as that of single internal mammary artery—coronary artery anastomoses. The left internal mammary artery is best used sequentially for second diagonal—anterior descending combinations with the side-to-side anastomosis on the first or second diagonal and the end-to-side component on the anterior descending. This sequence may be reversed when the anterior descending is the same size or smaller than the diagonal. Another good combination is two relatively high circumflex branches. When the left internal mammary artery is used for sequential purposes, the left pericardial leaf should either be divided to within 1 cm from the left phrenic nerve or the arterial graft may be passed through a rent in the left pericardial leaf. The same avenue of entry is useful for the right internal mammary artery when it is passed over the hilus and through the pericardium to reach branches of the right coronary artery. Internal mammary artery grafts must be redundant and should be sutured to the epicardium. Failure to sew the thoracic artery pedicle down may result in its adherence to the overlying chest wall, which causes anastomotic stricture.

Bilateral internal mammary artery grafting is performed in approximately 30 to 40 percent of our patients, depending upon indications and preference of the surgeon. Younger patients are the best candidates for bilateral arterial grafting, and these conduits should be used to graft the most important coronary arteries. Generally, we avoid crossing the midline with the right internal mammary pedicle, unless it is unlikely that the patient will ever need another operation. In reoperations, injury to the right internal mammary artery pedicle as it passes under the sternum frequently occurs during re-entry.

The right internal mammary artery, especially in men, is useful for the distal right coronary branches, but should be performed to this vessel only when it is dominant and severely narrowed, not totally occluded and receiving collaterals from the left coronary system. A variety of other uses can be found for the right internal mammary artery. It can be passed across the midline to the anterior descending artery if reoperation is unlikely. The right pedicle may be passed through the transverse sinus to graft a lateral circumflex as long as the vessel lies close to the left atrial appendage. Circumflex vessels that lie more distally generally cannot be reached by a graft through the transverse sinus. The pedicle passed through the transverse sinus should be relatively thin so that it is not stuffed into the narrow aperture with resultant occlusion of the artery from external pressure. Furthermore, the surgeon must guard against twisting of the pedicle as it transverses the sinus. Some reports indicate that transverse sinus arterial grafts have a lower patency. The same may be said for the right internal mammary artery applied elsewhere, but we believe that it is inherently as good a conduit as the left. The slightly lower patency reported by several groups for the right internal mammary artery is probably related to grafting technique and a pedicle that is stretched to reach a distal point of anastomosis.

The free internal mammary artery graft is useful to avoid crossing the midline and jeopardizing arterial viability during reoperation; it also has greater versatility. In contrast to in situ internal mammary artery grafts, the free pedicle reaches all coronary arterial branches. It may be used as a sequential graft. Recatheterization after 5 years shows a patency comparable to that of the in situ internal mammary artery graft and, similarly, there are no wall alterations to suggest the occurrence of late graft atherosclerosis.

When internal mammary artery grafts are used, they are often constructed last in the grafting sequence to avoid anastomotic disruption while the left ventricle is manipulated for exposure to perform vein grafts. Free arterial grafts are performed last in sequence, and we prefer to construct the distal anastomosis first, followed by the proximal anastomosis. The free internal mammary artery to aortic anastomosis is best constructed with continuous 6–0 polypropylene except when the aortic wall is thick from atherosclerosis. In those cases, it seems better to create the proximal anastomosis either on the hood of a vein graft or to graft a patch of saphenous vein into a 4.0- or 4.5-mm oval aortic opening and then to sew the free graft into a smaller opening within the vein patch.

The saphenous vein is still an excellent conduit and works well in the aortocoronary position, but its durability is compromised by the formation of vein graft atherosclerosis. Serial studies on its patency show that approximately half of vein grafts are closed by the tenth postoperative year (Fig. 1), and of those that remain open, approximately half show wall alterations consistent with atherosclerosis. Vein graft atherosclerosis has become the leading indication for reoperation. Still, the vein graft has many uses and is more versatile than any arterial graft. A number of secondary targets may be grafted by either individual or sequential aortocoronary vein grafts. These include distal circumflex branches, totally obstructed vessels, endarterectomized coronary arteries, diagonal branches not included in arterial grafting, and grafts in unstable emergency patients and the very elderly. A number of situations are not conducive to use of internal mammary artery graft, and hence the vein graft becomes the

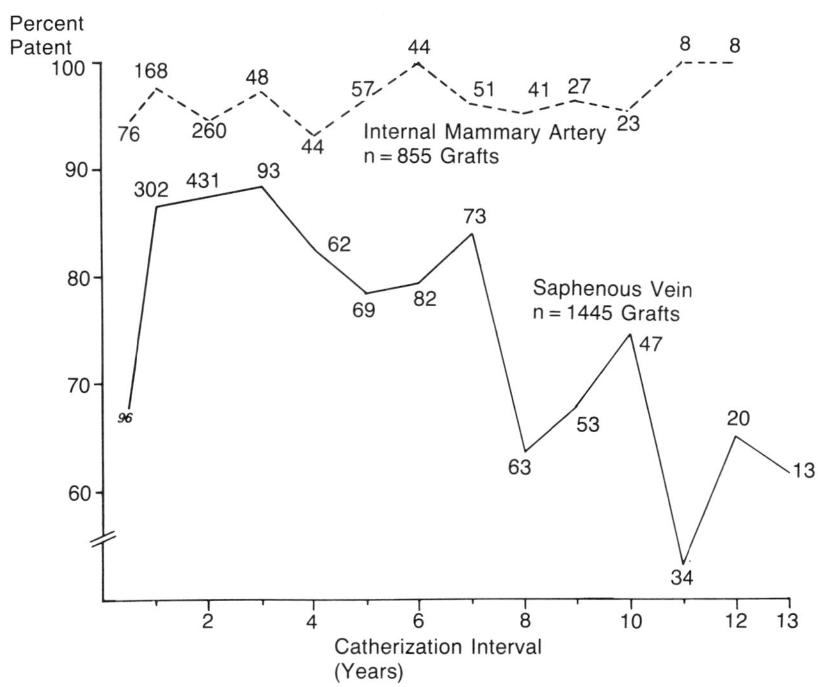

Figure 1 The patency of internal thoracic (mammary) artery and saphenous vein grafts to the anterior descending coronary artery at 1-year intervals. The number of patients restudied at each interval is noted. (Reprinted by permission from Loop FD, Lytle BW, Cosgrove DM, et al. Influence of the internal mammary artery graft on 10-year survival and other cardiac events. N Engl J Med 1986; 314:1–6.)

graft of choice: (1) extensive brachiocephalic disease; (2) previous chest wall irradiation; (3) a previous mastectomy resulting in diminished internal mammary artery size; (4) emergency operations in unstable patients; (5) poor left ventricular function; and (6) some combined higher risk operations, such as valve, carotid endarterectomy, or ventricular aneurysmectomy combined with coronary bypass grafting.

In summary, performance of distal anastomoses first in coronary artery grafting may be accomplished routinely because of improvements in myocardial protection. Currently, it is our preference to perform one aortocoronary graft completely, administer cardioplegia, and then proceed to the next graft. Present myocardial protection techniques permit all grafting to be performed under one period of cross-clamping, which includes all proximal anastomoses. In reoperations, vein graft aortic anastomoses are much easier to perform with the aorta fully cross-clamped. This technique is carried over to primary revascularization cases. We find it technically easier, and it eliminates the need for application of a side-biting or tangential vascular clamp.

SUGGESTED READING

Chesebro JH, Fuster V, Elveback LR, et al. Benefit effect of dipyridamole and aspirin on late vein-graft patency after coronary bypass operations. N Engl J Med 1984; 310:209–214.

Loop FD. Use of the *in situ* and free internal thoracic artery for myocardial revascularization. J Cardiac Surg 1986; 1:205–216.

Loop FD, Lytle BW, Cosgrove DM, et al. Free (aorta-coronary) internal mammary artery graft: Late results. J Thorac Cardiovasc Surg 1986; 92:827–831.

Loop FD, Lytle BW, Cosgrove DM, et al. Influence of the internal mammary artery graft on 10-year survival and other cardiac events. N Engl J Med 1986; 314:1–6.

Lytle BW, Loop FD, Cosgrove DM, et al. Long-term (5 to 12 years) serial studies of internal mammary artery and saphenous vein coronary bypass grafts. J Thorac Cardiovasc Surg 1985; 89:248–258.

CORONARY REVASCULARIZATION: PROXIMAL ANASTOMOSES PRECEDING DISTAL ANASTOMOSES

MARSHALL L. JACOBS, M.D.

To achieve satisfactory results in coronary bypass surgery, it is important to accomplish complete revascularization and to minimize ischemic injury to the myocardium during the surgical procedure. A variety of operative techniques have been associated with satisfactory outcome. At our institution (Massachusetts General Hospital), where a large segment of the clinical population is made up of patients with unstable angina, preinfarction angina, acute myocardial infarction, and postinfarction angina, we have evolved a surgical technique in which sequential revascularization of myocardial zones is accomplished in an order based upon the severity of obstructive lesions and risk of myocardial jeopardy of each zone, with delivery of hypothermic cardioplegic solution after the construction of each graft. This is accomplished by completing all proximal anastomoses first and then constructing distal anastomoses in a sequence based on the severity of the coronary obstructive lesions and the territory of clinical ischemia.

TECHNIQUE

While the greater saphenous vein is exposed and removed from the leg, midline sternotomy is performed. The opened pericardium is tacked to the wound edges, and heparin is given intravenously. The distal ascending aorta is cannulated for perfusion. The venae cavae are either cannulated individually via the right atrium or a large two-stage cannula is passed into the right atrium and inferior cava. Appropriate lengths of the prepared saphenous vein are selected for grafts. A Satinsky side-biting clamp is placed on the ascending aorta to exclude a segment of aorta from which buttons of aortic wall are excised. Segments of vein are anastomosed to the aorta with continuous 5–0 monofilament suture. Separate applications of the partially occluding clamp to the right and left sides of the ascending aorta are often required when three or more proximal anastomoses are constructed. During the completion of the final proximal anastomosis, hypothermic bypass is initiated, and the patient is gradually cooled to a core temperature (measured in the nasopharynx) of 25° C. During cooling, a pursestring suture is placed near the junction of the right superior pulmonary vein with the left atrium, so that a left ventricular vent can later be introduced. Two polyvinyl catheters are inserted in the ascending aorta, one for the delivery of cardioplegic solution and one for monitoring the pressure at which the coronary arteries are perfused with the solution. During the period of perfusion at 25° C, the systemic flow rate is generally kept at or above 1.6 L per minute per square meter of body surface area.

Ventricular fibrillation generally occurs spontaneously when the core temperature is between 30° and 25° C. At this point, the left ventricular vent is inserted to prevent distention of the heart. The coronary arteries are then examined, and sites for anastomoses are selected and prepared by incision of the epicardium and epicardial fat. The sequence in which distal anastomoses will be accomplished is determined at this point. Regions where clinical ischemia was documented preoperatively and regions distal to critical stenoses in principal vessels are grafted first. Vessels with less critical disease and smaller vessels that are grafted to achieve complete revascularization are grafted last. For a time, we based our sequence of grafting on a temperature map of the myocardium that was determined during the delivery of the initial dose of cardioplegic solution. The solution, which is cooled to 4° C, was infused into the aortic root at a pressure of 70 to 100 mm Hg, and myocardial temperatures in the midwall of the anterior, lateral, and inferior zones of left ventricular myocardium were monitored with myocardial thermistors. The areas where the least satisfactory myocardial cooling was achieved were revascularized first, based on the assumption that myocardial protection can be expected to be least satisfactory in these areas. A high degree of success was achieved with this method, as evidenced by good preservation of ventricular function and a low incidence of perioperative infarction. We found that the sequence suggested by temperature mapping could reliably be predicted by analysis of the angiogram and preoperative clinical events. For that reason, myocardial temperature mapping is no longer a routine part of our technique for revascularization.

After application of the aortic cross-clamp, an initial dose of cold cardioplegic solution (750 to 1,000 ml) is delivered into the aortic root by roller pump, the rate of delivery being determined by pressure in the aortic root. As mentioned above, we try to achieve a coronary perfusion pressure of 70 to 100 mm Hg. Topical myocardial cooling may be added as well, with a continuous drip of iced lactated Ringer's solution into the pericardial well. An additional dose of cardioplegia (300 to 700 ml) is delivered into the aortic root after the completion of each distal anastomosis. In this way, myocardial protection of regions beyond critical coronary artery stenoses is optimized. Each successive dose of cardioplegia is delivered not only into the native coronary ostia but also into the vein grafts and thus to each zone of myocardium as soon as it has been revascularized. Systemic warming is begun while the last distal anastomosis is being constructed.

In instances in which myocardial ischemia is difficult to control in the prebypass period and in patients who have severe atherosclerotic changes or areas of calcification in the aortic root or marked dilatation of the aortic root, the technique is modified such that bypass may be established prior to construction of the proximal anastomoses. Systemic cooling is accomplished while the vein grafts are being anastomosed to the ascending aorta. This allows the surgeon to have precise control over the aortic pressure during such manipulations as application of and removal of the side-biting clamp. In general, this alteration in sequence adds no more than 20 minutes to the total bypass time.

Use of an internal mammary artery to revascularize the left anterior descending artery may impact on the operative strategy. Since cardioplegic solution cannot be delivered through the internal mammary graft and since perfusion of the myocardium through the open mammary graft results in washout of cardioplegia and warming of the myocardium, the anastomosis of internal mammary artery to coronary artery is generally performed last. To optimize myocardial protection to the region that will be perfused by the internal mammary artery, a vein graft to an anterior wall vessel may be constructed early in the sequence. For example, if one chooses to revascularize a left anterior descending artery with an internal mammary artery, early in the operation myocardial protection of the anterior wall of the left ventricle can be enhanced by an anastomosis of a saphenous vein graft to a diagonal artery. In this way, cardioplegic solution is delivered to the myocardium beyond the stenosis of the left anterior descending artery.

This approach to coronary revascularization is adaptable to combined procedures such as coronary bypass grafting with valve replacement or aneurysmectomy. Construction of proximal anastomoses first, followed by the distal anastomoses and finally by the noncoronary portion of the operation, affords optimal myocardial protection during these potentially lengthy procedures. Operative strategies that involve construction of the proximal anastomoses after removal of the aortic cross-clamp of necessity involve a period of time during which the heart is reperfused and rewarmed but not yet revascularized. The success of the technique herein described, we believe, is based on optimal delivery of cardioplegic solution to ischemic zones and completion of revascularization prior to reperfusion.

SUGGESTED READING

Akins CW, Buckley MJ, Daggett WM, Hilgenberg AD, Austen WG. Myocardial revascularization with combined aortic and mitral valve replacements. J Thorac Cardiovasc Surg 1985; 90:272-277.

Daggett WM, Randolph JD, Jacobs ML, O'Keefe DD, Geffin GA, Swinskin LA, Boggs BR, Austen WG. The superiority of cold oxygenated diluted blood cardioplegia. Ann Thorac Surg 1987; 43:397–402.

Nugent WC, Weintraub RM, Thurer RL, Levine FH. Aortic valve replacement and coronary bypass in patients with severe stenosis of the left main coronary. Ann Thorac Surg 1983; 35:562-564.

Toal KW, Bodenhamer RM, Daggett WM. Myocardial temperature mapping in patients with left main coronary artery disease. J Cardiovasc Surg 1986; 27:588-594.

VanderSalm TJ, Okike ON, Cutler BS, Paraskos JA, Ferulo J, Daggett WM. Improved myocardial preservation by improved distribution of cardioplegic solutions. J Thorac Cardiovasc Surg 1982; 83:767-771.

CORONARY SURGERY WITHOUT CARDIOPLEGIA

CARY W. AKINS, M.D.

Surgical revascularization of the myocardium remains the cornerstone of treatment for patients who have significant symptomatic ischemic heart disease, significant obstructing lesions of the left main coronary artery, or triple-vessel disease, or double- or single-vessel disease in which large amounts of myocardium are at risk. Experience with this procedure over the past decade has demonstrated surprisingly low mortality rates, low perioperative infarction rates, and excellent symptomatic results.

Although the majority of cardiac surgeons have converted to some form of hypothermic potassium cardioplegic arrest for myocardial preservation during coronary revascularization, I continue to use a modified form of hypothermic fibrillatory arrest. The same technique is applicable for left ventricular aneurysm resection. The only contraindication to using this technique is significant aortic insufficiency; however, if the aortic insufficiency is severe enough to compromise this method, it probably will require valve replacement.

TECHNIQUE OF HYPOTHERMIC FIBRILLATORY ARREST

Basically the technique of hypothermic fibrillatory arrest arises from a simple hydraulic argument: if the patient can be controlled in a nonischemic state preoperatively, then in the operating room, as long as a perfusion gradient across the myocardium is maintained at a level at least as good as the patient's normal level and the demands for myocardial oxygen consumption are reduced by systemic cooling, the myocardium ought to survive until the ischemic areas can be revascularized.

The technique of operation is based on several principles: (1) proximal vein-to-aorta anastomoses before bypass, (2) systemic hypothermia to 25 to 28° C, (3) local pericardial cooling, (4) maintenance of perfusion pressure at 80 to 100 mm Hg, (5) elective ventricular fibrillation, (6) routine left ventricular venting, (7) avoidance of aortic cross-clamping, (8) local vessel occlusion for vein-to-coronary anastomoses, (9) grafting of the most ischemic zone first, (10) complete revascularization, and (11) addition of mannitol to the bypass priming solution.

There are certain potential advantages of this technique over those associated with hypothermic potassium cardioplegic arrest. One is the avoidance of aortic cross-clamping, which carries a small but definable risk of damage to the ascending aorta, particularly with a heavily calcified aorta. Also, the degree of systemic hypothermia of 25 to 28° C is generally less than that used for cardioplegia techniques, and therefore cooling and rewarming times are shortened. Because the proximal anastomoses are performed prior to the institution of bypass, as each distal anastomosis is completed, that area of the myocardium is now perfused with oxygenated blood. Finally, the technique is particularly useful for emergency revascularization due to acute coronary occlusion, when imposing global cardiac ischemia with an aortic cross-clamp is deleterious to the heart, which already has severe regional ischemia.

Preoperative Preparation

The planning of the revascularization procedure should be completed in detail before the patient arrives in the operating room. The surgeon should decide preoperatively which vessels he plans to revascularize and which conduits he plans to use for each arterial segment. A current coronary arteriogram, performed within at least 6 months, is required. Any area of myocardium that moves must have its blood supply identified. This can, for example, be a problem when anterior wall motion is preserved despite a left anterior descending occlusion, and no distal left anterior descending filling is visible during left coronary angiography. Careful search for collateral blood supply to the left anterior descending artery, especially from the conus branch of the right coronary artery, is required to identify a graftable segment.

Operative Procedure

Vein is harvested from the groin to the calf in most settings. The left internal mammary artery is usually harvested from the underside of the left chest wall and is utilized now in over 90 percent of elective revascularization procedures. I do not routinely use bilateral internal mammary grafts, nor do I regularly use mammary arteries for sequential grafts.

After the vein is harvested, it is carefully distended with the patient's own heparinized blood. Appropriate lengths of vein are measured and divided according to the revascularization plan established before the operation. I generally use a separate piece of vein for each of the three major arterial segments; the right, the left anterior descending, and the circumflex systems. On certain occasions one piece of vein may be used for two systems. The left internal mammary graft is used most commonly for the left anterior descending, its first large diagonal, or the ramus intermedius coronary artery. When sufficient greater saphenous vein cannot be found, my choices of alternate conduits include lesser saphenous vein, the right internal mammary artery or, rarely, thin-walled Goretex.

The operative procedure is begun by heparinization of the patient and cannulation of the ascending aorta. Proximal anastomoses are then performed over a side-biting clamp utilizing one suture of 5-0 polypropylene after a small button of aortic tissue has been removed with a Karp punch.

Cannulation of the atrium for venous drainage is delayed until the proximal anastomoses are completed in order to avoid the onset of atrial fibrillation that may be caused by manipulation of the atrium. Upon completion of the proximal anastomoses, inferior and superior vena caval cannulas are inserted. The patient is placed on cardiopulmonary bypass and cooled systemically to 25 to 28° C. Iced Ringer's lactate solution is dripped over the heart until it fibrillates. The left ventricle is vented via the right superior pulmonary vein utilizing a special vent catheter with a side lumen that directly monitors left ventricular pressure for the perfusionist, who regulates vent flow. The mean aortic perfusion pressure is maintained between 80 to 100 mm Hg by alterations in pump flow or the administration of phenylephrine or sodium nitroprusside.

The goal of the revascularization is to bypass all arteries 1 mm in size or larger that are deemed significantly obstructed. The definition of significant obstruction is dependent not only on diameter reduction by a stenosis but also on the length of stenotic areas and the presence of serial sequential lesions. Those areas of the myocardium that are deemed to be the most ischemic are revascularized first. This technique allows the performance of internal mammary grafts at any time during the procedure and not necessarily at the end. In situations in which occluded arteries are fed by collaterals from other diseased arteries, I generally graft the occluded artery first to provide retrograde flow through the collaterals to the unoccluded artery, so that the myocardium it serves will be perfused while that anastomosis is being performed.

The arterial segment that is judged to be most ischemic is first identified and the area for the anastomosis chosen. Hollow vinyl tapes for proximal and distal control are placed around the artery above and below the area of anastomosis, incorporating some adventitial tissue to minimize arterial damage, and secured to the drapes. An arteriotomy is made, and the inner diameter of the artery is sized with calibrated probes. For sequential anastomoses special care is taken to make sure that the venotomy allows the vein to lie in a smooth course over the artery on its way to the distal anastomosis. The length of a coronary arteriotomy is determined in part by the amount of disease in that coronary, the size of the conduit, and the angle at which the conduit approaches the artery. The usual length is approximately 5 to 10 mm. Arteriotomies for internal mammary grafts are somewhat shorter.

All distal anastomoses are performed using 7-0 polypropylene suture with either five or six stitches and at least two or three interrupted sutures at the apex of every anastomosis. Frequently, the back wall is run in an open fashion to provide the best exposure during the beginning of anastomosis. Before the final suture is tied down, the anastomosis is probed to ensure patency, and blood is vented from the vein graft to avoid embolizing air.

Rewarming is initiated during the final distal anastomosis. Defibrillation is accomplished once the systemic venous return temperature has reached 32° C. Two atrial and two ventricular pacing wires are left on the heart. A left atrial pressure monitoring catheter is inserted through the vent purse-string in the pulmonary vein. The pericardium is routinely left open.

Postoperative Management

In accordance with our current conviction that blood conservation is an important facet of cardiac surgery, the chest tubes left in the pericardial space are connected to an autotransfusion system that is utilized for the first 24 hours. Normovolemic anemia, often to a hematocrit of 20 ml per deciliter, is accepted as long as the patient is well revascularized and has no significant symptoms. Temporary atrial and ventricular pacing wires are routinely removed on the fifth postoperative day, and the patient is discharged a day or two later.

RESULTS OF SURGERY

The results of surgery utilizing this technique have been uniformly satisfactory. For the last 1,300 patients who underwent nonemergency bypass grafting, including those with reoperative revascularization, the mortality rate has been 0.3 percent with a perioperative new Q-wave infarction rate of 0.8 percent.

SUGGESTED READING

Akins CW. Noncardioplegic myocardial preservation for coronary revascularization. J Thorac Cardiovasc Surg 1984; 88:174–181.

Akins CW. Resection of left ventricular aneurysm during hypothermic fibrillatory arrest without aortic occlusion. J Thorac Cardiovasc Surg 1986; 91:610–618.

Akins CW. Early and late results following emergency isolated myocardial revascularization during hypothermic fibrillatory arrest. Ann Thorac Surg 1987; 43:131–137.

Akins CW, Carroll DL. Event-free survival following elective isolated myocardial revascularization during hypothermic fibrillatory arrest. Ann Thorac Surg 1987; 43:628–633.

REOPERATION FOR CORONARY ARTERY DISEASE

DELOS M. COSGROVE III, M.D.

As the number of patients who have undergone primary myocardial revascularization continues to burgeon, potential candidates for a secondary myocardial revascularization procedure have increased exponentially. In the last decade, the number of secondary myocardial revascularizations at The Cleveland Clinic has increased by 435 percent. Currently, 412 reoperative myocardial revascularization procedures represent 18 percent of our total revascularization procedures per year. Assuming that the number of primary procedures remains constant, it can be estimated that approximately 25,000 reoperations for myocardial revascularization will be done in the United States in 1990.

INDICATIONS AND CONTRAINDICATIONS

Percutaneous transluminal coronary angioplasty is a potential alternative to reoperation in patients with stenotic grafts or progression of disease in the native circulation. This option has limited applicability because of the poor long-term results of dilation of stenotic grafts and the potential for embolization of atherosclerotic debris from the vein graft into the native circulation. Percutaneous transluminal coronary angioplasty of the native circulation or of vein grafts in postoperative patients has the added disadvantage of the inability to provide immediate cardiac surgical correction of an anatomic defect produced by this procedure.

The indications for reoperation can be angiographically divided into reoperation for graft failure, progression of disease in the native circulation, and a combination of the two. From 1967 to 1978, 55 percent of our patients were reoperated on for progression of disease in the native circulation. Recently this has been a much less frequent indication, with graft failure, alone or combined, now accounting for 82 percent of reoperative procedures.

Indications for reoperation are the same as those for primary operation, with decisions being made on the basis of the patient's general clinical status, presence of concurrent life-threatening diseases, functional class of angina, coronary anatomy, and left ventricular function. The presence of a patent internal mammary artery graft is not considered a contraindication. The presence of a stenotic vein graft has particular importance in the decision-making process in patients with previous vein grafts. Follow-up of patients with patent but stenotic vein grafts at 1 year demonstrated that 60 percent of these grafts progressed to complete occlusion at a mean follow-up time of 7 years. In a series of vein grafts found to be stenotic but open at a mean time of 7 years, 3 years later 39 percent remained stenotic, stenosis increased in 33 percent, and 28 percent went on to complete occlusion. In 80 patients found to have stenotic vein grafts, the event-free survival was 49 percent at 5 years. Of these 80 patients, 21 percent had myocardial infarction, 26 percent underwent reoperation, and 26 percent died. This suggests that stenotic vein grafts have an unstable natural history and carry a poor prognosis for both graft patency and clinical result. It is therefore important that the presence of a stenotic vein graft be weighed in the decision-making process when reoperation is considered.

Emergency reoperative myocardial revascularization should be avoided. Intensive medical therapy, including Swan-Ganz catheter monitoring, continuous arterial pressure monitoring, and intra-aortic balloon counterpulsation, should be used to alleviate ischemia so that reoperation can be undertaken as an elective procedure.

PERIOPERATIVE MANAGEMENT

Preoperative planning takes on increased importance in patients undergoing reoperative procedures. Drugs affecting platelet function, particularly salicylates, should be discontinued at least 1 week preoperatively. Preoperative banking of autologous blood is advantageous whenever possible.

Anesthetic management is of increased importance in reoperation because the interval from induction of anesthesia to initiation of cardiopulmonary bypass, a period of potential silent ischemia, is increased. A Swan-Ganz catheter and close monitoring of electrocardiographic tracings, including the precordial lead V_5, are valuable adjuncts to help monitor the presence of ischemia.

The lateral chest film shows the proximity of vital cardiac structures to the sternum and can help predict the approximate location of a patent internal mammary artery graft. This helps to evaluate the safety of re-entry. The coronary arteriogram can identify the presence of a patent internal mammary artery graft immediately below the midline of the sternum. In high-risk situations, it is prudent to expose the femoral vessels prior to sternotomy so that cannulation and cardiopulmonary support are readily available in case of hemorrhage at the time of re-entry. If major hemorrhage is encountered during re-entry, cardiopulmonary bypass should be initiated via the femoral vessels and systemic cooling begun. This will reduce blood loss and the potential for myocardial ischemia and facilitate dissection of the heart.

The use of the oscillating saw has greatly reduced the incidence of damage to cardiac structures. The outer table of the sternum is opened first. Upward traction is then exerted on the sternum and the lungs are deflated, allowing cardiac structures to fall posteriorly away from the sternum. The posterior table is opened, and the sternum is dissected from the heart and great vessels using the cautery. The pericardium is incised parallel to the left anterior descending coronary artery. The dissection of the left ventricle is carried out after administration of cardioplegia by sweeping of the surgeon's hand posteriorly and laterally around the apex. An occasional patient may present for reoperation requiring only grafts to the circumflex artery or to a posterior ventricular branch of the right coronary artery. In such situations, a left thoracotomy incision with cardiopulmonary bypass via the femoral vessels provides easy access to the lateral wall of the heart and avoids the potential complications of resternotomy; proximal graft anastomoses in this situation can be placed to the descending thoracic aorta or to the subclavian artery.

Cannulation of the right atrium for venous return may prove hazardous if an atherosclerotic vein graft overlies the atrium. In this situation, a long Silastic catheter placed through the femoral vein allows the patient to be placed on cardiopulmonary bypass at flows up to 3 L per minute. If venous return is inadequate, a second venous cannula may be added after the atherosclerotic vein graft has been interrupted.

The method of treating old patent vein grafts has been controversial, but increasing evidence suggests that all grafts should be replaced at the time of reoperation. Marshall recently demonstrated that angiography underestimates the extent of atherosclerotic involvement of patent vein grafts. He noted that 12 of 13 vein grafts more than 3 years old demonstrated significant atheromatous material covering an average of 35 percent of the intimal surface of the vein grafts, and he recommends replacing all vein grafts more than 3 years old to prevent embolization. The clinical benefit of this approach was demonstrated by Grondin, who significantly reduced the operative mortality rate and incidence of perioperative myocardial infarction by dividing all patent vein grafts at the time of reoperation.

The method for dealing with atherosclerotic vein grafts has been standardized. A "no-touch" technique is employed for all vein grafts. The patient is placed on cardiopulmonary bypass and cooled systemically to 25° C, the aorta cross-clamped, and cardioplegic solution injected. After discontinuation of cardioplegia infusion, and with no antegrade or retrograde flow through the coronary grafts, a scalpel is used to transect the vein graft proximally. The vein grafts are divided distally just prior to the anastomosis to prevent embolization from the vein graft during manipulation. Vein grafts are not clipped or suture ligated in continuity, as this may squeeze atherosclerotic debris into the distal coronary tree. Sequential grafts with thrombosed portions have a similar potential for thrombosis and should be completely replaced. Distal anastomoses are performed first, followed by proximal anastomoses, which are performed with the aorta clamped. The aortic clamp is then removed, allowing blood to flush atherosclerotic debris antegrade and retrograde out of the remaining old vein graft remnants. The graft remnants are then suture ligated.

The internal mammary artery graft is the conduit of choice and is used in 60 percent of the patients undergoing reoperation. Caution is advised when replacing a stenotic vein graft that supplies a large totally obstructed artery. The internal mammary artery may not be able to immediately supply adequate flow, and ischemia may result. When venous conduit is difficult to obtain, the lesser saphenous system is usually present and is of excellent quality. Recent experience with the right gastroepiploic artery suggests that this may be a conduit with long-term patency approaching that of the internal mammary artery. Cephalic vein and Goretex are not used because of their poor long-term patency. There has not yet been sufficient experience to render an opinion regarding the usefulness of cryopreserved venous conduits.

Space on the ascending aorta may be at a premium following previous grafting. The most proximal portion of the vein graft is seldom involved in the atherosclerotic process, and transection of the graft, leaving only a small rim of vein graft, provides an excellent site for proximal anastomosis.

Reoperation in patients with patent internal mammary artery grafts is becoming an increasingly prevalent problem as use of the internal mammary artery at primary operation is increasing. The potential for injury to the internal mammary artery is decreased if, at the time of the original operation, the pericardium is notched, allowing the graft to fall posteriorly away from the sternum. A right internal mammary artery graft crossing the midline is at considerable risk at reoperation. In young patients and patients with a strong possibility of reoperation, use of the right internal mammary artery as a free graft avoids crossing the midline and the associated risk of injury at subsequent reoperation. The internal mammary artery used in this manner has been demonstrated to have a high patency rate and is a graft that is less likely to become atherosclerotic, as compared with vein grafts.

Patients with patent internal mammary artery grafts are approached in a manner similar to that in other coronary reoperations. Two approaches to managing the patent internal mammary artery are then possible. It may be dissected out and clamped, or, more commonly, not exposed at all. In the latter situation, the patient is cooled systemically to 22° C, and pump flow is decreased. This latter maneuver decreases coronary blood flow, facilitating distal anastomoses and preventing rewarming of the myocardium.

Hemostasis is obtained by controlling major bleeding prior to discontinuation of cardiopulmonary bypass. The free edge of the pericardium is run with a continuous suture to enhance hemostasis. Administration of platelets or fresh frozen plasma is not routinely practiced. Fibrin sealant is a useful adjunct to help control diffuse capillary bleeding. The intraoperative collection, processing, and autotransfusion of blood from the operative field have greatly helped to reduce transfusion requirements. Postoperatively shed mediastinal blood is collected in the cardiotomy reservoir and transfused without processing. Careful evaluation of this method of blood conservation has demonstrated no adverse effect on coagulation.

RESULTS

An extensive analysis of the results of reoperative coronary artery surgery was reported by Lytle. Of 1,500 patients operated on between 1967 and 1984, there were 51 deaths, resulting in a 3.4 percent operative mortality rate. Operative mortality rate remained constant throughout that period, as did the perioperative myocardial infarction rate of 8 percent. There was a marked decrease in the reoperation for bleeding rate from 11 percent in the first portion of the series to 4.2 percent in 1982 through 1984 and a similar reduction in the use of blood from 8 U to 2 U in the more recent time frame. In the subset of patients operated on between 1982 and 1984, 81 percent of the deaths were felt to be of cardiac origin. Complications of repeat sternotomy contributed to death in three cases, and four cases of embolization of atherosclerotic debris were noted at operation or postmortem study.

Logistic regression analysis identified left main artery disease, New York Heart Association Functional Class III–IV, and incomplete revascularization at the time of reoperation as the principal factors adversely affecting surgical outcome. Two hundred and fifty-six patients underwent coronary angiography at a mean interval of 39 months postoperatively. Of 349 vein grafts, 70 percent were patent without stenosis. Eighty-nine left internal mammary artery grafts were similarly studied. Ninety-one percent of those were patent with no stenosis.

Reoperative myocardial revascularization for recurrent angina can be accomplished with low morbidity and mortality rates but requires careful preoperative planning and meticulous attention to intraoperative technique.

SUGGESTED READING

Cosgrove DM. Reoperation in patients with patent grafts. J Cardiac Surg 1987; 2:337–342.

Faro RS, Javid H, Najafi H, Serry C. Left thoracotomy for reoperation for coronary revascularization. J Thorac Cardiovasc Surg 1982; 84:453–455.

Grondin DM, Pomar JL, Hebert Y, Bosch X, Santos JM, Enjalbart M, Campeau L. Reoperation in patients with patent atherosclerotic coronary vein grafts. A different approach to a different disease. J Thorac Cardiovasc Surg 1984; 87:379–385.

Lytle BW, Loop FD, Cosgrove DM, Taylor PC, Goormastic M, Peper W, Gill CC, Golding LAR, Stewart RW. Fifteen hundred coronary reoperations: results and determinants of early and late survival. J Thorac Cardiovasc Surg 1987; 93:847–859.

Marshall WG Jr, Saffitz J, Kouchoukos NT. Management during reoperation of aortocoronary saphenous vein grafts with minimal atherosclerosis by angiography. Ann Thorac Surg 1986; 42:163–167.

CORONARY ARTERY SPASM

JOHN R. McCORMICK, M.D.
ARTHUR J. ROBERTS, M.D.

The prevalence of coronary artery spasm as an important pathophysiologic mechanism in patients with coronary heart disease is uncertain. Coronary artery spasm may contribute to a spectrum of clinical presentations, ranging from the patient with normal coronary arteries and variant angina of a stable nature, to the patient with multivessel atherosclerotic coronary artery disease with superimposed coronary artery spasm producing thrombosis and myocardial infarction. In addition, the diagnosis is often imprecise. For example, is the cause of unstable angina occurring at rest frequently coronary artery spasm or some other mechanism? Thus, we must define the subgroups of patients with coronary heart disease that we wish to include within the topic coronary artery spasm.

Prinzmetal, in 1959, identified a group of patients with angina at rest and transient S-T segment elevation and termed the syndrome variant angina. The etiology was thought to be coronary artery spasm. Subsequently, the concept of coronary artery spasm achieved prominence in many investigators' minds to explain the pathogenesis of other clinical presentations of coronary heart disease. We consider that coronary artery spasm occurs in a clinical situation in which angina is more likely to be precipitated by a decreased coronary blood flow than by an increased myocardial oxygen demand. Using this definition, we include within the term coronary artery spasm subgroups of coronary heart patients with (1) classic variant angina, (2) unstable angina with pain at rest and transient, S-T segment elevation or depression, (3) postmyocardial infarction unstable angina meeting the same criteria, and (4) significant S-T segment elevation and hemodynamic compromise after coronary artery bypass graft surgery.

THERAPEUTIC ALTERNATIVES

Stable Classic Variant Angina

Pharmacologic management is the mainstay of treatment. Ninety percent of patients are successfully managed with nitrates and calcium channel blockers, either nifedipine, verapamil, or diltiazem. Beta-adrenergic blockers often have an adverse effect but may be required to decrease myocardial oxygen demand if hemodynamically important fixed coronary artery stenoses are present. Coronary bypass surgery is indicated when important symptoms persist and coronary arteriography demonstrates greater than or equal to 70 percent fixed stenoses in one or more vessels. It is unsuccessful in the few patients with variant angina and normal coronary arteries. Partial sympathetic denervation of the heart as an adjunct to coronary bypass grafting may be considered. Percutaneous transluminal coronary angioplasty represents an alternative method of revascularization and is a competitive procedure to coronary bypass grafting for the patient with single or double vessel coronary artery stenoses.

Unstable Angina

Coronary artery spasm may cause pre- or postmyocardial infarction unstable angina with associated transient S-T segment changes. The diagnosis of spasm in these patients may be elusive, especially if there is a significant amount of concomitant fixed stenoses. The diagnosis

TABLE 1 Coronary Artery Spasm: Results of Surgical Treatment

	University of Florida	*Boston University Medical Center*		
		Stable	*Unstable*	*Postinfarction*
Number of patients	20	9	31	12
Intra-aortic balloon pump	6	0	11	10
Early deaths	1	0	0	3
Late deaths	0	0	0	0
Early myocardial infarction	2	1	6	2
Late myocardial infarction	1	0	2	0
Recurrent angina	6	3*	7*	2*

* Twelve patients in the Boston University Medical Center series had angina at late follow-up examination. Eight were Class 1; two Class 2; and two were Class 3 (Canadian Heart Association).

should be suspected in patients with angina at rest and transient S-T segment elevations. These patients should be admitted to a coronary care unit for intensive pharmacologic management and hemodynamic monitoring. Many require intravenous nitroglycerin to decrease the episodes of unstable angina. If the patient's unstable angina remains refractory to maximum medical therapy, we recommend percutaneous intra-aortic balloon insertion, which is almost uniformly successful in eliminating the unstable angina episodes. All patients should promptly undergo cardiac catheterization to define coronary anatomy, and most will be found suitable for revascularization by either percutaneous transluminal coronary angioplasty or coronary bypass grafting.

Coronary Artery Spasm Postcoronary Bypass Grafting

This complication occurs in less than 1 percent of surgical patients, may produce severe hemodynamic compromise, and is associated with a high mortality rate. The clinical problem is to distinguish between those patients who are experiencing coronary artery spasm and those who are evolving a myocardial infarction from some other cause. If there is S-T segment elevation in the electrocardiographic distribution of a coronary artery that was not diseased and not bypassed, spasm is a likely etiology. S-T segment elevation in the electrocardiographic distribution of a bypassed coronary artery may be caused by spasm in the conduit or the distal native coronary artery. Therapy with intravenous nitroglycerin may be ineffective, and treatment in the operating room must then consist of boluses of intracoronary nitroglycerin given down the bypass grafts (0.1- to 1.0-mg bolus as frequently as required) until the spasm is relieved. If cardiac arrest is imminent in the intensive care unit, the sternotomy incision may be opened and nitroglycerin given directly as described above. Otherwise, emergency cardiac catheterization confirms the diagnosis and permits intracoronary nitroglycerin infusion. Oral nifedipine should also be given (10 mg sublingually during the acute episode); it may be given intraoperatively and should be continued indefinitely.

RESULTS OF SURGICAL TREATMENT

Prior to about 1980, authors generally reported unfavorable results with the surgical treatment of patients with coronary artery spasm, particularly in contrast to the results obtained in chronic stable effort-related angina. However, recent series have demonstrated a more favorable outcome. Our surgical experience at the University of Florida and Boston University Medical Center is summarized in Table 1.

The number of patients is small, but nevertheless, the results obtained support the conclusion that surgical treatment in patients with coronary artery spasm is nearly as effective as coronary bypass surgery in patients in whom spasm is absent. However, the perioperative infarction rate and the incidence of recurrent postoperative angina are higher in the coronary spasm group. Note should be made of the frequent use of the intra-aortic balloon at both institutions (27 out of 72 patients), which we think contributes significantly to the safety of the perioperative management of the unstable patient with coronary artery spasm.

Partial sympathetic denervation as an adjunct to coronary bypass grafting has been advocated by a few groups, with purportedly improved results. We find the data unconvincing, and our understanding of the pathogenesis of coronary artery spasm does not, even theoretically, influence us to use this technique.

SUGGESTED READING

Buxton AE. Perioperative coronary artery spasm. In: Roberts AJ, Conti CR, eds. Current surgery of the heart. Philadelphia: JB Lippincott, 1987:117.

Buxton AE, Goldberg S, Harken A, et al. Coronary-artery spasm as a cause of perioperative myocardial infarction. Jpn Heart J 1984; 25:275–281.

Buxton AE, Hirshfeld JW Jr, Untereker WJ, et al. Perioperative coronary arterial spasm: long-term follow-up. Am J Cardiol 1982; 50:444–451.

Faro RS, Pepine CJ, Roberts AR. Coronary artery spasm: clinical spectrum and results of medical and surgical therapy. In: Roberts AJ, ed. Difficult problems in adult cardiac surgery. Chicago:Year Book, 1985:65.

Schick EC Jr, Davis Z, Lavery RM, et al. Surgical therapy for Prinzmetal's variant angina. Ann Thorac Surg 1982; 33:359–364.

CORONARY REVASCULARIZATION DURING ACUTE MYOCARDIAL INFARCTION

SAMUEL L. SELINGER, M.D.

Catheterization of patients in the first hours following onset of myocardial infarction has demonstrated an 80 percent acute total coronary occlusion rate when chronic coronary disease is converted to transmural myocardial infarction (TMI). Acute evolving myocardial infarction then continues to recruit cell populations until the process is terminated by myocardial scar formation or complicated by continued ischemia, heart failure, and frequently mortality. Most hospital deaths from myocardial infarction are secondary to left ventricular failure. Mortality in hospital survivors is usually related to impaired ventricular function and subsequent ischemic events.

Our approach in Spokane, Washington, since mid-1972 has aimed at resupplying oxygen to the myocardium by administration of adequate coronary blood flow to all ischemic areas. Early myocardial reperfusion was achieved with coronary artery bypass surgery. More recently thrombolytic and/or angioplastic techniques have been added in an attempt at myocardial revascularization.

GOALS

The goals of early coronary artery bypass graft surgery in acute evolving myocardial infarction are to restore adequate blood flow, limit myocardial damage, and offer long-term protection from subsequent ischemia. Since evolving necrosis occurs rapidly, the goal is to be on cardiopulmonary bypass within 6 hours of the onset of pain. This time limit is occasionally extended to 8 hours, particularly in young patients who are suffering from anterior myocardial infarction, in whom the distal left anterior descending artery is visualized by collateral flow. Patients with infarctions due to small coronary artery branch occlusions (circumflex, small right, or diagonals) are not surgical candidates.

Until recently, patients with single as well as multivessel disease were all approached with surgical revascularization. Currently, attempts are being made to open single vessel left anterior descending or right coronary lesions with angioplasty techniques or thrombolytic therapy or both. If these are unsuccessful, the patient may still be a surgical candidate. In general, patients are not turned down because of age, arrhythmias, pulmonary edema, cardiogenic shock, or prior cardiac surgery.

TECHNIQUES

Intra-aortic balloon pump support is used preoperatively when there is shock or anticipated delay in proceeding to the operating room. High-risk patients (prior myocardial infarction in a separate region of the heart, left ventricular end-diastolic pressure greater than 25 mm Hg, cardiac index less than 2, ejection fraction less that 30 percent) have an arterial sheath left in place at the time of cardiac catheterization through which a percutaneous balloon can be introduced if necessary. Emphasis is placed on proceeding rapidly with the heart catheterization and then to cardiopulmonary bypass as soon as possible.

Cardiopulmonary bypass is achieved by ascending aortic cannulation and venous drainage with a single, two-stage atrial cannula through the right atrial appendage. Systemic hypothermia to 24° C is used, unless only a single coronary artery bypass is required. Additional myocardial cooling is achieved with topical 4° C Ringer's and then 4° C oxygenated potassium cardioplegic solution. The major coronary artery supplying the area of infarction is grafted first distally and then proximally. Additional cardioplegia is introduced to achieve cardioplegic arrest beyond the occlusion. In cases of total occlusion of the left anterior descending with poor visualization of the distal artery, it is usually prudent to graft the major diagonal vessel as well. Other major vessels with significant obstructions are then grafted in a similar fashion. Although internal mammary artery grafts provide a better long-term conduit than saphenous veins, the additional time to take down the internal mammary artery is not usually justified in the face of acute progressive myocardial necrosis, with the main exception being the lack of available vein conduits. We do not routinely explore the proximal artery for thrombus but remove the thrombus if it appears at the arteriotomy site. The aorta is vented through the cardioplegia needle whenever cardioplegia is not being delivered. Atrial and ventricular pacing wires and a left atrial pressure line are always placed. The pericardium is drained and closed. Persistent postoperative hypotension in the presence of adequate right and left ventricular filling pressures is initially treated with an intra-aortic balloon pump, then inotropic agents.

RESULTS

If early reperfusion of acute evolving myocardial infarction can limit the extent of infarction, there should be lower mortality in comparison to patients treated with conventional therapy, preservation of ventricular function, and a low incidence of subsequent ischemia. Our results are based on concurrent nonrandomized clinical studies of comparable groups undergoing surgical reperfusion and conventional therapy.

Mortality

Medical and surgical groups were similar in age, evidence of previous myocardial infarction, coronary anatomy, and clinical classification. In-hospital mortality of the conventionally treated group was 11.5 percent compared with 5.8 percent for the surgical group. If shock patients are excluded, medical mortality was 9.3 percent, significantly different than the surgical mortality of 1.2 percent.

Early surgery within 6 hours of symptom onset had a 2 percent in-hospital mortality compared with 11.5 percent for conventional therapy. At 36 months mean follow-up, the mortality difference widened to 6 percent versus 20.5 percent. At 10 years mean follow-up, the mortality was 18 percent for the surgery group compared with 40 percent for the conventional group. These data suggest that early reperfusion results in significantly lower in-hospital and long-term mortality than does conventional therapy.

Acute anterior myocardial infarction has a higher mortality than inferior myocardial infarction. In-hospital mortality for surgically treated anterior myocardial infarction patients was 7 percent and for conventionally treated patients, 16.5 percent. Surgical revascularization of anterior myocardial infarction without shock resulted in a mortality of 1.3 percent. The mortality difference at 10 years mean follow-up was 28 percent for early surgical revascularization and 50 percent for conventional therapy of acute anterior myocardial infarction. Unlike the findings for early revascularization, there was no significant in-hospital mortality difference between late revascularization and conventional therapy of anterior myocardial infarction. However, at 10-year mean follow-up, late (6 to 24 hour) revascularization, like early reperfusion, was significantly better than conventional treatment. Thus, coronary artery bypass grafting would appear to provide excellent long-term protection in anterior myocardial infarctions, even if performed later than 6 hours.

Left Ventricular Function

If early reperfusion results in salvage of myocardial muscle, this should be reflected in wall motion studies. Patients with early revascularization were placed on bypass in a mean of 4.8 hours compared with 9.2 hours for late revascularization patients. The early group had a significantly better mean initial ejection fraction (48 percent versus 42 percent), which then improved significantly to a mean of 53 percent. Late revascularization failed to significantly improve global ejection fraction. Additionally, in early reperfusion, the regional ventricular function was more likely to improve in the segments affected by the infarction process. Those patients who did respond in the late group exhibited either nontotal coronary occlusion of the left anterior descending artery or major coronary collateral perfusion distal to the occluded vessel. Thus, there was significant improvement in global and regional function in patients with anterior transmural myocardial infarction who received reperfusion within 6 hours of symptom onset. Contractile impairment below the normal range frequently remained, however, even if reperfusion was performed early.

Anginal Classification

Significant angina pectoris has been reported to occur in 40 to 50 percent of conventionally managed patients following myocardial infarction. Six-year follow-up studies of surgically treated acute myocardial infarction indicates that 70 percent of the patients are free of any angina, and 25 percent reported angina only with maximum exercise. Thus, coronary artery bypass for acute myocardial infarction appears to offer sustained relief of chest pain and avoidance of postinfarction angina in most patients.

NONTRANSMURAL MYOCARDIAL INFARCTION

Although short-term survival of patients with nontransmural myocardial infarction is better than for those suffering from transmural myocardial infarction, these patients have a similar long-term mortality. Coronary angiography in nontransmural myocardial infarction reveals a higher prevalence of triple-vessel disease and less total occlusion than is found in transmural myocardial infarction. Despite more multivessel involvement, in-hospital mortality for surgical reperfusion of nontransmural myocardial infarction (3 percent) was lower than in the transmural myocardial infarction group. At a mean follow-up time of 4.3 years, total mortality was only 6.5 percent. Even nontransmural myocardial infarction subset patients with triple-vessel disease that was revascularized experienced a 4.2 percent in-hospital mortality and an 8.4 percent total mortality at 4.3 years mean. Fairly stable survival curves indicate that bypass surgery in the presence of multivessel disease offers some protection against subsequent fatal cardiac events. As in the previously discussed transmural group, mortality with surgical treatment in this group was lower than in those receiving conventional therapy for nontransmural myocardial infarction. With its lower level of early myocardial damage, nontransmural myocardial infarction offers superb potential for myocardial preservation, even with multivessel disease.

ALTERNATIVES IN REPERFUSION THERAPY

The current techniques for early coronary reperfusion include thrombolytic therapy, angioplasty, and surgery. The availability and current growth of angioplasty and thrombolytic therapy have certainly changed the patient population that we are surgically revascularizing. Angioplasty, which can be performed at the initial cardiac catheterization, has been particularly suitable for single-vessel disease; in multivessel disease, it is usually performed on the artery of the distribution that is ischemic, leaving other critically narrowed arteries to subsequent therapy. Today, the major patient population that we are surgically revascularizing on an acute basis includes patients with multivessel disease with the acute artery totally occluded; additionally, we are revascularizing some patients with a totally occluded single vessel if this vessel has not responded to angioplasty dilation. The addition of angioplasty in the treatment of acute infarction usually means that if the patient is subsequently referred to surgery because of angioplasty failure, the time from infarction onset until cardiopulmonary bypass is prolonged, possibly increasing morbidity and mortality.

We have early experience with patients who have required surgery following failed thrombolytic therapy. We have revascularized a few patients acutely following intracoronary administration of up to 250,000 units of streptokinase, but we prefer not to operate acutely if a higher dose has been used.

Coronary bypass surgery can be performed on all vessels with major occlusions with low reocclusion rates. It is particularly suitable for multivessel disease, the single occluded left anterior descending artery unresponsive to other therapy, and patients who are too unstable from cardiogenic shock or multiple life-threatening arrhythmias for other therapy.

CONCLUSION

Early surgical revascularization of acute myocardial infarction can be performed with low mortality and morbidity. Long-term follow-up evaluation indicates low rates of angina, reinfarction, and death as well as improved global and regional ejection fractions in those patients who have been revascularized within 6 hours of symptom onset. These long-term results are consistent with revascularization on a less emergent basis, confirming the concept of total revascularization.

Recently, angioplasty and thrombolysis techniques have been developed to provide reperfusion (but not necessarily total revascularization). These therapies are all potentially complementary but must be applied early to be effective. Our results support the concept that contractile impairment at the time of successful intervention is a major determinant not only of short-term mortality but also of long-term progressive mortality. The determination of which therapy or combination of therapies will result in the lowest mortality and morbidity remains a major challenge.

SUGGESTED READING

Berg R Jr, Selinger SL, Leonard JJ, Coleman WS, DeWood MA. Acute evolving myocardial infarction a surgical emergency. Thorac Cardiovasc 1984; 88:902–906.

DeWood MA, Spores J, Berg R Jr, Kendall RW, Grunwald RP, Selinger SL, Hensley GR, Sutherland KI, Shields JP. Acute myocardial infarction: a decade of experience with surgical reperfusion in 701 patients. Circulation 1983; Suppl III:13–24.

DeWood MA, Spores J, Heit J, Berg R Jr, Selinger SL, Rudy LW, Hensley GR, Shields JP. Anterior transmural myocardial infarction. The effects of surgical reperfusion on global and regional left ventricular function. J Am Coll Cardiol 1983; 1:1223–1234.

Selinger SL, Berg R Jr, Leonard JJ, Coleman WS, DeWood MA. Surgical intervention in acute myocardial infarction. Bull Tex Heart Instit 1984; 11:44–51.

Selinger SL, Berg R Jr, Leonard JJ, Coleman WS, DeWood MA. Coronary bypass surgery in evolving acute myocardial infarction. In: Roberts A, ed. Difficult problems in adult cardiac surgery. Chicago: Year Book, 1985.

CARDIOGENIC SHOCK

JOHN M. MORAN, M.D.
ARUN K. SINGH, M.D., F.R.C.S.(C)

Circulatory shock is a condition caused by reduction in blood flow to various bodily tissues, which in turn results in inadequate oxygen delivery to meet metabolic demands; this occurs in spite of physiologic compensatory mechanisms. "Cardiogenic shock" is a term used to describe such a clinical condition, which results from inadequate pumping function of the heart. Cardiogenic shock is most often caused by transmural myocardial infarction, but it may also result from other causes of cardiac dysfunction, including myocarditis, pulmonary embolism, cardiac tamponade, and intractable ventricular arrhythmias. Acute transmural myocardial infarction is followed in 10 to 15 percent of cases by cardiogenic shock, which in turn carries a mortality rate of 75 to 100 percent if not properly treated. The emphasis in this chapter is on the prompt institution of various treatment alternatives that may interrupt the cycle of infarct extension, further reduction of cardiac output, additional decreases in tissue perfusion, and further extension of infarction. A plan of action based on a knowledge of cardiac physiology and pharmacology helps to decrease mortality in this highly lethal disease.

INITIAL MANAGEMENT

The prompt institution of monitoring, usually in the emergency room setting, is the first and immediate priority. A baseline 12-lead electrocardiogram followed by institution of on-line electrocardiographic monitoring, establishment of venous access for monitoring of central pressure and drug administration, and insertion of a Foley catheter, an intra-arterial needle, and a pulmonary artery catheter (Swan-Ganz) should all be done quickly when cardiogenic shock is suspect or evident. If significant bradycardia or heart block is present, either a transvenous pacing catheter or a pacing Swan-Ganz catheter should be placed. Baseline arterial blood gas and electrolyte determinations should be obtained. An adequate airway must be assured and oxygen delivered initially by face mask. If ventilation is inadequate with a Pco_2 greater than 50 mm Hg, or if the patient is desaturated while breathing supplemental oxygen, careful endotracheal intubation and mechanical ventilation should be considered. Positive end expiratory pressure should b~ added as needed to improve oxygenation.

An initial chest x-ray film should be obtained to assess the presence of pulmonary congestion and pleural effusion. If the cardiac index is below 2 L per minute per square meter and the pulmonary vasculature is not congested, intravascular volume expansion is the first line of treatment (to be discussed). However, if the lung fields are congested while the patient is in a low output state, inotropic agents, vasodilators, diuretics, and possibly the intra-aortic balloon pump must be considered, in that order. If the patient is relatively unstable with hypotension, the blood pressure can be raised by infusion of norepinephrine or dopamine or both, which can be titrated up or down as further diagnostic information and cardiac output data become available.

Intravascular volume depletion that may accompany cardiogenic shock may require vigorous therapy. Volume replacement should be directed by the pulmonary capillary wedge pressure, which, if below 15 mm Hg, should indicate volume replacement to the point of achieving a pressure of approximately 20 mm Hg. Five percent albumin or hetastarch is preferred to increase intravascular volume. Once intravascular volume is satisfactory, further drug therapy or mechanical support or both should be considered if needed. Low doses of morphine sulfate (4 to 8 mg) should be given intravenously for pain control and to alleviate anxiety, thus minimizing sympathetic overstimulation and its deleterious effects on heart rate and systemic vascular resistance.

DRUG THERAPY FOR CARDIOGENIC SHOCK

Considerations for drug therapy in cardiogenic shock include inotropic and vasoactive agents. Dopamine is one of the most widely used therapeutic agents in treating cardiogenic shock because of its unique spectrum of action. At low doses (2 to 5 μg per kilogram per minute) it produces vasodilation of the splanchnic, renal, coronary, and cerebrovascular circulatory beds. At higher doses (6 to 15 μg per kilogram per minute) it increases myocardial contractility by virtue of beta-stimulation. At even higher doses (20 μg per kilogram per minute), it becomes a generalized alpha-stimulating agent, causing peripheral vasoconstriction. For use in cardiogenic shock, 10 to 15 μg per kilogram per minute often increases cardiac output with little effect on peripheral resistance; it has beneficial vasodilatory effects on renal blood flow, which may be of major significance under these circumstances. At higher doses, it may adversely affect myocardial oxygen consumption with the risk of extending myocardial damage and arrhythmias; hence, it is important to use the lowest possible dose that will produce satisfactory hemodynamic improvement.

Norepinephrine may also produce beta$_1$ as well as alpha actions. At low doses, beta activity predominates, whereas at higher doses it may produce vasoconstriction. This agent is generally used to manage hypotension, particularly early in the course of management while further invasive hemodynamic monitoring is being achieved. The usual initial dose is 2 to 8 μg per minute, administered through a central catheter.

Dobutamine is a relatively new agent that acts primarily on beta$_1$ adrenergic receptors. It may be an alternative to dopamine, and it may produce fewer chronotropic and arrhythmogenic effects.

Isoproterenol is a pure beta adrenergic agonist that augments myocardial contractility and increases heart rate. It causes peripheral vasodilation and thus may lower blood pressure in spite of improving cardiac output. It has been well documented that its potent inotropic and chronotropic effects actually increase myocardial oxygen demand and may lead to extension of myocardial necrosis; it also may be arrhythmogenic. For these reasons, isoproterenol is rarely useful in the treatment of cardiogenic shock.

Epinephrine is also a potent beta- agonist that causes splanchnic and renal vasoconstriction and thus has an unfavorable influence on the redistribution of cardiac output. In higher doses it may also be arrhythmogenic and thus potentially hazardous for the treatment of cardiogenic shock.

In summary, the initial choices for inotropic therapy in cardiogenic shock are first dopamine, followed by norepinephrine, if needed; both of these drugs exert potent inotropic effects and can favorably affect the redistribution of blood flow toward the heart, brain, and kidney. It must be remembered that not all patients react in a predictable fashion in cardiogenic shock and that there must be ample latitude for switching drugs empirically to find the most beneficial effects on cardiac output and systemic vascular resistance in any given patient.

The need for diuretic therapy should be considered when treatment of hypovolemia and hypotension makes its use safe. If given prematurely, diuretics may only worsen tissue perfusion and the shock state. The most commonly used intravenous drugs include furosemide and ethacrynic acid. The lowest dose that results in a desired response should be used, and a urinary output of 40 to 50 ml per minute is sufficient. These drugs have potent effects in diminishing pulmonary congestion and in reducing myocardial oxygen demand by decreasing heart size.

There is little room for digitalization in acute cardiogenic shock; the maximum inotropic effect of digitalis is less than that of catecholamines, and in the low output state, hypoxia and acidosis may predispose to digitalis-induced arrhythmias. However, digitalis is indicated for treating supraventricular arrhythmias, and this is probably the only setting in which it should be used acutely.

The physiologic basis for vasodilator therapy in cardiogenic shock is to alter cardiac preload and afterload in a manner that favorably affects myocardial oxygen supply and demand and possibly to reduce the extent of infarction. Vasodilator therapy should not be used routinely, but may be of benefit in patients without severe hypotension and with evidence of excessive vasoconstriction despite adequate volume replacement. In addition, in cardiogenic shock associated with severe, acute mitral regurgitation, vasodilator therapy may help reduce the regurgitant fraction and improve forward cardiac output. The most commonly used drug for this purpose is nitroprusside, which acts directly on vascular smooth muscle, causing both arterial and venous dilatation. The drug is administered intravenously through a central line starting at 0.5 μg per kilogram per minute and gradually increasing as dictated by hemodynamic measurements and clinical response.

TREATMENT OF ARRHYTHMIAS

Any arrhythmia that occurs in a patient with cardiogenic shock can cause further hemodynamic deterioration unless it is promptly treated. Arrhythmias seen in this setting run the entire gamut of atrial and ventricular dysrhythmias, from sinus tachycardia to torsade de pointes and ventricular fibrillation. All are treatable, and usually successfully so, unless the extent of left ventricular damage is so severe as to preclude survival. The mainstay of treatment for ventricular ectopia or bursts of ventricular tachycardia is lidocaine, as an intravenous bolus dose of 50 to 100 mg, followed by an infusion at 2 to 4 mg per minute. If this is ineffective, intravenous procainamide or disopyramide may be utilized. If these agents are ineffective or only partially effective, the use of intravenous amiodarone should be considered. Atrial dysrhythmias including fibrillation may precede or follow the development of cardiogenic shock. All have a deleterious effect on cardiac output and should be corrected as soon as possible by the use of the usual pharmacologic methods or, if needed, by cardioversion. If complete heart block develops, atrioventricular sequential pacing is extremely effective in improving the hemodynamic situation. Occasionally in a patient who can otherwise be treated successfully for cardiogenic shock, recurrent and intractable ventricular tachycardia may emerge as a primary problem. The need for specific antiarrythmic surgery is unusual but not rare within the first 2 weeks after myocardial infarction. Ideally, this takes the form of intraoperative mapping and endocardial resection of the postinfarction scar, after appropriate electrophysiologic studies have been performed in the laboratory; details of these techniques are outlined in the chapter *Recurrent Ventricular Tachycardia: Surgical Management.*

MECHANICAL CIRCULATORY ASSISTANCE

Consideration of intra-aortic balloon pumping (IABP) should enter the plan of action for treatment of cardiogenic shock at an early stage if the previously mentioned resuscitative pharmacologic measures are either minimally or not effective. This modality is readily available in most major medical centers and, where it is not available, rapid transporation of the patient to such a center should be arranged. Because of the surgical implications of cardiogenic shock, all efforts should be made to transfer such patients to an institution where cardiac surgery can be promptly performed if necessary.

Over the past 2 decades a variety of methods of mechanical circulatory assistance have been investigated. In addition to IABP these have included partial cardiopulmonary bypass with extracorporeal membrane oxygenation, left ventricular assist devices on occasion adapted to assist the failing right ventricle, use of the total artificial heart, and cardiac transplantation.

Approximately half the patients with inferior myocardial infarction have significant right ventricular involvement. Cardiogenic shock due primarily to right ventricular infarction may occur in up to 5 percent of all patients with infarctions and manifests with much the same clinical picture; in its most pure form, pulmonary capillary wedge pressures may be normal, whereas central venous pressure may reach 20 to 25 mm Hg. Bradycardias are common, including heart block, and atrioventricular sequential pacing may be effective. There has recently been a developing interest in pulmonary artery balloon counterpulsation to assist the failing right side of the heart when all the usual methods fail. There is growing awareness that effective pulmonary artery balloon counterpulsation may take over approximately half the function of the right ventricle, much as IABP does for the left ventricle. The device has been utilized on occasion in the perioperative setting when right-sided heart failure has been accurately diagnosed; an intra-aortic balloon has been placed in the pulmonary artery via a graft sewn to the pulmonary artery. Work is proceeding on a pulmonary artery balloon that is tailored anatomically to the human pulmonary artery and on percutaneous methods of inserting such a balloon designed for use in the nonoperative setting.

ANGIOPLASTY AND THROMBOLYTIC THERAPY

Balloon angioplasty for selected patients with appropriate coronary anatomy has been widely practiced in recent years. There are early reports of patients who have been resuscitated from a shock state, some of whom have subsequently gone on to surgery. Similarly, there are isolated reports of patients who have undergone thrombolytic therapy with streptokinase and experienced reversal of potentially lethal cardiogenic shock. Studies are currently under way that are designed to evaluate the combination of these methods in the treatment of early myocardial infarction with and without shock. The results to date are inconclusive.

EMERGENCY SURGERY FOR CARDIOGENIC SHOCK

Patients who have not responded well to the foregoing methods of treatment of cardiogenic shock should be considered for urgent surgery following cardiac catheterization and coronary angiography. Cardiac catheterization in acutely ill patients in cardiogenic shock, with IABP, can be done safely. The value of this study is apparent when it is realized that over 50 percent of patients undergoing catheterization become surgical candidates. The surgically remediable conditions that may be revealed by catheterization include:

1. Proximal coronary stenoses with good quality bypassable distal vessels. Variable degrees of ventricular dysfunction are present, and considerable judgment is required to distinguish reversible akinesis due to a "stunned" myocardium from irreversible transmural infarction. Often a thallium perfusion scan helps to distinguish viable from dead myocardium in this respect. Early surgery in this difficult group of patients produces at least 50 percent survival, and if revascularization is carried out within 12 to 16 hours after the onset of symptoms, survival can approach 75 to 80 percent.
2. Significant mitral insufficiency. This may be due to papillary muscle dysfunction, papillary muscle rupture,

or simply to left ventricular dilation with consequent dilatation of the mitral valve annulus and central regurgitation. Particularly in the case of papillary muscle rupture, the onset of cardiogenic shock may be catastrophic; nearly 70 percent of patients die within 24 hours. Aggressive treatment with IABP support and emergency operation produces early survival approaching 70 percent, with early and late results dependent on preoperative ventricular function. The early surgical management of acute mitral regurgitation is discussed further in the chapter *Acute and Chronic Mitral Regurgitation in the Ischemic Heart.*

3. Rupture of the interventricular septum. Frank cardiogenic shock occurs in at least 50 percent of these patients. Short-term improvement can be achieved with IABP support, but urgent operation is required as soon as the diagnosis has been made. With contemporary techniques of surgery and myocardial protection, survival rates as high as 67 percent have been reported. This is outlined further in the next chapter.
4. Free wall myocardial rupture and/or false ventricular aneurysm. If the typical syndrome of rupture with tamponade occurs, surgery may be performed as a salvage attempt, without cardiac catheterization, and with a high operative mortality rate.

Unfortunately, in up to half of the patients undergoing cardiac catheterization for cardiogenic shock, global hypokinesis or severe distal disease or both are encountered, and therefore surgery may be contraindicated. In the various groups of patients who are candidates for surgery, the results are sufficiently satisfactory to encourage continuing efforts and aggressive surgical therapy. Important points that have emerged are early surgery rather than delay, since there is often little improvement with medical treatment and deterioration of vital organ function occurs; an aggressive approach designed not only to correct mechanical lesions but also to provide for complete revascularization; and, frequently, mechanical support during the perioperative period.

SUGGESTED READING

Buckley MJ. Surgery for acute myocardial infarction: evolution and current status. In: Moran JM, Michaelis LL, eds. Surgery for the complications of myocardial infarction. New York: Grune & Stratton, 1980:247.

Dunkman WB, Leinbach RC, Buckley MJ, et al. Clinical and hemodynamic results of intraaortic balloon pumping and surgery for cardiogenic shock. Circulation 1972; 46:465–477.

Johnson SA, Scanlon PJ, Loeb HS, et al. Treatment of cardiogenic shock in myocardial infarction by intra-aortic counterpulsation and surgery. Am J Med 1977; 62:687–692.

Laks H, Rosenkranz E, Buckberg GD. Surgical treatment of cardiogenic shock after myocardial infarction. Circulation 1986; 74(Suppl III):11–16.

Mueller HS, Evans RJ, Ayers SM. Effects of dopamine on hemodynamics and myocardial metabolism in shock following acute myocardial infarction in man. Circulation 1978; 57:361–365.

POSTINFARCTION VENTRICULAR SEPTAL RUPTURE

MARSHALL L. JACOBS, M.D.
WILLARD M. DAGGETT Jr., M.D.

Ventricular septal rupture occurs through a zone of necrotic myocardium, complicating acute myocardial infarction in 1 to 2 percent of cases. It is most likely to occur within the first 10 to 14 days following infarction. In the majority of cases, septal rupture occurs as a complication of an individual's first myocardial infarction.

The recognition that postinfarction ventricular septal rupture usually constitutes a surgical emergency has been associated with increasingly favorable results in the management of this difficult lesion. Historical references indicate that without aggressive surgical management, approximately one-fourth of patients die within the first 24 hours, more than one-half die within the first week, and more than three-quarters die within the first month. Having adopted an approach that involves early surgical correction, we have achieved and reported a 75 percent hospital survival rate among patients treated since 1975.

PREOPERATIVE ASSESSMENT

The presence of a new systolic murmur or the sudden onset of congestive heart failure within the first week to 10 days following an acute myocardial infarction should raise the suspicion of ventricular septal rupture. Approximately one-half of patients have recurrent chest pain, and about one-half are noted to be in cardiogenic shock. The differential diagnosis includes postinfarction ventricular septal rupture and acute mitral regurgitation secondary to papillary muscle rupture. Right heart catheterization with a Swan-Ganz catheter is useful in differentiating between these two problems and in monitoring the patient's hemodynamics. An oxygen saturation step-up from right atrium to pulmonary artery is noted. The use of pharmacologic therapy to improve cardiac output is adjunctive. In our experience the institution of intra-aortic balloon pump support, which increases cardiac output and coronary perfusion pressure and decreases the left-to-right shunt, is the mainstay of preoperative therapy. Patients are taken expeditiously to the cardiac catheterization laboratory, where left heart catheterization with ventriculography and coronary angiography are performed to clarify issues of ventricular wall motion, coronary obstructive lesions, and valvular dysfunction, and to confirm the diagnosis of ventricular septal rupture. Early operation for patients with hemodynamic instability is essential to achieve the best operative survival. Gaudiani, Hill, and others have similarly stressed the importance of early surgical intervention before the development of multisystem failure.

OPERATIVE TECHNIQUE

Techniques for closure of postinfarction ventricular septal rupture have evolved based on the following eight principles: (1) expeditious establishment of hypothermic total cardiopulmonary bypass and meticulous attention to myocardial protection; (2) transinfarction approach to the ventricular septal defect with the site of left ventriculotomy determined by the location of transmural infarction; (3) thorough debridement of the left ventricular margins of the infarct back to viable muscle to prevent delayed rupture of the ventricular closure; (4) conservative debridement of right ventricular muscle as required for complete visualization of the margins of the ventricular septal defect; (5) inspection of the papillary muscles and concomitant replacement of the mitral valve only if there is frank papillary muscle rupture; (6) closure of the ventricular septal defect without tension, which in most instances requires the use of prosthetic material; (7) closure of the infarctectomy without tension with generous use of prosthetic material as necessary and epicardial placement of the patch to the free wall to avoid strain on the friable endocardial tissue; and (8) buttressing of suture lines with pledgets or strips of Teflon felt or similar material to prevent sutures from cutting through friable muscle. Details of the surgical techniques for anterior, apical, and inferoposterior defects all adhere to these eight principles.

Anterior Defects

Small anterior septal defects can be closed by approximation of the septum to the right ventricular free wall, using a row of interrupted mattress sutures buttressed with strips of Teflon felt. Closure of the ventriculotomy is accomplished with a similar row of mattress sutures and Teflon felt strips. Larger anterior septal defects require a prosthetic patch to avoid tension, which could lead to disruption of the repair (Fig. 1). Felt pledgeted sutures are placed through the remaining septum and through the right ventricular free wall. Each is then passed through the patch and through an additional pledget before all are tied. The patch is thus secured on the left ventricular side of the septum. The remaining infarctectomy defect in the anterior wall of the left ventricle is closed by approximating the edges of the ventriculotomy with interrupted mattress sutures buttressed with strips of Teflon felt. An additional over-and-over suture assures hemostasis.

Apical Defects

After incision through the area of apical infarction, the debridement of necrotic myocardium results in amputation of the apical portion of the left ventricle and septum. In most instances, the reconstruction can be accomplished by simple reapproximation of the remaining margins of the right and left ventricular free walls to the apical septum. A row of interrupted mattress sutures is placed through a strip of felt, the left ventricular wall, a second strip of felt, the septum, a third strip of felt, the right ventricular wall, and a fourth strip of felt. The sutures are then tied, and the repair is completed with an additional over-and-over running suture.

Inferoposterior Septal Defects

Occurrence of ventricular septal rupture following inferior infarction has been associated with higher mortality than anterior infarction because of the greater technical challenge of successfully managing inferoposterior defects. Early attempts at primary closure were associated with a higher incidence of failure due to intraoperative or early postoperative disruption of the repair. The soft myocardium would not hold even buttressed sutures that of necessity were tied under tension. Analysis of such early experiences led to the evolution of the eight principles previously outlined. An operative technique has been devised by Daggett based on these principles, which has resulted in dramatic improvement in operative survival of patients with inferoposterior septal rupture. Retraction of the heart and inspection of the inferior wall are accomplished before crossclamping. Then, after cardioplegic arrest, the left ventricular portion of the infarct is excised, affording visualization of the septal defect. Left-sided papillary muscles are inspected. If there is frank necrosis or rupture of a papillary muscle, mitral valve replacement is accomplished through a conventional left atrial approach to avoid tearing of ventricular muscle during exposure of the mitral valve. In most instances, the papillary muscles and mitral chordal apparatus are intact. All infarcted left

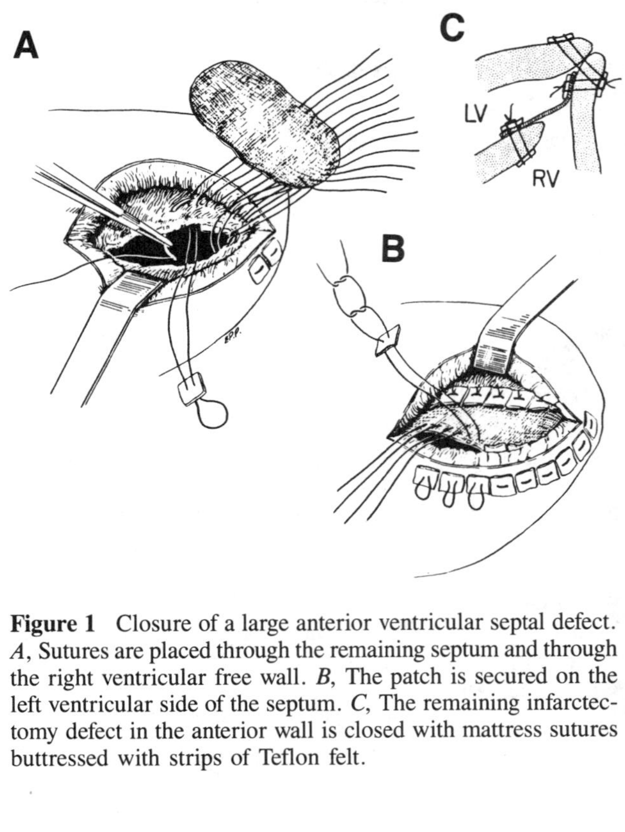

Figure 1 Closure of a large anterior ventricular septal defect. *A*, Sutures are placed through the remaining septum and through the right ventricular free wall. *B*, The patch is secured on the left ventricular side of the septum. *C*, The remaining infarctectomy defect in the anterior wall is closed with mattress sutures buttressed with strips of Teflon felt.

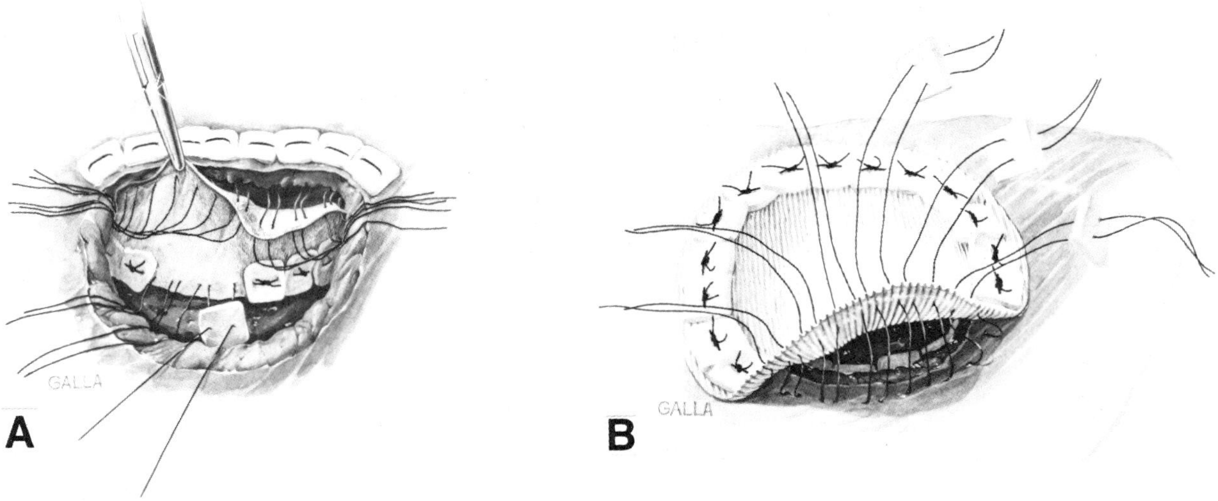

Figure 2 Closure of a large inferior ventricular septal defect. *A*, A prosthetic septal patch is secured with pledgeted mattress sutures. *B*, The infarctectomy is closed with a second patch of prosthetic material.

ventricular muscle should be debrided. Debridement of right ventricular muscle is more conservative. Delayed right ventricular rupture has not been a problem.

The smallest inferior septal defects can be closed by approximating the septum to the right ventricular free wall using mattress sutures and strips of felt. Larger defects require a prosthetic septal patch (Fig. 2). Pledgeted mattress sutures are placed from the right ventricular side of the septum and from the epicardial side of the right ventricular free wall. All sutures are passed through the perimeter of the patch and through additional pledgets before they are tied. Thus, again, the patch is secured to the left side of the interventricular septum. To avoid tension, the infarctectomy must be closed with a second epicardial patch of prosthetic material. Felt pledgeted mattress sutures are placed around the perimeter of the infarctectomy, having been placed from the endocardial to the epicardial surface of the ventricles. In the region where the septal patch joins the right ventricle, this row of sutures is passed through the septal patch and then out through the epicardial surface of the right ventricle. A woven Dacron patch that has been preclotted by heat fixation with serum albumin is tailored to overlap the infarctectomy. The sutures are passed through the edge of that patch and tied over additional pledgets. This results in epicardial placement of the patch, avoiding strain on the friable endocardial tissue.

Associated Coronary Bypass Surgery

In general, major coronary arteries not associated with the region of acute infarction are bypassed at the time of repair if they have high-grade stenoses and if the distal vessels are of satisfactory quality. To preserve anterior right ventricular function in patients with very proximal occlusion of the right coronary artery, we recommend direct revascularization of the acute marginal branch of this artery if it is not in continuity with more distal right coronary grafts.

RESULTS

An aggressive, early operative approach has resulted in overall hospital survival of 75 percent in our institution. The survival of patients with cardiogenic shock has improved dramatically to approximately 67 percent by comparison to earlier experiences in which surgery was often delayed. Anatomic location of the septal defect has remained a significant determinant of hospital mortality. Surgically treated anterior septal ruptures had a 15 percent hospital mortality rate; posterior defects resulted in a 34 percent mortality rate.

Long-term results are favorable; for patients surviving hospitalization, approximately 85 percent are alive at 5 years, with most patients in New York Heart Association Functional Class I or II.

SUGGESTED READING

Daggett WM. Surgical technique for early repair of posterior ventricular septal rupture. J Thorac Cardiovasc Surg 1982; 84:219–223.

Daggett WM, Buckley MJ, Akins CW, Leinback RC, Gold HK, Block PC, Austen WG. Improved results of surgical management of postinfarction ventricular septal rupture. Ann Surg 1982; 196:269–277.

Gaudiani VA, Miller DC, Stinson EB, et al. Postinfarction ventricular septal defect: an argument for early operation. Surgery 1981; 89:48–55.

Heitmiller R, Jacobs ML, Dagget WM. Surgical management of postinfarction ventricular septal rupture. Ann Thorac Surg 1986; 41:683–691.

Hill D, Lary D, Kerth W, Gerbode F. Acquired ventricular septal defects. J Thorac Cardiovasc Surg 1975; 70:440–450.

Sanders RJ, Kern WH, Blount SG. Perforation of the interventricular septum complicating myocardial infarction. Am Heart J 1956; 51:736–748.

COMBINED CAROTID AND CORONARY ARTERY DISEASE

ELLIS L. JONES, M.D.

The relationship between extracranial carotid disease and coronary artery disease is reflected by the incidence of myocardial infarction following carotid endarterectomy and by the devastating effects of neurologic injury that sometimes occur after routine coronary bypass surgery. The incidence of significant carotid disease in candidates for myocardial revascularization has been reported to be between 5 and 15 percent. Because of the association between carotid and coronary disease, the fear of infarction following isolated carotid endarterectomy, and the concern for neurologic injury after coronary bypass, there has been a recent trend to standardize the surgical approach to patients with both conditions. Some surgeons have advocated combined operations, anticipating that risk and mortality factors will be similar to those of coronary or carotid surgery alone; others have recommended the staging of certain categories of patients with coronary and carotid disease and combining operations only when definite clinical indications exist.

HISTORIC PERSPECTIVE AND CLINICAL EVALUATION

Fatal myocardial infarction after isolated carotid endarterectomy has been reported to occur with a frequency that varies from 1 percent in patients without history of coronary disease to 7 percent in patients with known coronary disease, and even as high as 17 percent in patients with unstable angina.

Perioperative stroke constitutes a major potential risk of both carotid endarterectomy and myocardial revascularization; in experienced hands, this risk should not exceed 2 to 3 percent following isolated endarterectomy. The reported incidence of neurologic injury after coronary bypass is just under 1 percent in our own series of patients having coronary surgery alone; this incidence rises with the increasing age of the bypass patient population. The etiology of perioperative stroke may include several factors: reduced flow through extra- or intracranial vessels, emboli from ulcerated carotid artery plaque, or emboli from the heart or aorta. Because of confusion regarding the etiology of stroke, patients with a positive neurologic history or asymptomatic cervical bruit found at the time of elective hospital admission have produced justifiable concern in organizing a protocol for preoperative evaluation and treatment. A number of studies have failed to demonstrate a direct relationship between cervical bruit, severity of carotid disease, and the incidence of perioperative stroke. Some of the confusion may be attributed to the fact that only half of the preoperative patients found to have asymptomatic cervical bruits have significant carotid stenosis, and in some patients who have no clinical signs or symptoms, severe carotid occlusive disease may exist. Fear of perioperative stroke secondary to low flow states through obstructed carotid arteries has been responsible for the development of numerous noninvasive tests to detect significant carotid disease. However, once such obstructions have been found, there has continued to be confusion regarding the optimal method of management.

Noninvasive tests now used for evaluation of carotid bruits are real-time B-mode scans, carotid phonoangiography, ophthalmosonometry, pulsed and continuous wave Doppler, and ocular pneumoplethysmography. The latter two tests have been the most helpful in my experience. In experienced hands, noninvasive evaluation of cervical bruits is capable of detecting a reduction of 75 percent or greater of cross-sectional lumen with a sensitivity of 90 percent.

The recognition, diagnosis, and management of carotid disease in patients undergoing coronary bypass surgery have undergone significant change over the past several years. With the ever-increasing mean patient age characteristic of most reported series, occurrence of perioperative stroke has become a considerable problem. Numerous tests, invasive and noninvasive, have been suggested to rule out occult extracranial cerebrovascular obstructions. Unfortunately, in unstable patients, extensive testing, particularly employing arteriography, can be dangerous, and the procedure itself may cause embolism and stroke in those patients with aortic atherosclerotic plaques.

The exact etiology of perioperative stroke is not yet clear. It is probable that there has been a subtle change in the etiology, with most older published series reporting stroke as a direct consequence of dislodgment of embolic debris from a diseased ascending aorta. With progressive experience and refinement in operative technique, today a significant number of these neurologic events occur because of occult lesions of the carotid arteries, intracerebral vessels, or left ventricular endocardium. All three types of lesions are known to increase in incidence with an aging patient population that often has multisystem vascular disease. As older and sicker patients have undergone coronary revascularization procedures, the incidence of perioperative stroke appears to be occurring at an accelerated rate. Many patients are too unstable to undergo standard arteriographic tests, and the need for safe, rapid, noninvasive procedures is readily apparent. Recently, Goodson, Flanigan, and colleagues have shown a greater correlation between duplex ultrasonography and operative findings at the time of carotid endarterectomy than that found with carotid arteriography. Even ulcerated carotid plaque was more readily identified with duplex scanning than with arteriography. If such data can be substantiated, standard procedures may soon be to test noninvasively asymptomatic individuals felt to be at increased risk for perioperative stroke, e.g., the elderly and all patients with carotid bruits. Certainly, all patients with even a suggested history of stroke or with transient ischemic attack symptoms should have some type of investigative study. In the past, patients with abnormal noninvasive testing findings (ocular plethysmography, Doppler) have been referred directly for carotid arteriography to validate the degree of stenosis. With refinement in duplex scanning, this second step may no longer be necessary.

At the present time, an acceptable approach to the asymptomatic patient with suspected cerebral vascular disease and proven coronary artery obstruction is to perform noninvasive testing of the extracranial carotid vessels (that is, ocular plethysmography, Doppler), and if the results are abnormal, to proceed directly to carotid arteriography. In those with prior or current neurologic symptoms (stroke or transient ischemic attack), noninvasive tests may also be performed, but at present intracerebral as well as extracerebral arteriographic evaluation will be necessary before any cardiac operation is carried out. A judgment as to which obstructions are hemodynamically significant is difficult but probably can best be made by combining the findings of both the noninvasive and arteriographic tests. In those patients with symptoms but without hemodynamically significant extracranial carotid obstruction according to noninvasive testing, a thorough evaluation of intracerebral vascular anatomy should be performed with an arteriographic procedure. Any patient having symptoms thought to be related to proven ulcerated carotid plaque should have combined endarterectomy and coronary bypass to avoid cerebral embolization.

Asymptomatic cervical bruits are present in approximately 10 percent of patients presenting for coronary bypass surgery and approximately one-half have carotid stenosis as shown on noninvasive testing. All data available from our own experience in years past have supported the contention that cervical bruits do not effectively identify subgroups of cardiac patients at increased risk for perioperative stroke. As will be discussed later, however, this concept may be changing. It is probable that if Doppler flows demonstrate obstruction that is greater than 50 percent lumen diameter (greater than 75 percent reduction in lumen cross-sectional area), the stroke rate is slightly increased. Among patients with abnormal ocular pneumoplethysmography results, approximately two-thirds are found to have significant carotid artery stenosis. Significant carotid stenosis is found in approximately one-third of patients without cervical bruits but with abnormal ocular pneumoplethysmography. Asymptomatic patients without hemodynamically significant carotid disease verified by ocular pneumoplethsmography can be spared cerebral angiography.

Until recently, it was my impression that except for patients with extensive bilateral carotid disease, most cerebral vascular injuries following routine coronary bypass have been unrelated to occult extra- or intracranial cerebral vascular obstruction, as was once thought. The superb autoregulatory mechanism of the cerebral circulation, the use of systemic hypothermia, and the salutory effects of hemodilution appear to be sufficient to protect the brain from low-flow states that might theoretically occur when the extracranial circulation is obstructed or even occluded. With the marked increase in patient population age that has been seen in the last several years and the increased incidence of neurologic injury that has accompanied this age increase, it may be that occult carotid or cerebrovascular disease will prove to be a major contributor to perioperative stroke. Because of the devastating consequences that stroke brings to both patient and family, for medicolegal and ethical reasons a thorough neurologic evaluation should be performed in this population prior to a contemplated coronary surgical procedure.

In my own experience the almost 9 percent incidence of perioperative stroke in patients with a prior history of stroke or transient cerebral ischemic attack who had coronary bypass *only* would suggest that these patients be treated differently and should have the most careful and thorough preoperative evaluation (including angiography) prior to elective bypass surgery. When significant carotid vascular disease is found in these patients, a combined carotid and coronary operation should be performed.

When coronary bypass and carotid endarterectomy are combined, our hospital mortality is approximately 3 percent compared with less than 1 percent for patients having isolated coronary bypass during this same time interval. The incidence of stroke after each procedure was 1.5 percent and 0.5 percent, respectively. These differences are not statistically significant. Primary contributory factors to the development of stroke appear to be advanced age and the presence of extensive atherosclerosis in the ascending aorta. The latter finding implies an embolic etiology for the stroke event.

RECOMMENDATIONS FOR MANAGEMENT

Based on past experience, the following recommendations can be made for the treatment of patients with both carotid and coronary atherosclerotic disease. A simultaneous carotid-coronary operation is performed when there is symptomatic neurologic disease (transient ischemic attacks or prior stroke) and significant carotid vascular obstruction associated with unstable angina pectoris, significant left main artery obstruction, or diffuse multivessel disease. Although the evidence is not substantial, I have also recommended the combined approach in the elderly (older than 70 years) and in patients less than 50 years of age found to have asymptomatic, anatomically significant carotid vascular disease. In the former group, extracranial vascular obstruction has an increased likelihood of being associated with intracerebral arterial disease, and the combined effect of the two could potentially cause reduced cerebral blood flow during cardiopulmonary bypass. However, this supposition is totally unproved at the present time. In patients less than 50 years old, the combined approach may be justified by the extended longevity of most of these patients who have an increased likelihood of later symptoms secondary to extracranial carotid vascular obstruction.

A simultaneous approach to carotid and coronary disease is also recommeded whenever bilateral carotid and severe or unstable coronary artery disease coexist. However, the treatment of bilateral extracranial carotid vascular obstruction presents several difficult problems. For patients with unstable angina and bilateral carotid disease the operative risk is high, with death, cerebral accident, or transient deficit reported in as many as 20 percent. Patients with unstable angina and severe bilateral carotid disease should be treated by first performing endarterectomy on the carotid, which contributes the majority of cerebral blood flow, and then coronary bypass as part of the combined procedure. The second carotid obstruction can be treated surgically as an isolated procedure at a later date if indicated.

Preference for the staged approach, i.e., performing the carotid endarterectomy first followed at some later date by myocardial revascularization, should be exercised only when the patient has clinically stable angina pectoris. In this setting, patients having transient ischemic attacks associated with significant carotid disease, complicated carotid revascularization procedures, or significant bilateral carotid disease should have the carotid portion of the operation performed first as a separate procedure. Complicated carotid revascularization procedures may frequently be necessary when there is restenosis of a prior endarterectomy site. In this situation, operating time and the extent of the grafting procedures are less predictable, and it is probably best to do the operation as a staged procedure whenever possible.

Coronary artery bypass may be performed as the only procedure in most situations when there is discovery of an asymptomatic cervical bruit associated with a moderate degree of unilateral carotid obstruction or less. My approach to patients with very unstable angina and asymptomatic cervical bruit has been to treat the situation with coronary bypass alone, and this has produced no significant increase in stroke rate. In many of these patients with cervical bruit, coronary bypass was performed without the benefit of prior cerebral or carotid angiography. Patients with prior stroke and very unstable angina may be similarly treated, although the stroke rate probably will be increased. In this latter situation the risk of stroke attendant on extensive diagnostic cerebral arteriographic studies during a time of cardiac instability is probably higher than the risk of stroke following myocardial revascularization alone.

SUGGESTED READING

Barnes RW, Marszalek PB, Rittgers SE. Asymptomatic carotid disease in preoperative patients. Stroke 1980; 11:136.

Craver JM, Murphy DA, Jones EL, et al. Concomitant carotid and coronary artery reconstruction. Ann Surg 1982; 195:712–720.

Goodson SF, Flanigan DP, Bishara RA, et al. Can carotid duplex scanning supplant arteriography in patients with focal carotid territory symptoms? J Vasc Surg 1987; 5:551–557.

Hertzer NR, Loop FD, Taylor PC. Staged and combined surgical approach to simultaneous carotid and coronary vascular disease. Surgery 1978; 84:803–811.

Schwartz RL, Garrett JR, Karp RB, Kouchoukos NT. Simultaneous myocardial revascularization and carotid endarterectomy. Circulation 1982; 66:(Suppl 1):97–101.

VENTRICULAR ANEURYSM

ELDRED D. MUNDTH, M.D.

In most instances left ventricular aneurysm occurs as a result of a previous transmural myocardial infarction and is associated with significant coronary artery occlusive disease. Clinical manifestations range from symptomatic congestive heart failure, angina, arterial embolism, ventricular ectopy, and tachyarrhythmias to totally asymptomatic. Because of the frequency of significant multivessel coronary artery disease and myocardial ischemia, angina is a frequent symptom; approximately 75 percent of patients considered for surgical treatment of left ventricular aneurysm require concomitant coronary artery bypass revascularization. Actual rupture of a true left ventricular aneurysm is rare but is a known potentially fatal complication of postinfarction left ventricular false (pseudo-) aneurysm.

INDICATIONS FOR SURGERY AND PATIENT SELECTION

Delineation of the criteria for diagnosis is important in determining the indications for surgery in the treatment of left ventricular aneurysm. The criteria are based upon the ventriculographic demonstration of a focal or regional left ventricular wall aneurysm, characterized by an akinetic segment with dyskinetic systolic paradoxic bulging with or without evidence of mural thrombus. Differentiation is made between segmental wall akinesis and true aneurysm, as defined above.

Currently, the indications for surgical resection of left ventricular aneurysm with concurrent coronary artery bypass revascularization when required are as follows:

1. Angina, particularly when associated with multivessel coronary artery disease, refractoriness of symptoms to medical therapy, or significant global left ventricular dysfunction;
2. Congestive heart failure or a combination of angina and congestive heart failure;
3. Systemic arterial emboli;
4. Ventricular tachyarrhythmias that are refractory to antiarrhythmic drug therapy; this may require electrophysiologic studies and map-guided endocardial resection, as discussed in the chapter on *Recurrent Ventricular Tachycardia: Surgical Management;*
5. Asymptomatic patient with multivessel coronary artery disease and significant global left ventricular dysfunction.

Significant global left ventricular dysfunction is defined in terms of objective physiologic parameters, including left ventricular ejection fraction of less than 40 percent, left ventricular end-diastolic pressure greater than 15 mm Hg, increased left ventricular end-diastolic volume, and reduced cardiac index, less than 2.5 L per minute per square meter of body surface.

Contraindications for surgical management of left ventricular aneurysm are relatively few for symptomatic patients. The primary relative contraindication is severe overall left ventricular dysfunction when the ejection fraction of the nonaneurysmal left ventricular wall segments is less than 30 percent. The operative mortality is significantly increased (higher than 10 percent) and the postoperative functional benefit greatly decreased in this group of patients, who usually present with severe congestive heart failure, low cardiac output, and frequently without associated angina.

Because of the lack of prospectively randomized studies comparing the effect on longevity of surgical versus medical treatment in asymptomatic patients, the selection of patients for surgical treatment in this category remains an individual judgment based upon location and extent of coronary artery disease, age, results of stress thallium perfusion scanning, and findings of studies of contractile segmental wall ejection fraction.

False (pseudo-) left ventricular aneurysms demonstrated by left ventriculography and confirmed by two-dimensional echocardiography constitute an indication for surgical treatment because of the propensity for rupture, particularly if associated with a history of recent myocardial infarction.

SURGICAL APPROACH AND OPERATIVE TECHNIQUES

Preoperative preparation must cover a complete diagnostic evaluation, including selective coronary arteriography, biplane left ventriculography, calculations of global ejection fraction and ejection fraction of the nonaneurysmal contractile portion, measurement of hemodynamic indices of left ventricular end-diastolic pressure and cardiac index, and notation of whether significant mitral regurgitation is present. Noninvasive studies, including two-dimensional echocardiography and stress thallium perfusion scanning, are most helpful in assessing septal motion and the presence of intracavitary thrombus or false aneurysm and in determining ischemic but viable myocardial regions that might benefit significantly from appropriate coronary artery revascularization.

Careful preoperative management, particularly during induction of anesthesia, is extremely important in patients with unstable myocardial ischemia and severe left ventricular dysfunction. Careful attention must be paid to preventing an excessive rise in arterial afterload or in left ventricular filling pressure (preload). This may result in increased left ventricular end-diastolic pressure, increase in left ventricular end-diastolic volume, and, consequently, in increased wall tension with concomitant increase in the myocardial oxygen consumption requirement (Laplace's law). If these hemodynamic changes occur, a vicious cycle of myocardial ischemia and progressive left ventricular dysfunction can take place, greatly increasing the risks of surgery. Management of these patients requires maintaining them on intravenous nitroglycerin ranging from 0.5 to 3 μg per kilogram per minute, with careful monitoring of the pulmonary artery diastolic pressure, cardiac output index, and mixed venous oxygen saturation, as well as arterial pressure. A 2-lead electrocardiogram (including an apical precordial lead), central venous pressure, and urinary output are also monitored. For those patients who have severe overall left ventricular dysfunction or unstable myocardial ischemia or both, the use of elective prophylactic intra-aortic balloon assistance preoperatively must be considered.

The surgical approach is through a standard median sternotomy incision. Because of the frequency of dense pericardial adhesions, dissection of the adhesions is reserved until after institution of cardiopulmonary bypass to reduce the risk of systemic emboli. Following dissection of pericardial adhesions, systemic hypothermia to 26°C is achieved, the aorta is cross-clamped, and cold (4°C to 8°C) hyperkalemic blood cardioplegia containing lidocaine is infused into the aortic root, achieving prompt cessation of cardiac electromechanical activity. In some cases, extensive calcification is present in the wall of the aneurysm, with extremely dense adhesion to the pericardium. In this situation, my preference is not to attempt to dissect the calcified aneurysm free from the pericardium but rather to achieve total hypothermic cardioplegic arrest and then make a ventriculotomy and separate the aneurysm from the ventricular wall–pericardial attachment, leaving the densely adherent, calcified aneurysmal wall attached to the pericardium. The additional aneurysmal wall is then resected as required. Supplemental cardioplegia is administered as required, depending upon the cross-clamp global ischemia time. Left ventricular venting is generally used with a preformed angled No. 22 F vent catheter carefully placed in the left ventricle via a pursestring suture in the right superior pulmonary vein after total cardioplegia has been accomplished. Venting of the left ventricle can effectively assist in delineating the anatomic extent of the aneurysm as a result of the "dimpling" of the aneurysmal transmural thinned-out scar tissue (Fig. 1A). A ventriculotomy incision is made linearly in the direction of the major longitudinal axis of the aneurysm, which in the case of the more common anteroapical wall aneurysm is parallel to the course of the left anterior descending coronary artery. Occasionally, with the less common posterior wall aneurysms, this will be a transverse incision. Allis clamps are placed on the edges of the aneurysmal wall, facilitating exposure of the aneurysm and left ventricular chamber. A moist surgical sponge is carefully placed deep within the ventricular chamber covering the left ventricular outflow tract and aortic and mitral valves, so that any thrombus or debris from resection of the aneurysm can be readily removed on completion of the resection. Removal of mural thrombus is facilitated by use of sponge forceps initially, followed by gentle wiping from inside out of the left ventricular chamber using a moist sponge (Fig. 1B). Following this and removal of the sponge from the left ventricular chamber, it is helpful to palpate the extent of the thin-walled aneurysm, grasping the aneurysm wall with the palpating thumb inside the chamber and the fingers outside so as to approximately define a 1- to 1.5-cm rim of scar that is left for suture closure of the ventriculotomy. Although

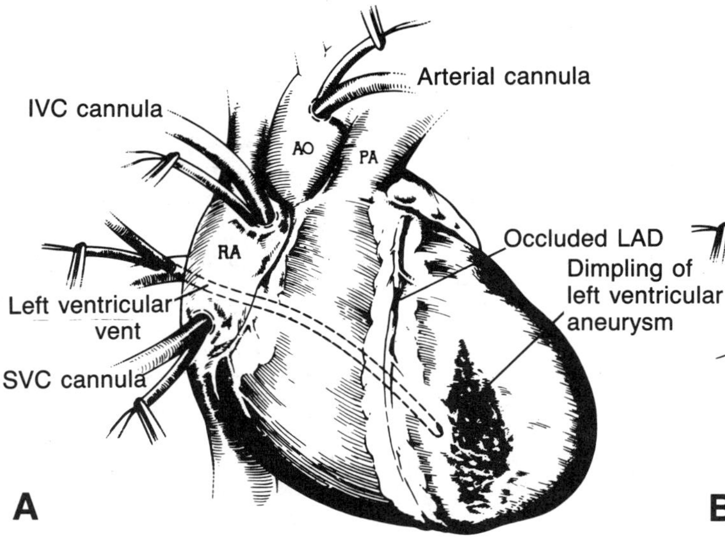

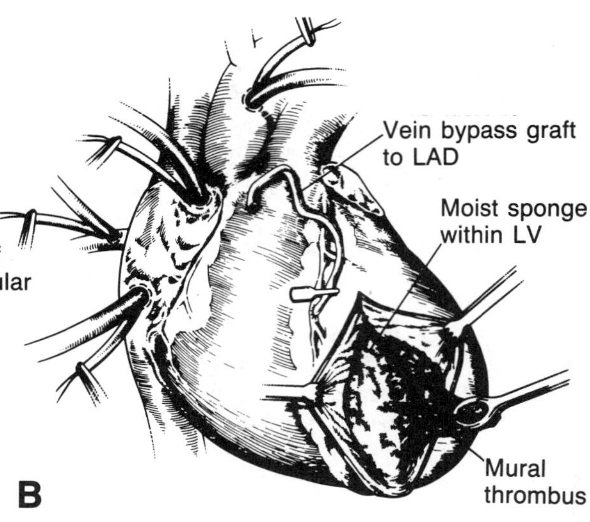

Figure 1 *A,* ''Dimpling'' of left ventricular wall on cardiopulmonary bypass with left ventricle vented in patient with anterolateral left ventricular aneurysm. The invaginated, or ''dimpled,'' left ventricular wall assists in delineation of the extent of the aneurysm, facilitating placement of the initial ventriculotomy incision and defining the limits of resection. *B,* Illustration of mural thrombus in an anterolateral left ventricular aneurysm after initial ventriculotomy. Sponge forceps are used to gently tease away the mural thrombus after carefully placing a moist sponge in the left ventricular chamber to prevent thrombotic debris from falling into ventricular trabecular recesses during removal of the mural thrombus. Also illustrated is a saphenous vein bypass with the distal anastomosis completed to the left anterior descending artery (LAD).

aneurysm of the posterior-inferior wall is relatively uncommon, the surgical techniques for resection and repair are similar to the technique described earlier for anterolateral aneurysm repair. On rare occasions, the aneurysm may involve a posterior papillary muscle so that complete resection results in detachment of the ventricular wall attachment of the papillary muscle. In most of these cases, preoperative cardiac catheterization will show significant (3 to 4+) mitral regurgitation. Appropriate surgical management of mitral regurgitation may require mitral valve replacement, particularly if scar tissue replaces most of the papillary muscle, and this can be accomplished readily through the ventriculotomy. In selected cases, the mitral valve can be effectively preserved by suture reattachment of the base of the papillary muscle to the free ventricular wall. For the repair, Teflon felt-backed mattress sutures of 3–0 Dacron-Teflon material are used (Fig. 2A).

Ventriculotomy closure is accomplished using a double-layer suture technique over 1.5-cm wide Teflon felt strips; the initial layer is a running horizontal mattress suture of 0 Teflon-coated Dacron material, and the second layer is a simple running over-and-over suture of the same material (Fig. 2B).

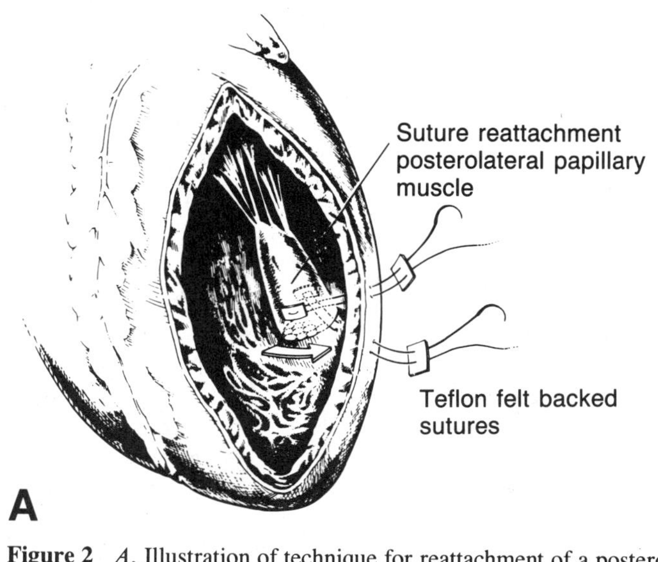

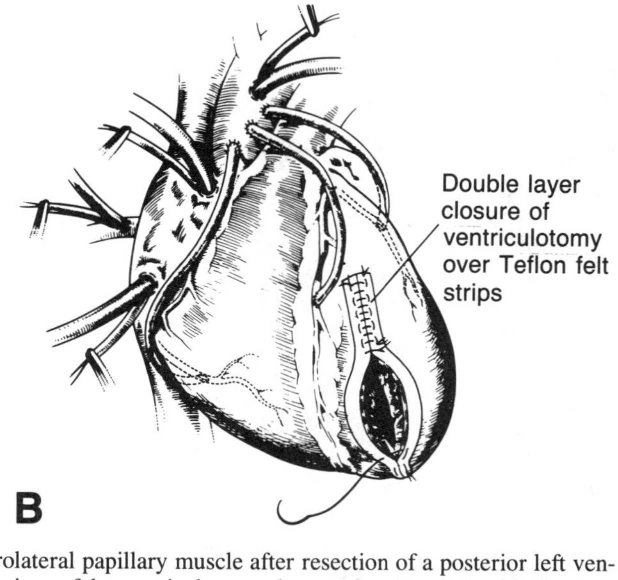

Figure 2 *A,* Illustration of technique for reattachment of a posterolateral papillary muscle after resection of a posterior left ventricular aneurysm involving the base of the papillary muscle. *B,* Technique of the ventriculotomy closure after completion of aneurysm resection, mural thrombectomy and triple aortocoronary artery bypass (see text).

Left ventricular false aneurysms are managed similarly in terms of surgical technical aspects. Although the false aneurysm may be of considerable size, in most instances the neck of the pseudoaneurysm is relatively small. In some cases the actual false aneurysm may be relatively small and difficult to delineate intraoperatively while the heart is decompressed on cardiopulmonary bypass. To delineate the location and extent of a small false aneurysm, I have found it useful to fill the left ventricle with cold saline solution via the vent catheter, which causes a protrusion of the false aneurysm and allows accurate delineation of the aneurysm itself as well as of its neck. Resection of a false aneurysm and suture closure of the ventriculotomy are identical to the procedures described for true left ventricular aneurysms.

With continued cold cardioplegia, required coronary artery bypass grafts are constructed at this time using reversed saphenous vein segments. Frequently, the left internal mammary artery is used, particularly for bypass of a medium or smaller caliber distal left anterior descending coronary artery. In the latter case, the internal mammary artery would have been dissected free of the chest wall, ready for use prior to instituting cardiopulmonary bypass. In general, I prefer to perform the distal vein graft–coronary artery anastomoses first, with the proximal aortic anastomoses accomplished during rewarming on cardiopulmonary bypass. The decision of whether concomitant coronary artery bypass should accompany aneurysm resection is based upon (1) whether there are significant stenoses (diameter reduction of more than or equal to 50 percent), (2) symptoms of angina or thallium scan evidence of ischemic but reperfused areas of myocardium, (3) acceptable distal vessel run-off, as estimated from the preoperative coronary arteriogram, later confirmed by intraoperative inspection of the vessel, (4) significant stenosis in a coronary vessel supplying a dysfunctional segment of left ventricular wall shown to be ischemic with reperfusion on thallium scan, and (5) the angiographic demonstration of a patent distal vessel (proximally occluded) with distribution to the aneurysm (e.g., left anterior descending) with evidence of patent significant branches to viable myocardium (e.g., septal branches). In cases of large anteroapical left ventricular aneurysms, bypass of significantly narrowed posterior and posterolateral wall vessels may be very important in achieving improved global left ventricular function postoperatively, particularly when there is evidence of preoperative ischemic dysfunction.

Care must be taken prior to weaning from cardiopulmonary bypass that both the aortic root and left ventricular apex are thoroughly air-vented; this is done using a large-bore needle with the patient in the Trendelenburg position. We have used the cardioplegia site for ascending aorta venting and insist on accomplishing venting before spontaneous contraction and left ventricular ejection occur.

In all cases we prefer placing both temporary epicardial atrial and ventricular pacing wires, along with a left atrial pressure catheter monitoring line (inserted through the vent site pursestring suture in the right superior pulmonary vein) in addition to the pulmonary artery catheter and arterial pressure line. We have found the use of a fiberoptic pulmonary artery catheter with on-line continuous computer monitoring of the pulmonary venous oxygen saturation most helpful in the early postoperative period, particularly in patients with marginal preoperative left ventricular function. I feel it is important to maintain optimal levels of left ventricular preload (mean left atrial pressure) and left ventricular afterload (mean arterial pressure and systemic vascular resistance, SVR*) in the early postoperative phase. Excessive levels of preload or afterload may lead to deterioration of left ventricular function within the first 24 to 48 hours postoperatively since left ventricular compliance is usually significantly reduced, particularly in this group of patients. In most cases, the postoperative patient initially is maintained on intravenous nitroglycerin in the range of 0.5 to 3 μg per kilogram per minute, and an attempt is made to maintain the cardiac index at greater than or equal to 2.3 L per minute per square meter of body surface at left atrial pressures in the range of 6 to 14 mm Hg. Because of overall left ventricular dysfunction, inotropic agents may be required initially to maintain acceptable hemodynamic indices. Dobutamine in a dosage range of 3 to 7.5 μg per kilogram per minute is usually effective. If, despite pharmacologic inotropic support, the hemodynamic indices are marginal, circulatory assistance with an intra-aortic balloon pump is indicated.

Not infrequently in these situations the intra-aortic balloon pump will have been inserted preoperatively because of known marginal left ventricular function. I feel it is very important not to allow progressive hemodynamic deterioration with falling cardiac output, hypotension, rising mean left atrial pressure, and increasing inotropic support requirements before instituting effective circulatory assistance with intra-aortic balloon pumping. Our experience has been that the salvage rate and functional results of patients who have required intra-aortic balloon pump assistance are excellent despite the critical nature of left ventricular dysfunction.

In general, postoperative anticoagulation therapy is restricted to patients in whom significant mural thrombus is encountered and no specific contraindications exist. Many patients have concomitant coronary artery bypass revascularization, and if significant mural thrombus is not found and anticoagulation not started, antiplatelet aggregating drug therapy (acetylsalicylic acid plus dipyridamole) is started early postoperatively in the absence of specific contraindications. Our general policy in patients who have been anticoagulated with warfarin sodium is to switch them to antiplatelet drug therapy at 3 to 4 months postoperatively.

---

* $SVR = \frac{MAP - CVP}{C.O.} \times 80$, where

MAP = mean arterial pressure
CVP = central venous pressure
C.O. = cardiac output
normal range 1,000 to 1,400

Arrhythmias, including ventricular irritability, are not uncommon postoperatively in patients undergoing left ventricular aneurysmectomy. Arrhythmias are treated with specific antiarrhythmic drugs when indicated. Our policy is to routinely wean the patient from cardiopulmonary bypass on intravenous lidocaine at 2 mg per minute, with gradual weaning from 24 to 48 hours postoperatively. It is also extremely useful to place both temporary atrial and ventricular epicardial pacing wires. Maintenance of normal atrioventricular transport at an optimum heart rate (75 to 90 per minute) postoperatively by atrial pacing or atrioventricular sequential pacing where required is important to optimize cardiac output and left ventricular function. The temporary pacing wires are generally removed on the fifth postoperative day. A permanent pacemaker is usually not required.

RESULTS OF SURGERY

The dominant variable determining operative risk and late mortality is the status of preoperative left ventricular function. Preoperative poor overall left ventricular function increases the operative risk and late mortality substantially. The overall operative mortality in our experience has been less than 5 percent, which compares favorably to the figure of 8 or 9 percent reported in the literature. In our experience the operative mortality is less than 3 percent in the group of patients with an ejection fraction of greater than 30 percent of the nonaneurysmal left ventricular wall segments. Late mortality overall in patients undergoing left ventricular aneurysmectomy is approximately 5 percent per year or 75 percent 5-year survival. Other factors that have an adverse effect on operative and late mortality are multivessel coronary disease associated with congestive heart failure, unstable ventricular ectopy preoperatively, and incompleteness of myocardial revascularization. Long-term survival is greatly improved in the group of patients undergoing left ventricular aneurysmectomy in whom (1) angina rather than congestive heart failure is the prominent presenting symptom, (2) single- or two-vessel disease is present rather than extensive multivessel disease, and (3) revascularization is complete. Five-year survival in this group of patients approaches 85 percent. In asymptomatic patients, the 5-year survival is slightly over 90 percent.

Good or excellent functional results can be expected in 90 percent of patients with aneurysm resection and complete revascularization. In our experience, 70 percent of patients are asymptomatic, with the great majority being able to return to their previous work with minimal, if any, activity restrictions.

Since the available data indicate that the 5-year survival of patients with angiographically proved left ventricular aneurysm treated medically is approximately 50 percent, there is a fairly cogent indication for elective surgery even in the asymptomatic patient. Although a prospectively randomized study comparing longevity of medically versus surgically treated patients is not available, current data suggest that life expectancy is improved with surgical management in properly selected patients with left ventricular aneurysm.

SUGGESTED READING

Akins CW. Resection of left ventricular aneurysm during hypothermic fibrillatory arrest without aortic occlusion. J Thorac Cardiovasc Surg 1986; 91:610–618.

Barratt-Boyes BG, White HD, Agnew JM, Pemberton JR, Wild CJ. The results of surgical treatment of left ventricular aneurysms. An assessment of the risk factors affecting early and late mortality. J Thorac Cardiovasc Surg 1984; 87:87–98.

Cosgrove DN, Loop FD, Irrazaval MJ, et al. Determinants of long-term survival after ventricular aneurysmectomy. Ann Thorac Surg 1978; 26:357–363.

Mundth ED. Left ventricular aneurysmectomy. In: Cohn LH, ed. Modern technics in surgery, cardiac/thoracic surgery. New York: Futura Publishing Co, 1979:1.

Reddy SB, Cooley DA, Duncan JM, Norman JC. Left ventricular aneurysm. Twenty-year surgical experience with 1,572 patients at the Texas Heart Institute. Cardiovasc Dis Bull Tex Health Inst 1981; 8:165–186.

DIFFUSE CORONARY ARTERY DISEASE

W. DUDLEY JOHNSON, M.D.
JEROLD B. BRENOWITZ, M.D.
SAED F. SAEDI, M.D.
KENNETH L. KAYSER, M.S.

Coronary artery bypass (CAB) surgery is commonly refused to severely symptomatic patients with diffusely diseased coronary arteries, many of whom would otherwise be suitable surgical candidates. Although there are no precise data on the size of this group of patients, the CASS investigators have estimated that as many as 4.9 percent of the subjects in their study have "no graftable arteries" at all. In addition, there are no generally accepted criteria to define diffuse coronary artery disease. In our opinion, a patient who has multiple localized obstructions that can be bypassed with any number of conventional grafts does not have diffuse disease. A diffusely diseased artery is totally or nearly totally atherosclerotic, particularly in the distal portions of the vessel and its side branches, such that a bypass to any region of the coronary artery would fail to provide adequate flow to most of the vessel (Fig. 1).

In an attempt to deal more effectively with diffusely diseased coronary arteries, we began to perform right coronary artery endarterectomies in 1969 and endarterectomies of the left coronary artery in 1974. Because of the nature

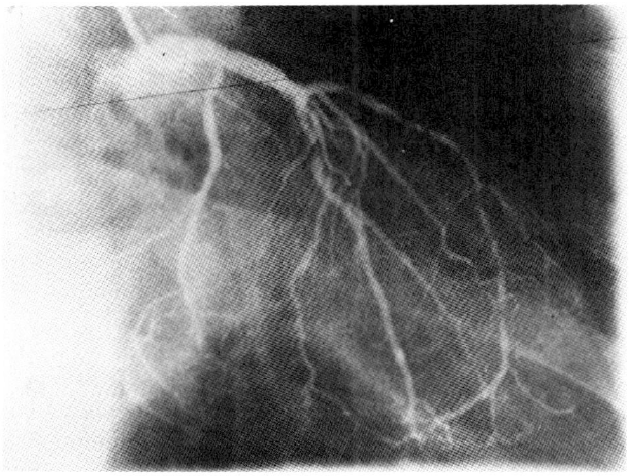

Figure 1 Diffuse atheromatous disease in the left anterior descending artery with multiple critical obstructions, including a diffusely diseased diagonal branch.

of our referral practice, we have performed coronary artery endarterectomies with increasing frequency, and since 1978 we have entered all coronary artery endarterectomies in our data registry. From January 1, 1978, through December 31, 1986, 5,005 CAB operations were performed: 25.1 percent required one coronary endarterectomy and an additional 24.9 percent required two or more endarterectomies. There is even a subgroup of 144 patients with diffuse triple vessel disease who required endarterectomy and reconstruction of their left anterior descending artery, circumflex artery, and right coronary artery. The results of our entire experience with coronary artery endarterectomy, with particular emphasis on the long-term clinical results and long-term graft patency, have been reported and will be summarized below.

Our rationale for performing endarterectomy in diffusely diseased coronary arteries is to attempt as complete a revascularization as possible for all viable myocardium. The value of complete revascularization is well documented in numerous studies. Relief of symptoms, freedom from repeat surgery, and survival are all adversely affected by incomplete revascularization. Lawrie and associates studied 1,274 men with double and triple vessel disease who had CAB surgey. One of the variables that best predicted late mortality was the number of diseased but ungrafted arteries. The presence of residual lesions in the left anterior descending artery was the most important predictor of late cardiac death in their series. Schaff and co-workers studied the 10- to 12-year results of CAB surgery in 500 patients. The presence of diseased but ungrafted arteries was the most significant predictor of late cardiac events, including cardiac-related death, recurrence of angina, myocardial infarction, and repeat CAB surgery.

Much has been learned technically from our endarterectomy experience; a few basic principles will be mentioned here. All atheromatous material must be removed from the artery distal to the arteriotomy site. If the distal intima does not come out cleanly, complete with fine tapered ends, one of two approaches must be used. In one, the arteriotomy is extended and the end of the intima is identified and again carefully extracted; the process is repeated until all diseased intima is removed. A second approach is to make a second opening in the coronary artery, complete the endarterectomy, and close this opening with a separate vein graft or a vein patch. A simple, relatively short opening is often adequate to remove all diseased intima from the right coronary artery, but a short incision is rarely adequate to clean out a major branch of the left coronary system. To do a left coronary artery endarterectomy, usually a long incision is made in the artery and the atheromatous material is carefully removed under direct vision. Each side branch is identified. The atheromatous material is carefully extracted from each branch, one at a time. A saphenous vein is then split lengthwise and attached over the entire length of the arteriotomy. The vein's proximal end is attached as a bypass to the aorta. For an endarterectomy of a totally diseased left anterior descending artery, an arteriotomy of 10 to 15 cm is nearly always required. Somewhat shorter incisions are adequate for large diagonal and circumflex branches. Rather than simply calling these procedures endarterectomy, we prefer a more realistic term to describe them: coronary artery reconstruction.

In our series of 144 patients who required triple vessel endarterectomies and reconstruction, the average pump time was 342 minutes with an average aortic cross-clamp time of 195 minutes. Despite the length of time on bypass, only one patient in that series (0.7 percent) suffered a permanent neurologic injury, and one additional patient developed postoperative renal failure requiring dialysis. The current techniques of perfusion and myocardial preservation allow sufficient time to perform these complex operations safely as long as the technical aspects of the procedure can be completed satisfactorily.

All patients undergoing CAB surgery were placed into one of three groups: those with conventional grafts only (group A), those in whom one graft was placed to a vessel that required endarterectomy and reconstruction (group B), and those in whom two or more endarterectomies were done (group C).

Furthermore, the operative mortality within each group was stratified based on the presence of well-established preoperative risk factors: age greater than 70 years, repeat CAB surgery, insulin-dependent diabetes mellitus, female sex, and severe left ventricular dysfunction (ejection fraction less than 0.35). When analyzing our mortality data, two patterns clearly emerge. First, patients with diffusely diseased coronary arteries that required multiple endarterectomies had a significantly increased mortality, both early and late. Perhaps more importantly, however, the number of preoperative risk factors other than diffuse disease severely affected survival, particularly in patients with multiple (more than two) risk factors (Table 1). The operative mortality ranged from 0.5 percent in 1,134 low risk patients who did not require endarterectomy to 26.9 percent in the highest risk group of patients with multiple preoperative risk factors who required multiple coronary artery endarterectomies. Similar trends are seen with long-term survival (Table 2).

TABLE 1 Thirty-Day Mortality*

Number of Risk Factors	*Group A*	*Group B*	*Group C*
0	6/1,134 (0.5%)	8/471 (1.7%)	32/594 (5.4%)
1	31/908 (3.4%)	27/514 (5.3%)	45/455 (9.9%)
2 or more	62/462 (13.4%)	44/270 (16.3%)	53/197 (26.9%)
Total	99/2,504 (4.0%)	79/1,255 (6.3%)	130/1,246 (10.4%)

* Entire group: 308 deaths/5,005 patients (6.2 percent)
From Brenowitz JB, Kayser KL, Johnson WD. Results of coronary artery endarterectomy and reconstruction. J Thorac Cardiovasc Surg 1988; 95:4.

TABLE 2 Five-Year Survival

Number of Risk Factors	*Group A*	*Group B*	*Group C*
0	92.0%	92.2%	83.8%
1	83.8%	74.4%	73.5%
2 or more	62.2%	54.1%	36.8%

Adapted from Brenowitz JB, Kayser KL, Johnson WD. Results of coronary artery endarterectomy and reconstruction. J Thorac Cardiovasc Surg 1988; 95:6.

TABLE 3 Early Graft Patency (940 Patients)

	Endarterectomy Grafts	*Conventional Grafts*
Right coronary artery	318/356 (89.3%)	671/719 (93.3%)
Left anterior descending artery	381/427 (89.2%)	886/1003 (88.3%)
Circumflex artery	102/118 (86.4%)	893/1003 (89.0%)

Adapted from Brenowitz JB, Kayser KL, Johnson WD. Results of coronary artery endarterectomy and reconstruction. J Thorac Cardiovasc Surg 1988; 95:5.

There was no significant difference in the early patency of endarterectomy grafts (88.9 percent) when compared with the early patency of conventional grafts (90.5 percent). This was true for the entire series, as well as when grafts to the left anterior descending, circumflex or right coronary artery were considered individually (Table 3). Late graft patency in 288 symptomatic patients was similar when endarterectomy (71.7 percent) and conventional (75.8 percent) vein grafts were compared (Table 4). Our early patency results certainly compare favorably with those of other published series. Although our long-term follow-up of endarterectomy grafts only averages 31.4 months, all of the patients restudied were symptomatic, and the 71.7 percent patency rate is similar to that found in literature reports for conventional grafts and exceeds the results of other series of endarterectomy grafts. More importantly, there was no demonstrable difference between late endarterectomy and late conventional vein graft patency in our series. These results appear to verify the long-term durability of endarterectomy grafts in our experience.

TABLE 4 Late Graft Patency (288 Patients)

	Endarterectomy Grafts (Angina 31.4 mo)	*Conventional Grafts (Angina 38.8 mo)*
Right coronary artery	57/82 (69.5%)	183/236 (77.5%)
Left anterior descending artery	69/95 (72.6%)	250/326 (76.7%)
Circumflex artery	11/14 (78.6%)	211/288 (73.3%)

Adapted from Brenowitz JB, Kayser KL, Johnson WD. Results of coronary artery endarterectomy and reconstruction. J Thorac Cardiovasc Surg 1988; 95:5.

TABLE 5 Current Anginal Status*

	No Angina	*Angina*
Group A: 1,575 patients; average 67.8 mo	1,121 (71.1%)	Class I–II 382 (24.3%) Class III–IV 72 (4.6%)
Group B: 747 patients; average 51.4 mo	504 (67.5%)	Class I–II 208 (27.8%) Class III–IV 35 (4.7%)
Group C: 689 patients; average 43.9 mo	457 (66.3%)	Class I–II 204 (29.6%) Class III–IV 28 (4.1%)
All endarterectomy patients 1,436 patients; average 47.8 mo	961 (66.9%)	Class I–II 412 (28.7%) Class III–IV 63 (4.4%)

* 3,011 patients; average follow-up, 58.3 months.
From Brenowitz JB, Kayser KL, Johnson WD. Results of coronary artery endarterectomy and reconstruction. J Thorac Cardiovasc Surg 1988; 95:7.

Finally there is a slight but significant decrease in long-term angina relief in patients requiring endarterectomies, although there is no real difference between those with one endarterectomy and those with multiple endarterectomies (Table 5). Almost 67 percent of the endarterectomy patients were asymptomatic, with an average follow-up of 47.8 months and with only 4.4 percent having Class III–IV angina. The results are only slightly better in patients with conventional grafts only (71 percent asymptomatic, 4.6 percent Class III–IV, average 67.8 months), clearly demonstrating beneficial long-term symptomatic relief in patients, irrespective of the number of endarterectomies required.

In conclusion, the early results, long-term survival, persistent relief of angina, and long-term graft patency data all confirm that our techniques of coronary artery endarterectomy and reconstruction provide lasting relief to patients with severe diffuse coronary artery disease.

SUGGESTED READING

Brenowitz JB, Kayser KL, Johnson WD. Triple vessel coronary artery endarterectomy and reconstruction. J Am Coll Cardiol, submitted for publication April 1988.

Brenowitz JB, Kayser KL, Johnson WD. Results of coronary artery endarterectomy and reconstruction. J Thorac Cardiovasc Surg 1988; 95:1–10.

CASS Principal Investigators and Their Associates. Coronary artery study (CASS): A randomized trial of coronary artery bypass surgery. Survival data. Circulation 1983; 68:939–950.

Lawrie GM, Morris GC, Silvers A, et al. The influence of residual disease after coronary bypass on the 5-year survival rate of 1274 men with coronary artery disease. Circulation 1982; 66:717–723.

Schaff HV, Gersh BJ, Pluth JR, et al. Survival and functional status after coronary artery bypass grafting: results 10 to 12 years after surgery in 500 patients. Circulation 1983; 68(Suppl II):200–204.

RECURRENT VENTRICULAR TACHYCARDIA AND FIBRILLATION: THE AUTOMATIC INTERNAL DEFIBRILLATOR

EDWARD B. STINSON, M.D.
CHARLES D. SWERDLOW, M.D.

The automatic implantable cardioverter defibrillator (AICD) represents a notable product of biomedical engineering that provides a powerful tool in the management of patients with life-threatening ventricular arrhythmias. A decade of orderly experimentation and development preceded its introduction into clinical use in 1980. The earliest version of the only clinical unit commercially available at present* was designed principally to recognize and terminate ventricular fibrillation. Sensing of ventricular fibrillation was based on a probability density function that identified the arrhythmia by virtue of a low likelihood of isoelectric activity in the transcardiac electrogram obtained through the implanted defibrillation electrodes. This technique of morphology sensing was highly specific but not satisfactorily sensitive for the detection of ventricular tachycardia, the type of arrhythmia now recognized as most commonly responsible for initiating episodes of cardiac arrest. Rate counting capability, utilizing a separate ventricular bipolar electrode array, was therefore incorporated into the AICD system. This provided for electronic recognition of ventricular tachyarrhythmias that were not sinusoidal or continuously oscillating but whose rate exceeded a preset threshold. Devices available at present employ either a combination of both morphology and rate sensing or rate counting alone. We have found the latter modification to be highly reliable for rapid detection of ventricular tachycardia or fibrillation and prefer it, but many patients require drug treatment to prevent ventricular rates during sinus tachycardia or supraventricular arrhythmias from exceeding the preset rate cutoff.

* Cardiac Pacemakers Inc, St. Paul, MN.

DEVICE DESCRIPTION AND FUNCTION

The components of the AICD consist of a pulse generator, a bipolar lead system for rate sensing (right ventricular endocardial catheter or direct epicardial screw-on electrodes), and two electrodes for delivery of shocks and monitoring of transcardiac electrogram morphology. The pulse generator is substantially larger than current pacemakers; its dimensions are 10.8 × 7.6 × 2.0 cm with a displacement volume of 148 cc (weight 250 g). The lithium batteries and energy storage capacitors are contained in the lower portion of the titanium casing beneath the electronic module; integral with the top is an epoxy header with four lead receptacles and standard terminal pin settings. A raised disk on the front of the casing indicates the location of a piezoelectric crystal that emits audible tones for assessment of device status (active or inactive) and sensing function during application of a doughnut-shaped magnet over the microcircuitry; at implantation this side should be positioned anteriorly.

Two lead configurations for delivery of defibrillating shocks are available. One consists of a combination of a superior vena caval (transvenous) spring-coil electrode that serves as the anode and a rectangular titanium mesh patch (cathode) secured in the region of the left ventricular apex. Alternatively, two patch electrodes (standard or large size, or one of each) may be used in either intrapericardial or extrapericardial locations. We have found that the patch-

patch combination generally results in lower energy requirements for defibrillation, and we employ it almost routinely. Either a limited left thoracotomy or a sternotomy incision (in the case of concomitant cardiac surgical procedures) facilitates proper positioning of the double-patch configuration, as discussed below.

Upon detection of ventricular arrhythmia by rate-morphology criteria or rate sensing alone, the device initiates a charging cycle that requires 5 to 15 seconds. The capacitors then deliver a truncated exponential defibrillating pulse of 23 to 28 joules, synchronized with the bipolar electrogram. The sequence of sensing and charging requires a total elapsed time of 10 to 35 seconds. After delivery of a countershock, the unit continues to monitor the cardiac rhythm, and if a tachyarrhythmia that satisfies the detection algorithm persists, it will recycle through additional sensing and charging periods for a total of four shocks. Energy delivery for the second and subsequent rescue shocks is automatically increased to 28 to 37 joules. High energy units that provide 28 to 37 joules for every pulse in the sequence are available. Automatic resetting of the pulse generator into an active mode requires restoration for at least 35 seconds of a monitored rhythm that does *not* satisfy the sensing criteria and therefore does not activate a charging cycle (e.g., sinus rhythm, bradycardia, or asystole). The device has a battery life sufficient for approximately 2 to 3 years of monitoring if few shocks are delivered or the capability to deliver in excess of 100 shocks.

PATIENT SELECTION AND EVALUATION

The accumulation of clinical experience and evidence of efficacy has gradually led to substantial liberalization of the indications for AICD implantation. We now consider patients who have had sustained ventricular tachycardia or fibrillation as potentially appropriate candidates if antiarrhythmic drugs are judged ineffective, cause unacceptable toxicity, or cannot be evaluated adequately by electropharmacologic testing or noninvasive monitoring. An acute precipitating event such as myocardial infarction, drug toxicity, or electrolyte imbalance should not be responsible for the ventricular tachyarrhythmia. There should be no separate systemic illness that would preclude or seriously limit rehabilitation. The lower age limit is dictated by body size because of the relatively large bulk of the currently available device. The AICD is not appropriate for patients who continue to have frequent episodes of sustained ventricular tachycardia or nonsustained tachycardia longer than 5 seconds despite antiarrhythmic drug therapy.

Full cardiac evaluation, including catheterization, coronary arteriography, and left ventriculography, should be completed preoperatively, since the majority of candidates for AICD implantation have coronary artery disease with prior myocardial infarction. In our experience, approximately 75 percent of patients have had ischemic heart disease, 20 percent some other form of recognized cardiac abnormality such as cardiomyopathy or valvular deformity, and the residual 5 percent have had no identifiable structural heart disease. For patients with separate lesions warranting operative treatment, placement of defibrillating and rate sensing leads is performed at the time of sternotomy; implantation of the pulse generator is often delayed, however, because of the potential for the principal cardiac procedure to alter electrophysiologic behavior and responsiveness to antiarrhythmic drugs. For patients with recurrent ventricular tachycardia only in whom the clinical presentation, cardiac pathology, and electrophysiologic studies indicate a high likelihood of success for a primary ablative approach (subendocardial resection or cryoablation), the question of concomitant AICD implantation remains problematic. At present, our practice is to place defibrillating patch electrodes at the time of the principal procedure in nearly all such patients; exceptions include those with monomorphic ventricular tachycardia and intraoperative mapping data that clearly delineate an arrhythmia mechanism that can be reliably ablated.

OPERATIVE PROCEDURE

General anesthesia is required for implantation of the currently available AICD system. Anesthetic techniques are similar to those employed for most cardiac surgical patients. Antiarrhythmic drugs, however, should not be given intraoperatively before AICD testing because they may alter defibrillation thresholds, and the anesthetic regimen should be designed to prevent surges in sympathetic nervous system activity and to avoid depression of myocardial contractile function. We also usually delay insertion of a pulmonary artery flotation balloon catheter because of the potential for mechanical stimulation of ventricular arrhythmias. A reliable external defibrillation system is mandatory; we have found an anterior-posterior electrode system with the stationary posterior "paddle" positioned before skin preparation and draping to be satisfactory. Standard leads are attached externally for recording of the electrocardiogram.

Various approaches have been used for implantation of defibrillating and rate sensing electrodes, including median sternotomy, limited anterior left thoracotomy, and subxiphoid and subcostal incisions. The pulse generator itself is placed in a deep subcutaneous position in the midabdomen, usually in the left periumbilical region. We have employed a short (5-inch) left anterior thoracotomy incision in all cases that have not involved a simultaneous cardiac procedure. This is usually preferable to a repeat sternotomy in patients who have had prior cardiac operations and avoids intrapericardial insertion of defibrillating electrodes in patients who may require a subsequent cardiac procedure. Another major reason for this approach is that it facilitates positioning of two extrapericardial patch electrodes so as to interpose the maximum ventricular mass between them.

The cathodal patch is positioned over the posterior basal portion of the left ventricle and secured to the outside of the parietal pericardium with sutures placed through the edges of the Silastic backing of the patch electrode. The type of suture is probably not important; we have used both absorbable and nonabsorbable sutures and have never observed postoperative patch electrode migration. Occasionally, proper placement of this electrode sufficiently posteriorly requires dissection and freeing up of the phrenic nerve and associated vessels from the pericardium. We have not identified chronic phrenic nerve dysfunction attributable to contact with the electrode, but this has been reported by others. Placement of the opposite patch electrode requires partial dissection of anterior and apical portions of the pericardium from the sternopericardial ligamentous attachments and the anterior left hemidiaphragm. Into the space thus created, the rectangular patch should be secured without angular distortion. Standard or large patches or a combination may be used according to anatomic conditions, but satisfactory defibrillating capability must be confirmed.

The coil-patch defibrillating electrode configuration requires transvenous insertion of the coil electrode (anode) through the left subclavian vein using standard introducer technique. Under fluoroscopy the tip of the electrode is advanced into the mid right atrium, and the cable is then anchored with a sleeve stabilizer at the site of insertion to prevent migration. The cathodal patch electrode is sutured to the external surface of the pericardium in the region of the left ventricular apex.

For bipolar rate counting, either two screw-on epicardial electrodes may be applied through a 1- to 2-cm pericardiotomy or a transvenous bipolar right ventricular endocardial catheter may be inserted through the left subclavian vein and tunneled to the generator pouch. Epicardial electrodes should be closely spaced (1 to 1.5 cm) and inserted into healthy myocardium in order to provide high signal quality (greater than 5 mV) and to avoid artificial rate counting in the presence of severe intraventricular conduction delay.

It is also useful to attach to the left ventricle two temporary epicardial pacing wires that are exteriorized through the incision or an adjacent interspace. These are used both intraoperatively and postoperatively for arrhythmia induction, thereby avoiding the passage of high currents through the permanent rate counting electrodes with consequent potential degradation of signal quality and elevation of pacing thresholds (a future option) due to local fibrosis.

The requirement for cardiac pacing poses special problems. Because of the automatic gain control incorporated in the AICD sensing circuitry, a high-amplitude pacing signal may be preferentially sensed, thereby leading to erratic detection of arrhythmias. A bipolar pacing system is therefore mandatory, and this may require conversion of an already established unipolar pacemaker; the output of the pacemaker should be programed to a level as low as practicable and sensitivity adjusted to maximal. The rate counting and pacing electrodes should be positioned as far apart as possible.

After application of the electrodes and sensing leads, defibrillating capability at energy levels of 20 joules or less should be confirmed, using an external cardioverter-defibrillator device that allows for operator control of energy settings and triggering of shocks. During threshold testing it is important to ensure firm contact between patch electrodes and the myocardium or pericardium by packing with sponges. Confirmation of defibrillating capability is necessary both for patients with clinical ventricular tachycardia and those with clinical ventricular fibrillation because of the potential for acceleration of ventricular tachycardia to fibrillation by an ineffective shock despite synchronization to the local bipolar electrogram. Fibrillation is induced with a rectified AC current delivered through the temporary epicardial pacing wires. Inability to defibrillate at acceptable energy thresholds requires reconfiguration of the electrode system (e.g., repositioning of patches or conversion of a coil-patch system to a double-patch technique). The leads are then tunneled through the diaphragm beneath the left costal margin to a deep subcutaneous pocket fashioned in the left periumbilical region; all of the leads can be passed simultaneously using a chest tube.

After appropriate connections to the generator are made, the unit is activated with a magnet, and its ability to sense and terminate a tachyarrhythmia is documented. In patients with ventricular tachycardia, an arrhythmia similar in rate and morphology to the clinical arrhythmia should be induced by programed stimulation using the temporary pacing wires. A special telemetry receiver probe connected to an external read-out unit allows monitoring of device function in terms of sensing and charging times, and direct attachments to the lead set screws with special adapters permit continued recording of bipolar and transcardiac electrode signals. Internal filters blind the device to rectified AC current, but during delivery of programed stimuli the magnet must be applied to obviate artificial initiation of a charging cycle. The details of magnet application for device activation, inactivation, and interrogation are included in the manufacturer's user manual. After confirmation of proper device function, the set screws must be capped to prevent sensing of myoelectric potentials that can initiate a discharge cycle. The generator is then inactivated to eliminate interference by radiofrequency current associated with use of electrocautery during closure of the incision. Details of wound closure are routine, with particular attention to avoidance of kinking of the cables and obliteration of dead space in the generator pocket.

The series of steps involved in AICD implantation in conjuntion with other cardiac surgical procedures is conceptually identical to that described above. We have routinely used a double-patch technique and have usually positioned the electrodes within the pericardium. The likelihood of coronary artery bypass graft closure caused by intrapericardial patches is unknown. We have confirmed continued graft patency without distortion in several patients. Nevertheless, it seems prudent to avoid contact between patch electrodes and bypass grafts insofar as possible; this may require replacement of one or both patches on the external surface of the pericardium. The patches are sutured to the pericardium, not the myocardium, whether inside or outside. The placement of defibrillating electrodes and sensing leads and confirmation of satisfactory arrhythmia detection and conversion energy thresholds should be carried out after the primary procedure and resuscitation of the heart, but before discontinuation of cardiopulmonary bypass in order to avoid critical hemodynamic compromise. In some patients the final decision to proceed with generator implantation may be delayed for several days postoperatively in order to allow further electrophysiologic testing under conditions that more closely resemble the expected chronic situation. In this case the ends of the defibrillating and sensing cables are tunneled into a small subcutaneous pocket in the left upper quadrant and capped. Retesting and generator insertion are carried out in a second-stage procedure if indicated.

AICD implantation in children poses special problems because of the size of the device currently available. We have installed a complete system without difficulty in a teenager who weighed 49 kg, but implantation in infants and small children is impractical at present. In the near future, however, small AICD devices can be expected.

We believe that the sequence of intraoperative management as described above is best carried out as a fully collaborative effort by surgeon and electrophysiologist. The electrophysiologist has evaluated the patient preoperatively and has designed a program of continuing antiarrhythmic treatment that includes AICD implantation. Adjunctive drug therapy significantly influences the choice of rate thresholds, the reliability of morphology sensing, and the acceptability of defibrillating energy thresholds in marginal cases. The last involves a substantial element of judgment best exerted within the context of total evaluation of the type of underlying disease, concomitant drug therapy, and future expectations regarding disease progression and its management.

EARLY POSTOPERATIVE CARE AND COMPLICATIONS

In the immediate postoperative period, the principles of management are similar to those used for cardiac surgical patients in general, with particular attention to continuous monitoring of cardiac rhythm and administration of antiarrhythmic drugs, if indicated. Patients with seriously compromised left ventricular function require the full spectrum of intensive care, including ventilatory support and pharmacologic control of cardiac performance with inotropic and vasoactive agents.

Complications particular to recipients of AICD devices include infection involving one or more components of the AICD system, migration of a transvenous lead, device malfunction, and precipitation or exacerbation of antiarrhythmic drug toxicity. Because of the large combined surface area of the AICD components, we feel that prophylactic administration of antibiotics is indicated; wide-spectrum coverage identical to that used in patients undergoing valve replacement is employed for a minimum of 48 hours, beginning intraoperatively. Infection almost always requires explantation of the system according to principles established in pacemaker technology. Migration of the transvenous coil electrode is unusual and can be prevented with a lead stabilizer sleeve. If transthoracic defibrillation is required in the early postoperative period, the external defibrillating electrodes should be positioned so that the current path does not include the epicardial patch electrodes, which may diminish transcardiac current flow. Early postoperative AICD generator malfunction is very rare if standard preimplantation quality assurance evaluation has been followed. All of the adverse side effects associated with antiarrhythmic drugs may be encountered early in the postoperative period. For this reason, continued close collaboration between surgeon and electrophysiologist in patient care is desirable. Worthy of special mention is pulmonary toxicity caused by amiodarone, a drug used with increasing frequency. Pneumonitis caused by this agent is expressed functionally in loss of effective gas exchange surface area and decreased lung capacity. Operative risk is probably increased by preexisting amiodarone toxicity. One of our patients died 10 days postoperatively of pulmonary insufficiency attributable to this complication. If amiodarone-induced pulmonary toxicity is recognized preoperatively, the drug should be discontinued and operation delayed until pulmonary function improves.

Before transfer of the patient from the intensive care unit, the AICD should be activated and its monitoring function confirmed, since the quality of subsequent inhospital arrhythmia detection and response by external systems may be less secure. During the remainder of hospitalization the regimen of concomitant drug therapy, if indicated, is stabilized. Shortly before discharge, a final electrophysiologic study should be carried out. This is limited to the induction of the patient's primary clinical arrhythmia by programed stimulation or AC current, as appropriate, using the exteriorized temporary pacing wires placed at operation. The purpose of this study is to confirm the appropriate sensing and cardioverting-defibrillating capability of the device and to allow patients not rendered unconscious by their arrhythmia to experience a shock while awake under controlled conditions (including psychological assurance).

LONG-TERM FOLLOW-UP

Orderly postoperative follow-up after AICD implantation requires detailed evaluation of device status at standard intervals. An external probe unit is used in conjunction with a magnet to interrogate the AICD. Brief application of the magnet initiates a charging cycle with subsequent discharge of the capacitors through an internal load. A radiofrequency telemetry channel in the device transmits a signal that is decoded by the external probe to read out both the charging time and the cumulative number of shocks delivered. Magnet application also allows confirmation of active device status and monitoring function by virtue of an audio signal, as noted above. The total battery life of the generator is nominally a minimum 0.55 ampere hours; this should provide 2 to 3 years of monitoring function if relatively few shocks are delivered. In practice, however, elective generator replacement is scheduled on the basis of serial measurements of capacitor charging times that lengthen with battery depletion. At the time of generator replacement, sensing lead signal quality and defibrillation thresholds are reassessed as during the primary procedure.

An important component of long-term treatment is the management of concomitant antiarrhythmic drug therapy. The reasons for continued administration of such agents includes excessively frequent episodes of sustained ventricular tachycardia, nonsustained ventricular tachycardia, atrial fibrillation or other supraventricular tachycardia, and sinus tachycardia. Nearly 90 percent of our patients have received antiarrhythmic drugs after AICD implantation. Close attention to other aspects of cardiac care must also be rendered, since approximately 85 percent of recipients of the device have structural heart disease with clinically significant ventricular dysfunction.

Device explantation has rarely been required. In two of our patients with marginally acceptable defibrillation thresholds at operation, predischarge testing showed that the shock during induced ventricular tachycardia accelerated the arrhythmia to fibrillation and subsequent rescue shocks were ineffective; the devices were therefore removed. Explantation was carried out in another patient who received an early version of the AICD that relied solely on the probability density function (not rate counting). Ventricular tachycardia in this patient was uniform with significant isoelectric components and was not reliably sensed. Finally, one patient required removal of the generator because of late postoperative infection of the subcutaneous pocket.

RESULTS OF AICD IMPLANTATION

The mortality rate attributable to sudden death after implantation of an AICD appears to be remarkably low in the short to intermediate term (1 to 5 years). Proof of efficacy of this treatment, however, has not and probably will not be forthcoming in the form of controlled studies. At present, only inferential evidence is available from comparative analysis of the survival experience of patients treated with antiarrhythmic drugs. In our experience, patients with recurrent and serious ventricular tachyarrhythmias for whom an efficacious antiarrhythmic agent cannot be identified by electrophysiologic study have sustained a 1-year mortality rate of 26 percent for sudden death and 40 percent for any cardiac death without AKD implantation. Other studies have confirmed the extremely poor prognosis for such patients who resemble, in large part, those whom we have selected for AICD implantation in terms of age, underlying cardiac disease, clinical arrhythmia history, and quality of left ventricular function.

In contrast, the 1-year mortality rate for sudden death in patients treated with an AICD at our institution has been 5 percent or less in repeated analyses at various stages of our experience. Other centers have reported equally impressive results. Table 1 summarizes mortality rates for both sudden death and total cardiac death through 5 years postoperatively in a combined series of 207 patients from Stanford University Medical Center and Sequoia Hospital.*

FUTURE DEVELOPMENTS

A major clinical problem with AICD units to date consists of the inability to determine with certainty the underlying cardiac rhythm at the time of device discharge. Thus, in patients receiving relatively frequent shocks, prolonged external monitoring may be necessary to confirm appropriate device function and to refine drug therapy in those patients with supraventricular arrhythmias that trigger the unit. In future versions of the automatic system, this problem will yield to incorporation of a memory feature. Other developments will include further downsizing of the generator, programability of shock energy setting, and sensing features such as recognition of regularity and abruptness of onset of tachycardia as well as rate thresholds. Programable VVI and antitachycardia pacing capability will also be included, and different modes of shock delivery such as sequential pulsing will be evaluated. It is also likely that different defibrillating electrode configurations such as catheter systems will be perfected, thereby reducing the magnitude of the operative procedure required for implantation.

Some of these considerations represent relatively straightforward problems in electrical engineering. Others will depend upon more advanced understanding of basic

* Data furnished in part by Dr. Roger A. Winkle (personal communication).

TABLE 1 Life Table Analysis of Survival Rates After AICD Implantation in 207 Patients

Postoperative interval (Years)	*Number at Risk*	*Sudden (Arrhythmia)**	*All Cardiac**
0–1	207	97.9% (± 1.2)	91.5% (± 2.1)
1–2	116	95.5% (± 2.0)	85.6% (± 3.1)
2–3	80	93.7% (± 2.7)	82.8% (± 3.6)
3–4	54	93.7% (± 2.7)	82.8% (± 3.6)
4–5	26	93.7% (± 2.7)	82.8% (± 3.6)

* Freedom from event.

aspects of cardiac electrophysiology. It is reasonable to expect smaller, smarter, and longer-lived versions of the AICD in the near future. Even the current first-generation device, however, provides a powerful new tool in the management of life-threatening ventricular arrhythmias.

SUGGESTED READING

Echt DS, Armstrong K, Schmidt P, Oyer PE, Stinson EB, Winkle RA. Clinical experience, complications, and survival in 70 patients with the automatic implantable cardioverter/defibrillator. Circulation 1985; 71:289–296.

Mirowski M, Reid PR, Mower MM, Watkins L, Gott VL, Schauble JF, Langer A, Heilman MS, Kolenik SA, Fischell RE, Weisfeldt ML. Termination of malignant ventricular arrhythmias with an implanted automatic defibrillator in human beings. N Engl J Med 1980; 303:322–324.

Mirowski M, Reid PR, Winkle RA, Mower MM, Watkins L, Stinson EB, Griffith LSC, Kallman CH, Weisfeldt ML. Mortality in patients with implanted automatic defibrillators. Ann Intern Med 1983; 98:585–588.

Winkle RA, Bach SM Jr, Echt DS, Swerdlow CD, Imran M, Mason JW, Oyer PE, Stinson EB. The automatic implantable defibrillator; local ventricular bipolar sensing to detect ventricular tachycardia and fibrillation. Am J Cardiol 1983; 52:265–270.

Winkle RA, Mead RH, Ruder MA, Schmidt P, Stinson EB, Buch WS, Gaudiani V. Five year experience with the automatic implantable defibrillator in 157 patients. J Am Coll Cardiol 1987; 9:167A.

Winkle RA, Stinson EB, Echt DS, Mead RH, Schmidt P. Practical aspects of automatic cardioverter/defibrillator implantation. Am Heart J 1984; 108:1315–1346.

RECURRENT VENTRICULAR TACHYCARDIA: SURGICAL MANAGEMENT

ALDEN H. HARKEN, M.D.

Although ventricular tachyarrhythmias are common, surgical therapy is usually unnecessary. To put this in perspective, however, coronary artery disease is present in almost all adult patients treated by surgeons in the United States. Myocardial ischemic damage creates the electroanatomic substrate requisite for re-entrant ventricular tachyarrhythmias. Perhaps 5 to 10 percent of survivors of myocardial infarction develop sustained ventricular tachycardia; the annual prevalance of clinically significant ventricular tachycardia in this cohort may approach 50 percent, with half of these patients sustaining fatal episodes. Thus, approximately 400,000 Americans die of postinfarction ventricular tachyarrhythmias each year. The problem is considerable; so is our ignorance concerning rational pharmacologic and surgical therapy.

PHARMACOLOGY OF ANTIARRHYTHMIC DRUGS

It is essential that surgeons have some appreciation for the pharmacology and pharmacokinetics of antiarrhythmic drugs, in that they will almost never see a patient until he or she has been pushed to the limits of polypharmacy. Unlike the surgical approach to supraventricular arrhythmias, in which a neat, accessory anatomic structure can frequently be identified and ablated, the surgery for ventricular tachyarrhythmias is based on fabrication and supposition. Patients do not become surgical candidates until they have failed maximal medical therapy. By the time surgeons see such patients, therefore, their myocardial cells are reeling from multiple channel blockers, conduction depressants, and negative inotropes.

Many observers have acknowledged that pharmacologic therapy for the patient with ventricular tachyarrhythmias cannot be developed logically and predictably. Recurrent, inducible ventricular tachyarrhythmias are by definition re-entrant. We now believe that the individual pathways involved in the tachycardia circuit are microareas of heterogeneous ischemic myocardial damage. Electrical ventricular activation normally occurs very rapidly—an impulse travels perhaps 2 to 3 m per second. Ischemic damage tends to slow this conduction dramatically. Similarly, there may be frequency-dependent block, which when immersed in a heterogeneous bed of myocardial scar can promote and sustain an impulse that may travel along one arm of a re-entrant circuit sufficiently slowly that the origin has a chance to be repolarized prior to its return. In some re-entry loops, propagation may be dependent on slow calcium channel activity, and in others it may depend on fast sodium channels. Indeed, the re-entrant circuit itself may not be stable. Most antiarrhythmic drugs slow conduction and therefore may be proarrhythmic. Damaged myocardial and Purkinje tissues generally depolarize when they become ischemic. The diastolic membrane potential of these cells is almost certainly influenced by the nature and degree of damage from reperfusion and intramyocardial scar. When this complex electroanatomic swamp is modified by the autonomic nervous system, heterogeneous blood flow, variable drug concentrations, active and inactive membrane channel states, diastolic membrane potential, and heart rate, a very unstable substrate for ventricular tachyarrhythmias exists. These multiple variables explain the unpredictability of the micro re-entry circuit. Successful pharmacologic antiarrhythmic therapy probably unselectively makes "sick cells sicker." Because conduction is further depressed, the re-entrant loop is no longer successfully maintained. The surgeon has a huge therapeutic advantage. All changes in refractory time, conduction velocity, or anatomic pattern may destabilize the re-entry circuit. Like the cardiologist, who manipulates the circuit indirectly, the surgeon's goal is to excise or disengage this circuit from the rest of the functioning myocardium.

PROGRAMMED ELECTRICAL STIMULATION

All patients are subject to electrophysiologic testing with programmed electrical stimulation prior to surgery. This is the mechanism by which the antiarrhythmic efficacy can be tested efficiently in the hospital. When drugs fail, it is extraordinarily helpful to have a preoperative "catheter map" performed in the electrophysiology laboratory. The tachycardia is induced with programmed electrical stimulation. The earliest area of ventricular activation during each cycle is assessed with a sensing catheter in the left ventricle. If the origin of a circuit can be localized to the anterior, lateral, posterior, or septal portion of the left ventricle and then this localization can be identified as apical or basilar, this is very advantageous for the surgeon. Approximately 10 percent of the time, the clinical tachycardia cannot be induced in the operating room. A very effective directed surgical procedure can be accomplished with this preoperative localization alone.

Intraoperative mapping is also accomplished in all patients for more precise localization. A transvenous pacing catheter is placed on the diaphragmatic surface of the right ventricle either the night prior to or the morning of surgery.

Programmed stimulation is based on the insertion of a paced extra stimulus into the micro re-entrant circuit. This is possible by virtue of frequency-dependent conduction block. A train of six paced electrical stimuli captures the ventricle. Single, double, or triple extra stimuli are then rapidly applied to the ventricle at progressively shorter pacing intervals. With progressive cycle shortening, the impulse may be blocked down one arm of a re-entrant circuit, permitting the same impulse to travel along the alternate pathway and return along the "blocked" route sufficiently slowly such that the origin will have had a chance to repolarize—thus permitting re-excitation and re-entry.

INTRAOPERATIVE MAPPING

Following cannulation for cardiopulmonary bypass, a reference "plunge" electrode is placed on the left lateral free wall of the ventricle (adjacent to a circumflex marginal vessel). The anterior right ventricle is thinner and therefore a more difficult area from which to obtain a good signal. In addition, if the reference electrode is placed on the anterior right ventricular surface, it tends to be dislodged during manipulation of the heart. The transvenous pacing catheter has been placed previously. Three mapping techniques may be utilized.

Activation Sequence Mapping. With programmed stimulation from the right ventricular pacing catheter, intraoperative sustained ventricular tachycardia may be induced 80 to 90 percent of the time. Occasionally, it is necessary to pace through the left ventricular reference electrode. We no longer map the epicardium. Normothermic cardiopulmonary bypass is initiated. The left ventricular aneurysm or area of infarction is opened, and ventricular tachycardia is induced. Note that when the heart is 'tipped up" so that the surgeon can access the left ventricular endocardium, the morphology of the tachycardia will change. For several dozen patients, we chased this as a "new" tachycardia. An arbitrary map is then created, with noon, 3 o'clock, 6 o'clock, and 9 o'clock being readily identifiable anatomic structures around the circumference of the ventriculotomy. The exploring electrode is then moved circumferentially around the ventriculotomy, initially at its edge. Upon completion of the initial circumference, the exploring electrode is moved 1 cm in from the edge, and an additional circumference is completed. Usually, this can be accomplished at four or five 1-cm intervals into the left ventricle. To complete a full map usually takes 2 to 3 minutes. In activation sequence mapping, look for the earliest site of ventricular origin in each tachycardia complex. That site is the location where the electrogram during each QRS complex actually precedes the electrical signal at the limb leads. We assume that this earliest site is either the origin or some obligatory part of the re-entrant tachycardia circuit.

Sinus Rhythm Mapping. In moving the exploring electrode around the endocardial surface, there will be areas, usually close to the scar, that exhibit continuous, low voltage, fragmented electrical activity tailing off the QRS complex. Some observers believe that this continuous electrical activity during ventricular tachycardia represents the re-entrant circuit. I believe that it is pathologic but does not necessarily represent activity that engages the rest of the contractile portion of the left ventricle. Therefore, sinus rhythm mapping is sensitive but is not specific.

Pace Mapping. Conceptually, this technique is very appealing. It does not require the induction of ventricular tachycardia. Instead of recording from the exploring electrode, a pacing impulse is inserted through the exploring electrode. When a QRS morphology is produced in the limb leads that mimics the clinical tachycardia morphology, it is assumed that the origin and tachycardia circuits must be similar. There are two problems with this practice. First, manipulation of the heart intraoperatively makes correlation with the clinical tachycardia QRS morphology difficult. Second, substantially different pace maps may be produced by pacing at closely adjacent sites, presumably by virtue of differing exit circuits. We therefore rely heavily on activation sequence mapping.

OPERATIVE TECHNIQUE

We have encouraged our anesthesiologists to use a nitrous oxide–narcotic technique. This has proved to be less negatively inotropic than inhalational agents. Because most patients with ventricular tachycardia have poor ventricular function, it is an advantage to use a less depressant anesthetic.

All patients undergoing surgery for ventricular tachycardia have a pulmonary artery catheter placed just prior to surgery, in the operating room. Again, the anesthesiologist may defer this procedure for fear of inducing ventricular tachycardia during catheter transit of the right ventricle. In the past 100 patients, we have induced ventricular tachycardia only on two occasions during placement of the pulmonary artery catheter. In both instances, it was very easy to break this tachycardia by pacing from the transvenous right ventricular pacing catheter. Again, these patients have poor ventricular function, and hemodynamic monitoring from a pulmonary artery catheter is invaluable when weaning them from cardiopulmonary bypass.

A standard median sternotomy incision is used whether or not the patient has had previous cardiac surgery. We no longer map the epicardium, and therefore we proceed directly to normothermic cardiopulmonary bypass with a single aortic and a single venous cannula. During normothermic cardiopulmonary bypass, the left ventricle is tipped up and opened. A common concern at this point is air embolism. Because the aorta exhibits normal perfusion pressure (60 to 80 mm Hg) and the decompressed open left ventricle exhibits atmospheric pressure (0 mm Hg), there is no way that air or clot can "swim upstream" through the aortic valve to produce an embolus. Upon opening the left ventricle, intraventricular clot is encountered almost 50 percent of the time. It is most efficient to remove this clot prior to mapping. Gross clot is removed and micro-aggregates are then wiped free with an unfolded sponge on the finger. Do not complete the aneurysmectomy at this time. The fibrous edges of the aneurysm are easy to grasp with an Allis clamp and may be excised later, leaving a smooth surface for ventricular closure.

After mapping is complete, the systemic bypass temperature is dropped to 25° C and blood cardioplegia is infused through the aortic root. Some surgeons can operate on a moving target, but I feel that control is better in an arrested heart. Although it is tempting to complete the aneurysmectomy at this time, it is not advisable. The plane of endocardial resection is easiest to initiate in the fibrous scar of the aneurysm. The endocardial peel is characteristically 1 to 2 mm thick and is carried down beyond the fibrous edge of the endocardial scar out on to apparently normal myocardium. A typical endocardial excision encompasses a 5 × 5 cm endocardial zone. If concomitant coronary bypass surgery is indicated, it should be accomplished at this time. The open left ventricle produces a nicely decompressed heart. Additionally, cold solution may periodically be poured directly into the left ventricle both to cool the endocardium and to wash out microaggregates.

The aneurysm is then resected, and the left ventricle is closed using a 0 nonabsorbable monofilament suture in an everting mattress and then over-and-over fashion along large felt pledgets. The left ventricle is evacuated of air. After rewarming the patient systemically, we now reperfuse the myocardium with warm hypocalcemic, hyperkalemic blood cardioplegia prior to removing the aortic cross-clamp.

Two special problems deserve discussion. When the tachycardia origin or earliest area of ventricular activation derives from the base of the papillary muscle or deep within the septum, I excise as much endocardium as I dare and then cryoablate the offending but structurally important portion of myocardium with a 1.5-cm cyroprobe cooled to −70° C for 3 minutes. When the origin proves to be the base of the papillary muscle (which it frequently is with inferior myocardial infarctions), in addition to freezing, I perform an encircling endocardial excision around the base of that papillary muscle. We have no evidence of efficacy, but it is conceptually appealing and makes me feel better. Having seen many infarcted, fibrotic (but structurally intact) papillary muscles, I am now convinced that a papillary muscle does not need to be viable in order to be mechanically effective and am therefore quite aggressive with the cyroprobe if it is believed that the tachycardia circuit involves this structure.

POSTOPERATIVE CARE

These patients are very sick, and those in particular who have been on amiodarone require catecholamine support postoperatively. Always warn patients and their families that patients will have cardiac arrhythmias in the early postoperative period, so that they will not think the operation was unsuccessful when the arrhythmias occur. Superventricular arrhythmias are extraordinarily common, and bursts of automatic ventricular activity are also frequent. I am convinced that this is based on extraordinarily high catecholamine levels, and I know these do not correlate with postoperative electrophysiologic testing. Occasionally, patients look extraordinarily good on the afternoon following surgery, and the temptation is to extubate them that evening. Again, perhaps due to the catecholamine levels, automatic rhythm disorders can be frequent that evening. Even in the hemodynamically stable patient, it is helpful to have total control of the airway when these abrupt rhythm disorders occur. They are sufficiently frequent that I now insist on controlled ventilation through the first postoperative night even in stable patients.

The rest of the postoperative course is handled exactly like that for a left ventricular aneurysmectomy with or without coronary bypass grafting. Of course, the electrocardiogram will exhibit myocardial injury. For anyone who has seen the extent of endocardial resection and left ventricular aneurysmectomy, this comes as no surprise. The cardiologist should not tell the Intensive Care Unit nurses or the patient's family that the patient has had a perioperative infarction after seeing this injury current on the postoperative electrocardiogram.

POSTOPERATIVE ELECTROPHYSIOLOGIC TESTING

We believe that it is essential for the patient to undergo a full electrophysiologic study (EPS) in the catheterization laboratory 7 to 10 days postoperatively. Again, these results frequently do not correlate with the rhythms seen in the early postoperative period. Patients with nonsustained ventricular tachycardia in the early postoperative period may have a completely clean EPS study with no inducible arrhythmias. Conversely, patients with a completely benign postoperative course may have inducible arrhythmias. The prognostic value of the EPS test, we believe, is sufficiently good to tailor further pharmacologic therapy. In our experience, there has been a 9 percent

30-day operative mortality. Two-thirds of the remaining patients are "noninducible" without antiarrhythmic agents. The residual 25 percent are responsive to antiarrhythmic therapy postoperatively, although they were not prior to surgery. Less than 5 percent of patients are "electrical failures." These patients (usually those with multiple preoperative tachycardia morphologies) may be predictable. In this patient population, an automatic internal defibrillator may be appropriate, as outlined in the preceding chapter.

SUGGESTED READING

Cox JL, Holman WL, Cain ME. Cryosurgical treatment of atrioventricular node reentrant tachycardia. Circulation 1987; 76:6–14.

Boineau JP, Cox JL. Slow ventricular activation in acute myocardial infarction: a source of reentrant premature ventricular contractions. Circulation 1973; 48:702–713.

Harken AH, Horowitz LN, Josephson ME. Comparison of standard aneurysmectomy and aneurysmectomy with directed endocardial resection for the treatment of recurrent sustained ventricular tachycardia. J Thorac Cardiovasc Surg 1980; 80:527–534.

Martin JL, Untereker WJ, Harken AH, Horowitz LN, Josephson ME. Aneurysmectomy and endocardial resection for ventricular tachycardia: favorable hemodynamic and antiarrhythmic results in patients with global left ventricular dysfunction. Am Heart J 1982; 103:960–965.

I CONGENITAL ANOMALIES

CORONARY ARTERY ANOMALIES

JAMES E. LOWE, M.D.

Congenital coronary arterial malformations have long been recognized, but the frequency of such reports in the literature has increased greatly since the introduction of selective coronary arteriography in 1959. Major anomalies amenable to surgical correction include anomalous origin of either the left or right coronary artery from the pulmonary artery, congenital coronary fistulas, congenital aneurysms of the coronary arteries, and congenital membranous obstruction of the ostium of the left main coronary artery. Minor anomalies, in which there is variation in the origin of the coronary arteries from the aorta with normal distal circulation, and secondary anomalies, associated with congenital heart defects such as transposition of the great vessels, truncus arteriosus, and tetralogy of Fallot, seldom require surgical intervention. This review summarizes the clinical manifestations, evaluation, and surgical management of patients with major coronary anomalies, including congenital origin of either the left or right coronary artery from the pulmonary artery, congenital coronary fistulas, congenital coronary aneurysms, and membranous obstruction of the ostium of the left main coronary artery.

Based on our experience and supported by that of others, we recommend that most patients with major congenital coronary arterial malformations be considered candidates for surgical correction. In most instances, the natural history of these lesions is not associated with a normal life expectancy, with the possible exception of congenital origin of the right coronary artery from the pulmonary artery. Since these malformations can now be safely corrected with gratifying long-term results, surgical intervention should be strongly recommended once a precise diagnosis has been established.

PREFERRED APPROACH AND THERAPEUTIC ALTERNATIVES

Successful surgical management of patients with congenital coronary arterial malformations depends on a thorough preoperative evaluation, with precise definition of the anatomy and pathophysiology of the anomaly at the time of cardiac catheterization. Coronary artery fistulas, origin of the right coronary from the pulmonary artery, coronary aneurysms, or membranous obstruction of the ostium of the left main coronary is best approached through a median sternotomy incision. Since there are several surgical alternatives for the management of patients with origin of the left coronary artery from the pulmonary artery, the incision chosen depends on the procedure planned.

Origin of the Left Coronary Artery from the Pulmonary Artery. Two basic approaches are available in the surgical treatment of origin of the left coronary from the pulmonary artery. Simple ligation at the site of origin from the pulmonary artery is effective treatment if enough collaterals from the right coronary exist to supply the left coronary system adequately. This approach is usually reserved for small infants in whom the left coronary artery is too small for a direct anastomosis. Ligation prevents the steal of right coronary artery collateral flow into the low-pressure pulmonary artery system. The major disadvantage of this form of therapy is that the patient has a one coronary artery system. The long-term fate of even large collaterals from the right coronary is unknown, and atherosclerotic coronary artery disease later in life involving the right coronary would affect flow throughout the entire coronary system. Simple ligation, however, may be lifesaving, and reconstruction of a two coronary system can be accomplished at a later time.

If collateral flow from the coronary artery is inadequate or if the patient has large enough vessels, the initial repair can be designed to reconstruct a two coronary artery system. The adequacy of collateral flow from the right coronary artery is best assessed at the time of operation; temporary occlusion of the left coronary artery at its origin from the left pulmonary artery should result in a significant increase in arterial pressure measured within the left coronary artery and an improvement in ventricular function. If coronary blood flow is assessed to be inadequate, a bypass procedure is indicated. At present, this is best accomplished by either ligation and saphenous vein bypass grafting or ligation and left or right subclavian to left coronary anastomosis. In younger children and infants the latter procedure has technical advantages, since in this group the subclavian artery is usually larger than autologous saphenous vein. Subclavian artery to left coronary artery bypass can be performed with or without cardiopulmonary bypass, whereas saphenous vein bypass grafting is performed using cardiopulmonary bypass.

Simple ligation is best accomplished through a left third interspace anterior thoracotomy. The pericardium is opened with particular care to avoid stretching or contusing the phrenic nerve. Careful dissection near the posterior sinus of Valsalva of the pulmonary artery is necessary to assure that the origin is identified. The left coronary artery is then clamped at its origin, and if this is tolerated, it is permanently obliterated with multiple transfixion sutures and divided. Left subclavian to left coronary artery anastomosis is also done through this incision, and the anastomosis is accomplished using interrupted sutures of 7–0 Prolene. If a two coronary system is to be reconstructed using saphenous vein, a median sternotomy incision is made, and the procedure is usually done with cardiopulmonary bypass.

Origin of the Right Coronary from the Pulmonary Artery. This rare anomaly usually produces no symptoms, and therefore few patients come to surgical treatment. The only such case reported thus far was successfully managed by removal of the anomalous right coronary with a cuff of pulmonary artery, followed by successful reimplantation into the ascending aorta. This represents the ideal form of treatment. Alternatives include simple ligation at the site of anomalous origin with or without saphenous vein bypass grafting.

Coronary Artery Fistulas. Since patients with coronary artery fistulas have had a precise and detailed angiographic demonstration of the involved coronary artery, the recipient cardiac chamber, and the exact site of communication, it can often be anticipated preoperatively whether cardiopulmonary bypass will be required. Patients with a single communication that is easily dissected out usually do not require bypass for suture obliteration. However, in patients with multiple communications or large tortuous draining channels, the fistula is best obliterated by opening the recipient cardiac chamber during cardiopulmonary bypass to completely close all fistulous tracts. Finally, if fistula obliteration in any way jeopardizes coronary artery flow, a saphenous vein bypass graft is inserted during cardiopulmonary bypass under hypothermic potassium cardioplegia. In general, therefore, these procedures are always planned with at least pump standby.

After a median sternotomy incision is made, a pericardial cradle is created, and the fistulous communication is dissected and obliterated using multiple transfixion sutures of nonabsorbable material. If a cardiac chamber or the main pulmonary artery must be opened in order to close larger or multiple fistulous tracts, cardiopulmonary bypass is instituted. An arterial perfusion cannula is inserted into the ascending aorta or femoral artery and venous return cannulas into the superior and inferior venae cavae. Tapes are placed around both inferior and superior venal cavae. If the right atrium, right ventricle, or pulmonary artery is opened, the tapes are snugged up around the venous cannulas to eliminate all blood return to the right side of the heart except for coronary sinus flow. The heart is then made to fibrillate, and the recipient cardiac chamber is opened. If the fistulous communication communicates with the left side of the heart, and obliteration requires opening the left atrium or left ventricle, or if saphenous vein bypass grafting is planned, the aorta is cross-clamped under cold potassium cardioplegia and topical hypothermia. After operative repair, intraoperative shunt curves are obtained to prove there is no evidence of a residual left-to-right shunt.

Coronary Artery Aneurysms. This rare condition is usually asymptomatic and is discovered after a major complication such as embolization with infarction, sudden rupture into the pericardial cavity, or rupture into a cardiac chamber with fistula formation. In patients who initially survive and can be studied, the aneurysm is best treated by excision and saphenous vein interposition grafting. The entire aneurysm is excised on cardiopulmonary bypass, and an interposition graft of saphenous vein is placed using a continuous 7–0 nonabsorbable suture. Another surgical option would be proximal and distal ligation of the aneurysm with saphenous vein or internal mammary artery bypass grafting. The correct treatment for those patients who are incidentally found to have asymptomatic coronary artery aneurysms is unknown. However, if they are large and there is evidence of thrombus, the possibility of distal embolization and acute myocardial infarction should be considered, and in select patients elective operative repair should be undertaken.

Membranous Obstruction of the Ostium of the Left Main Coronary Artery. Simple excision of the obstructing membrane via an aortotomy is effective treatment of this exceedingly rare malformation. More difficult than the surgical correction is recognizing this entity preoperatively. Although it is rarely encountered, this malformation underscores the importance of a careful preoperative evaluation of the origin and distribution of the coronary arteries in patients with complex congenital heart disease.

PROS AND CONS OF TREATMENT

After a detailed preoperative assessment, successful surgical repair of congenital coronary arterial malformations can be achieved with gratifying long-term results and an acceptable operative mortality in view of the natural history of most of these conditions.

We have personally evaluated 35 patients with anomalous origin of the left coronary artery from the pulmonary artery, and 25 have been treated surgically. These 20 female and 15 male patients ranged in age from 1 month to 61 years. Nineteen of them had severe congestive heart failure, five had angina, and two infants came to our attention because of failure to thrive. The remaining nine patients came for evaluation of cardiac murmurs of uncertain cause, cardiomegaly, or unexplained dyspnea. All 10 patients not operated on died within several hours to several months after diagnosis. Of the 25 patients who had surgical repair, 14 had simple ligation at the origin of the left coronary from the pulmonary artery, resulting in five operative deaths (36 percent). Six patients have been treated with ligation followed by saphenous vein bypass grafting, with no operative deaths. One patient was treated with ligation and left subclavian to left coronary anastomosis and has done well. Prior to corrective operations, early in our experience, two patients were treated with de-epicardialization and are long-term survivors. De-epicardialization was accomplished by applying phenol over the epicardial surface of the left ventricle in an effort to promote the development of collaterals through the inflammatory healing process. One early patient had pulmonary to aortic anastomosis and died shortly after operation, and one patient died during thoracotomy before a planned simple ligation. Among these 25 patients there were seven deaths, an overall operative mortality rate of 28 percent. In view of the 95 to 100 percent mortality in those not treated surgically, surgical therapy is definitely indicated.

In patients who survive beyond the age of 1 year, the proper form of treatment is controversial. Some have been successfully treated by ligation of the left coronary artery, and others have been treated by anastomosis of the left coronary artery to the aorta, either directly or by venous autograft or prosthetic graft. Although the single best form of surgical therapy for this disorder is unknown, simple ligation in the newborn with adequate right coronary artery collateral flow is generally recommended. In older infants, children, or newborns with inadequate flow, our procedure of choice is ligation and immediate left or right subclavian artery to left coronary reanastomosis. In older children or adults, a two coronary system can also be reconstructed using saphenous vein or internal mammary artery bypass grafting. It should be emphasized, however, that although our initial experience (as well as that of others) with subclavian to left coronary anastomosis and saphenous vein interposition grafting has been good, the long-term results in significant numbers of patients are as yet unknown. In patients with adequate collateral flow from the right coronary to the left coronary system, immediate reconstruction assumes that vein graft or subclavian shunt flow is greater than intrinsic collateral flow. If this is not the case, the hemodynamics continue to favor collateral flow into the left coronary arterial system, which may result in subsequent vein graft or subclavian shunt failure. Clinically, patients may continue to do well even with occluded vein grafts or subclavian shunts because of adequate right coronary collateral flow.

Thirty patients with congenital coronary artery fistulas have been evaluated at the Duke University Medical Center. These patients ranged in age from 6 weeks to 76 years, with a mean of 32 years and equal distribution among males and females. Half the patients came to surgical attention because of symptoms such as congestive heart failure, angina, or failure to thrive. The remainder were asymptomatic and came to operation after evaluation of asymptomatic heart murmurs or cardiomegaly found on a routine chest film. Twenty-three of these patients have had operative repair. All procedures were done through a median sternotomy, and 14 patients had suture obliteration of the fistula without bypass (61 percent). Seven patients had cardiopulmonary bypass in order to open the recipient cardiac chamber and successfully occlude multiple draining fistulous tracts (30 percent). Two patients had saphenous vein bypass grafting after fistula obliteration in order to reconstitute distal coronary flow (9 percent). The mean time of follow-up for these 23 patients has been 10 years. There were no operative deaths and all patients are well, without evidence of recurrent fistula formation, although one patient with a complex fistula of the circumflex coronary artery to right ventricle has a small residual shunt.

Results of surgical treatment of congenital coronary artery aneurysms depend on the degree of left ventricular dysfunction resulting from the complication that brings the patient to surgical attention. Too few of these patients have been treated surgically to allow comment on long-term results. Similarly, little is known about the rare patient with surgically treated anomalous origin of the right coronary artery from the pulmonary artery, although successful repair has been reported.

Two patients with membranous obstruction of the ostium of the left main coronary artery have recently had successful repairs. This is perhaps the rarest of the congenital coronary malformations amenable to surgical treatment, but more cases may be recognized with careful preoperative evaluation of the origin and distribution of the coronary arteries in patients with complex congenital heart disease.

Because of the markedly reduced life expectancy of patients with major congenital coronary arterial malformations, most should be considered candidates for surgical correction. The appropriate operation is chosen after thorough preoperative evaluation precisely defines the anatomy and pathophysiology of the condition. Appropriate surgical intervention yields gratifying long-term results, with a low operative mortality compared with the mortality observed in untreated patients.

SUGGESTED READING

Josa M, Danielson GK, Weidman WH, et al. Congenital ostial membrane of left main coronary artery. J Thorac Cardiovasc Surg 1981; 81:338–346.

Lowe JE, Oldham HN Jr, Sabiston DC Jr. Surgical management of congenital coronary artery fistulas. Ann Surg 1981; 194:373–380.

Lowe JE, Sabiston DC Jr. Congenital coronary malformation. In: Cohn L, ed. Modern technics in surgery, cardiac-thoracic surgery. Mt. Kisko, NY. Futura Publishing Co, 1981:17.

Pinsky WW, Fagan LR, Mudd JF, et al. Subclavian-coronary artery anastomosis in infancy for the Bland-White-Garland syndrome: a three-year and five-year follow-up. J Thorac Cardiovasc Surg 1976; 72:15–20.

Sabiston DC Jr, Neill CA, Taussig HB. The direction of blood flow in anomalous left coronary artery arising from the pulmonary artery. Circulation 1960; 22:591–597.

PRIMUM ATRIAL SEPTAL DEFECTS

RAYMOND LEE, M.D.
GUS J. VLAHAKES, M.D.

Ostium primum atrial septal defect represents one end of the spectrum of atrioventricular canal defects. This congenital abnormality is the result of incomplete development of the superior and inferior endocardial cushions rather than an inherent defect of the atrial septum secundum itself. The result of this incomplete development is a deficiency of atrial septum primum; this results in a large, low-lying atrial septal defect (ASD) that lies just superior to separately formed mitral and tricuspid valves and an intact ventricular septum and is bounded posterosuperiorly by the free edge of the atrial septum secundum. In two-thirds of primum ASDs, the endocardial cushion defect also results in a cleft in the anterior mitral leaflet, and in one-third in an additional cleft in the tricuspid septal leaflet. It is the mitral cleft and the 30 percent incidence of mitral insufficiency that set primum ASDs apart clinically from the more common secundum ASDs. As discussed later, it is also the low-lying position of the defect that sets primum defects apart surgically from the secundum ASD. The left-to-right shunt, which is usually large and produces volume overloading of the right ventricle, may be made even larger by any mitral regurgitant flow, some of which may be directed into the right atrium. Some patients, particularly neonates with this defect, may also have a small left ventricle that may be less compliant, thus requiring higher filling pressures that exacerbate the left-to-right shunt.

CLINICAL FEATURES

Unlike patients with secundum ASDs who tend to be asymptomatic and whose lesions tend to go undetected until they reach school age, patients with primum ASDs may have their lesions discovered in infancy as a result of the prominence of cardiac murmurs and the higher frequency of symptoms caused by congestive heart failure and sometimes mitral insufficiency. Sixty percent of patients are symptomatic, exhibiting dyspnea on exertion, fatigue, or recurrent respiratory infections. Growth failure is common, and congestive heart failure occurs in 20 percent of all patients; when congestive heart failure is present, 84 percent of these patients are less than 6 years of age. The severity of symptoms generally depends on the degree of mitral regurgitation. Pulmonary artery hypertension rarely develops before late adolescence and tends to occur at an end stage. However, when it occurs, right-sided filling pressures may exceed those on the left, resulting in a right-to-left shunt with right-sided heart failure and cyanosis.

On physical examination the precordium is hyperactive, with prominent pulsations representing increased right ventricular volume overload. On auscultation the first sound is usually normal, the second sound is split and fixed in relation to respiration, which represents delayed pulmonary valve closure, and a third sound may be present in the setting of right ventricular failure. A systolic ejection murmur over the left upper sternal border radiating to the upper lung fields, a holosystolic murmur radiating to the axillae, and a low-pitched mid-diastolic murmur at the lower left sternal border represent increased pulmonary blood flow, mitral regurgitation, and increased flow through the tricuspid valve, respectively.

Electrocardiogram

The electrocardiogram is fairly diagnostic for a lesion produced by a failure of endocardial cushion development and helps to distinguish primum from secundum ASDs; there is a left-shifted QRS axis in the frontal plane and a characteristic vectorcardiogram. The left axis deviation of the QRS axis does not correlate with chamber size or pressures but is thought to be due to a primary abnormality of the conduction system, since it persists after surgical repair. The typical vectorcardiogram lies above the isoelectric line with a counterclockwise directed loop. There may be P-wave changes indicative of atrial enlargement, first-degree heart block reflecting increased internodal conduction time, right ventricular hypertrophy, and an rsR′ pattern suggesting a complete or incomplete right bundle branch block due to delayed right ventricular depolarization. Evidence of left ventricular hypertrophy may appear in the presence of significant mitral regurgitation.

Chest X-Ray Film

The cardiac silhouette is usually enlarged mainly due to dilatation of the right atrium and right ventricle with an average cardiothoracic ratio of 0.60. The pulmonary artery is markedly dilated, and the pulmonary vascular markings are greatly increased. In the presence of mitral regurgitation, the left atrium and left ventricle may also appear enlarged.

Echocardiography

The most notable echocardiographic feature is the conspicuous absence of echoes in the lower atrial septum, which is normally relatively thick and easily imaged. The cleft anterior mitral leaflet is also characteristic. In the short-axis parasternal projection, the normal "fish-mouth" appearance of the mitral valve in diastole is transformed by the cleft anterior leaflet to look like a horseshoe. Other features, seen in the M-mode, are narrowing of the left ventricular outflow tract and inferior displacement of the atrioventricular valves toward their corresponding ventricular apices.

Cardiac Catheterization

Catheterization studies are useful not only for confirming the diagnosis of primum ASD but also for identifying other cardiac anomalies such as partial anomalous pulmonary venous connection or persistent left-sided superior vena cava, which would influence operative therapy. A left-to-right shunt is easily demonstrated by a significant oxygen saturation step-up in the right atrium compared to that in the high superior vena cava. Another characteristic feature of primum ASD, as in other types of atrioventricular canal defects, is the typical gooseneck deformity of the left ventricular outflow tract caused by the abnormal attachments of the mitral valve to the ventricular septum, which make the outflow tract narrow and elongated. Right ventricular and pulmonary artery pressures are highly variable but may be slightly elevated, depending on the size of the shunt and the pulmonary vascular resistance.

DIFFERENTIAL DIAGNOSIS

The spectrum of anomalies considered in a patient presenting with primum ASD include secundum ASD, anomalous pulmonary venous return, common atrium, and other variants of partial atrioventricular canal. The electrocardiogram and vectorcardiogram usually can eliminate secundum ASD and/or anomalous pulmonary venous connection because both generally have right axis deviation of the QRS axis in the frontal plane with a clockwise-directed vectorcardiogram loop. Echocardiography and cardiac catheterization have proved invaluable in differentiating primum ASD from other lesions.

INDICATIONS FOR SURGERY

Most of the data on patients who have not undergone surgical correction show that they exhibit serious clinical deterioration by the fourth decade of life. Somerville reported a 54 percent incidence of death or severe symptoms in patients over 30 years old, with the most common cause of death or severe symptoms being severe mitral regurgitation (22 percent) or serious arrhythmias (56 percent). In fact, although arrhythmias are reported to be relatively uncommon (25 percent) under the age of 30 years, they increase dramatically in patients over 30 years, with an 80 percent incidence in those between the ages of 40 and 50 years. The mean age at death of patients with primum ASDs is 35 years, whereas the mean age at death for patients with secundum ASDs is 55 years. In a study of 144 patients with uncorrected primum ASDs, Weyn found only eight patients older than 30 years.

Surgical correction should be performed electively when patients are preschool age. If, however, patients are symptomatic from congestive heart failure or if growth failure occurs, operation is scheduled at the time of diagnosis. In the select group of patients with mitral insufficiency who may or may not be symptomatic, surgery is scheduled at diagnosis in an attempt to prevent the worsening of the condition with time. The surgical therapy depends on whether the insufficiency is in the central orifice or through the cleft in the anterior leaflet.

SURGICAL THERAPY

The approach is via a median sternotomy incision. The pericardium is eccentrically opened and a patch of pericardium is first cleaned of extraneous tissue and saved on a sponge soaked with saline. The heart is then examined to detect any other congenital anomalies. Cardiopulmonary bypass is established with direct bicaval cannulation and ascending aortic perfusion. Alternatively, in children less than 8 to 10 kg, deep hypothermia and circulatory arrest are employed. The aorta is then cross-clamped, and cold cardioplegia is infused. The right atrium is incised obliquely, exposing the defect; the mitral valve is visualized across the defect (Fig. 1). The left ventricle is then filled with cold saline across the mitral annulus in order to examine the mitral valve during passive distention of the left ventricle for evidence of insufficiency. We close the mitral cleft, the superior and inferior elements of the anterior leaflet are approximated starting nearest their septal attachments with interrupted 5–0 polypropylene sutures until the insufficiency through the cleft is minimized (Fig. 2). Great care is taken to avoid excessively closing the cleft, which may distort the central approximation leaflet tissue and thereby create or exacerbate central regurgitation. In the case of an infant or child with moderate to severe central mitral insufficiency, plicating annuloplasty sutures are placed at the commissures in an attempt to decrease the parietal circumference; however, care must be taken not to excessively plicate the mitral annulus. It is easy to make the valve relatively stenotic in a child; the goal should be improvement rather than complete elimination of regurgitation in the younger age groups. In an adult patient with regurgitation, a Carpentier annuloplasty ring is preferred to restore mitral annular geometry and is effective in controlling central regurgitation. Only rarely is mitral valve replacement needed.

In order to close the ASD as well as to avoid injuring the conduction system with suture lines, an understanding of the anatomy of the atrioventricular conduction system

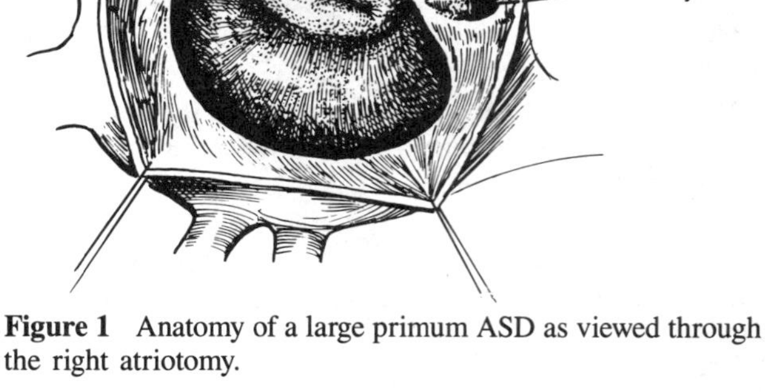

Figure 1 Anatomy of a large primum ASD as viewed through the right atriotomy.

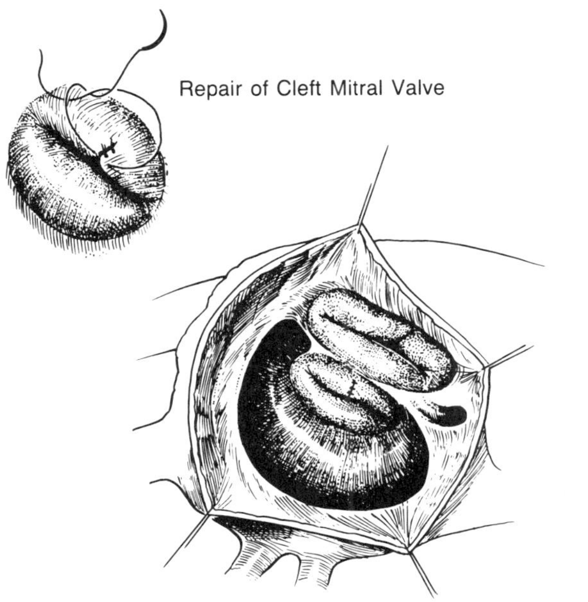

Figure 2 Repair of the cleft in the anterior leaflet of the mitral valve. Only three sutures are used here; if the sutures are placed too close to the central orifice, they may distort the coapting surface of the anterior leaflet and produce or exacerbate central regurgitation.

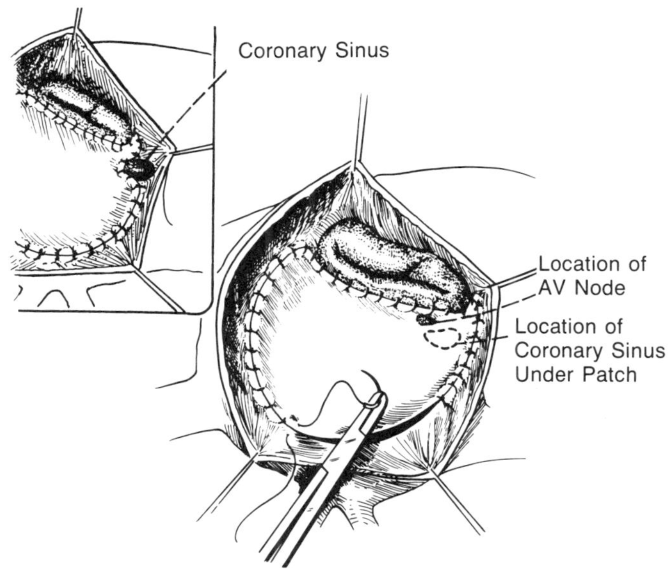

Figure 3 Placement of the pericardial patch to close the defect. The patch suture line is brought widely around the coronary sinus to avoid the conduction system. The inset shows how the technique is varied in instances of persistent left superior vena cava; the suture line is brought posteriorly to clear the conduction system, then into the coronary sinus, along its medial wall.

is crucial. The classic work of Lev in 1958 documented the anatomy of the conduction system in the case of primum ASD; in this lesion the atrioventricular node may be displaced from its usual position in the triangle of Koch to a location bounded by the coronary sinus, the lower edge of the atrial septum, and the tricuspid valve leaflet. Using this information, the pericardial patch is trimmed to cover the atrial septal defect as well as the coronary sinus. In this manner, the lower edge of the patch is sutured with a continuous 4–0 polypropylene suture along the insertion of the tricuspid septal leaflet, with most of the suture material passing through the leaflet tissue itself; the suture line is then carried widely around the coronary sinus. This avoids the conduction system and does not interfere with the mitral valve (Fig. 3). It does, however, create a small right-to-left shunt, as the coronary sinus now is directed into the left atrium. Normally, this poses no problems. However, if there is a persistent left-sided superior vena cava draining into the coronary sinus, the degree of right-to-left shunting would become unacceptable; to avoid this in these cases as well as to avoid the conduction system in the repair, the inferior suture line is then brought posteriorly inside the usually much larger coronary sinus along its medial wall (inset, Fig. 3). This avoids both the conduction system and an unacceptable right-to-left shunt.

RESULTS AND COMPLICATIONS

At the Massachusetts General Hospital, 65 patients with primum ASD have been diagnosed and surgically treated since the late 1960s. The surgical results have been excellent, with no operative mortality; one patient required late mitral valve replacement. Using the surgical technique described above, there have been no cases of complete heart block, compared with a reported 7 percent incidence with techniques that make no attempt to avoid the conduction system. Although patients rarely require mitral valve replacement at first presentation, approximately 10 percent of surgically treated patients are reported to require mitral valve replacement at an average of 10 years after repair. The operative mortality reported with other techniques varies from 4 to 11 percent. The main causes of death or severe symptoms in these cases are a low cardiac output state and serious arrhythmias. Because it avoids the conduction system and the mitral valve, we feel our technique results in an improved operative mortality, a low incidence of heart block, and fewer arrhythmia complications. Closure of the mitral valve cleft at the time of repair may decrease the incidence of late mitral regurgitation requiring valve replacement.

SUGGESTED READING

Lev M. The architecture of the conduction system in congenital heart disease: I. Common atrioventricular orifice. Arch Pathol 1958; 65:174–191.

Levy S, Blondeau P, Dubost C. Long-term follow-up after surgical correction of the partial form of common atrioventricular canal (ostium primum). J Thorac Cardiovasc Surg 1974; 67:353–363.

Losay J, Rosenthal A, Castenada AR, Bernhard WH, Nadas AS. Repair of atrial septal defect: results, course, and prognosis. J Thorac Cardiovasc Surg 1978; 75:248–254.

Sommerville J. Ostium primum defect: factors causing deterioration in the natural history. Br Heart J 1965; 27:413–419.

Weyn AS, Bartle SH, Nolan TB, Dammann JF. Atrial septal defect-primum type. Circulation 1965; 32(Suppl. III):13–23.

SECUNDUM ATRIAL SEPTAL DEFECTS

EDWARD D. VERRIER, M.D.

Secundum atrial septal defect is one of the most common congenital heart defects and was one of the first lesions directly repaired using cardiopulmonary bypass. There are three basic types of defects occurring in the atrial septum: the ostium secundum, the sinus venosus, and the ostium primum. The ostium secundum defects are caused by developmental failure of the septum primum and range from a small, persistent foramen ovale in the upper third of the septum to a large, sometimes trabeculated defect extending down to the inferior vena cava. Sinus venosus defects occur at the junction of the superior vena cava and right atrium but may also extend inferiorly across the septum. This defect is almost always associated with anomalous drainage of the right superior pulmonary veins, which usually enter at the junction of the superior vena cava and right atrium. The ostium primum defect is caused by a deficiency in the atrioventricular septum and is discussed in the preceding chapter. The ostium primum, secundum, and sinus venosus defects may coexist or there may be multiple fenestrations of septal tissue extending across the defects. Very rarely, either the entire septum fails to develop, resulting in a common atrium, or a very small defect may be present directly in the coronary sinus.

Repair of a secundum atrial septal defect is necessary to correct left-to-right shunting of blood across the atrial septum. Left atrial pressure is normally slightly higher than right atrial pressure, causing this left-to-right shunt through the atrial septal defect. If the defect is large enough for equalization of pressures between the two atrial chambers, the extent of shunting is determined by the relative compliances of the right and left ventricles during diastole or the relative resistances of the pulmonary and systemic vascular beds. Since the diastolic compliance of the left ventricle is usually less than that of the right ventricle, and since systemic vascular resistance is higher than pulmonary vascular resistance, both factors increase the left-to-right shunt through the atrial septal defect. Excessive pulmonary blood flow and volume overload of the right ventricle ensue.

Uncomplicated atrial septal defects rarely cause severe symptoms in infancy, although occasionally severe congestive heart failure develops. More commonly, the excessive pulmonary blood flow is well tolerated, and these children remain asymptomatic. There is also little likelihood that pulmonary vascular obstructive disease will develop as a result of an atrial septal defect for many years. However, the natural history of atrial septal defects has been inferred from numerous retrospective studies and a few serial studies of patients not operated on. The average life expectancy of a person with an atrial septal defect is reduced to about 50 years, and congestive heart failure or atrial arrhythmias frequently develop in the third or fourth decade of life. Therefore, we recommend repair for uncomplicated atrial septal defects as an elective procedure in any patient with evidence of a left-to-right blood flow shunt in excess of 1.5 to 1. We prefer to repair this lesion in asymptomatic children before they start school, usually when they are between 4 and 6 years of age. In the unusual symptomatic infant who does not respond promptly to medical therapy, the defect should also be repaired. In addition, atrial septal defects are frequently closed as part of a total repair involving other more complex congenital heart anomalies.

DIAGNOSIS

Since most patients are asymptomatic, the diagnosis is suspected by hearing a murmur in a child during a preschool examination. Occasionally some children present with either fatigue or dyspnea on exertion and more rarely with severe congestive heart failure, syncope, or hemoptysis. The diagnosis can frequently be confirmed by M-mode echocardiography, which shows reverse septal motion and a dilated right ventricle. Two-dimensional echocardiography can better visualize the actual defect in the atrial septum, estimate size, and determine the presence or absence of anomalous pulmonary veins. Cardiac catheterization is done routinely only when the diagnosis is unclear according to echocardiography. If associated anomalies, anomalous pulmonary venous drainage, or pulmonary hypertension is suspected, cardiac catheterization is indicated.

SURGICAL TREATMENT

At surgery, we routinely place only one large, well-secured intravenous and one percutaneous intra-arterial line. No central venous, left atrial, Swan-Ganz, or Foley catheters are necessary.

Since secundum atrial septal defects occur approximately twice as often in females as in males, the choice of incision may have cosmetic implications. Many surgeons prefer a right anterolateral thoracotomy incision, particularly in older girls, since the incision can be made beneath the breast tissue. This incision provides good exposure of the right atrium but permits less flexibility in the event that other associated anomalies are present. If the incision is too high in the skin anteriorly beneath the right nipple, it has the potential to leave a scar across tissue that may later become part of the breast. The position of this incision may be difficult to anticipate in a younger prepubertal girl. If it is selected, the fifth or sixth intercostal space is opened, and the pericardium is entered anterior to the phrenic nerve.

The second possible incision used for cosmetic reasons is the bilateral submammary one. A single transverse incision is made below both breasts and a large subcutaneous flap is developed superiorly to the sternal notch. The sternum is then transected in the midline. This technique has the same disadvantage as the right anterolateral thoracotomy incision in that it may be misplaced into tissue that will later develop into breast. There is also concern among some surgeons that wound complications are more possible after this extensive dissection. Since a median sternotomy is performed, however, more flexibility is possible once the sternum is transected.

At the University of California (San Francisco), we prefer a standard median sternotomy incision. In girls we prefer to make this incision low and short and then only to transect the sternum partially, from the xiphoid process proximal to the manubrium. This brings the incision much lower for better cosmesis but allows the flexibility to extend the incision cephalad in order to completely transect the sternum if exposure is inadequate or a more complicated intracardiac anomaly is found. Once the sternum is partially transected from the xiphoid proximal to the angle of Louis, a Hemelstine retractor is inserted, and the sternum is gently opened. This usually allows adequate access to the ascending aorta for arterial cannulation and good exposure of the right atrium for bicaval venous cannulation and placement of caval tapes.

The heart, great vessels, and venous connections are carefully inspected once the pericardium is opened, and a pericardial cradle is created. This inspection may be particularly important if one is operating without prior cardiac catheterization. The right atrium and ventricle should appear enlarged consistent with volume overload secondary to the left-to-right atrial shunt. The left atrium and left ventricle should be normal. The great vessel position should be normal, with an enlarged pulmonary artery but no patent ductus arteriosus. The size of the right-sided superior vena cava should be noted, since a small superior vena cava or transverse innominate vein may signify a left-sided superior vena cava. This anomalous vessel should also be sought for in the fold of Marshall, since this vessel enters the coronary sinus next to the left atrium. Failure to recognize the presence of a left-sided superior vena cava may influence the ability to later visualize the septal defect because of the large venous return coming through the coronary sinus. Finally, the pulmonary venous anatomy is carefully noted, particularly on the right side at the junction of the superior vena cava and the right atrium.

Once pursestring sutures are placed, heparin (3 mg per kilogram) is given intravenously or directly in the right atrium. Arterial cannulation is usually in the ascending aorta. In some older children who undergo a right anterior thoracotomy, cannulation also may be accomplished through the right femoral or iliac artery. Venous cannulation is dependent upon the position of the atrial septal defect, the size of the patient, whether or not associated anomalies are present, a left-sided superior vena cava, and surgeon preference. Either straight or right-angled bicaval venous cannulas are usually used. The superior vena cava cannula may be inserted through the right atrium and directed into the vessel or inserted directly into the superior vena cava (right-angled cannula). The right-angled cannula is particularly helpful for more complex forms of secundum atrial septal defects high in the septum such as the sinus venosus type or those involving partial anomalous pulmonary venous drainage. The inferior vena cava cannula may also be inserted through the right atrial appendage (straight cannula) or at the inferior vena caval and right atrial junction (right-angled cannula). Caval tapes are routinely used to minimize systemic venous blood return into the right atrium and to avoid sucking air into the venous return circuit. For a smaller patent foramen ovale or secundum atrial septal defect, a single standard straight cannula can be used to drain inferior vena caval blood, and the cardiotomy sucker can be placed into the superior vena cava once the right atrium is opened. This alternative technique of venous cannulation may be particularly helpful in small infants or when associated anomalies are being corrected that only require a single venous cannula.

Once atrial and venous cannulation is complete, normothermic cardiopulmonary bypass is instituted. In order to avoid air embolism, which is the most worrisome complication of this repair, we fibrillate the heart using an external fibrillator on the surface of the right ventricle. Routinely the patient's temperature is allowed to drift down to 33 to 34 °C while the defect is being repaired. The patient is then systemically rewarmed during right atrial closure. For sinus venosus defects or other more complex lesions, moderate hypothermia (28 °C) is often added to the fibrillatory technique. We almost never use cardioplegic arrest.

OPERATIVE TECHNIQUE

The right atrium is opened using an oblique incision, taking care not to injure the sinoatrial node. The internal anatomy of the right atrium is then inspected for the following:

1. the size and location of the atrial septal defect;
2. the relation of the atrial septal defect to the superior and inferior venae cavae;
3. the size and location of the coronary sinus;
4. the amount of blood returning to the field through the coronary sinus (? anomalous superior vena cava);
5. entry points of the pulmonary veins, particularly those on the right side;
6. the location of the atrioventricular node; and
7. the presence or absence of fenestrations crossing the atrial septal defect.

A cardiotomy sucker is used to remove excess blood in the right atrium in order to obtain good visualization of the anatomy. This sucker is not routinely placed across the defect and into the left atrium, as this maneuver could leave residual air in the left atrium.

A patent foramen ovale or a very small ostium secundum defect may be closed by a direct suture technique. We use a double layer of 3–0, 4–0, or 5–0 Prolene sutures. We believe it is particularly important not to close the defect under tension because a residual defect may result. Therefore, most standard ostium secundum defects are patched using a Teflon felt material. We routinely use Teflon felt because it is easy to handle and is rapidly covered with vascular endothelium. Occasionally pericardium is used, particularly in more complex lesions, such as an ostium primum defect. Bovine pericardium has also been used for exceptionally large lesions such as a common atrium.

We start the suture line with a mattress stitch in the most inferior, lower corner of the atrial septal defect. Care must be used to place this suture carefully, as the inferior vena cava cannula and eustachian valve may interfere with visualization of this corner of the defect. A simple over-and-over stitch is used around the rim of the atrial septal defect, bringing both limbs of the double-stranded suture up to the defect's highest point. If the atrial septal defect has multiple fenestrations, care is used to ensure that the patch closes all of them. When the patch closure is almost complete, the anesthesiologist gently inflates the lung to expel any residual air caught in the pulmonary veins or left atrium, and then the stitch is tied. We then place an aortic needle vent into the ascending aorta to remove any further residual air prior to defibrillation. Once the atrial septal defect is closed, the fibrillator is removed and the right atrial incision is closed with a 4–0 or 5–0 Prolene suture in two layers. Usually the heart will spontaneously defibrillate into normal sinus rhythm once the fibrillator is removed and rewarming is started. Occasionally the heart is defibrillated with 5 to 10 watt seconds of electrical current. The caval tapes are removed, and the patient is weaned from cardiopulmonary support once rewarming is complete.

SINUS VENOSUS DEFECT

Adequate exposure of the superior vena caval-right atrial junction is important in the sinus venosus defect in order to have adequate visualization of the orifices of the right superior pulmonary veins. In many sinus venosus atrial septal defects, a standard oblique right atrial incision can be used, particularly if the anomalous pulmonary vein enters low at the superior vena caval-right atrial junction. Care must be used not to injure the sinoatrial node or sinoatrial nodal artery, but to still have adequate visualization of the atrial septal defect and pulmonary veins. To ensure exposure, the atrium is frequently opened more posteriorly between the sinus node and the interatrial groove. This longitudinal incision may then be extended superiorly along the vena cava. Occasionally it may be necessary to actually enlarge the atrial septal defect in order to create a large, nonrestrictive channel between the superior pulmonary veins and the left atrium. Pericardium is used almost exclusively for this intra-atrial patch. The pericardial patch is sutured with a running 4–0 or 5–0 Prolene suture and is usually begun around the orifice of the superior pulmonary vein and brought laterally around the atrial septal defect. A second pericardial patch may then be required in order to enlarge the superior vena cava itself. The necessity for the second patch depends on the degree of bulging required to achieve an adequate opening between the superior pulmonary vein and the left atrium.

POSTOPERATIVE CARE

These children routinely require minimal postoperative care and frequently return to a monitored bed on the floor rather than to the intensive care unit. We do not routinely sedate the child or find it necessary to give large systemic doses of analgesics. Most children are extubated in the operating room or postanesthetic recovery room. The anterior mediastinal tube is left in place until the next morning. The child is usually discharged from the hospital in 5 days.

RESULTS

These lesions may be repaired with very low surgical risk. Over the 3-year period of 1984 to 1986, we repaired 93 atrial septal defects of the simple ostium secundum or sinus venosus type. In that group, there was no morbidity or mortality. During that period, there were 25 patients operated on for "complex" atrial septal defects, which included concomitant pulmonic stenosis or ventricular septal defect. In this group there was one death of a child operated on for severe tricuspid regurgitation and atrial septal defect; he had had a previous conduit placed and a ventricular septal defect closed. He died postoperatively of right ventricular failure.

SUGGESTED READING

Harvorth SG. Pulmonary vascular disease in atrial septal defect in childhood. Am J Cardiol 1983; 51:265–272.

Kirklin JW, Swan HJC, et al. Anatomic, physiologic, and surgical considerations in repair of interatrial communications in man. J Thorac Cardiovasc Surg 1955; 29:37–53.

Spangler JG, Feldt RH, et al. Secundum atrial septal defect encountered in infancy. J Thorac Cardiovasc Surg 1976; 71:398–401.

Stewart S, Alexson C, et al. Early and late results of repair of partial anomalous pulmonary venous connection to the superior vena cava with a pericardial baffle. Ann Thorac Surg 1986; 41:498–501.

Williams WH, Zorn-Chilton S, et al. Extracardiac atrial pedicle conduit repair of partial anomalous pulmonary venous connection to the superior vena cava in children. Ann Thorac Surg 1986; 38:345–355.

TRUNCUS ARTERIOSUS

KEVIN TURLEY, M.D.

Truncus arteriosus is a rare congenital cardiac lesion occurring in less than 1 percent of infants born with congenital heart disease. It is a condition in which the main pulmonary truncus is not related to the right ventricle but arises from a separate site on the aorta. The embryology of this lesion is important in understanding the approach to surgical repair and the possible anatomic configurations that may influence and complicate such repair. The development of the main pulmonary trunk is related to the development of the proximal portion of the second through sixth aortic arches. These arches form the right and left pulmonary arteries, and when they fuse, a transverse pulmonary artery and a ductus arteriosus are formed. As the truncus rotates in infancy, a spiral septum develops that separates the common trunk into a pulmonary and an aortic component. If this does not occur, the main pulmonary artery does not separate, and no connection occurs between the transverse sixth arch and a separate main pulmonary artery. Thus, a transverse vessel connects directly to the common trunk. The embryologic description of Van Praagh, A1 to A4, defines the various configurations and subsets. The most common forms of truncus arteriosus are types A1 and A2, and are the types for which surgical repair is most commonly possible. Approaches to the other forms are complicated by the location of the pulmonary arterial segments and associated lesions, as in A4, in which an interrupted aortic arch and a small anterior aorta are present.

CLINICAL AND PHYSIOLOGIC PRESENTATION

The clinical presentation of truncus arteriosus is determined by the degree of pulmonary blood flow and by the presence of truncal valve insufficiency. In the neonatal period, pulmonary vascular resistance often remains elevated, and congestive heart failure may not be noted during this period. In some patients severe congestive heart failure is present from birth, and respiratory support is necessary, even in early infancy.

More commonly, after the first several weeks of life, pulmonary resistance decreases, pulmonary flow increases, and high output failure ensues. Rarely, patients present with a high pulmonary resistance from birth and never experience a drop in that resistance; these infants usually develop cyanosis, have good weight gain and growth in their early months of life, and eventually are inoperable because of progressive elevation of pulmonary vascular resistance. This group should be differentiated from an equally rare subset of infants born with stenosis at the origin of the pulmonary arteries; in these patients pulmonary blood flow is restricted, and consequently pulmonary vascular resistance is low. They likewise experience cyanosis, good weight gain, and growth in the early months of life, but if the pulmonary vascular bed develops, they are excellent candidates for repair.

The physiologic presentation and anatomic substrate define the timing and surgical approach. As previously noted, a small group of patients demonstrates severe congestive heart failure from birth and requires intervention despite maximal management. In these neonates attempts at direct anastomosis, or a tube-graft placement, may be successful. The size of the patient influences the method of repair since until recently only prosthetic conduits were available, and the smallest heterograft was a 12-mm conduit. If a low resistance is present, the use of a nonvalve conduit is possible. However, most commonly, a reactive pulmonary bed exists, and the presence of a pulmonic valve has, in our experience, markedly improved survival. The critical minimum systemic saturation of 83 percent in those patients without pulmonary arterial stenosis has been critical to operability. In patients in whom such stenosis is absent, a saturation below this level defines severe pulmonary hypertension, and attempts at repair in such individuals are doomed to failure.

Complicating anatomic considerations that increase the risk of surgical repair include: severe truncal valve insufficiency, which often is improved by the resection of the pulmonary component of the trunk and closure of the defect; truncal stenosis with a grossly dysmorphic valve, which carries an extremely high mortality in early infancy; severe override of the trunk, with potential subaortic stenosis; transcristal type ventricular septal defect, present in approximately 10 percent of our series; or a small left ventricular cavity. The type of lesion and associated anomalies, such as single pulmonary artery or interrupted arch, likewise increase the risk of repair. With each of these additional anomalies, in our experience pulmonary hypertension may be more rapidly progressive.

THERAPEUTIC ALTERNATIVES

The natural history of truncus arteriosus, if unrepaired in infancy, demonstrates that of 100 infants at birth, 75 percent die in the first year. Of the 25 remaining children, 35 percent become inoperable by age 4 or 5 because of pulmonary vascular disease. Of the 16 who are still operable at age 4 to 5, there is a 5 percent operative mortality. Of the 15 patients who survive the operation, 20 percent progress to late pulmonary vascular disease. Thus only 12 of the original 100 can be expected to live relatively normal lives.

The next alternative is pulmonary arterial banding. The natural history demonstrates that, of 100 patients, 50 percent die at the time of banding. Of those remaining, 10 percent die between 1 and 5 years of age, and of the 45 still alive, 9 percent die following band removal and repair. Finally, of the remaining 40 patients, 25 percent develop late pulmonary vascular disease, yielding only 30 relatively normal individuals. Therefore the final alternative of surgical repair in early infancy has been used at the University of California, San Francisco, since 1974.

DIAGNOSIS AND EVALUATION

The most common clinical features noted in infants born with truncus arteriosus and presenting from 1 to 2 months of age relate to the increased pulmonary blood flow and severe congestive heart failure. Such patients have a hyperactive circulation, liver enlargement, rales and wheezes, and peripheral pulses that are brisk and bounding. The skin is pale, sweating is common, and most are emaciated. The cardiac examination shows a hyperkinetic heart, a loud, single-second sound, and usually a systolic murmur. A clearly continuous murmur can be heard in infants with ostial stenosis of the pulmonary trunk and increased pulmonary blood flow. A diastolic murmur usually is due to truncal valve incompetence and is a significant prognostic finding.

The x-ray examination usually shows cardiomegaly and increased vascularity, and the electrocardiogram demonstrates biventricular or right ventricular hypertrophy. Findings on echocardiography and angiography are diagnostic of the anomaly. Estimation of pulmonary to systemic blood flow is difficult, as is estimation of the pulmonary resistance. However, a root angiogram will rule out persistent ductus arteriosus or aortopulmonary window and define the presence of interrupted aortic arch.

Critical in this evaluation are the location of the exit of the pulmonary trunk from the ascending aorta, the degree of truncal valve incompetence, and the location of the coronary arteries. With this information a surgical approach can be planned, and anatomic factors influencing the prognosis can be elucidated.

Initial medical management of infants with truncus is accomplished with the use of diuretics and digitalis, and, on many occasions, with ventilatory support. Tracheostomy should be avoided because it complicates the mediastinal surgical field and does not improve long-term results, as operative repair can be performed in early infancy, obviating the need for long-term respiratory support.

SURGICAL MANAGEMENT

At our institution since 1974 the age of early correction has decreased from 6 months to approximately 6 weeks in an attempt to minimize the problem of pulmonary vascular disease without increasing surgical mortality. Physiologic correction of truncus arteriosus is performed through a median sternotomy incision. Under general anesthesia, a radial arterial pressure monitoring line is placed and a standard intravenous system is placed in a peripheral vein. Pursestring sutures are placed high on the ascending aorta at the origin of the innominate artery, in the right atrial appendage, and a snare is placed about the pulmonary arterial trunk. Heparin is administered, the patient is cannulated, and cardiopulmonary bypass is instituted. The snare around the pulmonary trunk is tightened, and the pulmonary arteries are occluded. Oxygenated blood prime has been precooled to 4 to 8° C, and body temperature is rapidly reduced with bypass until it reaches approximately 20° C. The aorta is cross-clamped, and the pulmonary trunk is separated from the underside of the aorta. The aortotomy is then closed primarily, care being taken to avoid injury to the truncal valve or coronary arteries. The right ventricle is then opened near the truncal valve, and the truncal valve is inspected and made incompetent as the aortic clamp is released. The degree of truncal valve incompetence is then assessed. Rarely, severe truncal valve incompetence may be present, and valve replacement may be necessary. The ventricular septal defect is then closed. If a transcristal defect is present, care must be taken to avoid the conduction system, and a patch should be placed to the right side of the septum. If the usual truncal defect is present, a continuous suture technique is used. The perfusate is rewarmed, and the distal anastomosis to the pulmonary arterial segments is performed, a cuff of tissue having been created in the resection of the pulmonary artery.

Finally, the proximal right ventricular to conduit anastomosis is performed. If a Dacron-valved conduit is used, the heterograft valve with its ring is placed as far distally as possible toward the pulmonary artery to avoid encroachment upon the sternum or the coronary arteries and the possibility of compression of adjacent structures. It is further reinforced with Teflon felt in its proximal anastomosis to the ventricle.

Since 1985 ten aortic homografts, sizes 13 to 17 mm, have been used in primary repair of truncus arteriosus. With this technique the anterior leaflet of the mitral valve is used to patch the ventriculotomy, and no Teflon felt reinforcement is necessary. In only one of these cases has reoperation for hemorrhage from the graft been necessary. This is significantly different from the 25 to 40 percent reoperation rate noted with the use of Dacron conduits. Following completion of the repair and rewarming to 37° C, the patient is weaned from cardiopulmonary support, spontaneous defibrillation having occurred in 90 percent of patients, and electrical defibrillation is used in the remainder. The chest is then closed. On rare occasions conduits, especially of the Dacron type, may be compressed by the sternum, reducing cardiac output. If this occurs, closure of the skin can be accomplished and the child maintained on mechanical ventilatory support; delayed sternal closure may be performed 3 to 4 days later. Overall mortality in types 1 and 2 truncus arteriosus in our series of patients less than 6 months of age has been 15 percent using these techniques.

Surgical repair of truncus in older children is determined by the degree of pulmonary vascular resistance. If the resistance is elevated, when arterial oxygen saturation is below 83 percent, the likelihood of success or of significant reduction of pulmonary vascular resistance is unlikely. Unlike this group, in infants in whom pulmonary vascular resistance is elevated in early infancy (less than 6 months of age), the likelihood of resistance dropping is high, and at reoperation 85 percent of those in whom the initial resistance was elevated demonstrated a low pulmonary artery pressure.

LONG-TERM MANAGEMENT

Following repair in early infancy, reoperation for conduit replacement is part of the planned approach to this disease. The size of the initial conduit, the type of conduit, and the anatomic substrate determine the life expectancy of the conduit and the potential for successful replacement. If good pulmonary artery growth occurs, conduit size and the levels of potential obstruction—proximal anastomosis, proximal conduit, valve, distal conduit, or distal anastomosis—will determine the timing of reoperation, and an excellent result can be expected. If pulmonary arterial growth does not occur or if branched stenosis occurs, the results may be adversely affected; continued obstruction despite attempts at patch angioplasty or dilation is common.

When a Dacron conduit is used, its size is critical. In a review of our experience employing a 12-mm conduit (the smallest conduit manufactured and used in the smallest infants with the most diminutive pulmonary arterial systems), the mean time to reoperation was 49 months. In several of these patients, pulmonary arterial growth did not occur, especially in those with true type 2 lesions (separate orifice of the right and left pulmonary arteries). In several such patients the proximal anastomosis, proximal and distal conduit, and the valve all appeared relatively unobstructed; attempts at transluminal angioplasty of the distal pulmonary arterial tree prior to reoperation may benefit such patients.

In the most recent series of aortic homograft repairs, a larger homograft, 13 to 17 mm, could be placed, and long-term patency should be expected without the development of pseudointimal proliferation. Experience at many centers has demonstrated the development of mild valvar insufficiency in such patients; however, pseudointimal proliferation has been absent. Proximal or distal anastomotic stenosis in homograft recipients should represent a technical problem at the time of the initial operation as opposed to subsequent ingrowth as seen in patients with Dacron conduits. Fourteen of our recent conduit replacements have been accomplished using aortic homografts. No deaths have occurred in these patients, and the homograft has functioned as an excellent replacement conduit.

The major postoperative complication in the repair of truncus arteriosus in early infancy is hemorrhage, which has been obviated through the use of the aortic homograft technique. However, early reoperation may be indicated in this group since the total mediastinal volume is low and the conduits themselves occupy a large portion of this volume. Tamponade can occur with a minimal volume in this group. Thus, if it is suspected, the lower portion of the incision is opened to evaluate this problem if low cardiac output develops in the presence of hemorrhage.

The patient is mechanically ventilated with a CO_2 in the range of 30 mm Hg and pH in the range of 7.50; sedation is achieved using a fentanyl anesthetic technique to minimize the reactivity of the pulmonary circulation. Special care must be taken that adequate sedation has been accomplished without paralysis, so that stimuli such as routine suction do not initiate a pulmonary hypertensive crisis during the early postoperative period.

The repair of truncus arteriosus in early infancy must be viewed as a lifetime commitment on the part of the surgeon. The availability of aortic homografts has allowed us to conjecture that conduit changes will be less frequent and the chance of mechanical prosthetic obstruction less of a problem. Late results demonstrate the absence of pulmonary vascular disease and good growth of pulmonary arteries in these patients; however, continued vigilance in the truncus group is necessary. Since the nature of infant repair is one that produces a lifetime surgical illness, it would follow that initial surgical repair is but a part of the overall management. Continued improvements will decrease the need for intervention later in life.

SUGGESTED READING

Boyce SW, Turley K, Yee ES, Verrier ED, Ebert P. The fate of the 12-mm porcine valved conduit from the right ventricle to the pulmonary artery. J Thorac Cardiovasc Surg 1988; 95:201–207.

Ebert PA, Turley K, Stanger P, Hoffman JIE, Heymann MA, Rudolph AM. Surgical treatment of truncus arteriosus in the first 6 months of life. Ann Surg 1984; 200:451–456.

Oldham HN Jr, Kakos GS, Jarmakani MM, Sabiston DC Jr. Pulmonary artery banding in infants with complex congenital heart defects. Ann Thorac Surg 1972; 13:342–350.

Van Praagh R, Van Praagh S. The anatomy of common aorticopulmonary trunk (truncus arteriosus communis) and its embryologic implications: a study of 57 necrosy cases. Am J Cardiol 1965; 16:406–425.

PALLIATION IN CONGENITAL HEART DISEASE

MARC R. DE LEVAL, M.D.

Many radical surgical repairs are actually palliative procedures, either because additional surgery is required or because they have not restored a normal circulation. Prosthetic valve replacements in infancy and childhood, repairs involving extracardiac valved conduits, and the Fontan operation are some examples. In this chapter we consider as palliative procedures operations that do not intend to be so-called complete repairs. Most of these procedures are performed in infants and their goals are: (1) to improve the patient's condition, allowing growth to occur, and to temporize until a corrective procedure can be done with lower risk at a later age; (2) to alter the patient's hemodynamics so he or she is a suitable candidate for corrective surgery; or (3) to improve the hemodynamics in the case of noncorrectable lesions (definitive palliation).

The main objectives of palliative surgery are (1) to decrease pulmonary blood flow, (2) to increase pulmonary blood flow, (3) to improve intracardiac mixing or, (4) to prepare for a future Fontan's operation.

OPERATIONS TO DECREASE PULMONARY BLOOD FLOW

Procedures to decrease pulmonary blood flow include pulmonary artery banding and creation of pulmonary atresia with a systemic-to-pulmonary artery shunt. The latter is discussed with the Norwood procedure.

Banding or constriction of the pulmonary artery was first suggested as a treatment for intractable heart failure in infants with a large left-to-right shunt at the ventricular level. Many of these patients had a large ventricular septal defect, and they are now candidates for radical repair.

The current indications for banding of the pulmonary artery are:

1. Complex ventricular septal defect, including (a) multiple ventricular septal defects, (b) ventricular septal defect with straddling and/or overriding atrioventricular valve, and (c) large ventricular septal defect and coarctation of the aorta. In this group are also included patients with interrupted aortic arch, for whom we sometimes prefer reestablishing continuity between the ascending and descending aorta with banding of the pulmonary artery rather than a complete repair. This would be the case particularly when there is a significant deviation of the infundibular septum such that the closure of the ventricular septal defect could contribute or enhance a left ventricular outflow tract obstruction. The last indication is (d) ventricular septal defect with a small right or left ventricle.
2. Double-inlet ventricles and absence of right or left atrioventricular connection with high pulmonary blood flow. The same applies for cases of double-outlet ventricles and corrected transposition with ventricular septal defect and pulmonary hypertension.
3. Transposition of the great arteries with ventricular septal defect is at present usually considered for arterial switch with closure of the ventricular septal defect. Patients with persistent truncus arteriosus or complete atrioventricular septal defect requiring surgery in infancy are also candidates for primary radical repair.

There is one additional indication for banding of the pulmonary artery with which we have no personal experience—constriction of the pulmonary artery in simple transposition of the great arteries, which attempts to prepare the left ventricle to serve the systemic circulation.

The operation is performed through a left lateral thoracotomy incision in the third or fourth intercostal space. A right thoracotomy incision might be used if an additional procedure such as a Blalock-Hanlon septectomy is performed at the same time.

The left lung is first retracted anteriorly, and the ductus arteriosus is routinely dissected and ligated. This must be done even if the ductus arteriosus has not been demonstrated to be patent preoperatively, as it can be easily missed in patients with systemic pressure in the pulmonary artery.

Next the pericardial sac is opened in front of the phrenic nerve. The incision has to be carried out anteriorly in the superior aspect of the mediastinum beneath the thymus gland to stay well away from the phrenic nerve. Phrenic nerve palsy is one of the main complications following banding of the pulmonary artery. Stay sutures are placed on the edges of the pericardial sac. Then the dissection has to be carried out between the aorta and the pulmonary artery so as to open a plane for passage of the banding material. This maneuver can be facilitated by placing a traction suture on the tip of the left atrial appendage. The pulmonary artery is then retracted to the left in order to expose the pericardial reflection between the aorta and the pulmonary artery. This structure often contains small vessels, which are carefully electrocoagulated before the incision is made. Next an angled clamped is passed from the left to the right between the aorta and the pulmonary artery, and a heavy (1 to 2 mm) braided silk is passed around the pulmonary artery. During this maneuver care must be taken not to damage the origin of the left coronary artery. If this dissection proves difficult, the ligature may be passed more easily by subtraction, first through the transverse sinus and then between the aorta and the pulmonary artery. The position of the ligature should be carefully checked, making sure that it has been passed around the main pulmonary artery and not just around the left pulmonary artery. A pressure monitoring needle is then placed in the distal pulmonary artery and the constrictive device is slowly tightened around the pulmonary artery. To assess the optimal degree of constriction, the patient is ventilated on 50 percent oxygen. The systemic arterial and distal pulmonary arterial pressures are carefully watched (Fig. 1). The optimal pulmonary-to-systemic arterial pressure ratio is usually between 0.5 and 0.3. The arterial Po_2 has to be checked. It is useful to look at the color of the left atrial appendage, which is a good indicator of the pulmonary blood flow. If the appendage becomes blue, assuming that the lungs are well ventilated, this indicates that the pulmonary blood flow is insufficient and the band is too tight.

The mortality for banding of the pulmonary artery depends on the underlying lesions and can range from less than 10 percent to greater than 70 percent.

OPERATIONS TO INCREASE PULMONARY BLOOD FLOW

These procedures include systemic to pulmonary or cavopulmonary shunts, palliative relief of right ventricular outflow tract obstruction, and remodeling of the peripheral pulmonary circulation.

Shunt Procedures

Originally introduced by Blalock and Taussig in 1945 as a treatment of tetralogy of Fallot, shunt procedures are currently often indicated for more complex congenital cardiac defects.

In our institution (The Hospital for Sick Children, London), we continue to perform shunts on infants with tetralogy of Fallot who require surgery under the age of 6 months. Pulmonary atresia with or without ventricular septal defect, double-outlet ventricles, double-inlet ventricles, and absent atrioventricular connection with reduced pulmonary blood flow are the main indications for shunt operations.

Systemic-to-pulmonary arterial shunts can be peripheral or central.

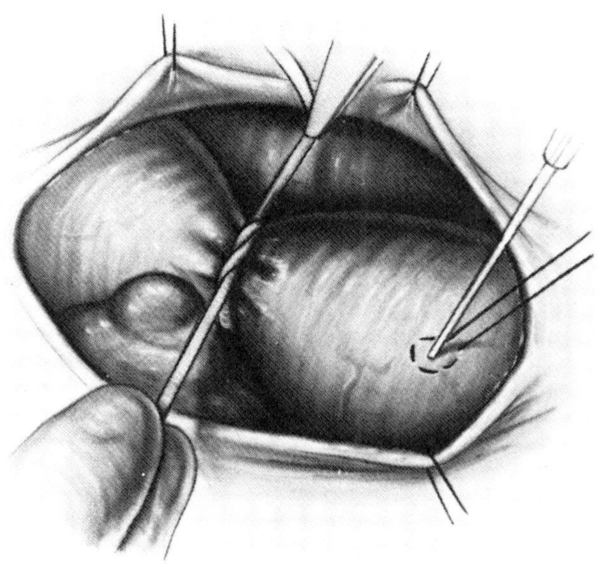

Figure 1 Technique of pulmonary artery banding with measurement of distal pulmonary artery pressure.

Peripheral shunts include the Blalock-Taussig shunt, the Pott's anastomosis, the Waterston shunt, and the prosthetic subclavian artery to pulmonary artery shunt (modified Blalock-Taussig shunt). The Blalock-Taussig shunt is performed on the side of the innominate artery; it appears to provide the optimal palliation and has remained the standard shunt procedure. Distortion of the peripheral pulmonary arteries is the main disadvantage of all peripheral shunts. This complication was frequently seen following the direct aortopulmonary anastomosis (Pott's and Waterston), which in addition made it difficult to adjust the pulmonary blood flow. Both of these shunt procedures have now been almost completely abandoned in our institution. The classic Blalock-Taussig shunt performed in the neonatal period often tends to kink the pulmonary artery, which is pulled up by the subclavian artery. If the prosthesis utilized for the modified Blalock-Taussig shunt has a greater diameter than the subclavian artery, the flow through the shunt is, in theory, limited by the diameter of the subclavian artery, and there is a potential for increasing flow as the patient grows. The modified Blalock-Taussig shunt is equally successful on either side of the aortic arch. The potential risk of late distortion of the distal pulmonary arteries persists.

The classic and the modified Blalock-Taussig shunts are performed through a lateral thoracotomy incision through the fourth intercostal space. The lung is retracted posteriorly so as to place the pulmonary artery on a little tension. The periarterial plane of cleavage that results in easy anatomic dissection is close to the vessel wall. It is important to identify the main branch of the pulmonary artery rather than its upper lobe branch. The dissection of the pulmonary artery is carried well medially to free an adequate length. Attention is then paid to the subclavian artery. The mediastinal pleura is incised. For the classic Blalock-Taussig shunt, a more extensive dissection of the mediastinum is required. A groove is created by blunt dissection between the trachea and the superior vena cava. The azygos and any venous branches crossing the subclavian artery are doubly ligated and divided. After careful identification of the vagus nerve and its recurrent branch, dissection is carried out on the subclavian artery. The branches of the subclavian artery often arise close together. They are all doubly ligated and divided. The artery is then occluded proximally with a vascular clamp and divided distally just proximal to the distal ligatures. Next the subclavian artery is passed beneath the vagus nerve and its recurrent branch. Ample blunt dissection of the innominate and carotid arteries and the creation of a deep groove between the superior vena cava and the trachea provide more mobility to the subclavian artery and enough length to prevent undue tension on the pulmonary artery. The pulmonary artery is then occluded proximally with a vascular clamp and distally with a tourniquet snared on the peripheral branches. A transverse incision is made on the anterosuperior aspect of the pulmonary artery, and the subclavian to pulmonary artery anastomosis is performed with continuous sutures of fine polypropylene (6–0 to 7–0) (Fig. 2).

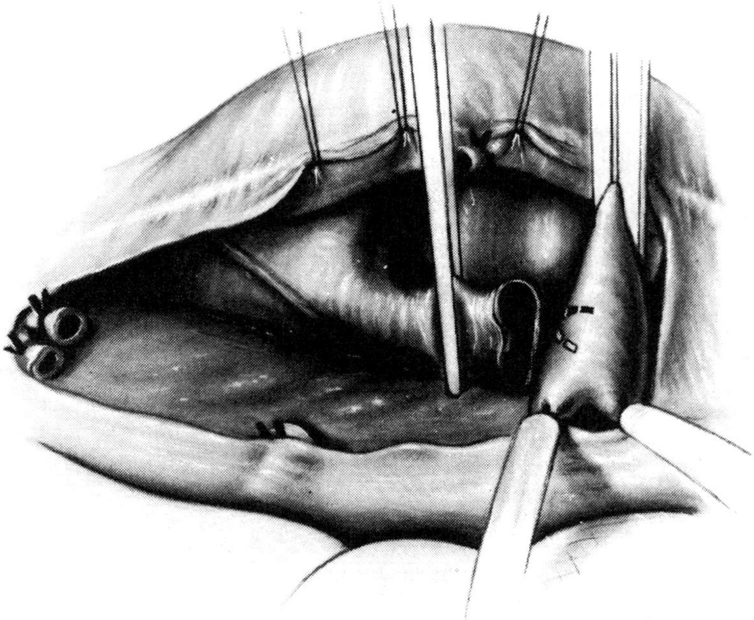

Figure 2 Preparation for subclavian-to-pulmonary artery anastomosis. Note the transverse incision in the pulmonary artery.

For the modified Blalock-Taussig shunt, the mediastinal dissection is limited to the origin of the subclavian artery, around which a tape is passed so as to pull it anteriorly and facilitate its isolation into a vascular clamp of the Cooley type. A longitudinal incision is made on the subclavian artery, and an obliquely trimmed expanded polytetrafluoroethylene prosthesis is anastomosed side-to-end with a continuous suture of 6–0 or 7–0 Prolene. A 5-mm graft is used in small infants and a 6-mm graft in bigger children. The length of the graft is adjusted so that it lies straight along the mediastinum without traction on the pulmonary artery. When the anastomosis between the prosthesis and the subclavian artery is completed, the subclavian clamp is released so as to fill the prosthesis with blood. The clamp is then reapplied on the subclavian artery, the graft is flushed with saline, removing all blood clots, and 1 mg per kilogram of heparin is given intravenously. The pulmonary artery is then isolated between the vascular clamp and distal tourniquets and the prosthesis is anastomosed to the subclavian artery, as for the classic Blalock-Taussig shunt (Fig. 3).

Central shunts interposing prosthetic grafts between the descending aorta and the main pulmonary artery have the theoretical advantage of producing less distortion of the pulmonary arteries, and this might be important for small pulmonary arteries or when the shunt is performed in early infancy. Such shunts have the disadvantages, however, of necessitating the opening of the pericardial sac. Furthermore, small-diameter prostheses have to be utilized in small infants to prevent flooding of the lungs, thus limiting the period of satisfactory palliation. Central shunts are performed on cardiopulmonary bypass if it is expected that the occlusion of the main pulmonary artery is likely to produce intolerable hypoxemia during the shunt procedure.

Caval-pulmonary anastomosis (Glenn's operation) has been performed only occasionally in our institution over the last 15 years. This shunt has the theoretical advantage of not overloading the ventricles and might still have a place in the concept of the Fontan circulation, either as a palliative procedure or as part of the Fontan operation itself.

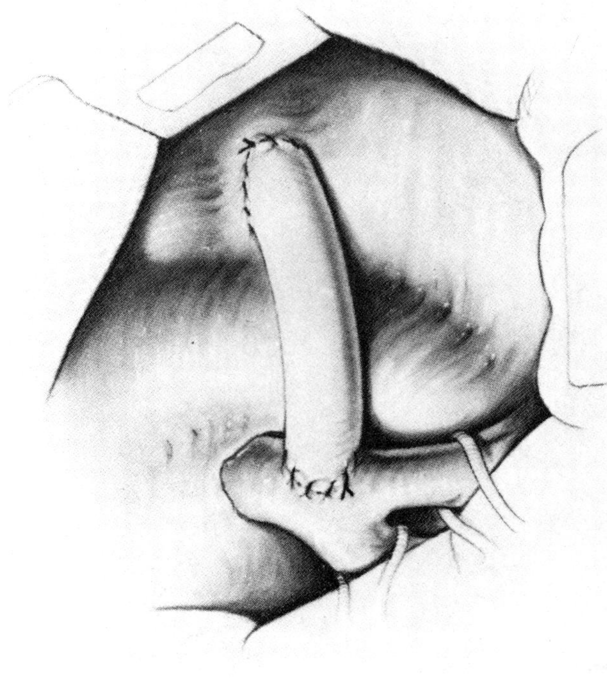

Figure 3 Modified Blalock-Taussig shunt.

Relief of Right Ventricular Outflow Obstruction

Pulmonary Valvotomy

Critical pulmonary stenosis or pulmonary atresia with intact ventricular septum in the neonatal period is the main indication for pulmonary valvotomy. The operation can be a closed transventricular valvotomy (Brock's procedure), a transpulmonary valvotomy from a left thoracotomy incision, or a pulmonary valvotomy under inflow occlusion. Pulmonary valvotomy is indicated for patients who have a right ventricular chamber worth preserving, and the procedure can be performed in isolation or in combination with a systemic-to-pulmonary artery shunt.

The Brock procedure is performed through a midline sternotomy incision. A pursestring suture is placed on the body of the right ventricle, and Brock's knives of increasing sizes are passed through the pursestring into the right ventricle through the pulmonary valve. This is followed by dilation of the pulmonary valve orifice with Brock's dilators.

For a number of years we have performed transpulmonary valvotomies through a left thoracotomy incision in conjunction with a systemic-to-pulmonary artery shunt. The procedure consists of clamping the main pulmonary artery proximal to its bifurcation, opening the main pulmonary artery, and performing the valvotomy from above. The long-term results have been rather poor, with a fairly high incidence of restenosis of the pulmonary valve. For that reason, we currently prefer the technique of pulmonary valvotomy with partial or complete excision of the pulmonary valve under inflow occlusion. The operation is performed through a midline sternotomy incision, snares are passed around both cavae, and a side-biting clamp is applied on the main pulmonary artery, on which a vertical arteriotomy incision is made. The caval tapes are then snugged down. A Castaneda clamp is passed through the transverse sinus so as to occlude the aorta and the distal main pulmonary artery, including the patent ductus arteriosus. The side-biting clamp on the main pulmonary artery is released, and the valvotomy with valvectomy is performed. The side-biting clamp is then reapplied on the main pulmonary artery when the caval tapes and the aortic clamp have been released. The long-term results of this procedure have been more satisfactory than those of the Brock procedure, although they rarely provide complete relief of the right ventricular outflow tract obstruction, in which there is often a muscular subvalvar component in the anterior aspect of the right ventricular outflow tract.

Transannular Patch and Right Ventricle to Pulmonary Artery Conduit

These procedures are indicated as palliation for extreme forms of tetralogy of Fallot with hypoplastic pulmonary arteries and more commonly for cases of pulmonary atresia, ventricular septal defect, and small or hypoplastic central pulmonary arteries. Compared with a peripheral shunt, these procedures have the advantage of producing less distortion of the pulmonary arteries, providing a more even flow to both lungs, and perhaps providing a better stimulus for the arteries to grow while they are subjected to a wider pulse pressure once connected to the right ventricle.

The operation is performed through a midline sternotomy incision, usually on cardiopulmonary bypass. An alternative technique of partial enlargement of the right ventricular outflow tract without cardiopulmonary bypass has been described, but we have no personal experience with this procedure.

Remodeling of Peripheral Pulmonary Arterial Circulation

These procedures are indicated for cases of complex pulmonary atresia with ventricular septal defect and multifocal pulmonary blood supply. In this condition part or all pulmonary segments are perfused via large collateral arteries, and the purpose of the palliative treatment is not only to increase the pulmonary blood flow but also to connect two or more of these vessels together in the hope of an eventual connection of the right ventricle with as many bronchopulmonary segments as possible. Technically, these so-called unifocalizations have consisted of (a) connecting the central pulmonary arteries and collateral arteries to a subclavian artery with a bifurcated prosthetic graft; (b) performing a systemic-to-pulmonary artery shunt on a large collateral artery normally connected to a central pulmonary artery; or (c) connecting the central pulmonary arteries with a large collateral artery directly, or by interposition of a prosthesis (Fig. 4). Occasionally we have also enlarged localized stenoses at the origin of some of these collateral vessels. We have recently analyzed the long-term results of these attempts to unifocalize the pulmonary blood supply, and they have been disappointing. Very few patients underwent a successful complete repair. We would currently recommend unifocalization only as a palliative measure to increase pulmonary blood flow in patients with cyanosis but not for the sole purpose of an eventual complete repair.

PROCEDURES TO IMPROVE INTRACARDIAC MIXING

These procedures include the atrial septectomy and the palliative atrial switch operation.

Atrial Septectomy

This was first described by Blalock and Hanlon as a treatment of transposition of the great arteries in which survival depends on effective mixing of the systemic and the pulmonary venous blood. The introduction of the balloon atrial septostomy by Rashkind and Miller has greatly reduced the indications for the surgical septectomy in transposition of the great arteries. In simple transposition of the great arteries, we would rather proceed with an intracardiac repair than a surgical septectomy in the case

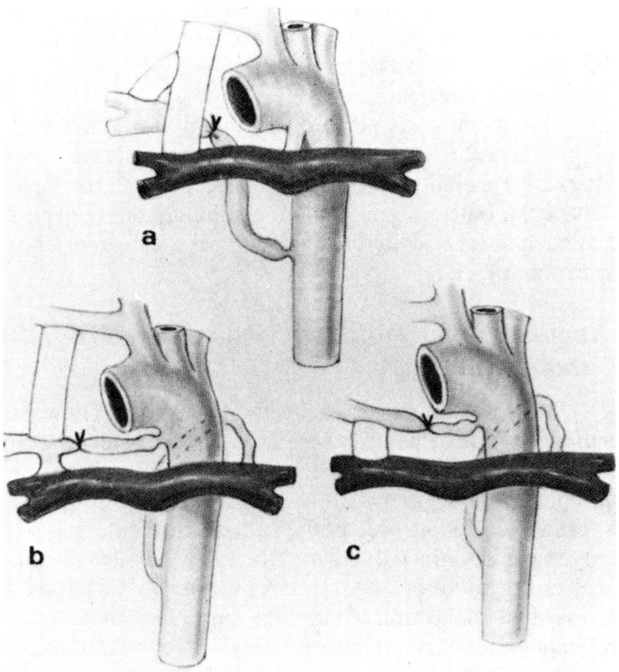

Figure 4 Techniques for remodeling the peripheral pulmonary arterial circulation. *A*, Connection of the central pulmonary and collateral arteries to a subclavian artery with a bifurcated prosthetic graft. *B*, A systemic-to-pulmonary artery shunt on a collateral artery normally connected to a central pulmonary artery. *C*, Connecting the central pulmonary arteries to a large collateral artery with interposition of a prosthesis.

of failure of the balloon septostomy. In complex transpositions of the great arteries and particularly in cases of transposition with ventricular septal defect and pulmonary stenosis, we often perform an atrial septectomy in addition to the systemic-to-pulmonary shunt if the interatrial septum is intact. This is because better mixing is achieved when it takes place at the atrial level, even in the presence of a ventricular septal defect. Atrial septectomies are currently more often indicated for cases of absent atrioventricular valve connections or atrioventricular valve atresia with restrictive atrial septal defect. Technically the Blalock-Hanlon septectomy continues to be our procedure of choice. This is performed through a right lateral thoracotomy incision in the fifth intercostal space. The pericardium is incised behind the phrenic nerve. Ligatures are passed around the right pulmonary artery and the right upper and right lower pulmonary veins. A partial occlusion clamp is then applied so as to exclude a portion of each atrium across the atrial septum. Parallel incisions are made above and below the interatrial groove. The interatrial septum is then grasped with artery forceps. The septum is pulled out while the vascular clamp is released, and it is then excised (Fig. 5).

In some institutions the atrial septectomy is performed under inflow occlusion or on cardiopulmonary bypass. We have no experience of the former procedure, and we occasionally perform the septectomy on cardiopulmonary bypass mainly if an additional procedure is required.

Atrial Switch Procedure

A palliative Mustard's or Senning's operation is sometimes performed for patients with transposition of the great arteries who are not candidates for complete repair because of obstructive pulmonary vascular disease. A Mustard's or Senning's operation is performed, leaving, or sometimes creating, an intra- or extracardiac shunt to allow for a right-to-left shunt when the pulmonary vascular resistance increases beyond the systemic vascular resistance.

OPERATIONS TO PREPARE FOR A FONTAN'S PROCEDURE

Many patients have undergone a palliative operation before a Fontan's repair. Most often these are systemic-to-pulmonary artery shunts, occasionally banding of the pulmonary artery or atrial septectomy. Two additional palliative interventions have to be mentioned: the relief of subaortic obstruction and the Norwood operation for hypoplastic left-sided hearts.

Relief of Subaortic Obstruction

Patients with absent right atrioventricular connection or double-inlet left ventricle with transposition of the great arteries and high pulmonary blood flow who underwent banding of the pulmonary artery in infancy have a tendency to develop severe subaortic obstruction. It is now well documented that a Fontan's operation in the presence of severe ventricular hypertrophy is unlikely to succeed, and the subaortic obstruction has to be relieved or bypassed beforehand. It is often not technically feasible to directly resect the obstructing muscle. Alternatively, connection

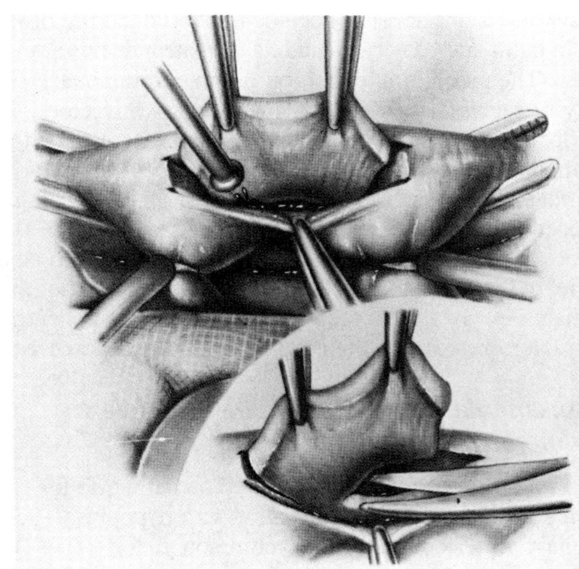

Figure 5 Technique of Blalock-Hanlon atrial septectomy. Parallel incisions are made in the atrial wall. The interatrial septum is grasped, pulled out, and excised.

of the main pulmonary artery with the side of the aorta (Damus-Kaye-Stansel procedure) might be the operation of choice. The pulmonary blood flow is then subsequently provided via a systemic-to-pulmonary artery shunt.

Norwood's Procedure

This is a palliative intervention that consists of using the main pulmonary artery as a systemic outflow for cases of hypoplastic left-sided heart syndrome. The right ventricle is therefore utilized as a systemic ventricle, and the pulmonary blood supply is provided via a systemic-to-pulmonary artery shunt. Details about this approach are given in the next chapter.

SUGGESTED READING

deLeval MR, McKay R, Jones M, Stark J, Macartney FJ. Modified Blalock-Taussig shunt. Use of subclavian artery orifice as flow regulator in prosthetic systemic to pulmonary artery shunts. J Thorac Cardiovasc Surg 1981; 81:112–119.

Kirklin JK, Blackstone EH, Kirklin JW, Pacifico AD, Bargeron LM. The Fontan operations. Ventricular hypertrophy, age and date of operations as risk factors. J Thorac Cardiovasc Surg 1986; 92:1049–1064.

Norwood WI, Lang P, Castaneda AR, Campbell DN. Experience with operations for hypoplastic left heart. J Thorac Cardiovasc Surg 1981; 82:511–518.

Stark J, deLeval M, eds. Surgery for congenital heart defects. London: Grune & Stratton, 1983.

HYPOPLASTIC LEFT-SIDED HEART SYNDROME

WILLIAM I. NORWOOD, M.D., Ph.D.
JOHN D. PIGOTT, M.D.

Hypoplastic left-sided heart syndrome is an anatomic constellation of congenital cardiac malformations characterized by aortic and mitral valve atresia or stenosis and marked hypoplasia or absence of the left ventricle. Consequently the ascending aorta and aortic arch are both functionally and structurally a branch of the thoracic aorta, with retrograde flow through the aortic arch and ascending aorta. Since the ascending aorta carries only coronary flow, it is correspondingly small (1 to 3 mm in diameter). In our series of patients with hypoplastic left-sided heart syndrome, 78 percent had normally related great arteries, 10 percent had double-outlet right ventricle and severe hypoplasia of the left ventricle, and 12 percent had malalignment of the atrioventricular canal with right ventricular dominance and hypoplasia of the left ventricle. This malformation is the fourth most common congenital cardiac anomaly presenting in the first year of life.

A physiologic consequence of this anatomy is that the systemic circulation is supported virtually in its entirety by flow through the ductus arteriosus. Pulmonary venous return passes through a patent foramen ovale or atrial septal defect to the right atrium, where mixing of pulmonary and systemic venous blood occurs. This physiology allows normal growth and development in utero. Newborns with hypoplastic left-sided heart syndrome are generally only mildly cyanotic with a PaO_2 of 50 mm Hg to 60 mm Hg, and cardiac disease may go unrecognized until development of pallor, limpness, and metabolic acidosis as a result of the natural closure of the ductus arteriosus. When this condition is unrecognized and untreated, virtually all infants die in the first days to weeks after birth. Most often, these neonates may be readily resuscitated with continuous infusion of prostaglandin E_1 to maintain patency of the ductus arteriosus and a bolus of sodium bicarbonate to reverse metabolic acidosis. Catecholamine support is rarely necessary and may increase pulmonary blood flow at the expense of the systemic circulation.

Recently, two approaches to the surgical management of hypoplastic left-sided heart syndrome have been advanced: reconstructive surgery or cardiac replacement. The rationale for reconstructive surgery is based on the fact that the lungs, coronary anatomy, and myocardial biochemistry are inherently normal in this condition. Thus, if one considers hypoplastic left-sided heart syndrome as one of several cardiac malformations with only one effective ventricle, a surgical approach may be devised leading to a modification of Fontan's procedure. It has been demonstrated that a good functional result following a Fontan's procedure can be expected when the pulmonary artery architecture is near normal, the pulmonary vascular-resistance is that of the normal mature lung, and ventricular function has been preserved (low end-diastolic pressure). However, since the systemic circulation in neonates with hypoplastic left-sided heart syndrome is dependent on the patency of the ductus arteriosus, which characteristically closes in the first days of life, surgery is urgently necessary. The pulmonary vascular resistance of the newborn is prohibitively high for a Fontan's procedure, and therefore staged surgical therapy is necessary. The general goals of the initial stage are to establish unobstructed systemic output from the right ventricle, to assure normal maturation of the pulmonary vasculature by regulating pulmonary arterial blood flow and pressure, and to assure a widely patent interatrial communication, thereby avoiding pulmonary venous hypertension. Although several approaches to these goals have been conceived, the surgical techniques outlined here are designed additionally to incorporate as much as possible the patient's own tissues and to avoid conduits or circumferential suture lines, thus minimizing the number of surgical interventions.

PALLIATION FOR HYPOPLASTIC LEFT-SIDED HEART SYNDROME (STAGE I)

The operating room is maintained at a temperature of 20° C to promote surface cooling of the patient. Induction of general anesthesia with pancuronium bromide (0.1 mg per kilogram) and fentanyl (25 μg per kilogram in 10 μg per kilogram increments) is achieved. The left radial artery is cannulated with a 22-gauge indwelling catheter and a urinary bladder drainage tube, a nasogastric tube, and nasopharyngeal, esophageal, and rectal temperature probes are placed. During this preparatory time, the rectal temperature typically decreases to 31° C to 33° C.

A conventional midline sternotomy incision is made, and excision of the thymus is undertaken to facilitate exposure of the diminutive aortic arch and its branch vessels. Cannulation for arterial infusion is most conveniently achieved in the proximal main pulmonary artery just above the sinuses of Valsalva by placing a single, diamond-shaped pursestring suture through a small rubber tourniquet. A No. 10 F aortic cannula is fitted with a rubber bumper about 3 or 4 mm from the tip. Following heparinization, a side-biting C-clamp is placed so as to exclude the pursestring suture, the pulmonary artery is incised, and the cannula is introduced. Threading of the cannula through the ductus arteriosus should be avoided, since it is unnecessary and requires excessive manipulation of the cardiovascular structures. A minimal amount of distortion, manipulation, and trauma to the delicate neonatal cardiovascular structures is essential to preserve anatomy and function. A No. 16 F venous cannula is placed through the right atrial appendage, and cardiopulmonary bypass is instituted. The right and left pulmonary arterial branches are rapidly exposed and occluded with 2–0 Tevdek tourniquets to assure systemic perfusion through the ductus arteriosus (Fig. 1). The infant is cooled to 20° C while

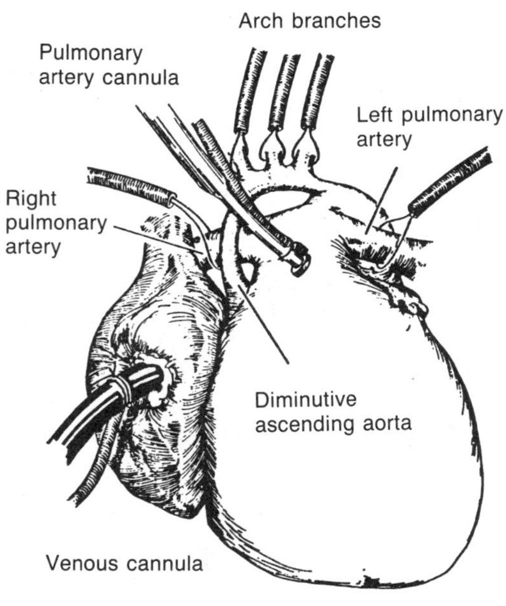

Figure 1 Exposure and cannulation for cardiopulmonary bypass.

monitoring esophageal, nasopharyngeal, and rectal temperatures. The rectal temperature generally decreases somewhat more slowly than the nasopharyngeal and esophageal temperatures, reaching 20° C after approximately 15 minutes of cardiopulmonary bypass. During this time, the branch vessels of the aortic arch are exposed and looped with 2–0 Tevdek tourniquets in preparation for circulatory arrest. Dissection is carried around the aortic arch onto the thoracic aorta in the posterior mediastinum. At this point the branch vessels of the aortic arch are occluded, the circulation is discontinued, and the blood is drained into the venous reservoir. The arterial and venous cannulas are removed and cardioplegia solution is infused through the pulmonary arterial cannulation site while the descending thoracic aorta is temporarily occluded. Through the right atrial cannulation site the septum primum is identified and excised (Fig. 2A). Attention is then turned to the main pulmonary artery, which has been dissected from the diminutive ascending aorta during the cooling phase of cardiopulmonary bypass. Adjacent to the takeoff of the right pulmonary artery, the main pulmonary artery is transected, and its distal stump is oversewn with a homograft patch using a running monofilament suture technique (Fig. 2B). Patch closure is recommended in order to better maintain continuity between the right and left pulmonary artery branches. The ductus arteriosus is then exposed, ligated, and transected at its entrance into the thoracic aorta. The aortic incision is carried distally 1 to 2 cm into the thoracic aorta and also proximally into the aortic arch and ascending aorta to the level of the rim of the transected proximal main pulmonary artery (Fig. 2C). Because the isthmus of the aorta and the aortic arch actually function as a branch of the main pulmonary artery-ductus-thoracic aorta continuum, the junction of the isthmus and thoracic aorta should be gusseted with a patch in order to minimize the development of distal aortic arch obstruction (Fig. 3A). Pulmonary homograft is used for this patch because it is thin, pliable, and hemostatic. Again, a monofilament running suture technique is used. At this point, we favor the construction of a short central shunt of 4-mm tube graft (PTFE) between the inferior aspect of the augmented aortic arch and the confluence of branch pulmonary arteries (Fig. 3B). The rationale for a central shunt is to obtain a more even distribution of flow and thus growth of the right and left pulmonary arteries. The remaining pulmonary homograft gusset is then carried to 5 mm above the end of the most proximal incision in the ascending aorta (Fig. 3C). The proximal anastomosis of the main pulmonary artery to the ascending aorta is begun with multiple interrupted fine monofilament sutures to avoid pursestringing of the inlet into the diminutive aortic root (Fig. 4A). The reconstruction is completed by anastomosis of the ascending aorta, main pulmonary artery, and pulmonary homograft, thus creating outflow from the right ventricle to the augmented aorta through the pulmonary valve (Fig. 4B). Cardiopulmonary bypass is reinstituted, and the patient is rewarmed to 37° C. The tourniquets on the branch vessels of the aortic arch are removed, but those on the branch pulmonary arteries remain until the patient is weaned from cardiopulmonary bypass. Following weaning from cardiopulmonary bypass,

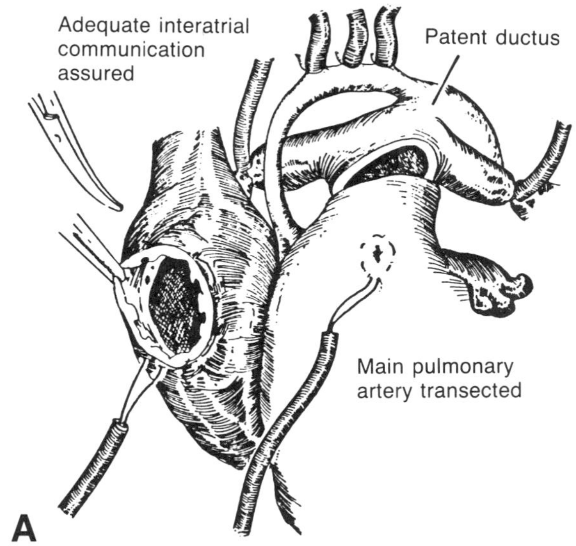

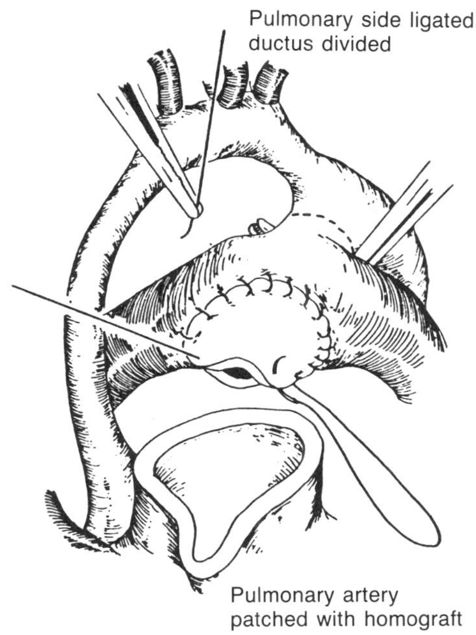

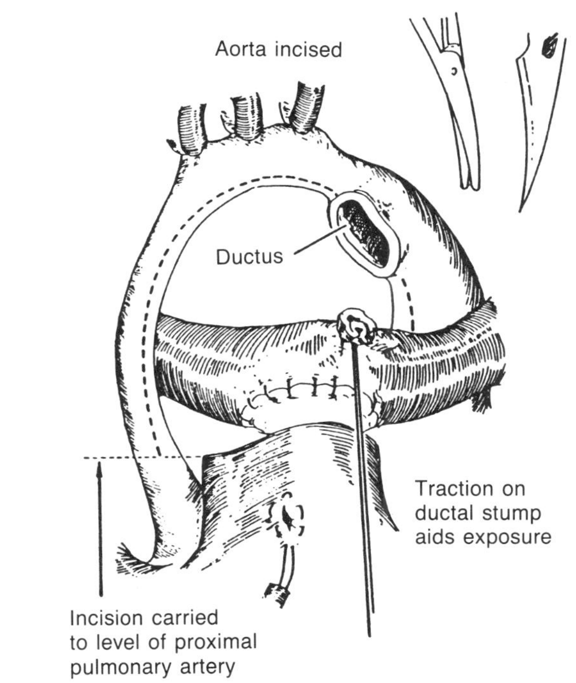

Figure 2 *A*, Cannulas are removed, the atrial septum is excised, and the pulmonary artery is divided. *B*, The pulmonary side of the ductus is ligated, and the ductus is divided. The pulmonary side of the transected pulmonary artery is patched with arterial homograft. *C*, The underside of the aortic arch is incised, carrying the incision proximally to the level of the proximal pulmonary artery.

the cannulas are removed and a pressure monitoring line is placed through the right atrial appendage cannulation site. Using the lowest possible mean airway pressure, ventilation is adjusted to maintain the P_{CO_2} between 20 and 30 mm Hg in order to minimize pulmonary vascular resistance. Generally the P_{O_2} ranges from 40 to 45 mm Hg. A PaO_2 of 50 mm Hg or higher suggests a large pulmonary to systemic flow ratio, which may result in inadequate systemic perfusion. The ventilator may be used to adjust the pulmonary to systemic flow ratio when this occurs by rapidly decreasing F_{IO_2} to 30 percent and allowing P_{CO_2} to increase to 40 mm Hg. Pharmacologic support is rarely necessary in the postoperative period.

FONTAN'S PROCEDURE (STAGE II)

Following the previously described palliative surgery, the right ventricle is subjected to both a volume and pressure load. With a view to long-term preservation of ventricular function, assessment for suitability for Fontan's procedure is undertaken at 12 to 18 months of age. At this age, the pulmonary resistance is likely to be low (< 2.5 Wood's units) and ventricular end-diastolic pressure normal (<7 to 8 mm Hg), and the following surgery may then be planned.

The heart is exposed through a midline sternotomy incision, and cannulation for cardiopulmonary bypass is achieved by placement of an arterial cannula in the ascending aorta and a single venous cannula through the right atrial appendage. The systemic to pulmonary artery shunt is exposed and occluded as cardiopulmonary bypass is instituted, and the patient's core temperature is reduced to 20° C. During this cooling phase on cardiopulmonary bypass, the right and left pulmonary artery branches are exposed from pericardial reflection to pericardial reflection. This exposure is in preparation for widely augmenting the pulmonary arteries to avoid proximal pulmonary arterial obstruction from unrecognized irregularities in size (Fig. 5). The aorta is then cross-clamped, and cardioplegia solution is infused as the circulation is arrested and blood is drained into the venous reservoir. The pulmonary arteries are opened by a single incision extending from be-

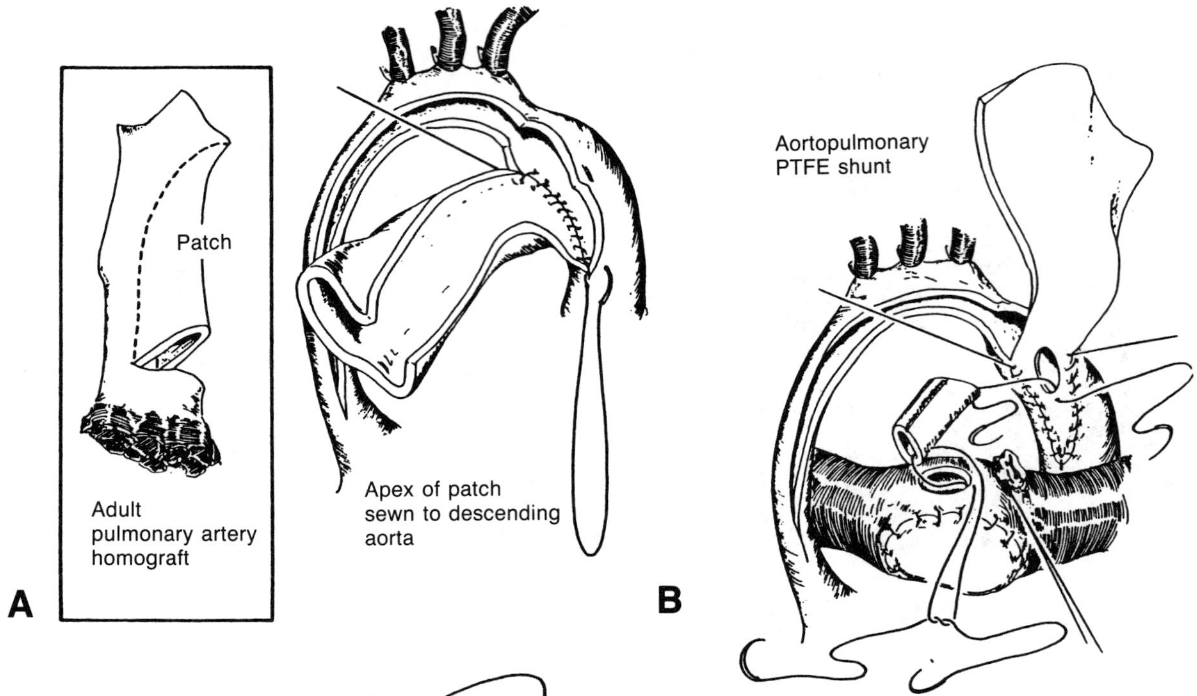

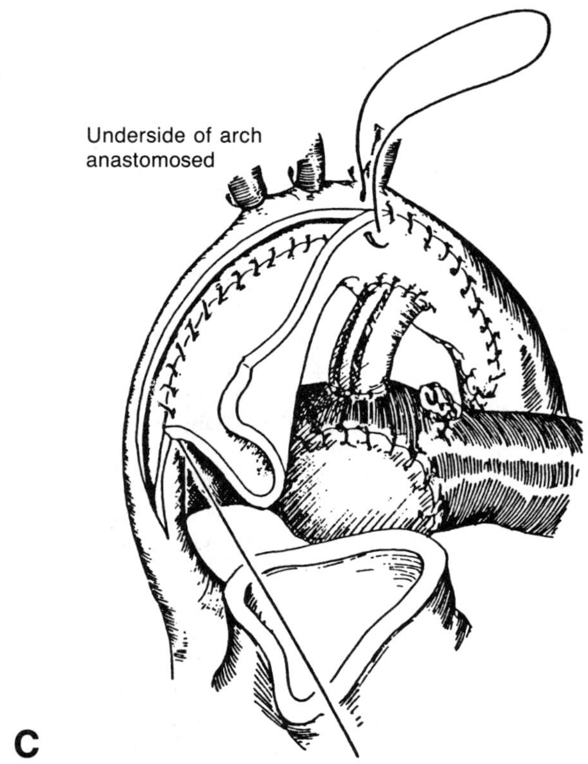

Figure 3 *A*, A patch of pulmonary artery homograft is cut as shown, and the apex of the patch is sewn to the descending aorta. *B*, An aortopulmonary shunt is created with a short segment of 4-mm diameter PTFE tube graft sewn between the pulmonary artery homograft and the central pulmonary artery. *C*, First the posterior portion and then the anterior portion of the aortic arch suture lines are completed.

hind the right superior vena cava across the midline to the left lower lobe branch (Figs. 6A and 6B). An incision in the right atrium is made from the sulcus terminalis superiorly to the right lateral insertion of the eustachian valve inferiorly (Fig. 7A). The interatrial communication is inspected and enlarged if possible. A final incision is then made in the dome of the right atrium adjacent to the right pulmonary artery, and this incision is carried into the posterior aspect of the right superior vena cava immediately adjacent to the most rightward aspect of the incision in the right pulmonary artery. A suture line is begun between the inferior lip of the incised right pulmonary artery and the posterior lip of the right superior vena cava–right atrial incision with running 5–0 monofilament suture (Fig. 7B). This provides the floor for the anastomosis of the systemic venous return to the pulmonary arterial tree. A piece of PTFE tubing 10 mm in diameter of sufficient length to extend from the inferior vena caval–right atrial junction to the right superior vena caval–right atrial junction is cut in half lengthwise for use as a baffle to channel inferior vena caval flow along the right lateral aspect of the right atrium to the superior anastomosis between the right atrium and the pulmonary arterial tree. The baffle is sutured with running 5–0 monofilament suture around the orifice of the inferior vena cava along the right lateral floor and free wall of the right atrium and around the patulous orifice in the superior dome of the right atrium (Fig. 8A). This particular baffling technique was introduced to minimize problems associated with tricuspid prolapse or regurgitation, or obstruction of pulmonary venous return to the right ventricle experienced early in this series with an alternate baffling technique. The construction of the systemic venous pulmonary arterial system is completed by gusseting the pulmonary arterial incision with an elongated triangular

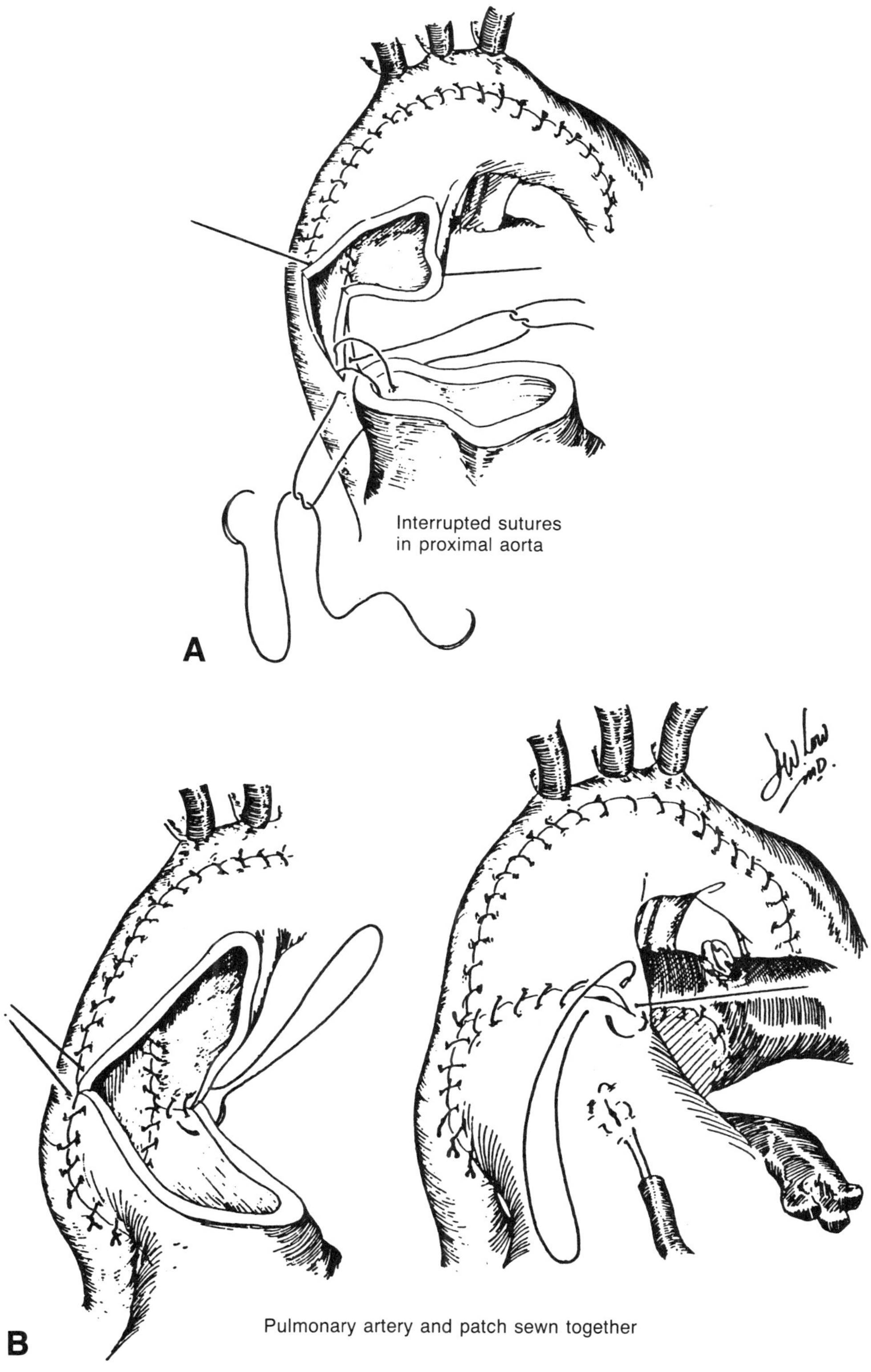

Figure 4 *A*, The pulmonary artery is then sewn to the proximal aorta. *B*, The suture line is completed by sewing the pulmonary artery to the homograft patch.

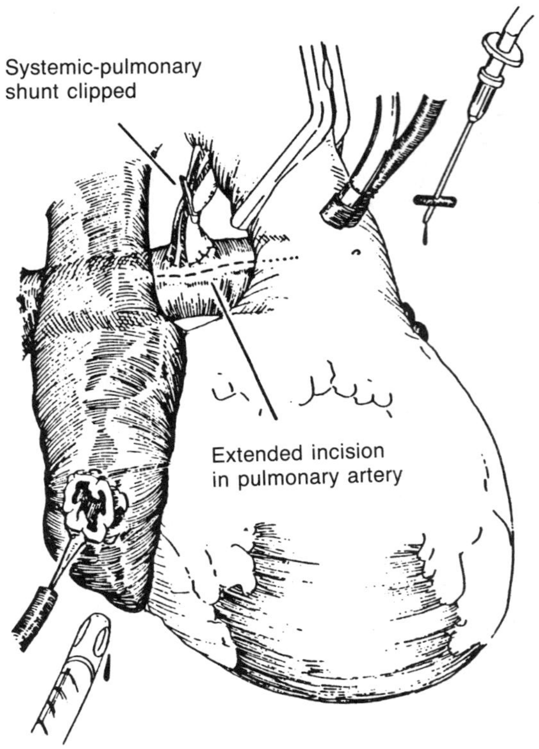

Figure 5 Preparation for a Fontan's procedure (Stage II). The aortopulmonary shunt is clamped as bypass is instituted; the aorta is cross-clamped, and cardioplegia is given. An incision is made in the pulmonary artery.

patch of pulmonary homograft material beginning on the left pulmonary artery with running 5–0 monofilament suture (Fig. 8B). As one approaches the right pulmonary artery and adjacent right superior vena cava, the base of the triangular pulmonary homograft patch is sutured onto the superior lip of the right superior vena caval-right atrial incision, providing a roof for the anastomosis (Fig. 9). The patient is placed back on cardiopulmonary bypass following closure of the initial right atriotomy with a running monofilament suture technique and rewarmed to 37° C. Placement of 18-gauge pressure monitoring catheters in the right pulmonary artery and through the right atrial appendage (now receiving exclusively pulmonary venous return) allows for postoperative assessment of right and left atrial pressures.

RESULTS

From October, 1984 through January, 1987, 115 newborns have undergone palliative surgery similar to that just described for hypoplastic left-sided heart syndrome at The Children's Hospital of Philadelphia. The hospital mortality among these patients was 28 percent. The 18-month actuarial survival is 62 percent, and to date, 29 patients have undergone application of Fontan's procedure for the treatment of hypoplastic left-sided heart syndrome. Among these 29 patients, there were nine early and one late deaths. The results continue to improve, both for initial palliation and later reconstructive surgery as we gain an ever increas-

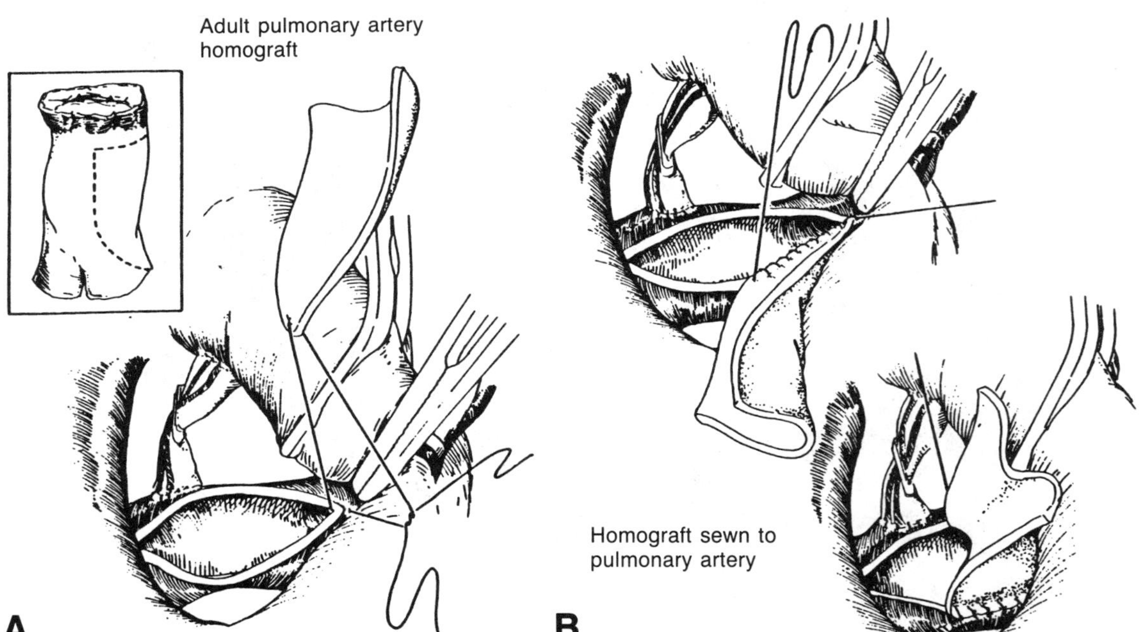

Figure 6 *A*, A patch of adult pulmonary artery homograft is cut as shown to augment the systemic venous pathway. *B*, The patch is sewn to the pulmonary artery as shown, beginning from the patient's left side.

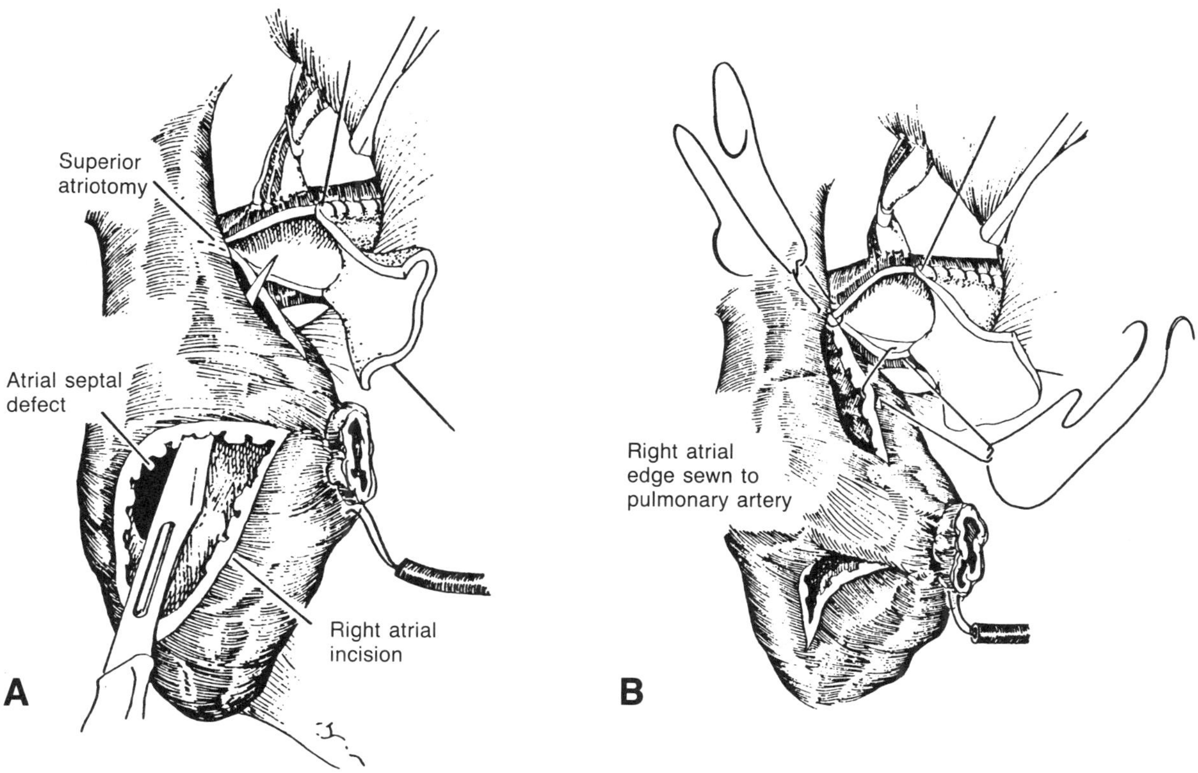

Figure 7 *A*, A superior atriotomy is performed via a right atrial incision. *B*, The right atrium is sewn to the augmented pulmonary artery beginning posteriorly.

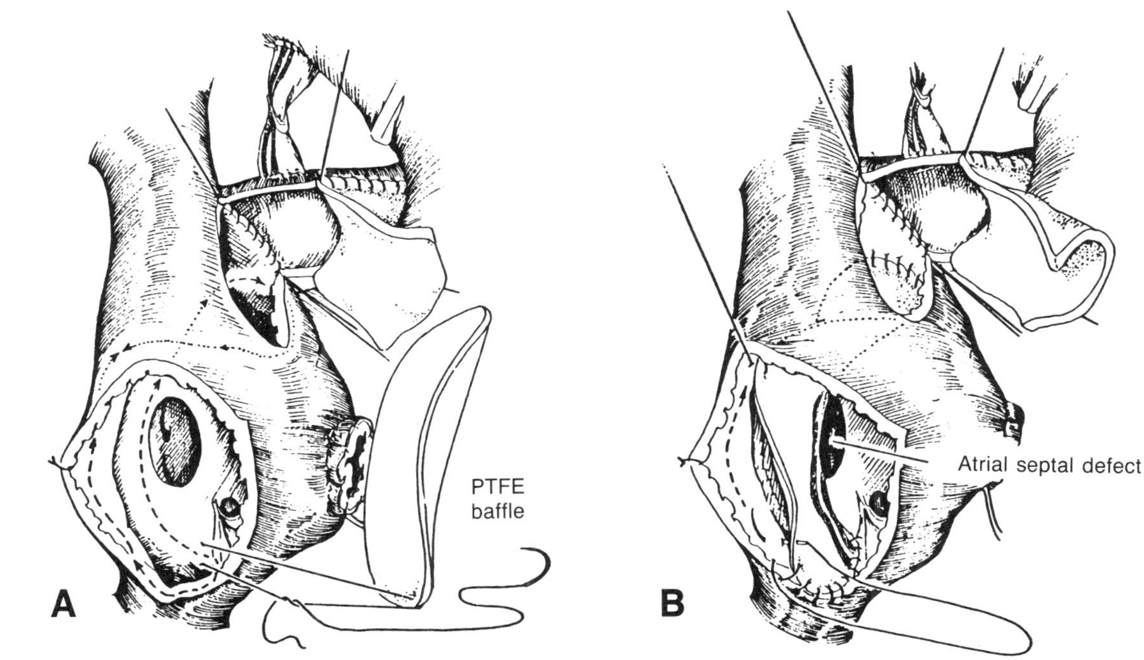

Figure 8 *A*, A PTFE baffle is then placed in the right atrium to direct left atrial blood across the atrial septal defect to the tricuspid valve. *B*, The atriopulmonary anastomosis is completed by sewing the pulmonary artery homograft to the right atrium anteriorly.

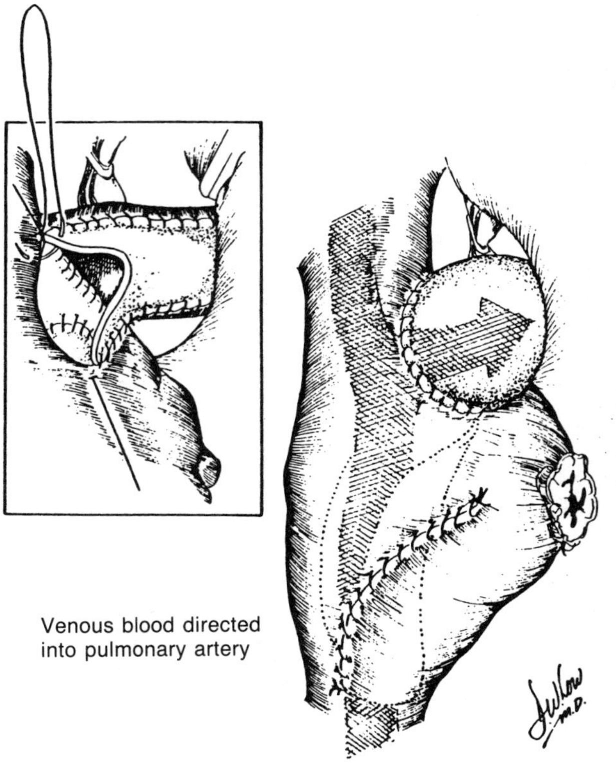

Figure 9 The right atrial incision is closed to complete the atriopulmonary pathway.

ing knowledge of the anatomy and physiology of this complex group of patients. What is outlined here as one approach for reconstructive surgery for this malformation will surely continue to evolve. However, this chapter provides a stepping stone for the surgical understanding of this malformation.

SUGGESTED READING

Doty DB, Marvin WJ Jr, Schieken RM, Lauer RM. Hypoplastic left heart syndrome: successful palliation with a new operation. J Thorac Cardiovasc Surg 1980; 80:148–152.

Helton JG, Aglira BA, Chin AJ, Murphy JD, Pigott JD, Norwood WI. Analysis of potential anatomical or physiological determinants of outcome of palliative surgery or physiological determinants of outcome of palliative surgery for hypoplastic left heart syndrome. Circulation 1986; 74(Suppl):70–76.

Noonan JA, Nadas AS. The hypoplastic left heart syndrome: an analysis of 101 cases. Pediatr Clin North Am 1958; 5:1029–1056.

Norwood WI, Lang P, Castaneda AR, Campbell DN. Experience with operations for hypoplastic left heart syndrome. J Thorac Cardiovasc Surg 1980; 82:511–519.

Norwood WI, Lang P, Hansen DD. Physiologic repair of aortic atresia-hypoplastic left heart syndrome. N Engl J Med 1983; 308:23–26.

VENTRICULAR SEPTAL DEFECT

JOHN E. MAYER Jr., M.D.

Ventricular septal defect is among the most common congenital defects of the heart, occurring with an incidence of 1.5 to 2.5 per 1,000 live births, and it was among the earliest of the congenital defects to be repaired with extracorporeal circulation. This defect is a common cause of heart failure and failure to thrive in infancy, and the mortality rate approaches 10 percent within the first year of life for those in severe congestive heart failure. In addition, in patients with large defects, there is a significant risk of developing irreversible pulmonary vascular disease if the defects are not repaired. Ventricular septal defects were first closed by Lillehei, Varco, and co-workers at the University of Minnesota in the early 1950s with remarkably good results, despite the fact that these efforts were among the first at open cardiac procedures. Subsequently, the advent of techniques of deep hypothermic circulatory arrest and continued improvements in anesthetic and postoperative management have made the surgical management of this defect increasingly safe.

This discussion will include isolated ventricular septal defects and those associated with coarctation and patent ductus, but will not address those ventricular septal defects that are part of a larger congenital defect complex, such as interrupted aortic arch, tetralogy of Fallot, atrioventricular canal, or truncus arteriosus.

THERAPEUTIC GOALS AND ALTERNATIVES

There are two major therapeutic goals in the management of ventricular septal defects. The first is to relieve the manifestations of congestive heart failure, including difficulty in feeding, tachypnea, poor weight gain, and recurrent respiratory infections, all of which are the result of excessive pulmonary blood flow due to left-to-right shunting at the ventricular level. A second goal is to prevent the development of irreversible pulmonary vascular obstructive disease, which results from excessive pulmonary artery pressure and blood flow in patients with large ventricular septal defects. Medical therapy with diuretics and digoxin frequently can reduce the congestive heart failure, although many patients still show subnormal weight gain. However, this period of medical therapy may allow for spontaneous reduction in size or even closure of some ventricular septal defects. The likelihood of spontaneous closure of these defects has been related to the age at which they are found as well as to their size and location. It has been stated that as many as 80 percent of ventricular septal defects seen in neonates at 1 month of age undergo spontaneous closure, whereas 50 percent of those seen in infants at 6 months of age spontaneously close. However, patients with large ventricular septal defects when measured angiographically have only a 5 to 10 percent chance of spontaneous closure. In addition, large subpulmonary ventricular septal defects or those in which there is malalignment between the infundibular and trabecular portions of the ventricular septum seem to be less likely to close spontaneously. There is no medical therapy, at present, that has any impact on the development of pulmonary vascular obstructive disease.

There are two surgical alternatives in the management of ventricular septal defect. The first and currently preferred approach for most ventricular septal defects is direct surgical closure. This approach has the advantages of being a curative procedure which, in the vast majority of cases, should be the patient's only operation and should effectively restore the heart to a near normal state. A second alternative is to band the pulmonary artery, thereby raising the resistance to flow through the pulmonary vascular bed, reducing the left-to-right shunt, and "protecting" the distal pulmonary vasculature from the high pressure and flow that were present from the ventricular septal defect. This option clearly has the disadvantage that it requires a second operation to close the ventricular septal defect and remove the pulmonary artery band. For this reason, and since closure of ventricular septal defects has become increasingly safe, it is not generally employed. However, there are circumstances, such as multiple ventricular septal defects ("Swiss cheese" ventricular septum) in which this procedure is still utilized. It is also used in some centers for management of coarctation of the aorta and large ventricular septal defect presenting within the first month or two of life.

PREFERRED APPROACH

The approach to the patient with a ventricular septal defect depends on a number of considerations, including the current clinical status, the location and size of the defect, the presence of associated cardiovascular defects, and the status of the pulmonary vascular bed. The patient with a small ventricular septal defect that has less than a 2 to 1 pulmonary-to-systemic flow ratio and normal pulmonary artery pressure and resistance does not require surgical intervention. The only exception to the nonsurgical management of small ventricular septal defects is in those patients who have associated aortic valvar incompetence. Frequently, these defects are subpulmonary (subarterial) in location, and the right coronary cusp of the aortic valve can prolapse. In patients with these defects, ventricular septal defect closure should be undertaken in an attempt to prevent progression of aortic valve insufficiency regardless of the size of the shunt. Not infrequently, the ventricular septal defect is partially sealed by the prolapsing aortic valve cusp and, in reality, the anatomic size of the true defect in the septum is relatively large, although "small" by shunt calculations. Patients with moderate-sized ventricular septal defects and greater than 2 to 1 pulmonary-to-systemic flow ratios but normal pulmonary artery pressures and resistance can generally be managed medically initially. However, those who have continuing subnormal growth and other manifestations of congestive heart failure by the time of 9 to 12 months of age should have elective operations at that time. Others have recommended delaying surgery until around 4 to 5 years of age, but this approach has the disadvantage of subjecting the left ventricle to a prolonged period of volume overload, with potentially damaging effects on late long-term function. For patients with large ventricular septal defects and poor response to medical therapy, surgical intervention is frequently necessary within the first 6 months. In our experience, age, per se, does not appear to be a risk factor in the management of these defects, and prompt closure is recommended for any patient with persistent congestive heart failure in this age group. Surgical intervention is also undertaken for patients who have evidence of elevated pulmonary vascular resistance within the first year of life. When defects are closed within this time frame, the chances for progressive pulmonary vascular obstructive disease are essentially reduced to zero.

Surgical approach to individual defects is determined primarily by the age and size of the patient and the location of the defect. Patients who weigh less than 8 to 10 kg are routinely repaired using the technique of profound hypothermia and circulatory arrest. Core cooling on cardiopulmonary bypass to rectal temperatures in the 18 to 20° C range is utilized, along with crystalloid cardioplegic protection of the myocardium. In older patients, standard cardiopulmonary bypass with moderate hypothermia (25° C) is utilized with crystalloid cardioplegic solution for myocardial protection. The majority of ventricular septal defects can be repaired by a right atrial approach, including perimembranous ventricular septal defects, inlet muscular ventricular septal defects, and some trabecular muscular septal defects. Apical muscular ventricular septal defects can occasionally be closed through a low right ventricular incision, but may require an apical left ventriculotomy in order to effect closure. Subpulmonary (subarterial) defects can be approached through the pulmonary valve annulus, thus avoiding any ventriculotomy incision. Alternatively, a right ventricular incision can be made over the infundibular area to expose these defects. Large anterior muscular ventricular septal defects also frequently require a right ventriculotomy. Dacron patches (Sauvage-U.S. Catheter Inc.) are generally used for closure of most defects, although patches of polytetrafluoroethylene (Goretex) have also been utilized. In general, the patches have been secured with multiple horizontal mattress sutures of Teflon-coated Dacron suture (Tevdek), which are reinforced with Teflon felt pledgets to keep them from pulling through. All of the sutures are placed initially, and traction on the previous suture frequently improves exposure for placement of the subsequent suture, particularly when the defect has an anterior extension beneath the anterior leaflet of the tricuspid valve. Those sutures are then passed, in order, through the margins of the patch, and it is tied down. In certain circumstances, a running monofilament suture (Prolene) is utilized. This technique is useful in perimembranous defects that extend into the inlet portion of the ventricular septum, where the defect is crossed by multiple chordal attachments of the septal leaflet of the tricuspid valve. In these circumstances, the running suture can be interwoven around the chordae. The suture line can then be reinforced with a few interrupted pledgeted sutures as well. Closure of ventricular septal defects requires an accurate knowledge of the location of the conduction system in order to avoid injury to it with resulting complete heart block. For membranous defects, the conduction tissue penetrates the ventricular septum at its posterior rim. In this area ventricular septal defect closure sutures are placed back from the edge of the defect and are fairly superficial. Sutures are also placed through the base of the septal leaflet of the tricuspid valve to avoid the exit of the conduction tissue from the atrioventricular node. For certain perimembranous defects with significant anterior extension or extension into the inlet septum, it is occasionally useful to detach part of either the anterior or the septal leaflets of the tricuspid valve near the annular level. This maneuver swings the overriding chordal attachments forward and out of the way and allows for better visualization in suture placement. In the situation of straddling chordal attachments from the tricuspid valve inserting into a left ventricular papillary muscle, it has been possible to detach these chordal attachments and reattach them to the right side of the ventricular septum. These defects are always of the inlet type. The conduction system appears to be more vulnerable to injury in these circumstances, and unfortunately there is an over 50 percent incidence of a complete heart block following repair of ventricular septal defects associated with straddling tricuspid valve.

Patients with coarctation of the aorta and ventricular septal defect generally present within the first 4 weeks of life in severe congestive heart failure. We have repaired the coarctation of the aorta as a primary procedure and have not routinely banded the pulmonary artery as some others have recommended. The subsequent course of the patient dictates management. If the patient can be weaned off the ventilator and maintains adequate oral nutrition with growth, closure of the ventricular septal defect is delayed, and the management of the patient is as outlined for isolated ventricular septal defect. However, these patients frequently are unable to maintain adequate nutrition following coarctation repair despite medical management, and in these situations the patient is returned to the operating room for ventricular septal defect closure. Some authors have recommended pulmonary artery banding for this combination of lesions, in addition to the repair of the coarctation, but this approach commits the patient to a second operation. A certain percentage of these patients have spontaneous closure of their ventricular septal defect and thus only require a repair of the coarctation. The type of ventricular septal defect, particularly when the infundibular and trabecular septa are malaligned, influences the likelihood of closure. We have not employed a primary repair of coarctation and ventricular septal defect through a midline sternal splitting approach.

PROS AND CONS OF TREATMENT

There are relatively few controversies regarding the management of ventricular septal defects. The question of pulmonary artery banding versus primary closure in patients within the first 6 months of life has generally been resolved in favor of primary closure. It is worthy of emphasis, however, that this approach should be utilized only in centers where there is significant experience of management of infants with congenital heart disease. A dedicated team of cardiologists, anesthesiologists, surgeons, and intensive care nurses is necessary in order to achieve optimal results. Accurate diagnosis by angiography and

TABLE 1 Repair of Ventricular Septal Defect in Infancy

Center		*Number*	*Deaths*	*%*
Green Lane	< 1 year old (1969–1982)	85	4	4.7
University of Alabama	< 1 year old (1974–1979)	35	1	2.8
Great Ormond Street		41	1	2.4
Children's, Boston	< 1 year old (1973-1981)	128	10	7.8

echocardiography is essential in planning and carrying out a successful operation.

By utilizing these techniques, excellent operative results can be obtained, as shown in Table 1. Since these results are obtainable in several centers, we feel justified in recommending the current approach.

SUGGESTED READING

Hoffman JIE, Rudolph AM. The natural history of ventricular septal defects with special reference to selection of patients for surgery. Adv Pediatr 1970; 17:57–79.

Kirklin JK, Castaneda AR, Keane JF, Fellows KE, Norwood WI. Surgical management of multiple ventricular septal defects. J Thorac Cardiovasc Surg 1980; 80:485–493.

Lev M. The architecture of the conduction system in congenital heart disease III. Ventricular septal defect. Arch Pathol 1960; 70:529.

Lillehi CW, Cohen M, Warden HE, Ziegler NR, Varco RL. The results of direct vision closure of ventricular septal defects by means of controlled cross circulation. Surg Gynecol Obstet 1955; 101:446.

Soto B, Becker AE, Moulaert AH, Lie JT, Anderson RH. Classification of ventricular septal defects. Br Heart J 1980; 43:332–343.

Yeager SB, Freed MD, Keane JF, Norwood WI, Castaneda AR. Primary surgical closure of ventricular septal defects in the first year of life: Results in 128 infants. JACC 1984; 3:1269–1276.

COARCTATION OF THE AORTA

JOHN L. MYERS, M.D.
DAVID B. CAMPBELL, M.D.
JOHN A. WALDHAUSEN, M.D.

Resection and end-to-end anastomosis for coarctation of the aorta were first performed in 1944 by Crafoord and Nylin and also by Gross and Hufnagel. Surgical repair in an infant was not reported until 1950.

Hemodynamic molding is the process by which blood vessels grow and develop around a flowing column of blood. Anomalies that alter the flow of blood through the heart can result in differential growth and development of the cardiac chambers, valves, and great vessels. Any process that increases the ratio of right and left ventricular outputs can result in decreased left ventricular output and abnormal growth and development of the aortic valve, aortic arch, aortic isthmus, and juxtaductal region of the aorta (Fig. 1).

Specific intracardiac anomalies, which can cause coarctation of the aorta based on the hemodynamic molding concept, are those that reduce output of the left side of the heart. Those clinically associated with coarctation of the aorta are ventricular septal defect, bicuspid aortic valve, congenital aortic stenosis, hypoplastic left ventricle, congenital mitral valve stenosis or atresia, a restrictive interatrial communication, and Taussig-Bing double outlet right ventricle. As might be expected, coarctation is quite rare among the lesions that reduce output of the right side of the heart, such as tetralogy of Fallot, pulmonary stenosis, and pulmonary atresia.

Generally there are two types of clinical manifestations. In infants, coarctation is usually preductal and is associated with isthmus hypoplasia as well as the intracardiac anomalies described earlier. These infants have severe congestive heart failure. Coarctation of the aorta in older patients is infrequently associated with other cardiac anomalies and is usually a discrete coarctation membrane at or just beyond the level of the ligamentum arteriosum (juxtaductal coarctation). With time, the aortic wall may grow unequally and cause a greater downward displacement of the lateral wall and coarctation

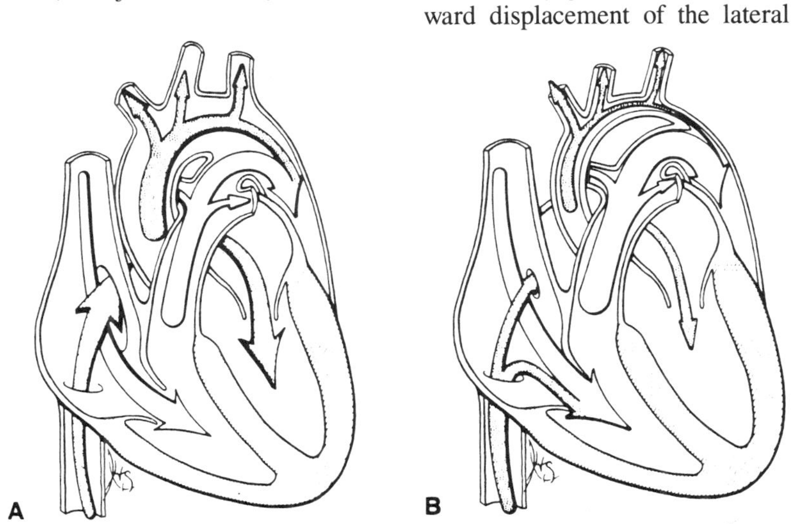

Figure 1 Fetal circulation. *A*, Normal fetal circulation with nearly equal output of the left and right ventricles. *B*, A restrictive foramen ovale results in increased pulmonary artery flow and decreased aortic flow, resulting in hypoplasia of the isthmus. (From Glenn W, et al, eds. Thoracic and cardiovascular surgery. 4th ed. Norwalk: Appleton & Lange, 1983.)

membrane compared with the medial wall that is held in place by the ligamentum arteriosum. This results in a "postductal" coarctation. In this latter group, consisting primarily of older children and young adults, the diagnosis is usually made incidentally when a patient is being evaluated for hypertension, headaches, epistaxis, lower extremity claudication, decreased femoral pulse, or heart failure.

PREFERRED APPROACH

Proper treatment of coarctation of the aorta is achieved by surgical procedures designed to eliminate the coarctation gradient. Aggressive medical management is essential for optimal preoperative preparation of these patients.

Newborns and Infants

Preoperative Management

Infants with coarctation of the aorta most frequently have severe congestive heart failure, signs of systemic hypoperfusion, and metabolic acidosis. During fetal life, the pulmonary arteries are in a parallel circuit with the ductus arteriosus and descending aorta. Thus, closure of the ductus arteriosus in infants with coarctation of the aorta causes a marked increase in the pulmonary arterial blood flow and a decrease in lower body (abdominal viscera and extremities) blood flow. The resulting increase in pulmonary venous return is delivered to the left ventricle, which is already compromised by the severe afterload caused by the coarctation. The end result is severe congestive heart failure and hypoperfusion of the abdominal viscera and lower body, which leads to metabolic acidosis, oliguria and further myocardial depression. Prompt, aggressive intervention is mandatory to improve systemic perfusion and correct metabolic acidosis. The use of prostaglandin E_1 is the most important advance in the preoperative management of these infants. The infusion of prostaglandin E_1 is begun at 0.1 to 0.2 μg per kilogram per minute. The dosage is then tapered by increments of 0.025 μg per kilogram per minute to a minimum of 0.05 μg per kilogram per minute as long as ductal patency is maintained. Opening the ductus arteriosus allows better perfusion of the abdominal viscera and the lower body, decreasing the production of lactic acid by improved tissue perfusion and allowing excretion of acid by improved renal perfusion. The increased blood flow through the opened ductus arteriosus also lessens the amount of pulmonary overperfusion, thus improving the left-sided congestive heart failure. Administration of dopamine is sometimes necessary for inotropic support of the compromised myocardium. An infusion of 3 to 5 μg per kilogram per minute is usually sufficient. Sodium bicarbonate is often required initially to improve the acidemia while systemic hypoperfusion is being corrected. Endotracheal intubation and mechanical ventilatory support are often helpful in babies with pulmonary edema. Hyperventilation is useful to further eliminate acid in the form of carbon dioxide. However, a low arterial P_{CO_2}, an elevated pH, and an increased F_{IO_2} promote a decrease in pulmonary vascular resistance. With an open ductus arteriosus, the amount of blood flow through the lungs and lower body is dependent upon the ratio of the vascular resistance in the respective vascular beds. Therefore, once ductal patency is established and acid base balance is optimized, the ventilatory support should be adjusted to maintain a P_{CO_2} of 35 to 40 mm Hg and the F_{IO_2} should be reduced to the lowest fraction permitting an arterial P_{O_2} of 25 to 35 mm Hg. This allows normalization of the pulmonary vascular resistance and reduction of the pulmonary overperfusion. When an infant's medical condition is satisfactory, prompt surgical intervention is mandatory.

Surgical Techniques

Infants Under 1 Year of Age

In infants of under 1 year, we prefer subclavian flap angioplasty and, in our experience, this has provided excellent short- and long-term results. It is performed through a fourth intercostal space posterolateral thoracotomy with dissection of the aorta and its branches from the left carotid to about 2 cm beyond the ductus arteriosus. The recurrent nerve is protected and the intercostal vessels are spared and controlled, if necessary, with Pott's ties. The subclavian artery is mobilized out to the origin of the vertebral artery, and both are ligated distal to this bifurcation (Fig. 2). The duct is ligated with No. 2 braided silk, and aortic cross-clamps are placed proximally between the left carotid and left subclavian arteries and distally approximately 2 cm distal to the ductus arteriosus. The subclavian artery is divided at the origin of the vertebral artery. A longitudinal incision is made in the aorta opposite the ductus and extended proximally across the coarctation, the isthmus, and into the subclavian artery (Fig. 3). The aortotomy is extended distally for at least

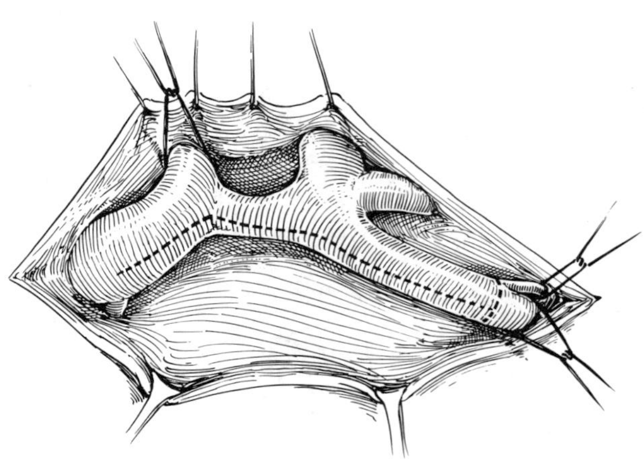

Figure 2 Repair of coarctation of the aorta using the subclavian flap technique. The operative exposure with ligatures around the ductus arteriosus, vertebral artery, and distal subclavian artery. The dotted line indicates the incision in the aorta and subclavian artery. (Modified from Waldhausen JA, Pierce WS, eds. Johnsons's surgery of the chest. 5th ed. Chicago: Year Book, 1985:303.)

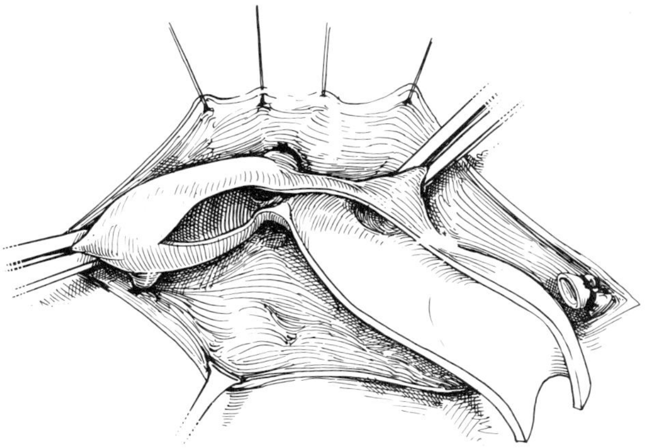

Figure 3 The incision is made distal to the ductus and extended proximally across the coarctation, isthmus, and divided subclavian artery. The coarctation membrane is then excised. (Modified from Waldhausen JA, Pierce WS, eds. Johnson's surgery of the chest. 5th ed. Chicago: Year Book, 1985:303.)

1 cm beyond the ductus. The coarctation shelf is excised with scissors, taking care that all the excess tissue is removed without injury to the aortic wall. Trimming or tapering of the subclavian flap should not be done and, in fact, is detrimental to the repair. A mattress suture of 5–0 or 6–0 monofilament absorbable suture material (PDS, Ethicon Inc.) is placed at the apex of the subclavian flap and the distal extent of the aortotomy (Fig. 4). The U-shaped repair is completed with a continuous suture of PDS (Fig. 5). If an absorbable suture material is not available, the flap should be sutured in place with interrupted sutures. Air is evacuated, and the aortic cross-clamps are removed. It is important to extend the aortotomy well beyond the area of coarctation to ensure that there is no residual narrowing. The subclavian artery is not dissected beyond the origin of the vertebral artery, since this may jeopardize collateral circulation to the arm. In our experience, no patient has suffered ischemic injury of the arm, and the subclavian artery has always been of adequate length to permit its use.

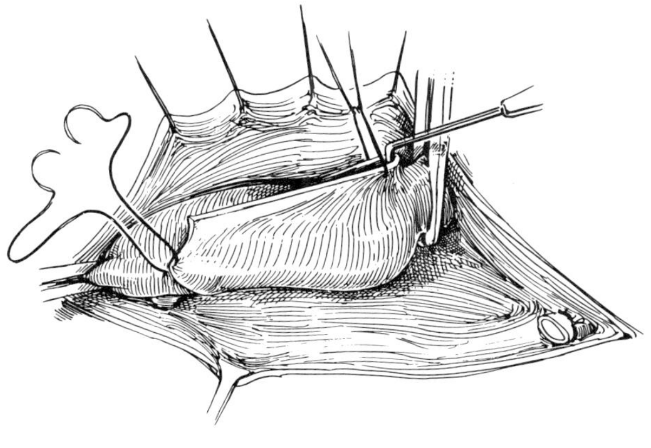

Figure 4 The flap is turned down into the aortic incision.

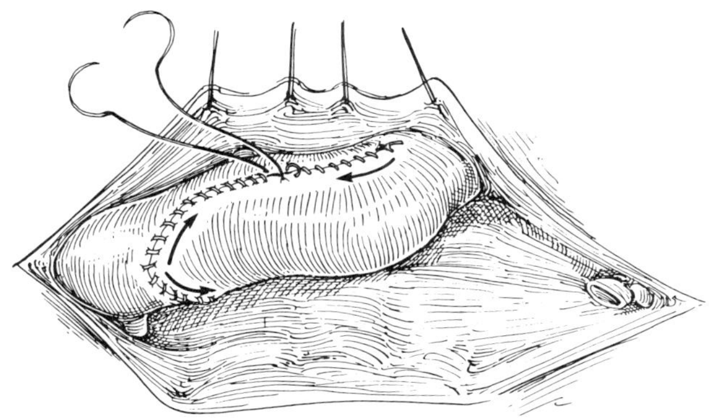

Figure 5 The complete subclavian flap repair.

Older Children (Older than 1 Year of Age) and Adults

After 1 year of age, treatment depends on the individual patient. If the isthmus is small or if the coarctation is long in a child of 2 or 3 years of age, the subclavian flap angioplasty is still utilized. After 12 months of age, however, our standard operation consists of resection and end-to-end anastomosis when the anatomy permits. We now avoid the use of synthetic graft material whenever possible. When used as a patch graft, such material has produced a high incidence of aneurysm formation opposite the patch. When used as a tubular graft, its main drawback has been lack of growth and the potential for infection. We perform resection of the coarctation and all juxtaductal tissue and mobilize the entire descending aorta and distal aortic arch. Repair is accomplished by end-to-end anastomosis using a continuous running suture of absorbable monofilament suture material (PDS) on the posterior row and interrupted PDS or polypropylene (Prolene) on the anterior row. We have managed a small number of patients with a very short coarctation with direct aortoplasty (longitudinal incision, excision of membrane, transverse closure). Early in our experience, 14 patients had prosthetic patch angioplasty. We no longer advocate this procedure because of aneurysm formation. Prosthetic graft interposition has been used in very long coarctations in which direct end-to-end anastomosis would result in excessive suture line tension.

RESULTS

The associated cardiac anomalies and mortality in infants are listed in Table 1. Table 2 lists the operative mortality as a function of age at operation. There have been only two deaths in 63 infants operated on in the first year of life. One newborn with coarctation and patent ductus arteriosus was operated on before prostaglandin E_1 was available for clinical use. This infant had severe congestive heart failure and metabolic acidosis preoperatively.

TABLE 1 Associated Cardiac Anomalies and Mortality in Infants

Anomalies	*Patients*	*Deaths (%)*
Coarctation alone	6	0 (0)
PDA		
All occurrences	50	0 (0)
With coarctation only	17	1 (6)
Primary intracardiac anomaly		
Simple VSD	18	0 (0)
Complex anomalies		
DORV (Taussig-Bing)	7	0 (0)
AV canal	5	0 (0)
TGA, VSD	5	0 (0)
Hypoplastic left ventricle	1	1 (100)
Valvular anomalies (AS, MR)	5	0 (0)
Total	63	2 (3)

PDA=patent ductus arteriosus; VSD=ventricular septal defect; DORV=double-outlet right ventricle; AV canal=atrioventricular canal; TGA=transposition of the great arteries; AS=aortic stenosis; MR=mitral regurgitation.

The other newborn had a hypoplastic left ventricle and was moribund at the time of operation. Of the 133 patients operated on for coarctation of the aorta, 63 patients (47 percent) were less than 1 year of age. Table 3 lists the operations in patients over 1 year of age. The overall operative mortality is 3 percent for all patients, irrespective of age. One patient (age 13) died from suture line dehiscence 12 hours postoperatively. Another patient (age 21) was operated on over 10 years ago and died at home 14 days after prosthetic patch angioplasty, an operation no longer recommended. Five patients had aortoplasties (longitudinal incision, excision of membrane, and transverse closure) with good results. This operation has only limited applicability. Eleven infants have undergone postoperative catheterization. Two residual gradients of over 5 mm Hg have been documented in four repairs performed with continuous nonabsorbable suture technique. Seven patients, who had subclavian flap angioplasty with

TABLE 2 Age at Operation and Mortality

Age at Operation	*Patients*	*Deaths (%)*
1–7 days	17	2 (12)
8–30 days	27	0 (0)
31–365 days	19	0 (0)
1–31 years	70	2 (3)
Total	133	4 (3)

TABLE 3 Operations in Patients Over One Year of Age

Type of Repair	*Patients*	*Death (%)*
Resection and end-to-end anastomosis	42	1 (2)
Prosthetic patch angioplasty	14	1 (7)
Subclavian flap angioplasty	6	0 (0)
Direct angioplasty	5	0 (0)
Interposition graft	3	0 (0)
Total	70	2 (3)

interrupted suture technique, had no gradients. All of the other infants have good femoral pulses and, clinically, no evidence of residual coarctation. Following repair in infancy, no systemic hypertension as measured in the right arm and no arm-to-leg gradients exceeding 10 mm Hg have been found in patients when examined 2 or more years after operation.

We now use a continuous suture technique with absorbable monofilament polydioxanone (PDS, Ethicon) in all subclavian flap angioplasty operations. This repair technique has been used for 21 patients, and the initial results are excellent.

In infants, aggressive preoperative preparation with prostaglandin E_1 infusions has allowed stabilization of neonates with profound cardiovascular decompensation. The low operative mortality rate and excellent late results have led us to recommend that coarctation of the aorta should be repaired at the time of diagnosis regardless of age or symptoms. Age is no longer a risk factor, and late hypertensive morbidity should be reduced by early successful repair. Absorbable vascular suture will be evaluated after long-term follow-up examinations are made.

SUGGESTED READING

Campbell DB, Waldhausen JA, Pierce WS, Whitman V, Fripp R. Should elective repair of coarctation of the aorta be done in infancy? J Thorac Cardiovasc Surg 1984; 88:929–938.

Fripp RR, Whitman V, Werner J, Nicholas GG, Waldhausen JA. Blood pressure response to exercise in children following the subclavian flap procedure for coarctation of the aorta. J Thorac Cardiovasc Surg 1983; 85:682–685.

Parr GVS, Waldhausen JA, Bharati S, et al. Coarctation in Taussig-Bing malformation of the heart. J Thorac Cardiovasc Surg 1983; 86: 280–287.

Rudolph AM, Heymann MA, Spitzhas N. Hemodynamic considerations in the development of narrowing of the aorta. Am J Cardiol 1972; 30:514–525.

Waldhausen JA, Nahrwold DL. Repair of coarctation of the aorta with a subclavian flap. J Thorac Cardiovasc Surg 1966; 51:532–533.

THE UNIVENTRICULAR HEART: ROLE OF VENTRICULAR SEPTATION

PAUL A. EBERT, M.D., F.A.C.S.

Partitioning of the univentricular heart has always been viewed as an ideal solution to this physiologic abnormality. Problems associated with partitioning have been the large intraventricular patch and its paradoxical motion, injury to the conduction system, the presence of pulmonary vascular disease, and location and positioning of the papillary muscles and chordae to the two atrioventricular valves. A high mortality rate in older children has limited enthusiasm for this procedure, and survivors were not found to be better functionally than patients with a Fontan's procedure and in many cases were more debilitated with a shorter life expectancy. A staged operation for partitioning of the single ventricle has been successful in small infants and is recommended if the anatomy permits.

The ideal patient for consideration of staged partitioning of the single ventricle is an infant in the first year of life with evidence of increased pulmonary circulation. An echocardiogram or cardiac catheterization should confirm the posterior location of the pulmonary artery adjacent to the tricuspid annulus and minimal if any evidence of a left-sided outflow tract chamber. The echocardiogram may substantiate that there is no crossing of posterior papillary muscles or chordae between the two atrioventricular valves. However, there is no definite way of proving this prior to the time of operative visualization of the ventricular chamber. There should be no evidence of infundibular or subpulmonic stenosis. Some infants may have had a previous pulmonary artery banding in the early weeks of life to control heart failure. This should not be a contraindication to staged partitioning. The main advantage of considering staging the partitioning is that a Teflon felt patch will become stiffer with less paradoxical movement. As well, the patches do not have to be sewn tightly in place, since there is no pressure differential across the residual ventricular septal defect, and injury to the conduction system is lessened by having to place fewer and less tightly tied sutures.

OPERATIVE APPROACH

The operation is performed through a medial sternotomy incision with institution of cardiopulmonary bypass by cannulation of the aorta and the right atrium. Total circulatory arrest is employed in the smaller infant, and direct cannulation of the vena cava in the larger infant. The right atrium is opened in an oblique or transverse fashion, and the internal anatomy of the heart is inspected through the tricuspid valve. One would hope to see the posterior papillary muscles of the mitral and tricuspid valves inserting on the back wall of the ventricle in such a fashion that a patch could easily be placed between them. The tricuspid annulus should be adjacent to the annulus of the pulmonary valve. A small triangular piece of Teflon felt is then fastened to the apex of the ventricle by placing sutures through the patch and then combining both of these sutures onto a single French eye needle and pulling it through the apex of the ventricle. The second suture can be placed at the most inferior portion of the junction of the two posterior papillary muscles and brought out directly through the posterior ventricle. A third and a fourth suture are then placed anteriorly, with care taken in all instances to avoid coronary vessels. These sutures are tied over a single narrow strip of Teflon felt or small individual pledgets of Teflon, and the patch is loosely approximated to the ventricle so the external Teflon strip or pledgets do not cut into the myocardium. An upper patch is fashioned in a semilunar manner so that it can be sutured between the aortic and pulmonary annulus, around to the anterior wall of the ventricle. A continuous suture technique is used between the pulmonary and aortic annuli, and then a similar technique to that for the lower patch is used on the free walls of the ventricle (Figure 1). A suture is placed through the patch, through the single eye of a French eye needle, and then pulled through the anterior wall. In the area posteriorly, one or two similar sutures are used to pull the patch to the posterior wall in order to avoid the normal area of the conduction system. Again, this patch does not have to be as tightly tied on the posterior wall of the ventricle, where conduction injury is more common. These two pieces of Teflon are separated with good communication (ventricular septal defect) between the newly created right and left ventricles, the atriotomy is closed, and the patient is rewarmed and taken off cardio-

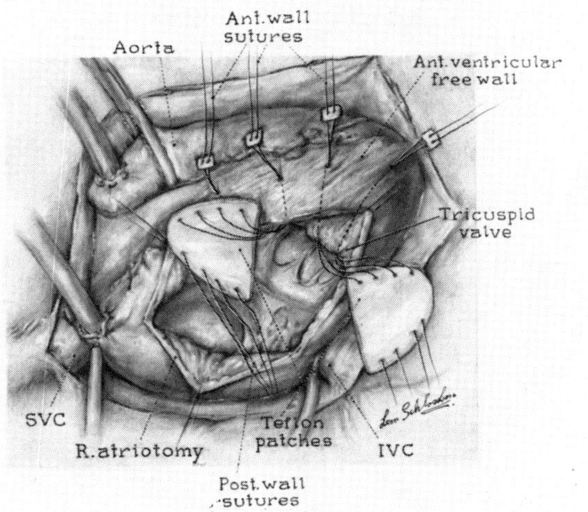

Figure 1 The two patches are being positioned in place. The lower patch is held by three or four sutures and is tied loosely in the apex. The upper patch has the continuous sutures between the aorta and pulmonary annulus. (From Ebert PA. Staged partitioning of single ventricle. J Thorac Cardiovasc Surg 1984; 88:908).

pulmonary bypass. If a pulmonary artery band was previously placed, it may be loosened or repositioned to accommodate more flow and allow for growth of the child; if one had not previously been placed and there is no evidence of pulmonary valve obstruction, then a band should be placed at this time and adjusted off cardiopulmonary bypass to produce a good thrill and a pressure gradient across the band.

The second stage of the procedure is elective and can be performed after 3 months. It is probably wise not to wait too long, because cyanosis and diminished pulmonary flow will also decrease cardiac chamber size and possibly make the postoperative course more difficult. Thus, the ventricular septal defect should be closed when the patches have stiffened and healed to the ventricle and there is still evidence of a left-to-right shunt through the ventricular septal defect.

The second operation is through the medial sternotomy incision. The child is placed on routine cardiopulmonary bypass with cannulations of the superior and inferior vena cava and the ascending aorta. The right atrium is opened, cardioplegia may or may not be employed at this point, and the ventricular septal defect is visualized through the tricuspid valve. The superior and inferior borders are Teflon, the anterior border is the anterior free wall of the ventricle, and the posterior border is that of the papillary muscle attachments of the atrioventricular valves. This is usually a rectangular-shaped defect. A piece of Teflon felt is cut, large enough to roll 5 to 6 mm of the posterior edge to the left ventricular side. The first sutures should be placed through the patch, 5 to 6 mm from its posterior edge and through the base of the Teflon on the inferior and superior portions of the defect. These are tied, allowing the flap of Teflon to fall into the left ventricular cavity posteriorly; thus a flap valve is created in this location, and no sutures are required in the posterior wall of the ventricle (Figure 2). The patch is sewn firmly to the Teflon superiorly and inferiorly, and several sutures are brought through the anterior wall of the ventricle, as in stage one of the procedure. It is recognized that there is no consistent location of the conduction system in the univentricular heart, but the commonest location seems to be in the posterior aspect of the tricuspid annulus, near where the bundle is located in normal patients. Thus, all sutures in this area can be eliminated in the second phase by securely anchoring the patch posteriorly to the superior and inferior pieces of previously placed Teflon. The band is removed from the pulmonary artery, and a generous patch is placed in the area of the pulmonary artery, or the segment is resected and the pulmonary artery is reconstituted in an end-to-end fashion.

POSTOPERATIVE MANAGEMENT

The postoperative management of these children has been relatively similar to that of any child having a moderately sized ventricular septal defect closure. Assuming sinus rhythm is present, a child would be ventilated for 24 hours and an attempt made at extubation the following morning. Management after the initial operation may be more difficult because there essentially is minimal change in the hemodynamics of the patient. Thus, the condition of the child prior to surgery would influence the postoperative management. If the child were in severe heart failure before operation, then application of a pulmonary artery band should improve the condition, but the effects of pulmonary overcirculation may still make respiratory management more difficult. Mechanical ventilation lasting from 1 to 6 days may be necessary after the first operation, depending entirely on the condition of the child. If a previous pulmonary artery band is in place, and the child is markedly cyanotic, then loosening of the band at the time of placement of the initial intraventricular patches may result in increased pulmonary circulation, which some-

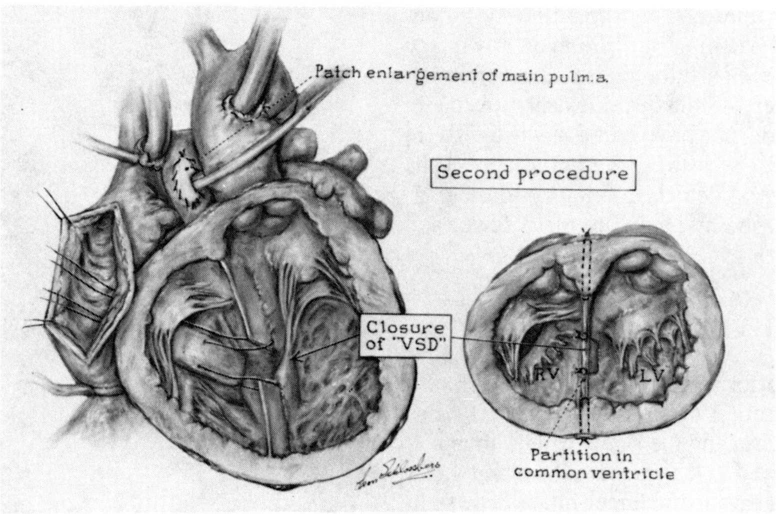

Figure 2 The completion of the ventricular septal defect closure at the time of the second operation. The tongue of the Teflon patch lies to the left side of the previously placed Teflon patches and thus does not require any sutures along the posterior wall of the heart. (From Ebert PA. Staged partitioning of single ventricle. J Thorac Cardiovasc Surg 1984; 88:908.)

times requires supportive ventilation for longer than usual. Heart failure, per se, and cardiotonic drugs have not been common accompaniments of staged partitioning.

RESULTS

I have performed both stages of ventricular septation in six patients, and all have survived to date. One child subsequently required conduit placement from the pulmonary ventricle to the pulmonary arteries because of gradual annular stenosis occurring over a 5-year period following septation. The annular stenosis in this patient appeared to be a natural progression of the patient's disease, since there was never any specific anatomic reason at the time of septation to suspect that the pulmonic annulus would have narrowed over 5 years.

In carefully selected candidates, septation may be an attractive option, as it creates two-ventricle physiology. I would point out that not many infants are actual candidates for this procedure because of the requirements that the pulmonary artery and the tricuspid annulus be somewhat adjacent and that it be possible to partition the ventricle so as to separate the mitral and tricuspid valves. However, if these anatomic requirements are met, septation is feasible and should be considered.

SUGGESTED READING

Doty DB, Schieken RM, Lauer RM. Septation of the univentricular heart. Transatrial approach. J Thorac Cardiovasc Surg 1979; 78:423–430.

Ebert PA. Staged partitioning of single ventricle. J Thorac Cardiovasc Surg 1984; 88:908–913.

McGoon DC, Danielson GK, Puga FJ. Univentricular heart. In: Glenn WL, Baue AE, Geha AS, Hammond GL, Laks H, eds. Thoracic and cardiovascular surgery. 4th ed. Norwalk, CT: Appleton-Century-Crofts, 1983.

INTERRUPTED AORTIC ARCH

RICHARD A. JONAS, M.D.

Posterior deviation of the conal (infundibular) septum relative to the muscular interventricular septum results in both a narrowing of the left ventricular outflow tract and creation of a posterior malalignment ventricular septal defect (VSD). It is suspected that the resultant decrease in blood ejected into the ascending aorta during in utero development can result in complete interruption of the aortic arch, most commonly between the left common carotid and left subclavian arteries. Up to two-thirds of patients with interrupted aortic arch have associated DiGeorge's syndrome. Associated cardiac problems can include truncus arteriosus, tricuspid atresia with transposition, or single ventricle. These complex malformations will not be considered here. Following birth, the neonate with interrupted aortic arch and VSD remains viable as long as the ductus arteriosus remains patent, allowing a right-to-left shunt to maintain lower body perfusion. The child may remain asymptomatic for several days, but as the ductus closes, the leg (and commonly left arm) pulses will diminish. The child will appear pale and poorly perfused, and some patients will be in respiratory distress as an attempt is made to compensate for a worsening metabolic acidosis. Renal function rapidly deteriorates, and there may also be major hepatic and mesenteric ischemic insults.

RESUSCITATION

Rapid diagnosis by 2-D echocardiogram followed by resuscitation of the neonate in the throes of ductal closure is essential to achieve satisfactory results for the management of this condition. Intravenous prostaglandin E_1 (PGE_1) should be started at a dose of 0.1 μg per kilogram per minute, preferably through an umbilical venous catheter. Placement of an umbilical arterial catheter, or, if this is not possible, of a dorsalis pedis or posterior tibial arterial catheter, allows direct monitoring of ductal patency. A normal arterial pulse contour should be visible within 1 to 2 hours of commencing administration of PGE_1. The child should be intubated and ventilated and appropriate bicarbonate given to correct metabolic acidosis. Since blood in both ventricles has a choice of passing to either the pulmonary or systemic circulation, it is important to maintain as high a level of pulmonary resistance relative to systemic resistance as possible. This can normally be achieved by ventilating with an FIO_2 of 21 percent and keeping arterial PCO_2 close to 40 mm Hg. Since neonatal pulmonary resistance is relatively high and can be further increased by appropriate ventilation, the child can now be maintained in a stable hemodynamic state to allow normalization of all parameters that were affected by the ischemic insult, particularly blood urea and creatinine levels. A low-dose (less than 10 μg per kilogram per minute) infusion of dopamine may be used to improve renal perfusion and cardiac output. A high calcium requirement as a manifestation of DiGeorge's syndrome is not uncommon and may necessitate a constant infusion. If sepsis is present, the child may require several days of appropriate intravenous antibiotic therapy preoperatively. In the majority of cases of interrupted aortic arch with VSD, 2-D echocardiography will provide adequate definition of the arch and VSD anatomy so that cardiac catheterization is usually unnecessary.

TREATMENT

Surgical management is the only treatment option for the neonate with interrupted aortic arch with VSD. In the vast majority of children in whom rapid diagnosis and resuscitation have been performed, surgery can be done electively with normal acid-base status and normal urea, creatinine, and electrolyte levels.

Reparative Surgery

Closure of the VSD and establishing aortic continuity create a physiologically normal circulation and avoid the secondary pathologic changes that can result from palliation. Repair also greatly simplifies the postoperative management and is therefore the surgical option of choice in the majority of cases. Aortic continuity can be established by conduit placement, but this should rarely be part of a reparative procedure. Usually a direct aortic anastomosis is satisfactory; previous concerns regarding growth of a circumferential aortic anastomosis appear to have been overemphasized in the light of data from the neonatal arterial switch experience and recent results for coarctation surgery.

Technique of Repair

With the child supine, approach is by median sternotomy. If a thymus is present, it is largely excised. Although single arterial cannulation of the pulmonary artery can result in satisfactory head cooling, this may not allow an adequate myocardial perfusion pressure during the cooling phase. Therefore, following heparinization, bypass is commenced with one arterial cannula in the ascending aorta and venous return via a single cannula in the right atrium. A second arterial cannula, on a Y-connector, is then inserted in the proximal main pulmonary artery. Pulmonary flow is controlled by fine tourniquets around the right and left pulmonary arteries. During cooling, tourniquets are placed loosely around the innominate, left common carotid, and left subclavian arteries. The ascending aorta, innominate artery, and left common carotid are fully mobilized. This is an important maneuver to avoid tension on the aortic anastomosis. A loose tie is placed around the patent ductus arteriosus. When the rectal temperature reaches 20° C, bypass is ceased and the tourniquets on the arch branches are tightened to avoid cerebral air embolism while the pulmonary artery tourniquets are removed. Cardioplegic solution is infused into the ascending aorta. All cannulas are removed. The ductus arteriosus is ligated and divided at its junction with the proximal descending aorta. It is important that no ductal tissue be left on the descending aorta, since this holds sutures poorly and may constrict and fibrose in time. Extensive mobilization of the descending aorta enables good visualization in this area and ensures a tension-free anastomosis. Excessive tension on the anastomosis can result in poor hemostasis, early and late anastomotic stenosis, and left bronchial compression. A direct anastomosis is fashioned to a longitudinal incision in the left side of the ascending aorta using continuous 6–0 PDS suture. Traction on the tourniquet around the left subclavian artery improves exposure of the descending aorta and minimizes tension on the anastomosis. After establishing proximal aortic to distal aortic continuity, the VSD is closed in the routine fashion with a Dacron patch, working through a right atriotomy and the tricuspid valve. Exposure is usually better than for a membranous VSD because of the posterior displacement of the conal septum. The foramen ovale is closed after filling the left side of the heart with saline, allowing air to vent through the aortic cannulation site in the ascending aorta. It is important that the arterial cannula be directly opposite the aortic anastomosis. This allows adequate retrograde coronary perfusion as well as antegrade perfusion, which may otherwise be a problem in the hypoplastic ascending aorta. The right atriotomy is closed, the ascending aorta and the right atrium are recannulated, and bypass is recommenced. The tourniquets on the head vessels are released. During rewarming, a left atrial line and ventricular pacing wire are inserted. A pulmonary artery line may also be inserted through the infundibulum of the right ventricle. Weaning from bypass may be assisted with inotropic support. Hemostasis is achieved with the assistance of thrombin-soaked Gelfoam and by transfusion with fresh blood, which should be irradiated if DiGeorge's syndrome is present.

Palliative Surgery

If diagnosis or resuscitation or both have been delayed, and the child has suffered a severe prolonged ischemic insult with failure to respond completely to resuscitative measures, it may occasionally be preferable to avoid the further insult of reparative surgery. However, since the child will not be physiologically normal after palliative surgery, postoperative management is more complex. Furthermore, the need for future surgery including conduit replacements makes palliative surgery a greatly inferior alternative to repair.

Technique of Surgical Palliation

The child is placed at 45 degrees left side up and is prepped and draped to allow for both median sternotomy and left thoracotomy incision. While the operation to be described can be performed through a single incision, in the author's opinion two incisions allow for minimal retraction of lungs, heart, and great vessels, which is essential in these metabolically compromised children.

Through a left lateral thoracotomy (fourth or fifth space) incision the left lung is gently retracted anteriorly. A side-biting clamp is placed on the descending aorta and the distal anastomosis to a 6- or 7-mm polytetrafluoroethylene (PTFE) tube is made. The conduit is controlled with a bulldog clamp and the side clamp is released.

A median sternotomy is performed. A ligature is placed loosely around the ductus arteriosus. The conduit is retrieved from the left chest, cut to length, and anastomosed to the ascending aorta in a side-biting clamp. The bulldog clamp is released. The ductus ligature is tied. The pulmonary artery is banded, usually achieving a transitory 15-mm increase in systemic systolic blood pressure while maintaining arterial saturation by pulse oximeter at greater than 80 percent.

POSTOPERATIVE MANAGEMENT

Repair

Management of the child who has undergone a technically sound reparative operation should be routine. There may be a continuing large calcium requirement, as observed during the preoperative resuscitation. Dopamine can usually be withdrawn over 24 to 48 hours, and ventilatory weaning proceeds as dictated by the child's blood gas status. Failure of the patient to progress rapidly should stimulate aggressive reinvestigation. A gradient between right arm and lower body should be carefully excluded. This is facilitated by the presence of an umbilical arterial line, often supplemented by placement of a right radial arterial line. The umbilical artery line is removed when the child is stable and starts enteral feeding. A residual VSD should be excluded by placement of a pulmonary arterial line in the operating room or by a careful 2-D echocardiogram. If a residual VSD is present, the magnitude of left-to-right shunt should be quantitated by cardiac catheterization. Cardiac catheterization will also exclude significant subaortic stenosis. This is particularly unusual in the neonatal period, although we have seen it develop over the next 1 to 2 years. If subaortic stenosis develops, it must be treated surgically by resection of the conal septum. This is not recommended as part of the initial procedure.

Palliation

Since the child who has undergone the conduit-pulmonary artery band procedure probably had multiple preoperative metabolic derangements, postoperative management is more complex and involves maximal support of all organ systems. Furthermore, since a VSD is still present, variations in the ratio of pulmonary to systemic vascular resistances continue to influence the distribution of cardiac output between these two vascular beds. Depending on the effectiveness of the pulmonary artery band, it may be necessary to either minimize pulmonary vascular resistance by hyperventilation with high concentration oxygen in the child who is slightly overbanded or to maximize pulmonary vascular resistance in the opposite case using techniques described for preoperative resuscitation. If such manipulations are inadequate, 2-D echocardiography with or without cardiac catheterization should be undertaken to assess band tightness. The threshold for cardiac catheterization should be lower if there is suspicion of a trans-conduit gradient.

The child who has undergone palliative surgery should be carefully monitored for the development of subaortic stenosis over the months following banding. A pulmonary artery band may stimulate hypertrophy of the conal septum, resulting in progressive subaortic stenosis. Closure of the VSD should be performed by 1 to 2 years of age before scarring at the band site has become severe. Conduit replacement is not usually required until 4 to 5 years of age, when a second conduit can be inserted. Occasionally, we have placed a third conduit in teenage children through a right thoracotomy, taking the conduit from the ascending to the descending aorta just above the diaphragm.

SURGICAL RESULTS

Between December 1983 and January 1987, the author has undertaken surgical management of interrupted aortic arch in 21 patients. There were three early deaths among six patients who had additional complex lesions such as hypoplastic left-sided heart syndrome or tricuspid atresia with transposition. There was one early death among 15 patients with interrupted aortic arch with VSD. The child who died had persistent metabolic acidosis despite the usual resuscitative measures and died from sepsis and hepatic failure 4 weeks postoperatively. Direct anastomosis and VSD closure have been achieved in seven out of the last eight patients.

While the surgery for interrupted aortic arch with VSD remains conceptually simple and the mobility and elasticity of neonatal tissues almost always ensure a tension-free aortic anastomosis, the essence of successful management of this condition remains rapid diagnosis and aggressive resuscitation to avoid permanent multiorgan ischemic damage to the neonate.

SUGGESTED READING

Barratt-Boyes BG, Nicholls TT, Brandt PWT, Neutze JM. Aortic arch interruption associated with patent ductus arteriosus, ventricular septal defect, and total anomalous pulmonary venous connection. J Thorac Cardiovasc Surg 1972; 63:367–373.

Celoria GC, Patton RB. Congenital absence of the aortic arch. Am Heart J 1959; 58:407–413.

Norwood WI, Lang P, Castaneda AR, Hougen TJ. Reparative operations for interrupted aortic arch with ventricular septal defect. J Thorac Cardiovasc Surg 1983; 86:832–837.

Trusler GA, Izukawa T. Interrupted aortic arch and ventricular septal defect. Direct repair through a median sternotomy incision in a 13 day old infant. J Thorac Cardiovasc Surg 1975; 69:126–131.

PATENT DUCTUS ARTERIOSUS

CONSTANTINE MAVROUDIS, M.D.

Patent ductus arteriosus (PDA) in low birth weight premature infants causing large left-to-right shunts has been associated with congestive heart failure, bronchopulmonary dysplasia, necrotizing enterocolitis, intracranial hemorrhage, and death. Expeditious surgical ligation of the PDA in these infants has improved lung compliance, decreased the duration of assisted ventilation, and increased nutritional utilization.

The introduction of indomethacin for pharmacologic constriction of the ductus arteriosus in 1976 proved useful in some premature infants. However, because of its toxicity, patients with hyperbilirubinemia, sepsis, coagulation deficiencies, and renal impairment may experience temporary or permanent deleterious changes in their already precarious clinical status, leaving surgical ligation as the method of choice to close the PDA.

PATIENT POPULATION

Two hundred and thirty-four patients underwent PDA ligation in the newborn intensive care unit at Kosair Children's Hospital in Louisville, Kentucky, over the 5-year period from July, 1981, through June, 1986. All patients were either born at the hospital or transferred from associated hospitals within a 200-mile radius. The mean gestational age of the infants was 29.1 weeks (range 25 to 35 weeks). The mean birth weight was 1,135 g (range 350 to 2,400 g). Forty-nine percent of patients weighed 1,000 g or less at birth. All patients had respiratory distress (P_{CO_2} >70 mm Hg and P_{O_2} <50 mm Hg with an inspired oxygen fraction of less than 50 percent) requiring assisted ventilation. All infants had endotracheal intubation and arterial blood gas monitoring. The patients who were suspected of having PDA were evaluated by all or a combination of the following methods: physical examination (with findings of systolic murmur, bounding peripheral pulses, and hyperactive precordium); echocardiographic measurement of the ratio between the left atrium and the aortic root sizes; ranged-gated Doppler study; and retrograde flush aortography. As a result of this evaluation, murmur and bounding pulses were found in 93 percent of patients. The echocardiogram showed an LA:Ao ratio greater than 1.2:1 in 78 percent of patients. The results of the Doppler study were positive in 81 percent of patients, and the aortograms were positive in 67 percent of a small number of patients in whom aortography was performed.

When PDA was diagnosed, a short trial of medical therapy was instituted with an attempt to wean the patient from the ventilator. If this attempt failed, surgical ligation was performed early on in the time period. When intravenous indomethacin became available, it was administered as long as patients had no contraindications. At the time of surgical ligation, the median age was 6 days (range 1 to 69 days) and the median weight was 1,102 g. In many instances, the infants were evaluated radiologically, and, when necessary, with aortography. Despite negative study results, surgical ligation was chosen in only three instances. All three infants weighed less than 700 g at the time of ligation; all of these patients subsequently died of causes unrelated to PDA ligation.

All of the 234 infants who underwent surgical ligation were critically ill and therefore at high risk. Despite this, some special preoperative complications were noted that were associated with a lower survival rate (Table 1). Thirty-three percent of the entire group had a history of at least one pneumothorax prior to operation. Ten percent had preoperative coagulation disorders and 5 percent showed signs of congestive heart failure. Other preoperative complications included persistent fetal circulation, the need for dopamine therapy, pulmonary hemorrhage, probable necrotizing enterocolitis, and cardiopulmonary arrest.

Surgical ligation of the patent ductus arteriosus was performed in an in-unit operating room; we advocate in-unit ductal ligation to minimize the risks of transportation, such as discontinuation of monitoring, temperature instability, and inadequate ventilation. The operating team included a scrub nurse, circulating nurse, the patient's intensive care nurse, an inhalation therapist, the surgeon, and his assistant. Morphine, 0.1 mg per kilogram of body weight, was administered intravenously, and the patient was placed in a right lateral decubitus position. Muscle paralysis was employed only when there was excessive patient activity. The patient was then taken to the operating room within the unit and prepared with betadine solution and draped. Ventilation was controlled by the inhalation therapist under the surgeon's guidance while blood pressure (arterial catheter or Doppler-assisted measurements) and pulse rate were monitored. Lidocaine (Xylocaine), 0.5 percent was infiltrated into the skin and a posterolateral thoracotomy was performed. The third interspace was entered and the lung was retracted anteriorly. The pleura was dissected away from the ductus arteriosus, and the transverse aortic arch, subclavian artery, descending aorta, vagus nerve, and recurrent laryngeal nerve were all identified. A small right-angle clamp was placed around the ductus arteriosus after adequate dissection was accomplished, and the ductus was ligated with one strand of 0 silk. The PDA was interrupted by a medium hemoclip (Fig. 1) under three circumstances: (1) when coagulopathy was so severe that it made excessive dissection dangerous, (2) when the patient's condition was so hemodynamically unstable that speed and minimal manipulation were mandatory, and (3) when the ductus arteriosus was inadvertently torn and the resultant bleeding had to be controlled. Pleural drainage was employed only in patients who had a preexisting pneumothorax or when the lung was injured on entry into the chest. Most of the time, pleural drainage was not employed; no patient required left pleural drainage postoperatively if a pneumothorax was not present preoperatively. Postoperatively, the patients were conscious and not paralyzed, which allowed the stabilization and weaning processes to be instituted immediately.

TABLE 1 Clinical Features of 194 Infants Who Underwent PDA Ligation

Variable	*Survivors (N = 152)*	*Nonsurvivors (N = 42)*	*Infants in Follow-up Study (N = 116)*
Mean gestational age (wk)	29.1	26.6	29.1
Mean birth weight (g)	1,193	1,003	1,232
≤ 1,000	57	26	45
> 1,000	95	16	71
M:F ratio	72:80 (1:1.1)	23:19 (1.2:1)	57:59 (1:1.03)
Mean age at ligation (§)	6.4†	4.9†	6.5*
Mean days in neonatal ICU‡	84 (11–324)	NA	86.6
Mean days to death‡	NA	37.3 (1–197)§	NA
Mean days of assisted ventilation	34.5	NA	37.4
Pneumothorax	46 (30.3%)	27 (64.3%)	34 (29.3%)
Intraventricular hemorrhage	58 (38.2%)	16 (38.1%)	47 (40.5%)
VP shunt for hydrocephalus	28	1	25
Bronchopulmonary dysplasia	91 (59.9%)	18 (60%)#	72 (62.1%)
Necrotizing enterocolitis	7 (4.6%)	6 (14.3%)	5 (4.3%)

* Does not include one patient who underwent ligation at 97 days.
† Does not include one patient who underwent ligation at 85 days.
‡ Numbers in parentheses are range.
§ Does not include one patient who died at 2 years of age.
# Refers to infants who survived at least 10 days.
ICU = intensive care unit; NA = not applicable; VP = ventriculoperitoneal.
From Wilkerson SA, Fleischaker J, Mavroudis C, Cook LN. Developmental sequelae in premature infants undergoing ligation of patent ductus arteriosus. Ann Thorac Surg 1985; 39:542.

RESULTS

None of the patients died as a direct result of PDA ligation. Life-threatening hemorrhage occurred in three patients and was immediately controlled. Eventually, all three patients were discharged from the hospital in satisfactory condition. The neonatal mortality rate* was 10.5 percent (overall mortality† was 17 percent). A preoperative pneumothorax proved to be a predictor of death. Thirty-two percent of patients with a preoperative pneumothorax eventually died, compared with 11 percent mortality among patients without a pneumothorax. Causes of death included acute renal failure, hepatic failure, severe hyaline membrane disease, coagulopathy, persistent fetal

* Neonatal mortality = deaths occurring within the first month of life.
† Overall mortality = total hospital deaths.

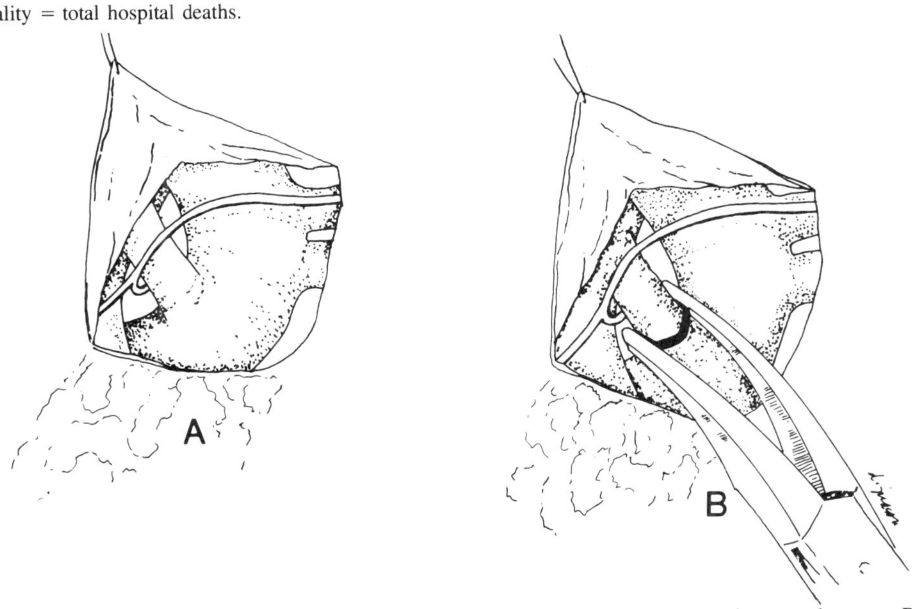

Figure 1 *A*, Arch of aorta, ductus arteriosus, vagus nerve, and recurrent laryngeal nerve. *B*, Application of hemoclip to the ductus arteriosus for interruption. (From Mavroudis C, Cook LN, Fleischaker JW, et al. Management of patent ductus arteriosus in the premature infant: indomethacin versus ligation. Ann Thorac Surg 1983; 36:563.)

circulation, intraventricular hemorrhage, and bronchopulmonary dysplasia. In general, patients who weighed more than 1,000 g had a better survival time and a shorter period of assisted ventilation (21 days versus 46 days) than patients weighing less than 1,000 g. One patient was found to have a left phrenic nerve injury for which no operative reason could be documented. This patient underwent diaphragmatic plication and eventually did well. Two patients developed superficial *Staphylococcus* wound infections that responded to local care and antibiotics.

One hundred and sixteen infants of this patient group were examined for developmental sequelae. Seven patients died before they were 3 years old—four from severe bronchopulmonary dysplasia and three from severe central nervous system dysfunction. Sixty-five percent of the remaining infants exhibited normal motor and mental development, although 58 percent showed some degree of postnatal growth retardation. There was no evidence of left arm dysfunction caused by the thoracic incision. None of the infants demonstrated recurrence of ductal patency. Mild sensorineural handicaps not expected to be of long-term significance were noted in 20 infants. Eighteen other infants (15.5 percent) were classified as having moderate to severe impairments, which may have substantial impact on development and ability to function. The clinical features of a portion of this study group are shown in Tables 2, 3, and 4.

MEDICAL VERSUS SURGICAL THERAPY

Since the introduction of indomethacin for pharmacologic closure of the PDA in 1976, there has been a constant controversy over the use of medical versus surgical therapy. The advantages of surgical therapy are low mor-

TABLE 2 Sensorineural Handicaps Among 18 Infants Exhibiting Moderate to Severe Impairment

Type of Handicap	*No. Patients*
Mental retardation*	
Mild	3
Moderate	10†
Severe	5
Sensory	
Visual impairment	7
Retrolental fibroplasia	4
Myopia	2
Other	1
Hearing impairment	4 (severe)
Motor	
Spastic quadriparesis	4 (all severe)
Spastic hemiparesis	4 (1 mild, 3 severe)
Spastic diplegia	7 (3 mild, 4 moderate)

* Mild to severe impairment was determined by the Bayley Mental Development Index or Psychomotor Development Index; mild is a score less than 84; moderate, less than 68; and severe, less than 50.
† Includes infant with Down syndrome.
From Wilkerson SA, Fleischaker J, Mavroudis C, Cook LN. Developmental sequelae in premature infants undergoing ligation of patent ductus arteriosus. Ann Thorac Surg 1985; 39:545.

TABLE 3 Incidence of Sensorineural Handicap by Birth Weight*

Birth Weight (g)	*Degree of Handicap*				*Total*
	Mild	*Moderate*	*Severe*	*Normal*	
601–700	0	0	1	1 (50.0)	2
701–800	4	3	1	6 (42.8)	14
801–900	4	3	0	9 (56.2)	16
901–1,000	2	0	2	9 (69.2)	13
1,001–1,200	1	2	1	18 (81.8)	22
1,201–1,500	4	2	1	15 (68.2)	22
1,501–2,000	3	1†	1	16 (76.2)	21
2,001–2,500	2	0	0	4 (66.7)	6
Total	20	11	7	78	116
		33%		67%	

* Numbers in parentheses are percentages.
† Infant with Down's syndrome.
From Wilkerson SA, Fleischaker J, Mavroudis C, Cook LN. Developmental sequelae in premature infants undergoing ligation of patent ductus arteriosus. Ann Thorac Surg 1985; 39:545.

TABLE 4 Relationship Between Intraventricular Hemorrhage and Sensorineural Handicaps in 116 Patients

	Developmental Status			
Variable	*Normal (N = 78)*	*Mild (N = 20)*	*Moderate (N = 11)*	*Severe (N = 7)*
Intraventricular hemorrhage				
(N = 47)	23	9	8	7
Grade* I (N = 18)	7	1	0	0
II (N = 13)	6	2	3	2
III (N = 13)	8	2	3	0
IV (N = 13)	3	3	2	5
Posthemorrhagic hydrocephalus				
(N = 25)	8	6	5	6

* Grade defined by Papile LA, Burstein J, Burstein R, et al: Incidence and evolution of subependymal and intraventricular hemorrhage: a study of infants with birth weights less than 1,500 g. J Pediatr 1978; 92:529.
From Wilkerson SA, Fleischaker J, Mavroudis C, Cook LN. Developmental sequelae in premature infants undergoing ligation of patent ductus arteriosus. Ann Thorac Surg 1985; 39:545.

bidity and mortality with quick, effective, and lasting ductal closure. The disadvantages are the risks of the operation, the infrequent but possible complications, and the potential long-term effects of thoracotomy. The advantage of indomethacin therapy is control of the PDA without the attendant risks of surgical intervention. The disadvantages of indomethacin therapy include its contraindications in infants with renal impairment, sepsis, coagulopathy, intracranial hemorrhage, and liver failure; its questionable efficacy in infants weighing more than 1,000 g; temporary ductus closure with reopening; and renal impairment, necrotizing enterocolitis, and other as yet unknown long-term effects.

Many studies have shown that surgical therapy for PDA ligation was associated with a significant decrease in necrotizing enterocolitis and mortality when compared with oral indomethacin therapy. Recently, intravenous indomethacin therapy has been shown to be as effective as oral therapy without the adverse effects of enterocolitis, bowel perforation, or hepatic failure. Because of the associated known toxicity of indomethacin and its unknown future complications, physicians have been hesitant to use the drug in neonates with renal impairment, sepsis, coagulopathy, intracranial hemorrhage, and liver failure. As many as 25 to 50 percent of patients have such preexisting conditions and are not candidates for indomethacin therapy. Under these circumstances, surgical ligation is indicated.

SUGGESTED READING

Edmunds LH Jr. Operation or indomethacin for the premature ductus (current review). Ann Thorac Surg 1978; 26:586–589.

Mavroudis C, Cook LN, Fleischaker JW, et al. Management of patent ductus arteriosus in the premature infant: indomethacin versus ligation. Ann Thorac Surg 1983; 36:561–566.

Mikhail M, Lee W, Toews W, et al. Surgical and medical experience with 734 premature infants with patent ductus arteriosus. J Thorac Cardiovasc Surg 1982; 83:349–357.

Oxnard SC, McGough EC, Jung AL, Ruttenberg HD. Ligation of the patent ductus arteriosus in the newborn intensive care unit. Ann Thorac Surg 1977; 23:564–567.

Wilkerson SA, Fleischaker J, Mavroudis C, Cook LN. Developmental sequelae in premature infants undergoing ligation of patent ductus arteriosus. Ann Thorac Surg 1985; 39:541–546.

TETRALOGY OF FALLOT

MARSHALL L. JACOBS, M.D.

The objective of improving systemic oxygen saturation in patients with tetralogy of Fallot (TOF) provided the motivation for the creation of several ingenious palliative procedures, including the Blalock-Taussig shunt (1945), the Potts anastomosis (1946), the closed pulmonary valvotomy (Brock, 1948), and the Waterston shunt (1962). Surgical correction of TOF was pioneered in 1954 by C.W. Lillehei; using controlled cross-circulation, he accomplished the first intracardiac repair of TOF with closure of the ventricular septal defect and relief of pulmonary stenosis. The technique of TOF repair has since evolved with considerable refinement, but the objectives remain the same: complete closure of the ventricular septal defect with preservation of sinus rhythm and relief of right ventricular outflow obstruction.

Although there is still controversy as to the desirability of initial palliation versus early total correction of TOF, it has been clearly demonstrated by Castaneda and others that in most patients with TOF, early repair can be accomplished with acceptably low operative risk and satisfactory early and late results. The need for a second surgical procedure is obviated in most instances, and the potential complications of shunt operations are avoided. There is evidence as well that left ventricular function after repair of TOF may be better in patients who undergo total correction in infancy than in those who are repaired at a later age. The therapeutic approach to patients with

TOF at this institution includes total correction whenever signs and symptoms warrant intervention. This includes infants with marked cyanosis, hypoxic spells, ductal dependency for pulmonary blood flow, and anatomically severe right ventricular obstruction. For children who do not require surgery in the first year of life on the basis of these indications, a corrective operation is recommended in the second or third year of life. Initial palliative operations are chosen only for infants with clearly defined anatomic contraindications to total correction. These include anomalous origin of the anterior descending coronary artery from the right coronary artery, multiple ventricular septal defects, or severely hypoplastic pulmonary arteries. (We have only encountered severely hypoplastic pulmonary arteries in infants with pulmonary atresia, ventricular septal defect, and multiple aortopulmonary collaterals. Pulmonary atresia per se does not constitute a contraindication to total surgical correction in infancy, particularly when there is a ductal or other unifocal source of pulmonary blood supply.)

PREOPERATIVE ASSESSMENT

Although two-dimensional echocardiography has permitted reliable noninvasive recognition of the pathologic anatomy of patients with TOF, all our patients are subjected to complete cardiac catheterization with biplane angiocardiography. Specific anatomic features delineated at catheterization include (1) the presence of single or multiple ventricular septal defects, (2) the degree of anatomic obstruction between the right ventricle and pulmonary artery, (3) the size of branch pulmonary arteries, (4) the presence of systemic sources of pulmonary blood supply, and (5) the sites of origin and course of the coronary arteries. Abnormalities of the atrioventricular valves in TOF with atrioventricular canal may be seen at ventriculography, but in general these are best evaluated by the echocardiogram. Neonates with TOF and severe systemic desaturation (SaO_2 <70 percent) are maintained on an intravenous infusion of prostaglandin E_1 to maintain patency of the ductus arteriosus and to improve oxygenation.

OPERATIVE TECHNIQUE

In neonates arterial blood pressure and blood gases are monitored with the use of an umbilical artery catheter. In all older infants and children, a radial artery is cannulated. Surgical approach is by median sternotomy. A graft of anterior pericardium is excised and stored in a saline soaked gauze for later use in the reconstruction of the right ventricular outflow tract. In general, the graft is trapezoidal in shape. In small infants the pericardium is incised along its diaphragmatic reflection. It is then cut just medial to the pleural reflection on each side up to the reflection of the pericardium over the great vessels, where it is cut in a direction parallel to the initial cut above the diaphragm. In general the width of the graft at the level of the aortic pericardial reflection is at least twice the diameter of the ascending aorta. Before correction is undertaken, the site of origin and course of the coronary arteries must be ascertained.

Operative technique in neonates and in infants weighing less than 10 kg includes core cooling with cardiopulmonary bypass and a period of hypothermic circulatory arrest. After heparinization, the distal ascending aorta is cannulated for perfusion, and a single venous cannula is inserted via the appendage of the right atrium. As cardiopulmonary bypass is initiated, the ductus arteriosus is ligated. A bubble oxygenator is used with a prime consisting of lactated Ringer's solution with either whole blood or packed red blood cells and serum albumin to achieve a hematocrit of 24 ml per deciliter during bypass. Flow is maintained at 100 to 150 ml per kilogram per minute and is continued until tympanic, esophageal, and rectal temperatures are all below 20° C. At this point, the aorta is cross-clamped, and perfusion is discontinued. Cold potassium blood cardioplegia solution (25 ml per kilogram) is infused into the aortic root. The venous cannula may then be removed.

A vertical incision is made in the distal portion of the right ventricular outflow tract. Because the infundibular septum may be significantly displaced anteriorly, leaving a very hypoplastic infundibular outflow tract, care must be exercised to incise only the right ventricular free wall and to avoid injury to the underlying infundibular septum. The incision is carried proximally only far enough to afford exposure of the ventricular septal defect. Only rarely do infants have significantly hypertrophied obstructing muscle bundles, but occasionally a hypertrophied bundle will bind the infundibular septum to the right ventricular free wall, and when present this should be divided. Excessive trimming of right ventricular muscle is avoided. If the pulmonary valve annulus is hypoplastic or atretic, the ventriculotomy incision is carried distally across the annulus onto the main pulmonary artery and at least to the origin of the left pulmonary artery. If fibromuscular atresia of the right ventricular outflow tract is encountered at the distal extent of the ventriculotomy, a longitudinal incision is made in the main pulmonary artery. This arteriotomy and the right ventriculotomy are joined by an incision that is carried through a partial thickness of the fibromuscular bridge between the ventricle and the pulmonary artery. The most commonly occurring ventricular septal defect in TOF is an anterior malalignment defect (Fig. 1). This is bordered superiorly by the infundibular septum, on the left and inferiorly by the limbs of the trabecula-septomarginalis, and on the right by the tricuspid annulus and the ventriculoinfundibular fold. A series of 5–0 Tevdek horizontal mattress sutures buttressed with pledgets of Teflon felt is placed around the defect. In general, the first suture is placed in the middle of the infundibular septum, and subsequent sutures are placed following a clockwise sequence. After placing sutures along the anterior and inferior rims of the defect, the septal leaflet of the tricuspid valve is gently retracted. Sutures along the posteroinferior aspect of the defect are placed a few millimeters from the actual rim of the defect, carefully staying on the right ventricular side of the septum, to avoid injury to the bundle of His. Sutures are then

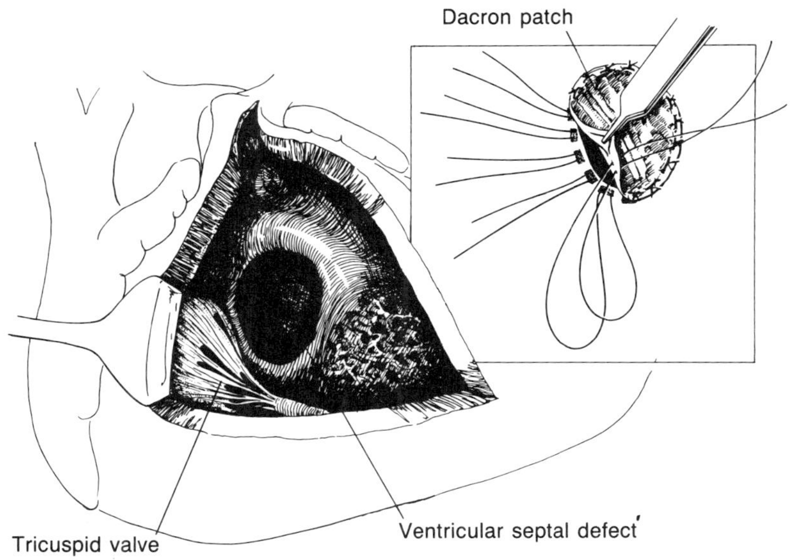

Figure 1 The malalignment ventricular septal defect is visualized through the right ventriculotomy. The incision is extended through the hypoplastic pulmonary annulus out onto the main pulmonary artery and to the point of origin of the left pulmonary artery. A Dacron patch (inset) is secured to the rim of the defect with Teflon felt pledgeted mattress sutures.

placed along the ventriculoinfundibular fold, around the aortic valve annulus, and up to the starting point on the infundibular septum. It is often helpful to infuse a second small dose of cardioplegic solution into the aortic root, to delineate the extent of the aortic valve and avoid injury to it. The sutures are then passed through the perimeter of a Dacron patch, which is tailored to a size slightly larger than that of the defect itself. Sutures are tied in the sequence in which they were placed, and all are cut.

Attention is directed to the reconstruction of the right ventricular outflow tract. The distal portion of the right ventricle and the main pulmonary artery are significantly augmented utilizing the graft of autologous pericardium (Fig. 2). As previously mentioned, in most infants the incision is carried out to the level of the origin of the left pulmonary artery. If there is stenosis of the origin of one or both pulmonary arteries, the incision is carried beyond the point of stenosis. No attempt is made to tailor the distal end of the pericardial graft. Intentional tapering of the graft to an eliptical or diamond shape can result in a significant residual pressure gradient between right ventricle and pulmonary artery. A continuous suture line with 5–0 monofilament suture is begun at the most distal point of the pulmonary arteriotomy and at the midpoint of the distal end (great vessel end) of the pericardial graft. The suture line is then carried along either side, to the proximal end of the right ventriculotomy. Some trimming of the pericardial graft is generally required at the ventricular end. The closure of the ventricular septal defect and the reconstruction of the right ventricular outflow tract can usually be completed during less than 60 minutes of hypothermic circulatory arrest. If more time is required, one has the option of resuming perfusion during suturing of the proximal portion of the right ventricular outflow patch. When bypass is resumed, and while the infant is being warmed, a small polyvinyl catheter is passed through a pursestring suture in the right ventricular outflow tract out into the pulmonary artery. A second catheter is placed in the left atrium via the right superior pulmonary vein. When the esophageal temperature reaches 37° C, bypass is discontinued. Many neonates benefit from a low dose infusion of dopamine (5 μg per kilogram per minute) during the early postoperative period to support right ventricular function. Since the foramen ovale remains patent, there may be mild systemic arterial desaturation due to right-to-left shunting at the atrial level while right ventricular function improves and pulmonary vascular resistance declines. Sedation and relaxation with narcotics and muscle relaxants are continued during the early

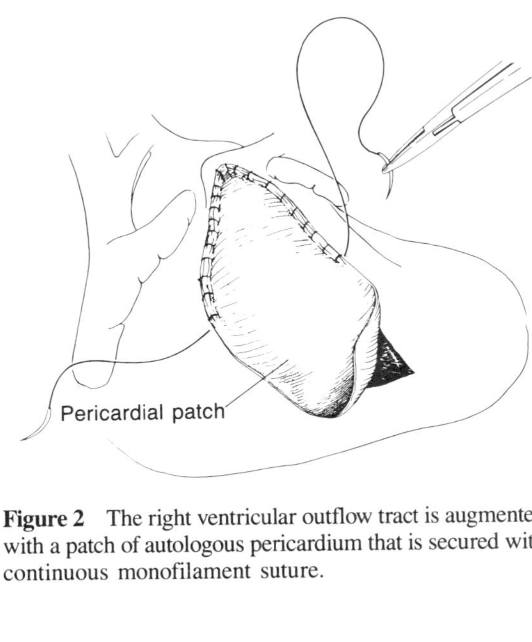

Figure 2 The right ventricular outflow tract is augmented with a patch of autologous pericardium that is secured with continuous monofilament suture.

postoperative period. A pullback of the pulmonary artery catheter during continuous pressure monitoring is performed to determine the degree of any residual gradient between the right ventricle and the pulmonary arteries. Most infants require 24 to 48 hours of postoperative ventilation before weaning can be accomplished. If the hemodynamics are unsatisfactory, echocardiography and/or recatheterization must be considered to delineate residual lesions.

The operative technique in children follows the same principles as that in infants. For children weighing more than 8 to 10 kg, conventional cardiopulmonary bypass with bicaval cannulation and moderate hypothermia (25 to 28° C) and multiple dose cardioplegia are utilized. Transannular incision and patching are much less frequently required in children who did not require surgery in infancy. That is to say that in most instances, the severity of early symptoms correlates with the degree of hypoplasia of the right ventricular outflow tract. Whenever possible, the integrity of the pulmonary annulus is maintained, with pulmonary valvotomy being accomplished via the right ventriculotomy or a separate pulmonary arteriotomy or both. When a transannular incision is required because of hypoplasia of the pulmonary valve annulus, some functional leaflet tissue may still be preserved. In older children, there is generally more hypertrophy of right ventricular muscle bundles. Relief of infundibular stenosis is accomplished by incision and partial excision of the hypertrophied bundles running from the infundibular septum to the right ventricular free wall. This is facilitated by gently passing a right-angled forceps behind the muscle bundles and carefully dividing each one. Adequate relief of muscular obstruction not only is necessary for relief of right ventricular outflow obstruction but is essential for adequate visualization of the ventricular septal defect. The technique for closure of the ventricular septal defect is the same as that described for infants. Augmentation of the right ventricular outflow tract in children can be accomplished with a graft of autologous pericardium or with a patch of Goretex or Dacron. In children with TOF with pulmonary atresia, an aortic homograft or dacron conduit with a porcine xenograft may be used to join the pulmonary arteries to the right ventricle. Unlike neonates, it is unusual for older children to require inotropic support after correction of TOF. A significant requirement for inotropic agents should raise the question of the presence of a residual defect, specifically a residual ventricular septal defect or residual right ventricular outflow gradient.

RESULTS

Between January 1985 and August 1987, we performed corrective operations for TOF on 28 infants and children. More than half were infants weighing less than 10 kg who underwent correction utilizing hypothermic circulatory arrest. For the total group, ages ranged from 1 day to 5 years. Included were four patients with TOF and pulmonary atresia (two of whom underwent total correction within the first 48 hours of life), one patient (age 3 years) with TOF and complete atrioventricular canal, one patient (age 3 years) with TOF and single pulmonary artery, and one patient (age 4 months) with TOF and absent pulmonary valve. Three patients who underwent corrective operations during this time period had undergone previous palliative procedures by means of a Blalock-Taussig shunt: one with anomalous origin of the anterior descending coronary artery from the right coronary artery (total correction at age 1 year), one with tracheoesophageal fistula (total correction at age 8 months), and one with multiple ventricular septal defects (total correction at age 3 years). There were no operative or late deaths. Complications included bleeding requiring re-exploration (one patient), seizures (one patient), residual ventricular septal defect without hemodynamically significant shunt (one patient), and late right ventricular failure requiring pulmonary valve xenograft implantation (one patient with TOF, pulmonary atresia, and multiple aortopulmonary collaterals). The last patient is currently in New York Heart Association functional Class II, and all other patients are in New York Heart Association functional Class I.

During the same time period, four patients underwent palliative operations for TOF including two Blalock-Taussig shunts (as indicated above). Two patients with pulmonary atresia, ventricular septal defect, multiple aortopulmonary collaterals, and hypoplasia of the pulmonary arteries (pseudotruncus) underwent palliative procedures. One received a nonvalved right ventricle to pulmonary artery conduit without ventricular septal defect closure and the other a right ventricle to pulmonary artery transannular patch without ventricular septal defect closure. These children both died.

We favor primary repair of TOF in symptomatic infants regardless of age, and elective repair of noncomplicated forms of TOF by the second or third year of life. Utilizing this approach, the results have been very satisfactory both in terms of low operative risk and with regard to freedom from symptoms. In our experience with a small number of infants with TOF and pulmonary atresia, those with unifocal (ductal) sources of pulmonary blood flow have achieved the same satisfactory results from early correction as have other symptomatic neonates with TOF.

SUGGESTED READING

Borow KM, Green LH, Castaneda AR, Keane JF. Left ventricular function after repair of tetralogy of Fallot and its relationship to age at surgery. Circulation 1980; 61:1150–1158.

Castaneda AR, Freed MD, Williams RG, Norwood WI. Repair of tetralogy of Fallot in infancy. J Thorac Cardiovasc Surg 1977; 74:372–381.

Jacobs ML, Vlahakes GJ. Complete atrioventricular canal associated with tetralogy of Fallot. Ann Thorac Surg 1987; 43:458–459.

Kirklin JW, Blackstone EH, Pacifico AD, Brown RN, Bargeron LM Jr. Routine primary repair vs two-stage repair of tetralogy of Fallot. Circulation 1979; 60:373–386.

Lillehei CW, Cohen M, Warden HE, Red RC, Aust JB, DeWall RA, Varco RL. Direct vision intracardiac surgical correction of the tetralogy of Fallot, pentalogy of Fallot, and pulmonary atresia defects; report of first ten cases. Ann Surg 1955; 142:418–445.

PULMONARY ATRESIA WITH INTACT VENTRICULAR SEPTUM

EDUARDO ARCINIEGAS, M.D.

Pulmonary atresia with intact ventricular septum is an uncommon congenital defect characterized by complete obstruction of the pulmonary valve, no ventricular septal defect, and varying degrees of right ventricular and tricuspid valve hypoplasia. The obstructed pulmonary valve usually consists of a tough, imperforate membrane. The right ventricular wall is generally markedly hypertrophied and may have associated diffuse fibrosis and endocardial fibroelastosis. The right ventricular cavity may be large (Greenwald type II or tripartite) but is more frequently small (Greenwald type I) because of absence of the trabecular portion, the infundibulum, or both. When the right ventricle is hypoplastic, intramyocardial sinusoids are often present that communicate with the coronary arteries and aorta and may contribute to myocardial ischemia and fibrosis. The tricuspid valve is commonly incompetent, and its size is proportional to that of the right ventricle. Right atrial enlargement and an interatrial communication are present in all cases. The pulmonary arteries are usually of normal or near-normal size and, in the neonatal period, they receive blood flow from the aorta through a patent ductus arteriosus that tends to close spontaneously during the first few days of life.

INITIAL MEDICAL MANAGEMENT

As soon as the presence of the defect is suspected, an intravenous infusion of prostaglandin E_1 is started to ensure ductal patency, increase pulmonary blood flow, and relieve hypoxemia and acidosis. The usual prostaglandin dosage of 0.05 to 0.1 μg per kilogram per minute is adjusted according to the levels of the patient's systemic arterial oxygen saturation to minimize the possibility of drug-induced apnea or hyperthermia. Endotracheal intubation, mechanically assisted ventilation, and intravenously administered sodium bicarbonate may also be necessary in the more critically hypoxic and acidotic infants. Simultaneously, the diagnosis is confirmed by two-dimensional echocardiography, cardiac catheterization, and cineangiography. To ensure unobstructed blood flow at the atrial level, balloon atrial septostomy is done in all but those patients with large right ventricular cavities.

SURGICAL MANAGEMENT

The initial surgical treatment is palliative and is required within the first few days of life in virtually all patients, prompted by the tendency of the ductus arteriosus to close spontaneously. The treatment goals are to provide a dependable source of pulmonary blood flow for relief of hypoxia and to decompress the right ventricle to give it additional potential for growth.

The available palliative procedures are systemic to pulmonary artery shunts and pulmonary valvulotomy, alone or in combination. The choice depends on the angiographic determination of the right ventricular cavity size, whether it is large or hypoplastic and, if the latter, on the presence or absence of a right ventricular outlet portion of infundibulum. Subsequent anatomic surgical correction by relief of the residual right ventricular outflow tract obstruction and closure of the atrial septal defect is possible only in patients with an adequately sized right ventricle and tricuspid valve. A modified Fontan's operation is the only available later option for patients with severe right ventricular and tricuspid valve hypoplasia, provided their pulmonary arteries are of a suitable size.

Large Right Ventricle. This subgroup comprises less than 10 percent of the patients. Initial treatment by pulmonary valvulotomy alone is usually successful in providing adequate pulmonary blood flow and decompressing the right ventricle and carries a risk of early postoperative death of less than 10 percent. Sometimes, however, associated significant infundibular obstruction may cause persistent or recurrent hypoxemia and may require the addition of a classic Blalock-Taussig shunt during the early postvalvulotomy period. Our preference is to perform a transventricular pulmonary valvulotomy through a midsternotomy without cardiopulmonary bypass. A small stab wound is made within the confines of a pledget-reinforced horizontal mattress suture placed in an avascular site in the mid-right ventricle and passed through a rubber tourniquet to minimize blood loss. Hegar's dilators are sequentially inserted through the stab wound, usually fracturing the valvular diaphragm with the 2- or 3-mm dilator. The valvular opening is then enlarged up to a 6- or 7-mm dilator, taking care not to perforate the right ventricle or the pulmonary artery. More recently, we have also clamped and opened the pulmonary artery trunk proximal to its bifurcation and, under direct vision, have removed a segment of the atretic valve while pushing the transventricular dilator firmly against it. This helps define the portion to be resected and prevents blood loss while the pulmonary arteriotomy is repaired.

Subsequent management includes hemodynamic reassessment by repeat cardiac catheterization at about 12 to 18 months of age. This is followed by relief of any residual right ventricular outflow tract obstruction by transannular outflow patching and closure of the atrial septal communication using cardiopulmonary bypass. Survival after the second stage operation may be anticipated in about 90 percent of the patients.

Hypoplastic Right Ventricle. All patients in this subgroup initially require a systemic-to-pulmonary artery shunt to establish a reliable source of pulmonary blood flow. The indication for a simultaneous transventricular pulmonary valvulotomy depends upon the presence or absence of a right ventricular infundibular or outlet portion.

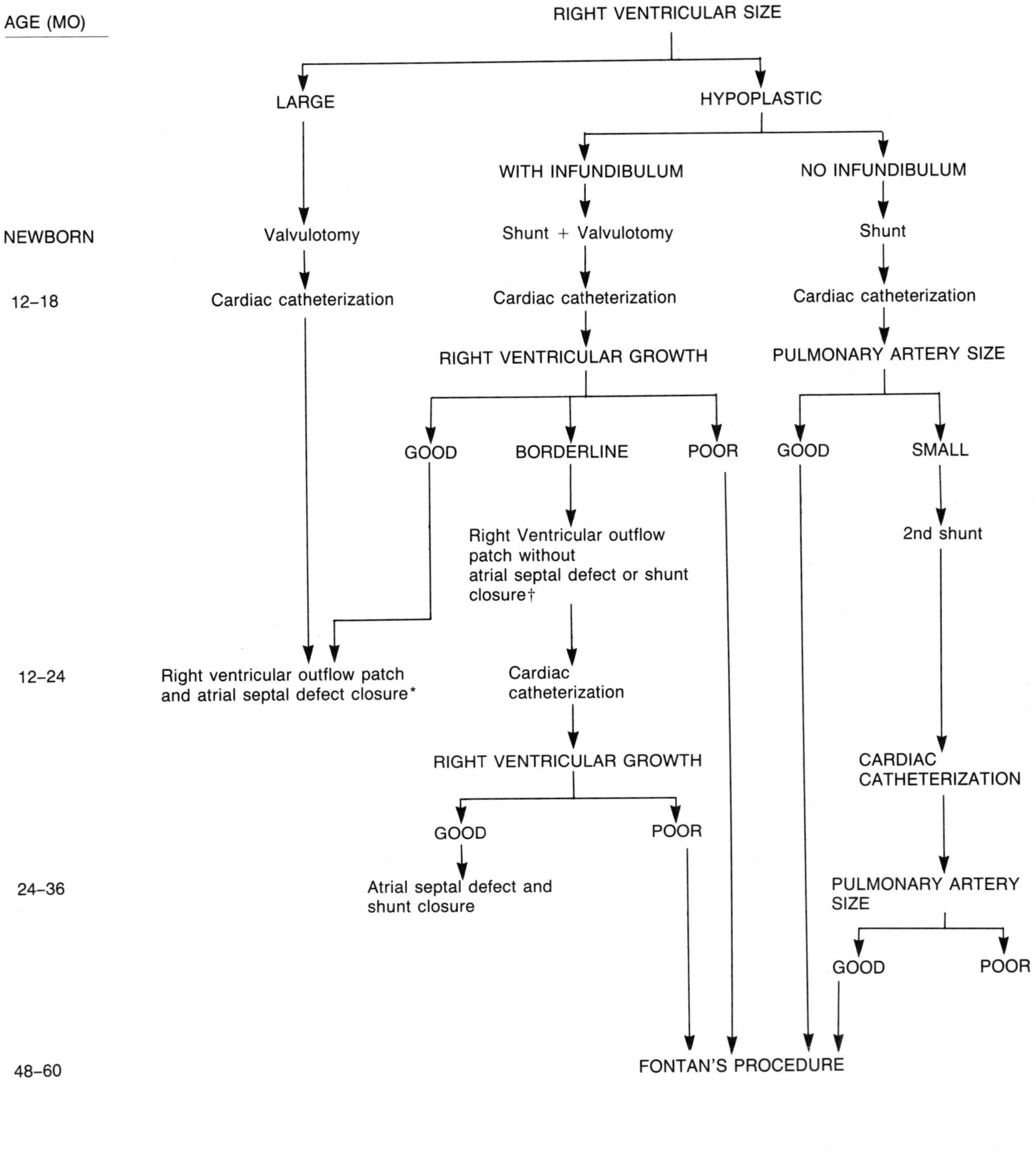

Figure 1 Summary of management of pulmonary atresia with intact ventricular septum. All patients, initially: prostaglandin E_1, 2-D echo cardiogram, cardiac catheterization, cineangiography, and balloon atrial septostomy (except in patients with large right ventricle.

* With shunt closure in patients with hypoplastic right ventricle.

† Complete repair is possible if temporary balloon closure of atrial septal defect is well tolerated.

Patients without a right ventricular infundibulum (approximately 10 percent of all patients) should undergo construction of a systemic-to-pulmonary artery shunt alone. Pulmonary valvulotomy is not possible in the absence of a right ventricular conus. Since these patients uniformly have a left-sided aorta, our choice is to perform a right-sided classic Blalock-Taussig shunt. Because the small and nondecompressed right ventricle has no growth potential, subsequent treatment consists of right ventricular exclusion and establishment of a Fontan-type circulation at about 4 to 5 years of age, provided the pulmonary arteries are of adequate caliber. An additional interim systemic-to-pulmonary artery shunt may be necessary to relieve recurrent hypoxemia and/or to promote further pulmonary arterial growth in patients with small pulmonary arteries.

Patients in whom a right ventricular infundibulum is present should receive a systemic-to-pulmonary artery shunt in combination with transventricular pulmonary valvulotomy without cardiopulmonary bypass in order to afford the right ventricle an opportunity for future growth. Our current policy in this situation (about 80 percent of all patients) is to perform a Waterston's shunt simultaneously with transventricular pulmonary valvulotomy through a bilateral third space anterior thoracotomy incision with sternal transection. A 2.5- to 3.0-mm Waterston's shunt, carefully constructed between precisely marked matching points in the aorta and right pulmonary artery, can be easily done with about 20 percent early postoperative mortality, a minimum of early and late complications, and little risk of pulmonary artery distortion or obstruction.

Subsequent management includes repeat cardiac catheterization and cardiac cineangiography at about 12 months of age to determine the adequacy of the right ventricular decompression and the right ventricular and tricuspid valve size. If right ventricular growth has been satisfactory, as judged by the right ventricular volume and tricuspid valve diameter, total intracardiac repair with cardiopulmonary bypass is done, which includes pericardial or prosthetic transannular patching, closure of the atrial septal defect, and interruption of any preexisting systemic-to-pulmonary artery shunts. A previous Waterston's shunt is routinely dismantled by detaching the right pulmonary artery from the aorta and enlarging it with a pericardial patch, if necessary.

When the right ventricular cavity remains small, further right ventricular growth may be obtained by insertion of a transannular patch and outflow tract muscle resection, using cardiopulmonary bypass, without closure of the atrial septal defect or the pre-existing systemic-to-pulmonary artery shunts. This may permit surgical atrial septal defect and shunt closure at a later date. Otherwise, right ventricular bypass by means of a modified Fontan's operation eventually will be necessary for "permanent palliation."

In patients with only moderate postvalvulotomy right ventricular growth and borderline tricuspid valve size, complete intracardiac repair employing cardiopulmonary bypass may be possible if temporary preoperative balloon occlusion of the atrial communication has been well tolerated. Otherwise, additional palliation by transannular patching without atrial septal defect closure is indicated, in the hope of further additional right ventricular cavity enlargement that may allow subsequent anatomic intracardiac correction.

Treatment of patients with large intramyocardial sinusoids and coronary-to-aortic connections may be problematic. Small and moderate communications may disappear or have no important hemodynamic effect following appropriate right ventricular decompression. The need for surgical obliteration of the right ventricular cavity in patients with larger communications and marked right ventricular hypoplasia is unclear at this time. However, in such patients, the right ventricle is defunctionalized and excluded by tricuspid valve suture at the time of a Fontan-type repair. In patients with larger right ventricles, it may be possible to identify and close by direct suture these communications within the right ventricular cavity at the time of intracardiac anatomic repair.

RESULTS

Pulmonary atresia with intact ventricular septum remains a major surgical challenge. However, current significant improved early and late postoperative results are attributable to a better understanding of the wide spectrum of the pathologic anatomy of this condition and to treatment protocols directed at maintaining adequate pulmonary blood flow while providing a potential for further growth of the hypoplastic right ventricle (see Fig. 1).

In an earlier era, operative mortality rates in excess of 50 percent were reported by numerous groups. However, with improved postoperative care and a greater understanding of the pathophysiology and potential for ventricular growth, mortality has now decreased and may vary from 7 to 10 percent after initial shunting or shunting plus pulmonary valvotomy. Approximately one-fourth of patients surviving initial surgery may require reoperation within the first few months or first few years of life. Reoperations are usually mandated by low pulmonary blood flow and cyanosis. Additional operations required include placement of an additional shunt, repeat valvulotomy, or placement of a transannular patch. These procedures may carry an additional 10 percent mortality risk.

Definitive correction later in life is also accompanied by a significant mortality. In infants who have sufficient right ventricular volume to permit valvulotomy or outflow patch repair earlier in life, a definitive repair by reconstruction of the right ventricular outflow tract may be associated with a mortality rate in excess of 25 percent. In children without adequate right ventricular function, in order to create in-series pulmonary and systemic circulations, a Fontan-type procedure is required for final correction. Because these patients may have abnormalities of left ventricular compliance, Fontan-type procedures in this setting may carry a significant risk of mortality (25 to 30 percent).

SUGGESTED READING

Cobanoglu A, Metzdorff MT, Pinson CW, Grunkemeier GL, Sunderland CO, Starr A. Valvulotomy for pulmonary atresia with intact ventricular septum. J Thorac Cardiovasc Surg 1985; 89:482–490.

deLeval M, Bull C, Stark J, Anderson RH, Taylor JFN, Macartney JF. Pulmonary atresia and intact ventricular septum: surgical management based on a revised classification. Circulation 1982; 66:272–280.

Kirklin JW, Barratt-Boyes BG. Pulmonary atresia with intact ventricular septum. In: Kirklin JW, Barratt-Boyes BG, eds. Cardiac surgery. New York: John Wiley & Sons, 1986:843.

Lewis AB, Wells W, Lindesmith GG. Evaluation and surgical treatment of pulmonary atresia with intact ventricular septum in infancy. Circulation 1983; 67:1318–1323.

Moulton AL, Bowman FO Jr, Edie RN, Hayes C, Ellis K, Malm JR. Pulmonary atresia with intact ventricular septum—a 16 year experience. J Thorac Cardiovasc Surg 1979; 78:527–536.

ATRIOVENTRICULAR CANAL DEFECT

SCOTT STEWART, M.D.

Patients who have complete atrioventricular canal defect generally have a marked increase in pulmonary blood flow and also may have, although uncommonly, significant mitral valve incompetence. Early operation is therefore recommended in order to reduce the risk of permanent pulmonary vascular injury occurring as a consequence of both pulmonary artery hypertension and pulmonary venous hypertension. Some groups continue to advise preliminary pulmonary artery banding in the neonate and complete repair at a later date. Although published results of this approach have been satisfactory, we, as well as others, prefer to undertake complete repair in infancy, since we believe that the operative mortality for this procedure at this age is at least as favorable as it is for the two-stage technique.

The single most important aspect of the preoperative evaluation is the determination of the relative size of the two ventricles. On rare occasions either the left or the right ventricle may be underdeveloped, negating the likelihood of a successful complete repair. Although we have had to make this determination at the time of a planned complete repair, it is much more desirable to have this information beforehand so that one may then proceed directly to a palliative procedure. The 2-D echocardiogram provides excellent information in this regard.

We believe that complete repair should be done before the age of 1 year. Currently, the mean age of our patients at the time of complete repair is about 6 months. We utilize continuous cardiopulmonary bypass at moderate hypothermia between 22 and 25° C. Most of the procedure is done at a low flow of 0.3 to 0.5 of full flow (2.2 L per minute per square meter of body surface) in order to reduce the bronchopulmonary collateral return to the left atrium.

After cardiopulmonary bypass is established and the caval tapes are secured, the right atrium is opened with a long transverse incision that begins at the base of the atrial appendage and passes between the cannulation site of the inferior vena cava and the right atrioventricular groove. Exposure is established by placing lateral stay sutures in the crista terminalis and medial stay sutures at 10 o'clock and 2 o'clock in the tricuspid valve annulus. The aortic cross-clamp is then positioned, and cold cardioplegia is established. The perfusion flow is reduced as low as is necessary to prevent any blood return to the left atrium. The size of the two ventricles is assessed to ascertain that complete repair is appropriate.

The ventricles are then distended with cold saline to bring the common atrioventricular leaflet tissue up into its closed position. The leaflet edges are always corrugated, and the interdigitations of the common anterior leaflet fit together with those of the common posterior leaflet. It is critical that the exact points of contact between the surfaces of the leading edges of the two leaflets are clearly identified. A 5–0 Prolene suture is placed through the common anterior and posterior leaflet tissue just to the right of the sagittal plane of the ventricular septum (Fig. 1). Several more sutures are usually placed between the common anterior and posterior leaflet components of the mitral valve tissue (see Fig. 1B). The leaflet tissue is not "unfurled" at its edge but is approximated by these sutures in exactly the manner in which the two surfaces meet. Intermittent distention of the ventricles is usually necessary in order to accurately coapt the leaflet tissue and thereby identify the exact position for each of these sutures. These sutures are never carried all the way to the tip of the leaflet tissue, and they usually extend only halfway to that point. We have never encountered mitral valve stenosis as a result of approximating this portion of the common anterior and posterior leaflets, but we have experienced mitral valve incompetence through this "cleft" when these leaflets have not been joined. A sump catheter now is placed within the left ventricle and the perfusion flow increased just to that point at which the collateral return to the left atrium is easily evacuated by the sump.

A 5–0 Prolene suture is placed through the corner of the tricuspid component of both the common anterior and posterior leaflets that constitute the tricuspid "septal" leaflet. These sutures are used to provide traction on the leaflet tissue after it has been divided. They are also helpful in identifying the leading edge of the leaflet, since once it has been divided, its correct orientation may be difficult to reestablish in the small infant.

The common anterior and posterior leaflets are divided back to the atrioventricular annulus along the right sagittal plane of the septum (see Fig. 1B). If the posterior leaflet

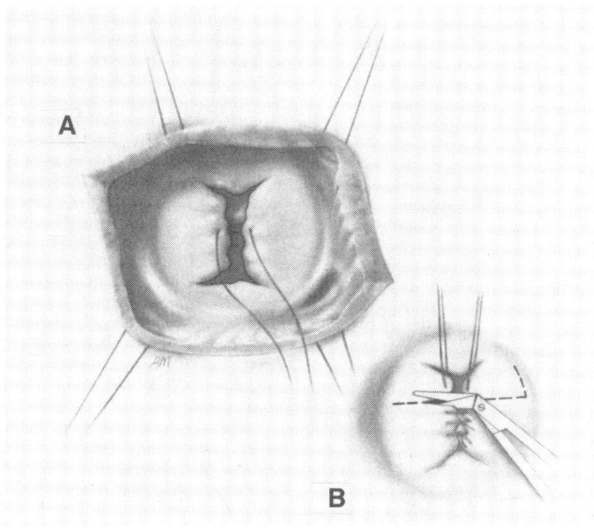

Figure 1 *A*, A 5–0 Prolene suture is placed through the common anterior and posterior leaflets in the sagittal plane of the septum. *B*, Several more sutures are placed in the "cleft" of the anterior leaflet of the mitral valve. Two stay sutures are placed through the edge of the tricuspid component of the common anterior and posterior leaflets. Those leaflets are then divided along the sagittal plane of the septum. A short anterior incision in the posterior leaflet significantly improves the exposure of the septum.

is attached to the top of the septum by a fused sheet of tissue without an underlying defect, then this leaflet does not have to be cut back. The previously placed traction sutures are now used to elevate the tricuspid tissue away from the septum and to expose the anterior and posterior limits of the ventricular septal defect (Fig. 2). Optimal exposure for the posterior corner of the defect is best achieved by a further incision of the common posterior leaflet in an anterior direction for 4 to 5 mm parallel to and a few millimeters away from the atrioventricular annulus (see Fig. 2). If there are numerous chordae from the tricuspid leaflet tissue to the crest of the septum that either inhibit exposure or will significantly complicate the suture line, they may be divided. This usually is not necessary.

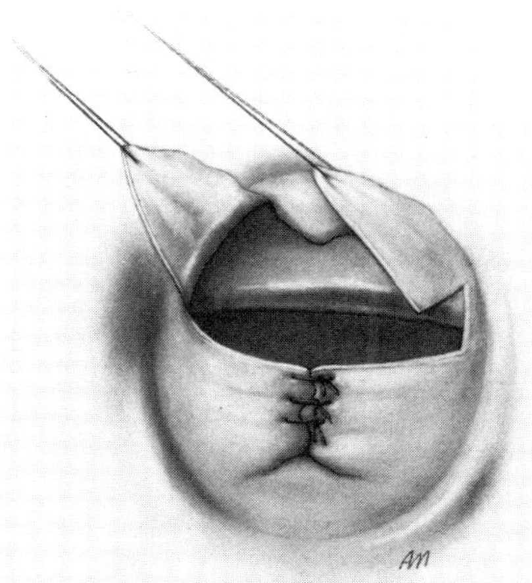

Figure 2 The stay sutures provide improved exposure to the septum and preserve the correct orientation of this delicate tissue.

A single patch of Dacron is used to close both the atrial and the ventricular components of the defect. It is trimmed to the exact width and shape required for the ventricular portion of the defect. It is left a little long so that the atrial portion may be trimmed to size when that segment is sewn into place. The patch is secured with two curved clamps to the towel drape just to the right of the sternotomy. Multiple interrupted 5–0 Prolene horizontal mattress sutures buttressed with pledgets are used to secure the patch to the right side of the ventricular septum. A small semicircular needle seems to work best within the confines of this limited space. The suture line begins at the anterior portion of the septal defect and proceeds to the posterior portion. Considerable care must be used to correctly estimate the spacing of these sutures so that one does not end up with either too much patch or too much septum. Attempts to correct this problem after the fact invariably result in distortion and incompetence of the atrioventricular leaflet tissue. The sutures may be placed relatively close to the crest of the septum until its midportion is reached, and then they must enter the right side of the septum progressively farther away from the crest in order to avoid the conduction tissue. After each suture has been placed through the septal tissue, it is passed through the patch material. The suture itself is then secured to the towel drape so that the most recently placed suture between the septum and the patch may be used for traction to set up the exposure for the next stitch. In this manner the suture line progresses from the anterior to the posterior portion of the defect. After all the sutures are placed, the patch is slid down into position and the sutures tied. In patients who have associated tetralogy of Fallot, the most anterior portion of the ventricular septal defect usually cannot be well visualized through the atrioventricular valve. This defect requires an anterior extension to the patch, which must be secured to the septum through the same ventriculotomy used to manage the right ventricular outflow tract obstruction. Generally at this point we lower the perfusion temperature to 8° C, release the aortic cross-clamp for about 5 minutes, and then replace the cross-clamp and instill a second dose of cold cardioplegia.

The short anterior incision in the posterior component of the tricuspid leaflet is closed with several interrupted 5–0 Prolene sutures. The leaflet tissue is now suspended onto the patch. A critical part of this maneuver is the placement of the leaflets at the correct level on the patch. That position can be best determined by identifying the upward limitation to movement of the leaflet tissue by those chordae that are attached to the septum. This will determine the level of the leaflet attachment to the patch. It is sometimes helpful to then mark that level on the patch, since once the suture line is begun, the exact mental reference point may be lost. The leaflet tissue is sutured to the patch with multiple interrupted horizontal mattress sutures, which are buttressed on the mitral side with small Dacron pledgets. The suture line begins anteriorly and proceeds posteriorly. The initial stay sutures that had been placed through the common anterior and posterior components of the tricuspid leaflet tissue are now used to set up those leaflets for this part of the suture line. They also prevent rotation of the leaflet tissue through 180 degrees. Each needle is driven through the mitral leaflet tissue, the patch, and then the tricuspid leaflet tissue. They are all placed before they are tied. Accurate spacing of the suture line is equally as important here as it was in placing the patch onto the ventricular septum. It is imperative that the anterior and posterior segments of leaflet tissue be neither too stretched out nor foreshortened onto the patch. After the leaflets have been suspended onto the patch, the left ventricle is again distended with cold saline to evaluate the competency of the mitral valve. The medial stay sutures must be released during this evaluation so that the valve is not distorted. The valve is almost always competent, although on occasion there may be a small central leak. We have never found it necessary to do a further procedure, such as a limited annuloplasty, in order to achieve a functionally satisfactory valve.

The patch is now secured to the atrial portion of the defect. We generally place the coronary sinus on the right side. The patch is secured to the posterior portion of the atrial septum with multiple horizontal mattress sutures, which are placed superficially in the endocardium and parallel with the anticipated course of the conduction tissue. Once the coronary sinus area has been passed, the aortic cross-clamp is released, and rewarming is begun. The remainder of the patch is trimmed and secured to the atrial septum with a running suture. Prior to completing that suture line, the aortic cross-clamp is momentarily positioned, the sump catheter removed, and the lungs expanded to expel air from the left side of the heart. The aortic cross-clamp is released and the right atrium closed. The caval tapes are released, and air is evacuated from the ascending aorta by a suction needle vent.

Monitoring catheters are left in both atria, and the pulmonary artery and pacing wires are placed on the right atrium and ventricle. Cardiopulmonary bypass is generally discontinued with a small infusion of dopamine.

The operative mortality for repair of simple complete atrioventricular canal defect has been 17 percent (7 out of 41) for our entire experience with this anomaly between the years 1973 and 1986. This number has been reduced considerably in recent years, in part coincident, we believe, with the introduction of cold cardioplegia in children in 1977. The mortality for the more complex forms, including associated tetralogy of Fallot, parachute mitral valve, and complex systemic and pulmonary venous anomalies, has remained at about 55 percent throughout this experience.

Complete heart block has occurred in only 2 percent (1 out of 50) patients. This was a patient with situs inversus, dextrocardia, absence of the coronary sinus, and systemic venous connection anomalies. Serious mitral valve incompetence after repair has occurred twice and, in both instances, the valve had not been secured to the patch with pledgets and the suture had cut through the leaflet tissue. This has not occurred since we modified our technique over 10 years ago.

SUGGESTED READING

Bender HW Jr, Hammon JW Jr, Hubbard SG, Muirhead J, Graham TP. Repair of atrioventricular canal malformation in the first year of life. J Thorac Cardiovasc Surg 1982; 84:515–522.

Rastelli GC, Ongley PA, Kirklin JW, McGoon DC. Surgical repair of the complete form of persistent common atrioventricular canal. J Thorac Cardiovasc Surg 1968; 55:299–308.

Stewart S, Harris P, Manning J. Complete endocardial cushion defect: the late results of repair using the single-patch technique. Ann Thorac Surg 1987; 39:234–237.

Studer M, Blackstone EH, Kirklin JW, et al. Determinants of early and late results of repair of atrioventricular septal (canal) defects. J Thorac Cardiovasc Surg 1982; 84:523–542.

TRICUSPID ATRESIA

ROBERT M. SADE, M.D.

Tricuspid atresia is defined by anatomic absence of the tricuspid valve and its orifice. The physiology of the lesion, however, is variable and is determined by associated malformations. Children with tricuspid atresia associated with increased pulmonary blood flow require treatment different from those with decreased pulmonary blood flow.

Because the right ventricle is severely hypoplastic in most forms of tricuspid atresia, only one ventricle is available for use as a pumping chamber. In 1971, Francis Fontan reported a corrective operation in three patients with tricuspid atresia, using the one available ventricle as a pump for the systemic circuit and connecting the right atrium directly to the pulmonary artery. This revolutionary concept is based on the physiologic fact that the pulmonary resistance is so low that it takes only a slight rise in systemic venous pressure to propel the systemic venous return through the pulmonary circuit into the left side of the heart. The Fontan concept now has stood the test of time, and it is widely accepted that such operations, collectively termed orthoterminal correction, are durable and effective treatment for children with tricuspid atresia. Low pulmonary vascular resistance is a prerequisite for this operation, and infants have elevated pulmonary vascular resistance that declines toward adult levels over the first few years of life. Therefore, because most patients with tricuspid atresia require surgical intervention during the first year of life, palliative surgery still retains a prominent place in the surgical management of tricuspid atresia.

PALLIATIVE SURGERY

Increased Pulmonary Blood Flow

About one-quarter of patients with tricuspid atresia have a moderate to large ventricular septal defect without severe pulmonary or subpulmonary stenosis. These patients have mild or no cyanosis. Most have balanced pulmonary blood flow requiring no treatment in early infancy or moderately increased pulmonary blood flow with congestive heart failure that responds well to digoxin and diuretics. These children tend to develop decreased size of the ventricular septal defect, with consequent decreasing pulmonary blood flow and increasing cyanosis over a few months or a few years. Treatment for them is then similar to that for the two-thirds of children with tricuspid atresia who start out life with severely decreased pulmonary blood flow (see next section).

A small number of children with tricuspid atresia, probably less than 5 percent, have a large ventricular septal defect with unrestricted pulmonary blood flow and congestive heart failure that cannot be controlled by medication. Failure of medical therapy with digoxin and diuretics usually is evidenced by continuing tachypnea, tachycardia, hepatomegaly, difficulty in feeding, and failure to thrive during infancy. Appropriate surgical intervention at this point is banding of the pulmonary artery. Protection of the pulmonary arterioles from the development of pulmonary vascular obstructive disease resulting from increased pulmonary blood flow is critically important to future corrective surgery; thus, in these infants the pulmonary artery band should be made as tight as the patient will tolerate. The number of patients who have undergone banding of the pulmonary artery is too small for meaningful survival statistics, but in general, the results should be similar to those of banding for other complex lesions (90 to 95 percent survival). The critical measures of success of banding are the pulmonary artery pressure and pulmonary vascular resistance, because they must be low enough to allow a safe corrective operation several years later.

Decreased Pulmonary Blood Flow

Most patients with tricuspid atresia require palliative surgery for severe hypoxia and cyanosis and consequent polycythemia during infancy. *Newborns* with tricuspid atresia and critical pulmonary stenosis or atresia usually become severely hypoxic when the ductus arteriosus closes on the first or second day of life. Effective palliation can be achieved immediately by infusion of prostaglandin E_1 at a rate of 0.05 to 0.1 μg per kilogram per minute, either intravenously or through an umbilical arterial catheter positioned at the aortic orifice of the ductus arteriosus. Hypoxia almost always is reversed within minutes after infusion is started. Long periods of prostaglandin infusion may be associated with progressively increasing lung water, pathologic changes in the pulmonary arteries, and friability of ductal and other vascular tissues, so an aortopulmonary shunt should be constructed after a day or two of infusion. The shunt we have found most durable and reliable in newborn infants is the modified Blalock-Taussig shunt, interposing a segment of 5- mm Goretex vascular graft between the side of the subclavian artery on the same side as the aortic arch, usually the left, and the side of the ipsilateral pulmonary artery.

In *older infants*, palliative operation is indicated when cyanotic spells or polycythemia (hemoglobin greater than 18 g per deciliter) is present. The modified 5-mm or 6-mm Goretex shunt, as described above, is the operation of choice for these children. After the age of 2 years, corrective surgery is indicated.

The Glenn shunt (cavopulmonary anastomosis) is no longer favored because of the late development of ventilation-perfusion imbalances and arteriovenous communications in the affected lung. Recent reintroduction of a modified shunt, connecting the cephalad end of the divided superior vena cava to the side of the right pulmonary artery, and allowing all the superior caval return to go to *both* capillary beds, may be a good palliative operation that is a first step toward later orthoterminal correction.

ORTHOTERMINAL CORRECTION

Timing of Operation

Since longstanding aortopulmonary shunts have deleterious effects on left ventricular function and pulmonary vasculature, both of which are critically important to the success of a Fontan-type procedure, elective correction is indicated when the pulmonary microvasculature has matured completely, around the age of 4 or 5 years. Corrective operation rather than palliation should be considered for patients over the age of 2 years who require surgery for the first time and patients of any age who have had a previous shunt that is beginning to fail (increasing cyanosis or hemoglobin greater than 18 g per deciliter).

Patient Selection

Fontan's criteria for a patient to undergo a corrective procedure are listed in Table 1. If these criteria are ob-

TABLE 1 Fontan's Criteria

Age > 4, < 15 years; weight > 13 kg
Sinus rhythm
Normal caval drainage
Normal or large right atrial volume
Pulmonary arterial mean pressure ≤ 15 mm Hg
Pulmonary resistance < 4 units × m²
Pulmonary branches of normal size*
Normal function of primitive ventricle (ejection fraction ≥ 0.60, end-diastolic pressure normal)
No mitral incompetence
No impairing effects of a previous shunt

served rigidly, the mortality rate following such a procedure should be less than 5 percent. None of the criteria, however, are inviolable. The more and the greater the degree to which these criteria are transgressed in a given patient, the greater the risk of the operation. Fairly wide variations from the physiologic criteria can be accepted if the cause of the abnormality is correctable; for example, pulmonary arterial pressure of 30 mm Hg and a resistance of 4 units may be acceptable if they are caused by mitral insufficiency that can be corrected by repair or replacement of the mitral valve at the time of corrective surgery. Because of the complex interrelations among pulmonary artery size, pressure, and resistance, left atrial pressure, and left ventricular function, it is difficult to pinpoint precise criteria that absolutely contraindicate operation.

Available Techniques

The aims of orthoterminal correction are to separate the pulmonary and systemic circuits and to connect the systemic venous drainage to the pulmonary arteries. The atrial septal communication always should be closed with a patch to avoid tension on the suture line and disruption leading to residual right-to-left shunt and cyanosis. Separation at the ventricular level can be achieved by closing the ventricular septal defect, which is necessary only when the right atrium is connected directly to the right ventricle, or, more commonly, by either dividing or ligating the pulmonary artery. A wide variety of methods has been used to connect the systemic venous drainage to the pulmonary artery. Although a valve was interposed between the right atrium and the pulmonary artery in almost all early variants, it now has become clear that satisfactory results can be obtained without the use of valves in the right heart circuit (Figs. 1 and 2). The tips of two mediastinal drainage tubes are left in the pleural spaces to provide drainage of hydrothorax that nearly always occurs postoperatively.

Postoperative Management

The most critical physiologic goals during the early postoperative period are maintaining an adequate right atrial-to-left atrial pressure gradient, a low pulmonary vascular resistance, and an efficiently functioning left ventricle. After termination of cardiopulmonary bypass, the right atrial pressure is kept in the range of 16 to 18 mm Hg. Respiratory alkalosis by hyperventilation is maintained to keep the pH in the range of 7.45 to 7.50. High pulmonary arterial pressure and respiratory alkalosis lower pulmonary vascular resistance and thereby increase cardiac output.

The left ventricle may be supported by the use of dobutamine (if high catecholamine doses are required) or dopamine (if low doses are required, for its renal arteriolar dilation effect), and nitroprusside (1 to 8 μg per kilogram per minute) to reduce afterload. In cases of a low cardiac output state requiring a high right atrial pressure, we have used a blood pressure cuff around the abdomen or MAST trousers to provide intermittent compression (30 seconds of inflation to 30 to 40 cm H_2O, and 30 seconds of deflation). We have found this to be helpful in maintaining relatively high systemic arterial perfusion pressure, while at the same time reducing accumulation of somatic edema and keeping ascites to a minimum.

Outcome of Orthoterminal Correction

Early mortality rate is related closely to preoperative physiology and anatomy, ranging from less than 5 percent in patients who satisfy all of Fontan's criteria to as high as 20 to 30 percent in patients whose conditions violate several of those criteria. It now appears that long-term quality of life is so much better after a Fontan-type procedure than after a palliative procedure that a relatively higher risk may be acceptable to many less than ideal candidates.

Morbidity early in the postoperative period may include low cardiac output state, pleural effusion and ascites, and arrhythmias. Low output is usually caused by marginal preoperative physiology or an inadequate venopulmonary anastomosis. It should be possible to overcome the low output state in most patients by observing the management principles outlined above, but reoperation to correct incomplete repair sometimes is needed. Pleural effusions are seen in virtually all patients after orthoterminal correction and require pleural drainage, usually for about a week. In the rare case of chronic pleural effusion, a Denver pleuroperitoneal shunt has been reported to be useful.

Arrhythmias may include virtually any supraventricular arrhythmia or heart block. Because of the critical importance of left ventricular function, it is important to maintain as normal a rhythm as possible. Temporary atrial and ventricular pacing wires should be left on all patients and arrhythmias treated vigorously, with both electrical manipulation and drugs.

A poor late result manifested as exercise intolerance often is related to poor preoperative hemodynamics with inadequate improvement postoperatively or to incomplete repair that may require reoperation. Any patient who is not doing as well as expected postoperatively should undergo cardiac catheterization to assess the adequacy of the surgical repair, and all patients should undergo catheterization at 1 to 2 years after operation. Fortunately, most patients have excellent exercise tolerance. Furthermore, at cardiac catheterization, most patients are able to double cardiac output during exercise, although ventricular volume and ejection fraction remain abnormal.

Unresolved Questions

Although it has been demonstrated clearly that Fontan's criteria for operability can be violated, both in number and degree, absolute limits of pulmonary artery size, pressure, and resistance, left ventricular end-diastolic and left atrial pressure, and age have not been determined.

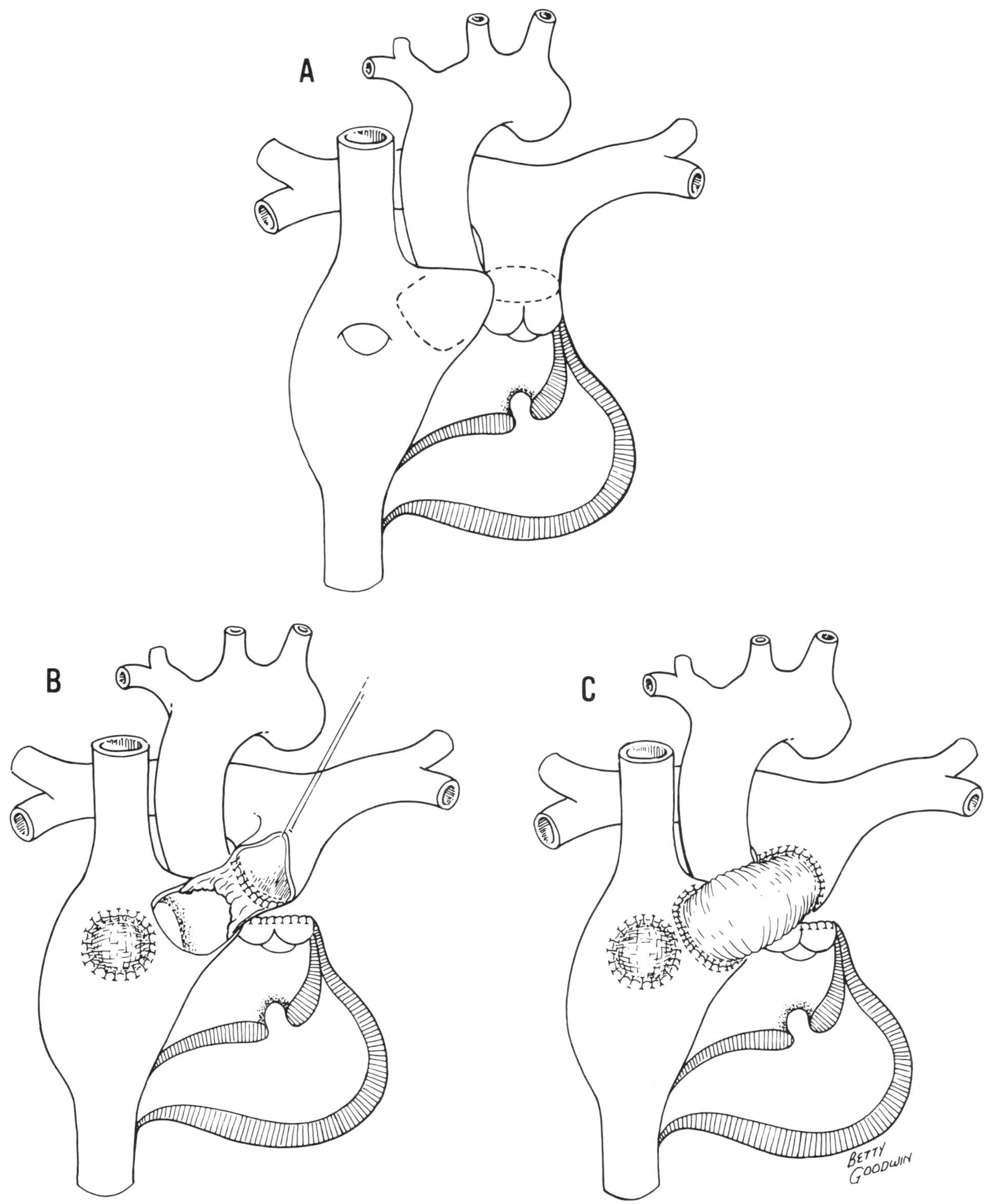

Figure 1 A frequently used repair when the great arteries are normally related. *A*, A rectangular flap is made in the right atrium based at the midportion of the atrial appendage; the pulmonary artery is transected immediately above the valve. *B*, The flap is reflected medially, and its most lateral free edge is sutured to the posterior edge of the pulmonary artery. The proximal stump of the pulmonary artery is oversewn, and the atrial septal communication is closed with a patch. *C*, The repair is completed by suturing a large patch over the atrial-pulmonary opening, thus completing the atriopulmonary conduit.

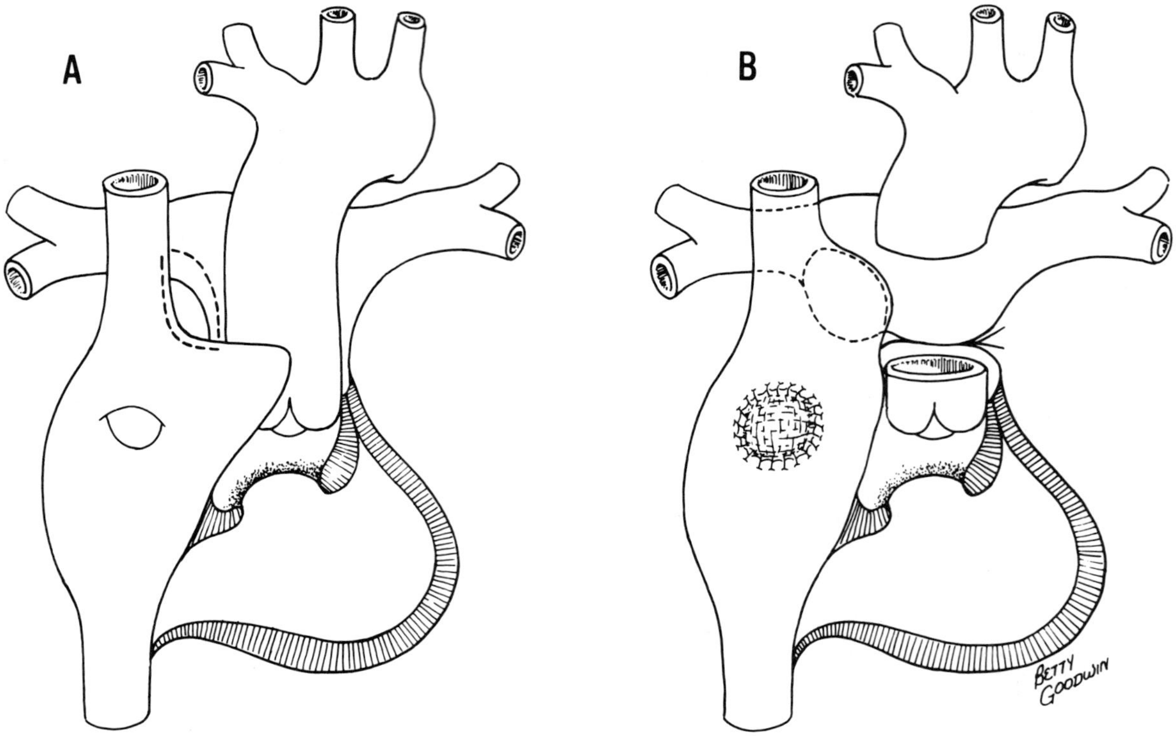

Figure 2 A commonly used repair when the great arteries are transposed. *A*, An incision is made on the cephalad edge of the atrial appendage into the superior vena cava to the level of the middle of the right pulmonary artery; a corresponding incision is made in the main pulmonary and right pulmonary arteries. *B*, The atrial septal defect is closed with a patch. The atrial opening is anastomosed to the pulmonary opening, creating a large atriopulmonary communication, and the main pulmonary artery is ligated.

Furthermore, follow-up has not been ongoing long enough in sufficient numbers of patients to determine accurately duration and quality of life. Thus, precise comparison with long-term results of palliative shunts is not possible. Early data strongly suggest that both quality of life and survival are improved markedly after a Fontan procedure, but much longer follow-up is needed.

Although most surgeons do not now use valves in the right heart circuit, there is suggestive evidence that the presence of both right atrial inflow and outflow valves may permit a more ventricle-like function for the right atrium than is possible without them, implying the possibility of better long-term results and expansion of the limits of preoperative physiology. The evidence is weak at this time, so the technical difficulties attending the use of such valves has inhibited most surgeons from using them until better documentation of their value is available. A related question is when, if ever, it is useful to include the right ventricle and intact pulmonary valve in the repair. In a few patients, the right ventricle may grow, but evidence that the growth is substantial enough and valve function useful enough to make this a worthwhile procedure is not yet available.

SUGGESTED READING

Behrendt DM, Rosenthal A. Cardiovascular status after repair by Fontan procedure. Ann Thorac Surg 1980; 29:322–330.

Fontan F, Baudet E. Surgical repair of tricuspid atresia. Thorax 1971; 26:240–248.

Fontan F, Deville C. Quaegebeur J, Ottenkamp J. Sourdille N, Choussat A, Brom GA. Repair of tricuspid atresia in 100 patients. J Thorac Cardiovasc Surg 1983; 85:647–660.

Kreutzer GO, Vargas FJ, Schlichter AJ, Laura JP, Suarez JC, Coronel AR, Kreutzer EA. Atriopulmonary anastomosis. J Thorac Cardiovasc Surg 1982; 83:427–436.

Laks H, Milliken JC, Perloff JK, Hellenbrand WE, George BL, Chin A, DiSessa TG, Williams RG. Experience with the Fontan procedure. J Thorac Cardiothorac Surg 1984; 88:939–951.

Mayer JE Jr, Helgason H, Jonas RA, Lang P, Vargas FJ, Cook N, Castaneda AR. Extending the limits for modified Fontan procedures. J Thorac Cardiovasc Surg 1986; 92:1021–1028.

THE DOUBLE-OUTLET RIGHT VENTRICLE

JAROSLAV F. STARK, M.D., F.R.C.S., F.A.C.S.
B. SETHIA, F.R.C.S.

Double-outlet right ventricle refers to the ventriculo-arterial connection in which one great artery and more than 50 percent of the other one arise from the right ventricle. Indications for surgery, timing of the operation, and the type of surgical procedure depend on several factors. These can be summarized as follows:

1. Atrioventricular concordance, discordance, or univentricular-atrioventricular connection.
2. Presence or absence of pulmonary stenosis.
3. The level of pulmonary arteriolar resistance.
4. The size and location of the ventricular septal defect and its relationship to the great arteries.
5. Presence or absence of other severe associated anomalies, such as overriding or straddling of the atrioventricular valves, or anomalies of pulmonary or systemic venous connections.

DIAGNOSIS

The presenting symptoms are those of either increased or decreased pulmonary blood flow. The symptoms and signs may be similar to those of high flow ventricular septal defect, to transposition of the great arteries with ventricular septal defect with or without pulmonary stenosis, or to tetralogy of Fallot.

In neonates and young infants, the diagnosis can be established on the basis of a clinical examination combined with chest x-ray, electrocardiogram, and cross-sectional echocardiography. We often proceed with palliative surgery on the basis of such an evaluation. Before corrective surgery, cardiac catheterization and angiocardiography must be used to evaluate the exact hemodynamics, especially the presence or absence of pulmonary vascular disease, and to ascertain the exact anatomic relationships and the presence or absence of other associated cardiac lesions.

The ventricular septal defect may be located anywhere in the interventricular septum. From the surgical point of view, the relationship between the ventricular septal defect and the great arteries is very important. We use Lev's classification of ventricular septal defect in double-outlet right ventricle: doubly committed, subaortic, subpulmonary, and noncommitted. The size of the ventricular septal defect is also important.

OPERATION PROCEDURES

Both palliative and corrective operations are used (Table 1). Palliative operations include systemic to pulmonary artery shunts, atrial septostomy or septectomy, and pulmonary artery banding.

Systemic to Pulmonary Shunt

If a shunt is indicated, we currently prefer a modified Blalock-Taussig shunt. The operation is performed through a full lateral thoracotomy incision, and a thin-walled Goretex graft is interposed between the subclavian artery and either the right or left pulmonary artery. We do not use a shunt smaller than 5 mm, which is usually adequate for most infants; a 6-mm shunt is used after about the age of 10 to 12 months. Before the pulmonary anastomosis is constructed, heparin 1 mg per kilogram is given, and this is not reversed at the end of the operation.

A classic Blalock-Taussig shunt on the side opposite the site of the aortic arch is another excellent option (right-sided shunt in left aortic arch and left-sided shunt in right aortic arch).

Atrial Septostomy or Septectomy

Patients with subpulmonary ventricular septal defect often have the physiology of patients with transposition of the great arteries and ventricular septal defect. Such patients benefit from better mixing at the atrial level, which can be achieved by creating or enlarging the interatrial communication. During the first 2 months of life, this is best done during cardiac catheterization using a balloon. In older patients a blade septostomy followed by balloon septostomy can be performed during cardiac catheterization. If these techniques fail, a surgical septectomy may be indicated. We prefer the Blalock-Hanlon technique of atrial septectomy to the inflow occlusion technique. The Blalock-Hanlon septectomy is performed through a right thoracotomy in the fifth intercostal space, and if the shunt operation is indicated at the same sitting, septectomy is performed first, followed by construction of a shunt. A standard technique is used. Before the clamp is applied on the atria and the pulmonary veins are snared, the lungs are hyperventilated for 2 to 3 minutes with 100 percent oxygen. Usually no more than 2 to 3 minutes of pulmonary artery or vein occlusion is required for this procedure.

Pulmonary Artery Banding

In some neonates with uncontrolled heart failure, pulmonary artery banding may be indicated. In patients with subaortic or doubly committed ventricular septal defect, a primary repair is usually preferred. However, under some special circumstances, such as in the presence of major associated congenital noncardiac anomalies (i.e., large exomphalos, tracheoesophageal fistula with esophageal atresia), pulmonary artery banding may be indicated. More often this procedure is used for patients with subpulmonary ventricular septal defect and high pulmonary blood flow during the first month or two of life. During the operation, the pulmonary arterial pressure is reduced to between 30 and 50 percent of systemic pressure. Arterial Po_2 should not be lowered below 30 mm Hg.

TABLE 1 Double-Outlet Right Ventricle

Palliative Operations	*Corrective Operations*
Systemic to pulmonary shunt	Tunnel left ventricle to aorta: without outflow patch/conduit with outflow patch/conduit
Pulmonary artery banding	
Atrial septostomy/septectomy	Tunnel left ventricle to pulmonary artery: with arterial switch with Damus-Kaye-Stansel procedure with Senning or Mustard procedure
	Closure of ventricular septal defect: with left ventricle pulmonary artery conduit and Senning or Mustard procedure
	Closure of pulmonary artery: atriopulmonary connection (Fontan's operation) and atrial septation

CORRECTIVE PROCEDURES

All corrective procedures are performed on cardiopulmonary bypass with systemic hypothermia, aortic cross-clamping, and crystalloid cardioplegia. In some infants, total circulatory arrest may be used, but in general we prefer to cannulate both cavae and use reduced flow rather than total circulatory arrest. Premedication and anesthesia do not differ from those for other operations for congenital heart defects. The use of monitoring lines and in-dwelling catheters is also routine. A midline sternotomy incision is used for all these operations. Whenever there is a possibility that an atrial repair (Mustard or Senning operation) may be utilized as part of the correction, venous cannulae are inserted directly into the superior and inferior venae cavae. Right-angled metal cannulae facilitate the direct cannulation, but the plastic Rygg's cannulae can also be used. We routinely start bypass with perfusate at 20 to 25° C, and during the initial phases of the operation, the patient is cooled systemically to this temperature. The anatomy is always assessed first through the right atrium and the tricuspid valve. If the possibility of using the Senning operation is being considered, the atrial incision is made just in front of the crista terminalis. Decompression of the left side of the heart is achieved by placing a sump through the foramen ovale; or if the intra-atrial septum is intact, a small incision is made in the fossa ovalis. We try to minimize the length of myocardial ischemia; therefore the original assessment and the final phases of the operation can be performed without aortic cross-clamping. When the aorta is cross-clamped, cardioplegia (St. Thomas' solution) is infused under pressure control into the root of the aorta and is recovered by a discard sucker from the coronary sinus. Then 30 ml per kilogram body weight is infused, and every 30 minutes a half-dose is repeated.

Before the aortic cross-clamp is removed, the sump is withdrawn from the left atrium and the lungs are inflated to expel air from the left atrium. The patent foramen ovale is then closed, the aortic clamp is removed while the perfusion is reduced, and the needle vent in the ascending aorta is put on high suction. While the patient is being fully rewarmed, various parts of the heart can be closed and conduits attached.

Discontinuation of bypass and the use of monitoring devices at this time and subsequently in the intensive care unit do not differ from other operations for congenital heart defects.

The type of corrective surgery depends on the type of ventricular septal defect and the presence or absence of pulmonary stenosis.

Connection of Left Ventricle Through Ventricular Septal Defect to Aorta

This type of repair is suitable for patients with subaortic or doubly committed ventricular septal defect. The anatomy is always assessed through the tricuspid valve because in some patients repair can be performed transatrially. In others the assessment facilitates the selection of the most appropriate ventriculotomy. The patch is cut from the tube of knitted or woven Dacron. This enables us to achieve a better geometry of the tunnel and avoids a too flat patch, which may cause subaortic obstruction. The ventricular septal defect may have to be enlarged, either by a simple incision or by partial excision of the muscle in the lateral superior margin of the defect. The patch can be attached either by a running stitch or by mattress stitches buttressed with Teflon pledgets. We usually combine both these techniques to achieve a quick and secure closure. In the area where the ventricular septal defect was enlarged, interrupted sutures are used, whereas the running stitch can easily be used through the base of the tricuspid valve and running across the ventricular-infundibular fold.

If pulmonary stenosis is present, it is relieved by a valvotomy. If infundibular obstruction is present, resection alone may be adequate, or an outflow tract patch may have to be placed. Under some circumstances, such as unfavorable distribution of the coronary arteries on the anterior surface of the right ventricle, the obstruction may have to be bypassed with a valved conduit. For the outflow tract patch, we generally prefer a pericardial patch, but a preclotted woven Dacron patch can also be used in older children. When a conduit is required, we use an antibiotic preserved aortic or pulmonary homograft, or in recent years, antibiotic sterilized and cryopreserved aortic or pulmonary artery homografts. We try to avoid Dacron extension to this homograft and prefer to use the anterior cusp of the mitral valve of the homograft for attachment to the right ventricle. If a longer conduit is needed, the homograft may be extended with knitted Dacron tube that is presealed with fibrin glue (Tisseel).

Connection of the Left Ventricle Through Ventricular Septal Defect to Pulmonary Artery

This operation is used for patients with a subpulmonary ventricular septal defect. In addition to constructing the tunnel from the left ventricle to the pulmonary artery, an arterial switch operation (Jatene's operation) is performed. The aorta is transected, and the coronary arteries are removed with the disks of the aortic wall. The pulmonary artery is also transected, the coronary arteries are transferred, and then the distal aorta is anastomosed to the proximal pulmonary artery and the distal pulmonary artery to the proximal aorta. The openings left after the excision of the coronary arteries are closed with pericardial patches. If the aorta is more or less anterior to the pulmonary artery, such as in transposition of the great arteries, it is useful to bring the aorta under the pulmonary bifurcation (Lecompte's maneuver). If, however, the vessels are side by side, as is the more common arrangement in patients with double-outlet right ventricle and subpulmonary ventricular septal defect, the proximal aorta is anastomosed on the junction of the main and right pulmonary arteries without performing Lecompte's maneuver.

Some surgeons prefer the Damus-Kaye-Stansel operation to the arterial switch, but we do not share their enthusiasm and prefer the switch operation for these patients. If the arterial switch operation cannot be performed, the left ventricle can still be connected to the pulmonary artery, and in addition, the circulation is switched at the atrial level by performing a standard Senning or Mustard procedure.

In some patients it may be possible to connect the left ventricle to the aorta, even when the ventricular septal defect is subpulmonary. Extensive resection of the infundibular septum is required, and the type of operation described by Kawashima or a Patrick-McGoon spiral patch can be used.

Left Ventricle to Pulmonary Artery Conduit

In some patients with uncommitted (remote) ventricular septal defect, it may be possible to enlarge the defect and then connect the left ventricle either to the aorta or to the pulmonary artery. If this is not possible, the ventricular septal defect may be closed, the left ventricle connected to the pulmonary artery with a valved conduit, and a Senning's operation performed. When a left ventricle to pulmonary artery conduit is used, we prefer an aortic homograft with a long extension of knitted Dacron tube presealed with Tisseel. The left pleural space is widely opened, and the conduit is placed in a long curve to avoid compression by the heart and to achieve a good attachment to the left ventricle without kinking. The anastomosis between the conduit and the left ventricle is reinforced with two Teflon strips for hemostasis. We do not use a metal intraventricular extension for this conduit.

Patients with Double-Outlet Right Ventricle with Hypoplasia of One of the Ventricles or with Straddling of One of the Atrioventricular Valves

Repair achieving a biventricular heart may not be possible. In such patients, when pulmonary stenosis is present, an atriopulmonary connection (modified Fontan's operation) is our operation of choice. We transect the pulmonary artery, oversew the pulmonary valve and the proximal pulmonary artery, and then perform a wide anastomosis between the main and right pulmonary arteries and the roof of the right and left atria. If there is any doubt about the adequacy of the left atrioventricular valve, it is advantageous to connect the pulmonary venous return, both to the mitral and to the tricuspid valves by septating the atria with a large patch. If the left atrioventricular valve is adequate, it may be easier to close the atrial septal defect and also to close the tricuspid valve with a patch. The patch for the tricuspid valve closure is placed above the coronary sinus to avoid any damage to the conduction system and also to protect the coronary sinus from the high venous pressure that is usually present in the right atrium following atriopulmonary connection.

TIMING OF THE OPERATION

The timing of the operation depends on the presence or absence of pulmonary stenosis and on the type and location of the ventricular septal defect. It is also influenced by the experience of the surgeon and the attitude of the department toward palliative versus corrective procedures.

The timing of the operation for patients with high pulmonary blood flow is shown in Figure 1. When congestive heart failure is controlled medically, repair can be delayed until about 6 months of age in subaortic and doubly committed ventricular septal defect. If the defect is subpulmonary, a balloon atrial septostomy is performed at the initial investigation, and the repair is delayed until the age of 3 to 6 months. In uncommitted (remote) ventricular septal defect, a balloon atrial septostomy is performed. Pulmonary artery banding should be done probably between 3 and 6 months of age. Because of the difficulties associated with the repair of double-outlet right ventricle and uncommitted ventricular septal defect, corrective surgery is delayed until the age of 3 to 5 years.

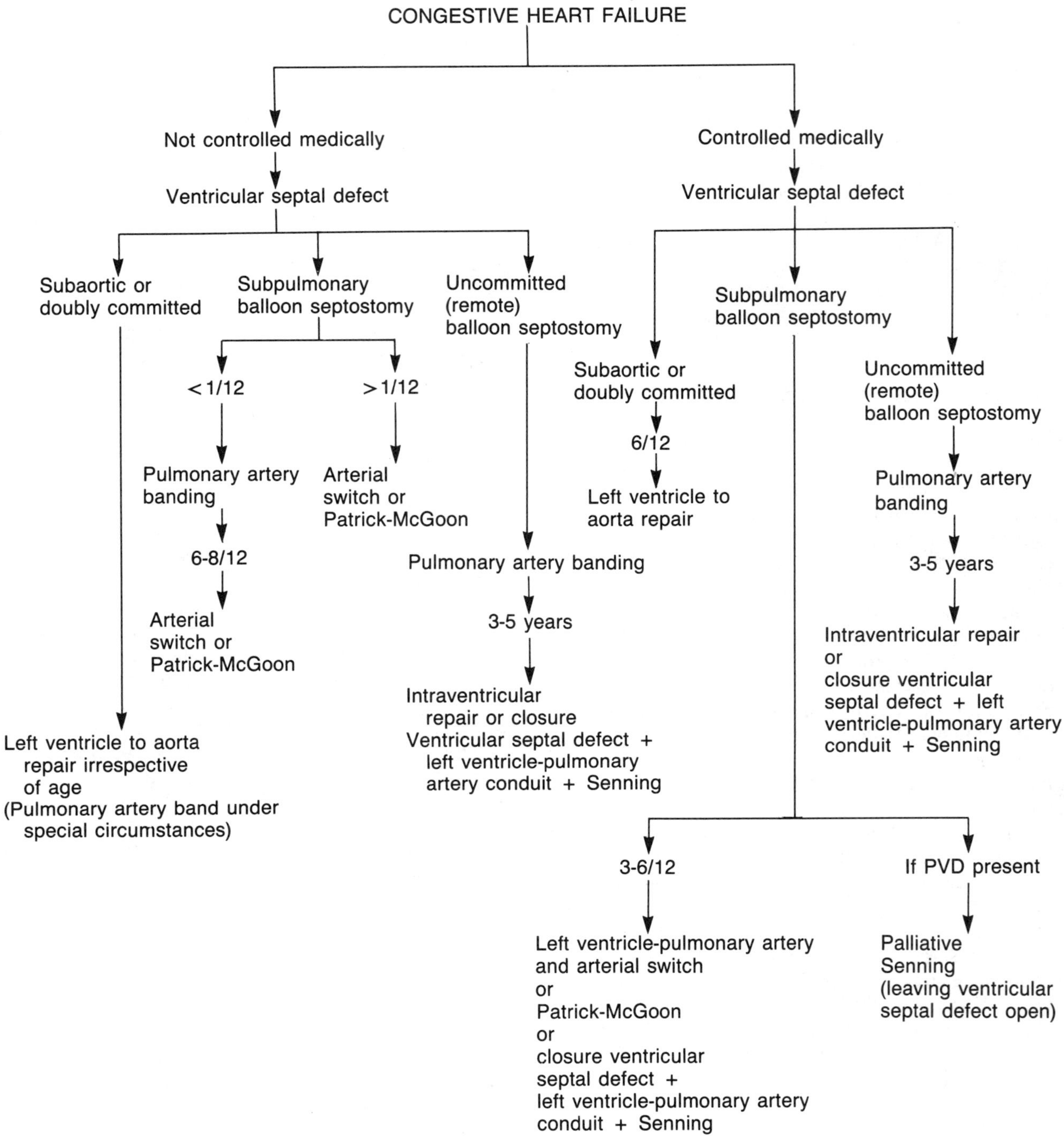

Figure 1 Double-outlet right ventricle: timing of surgery in patients without pulmonary stenosis.

If congestive heart failure is severe and not adequately controlled medically, we prefer to proceed with a complete repair irrespective of the age and weight of the patient in the presence of doubly committed or subaortic ventricular septal defect. In subpulmonary ventricular septal defect a balloon atrial septostomy is performed at the initial investigation, and this is followed by a pulmonary artery banding if the child is less than 1 month old. Over the age of 1 month, an arterial switch operation is our technique of choice. If the pulmonary artery was banded, an arterial switch or intraventricular repair (Patrick-McGoon) is scheduled for between 6 and 18 months of age. Patients in severe congestive heart failure and uncommitted (remote) ventricular septal defect have a balloon atrial septostomy followed by a pulmonary artery banding before the age of 3 months. Interventricular repair is delayed until the age of 3 to 5 years.

In patients with pulmonary stenosis (Fig. 2), timing of the operation again depends on the type of ventricular septal defect. In subaortic or doubly committed ventricular septal defect, a systemic to pulmonary shunt is preferred in patients less than 6 months old, whereas repair is considered after the age of 6 months. Patients with subpulmonary ventricular septal defect or uncommitted ventricular septal defect have balloon atrial septostomy initially. If cyanosis increases, a systemic to pulmonary shunt is indicated. Repair is delayed until the age of 3 to 5 years.

If the patient is only suited for an atriopulmonary connection, we prefer to wait until the age of 4 years but would not hesitate to proceed with surgery earlier if it is indicated.

RESULTS

Currently a survival rate of over 90 percent can be expected in patients with subaortic or doubly committed ventricular septal defect, whereas subpulmonary and noncommitted ventricular septal defects increase the risk to about 30 percent. Incremental risk factors are noncommitted (remote) ventricular septal defect, associated atrioventricular septal defect, younger age at operation, and the use of a transannular patch or a conduit.

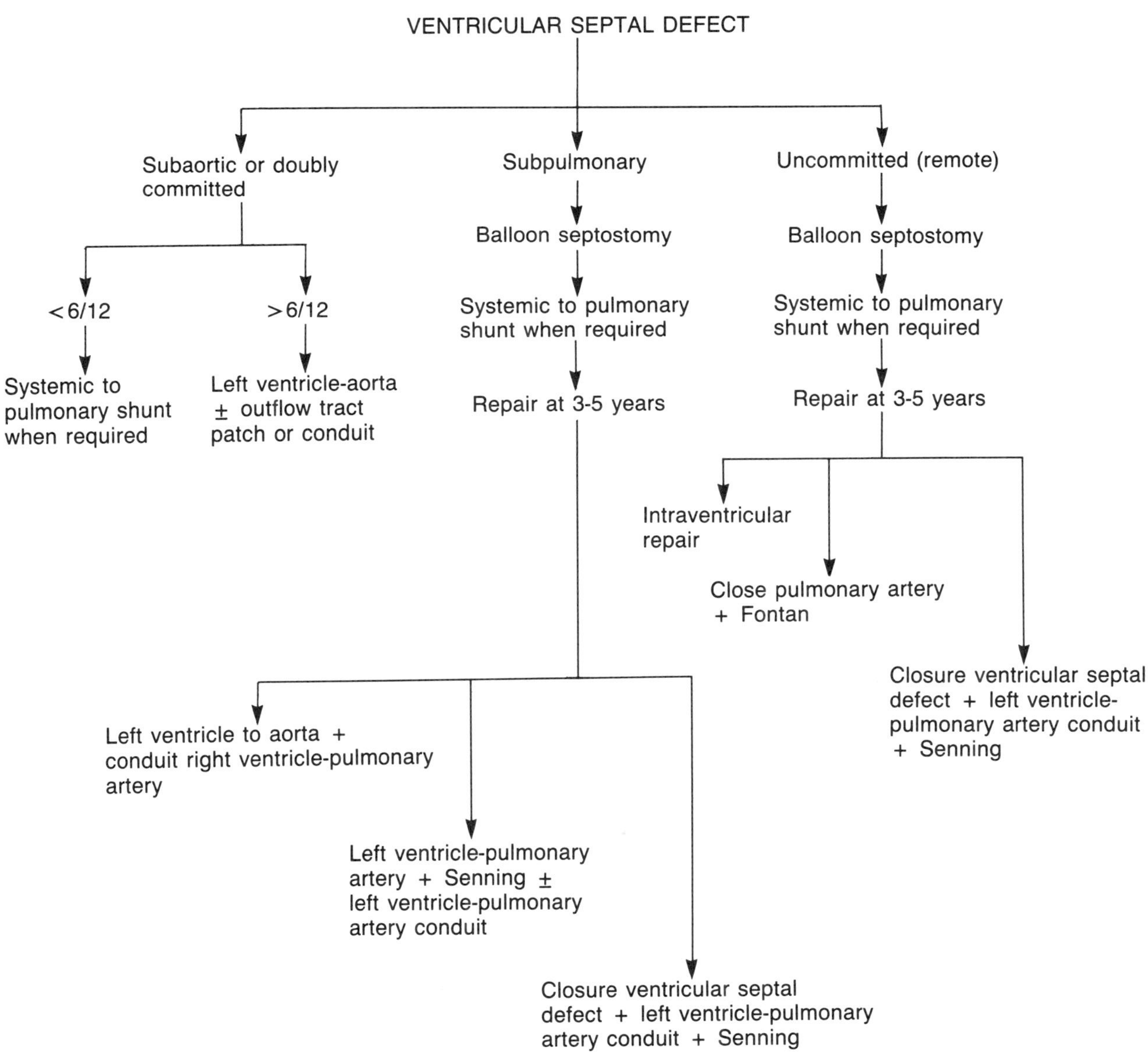

Figure 2 Double-outlet right ventricle: timing of surgery in patients with pulmonary stenosis.

SUGGESTED READING

Gomes MMR, Weidman WH, McGoon DC, Danielson GK. Double-outlet right ventricle without pulmonic stenosis. Surgical considerations and results of operation. Circulation 1971; 43 (Suppl I):31–36.
Gomes MMR, Weidman WH, McGoon DC, Danielson GK. Double-outlet right ventricle with pulmonic stenosis. Surgical considerations and results of operation. Circulation 1971; 43:889–894.
Kirklin JW, Barratt-Boyes BG, eds. Cardiac surgery. New York: John Wiley & Sons, 1986:1219.
Lev M, Bharati S, Meng CCL, Liberthson RR, Paul MH, Idriss F. A concept of double outlet right ventricle. J Thorac Cardiovasc Surg 1972; 64:271–281.
Stark J. Double-outlet ventricles. In: Stark J, deLeval M, eds. Surgery for congenital heart defects. London: Grune & Stratton, 1983:397.

CORRECTION OF TRANSPOSITION: THE SENNING PROCEDURE

ÅKE SENNING, M.D.

Many years ago, in an era in which cardiopulmonary bypass techniques were quite traumatic and circulatory physiology, myocardial preservation, and postoperative care were not nearly as well understood as they are today, clinical efforts were directed at palliative procedures in the treatment of transposition of the great arteries. The operative results in this era were disastrous. To achieve a "hemodynamic correction," the redirection of flow at the atrial level was done initially as a makeshift solution.

After an atrial switch has been performed, it is hoped that the two inflow chambers will function as conduits without obstruction to venous flow and have good reservoir capacity; they should grow with the child and adapt to the flow conditions. The surgical procedure should not cause arrhythmias, and there should be normal atrioventricular conduction allowing a normal atrial pumping function to be transferred through a normally functioning tricuspid ring and valve. Finally, we hope that the tricuspid valve will withstand systemic pressure over time and that the right ventricle will adapt itself to assume the load of the systemic circulation during a normal lifetime.

OPERATIVE TECHNIQUE

The surgical technique of the Senning atrial switch is described in detail in Sabiston and Spencer, *Gibbons Surgery of the Chest* (4th ed, 1983, pp 1153–1156). I will summarize the key features of the technique here.

The operation is performed through a standard median sternotomy, and cardiopulmonary bypass is used with patient cooling to between 17 and 22° C. In infants, deep hypothermia and circulatory arrest may be used, and in older children, direct superior vena cava and inferior vena cava cannulation may be used. The operation is started with a right atrial incision in front of the caval veins; this is outlined in Figure 1. The right atrial incision should have an extension into the atrial appendage to get enough length for the final suture line, as the upper part of it is sutured cranial to the sinus node on the superior vena cava. A second incision in the inner atrial groove should be extended by a perpendicular incision to the superior pulmonary vein right to the insertion of the pericardium to allow a sufficiently wide channel for pulmonary flow. Figure 2 demonstrates the surgeon's view into the atrium.

The incision in the atrial septum is made from the foramen ovale down to and into the coronary sinus to enlarge the atrial septal defect and to empty the coronary venous blood into the pulmonary circulation. No tissue from the atrial septum anterior to the foramen ovale is excised. In the anterior, superior portion of the septum, it is important to leave tissue to avoid injuring the arterial circulation to the sinus node and to spare the anterior conduction tissue between the sinus and the atrioventricular nodes. This incision in the atrial septum in the cranial direction is therefore done less far anteriorly and less cranially than during the early years of this procedure. The atrial septal flap, as shown in Figure 2, forms the roof of the pulmonary venous atrium. In our series of patients who had had prior extensive Blalock-Hanlon septectomy, a septal patch was needed at times, in which case autologous pericardium is preferred. Otherwise, an atrial septal patch is rarely necessary. The atrial septal flap is rotated posteriorly and is sutured in front of the left-sided pulmonary veins and behind the left atrial appendage. Thus, pulmonary venous drainage is isolated away from the mitral valve orifice (Fig. 3).

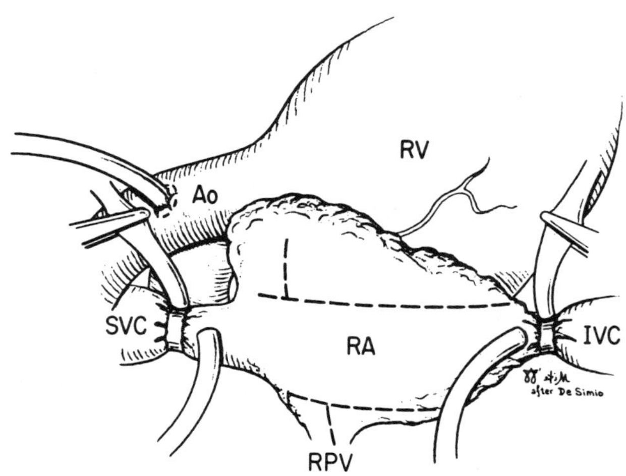

Figure 1 The atrial incisions for the Senning operation (Ao = aorta, RV = right ventricle, IVC = inferior vena cava, SVC = superior vena cava, RA = right atrium, RPV = right pulmonary vein). (Adapted from Sabiston DD Jr, Spencer FC. Gibbons surgery of the chest. 4th ed. Philadelphia: WB Saunders, 1983.)

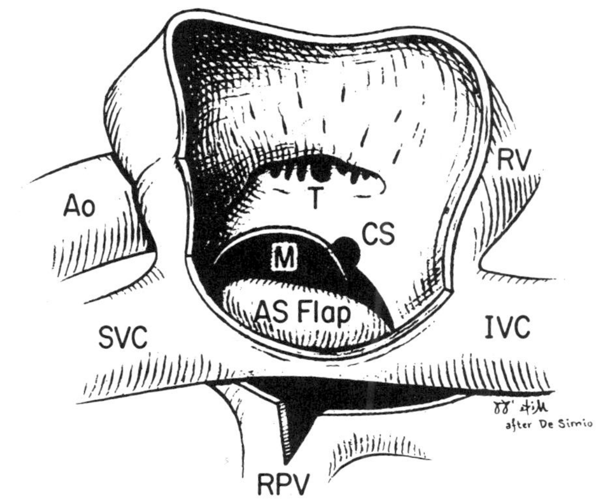

Figure 2 Surgeon's view into the atria (AS = atrial septum, CS = coronary sinus, T = tricuspid valve, M = mitral valve). (Adapted from Sabiston DD Jr, Spencer FC. Gibbons surgery of the chest. 4th ed. Philadelphia: WB Saunders, 1983.)

Next, the anterior edge of the posterior portion of the right atrial wall is brought anteriorly to the anterior edge of the atrial septal defect. This is indicated by dotted lines in Figure 3. The suture line is begun at the cranial end of the atrial wall and is carried inside the coronary sinus and down toward the inferior vena cava, as shown in Figure 4, panels A and B. This creates a tunnel that directs drainage from the superior vena cava and inferior vena cava across the mitral valve, thus isolating caval drainage from the tricuspid valve. The operation is then finished by completing the pulmonary venous pathway. The posterior edge of the anterior half of the right atrial wall is then sutured around the superior and inferior venae cavae, as indicated by the dotted lines in Figure 4, panel B. The suture line should pass above the sinoatrial node across the lower portion of the superior vena cava and onto the left atrial wall, thus completing the pulmonary venous pathway (Fig. 5).

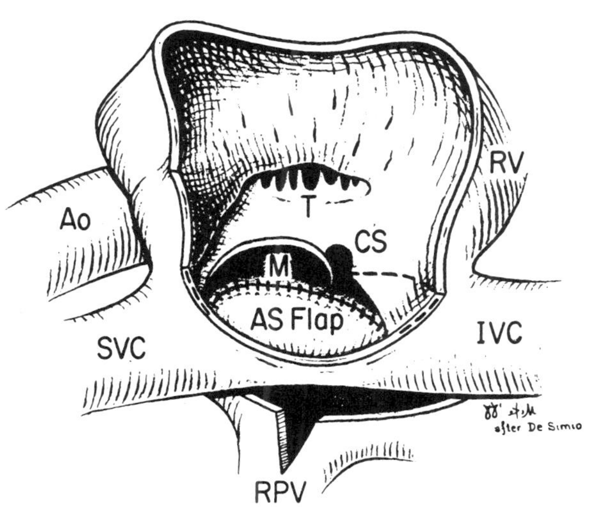

Figure 3 Suture of the atrial septal flap in front of the pulmonary veins to isolate pulmonary venous drainage from the mitral valve. (Abbreviations as in Figures 1 and 2). (Adapted from Sabiston DD Jr, Spencer FC. Gibbons surgery of the chest. 4th ed. Philadelphia: WB Saunders, 1983.)

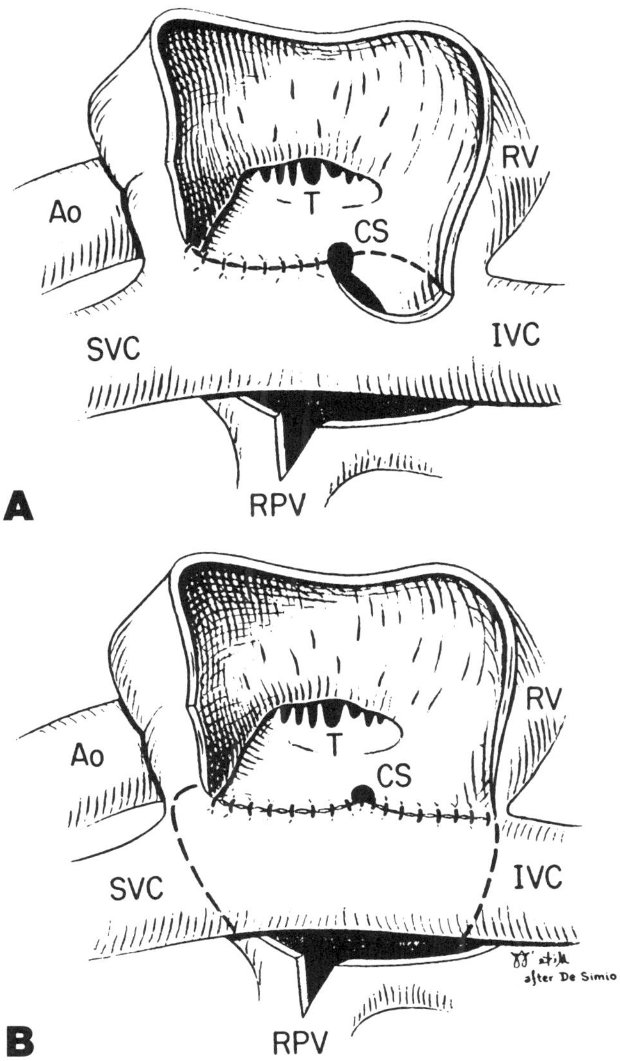

Figure 4 Creation of the systemic venous pathway to direct caval drainage to the mitral valve orifice. *A*, shows superior end of this suture line. *B*, shows completion of the pathway. Note that the suture line is carried into the posterior portion of the coronary sinus. Dotted lines indicate suture lines across cavae for completion of the pulmonary venous pathway. (Abbreviations as in Figures 1 and 2.) (Adapted from Sabiston DD Jr, Spencer FC. Gibbons surgery of the chest. 4th ed. Philadelphia: WB Saunders, 1983.)

In the few patients with juxtaposition of the atrial appendages, it may be necessary to enlarge the lateral wall of the pulmonary venous chamber with a piece of pericardium in situ. This means that the right atrial cut edge will be sutured to the pericardium to leave an adequate distance between the left and right atrial edges and thus to enlarge the pulmonary venous chamber. Before the suture line is completed, a small cannula for air removal may be inserted through the pulmonary venous chamber into the right ventricle. The patient is rewarmed, the ascending aorta is aspirated to remove air, and the aortic cross-clamp is removed. Bleeding is allowed to continue from the ascending aorta to permit exit of any remaining air.

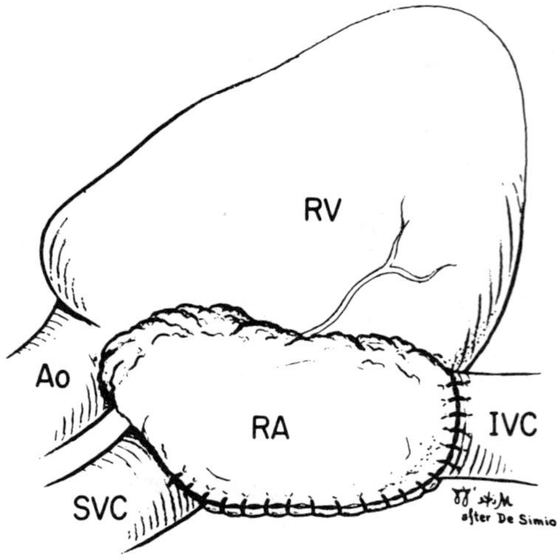

Figure 5 Completion of the pulmonary venous pathway by suture of the anterior half of the right atrial wall to the cut edge of the right pulmonary veins and left atrium. (Abbreviations as in Figures 1 and 2.) (Adapted from Sabiston DD Jr, Spencer FC. Gibbons surgery of the chest. 4th ed. Philadelphia: WB Saunders, 1983.)

RESULTS

In 1986 a consecutive series of 154 patients operated on between 1964 and 1975 had complete follow-up study. This patient population cannot be compared to present-day patients, as they were older and some had prior palliative procedures, such as a Blalock-Hanlon septectomy (94 patients) or banding of the pulmonary artery; in only a few patients was a Rashkind balloon septostomy done as the only palliative procedure. In earlier years prior to this series, perfusion techniques were less than optimal, and the diagnostic techniques were less well defined; the operative mortality rate was 6 percent for simple transposition, and in the "complicated" transposition group (ventricular septal defect and/or left ventricular outflow tract obstruction), nearly one-third of the patients died. The actuarial survival after operation showed that 92 percent of patients with simple transposition survived 10 years, and 89 percent of them reached 20 years. The late deaths were caused by cardiac insufficiency, infections, trauma, and sudden death without further diagnosis. In the group of "complicated" transpositions, 81 percent of the patients who survived surgery were alive at 10 years. Late deaths were caused by infection and endocarditis, valvular insufficiency, and heart failure. There were six sudden deaths, three of them of patients with myocardial impairment.

In the series of patients with simple transposition, there have been four reoperations for pulmonary valve stenosis, superior caval stenosis, and a superior caval vein connection to the pulmonary venous atrium. A more recent combined European series of 146 simple transposition cases revealed no caval obstructions. In our complex group, six patients were reoperated on for residual ventral septal defect, tricuspid insufficiency, pulmonary artery stenosis following debanding, and left ventricular outflow stenosis. All patients survived their reoperations.

Postoperative arrhythmias have been a problem following atrial switch procedures. Only 75 percent of patients are in sinus rhythm, and 14 percent have junctional rhythm. In our entire series of 220 patients surviving the operations between 1964 and 1984, there were two patients with complete heart block, but 14 pacemakers have been implanted to treat mainly bradyarrhythmias. Seven of them were implanted in the first postoperative year and the other seven between 2 and 16 years postoperatively.

Of the 111 survivors operated on in 1964 to 1975, 74 percent are classified New York Heart Association Class I, 25 percent Class II, and one patient Class III. Of course this classification is very subjective, as most patients are still children.

ATRIAL VERSUS ARTERIAL SWITCH

During the last few years, excellent results of the arterial switch procedures have been reported from several centers. This operation is now performed during the first days until 1 or 2 weeks after birth, and the mortality in the uncomplicated group with intact ventricular septum has decreased to a few percent. Late deaths and arrhythmias seem less common, and the functional status of the patients seems generally excellent.

Atrial or arterial switch may be performed in the first 2 weeks after birth and can be expected to have almost identical mortality rates. After an atrial repair, arrhythmias and, in a small percentage of patients, right-sided heart failure may follow. After the arterial repair, the neoaortic and the neopulmonary valves may become insufficient, but new postoperative arrhythmias are rare. For this reason, for infants less than 2 weeks old, I would recommend an arterial switch to decrease the incidence of arrhythmias and to leave the patient with a systemic left ventricle. After 1 month of age, infants should be treated with an atrial switch, unless the left ventricle has been conditioned to withstand the systemic load, e.g., by a large patent ductus or ventricular septal defect. The two-stage procedure (pulmonary artery banding followed by debanding and arterial switch) still seems to have a high operative mortality rate. Patients with pulmonary valve stenosis or anatomic left ventricular outflow tract obstruction are not good candidates for arterial switch and should have an atrial switch. Only two out of 55 patients in our series with left ventricular outflow tract obstruction required reoperation.

Newborns with transposition and a nonrestrictive ventricular septal defect and no left ventricular outflow tract obstruction should have correction with an arterial switch within the first 2 or 3 months, before pulmonary vascular disease or congestive heart failure has developed, as in this group the early and late mortality rates following atrial switch are too high.

Since no foreign material is used in a primary Senning procedure, the atrial chambers grow and contract almost normally. This is an advantage compared with the Mustard procedure. The two procedures are complicated by postoperative arrhythmias even if precautions are taken not to damage the conduction system. Lifelong follow-up of the patients is therefore necessary. During the first year, frequent electrocardiograms should be performed, and often a 24-hour electrocardiogram is required. In cases in which there is evidence of a significant bradyarrhythmia, pacemaker implantation should be considered.

In the next 5 to 6 years, it will be possible to judge more precisely the indications for the atrial versus the arterial switch, particularly as additional long-term data are obtained from the arterial switch operation. We should look toward further evolution in the clinical decision-making process with regard to the treatment of transposition of the great arteries.

SUGGESTED READING

Parenzan L, Locatelli G, Alfieri O, Villani M, Invernizzi G. The Senning operation for transposition of the great arteries. J Thorac Cardiovasc Surg 1977; 76:305–311.

Rubay JE, deHalleux C, Jaumin P, Moulin D, Kestens-Servaye Y, Lintermans J, Stijns M, Vliers A, Chalant CH. Long-term follow-up of the Senning operation for transposition of the great arteries in children under 3 months of age. J Thorac Cardiovasc Surg 1987; 94:75–81.

Senning Å. Surgical correction of transposition of the great vessels. Surgery 1959; 45:966–980.

Senning Å. Transposition av aorta och arteria pulmonalis. Opuscula Medica 1958; nr. 2.

Turley K, Ebert PA. Total correction of transposition of the great arteries. Conduction disturbances in infants younger than three months of age. J Thorac Cardiovasc Surg 1978; 76:312–320

Turley K, Wilson JM, Ebert PA. Atrial repairs of infant complex congenital heart disease. Emphasis on the first 3 months of life. Arch Surg 1980; 115:1335–1337.

CORRECTION OF TRANSPOSITION: ARTERIAL SWITCH PROCEDURE

ALDO R. CASTAÑEDA, M.D., Ph.D.

Transposition of the great arteries (TGA) is a congenital cardiac malformation in which the atrial-ventricular connection is concordant and the ventricular-arterial connection is discordant. TGA is the second most common congenital cardiac defect causing critical disease in infancy. Only 70 percent of infants with TGA and an intact ventricular septum (IVS) survive the first 2 months of life, and less than 5 percent reach the first year of life. Approximately 75 percent of children born with TGA have an essentially IVS; the remainder have either an associated hemodynamically significant ventricular septal defect (20 percent) or associated pulmonary or subpulmonary stenosis (5 percent) or both.

Senning in 1959 was the first to succeed at correcting TGA, basing the operation on Albert's intriguing principle of physiologic repair of TGA by rerouting pulmonary and systemic venous blood at the atrial level using autologous atrial flaps. However, a significant decrease in the risk of the operation only occurred after Mustard's (1964) modification of using an intra-atrial pericardial baffle to redirect pulmonary and systemic venous blood at the atrial level. In the meantime, the Senning operation has enjoyed a successful renaissance in many centers.

Hospital mortality after the atrial switch repair for simple TGA (either Mustard's or Senning's operation) has decreased continuously. In our own institution, the hospital mortality is now less than 2 percent, including in neonates. Five-year survival is approximately 90 percent and 10-year survival close to 85 percent. In view of these encouraging surgical results, why is there renewed interest in changing the surgical approach from an atrial inversion operation, or physiologic repair, to an arterial switch operation, or anatomic repair? Complications after atrial switch operations, particularly systemic or pulmonary venous pathway obstructions, are now much less common than 1 or 2 decades ago. However, of greater concern is the disquieting incidence of late rhythm disturbances after atrial inversion operation and also the question of whether the right ventricle can function over a normal life span as the systemic ventricle.

Although after an atrial switch operation for TGA and IVS most patients are initially in sinus rhythm, only approximately 50 percent remain in sinus rhythm 10 years after the operation. Late postoperative Holter monitoring, particularly during exercise, has unmasked important dysrhythmias, including premature atrial contractions, premature ventricular contractions, and junctional rhythms, in patients who otherwise have normal electrocardiograms. Not surprisingly, sudden death occurs more frequently in patients with these rhythm disturbances. The reasons for these arrhythmias are not clear. Although surgical trauma to the sinus node or its blood supply has been implicated, the interpretation of these findings is complicated by the fact that children with TGA are known to have rhythm disturbances before any surgery is performed.

With respect to the right ventricle's functioning as a systemic ventricle, there are a number of anatomic and physiologic data demonstrating that the left ventricle is better suited than the right one to function as a systemic pump. The ellipsoid-shaped and concentrically contracting normal left ventricle favors pressure work, whereas the normal right ventricle is crescent-shaped, has a large interior surface area to volume ratio, and its bellows-like contraction pattern seems better suited for pumping large volumes of blood against the low resistance pulmonary circuit. The right ventricle in patients with TGA is similar to the normal right ventricle and therefore should not function as efficiently as the systemic pump. Thus, the late response of the anatomic right ventricle's functioning as the systemic ventricle after atrial inversion procedures for TGA is of concern. In fact, right ventricular end diastolic and end-systolic volumes, right ventricular ejection fractions, and the response to afterload stress all have been found to be abnormal after atrial inversion procedures. Thus, the real and potential shortcomings of atrial inversion operations, as outlined above, are mostly responsible for the renewed interest in anatomic correction, or arterial switch operation (ASO).

Since the intracardiac structures are normal in-patients with TGA and IVS, it is not surprising that as soon as open heart surgery became available clinically, surgeons attempted to repair this complex malformation by switching the aorta and the pulmonary artery. In 1954, Mustard, in addition to switching the great arteries, also transferred the left coronary artery; however, he left the right coronary artery attached to the pulmonary circuit. These attempts and other trials did not succeed. Jatene and colleagues in São Paulo, Brazil, fortunately persisted in these efforts, and in 1975 they achieved the first successful ASO in an infant with TGA and ventricular septal defect (VSD). Although Aubert's ingenious attempts at retaining the left ventricle as a systemic ventricle in TGA without anatomically transferring the coronary arteries also proved successful, the Jatene technique has retained its original appeal and now is being used with increasing frequency.

In his initial report, Jatene limited the ASO concept to patients with TGA and VSD. He realized that in such patients the left ventricle soon would adapt to the decreasing resistance of the pulmonary circuit and therefore lose its capacity to pump against the high systemic resistance. However, since approximately 75 percent of all patients with TGA have an IVS, it seems clearly desirable to apply the arterial switch principle to this group of patients as well. In order to "prepare" the left ventricle for a subsequent arterial switch operation, Yacoub and associates first proposed to band the pulmonary artery in patients with TGA and IVS and to perform the arterial switch procedure as a second stage, several months later. To accomplish the same goal, that is, to offer an ASO to patients with TGA and IVS, we based our approach on the fact that intrauterine pulmonary and systemic resistances were nearly equal, and if the arterial switch operation were to be performed during the neonatal period, the left ventricle should still be capable of carrying a systemic workload. Early intervention therefore is necessary.

In patients with TGA and IVS, the left ventricular free-wall thickness is normal at birth but begins to decrease rapidly, paralleling the postnatal decrease in pulmonary vascular resistance. Baño and associates measured, at autopsy, left and right ventricular free-wall thickness in subjects with or without TGA. In TGA patients, the increase in right ventricular free-wall thickness is similar to the increase in left ventricular free-wall thickness of patients with normally related great arteries. Parenthetically, ventricular wall stress is directly proportional to intraventricular pressure and diameter and inversely proportional to wall thickness. Consequently, a dilated and thin-walled ventricle would be subject to high wall stress when faced with the increased resistance presented by the systemic circuit following an ASO.

The limits in left ventricular wall thickness or left ventricular pressure beyond which the left ventricle can be predicted to fail as a systemic pump have not been defined clinically with certainty; therefore, we have developed some empirical criteria. We have assumed that, during the first 14 days of life, virtually all patients have adequate left ventricular function after ASO, regardless of the preoperative left ventricular pressures. Beyond this age, we arbitrarily choose a preoperative left ventricular–right ventricular pressure ratio of 0.6 as the lower limit of acceptable left ventricular pressure. Two-dimensional echocardiography provides a noninvasive index of relative left and right ventricular pressures by outlining the ventricular septal position. When the ventricular septum bows towards the left, the left ventricular pressure is almost certainly low, and these patients are considered unfavorable candidates for the ASO unless the left ventricular–right ventricular pressure ratio measured at catheterization, or in the operating room, exceeds 0.6.

In addition to the assessment of left ventricular function, some anatomic contraindications to ASO also exist. For example, organic left ventricular outflow tract obstruction caused by subvalvar or valvar abnormalities precludes ASO in most instances. Hemodynamically significant mitral atrioventricular valve abnormalities may coexist in some patients with TGA and IVS, and these also would contraindicate performing ASO.

The pattern of coronary artery origin and distribution is somewhat variable in patients with TGA. Rarely do these anatomic variances constitute contraindications to the ASO. Most commonly, the right coronary artery arises from the right-facing sinus and the left coronary artery, including the circumflex branch, from the left-facing sinus. In the second most common variant, the circumflex coronary artery originates from the right coronary artery. Coronary artery transfer can prove difficult whenever the right coronary artery arises from the left-facing cusp (single leftsided origin) and passes anterior to the aorta, or likewise when the anterior descending coronary artery originates from the right-facing cusp. Coronary transfer occasionally can be more difficult when the aortopulmonary relationship is side by side rather than anteroposterior.

PREOPERATIVE ASSESSMENT

Detailed preoperative diagnosis of this defect is essential in order to obtain a successful outcome. Two-dimensional echocardiography usually can accurately define the diagnosis of TGA and can provide sufficient data about the presence of associated defects such as mitral valve or left ventricular outflow tract abnormalities, the position of the ventricular septum, and coronary artery patterns. Nevertheless, at this stage of our experience, we still insist on a cardiac catheterization in all patients, mostly to obtain direct measurements of right and left ventricular pressures and to rule out additional defects. An aortic injection is helpful in outlining the coronary arteries, but the final decision of suitability for transfer is made in the operating room. The indication for a balloon atrial septostomy at catheterization depends largely on the patient's metabolic condition and the projected timing of the operation. If acidosis is present, or if an operating room is not immediately available, or both, a balloon atrial septostomy is performed, and infusion of prostaglandin E_1 may be started to maintain ductal patency and improve oxygenation.

OPERATIVE TECHNIQUE

All neonates are subjected to deep hypothermic circulatory arrest, using core cooling to a rectal temperature of 20° C. During cooling, the ascending aorta and the pulmonary artery are cleared from each other, the ductus arteriosus is divided, and the right and left pulmonary arteries are mobilized well out into the hilus to the first pulmonary artery branches. At 20° C rectal temperature, the aorta is clamped, cardioplegic solution is injected, and the circulation is stopped. The ascending aorta is then transected, and the left and right coronary arteries are excised; the incision is begun at the free edge of the proximal aorta and is carried toward the base of the coronary sinus, well below the coronary ostium. As large a portion of aortic sinus wall as possible is excised to allow for growth of the coronary ostia and also to facilitate the aortic anastomosis. Then, the main pulmonary artery is transected proximal to its bifurcation, and the distal pulmonary artery is transferred anterior to the distal aorta (Lecompte's maneuver). A V-shaped excision of the pulmonary artery wall is made into both the left and right anterior sinuses of the neo-aorta. These incisions must not extend deeply into the sinuses, since this increases the distance across which the mobilized coronary artery must reach. The left coronary artery with its surrounding aortic wall then is sewn into the neo-aorta with continuous absorbable monofilament suture. A similar technique is used to transfer the right coronary artery into the right anterior sinus of the neo-aorta. When the circumflex coronary artery arises from the right coronary artery, the site of implantation is kept slightly higher to avoid kinking of the circumflex coronary artery. The proximal neo-aorta then is sewn end to end to the distal aorta with continuous monofilament absorbable suture. At this stage, the atrial septal defect is closed, the venous cannula is reinserted, the circulation is restarted, and the aorta is unclamped. Air must be vented through a separate stab incision in the distal aorta. All regions of the myocardium should be inspected early after the removal of the aortic clamp to ensure coronary patency and myocardial perfusion. Next is the reconstruction of the neo-pulmonary artery. The two coronary artery donor sites are filled with autogenous pericardium, and finally, the distal pulmonary artery is sewn to the proximal segment (neo-pulmonary artery) with continuous monofilament sutures. During rewarming to 36° C, a left atrial pressure monitoring line is inserted in the right superior pulmonary vein, and the right atrial line is placed through the right atrial appendage. Temporary ventricular pacing wires are sutured to the right ventricular surface.

Immediately after cardiopulmonary bypass, the use of fresh whole blood is important to minimize postoperative bleeding. Mechanical ventilation is used at least during the first 24 hours after surgery, or until the child is hemodynamically stable. During this period, all neonates are sedated heavily with intravenous narcotics and muscle relaxants. Arterial blood gases, electrolytes, calcium, glucose, and hematocrit are monitored frequently.

RESULT

Generally, the results of ASO for TGA and IVS have been favorable. There have been seven deaths in 59 neonates (11.8 percent). Most of the operative deaths have occurred early during our experience and were attributable to technical factors such as hemorrhage (one patient) or obstructed branches of the coronary arteries causing left ventricular failure (two patients). In two other neonates (older than 3 weeks of age), left ventricular failure with patent coronary arteries caused their deaths. In one, the preoperative echocardiogram showed deviation of the septum into the left ventricle, although the left ventricular pressure 1 week earlier had been equal to the systemic. Two other deaths were caused by pulmonary hemorrhage that occurred despite low left atrial pressures. The most favorable results have been in neonates under 10 days of age (in 51 patients, two deaths or 3.9 percent).

Recatheterization after operation has been carried out in 28 patients. One asymptomatic patient had an occluded left anterior descending artery. In this patient the right coronary and circumflex arteries arose from the right cusp. All coronary arteries were patent in the remaining 27 patients. In all, left ventricular function was normal, including left ventricular end-systolic and end-diastolic pressures and volumes and left ventricular ejection fraction. Hemodynamically significant main pulmonary artery stenosis was present in five patients. Four required reoperation (all successful), and the fifth patient underwent a balloon dilatation. We are quite certain that with more extensive mobilization of the pulmonary arteries, the incidence of this complication can be avoided or significantly reduced. So far no supravalvar aortic stenosis has been identified in any of the patients, and there has been no systemic semilunar valve regurgitation. All patients are in sinus rhythm.

Based on our own experience and the reports of others, ASO in the first few weeks of life can be recommended for children born with TGA and IVS. We must more accurately define the indices by which to judge the capacity of the left ventricle to function as the systemic pump in neonates and infants with TGA and IVS.

SUGGESTED READING

Aubert J, Pannetier A, Couvelly JP, et al. Transposition of the great arteries: new technique for anatomical correction. Br Heart J 1978; 40:204–208.

Bex JP, Lecompte Y, Baillot F, Hazan E. Anatomical correction of transposition of the great arteries. Ann Thorac Surg 1980; 29:86–88.
Castaneda AR, Norwood WI, Lang P, Sanders SP. Transposition of the great arteries and intact ventricular septum: anatomical repair in the neonate. Ann Thorac Surg 1984; 38:438–442.
Jatene AD, Fontes VF, Paulista PP, et al. Successful anatomic correction of transposition of the great vessels. A preliminary report. Arq Bras Cardiol 1975; 28:461–464.
Mustard WT, Chute AL, Keith JD, et al. A surgical approach to transposition of the great vessels with extracorporeal circuit. Surgery 1954; 36:39–51.
Yacoub MH, Radley-Smith R, Maclaurin R. Two-stage operation for anatomical correction of transposition of the great arteries with intact ventricular septum. Lancet 1977; 1:1275–1278.

WOLFF-PARKINSON-WHITE SYNDROME

GERARD M. GUIRAUDON, M.D., F.R.C.S.(C), F.A.C.C.
GEORGE J. KLEIN, M.D., F.R.C.P.(C), F.A.C.C.
ARJUN D. SHARMA, M.D., F.R.C.P.(C), F.A.C.C.

Wolff, Parkinson, and White originally described the syndrome of paroxysmal tachycardia in patients with a distinctive electrocardiographic abnormality of a short P-R interval, a widened QRS complex, and a slurred initial deflection, now known as the delta wave. The electrocardiographic abnormality and the arrhythmias are caused by an accessory atrioventricular pathway consisting of working myocardial tissue. This provides abnormal electrophysiologic continuity between the atria and the ventricles in the region of the atrioventricular annulus. The most important and prevalent arrhythmias associated with the Wolff-Parkinson-White (WPW) syndrome include atrial fibrillation with a rapid ventricular response as a result of conduction over the accessory pathway, and paroxysmal atrial tachycardia or atrial-ventricular re-entrant tachycardia utilizing the accessory pathway as part of the circuit. Ventricular fibrillation is known to occur in patients with the former arrhythmia. Multicatheter electrophysiologic studies using programmed stimulation and intracardiac recording are used to define the mechanisms of the observed arrhythmias and to establish their relationship to accessory pathways. The accessory pathways are also localized anatomically with the studies. The surgical correction of the syndrome involves the identification and ablation of the offending accessory pathway(s).

INDICATIONS FOR SURGERY

Operative correction is generally recommended for the following groups of patients: (1) the patient resuscitated from ventricular fibrillation as a result of atrial fibrillation with a rapid ventricular response over the accessory pathway; (2) the patient with recurrent, disabling arrhythmias refractory to reasonable medical management, (3) the patient with problematic arrhythmias who is undergoing cardiac surgery for nonrelated indications, and (4) as an alternative therapy to any patient facing a lifelong committment to antiarrhythmic medication or an implanted device (made possible as a result of the high success rate and low morbidity of operative correction).

Antiarrhythmic drug therapy is generally the initial therapeutic consideration. It is reasonable therapy when medication is efficacious, free of significant side effects, associated with good patient compliance, and relatively inexpensive. Amiodarone is particularly efficacious in treatment of the syndrome but should be used with great caution, especially in young patients, because of the frequent and sometimes serious adverse effects and the uncertain long-term adverse effects.

Specialized antitachycardia pacemaking devices are available for patients with paroxysmal atrial-ventricular re-entrant tachycardia. These pacemakers detect the occurrence of the arrhythmia and deliver a pacing sequence to terminate it. This is acceptable therapy in patients without a risk of a rapid ventricular response over the accessory pathway in the event of atrial fibrillation. Such devices are frequently more effective with concomitant medical therapy. It is our view that surgical correction is generally preferable to a lifelong commitment to a device that treats but does not prevent tachycardia.

Ablation of bundle of His intraoperatively or by means of a catheter prevents recurrent atrial-ventricular re-entrant tachycardia in patients in whom this is the primary problem. The procedure is not indicated in patients in whom atrial fibrillation with a rapid ventricular response over the accessory pathway is the primary or a potential problem. This procedure also leaves the patient with pacemaker dependency. In our opinion, this procedure is to be recommended rarely when a surgical correction is feasible.

Catheter ablation of accessory pathways has been attempted with variable success. Potentially serious problems such as atrial rupture, cardiac tamponade, and complete heart block have been reported. Nonetheless, this currently investigational technique is promising and may one day become a procedure of choice at least for some accessory pathway locations.

Accessory pathways are classified according to their attachment to the right or left ventricle as well as their course across the atrioventricular junction. The accessory pathway may attach to the left ventricular free wall (left free wall region, 60 percent), to the posterosuperior process of the left ventricle (posterior septal region, 24 percent), to the right ventricular free wall (right ventricular free wall region, 7 percent), and to the ventricular septal region (anterior septal region, 9 percent).

Surgical Technique: The Endocardial Approach

The region of interest (coronary sulcus and/or septal region) is approached endocardially via a right or left atriotomy similar to that used for tricuspid or mitral valve surgery. The atrium is incised along its attachment onto the atrioventricular annulus, and the atrioventricular fat pad is dissected and freed of its ventricular attachment. Approaches are designed for each of four general locations of the accessory pathway. The endocardial approach necessitates opening the heart and aortic cross-clamping combined with cold cardioplegic myocardial preservation; this technique is used for anterior septal accessory pathways.

Surgical Technique: The Epicardial Approach

The epicardial approach combines two steps: (1) dissection and mobilization of the atrioventricular fat pad with exposure of the atrioventricular junction, and (2) cryoablation of the atrioventricular junction (Fig. 1). This approach is carried out on the normothermic beating heart with or without normothermic cardiopulmonary bypass. The technique is used for left ventricular free wall, posterior septal, and right ventricular accessory pathways. It is not suitable for anterior septal accessory pathways, which are usually endocardial in the parahissian region. We approach the latter region from the endocardium after epicardial dissection of the right coronary fossa to facilitate identification of landmarks.

We have used the epicardial approach since July 1982 in 175 patients. Because the surgery is carried out on the normothermic beating heart, accessory pathway and bundle of His conduction can be monitored continuously, allowing immediate assessment at the moment of ablation.

All patients undergo electrophysiologic study to confirm the presence and location of the accessory pathway and its obligatory role in the genesis of the clinical arrhythmias. All patients have a stress test as well as an echocardiographic examination. Patients with associated cardiac structural abnormality undergo standard right- and left-sided heart catheterization and angiography. Patients over 40 years of age have routine left-sided heart catheterization with coronary angiography.

A median sternotomy incision was used in most of our patients. A left thoracotomy and a median sternotomy via a bilateral submammary incision are alternate exposures in rare selected cases.

We use a hand-held exploring electrode for intraoperative electrophysiologic mapping. Ventricular mapping during normal sinus rhythm or atrial pacing is confined to the base of the ventricle around the tricuspid and mitral valve annuli over 17 predetermined sites. Retrograde atrial mapping during reciprocating tachycardia or ventricular pacing is confined to the juxta-annular atrial wall at 17 corresponding sites.

The surgery carried out on the normothermic beating heart allows repetitive electrophysiologic testing and continuous monitoring of the electrocardiogram after each surgical step. Normothermic cardiopulmonary bypass is used when the heart has to be dislocated (left free wall accessory pathway) and when the septum is approached (anterior septal accessory pathways).

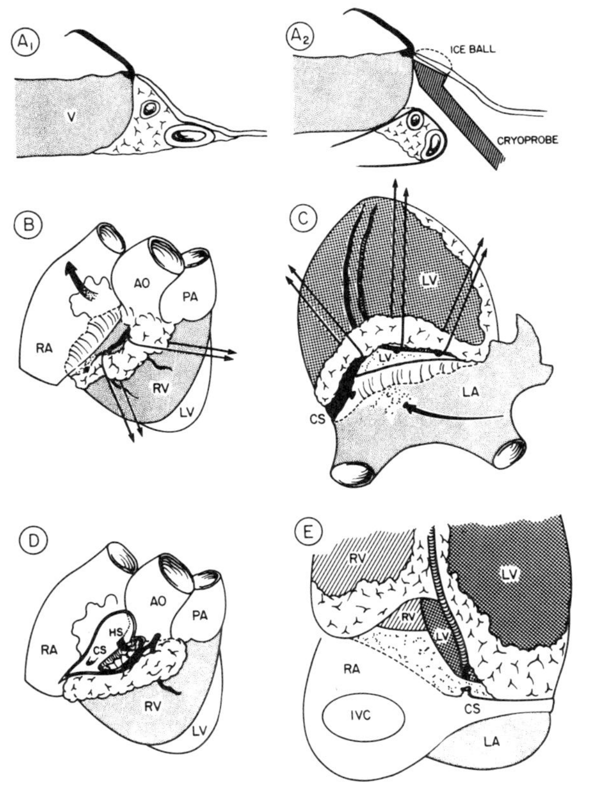

Figure 1 Surgical technique: *A*, Anatomy of the atrioventricular groove before (A_1) and after mobilization of the contents of the atrioventricular groove and application of the cryoprobe (A_2). *B*, Dissection of the right atrioventricular groove to approach the right free wall. *C*, Dislocation of the heart and dissection of the left atrioventricular groove to approach the left free wall. *D*, Dissection and exposure, including a right atriotomy, for anterior septal pathways. *E*, Dissection for posterior septal pathways. Note that a coronary venous tributary to the coronary sinus has been divided to facilitate exposure in this area. Key: Ao=aorta, CS=coronary sinus, HS=His bundle and membranous septum, IVC=inferior vena cava, LA=left atrium, RA=right atrium, PA = pulmonary artery, RV=right ventricle, and LV=left ventricle.

To attain consistent success during the first operation, complete ablation of all potential insertions of the accessory pathway onto either the ventricle or the atrium must be achieved. This includes the actual site of preexcitation as well as the adjacent areas.

Left ventricular, posterior septal, and right ventricular free wall accessory pathways course across the coronary sulcus. The atrioventricular fat pad is mobilized and the left atrioventricular junction is exposed, before cryoablation is carried out in the region of interest. The cryoprobe is applied to the atrium and onto the atrioventricular junction; freezing is accomplished at less than or equal to $-60°$ C for 2 minutes.

Anterior septal accessory pathways are mostly true septal and require a discrete approach of the membranous septum via an anterior right atriotomy along the tricuspid annulus.

PITFALLS AND POTENTIAL COMPLICATIONS

Injury to constituents of the coronary sulcus, such as a tear of the coronary sinus or of a cardiac vein, can occur; a coronary sinus diverticulum can be present in the posterior septal region (5 to 6 percent of cases) and may be injured. The circumflex coronary artery can be intramural (15 to 20 percent of cases) and easily injured. An atrial puncture may also occur.

The atrioventricular node and bundle of His are continuously monitored during dissection, and permanent heart block can be avoided.

A subendocardial accessory pathway may be present, coursing across the atrioventricular junction within the subendocardial layers. The persistence of accessory pathway conduction after adequate dissection of the atrioventricular sulcus suggests the presence of a subendocardial accessory pathway. On these rare occasions, we recommend combined epicardial and endocardial cryoablation. Most anterior septal pathways are subendocardial. Their proximity to the bundle of His requires discrete dissection of the septum.

MULTIPLE ACCESSORY PATHWAYS AND ASSOCIATED CARDIAC LESIONS

Multiple accessory pathways (7 percent of patients) are ablated in sequence.

The most common associated diseases are Ebstein's anomaly, coronary artery disease, and valvular disease. We perform accessory pathway ablation as the initial procedure with or without cardiopulmonary bypass and the associated procedure follows.

POSTOPERATIVE CARE

Before the chest is closed, a pair of temporary pacing wires is attached to each cardiac chamber; these are used for pacing and recording. Stimulation studies are performed 2 to 4 hours after surgery, 1 day and 5 to 7 days postoperatively. A daily 12-lead surface electrocardiogram is also obtained. Most patients are discharged 1 week after surgery.

Potential Postoperative Complications

Few complications have been observed in our experience, and no long-term effects. There was no mortality in a series of 175 patients.

Intraoperative and postoperative bleeding can occur either related to the median sternotomy or to coronary sulcus dissection.

Occasionally, accessory pathway conduction recurs in the postoperative period. A second unexpected accessory pathway may become manifest postoperatively in rare instances. Early reoperation may be necessary and is not associated with an increased surgical risk.

The risk of permanent heart block is minimal as well.

In all, surgical success approaches 99 percent, with no long-term complications.

CONCLUSION

The endocardial and epicardial approaches yield excellent results in terms of ablation of the accessory pathway. When the patient's anatomy permits, our preference is to use the epicardial approach. Its potential advantages include (1) continuous monitoring of pre-excitation during the dissection, allowing recognition of the moment of accessory pathway interruption and facilitating avoidance of inadvertent atrioventricular block with septal accessory pathways, and (2) cold cardioplegic cardiac arrest is not required; this also allows subsequent performance of concomitant procedures without adding to aortic cross-clamping and cardioplegic arrest time.

SUGGESTED READING

Gallagher JJ, Sealy WC, Cox JL, German LD, Kasell JH, Bardy GH, Packer DL. Results of surgery for preexcitation caused by accessory atrioventricular pathways in 267 consecutive cases. In: Josephson ME, Wellens HJJ, eds. Tachycardias—mechanisms, diagnosis, treatment. Philadelphia: Lea & Febiger, 1984:259.

Guiraudon GM, Klein GJ, Gulamhusein S, Jones DL, Yee R, Perkins DG, Jarvis E. Surgical repair of Wolff-Parkinson-White syndrome: a new closed-heart technique. Ann Thorac Surg 1984; 37:67–71.

Guiraudon GM, Klein GJ, Sharma AD, Jones DL. Surgical treatment of Wolff-Parkinson-White syndrome: the epicardial approach. In: Benditt DG, Benson DW, eds. Cardiac preexcitation syndromes. The Hague: Martinus Nijhoff Publishing, 1986:535.

Guiraudon GM, Klein GJ, Sharma AD, Milstein S, McLellan DG. Closed-heart technique for Wolff-Parkinson-White syndrome: further experience and potential limitations. Ann Thorac Surg 1986; 42:651-657.

Sealy WC, Hattler BG Jr, Blumenschein SD, Cobb FR. Surgical treatment of Wolff-Parkinson-White syndrome. Ann Thorac Surg 1969; 8:1–11.

VASCULAR RINGS

ALFRED A. deLORIMIER, M.D.

Aberrations in the formation of the embryonic double aortic system result in a variety of aortic arch anomalies. Persistence of all the segments results in a double aortic arch, whereas resorption of the right aortic arch between the right carotid and subclavian arteries produces an anomalous origin of the right subclavian artery from the distal left aorta. One of the most common anomalies occurs when the right proximal arch is incorporated into the left arch, resulting in a right innominate artery originating from the left aortic arch. Thus, the innominate artery traverses from left to right, compressing the trachea anteriorly.

Pulmonary artery sling occurs when the left pulmonary artery arises from the right pulmonary artery and encircles the right side of the trachea, coursing between the trachea and esophagus to supply the left lung.

Each of the anomalies becomes a problem when it compresses the trachea or the esophagus or both. Therefore, aortic rings and pulmonary slings produce symptoms of fixed airway obstruction consisting of inspiratory and expiratory wheezing, stridor, croup-like cough, recurrent pulmonary infections, and/or dysphagia. Apnea or an abortive sudden infant death syndrome has been related to vascular rings. Characteristically, the head and neck are held in hyperextension, and flexion of the head exaggerates the respiratory symptoms or may precipitate complete respiratory obstruction. The onset of symptoms is in early infancy in most of the patients, but there are instances in which airway compression is delayed until adulthood. Tracheomalacia and bronchomalacia are part of the anomaly; they are most severe adjacent to the anomalous vessels, but the malacia may extend to involve the entire trachea and occasionally the main bronchi.

INDICATIONS

The indication for operative correction is based upon symptoms produced by the airway compression. If anomalous anatomy is identified in the absence of symptoms, operative repair is not warranted unless a thoracotomy is necessary for some other indication. The development of symptoms beyond infancy and early childhood is exceptional.

DIAGNOSIS

The lateral chest roentgenogram shows distal tracheal compression in the anteroposterior direction. Except for the anomalous origin of the innominate or carotid artery, an esophagogram demonstrates indentation laterally and posteriorly at the level of T3 or T4. The definitive study is an arch aortogram in the anteroposterior and lateral projections. However, we prefer the cine computed tomography of the chest with intravenous contrast agent, which does not require anesthesia or sedation. Digital subtraction angiography, two-dimensional echocardiography, computed tomography, and magnetic resonance imaging are also valuable techniques to outline the anomalous anatomy. Flow-volume studies also identify fixed airway obstructions due to tracheomalacia that are intrathoracic or extrathoracic in position.

We find that bronchoscopy is an essential procedure preoperatively, and we use it intraoperatively following a correction of the obstructing vessel. Aortic rings produce tracheomalacia, and pulmonary slings are associated with stenotic complete tracheal rings that produce continuing airway obstruction in spite of relief of the vascular anomaly. The narrow, flexible fiberoptic bronchoscopes with video imaging and recording can be passed through an endotracheal tube, and this greatly facilitates identifying the severity of the airway obstruction. If there is a very narrow airway because of complete tracheal rings, which are associated with pulmonary artery sling, the preferred operation is probably tracheal resection. The left pulmonary artery may then be displaced to the left of the trachea rather than dividing the vessel and anastomosing it in a normal position.

SURGICAL TREATMENT

Double Aortic Arch

Through a fourth intercostal space posterolateral thoracotomy, the mediastinal pleura is incised anterior to the vagus nerve, and that part of the arch encircling the esophagus posteriorly is initially mobilized. The phrenic and recurrent laryngeal nerves are identified and preserved. The most narrowed portion of the double arch is dissected free of the surrounding mediastinal structures, and vascular clamps are placed proximal and distal to the narrowing of the vessels. If a narrowed segment between the ascending aorta and the carotid arteries (very rare) or between the carotid and subclavian arteries is encountered, the adequacy of blood flow in these vessels can be confirmed by Doppler determinations of blood pressures in both upper extremities before and after a clamp is applied to identify possible impairment of perfusion and, by inference, possible cerebral ischemia.

The narrowed portion of the arch is divided between the vascular clamps and oversewn with 4–0 or 5–0 nonabsorbable sutures. At the same time the ligamentum arteriosum or ductus arteriosus is divided. To ensure that fibrous tissues surrounding the esophagus and trachea are not contributing to continued narrowing, the vessels are dissected off the esophagus circumferentially. Most surgeons advocate extensive dissection of the major vessels off the trachea as well. However, tracheomalacia is characteristically a part of the anomaly, and we prefer to leave the fibrous attachments between the aorta and the trachea. The aorta may then be approximated to the posterior surface of the sternum, and the residual fibrous attachments to the trachea serve to pull it into an open position. In addition, we have reoperated on infants who have had division of a double aortic arch in whom the airway obstruction was not relieved because the divided end of the arch became adherent behind the esophagus, thereby resulting in a persistent constricting band. To avoid continued tracheal compression or tracheomalacia or recurrence of a constricting band, an aortopexy is accomplished by approximating the ascending aortic arch and the minor portion of the double aortic arch to the posterior sternum. Interrupted 3–0 nonabsorbable sutures are placed in the adventitia of the aorta and the periosteum of the posterior surface of the sternum. In this way, the trachea can be pulled to a widely patent position. A broader, more secure aortopexy can be accomplished by using a Dacron patch sutured to the ascending aorta. The patch covers the anterior 20 to 30 percent of the aortic circumference using multiple 4–0 nonabsorbable sutures to the adventitia. Then 2–0 or 3–0 nonabsorbable sutures in two or more rows are placed through the patch and the posterior sternal periosteum. Fiberoptic bronchoscopy is then performed to identify whether the tracheal lumen has been enlarged and whether persistent compression on the left or right anterior trachea warrants placement of additional aortopexy sutures to correct this.

Right-Sided Arch with Left Ligamentum Arteriosum

A right-sided aortic arch with a persistent left ligamentum can produce a constricting ring about the trachea and esophagus. Through a left fourth interspace thoracotomy, the ligamentum or ductus is divided and the esophagus is then mobilized circumferentially to relieve any fibrous constricting bands. The narrow diameter, flexible fiberoptic bronchoscope is then passed down the endotracheal tube to visualize the lower trachea and identify whether additional mobilization or aortopexy will be necessary to further enlarge the airway.

Anomalous Origin of the Innominate Artery

Compression of the trachea by an anomalous origin of the innominate artery (originating to the left of the trachea) from a left-sided arch is relieved by pulling the offending innominate artery anteriorly and away from the trachea. This is accomplished through a left fourth intercostal space thoracotomy. Once again, we do not dissect the fibrous attachments between the innominate artery and the trachea. As with aortopexy and the double aortic arch, a Dacron patch can be sutured to the innominate artery; this provides a broad, secure base for suture approximation of the innominate artery to the posterior sternal periosteum. The procedure will pull the collapsed trachea into an open position. Sometimes when sutures in the innominate adventitia are placed along the left side, the airway is distracted in an irregular configuration or only the left anterior portion of the trachea is opened and the right side remains compressed. The results of this procedure should be confirmed by fiberoptic bronchoscopy through the endotracheal tube before the chest is closed.

Anomalous Origin of Subclavian Artery

Dysphagia lusoria is a term used specifically for compression of the esophagus by the right subclavian artery originating anomalously from the distal left-sided aortic arch. Division of this vessel at its origin through a left thoracotomy incision has been advocated by most surgeons. There has been interest in using a right thoracotomy to divide the vessel at its origin with the intent of anastomosing it to the side of the aorta or carotid artery, in order to preserve optimum arterial supply to the right arm. However, it is often difficult to approximate the divided subclavian artery to the aorta and accomplish an anastomosis in small children. There are very few reports of ischemia to the arm because extensive collaterals usually develop, and therefore there is little reason to attempt anastomosis. However, the right thoracotomy approach is preferred by us because the subclavian artery can easily be pulled away from the retroesophageal position and sutured to the right of the esophagus. This maneuver avoids the reforming of a fibrous constricting band posterior to the esophagus after division of the vessel.

Right Aortic Arch and Left Ligamentum Arteriosum

Compression of the esophagus and the trachea due to a ductus arteriosus or ligamentum arteriosum from a right-sided aorta to left pulmonary artery is best approached by a left fourth intercostal space thoracotomy. After division of the ligamentum, the esophagus should be mobilized from fibrous bands. If tracheal compression from the aorta is evident by intraoperative fiberoptic bronchoscopy, an aortopexy may be necessary.

Pulmonary Sling

Anomalous origin of the left pulmonary artery may produce tracheal and right main bronchus compression and tracheomalacia, but in our experience, more frequently there is an association with complete tracheal rings. The trachea is usually elongated with more than the normal 13 or 14 tracheal rings. Bronchoscopy is imperative in order to assess whether the airway is compressed by the anomalous vessel or more likely if the compression is due to progressive, funneled narrowing by the complete rings from the cricoid cartilage to the carina.

If intrinsic tracheal ring narrowing is present, resection of the tracheal narrowing with displacement of the pulmonary artery to the left is the procedure of choice. In the case of an elongated trachea, a median sternotomy does not provide exposure to the distal trachea, and a right thoracotomy is preferred.

When the anomalous pulmonary artery is producing extrinsic compression, which is not associated with complete tracheal rings, a median sternotomy provides the best exposure to the pulmonary artery and its branches. A left fourth intercostal space thoracotomy may be used, but it is more difficult to gain access and divide the origin of the left pulmonary artery between the trachea and the esophagus, and the phrenic nerve frequently compromises the exposure. Anticoagulation with heparin, 1 mg per kilogram, is given intravenously to prevent thrombosis following division of the pulmonary artery. The left pulmonary artery is mobilized, then divided at its origin between clamps, and the proximal end is oversewn with fine nonabsorbable sutures. The left pulmonary artery is then brought to the left and anterior to the trachea and approximated to the main pulmonary artery where there is the least amount of tension. A partial occlusion clamp applied to the left lateral wall of the main pulmonary artery then allows a small portion of the vessel wall to be excised in an elliptical fashion. An end-to-side anastomosis is accomplished with a nonabsorbable running 5-0 suture in the posterior wall and interrupted fine silk sutures anteriorly to avoid stenosis from developing.

RESULTS

Morbidity from the surgical treatment of various anomalies comprising vascular rings is unusual. Recurrent laryngeal and phrenic nerve palsy develop from excessive traction on these nerves. Dissection in the posterior mediastinum may result in the division of the thoracic duct or its tributaries, producing chylothorax. Following division of anomalous vessels, vascular insufficiency of the upper extremities or of carotid artery distribution has not been described. More than 75 percent of the patients can be extubated at the termination of the procedure. However, 10 to 15 percent of those infants with associated tracheomalacia have been reported to require prolonged endotracheal tube or tracheostomy support of the malacic airway. Therefore, the use of intraoperative bronchoscopy and an aortopexy must be considered as part of the operative procedure. Occasionally, it is necessary to perform tracheal resection for localized tracheomalacia or to place a rib cartilage graft to support an extensive length of tracheomalacia. Many of these patients have stridor for months or years postoperatively because of the residual tracheomalacia. The mortality rate is less than 5 percent and this is usually due to associated congenital heart disease and occasionally to uncontrolled bleeding caused by the fracture of an exceptionally fragile vessel when it is clamped for suture ligation.

CONCLUSION

Most of the tracheal and esophageal compressions produced by aortic arch anomalies that result in encircling rings readily respond to the measures of simple division of the ring. However, there are any number of instances in which external compression remains or the trachea is intrinsically abnormal. Intraoperative bronchoscopy is a very important adjunct to evaluate the adequacy of the procedure. If intrinsic airway narrowing persists, it may be relieved by additional sutures in an aortopexy or innominate artery-pexy to the sternum. Otherwise, a definitive surgical repair of the intrinsic tracheal anomaly is required.

SUGGESTED READING

Arciniegas E, Hakami M, Hertzler JH, Farooki ZQ, Green WE. Surgical management of congenital vascular rings. J Thorac Cardiovasc Surg 1979; 77:721–727.

Julsrud PR, Ehman RL. Magnetic resonance imaging of vascular rings. Mayo Clin Proc 1986; 61:181–185.

Richardson JV, Doty DB, Rossi NP, Ehrenhaft JL. Operation for aortic arch anomalies. Ann Thorac Surg 1981; 31:426–432.

Roesler M, de Leval M, Chrispin A, Stark J. Surgical management of vascular ring. Ann Surg 1983; 197:139–146.

Tonkin IL, Gold RE, Moser D, Laster RE Jr. Evaluation of vascular rings with digital subtraction angiography. AJR 1984; 142:1287–1291.

SELECTION AND POST-OPERATIVE MANAGEMENT OF PROSTHETIC VALVES IN CHILDREN

DARRYL SHORE, F.R.C.S.

Following insertion of a prosthetic valve, the child or adolescent is subject to all the complications of valvular prostheses that apply in adults. However, in addition, there are problems specific to the child or adolescent that must be carefully considered when selecting valvular prostheses for use in this age group. These are:

1. Insertion of a prosthesis of adequate size.
2. Somatic growth of the individual, resulting in patient-valve mismatch.
3. The problem of long-term anticoagulation in childhood and adolescence.
4. Accelerated calcification of xenograft valves.

SELECTION OF VALVE SIZE

In one large retrospective study of valve replacement in children, when the sizes of prostheses inserted were closely examined, it was apparent that many of the valves were stenotic from the time of insertion. It is therefore essential when approaching valve replacement in a child or adolescent to have a knowledge of the appropriate normal valve area of the one being replaced according to the patient's weight or body surface area. This information is available from anatomic tables, and by using these guidelines and a knowledge of the effective orifice area for the size and type of prosthesis selected, the insertion of a valve of inadequate size can be avoided. A rational choice of prosthesis can then be made, and the need for annulus enlargement or for the insertion of a valve in the supra-annular position can be assessed.

SOMATIC GROWTH AND PATIENT-VALVE MISMATCH

An obvious problem associated with valve replacement in childhood and adolescence is that as body weight and surface area increase, transprosthetic gradients will increase. In fact, it is surprising how infrequently this problem has been reported, for the following reasons. (1) In some cases it has been possible to insert a prosthesis large enough to accommodate growth by the use of techniques for annulus enlargement, by the insertion of valves in the supra-annular position, or because dilation of the annulus has been part of the valvular pathology. (2) At times reoperation has been necessary prior to the time that it might be required as a result of somatic growth because of the occurrence of stenosis secondary to the accelerated calcification of tissue valves or because of pannus formation. However, the potential problem of increasing patient-valve mismatch that occurs with growth should influence surgical technique and choice of prosthesis.

It has also been reported that insertion of too large a mitral prosthesis can produce left ventricular outflow tract obstruction, most notably in cases of atrioventricular septal defect. Another complication of attempting to insert too large a prosthesis in the mitral position has been the production of atrioventricular dissociation.

LONG-TERM ANTICOAGULATION IN CHILDREN

Some authors have suggested that the thromboembolic complications of prosthetic valves occur less frequently in children and that the risks to the child of long-term anticoagulation are greater than those of thromboembolism. It is difficult to draw any conclusions from the data presented in the literature in support of the necessity for anticoagulation following insertion of a mechanical valve in children. This is largely because of variation among reported series in anticoagulation regimens, in the degree of therapeutic compliance (about which there is often little or no information), and in the use of antiplatelet drugs as alternatives to warfarin or dicumarol. Certainly there is no convincing evidence that the incidence of thromboembolic complications of valvular prostheses is lower in children than in adults. One previous claim that children in whom St. Jude Medical mechanical prostheses had been inserted could be maintained without warfarin or dicumarol therapy without an increase in the incidence of thromboembolic complications has been recently withdrawn. In my view, all patients in whom mechanical prostheses have been inserted should be on anticoagulation therapy with warfarin or dicumarol. However this is not always possible, for example in many third-world countries where medical supervision after surgery is not possible. In the selection of valves for use in children and adolescents, it should be borne in mind that long-term anticoagulation may seriously interfere with the normal activities of childhood. The child's personality, social background, and the likelihood of compliance with anticoagulant regimens should be considered. In addition, the teratogenic effect of anticoagulants should be borne in mind when replacing valves in adolescent females.

CHOICE OF PROSTHESIS IN CHILDREN AND ADOLESCENTS

Premature valve calcification in glutaraldehyde-preserved bioprostheses implanted in children has been widely reported, and thus, the use of these valves in pediatric and adolescent age groups has been largely abandoned. The onset of calcification in glutaraldehyde-preserved valve tissue has been delayed by preparation of the tissue with surfactant. This has been demonstrated in experimental animals, but so far such methods have not been shown to be clinically effective.

Aortic Valve Replacement

Antibiotic-sterilized or fresh aortic homograft valves inserted without a stent into the aortic position have an extended life when compared with commercial bioprostheses available at present. Excellent functional results and a probability of reoperation of 20 percent at 8 years make them a real alternative to mechanical prostheses for use in the aortic position, particularly in the small aortic root. If a mechanical valve is used, the St. Jude Medical valve prosthesis should be selected because in the aortic position it has been shown to have favorable hemodynamic function in the 19 mm and 21 mm sizes. In congenital aortic stenosis, supra-annular and annular enlargement may be necessary in order to insert a 19 mm valve. In patients with tunnel-like obstruction of the aortic ring and subaortic region, it may be necessary to incise the entire aortic root with its supravalvar component and to perform an aortic root replacement with an aortic homograft. An adult aortic homograft can usually be inserted and so will accommodate patient growth.

Mitral Valve Replacement

In children requiring mitral valve replacement, we prefer the St. Jude Medical mechanical prosthesis because of its low profile and good orifice-to-annulus ratio. Because there is no satisfactory method of enlarging the annulus unless aortic valve replacement is also performed, the valve may have to be placed in the supra-annular position, particularly in cases of congenital mitral stenosis. In cases of atrioventricular septal defect supra-annular positioning of the valve is advisable to avoid producing left ventricular outflow tract obstruction.

Tricuspid Valve Replacement

We feel the valve of choice for the tricuspid position is a stent-mounted aortic or pulmonary homograft valve. If these are not available, the St. Jude Medical valve should be selected for its optimal hemodynamic performance. In some series, but not all, good long-term results have been reported with the Starr-Edwards mechanical prosthesis in the tricuspid position.

Pulmonary Valve Replacement

The valve of choice for the pulmonary position is a homograft pulmonary or aortic valve.

POSTOPERATIVE MANAGEMENT

The management of the cardiovascular system proceeds along conventional lines, and a detailed description is outside the scope of this chapter. However, certain points are worthy of special mention:

1. All patients must have two atrial and ventricular pacing wires attached at the time of surgery.
2. In patients with long-standing mitral valve disease or an elevated pulmonary vascular resistance, a catheter should be left in the pulmonary artery to monitor pulmonary artery pressure.
3. In low output states, inadequate repair of associated congenital anomalies must be excluded by Doppler echocardiography or if necessary, by cardiac catheterization.
4. If valve malfunction is suspected as a cause of low output, this can usually be excluded by Doppler echocardiography. The transprosthetic gradients can be measured and regurgitant jets detected.
5. Dynamic subvalvular obstruction may be responsible for low output states after aortic valve replacement. This usually responds to expansion of the intravascular volume. Occasionally the use of beta-blockers may be necessary.

Long-Term Postoperative Management

All patients with mechanical prostheses are given a loading dose of warfarin on the evening of the first postoperative day. During the period of hospitalization, the maintenance dose is adjusted to maintain the INR between 2.5 and 3.5. Before the patient leaves the hospital, a Doppler echocardiographic study is performed to exclude any prosthetic valve malfunction and to measure any transprosthetic gradient. This provides a record that can be compared with those obtained at subsequent examinations. Valve malfunction can therefore be detected early and the timing of reoperations planned to avoid myocardial degeneration, pulmonary hypertension, or hepatic dysfunction. In patients in whom a St. Jude Medical valve has been inserted, it is possible to detect valve malfunction by cinefluoroscopic studies that measure minimal and maximal interleaflet angles. It has been reported that abnormal leaflet motion has been restored to normal by an alteration in anticoagulant therapy.

Serial electrocardiograms, and in older children, serial exercise testing, should be performed to follow the clinical course.

RESULTS

The selection of prosthetic valves for use in children and adolescents as outlined above is derived more from dissatisfaction with the results obtained with previously used prostheses rather than from good statistical evidence favoring one particular prosthetic valve.

Several problems are encountered in any analysis of results obtained after insertion of prosthetic valves in childhood with a view to comparing prosthetic valve performance. One of them relates to the wide variation in patient population. For example, the 24 percent hospital mortality rate reported in a Great Ormond Street series was considerably higher than that reported in contemporary series; however, in the first study the mean age of the patients was considerably lower and the percentage of patients with complex congenital heart disease was considerably higher. In a logistic analysis of the short-term risk factors, both young age and the complexity of the congenital heart disease independently increased the risk of hospital death. In none of the 12 patients who died was it possible to incriminate valve failure as the primary cause of death.

The characteristics of the patient population clearly also affect long-term results. In some cases it is difficult to be certain which is the primary cause of death, the underlying disease or valve malfunction, for example, when thromboembolic obstruction of a prosthetic valve occurs in the setting of a low output state. Differences in postoperative management, follow-up, and therapeutic compliance add to the difficulties. In the Great Ormond Street series, the chance of being free of a major thromboembolic episode at 5 years was 59±20 percent

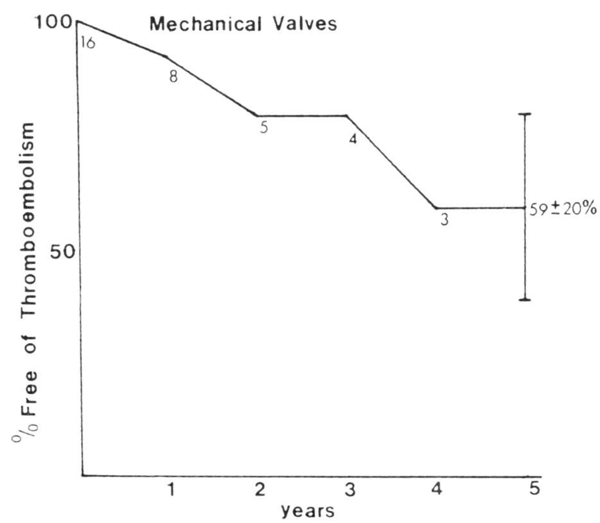

Figure 1 Actuarial freedom from thromboembolic complications, expressed as a percentage of total number of patients.

(Fig. 1), but at least three of the major thromboembolic episodes occurred in patients who were not on anticoagulation therapy. This high incidence of thromboembolic phenomena is in stark contrast to other reports that claim low thromboembolic rates after valve replacement in the pediatric age group. On the other hand, frequent hemorrhagic episodes reported by others were not seen in the Great Ormond Street series.

One type of valve failure that has not been difficult to define is the calcific degeneration of glutaraldehyde-preserved bioprostheses. In the analysis of the Great Ormond Street results, it was calculated that 5 years after insertion only 27±15 percent of bioprosthetic valves would not have been replaced (Fig. 2). There appears to be a sudden acceleration in bioprosthetic valve failure after 3 years. Many other reports have included identical data, and there have been additional reports of much earlier bioprosthetic valve degeneration. As stated previously, data such as these have led to most units abandoning the use of bioprosthetic valves in the pediatric and adolescent age groups. Because of the high incidence of thromboembolic rates with use of the Björk-Shiley valve and the high incidence of calcific degeneration of the bioprosthetic valves in the Great Ormond Street series in 1983, I adopted the use of the St. Jude Medical bileaflet valve in children because of its low profile, low thrombogenicity, and good annular-to-orifice ratio. All patients were maintained on warfarin after valve insertion. The fresh antibiotic-sterilized homograft was considered an alternative in the aortic position and was also used for pulmonary valve replacement. As yet the numbers involved in a small personal series of patients, 13 in all (three mitral, three pulmonary, and 6 aortic valve replacements, including three homografts) are too small and the follow-up period too short to produce any meaningful statistical results. However, the short-term results have encouraged us to continue with this policy of valve selection. There have been no late deaths and no documented thromboembolic episodes.

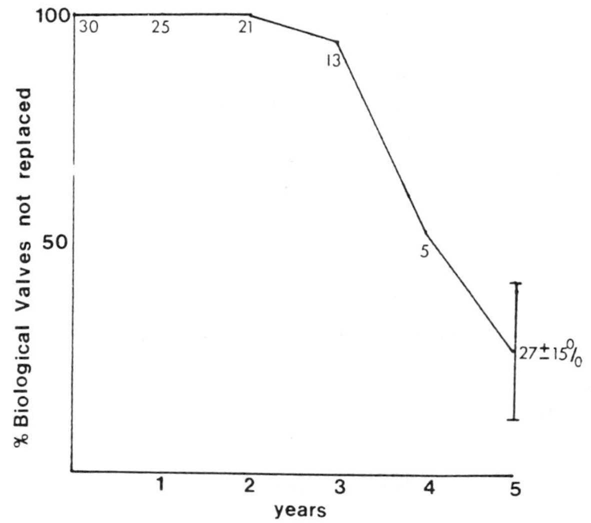

Figure 2 Percentage of patients who received bioprosthetic valves who have not had valves replaced, calculated by actuarial methods.

SUGGESTED READING

Crawford FA, Sade RM. The St. Jude Medical prosthesis in children without anticoagulation. Proceedings of the Fifth International Symposium on Heart Valves. Fort Lauderdale, Fla: April 1987.

Radley-Smith R, Fagan A, Yacoub M. An eleven year experience of fresh aortic homograft replacement in children. Am J Cardiol 1982; 49:1035.

Rowlatt JF, Rimoldi HJA, Lev M. The quantitative anatomy of the normal child's heart. Pediatr Clin North Am 1963; 10:499–588.

Shore DF, De Leval MR, Stark J. Valve replacement in children: biologic versus mechanical valves. Proceedings of the Second International Symposium on Cardiac Bioprostheses, Rome, 1982. Yorke Medical, 1982:238–247.

EXTRACORPOREAL MEMBRANE OXYGENATION FOR INFANTS AND CHILDREN

DANIEL P. RYAN, M.D.

In 1975 Bartlett and associates reported the first successful application of venoarterial extracorporeal membrane oxygenation (ECMO) in a newborn with meconium aspiration syndrome. Despite the discouraging results of the National Institutes of Health trial of ECMO in older patients, the efficacy of this technique in neonates has been demonstrated. At the present time ECMO has become a standard method of neonatal respiratory support in selected patients in over 40 centers across the United States.

INDICATIONS

Neonates who may be helped by this technique have persistent pulmonary hypertension of the newborn, also called persistent fetal circulation, as the major underlying pathophysiologic mechanism of respiratory failure regardless of the underlying disease process. The diseases that can lead to persistent pulmonary hypertension of the newborn include meconium aspiration, respiratory distress syndrome, congenital diaphragmatic hernia, primary pulmonary hypertension, and neonatal sepsis. The pulmonary vasculature in the neonate is very reactive to hypoxia, hypercarbia, and acidosis and responds with vasoconstriction. Increased pulmonary vascular resistance leads to reopening of the fetal shunts through the ductus arteriosus and the foramen ovale, resulting in significant right-to-left shunting; a cycle of worsening hypoxia and acidosis is thus started. The usual therapy consists of mechanical ventilation, pharmacologically induced paralysis, opiate sedation, induced respiratory alkalosis, and vasodilator therapy, but approximately 2 to 5 percent of neonates fail to respond. In addition, the use of high-pressure ventilation may paradoxically worsen the situation by decreasing venous return and cardiac output. High-pressure ventilation and high oxygen concentrations lead to barotrauma and oxygen toxicity that are both related to the development of chronic respiratory failure. ECMO, by providing tissue oxygenation and cardiac assist, can reverse the pulmonary vasospasm and support the child while the pulmonary pathology resolves, and at the same time, it avoids the deleterious effects of conventional treatment.

Retrospective criteria have been used to identify those neonates with respiratory failure who are at the highest risk of dying and are therefore candidates for ECMO. The two most commonly used methods are the postductal alveolar-arterial oxygen gradient ($D(A=a)O_2$) and an oxygenation index ($OI = [\text{mean airway pressure} \times FIO_2 \times 100]/PaO_2$) that takes into account the danger of high ventilator pressure. Having a $D(A\text{-}a)O_2$ of 620 mm Hg for 6 to 12 hours or an oxygenation index over 40 predicts a mortality of 85 percent in most centers. In addition, patients with acute deterioration or signs of severe barotrauma may be candidates before reaching these strict criteria levels.

Besides the neonatal population, there are occasional older children who may be helped by ECMO support. Some forms of viral pneumonia causing overwhelming respiratory failure have been treated with ECMO with occasional success. Children who are unable to be weaned from cardiopulmonary bypass or have acute deterioration following surgery for congenital heart disease also may be helped by ECMO. Nearly half of the patients who were treated with ECMO following cardiac surgery survived.

CONTRAINDICATIONS

The most common contraindication to ECMO support relates to the risk of intracranial hemorrhage. Early experience showed that the groups with the highest risk are the premature infants with a birth weight below 2 kg or an estimated gestational age of below 34 weeks. The presence of a pre-existing intracranial hemorrhage is also a contraindication because of the risk of extension due to the anticoagulation required. Other contraindications include profound neurologic impairment, congenital anomalies or conditions not compatible with meaningful quality of life, and irreversible lung disease such as severe bronchopulmonary dysplasia. Patients with congenital diaphragmatic hernia and severe pulmonary hypoplasia as defined by the lack of ever having adequate oxygenation are not candidates for ECMO support. Patients with major cardiac anomalies should be treated operatively, although they may be supported with ECMO until surgical correction or palliation can be achieved. Each patient being considered for ECMO support should undergo cranial ultrasonography and echocardiography to determine the presence of intracranial hemorrhage and structural heart defects.

TECHNIQUE

In the ECMO circuit venous blood is drained by gravity siphon from the right atrium to a small distensible bladder reservoir. The bladder volume is monitored by a servoregulator microswitch that turns off the roller pump if the venous drainage is inadequate for the pump flow. The pumping force is provided by an occlusive roller pump, and a silicone rubber membrane lung (Kolobow Sci-Med) is standard for long-term perfusion. In the neonatal population the 0.8 m^2 membrane lung is adequate for the anticipated maximal flows of 120 to 170 ml per kilogram per minute. The priming volume is approximately 400 ml or nearly twice the blood volume of the neonate; the priming solution is carefully adjusted for pH, temperature, hematocrit, and platelet count prior to initiating bypass.

The patients are placed on ECMO while in the neonatal intensive care area. The surgery is done under lidocaine anesthesia, fentanyl or morphine sedation, and muscle paralysis to prevent air embolism while the venous cannula is being placed. It is important to keep the head in a midline position during and just after cannulation to prevent kinking of the left internal jugular vein, which can cause severe intracranial venous hypertension and may contribute to cerebral edema and intracranial hemorrhage. Venoarterial access is gained through a right-sided neck approach via the internal jugular vein and the common carotid artery. The venous cannula is No. 12 to 16 F and is positioned so that the tip lies well within the right atrium. The right common carotid artery is ligated below the bifurcation, and a No. 8 to 12 F cannula is positioned with its tip just within the aortic arch. The cannula position is determined with the help of a chest x-ray film before starting bypass.

The neck dissection is done using good hemostasis to prevent late hemorrhage while the patient is anticoagulated. The neonate is given 100 U per kilogram of heparin prior to cannulation and is maintained on a heparin drip of 30 to 60 U per kilogram per hour to maintain the activated clotting time in the 220 to 240 sec range (normal 100 sec). After starting ECMO, the flow through the circuit is slowly increased until the infant is on full cardiopulmonary bypass. At this point the pressors are weaned and the ventilator settings are reduced to minimal values to provide "lung rest." Typical settings are FIO_2 of 0.25, peak inspiratory pressure of 20 mm Hg, positive end expiratory pressure of 5 mm Hg, and a rate of 15 breaths per minute. The infants are allowed to wake up and are sedated only as needed.

Blood flow through the circuit is maintained at a level to keep the venous saturation over 70 percent, indicating adequate tissue perfusion. The PaO_2 is maintained between 55 to 70 mm Hg and is adjusted by manipulating the ECMO blood flow rate. The PCO_2 is maintained between 35 and 45 mm Hg and is regulated by adding CO_2 to the gas flow to the membrane lung.

During the first 1 to 2 days of full ECMO support, the patient's pulmonary function worsens, as manifested by bilateral "white-out" of the lung fields on chest x-ray film and diminished breath sounds on examination. Over the next few days the lungs should clear. The ECMO flow is slowly weaned to a level of about 30 ml per minute as the lungs improve. The mean length of time on ECMO is 5 days, with a range of 3 to 16 days. When the infant is tolerating low flows, a trial off ECMO is done for 4 to 8 hours with the cannulas still in place. If no deterioration occurs, the cannulas are removed, again using local anesthesia and pharmacologic muscle paralysis. The vessels are ligated in the neck, and no repair is attempted because of the risk of embolism. Following removal from ECMO, the patients are usually weaned from the ventilator and extubated in 1 to 3 days.

RESULTS

The complications of ECMO are primarily related to the anticoagulation. Spontaneous intracranial hemorrhage and gastrointestinal and retroperitoneal bleeding have occurred. Tight control of the heparin dose by close monitoring of the activated clotting time on an hourly basis can prevent most of the problems. Bleeding may also occur at any previous surgical site, but it is seen most commonly in the neck. Hemorrhage is treated by lowering the activated clotting time to the 180 to 200 sec range and transfusing platelets to keep the count over 100,000 per mm^3 or more. Exploration of any surgical sites should be done to stop any continued local bleeding and is usually successful. In the case of intracranial hemorrhage, the only alternative is to rapidly wean the patient from ECMO and remove the cannulas before reversing the heparin. The rate of intracranial hemorrhage is 5 to 15 percent, and major bleeding from other sites occurs in 15 to 25 percent of patients.

Technical complications within the circuit have occurred with each component. Now that the system has become standardized, technical problems are uncommon. The oxygenators usually last 6 to 10 days before they need to be replaced. If a technical problem occurs, the infant is placed back on the high ventilator settings and taken off of ECMO until the problem is corrected, usually resulting in only a temporary period of instability and rarely causing the death of the child.

The other complications that have been seen are related to the state of the patient prior to starting ECMO. These include cardiac arrest, global myocardial dysfunction, renal failure, hepatic failure, fluid overload, and hypertension. The hypertension is related to a high renin state and is treated with vasodilators and captopril; it usually resolves by the time the patients are weaned from ECMO. Fluid overload and renal failure have been treated successfully with ultrafiltration or dialysis in the ECMO circuit.

The survival of patients treated with ECMO is now in the 85 to 90 percent range. The outcome is related to the primary diagnosis, with meconium aspiration approaching 100 percent survival and sepsis or congenital diaphragmatic hernia resulting in 55 to 70 percent survival.

The outlook for the survivors is also quite good. In follow-up studies the patients seem to fall into a normal distribution of all neonatal intensive care unit survivors, with normal test results in 70 to 80 percent of the children; 20 to 30 percent have mild to severe handicaps. The exact cause of the problems is not clear and may be related to the severe hypoxia and hypotension many of the patients have prior to starting ECMO support; it also may be due to the treatment itself. There have been only occasional reports of focal neurologic problems that can be related to the carotid artery and internal jugular vein ligation. Follow-up flow studies with noninvasive Doppler or radionuclide brain scans have been normal.

SUGGESTED READING

Bartlett RH, Gazzaniga AB, Jefferies MR, et al. Extracorporeal membrane oxygenation (ECMO) cardiopulmonary support in infancy. Trans Am Soc Artif Intern Organs 1976; 22:80–93.

Bartlett RH, Gazzangia A, Toomasian J, et al. Extracorporeal membrane oxygenation (ECMO) in neonatal respiratory failure: 100 cases. Ann Surg 1986; 204:236–245.

Bartlett RH, Roloff DW, Cornell RG, et al. Extracorporeal circulation in neonatal respiratory failure: a prospective randomized study. Pediatrics 1985; 76:479–487.

Hirschl RB, Bartlett RH. Extracorporeal membrane oxygenation support in cardiorespiratory failure. Adv Surg 1987; 21:189–212.

Kanter KR, Pennington G, Weber TR, et al. Extracorporeal membrane oxygenation support for postoperative cardiac support in children. J Thorac Cardiovasc Surg 1987; 93:27–35.

PERCUTANEOUS INTERVENTION IN CONGENITAL HEART DISEASE

JEAN S. KAN, M.D.

Transluminal balloon valvuloplasty has only recently been applied in the management of children with congenital heart disease. Based on the successful application of the technique in peripheral vascular and coronary artery disease and on preliminary research in animal models, several of the congenital cardiac malformations have been shown to be amenable to balloon angioplasty.

Indications for balloon angioplasty include (1) a simplified alternative to more invasive cardiac surgery (e.g., pulmonary valve stenosis, coarctation of the aorta, coarctation restenosis); (2) palliation in an attempt to defer surgical intervention until a later time (e.g., aortic valve stenosis, systemic to pulmonary artery shunt stenosis, restrictive atrial septal defect in transposition of the great arteries, or hypoplastic right-sided heart or hypoplastic left-sided heart); or (3) when surgical repair is uniformly unsuccessful (e.g., pulmonary vein stenosis).

Basic principles of balloon angioplasty in congenital heart disease are similar to those in other applications and include considerations such as selection of balloon size, inflation pressure, duration of inflation, and the need for immediate and long-term anticoagulation. The technique varies according to the lesion and the institution at which it is performed.

PULMONARY VALVE STENOSIS

The largest collective experience in balloon dilation procedures in congenital heart disease has been in the treatment of congenital pulmonary valve stenosis. Age of patients has been from the neonatal period to the eighth decade. The technique is the same for all ages. The dimension of the pulmonary valve annulus is measured from the cineangiogram with correction for magnification, using the angiographic catheter dimension to determine the magnification factor. Balloon size is selected at 100 to 125 percent of the annulus dimension. A No. 7 F flow directed catheter is positioned in the left pulmonary artery (LPA). A 0.035 inch exchange guidewire is advanced through the catheter and left in place in the LPA as the catheter is removed. The balloon catheter is advanced over the guidewire and positioned with the balloon straddling the stenotic valve. Arterial pressure is monitored through an indwelling arterial cannula. The balloon is inflated with dilute contrast medium (1:3 or less to decrease viscosity and increase the rate of inflation and deflation) until the "waisting" of the balloon by the stenotic valve is resolved. Contrast material is then rapidly withdrawn from the balloon; the inflation-deflation cycle is less than 6 seconds. If there is a delay in balloon evacuation or a fall in systemic blood pressure, the balloon may be advanced into the dilated main pulmonary artery as the evacuation process is completed. The balloon is then positioned across the valve and reinflated rapidly to verify the absence of "waisting," suggesting that the valve has been adequately opened.

Heparin (100 U per kilogram) is administered during the catheterization and balloon procedure. Long-term anticoagulation medication is not given.

Infundibular hypertrophy in cases of severe pulmonary stenosis (with suprasystemic right ventricular pressure) may result in acute outflow obstruction after a seemingly successful valvuloplasty—a situation also seen after surgical valvotomy described as "suicide right ventricle." Administration of propranolol prior to the valvuloplasty may prevent significant sequelae. A maintenance dosage of propranolol for several months after the procedure may be indicated to prevent obstruction as the muscular hypertrophy gradually regresses.

Dysplastic pulmonary valves as commonly seen in children with Noonan's syndrome do not appear to be amenable to balloon valvuloplasty and require surgical intervention.

Improvement in the systolic pressure gradient after balloon valvuloplasty appears to be comparable to that achieved after open heart surgery for pulmonary valve stenosis. Pulmonary valve regurgitation occurs infrequently and can be detected by Doppler 2-D echocardiography in only a few patients. The femoral vein through which the balloon was inserted was shown to be patent in those patients who had repeat catheterizations. There has been minor discomfort on insertion of the large balloon catheter into the femoral vein but no major complications. Rhythm disturbances include sinus bradycardia and premature ventricular contractions and may be managed by pacing or atropine administration.

Pulmonary valvuloplasty may be performed as an outpatient procedure.

AORTIC VALVE STENOSIS

Application of balloon valvuloplasty to aortic valve stenosis is an obvious extension of the technique. However, the potential for risk is considerable. Competence of the aortic valve after the valvuloplasty determines the interval until inevitable valve replacement is indicated. Balloon size is selected at 1 to 2 mm less than the annulus dimension to minimize the risk of annulus rupture and avulsion of the aortic valve. The large dilation balloon may not easily pass percutaneously into the femoral artery without injury to the vessel. Two smaller balloon catheters may be advanced from bilateral femoral arteries and positioned side by side across the stenotic aortic valve. In addition to minimizing injury to access vessels, the two-balloon technique provides for flow from the left ventricle to the aorta along the margins of the balloons during balloon inflation. Rapid inflation and deflation of the balloon are essential to avoid major disruption of the systemic pressure and flow. After valvuloplasty an aortogram is performed to assess the degree of aortic valve regurgitation.

Heparin (100 U per kilogram) is administered during the catheterization and valvuloplasty. Long-term anticoagulation is not maintained. Thrombolytic agents may be considered as an alternative to surgical exploration if there is evidence of diminished leg perfusion after the procedure.

After aortic valvuloplasty, patients are monitored for 24 hours in the intensive care unit.

Balloon valvuloplasty for aortic valve stenosis is still considered an investigational procedure and must be performed only with fully informed consent and institutional review board approval.

Potentially, one is able to titrate the degree of valve dilation to balance residual stenosis against valve regurgitation by hemodynamic and angiographic measurements between dilations by using progressively larger balloons. This is an opportunity not afforded the surgeon who must deal with a nonbeating heart. Further, as a palliative first-stage procedure for severe aortic stenosis, the balloon technique avoids the median sternotomy incision and subsequent adhesions; definitive surgery (valve replacement) may thereby be easier when performed some years later. The technique is particularly appealing in the critically ill neonate with severe aortic valve stenosis and in the elderly adult with calcific aortic stenosis, since open heart surgery may pose a particularly great risk in these populations. The advantage of percutaneous balloon valvuloplasty over surgical intervention in the young child or adolescent with moderately severe aortic stenosis is somewhat less clear.

Hemodynamic results after balloon aortic valvuloplasty appear to be comparable to those with surgical valvotomy, although there have not been controlled studies comparing the two approaches. Mild residual aortic valve stenosis and moderate aortic valve regurgitation are consistent with a good result. Follow-up by 2-D Doppler echocardiography establishes the long-term effectiveness of the procedure.

COARCTATION OF THE AORTA

Coarctation Restenosis

The pathology of coarctation restenosis of intimal proliferation makes this an attractive lesion for balloon dilation. Dimensions of the aorta are determined from the aortogram. The diameters of the aorta just proximal to the coarctation, at the coarctation, and just distal to the coarctation are measured. Balloon size is selected equal to the size of aorta proximal or distal, whichever is smaller (usually proximal) or equal to a multiple (three to four times) of the coarct segment. A guidewire is positioned across the obstruction. The balloon catheter is advanced over the guidewire and positioned with the balloon straddling the obstruction. The balloon is rapidly inflated and deflated and withdrawn, leaving the guidewire in place to allow reintroduction of the angiographic catheter. It is important never to cross a newly dilated vessel except along the previously positioned guidewire because of the risk of perforation. Postdilatation aortography demonstrates the degree of dilatation of the coarcted segment and the presence or absence of intimal or transluminal disruption.

Acute risk of rupture may be limited by surrounding scar tissue produced by the previous surgery.

Heparin is administered at the beginning of the procedure (100 U per kilogram). Long-term anticoagulation therapy has not been used.

Back and jaw pain have been described by patients during balloon inflation.

Results show marked angiographic and pressure gradient improvement with further improvements in the systolic pressure gradient over time attributed to remodeling at the coarctation site. The long-term risk of aneurysm formation is as yet unknown. Follow-up arm and leg blood pressure readings indicate the degree of residual obstruction. Magnetic resonance imaging, digital subtraction angiography, or direct angiography may be used to follow the architecture of the dilatation site.

Coarctation—Native

Unoperated coarctation of the aorta is less clearly an indication for balloon dilation and is an area of controversy. Several centers have reported excellent relief of obstruction using a technique identical to that for coarctation restenosis. One year follow-up studies have shown a variable presence of aneurysms at the dilatation site ranging from none to 64 percent occurrence. Long-term sequelae are unknown. At our center patients with previously unoperated coarctation of the aorta are referred for surgical correction.

BRANCH PULMONARY ARTERY STENOSIS

Severe stenosis of branch pulmonary arteries usually occurs as an associated malformation in tetralogy of Fallot but may appear as an isolated lesion, or as a complication of previous pulmonary artery surgery (e.g., pulmonary to systemic shunts). The response to balloon angioplasty is not uniform. The technique includes measurement of the proximal, stenotic, and distal pulmonary artery dimensions from the angiogram. Balloon selection at our institution is with a diameter no greater than the "normal" artery proximal or distal to the stenosis. However, the pulmonary artery appears to tolerate overdilation, and large balloons may be necessary to relieve the stenosis with resultant intimal and medial disruption. Sustained inflation (up to 1 minute) has been beneficial in some instances when brief rapid inflations failed to improve the stenosis.

Marked increase in pulmonary artery dimension and resultant elevation in distal pulmonary artery pressure have been demonstrated to cause transient pulmonary edema, which responds to diuretics and oxygen administration. Aneurysms of the pulmonary artery have been reported after overly vigorous dilation.

Advantages of balloon angioplasty over surgical treatment of these lesions relate to its ability to reach very distal lesions that may be difficult to approach surgically.

Heparin (100 U per kilogram) is administered during the diagnostic angiogram and in some patients aspirin and dipyridamole have been given for several months to diminish the risk of thrombus formation in small vessels.

VENOUS CHANNELS

Systemic Veins. Stenotic superior and inferior caval channels after otherwise successful surgical repairs for transposition of the great arteries and anomalous pulmonary venous return have been dilated using very large balloons.

Pulmonary Veins. Congenital pulmonary vein stenosis has thus far been shown not to be amenable to balloon dilation. However, surgery has also been uniformly unsuccessful in treating these lesions. Since severe pulmonary vein stenosis is a fatal abnormality if untreated, attempts at balloon dilation to develop a treatment approach are justified.

MISCELLANEOUS

In addition to the common application of balloon angioplasty described above, there is limited experience in dilation of restrictive atrial septal communication, stenotic systemic to pulmonary shunt, subaortic stenosis, and mitral valve stenosis. Other potential applications undoubtedly exist and depend on the creativity and facility of the individual performing the interventional catheterization to get the balloon to the area of narrowing. However, caution is advised, since not everything that can be dilated should be dilated.

RISKS

Risks of balloon angioplasty in the management of selected forms of congenital and acquired heart disease include rupture, bleeding, embolization of balloon material or clot, injury to access vessels, neurologic events, rhythm abnormalities, and death.

ADVANTAGES

For each angioplasty, advantages of the procedure must be considered to outweigh risks. Advantages of the percutaneous balloon technique include avoidance of general anesthesia, limited exposure to blood products (a particular concern of parents who worry about acquired immunodeficiency syndrome), shortened hospital stay (or totally outpatient procedure), cosmetic appeal of a percutaneous puncture in the groin compared with a chest incision, and considerable cost containment. Few families reject the balloon angioplasty, although it is unproved and still investigational, in favor of the more traditional surgical approach.

Balloon angioplasty is an appealing alternative to an open surgical procedure in the management of a select group of cardiac lesions. However, the long-term efficacy and relative risks and benefits compared with those of surgical correction have yet to be determined. Compulsive long-term follow-up and reporting are essential to determine the ultimate role of these procedures.

SUGGESTED READING

Cribier A, Saoudi N, Berland J, Savin T, Rocha P, Letac BE. Percutaneous transluminal valvuloplasty of acquired aortic stenosis in elderly patients: an alternative to valve replacement? Lancet 1986; 11:63–67.

Kan JS, White RI, Mitchell SE, Anderson JH, Gardner TJ. Percutaneous transluminal balloon valvuloplasty for pulmonary valve stenosis. Circulation 1984; 69:554–560.

Kan JS, White RI, Mitchell SE, Farmlett EJ, Donahoo JS, Gardner TJ. Treatment of restenosis of coarctation by percutaneous transluminal angioplasty. Circulation 1983; 68:1087–1094.

Lababid Z, Wu J-R, Walles JT. Percutaneous balloon aortic valvuloplasty: results in 23 patients. Am J Cardiol 1984; 53:194–197.

Lock JE, Bass JL, Castaneda-Zuniga WR, Fuhrman BP, Rashkind WJ, Lucas RV Jr. Dilation angioplasty of congenital or operative narrowings of venous channels. Circulation 1984; 70:457–464.

Lock JE, Castaneda-Zuniga WR, Fuhrman BP, Bass JL. Balloon dilation angioplasty of hypoplastic and stenotic pulmonary arteries. Circulation 1983; 67:962–967.

CARDIOPULMONARY BYPASS AND HYPOTHERMIC CIRCULATORY ARREST IN CONGENITAL HEART SURGERY

ALBERT D. PACIFICO, M.D.

The management of cardiopulmonary bypass (CPB), including the degree of hypothermia and the use of low-flow or circulatory arrest, should be tailored according to the complexity of the intracardiac repair, the size of the subject, and the anticipated duration of the procedure. Since 1972, we have used two types of support methods for infants and children. In the earlier years we employed surface cooling to 30 to 32° C, followed by CPB with a single venous cannula and core cooling to 20° C, which was accomplished by graded reduction of perfusate temperature. A period of hypothermic perfusion sufficient to ensure adequate caloric exchange was maintained. For example, in a 3-kg infant, total circulatory arrest was established after 15 to 20 minutes of hypothermic perfusion, reducing nasopharyngeal temperature to 20° C. The single venous cannula was removed from the right atrium, and the intracardiac procedure was performed completely during the arrest period. When the procedure was completed, the venous cannula was reinserted, CPB re-established, and the patient rewarmed. The approximate duration of cardiopulmonary bypass (the sum of that required for cooling and rewarming) for this technique was about 45 minutes, and an effort was made to keep the circulatory arrest time to within 45 to 60 minutes. The principal advantages of this method were the limited period of CPB and the performance of the intracardiac repair in a completely bloodless field uncluttered by venous cannulas. As time passed, this initial period of surface cooling was abandoned.

We have essentially abandoned the use of a single venous cannula with hypothermic circulatory arrest in the belief that (1) CPB with or without low flow is probably safer for cerebral protection than hypothermic circulatory arrest, (2) some degree of whole-body oxygen consumption continues even at 20° C (Fig. 1), and (3) comparably excellent intracardiac exposure can be provided when direct caval cannulation is used. The only exception is the special circumstance of a very small infant undergoing repair of total anomalous pulmonary venous connection. A detailed description of the method of support currently employed for congenital heart surgery follows.

TECHNIQUE

A median sternotomy incision is preferred for repair of all intracardiac defects. Ascending aortic cannulation is first accomplished using a thin-walled, short-tipped arterial cannula* sized to result in a transcannula gradient equal to or less than 100 mm Hg at full flow (2.5 L per minute per square meter of body surface area). Two venous cannulas are employed to separately cannulate each vena cava in all patients. Direct caval cannulation with appropriately sized thin-walled angled cannulas* (Fig. 2) reduces the clutter in the surgical field and provides superb access for intracardiac exposure of most defects via the right atrium. The size of the venous cannula is selected according to the flow rate shown in Table 1. The inferior vena caval pursestring suture is placed directly on the inferior vena cava (IVC) or at the caval-atrial junction and connected to a tourniquet with a fine plastic tube.* It is placed a bit rightward of the midline axis of the IVC. The superior vena caval pursestring suture is placed directly on the superior vena cava (SVC) as an oval in its longitudinal axis and similarly connected to a tourniquet. The SVC snare is placed before CPB by mobilizing the cava at the site of the right pulmonary artery using a 0 silk ligature, which is similarly connected to a tourniquet. The IVC snare is placed after establishing CPB in an effort to avoid prebypass myocardial depression. Following arterial cannulation, the IVC cannula is inserted and connected to the venous tubing via a Y-connector. The SVC cannula is then connected to the remaining limb of the Y-connector and occluded with a tubing clamp, after allowing the IVC cannula and Y-connector to fill with the patient's blood. CPB is established currently using a disposable bubble oxygenator with integral heat exchanger. The oxygenator size, priming volume, and arterial and venous tubing size are shown in Table 2. The oxygenator is ventilated with

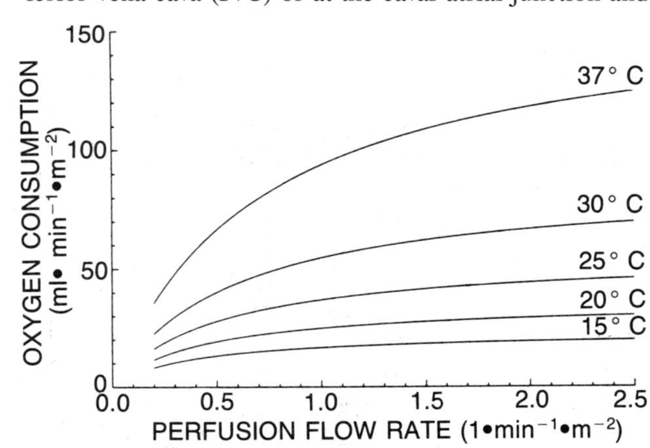

Figure 1 A nomogram of an equation describing the relation of whole body oxygen consumption (Vo_2) to perfusion flow rate and nasopharyngeal temperature. (From Kirklin JW, Barratt-Boyes BG. Cardiac surgery. New York: John Wiley & Sons, 1986, reproduced by permission.)

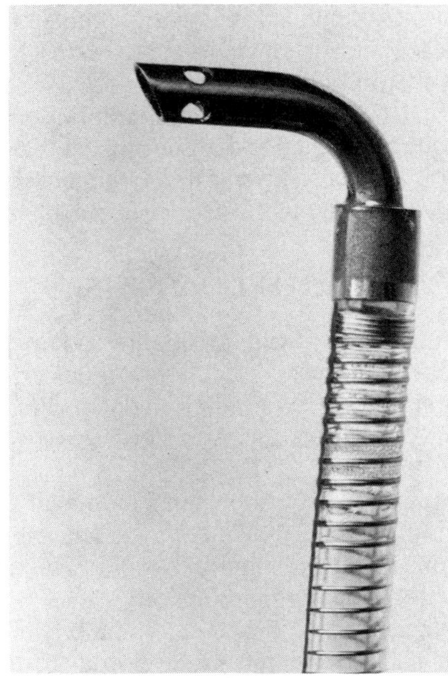

Figure 2 Photograph of a thin-walled No. 12 F DLP angled venous cannula. The outside diameter of the tip is 3.962 mm.

* DLP, Inc., Grand Rapids, MI.

TABLE 1 Venous Cannula* Flow Table

Total Flow (L/min)	*SVC (French Size)*	*IVC (French Size)*
<0.9	12	12
≥0.9<1.2	12	16
≥1.2<1.7	16	16
≥1.7<2.1	16	20
≥2.1<3.0	20	20
≥3.0<3.5	20	24
≥3.5<3.8	24	24
≥3.8	24	28

* DLP, Inc., Grand Rapids, MI.

TABLE 2 Details of Cardiopulmonary Bypass Apparatus

Oxygenator	*Flow (L/min)*	*Priming Volume (ml)*	*Tubing Diameter* *Arterial (inches)*	*Venous (inches)*
Adult	>2.5	1,500	3/8	1/2
Pediatric	>2.0≤2.5	800	3/8	3/8
Pediatric	>1.25≤2.0	600	1/4	3/8
Infant	>0.70≤1.25	500	1/4	3/8
Infant	≤0.70	500	1/4	1/4

100 percent oxygen using a gas-blood flow ratio of 1.5:1. Carbon dioxide is not employed. Chilled water is available in our operating rooms at 4° to 6° C, and together with warm water, it enters the mixing valve on the pump console. Water bath, perfusate, and nasopharyngeal temperatures are monitored. Initially, the water bath temperature is set at 25° C and later altered.

Table 3 shows the priming volume and its component solutions at various flow rates. The priming volume is kept low, and the surgeon is notified of any subsequent additions made by the perfusionist so he can monitor venous drainage. Although it occurs uncommonly, the IVC cannula can enter a hepatic vein with resultant reduction of its caval drainage. Blood is added for a calculated mixed hematocrit of 25 percent according to the formula:

$$\text{Mixed hematocrit} = \frac{\text{patient red cell volume (ml)} + \text{machine red blood cell volume (ml)}}{\text{patient BV} + \text{machine BV (ml)}}$$

where BV = blood volume. Patient blood volume is estimated from the formula [body weight (kg) • f • 1,000] where f = 0.08 for infants and children equal to or younger than 12 years of age and 0.065 for patients older than 12 years. This is converted to patient red cell volume by [patient BV][patient Hct]. Machine red blood cell volume is calculated from the formula:

$$\text{Machine red blood cell volume (ml)} = [(\text{mixed Hct})(\text{patient BV} + \text{machine BV})] - \text{patient red cell volume}$$

When a negative number is calculated, then additions of crystalloid to this value are permitted. When a positive number is calculated, then this amount of blood is added to the priming volume in place of crystalloid solution. Since cardioplegic solution is used in each operation, the priming volume of the cardioplegic reservoir (UAB system) or the anticipated volume of crystalloid cardioplegic solution (unless it is collected and discarded from the coronary sinus) should be added to the "machine BV" for accuracy. Hematocrit should be intermittently measured during the period of CPB and adjusted accordingly.

After establishing CPB at 25° C with only the IVC cannula in place, initially at a maximum flow rate of 1.6 L per minute per square meter of body surface area, the SVC cannula is inserted and "full flow" established at 2.0 to 2.5 L per minute per square meter of body surface area. The water bath is then adjusted to "coldest temperature" to permit initial cooling of the myocardium by the perfusate.

The temperature desired during most of the surgery is selected according to the specific procedure being performed, its estimated duration, and the degree of difficulty imposed by pulmonary venous return resulting from aortopulmonary collateral blood flow. In most procedures complete control of pulmonary venous return is obtained using a special disposable sump tip sucker,* which is introduced into the left atrium via the foramen ovale or a small intra-atrial defect created in the fossa ovalis. This permits optimal exposure working through a right atriotomy incision, which we prefer for repair of isolated ventricular septal defect (VSD), double-outlet right ventricle with subaortic VSD, classic tetralogy of Fallot, and repair of atrioventricular septal (canal) defects. The temperature is adjusted to 28° C and the flow to 1.6 L per minute per square meter of body surface area during the intracardiac repair. Lower flow or a short period of total circulatory arrest is unnecessary for these procedures, except in very unusual circumstances, and CPB is maintained throughout. During more complex operations, such as the arteri-

* DLP, Inc., Grand Rapids, MI.

TABLE 3 Components of Oxygenator Prime

Oxygenator	*Priming Volume (ml)*	*5% Dextrose Saline (ml)*	*Normosol-R (ml)*
Adult	1,500	500	1,000-BP*
Pediatric	800	100	700-BP
Pediatric	600	100	500-BP
Infant	500	100	400-BP

* BP=Blood prime.

TABLE 4 "Safe" Duration of Reduced Flow During Cardiopulmonary Bypass

Temperature (Nasopharyngeal)	*Flow (L/min/m²)*	*Duration (min)*
22° C	0.5	45
26° C	0.5	30
28° C	0.5	20

al switch repair of transposition of the great arteries, a temperature of 20 to 24° C is employed, which safely permits short periods of flow rate reduction to 0.5 L per minute per square meter of body surface area or total circulatory arrest (rarely used) to reduce the intracardiac return created by what can be a rather well-developed aortopulmonary collateral blood flow. Table 4 shows what we consider to be "safe" periods of low flow or circulatory arrest or both during hypothermic cardiopulmonary bypass.

Greater degrees of hypothermia are also of benefit in maintaining *myocardial hypothermia* during the period of aortic cross-clamping by reducing the ambient temperature and also the temperature of noncoronary myocardial collateral blood flow, which affects the rate of myocardial rewarming following the infusion of cold cardioplegic solution into the aortic root. The longer the duration of aortic cross-clamping, the more important these considerations become, and therefore greater degrees of systemic hypothermia are preferred when a longer period of aortic occlusion is expected.

Since 1977, we have preferred the use of cold sanguineous cardioplegia, which is infused at 4° C via a roller pump from a Gish cardioplegic reservoir at a rate of 150 ml per square meter of body surface area per minute for

TABLE 5 Management of Cardiopulmonary Bypass During the Arterial Switch Operation

Time (min)	*CPB Flow (L/min/m²)*	*Temperature*		*Surgical Maneuver*
		Water Bath	*Nasopharyngeal*	
0	1.6	25° C	37° C	On bypass; inset SVC cannula
1–2	2.2	4° C		Divide patent ductus arteriosus and complete mobilization of main and branch pulmonary arteries
3–4	2.2	4° C		Right atriotomy, insert sump vent across atrial septum
6–8	2.2	4° C		Clamp aorta; cardioplegia
10–35*	0.5–1.6	20–24° C	20–24° C	Divide aorta and main pulmonary artery; construct new aortic anastomosis and transfer coronary arteries
35–37*	0.5–1.6	20–24° C	20–24° C	Reinfuse cardioplegia
37–45*	0.5–1.6	20–24° C	20–24° C	Construct posterior aspect of new main pulmonary artery anastomosis
45–55	1.6	28° C		Suture patches to close defects left by coronary artery excision
65–73	2.2	42° C		Complete pulmonary artery anastomosis
74	2.2	42° C		Declamp aorta
75–80	2.2	42° C		Remove vent, close atrial septum and right atriotomy incision
81–93	2.2	42° C		De-air heart and obtain great artery hemostasis
94	0	42° C	37° C	Discontinue bypass

* Precise flow rate and water bath temperature selected according to magnitude of aortopulmonary and "noncoronary" collateral blood flow (see text).

TABLE 6 Management of Cardiopulmonary Bypass During Repair of a Complete Atrioventricular Canal Defect

Time (min)	*CPB Flow (L/min/m²)*	*Temperature*		*Surgical Maneuver*
		Water Bath	*Nasopharyngeal*	
0	1.6	25° C	37° C	On bypass; insert SVC cannula
1–2	2.2	4° C		Ligate patent ductus arteriosus
3–4	2.2	4° C		Right atriotomy; insert sump vent across atrial septum
5–7	2.2	4° C		Clamp aorta; cardioplegia
8–30	1.6	28° C	28° C	Assess valve architecture; place intraventricular Dacron patch and attach valve to crest of patch
31–33	1.6	28° C	28° C	Reinfuse cardioplegia
34–44	2.2	42° C		Place intra-atrial pericardial patch
45	2.2	42° C		Declamp aorta
46–55	2.2	42° C		Close right atriotomy and de-air heart
56	0	42° C	37° C	Discontinue bypass

TABLE 7 Management of Cardiopulmonary Bypass During Repair of Tetralogy of Fallot with Pulmonary Atresia and Large Aortopulmonary Arteries

Time (min)	*CPB Flow (L/min/m²)*	*Temperature*		*Surgical Maneuver*
		Bath	*Nasopharyngeal*	
0	2.2	25° C	37° C	On bypass
1–2	2.2	5° C		Vent left atrium
3	2.2	5° C		Open pleural space; ligate collateral arteries
6–10	2.2	5° C		Clamp aorta; cardioplegia
10–14	2.2	5° C		Right ventriculotomy
15	0.5	24° C	24° C	Close VSD
25*	0	24° C	24° C	Distal conduit anastomosis; reinject cardioplegia
35	2.2	32° C		Proximal conduit anastomosis
37	2.2	42° C		Proximal conduit anastomosis
46	2.2	42° C		Declamp aorta and de-air heart
57	0	42° C	37° C	Bypass discontinued

* Total circulatory arrest for 10 minutes.

2 minutes and repeated at 20 to 30 minute intervals. The cardioplegic reservoir is unprimed and after establishing CPB and allowing mixture of the perfusate prime with the patient's blood, an aliquot of 300 ml per square meter of body surface area is pumped from the oxygenator into the cardioplegic reservoir. To this is added 15 mEq per liter of KCl and 4 ml of sodium bicarbonate. The resultant solution has a potassium concentration of about 19 mEq per liter and provides effective electromechanical quiescence. Additional doses are reinfused at 20 to 30 minute intervals.

Tables 5 through 7 were constructed from recent operative reports to exemplify these techniques as employed during an arterial switch operation (Table 5), repair of a complete atrioventricular canal defect (Table 6), and repair of tetralogy of Fallot with pulmonary atresia and large aortopulmonary collateral arteries (Table 7).

SUGGESTED READING

Fox LS, Blackstone EH, Kirklin JW, Stewart RW, Samuelson PN. The relationship of whole body oxygen consumption to perfusion flow rate during hypothermic cardiopulmonary bypass. J Thorac Cardiovasc Surg 1982; 83:239–248.

Kirklin JW, Barratt-Boyes BG. Cardiac surgery. New York: John Wiley & Sons, 1986.

Kirklin JW, Lell WA, Baxley JG, Appelbaum A. Cardiopulmonary bypass for cardiac surgery. In: Sabiston DC Jr, Spencer FC, eds. Gibbons surgery of the chest. Philadelphia: WB Saunders 1976:845.

Kirklin JW, Pacifico AD, Hamner H, Allarde RR. Primary definitive intracardiac operations in infants: intraoperative support techniques. In: Kirklin JW, ed. Advances in cardiovascular surgery. New York: Grune & Stratton, 1973:86.

Pacifico AD. Low-flow bypass: the University of Alabama technique. In: Moulton AL, ed. Congenital heart surgery—current techniques and controversies. Pasadena: Appleton Davies, Inc, 1984:187.

EBSTEIN'S ANOMALY

JAMES K. KIRKLIN, M.D.
ALBERT D. PACIFICO, M.D.
JOHN W. KIRKLIN, M.D.

Ebstein's anomaly is a rare congenital cardiac malformation (it occurs in less than 1 percent of congenital cardiac defects), in which there is downward displacement of the septal and/or posterior tricuspid leaflets into the right ventricle. The leaflets are abnormally formed, and there is typically a large, sail-like anterior tricuspid leaflet. The right ventricle contains an atrialized portion (with an atrial pressure pulse contour and ventricular electrical potentials) proximal to the valve and a ventricularized distal portion. An interatrial communication is usually present, as is progressive and frequently massive right atrial dilatation. The right ventricle is typically dilated and thin-walled, with abnormalities of the muscle fibers. Pulmonary stenosis or atresia is present in less than one-third of cases. Wolff-Parkinson-White (WPW) syndrome is present in 5 to 10 percent of patients with Ebstein's anomaly.

When symptoms appear early in the patient's life (neonatal period), there is frequently severe cyanosis, marked right-sided congestive heart failure associated with severe tricuspid incompetence (occasionally with accompanying stenosis), and marked cardiomegaly. Most patients, however, do not become symptomatic until childhood or early adulthood, usually with mild dyspnea and fatigue. Cyanosis is common, as is progressive congestive heart failure. Paradoxical systemic emboli may occur in the presence of right-to-left shunting at the atrial level. Symptomatic supraventricular (occasionally with WPW syndrome) and ventricular arrhythmias are common. Sudden death accounts for approximately 20 percent of fatalities in patients with Ebstein's anomaly, presumably from ventricular or supraventricular arrhythmias. The most common cause of death is progressive heart failure, particularly when patients have advanced to New York Heart Association Class III or IV. The natural history for patients diagnosed after the first week of life is quite favorable, with nearly 60 percent surviving 20 years or more. Over half the patients over 25 years of age with Ebstein's anomaly are in Class I or II.

TREATMENT OPTIONS

Medical Therapy

Standard medical therapy for congestive heart failure is advised for symptomatic patients, and the prognosis for those in New York Heart Association Functional Class II is good. However, deterioration to Class III or IV is a poor prognostic sign, with most such patients dying within 2 to 3 years. At this advanced stage, medical therapy is generally ineffective except for the treatment of fluid retention. Antiarrhythmic therapy is occasionally helpful, particularly for atrial and ventricular arrhythmias unassociated with WPW.

In the neonatal period, high pulmonary vascular resistance exacerbates the tricuspid incompetence and resultant heart failure and accentuates right-to-left shunting at the atrial level. Intense medical therapy to relieve congestive heart failure, to lower pulmonary vascular resistance, and to treat cyanosis is necessary. If the patient survives the neonatal period, congestive heart failure usually improves in association with the falling pulmonary vascular resistance.

Surgery

The surgical options, depending upon the precise anatomic details, include tricuspid valve replacement, tricuspid valve annuloplasty, closure of the atrial septal defect, plication of the atrialized ventricle, excision of the right atrial wall, division of accessory bypass tracts, and relief of right ventricular outflow tract obstruction (Table 1). Under special circumstances, the Fontan operation may be advisable.

INDICATIONS FOR OPERATION

Congestive Heart Failure—New York Heart Association Class III or IV

Operation is generally advisable when patients with congestive heart failure reach New York Heart Association Class III or IV.

Moderate or Severe Cyanosis

In the presence of right-to-left shunting at the atrial level, progressive cyanosis may develop, usually accompanied by marked polycythemia. At this stage, operation is advisable, since only about 20 percent of such patients are alive after 10 years without operation.

Atrial Septal Defect with Left-to-Right Shunt and Pulmonary to Systemic Blood Flow Ratio (Qp:Qs) Greater Than 2

When the physiology is that of an isolated atrial septal defect, operation is advisable when symptoms of heart failure develop or when the Qp:Qs exceeds 2, even with mild symptoms.

WPW Syndrome with Debilitating Supraventricular Arrhythmias

When WPW syndrome is associated with severe and recurrent supraventricular tachycardia, or if the electrophysiologic studies indicate a life-threatening potential, operation is advisable and should include direct division of the right-sided accessory pathway.

TABLE 1 Surgical Options in Ebstein's Anomaly

Operative Procedure	*Comments*
Closure of atrial septal defect	Should be routine
Tricuspid valve replacement	Advisable in older children and adults when tricuspid regurgitation is moderate or severe
Tricuspid valve annuloplasty	Advisable in severely symptomatic infants and small children with moderate or severe tricuspid regurgitation if there is a large anterior leaflet
Plication of atrialized ventricle	Rarely necessary except when ventricle is aneurysmal and thin-walled with paradoxical motion
Excision of right atrial wall	Rarely necessary
Division of accessory Kent's bundle	Should be routine when indicated by pre-operative electrophysiologic studies
Relief of right ventricular outflow tract obstruction	Advisable when obstruction is present

Paradoxical Emboli

In view of the potential for serious stroke, operation is advisable in the presence of paradoxical emboli from a right-to-left interatrial shunt.

Progressive Cardiomegaly

The natural history appears somewhat less favorable in the presence of progressive increase in heart size. Thus, when progressive cardiomegaly is associated with other symptoms, operation is probably advisable.

TIMING OF SURGERY

Because of the favorable natural history for patients presenting with Ebstein's anomaly beyond the first week of life, most can be followed on medical therapy for many years. The median age at operation in the University of Alabama at Birmingham experience is about 20 years. Over half of the deaths that occur in patients with Ebstein's anomaly are associated with congestive heart failure, and Class IV heart failure is a major risk factor for mortality following operation. Patients should therefore be referred for operation before their condition progresses to the late stages of heart failure. The age at which operation is advised is highly variable and is dependent upon the criteria listed under Indications for Operation.

Preoperative Evaluation

Echocardiography and cardiac catheterization are essential to provide the anatomic details of the malformation. When an annuloplasty is being considered, the size of the anterior tricuspid leaflet and other details of the tricuspid valve anatomy can generally be ascertained by echocardiography. It is well known that intraoperative assessment of tricuspid incompetence by digital palpation can be misleading, particularly when incompetence is severe and there is no specific jet of incompetence. In general, right ventriculography is advised to preoperatively assess the degree of tricuspid incompetence. In addition, precise quantitation at cardiac catheterization of the magnitude of left-to-right shunting, if present, is important in the decision regarding operation in some patients. Formal electrophysiologic studies are recommended for any patient with a history of supraventricular dysrhythmias. If surgery is planned, any patient with documented WPW syndrome should have bypass tract division performed as part of the operation.

SURGICAL DETAILS

Valve Replacement

Replacement of the tricuspid valve is generally indicated when tricuspid valve incompetence is moderate or severe. Cardiopulmonary bypass is established with two venous cannulas, employing moderate systemic hypothermia (25 to 28° C) and cold cardioplegia for myocardial preservation. Working through the right atrium, the tricuspid valve leaflets are excised, leaving more of the base of the anterior and septal leaflets adjacent to the commissure near the point of penetration of the bundle of His. To minimize the risk of complete heart block, sutures are placed posterior to the atrioventricular node area and coronary sinus, as described by Barnard and Schrire. Interrupted pledgeted mattress sutures are used in this area. In the remainder of the suture line anteriorly (where sutures can be placed directly through the tricuspid annulus), either a continuous or an interrupted pledgeted technique is employed (Fig. 1). A mechanical prosthesis is the valve substitute of choice until approximately age 50 years. Thereafter, a stented porcine heterograft may be preferable, particularly after age 60.

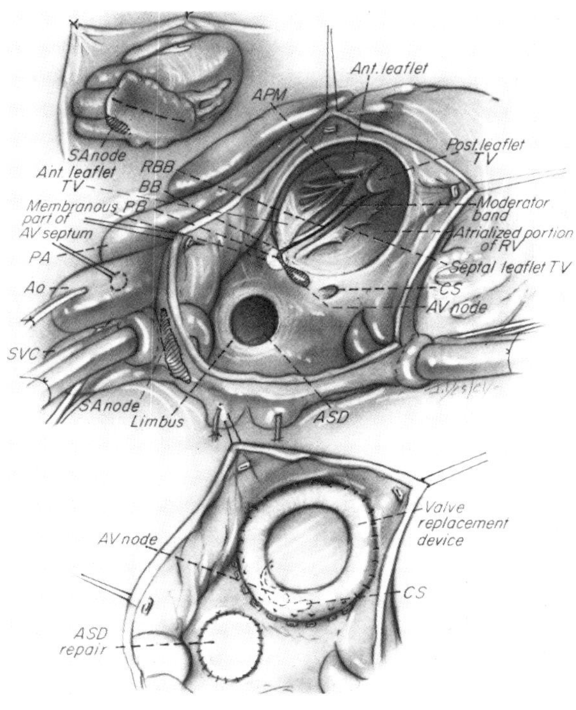

Figure 1 Replacement of the tricuspid valve and closure of the atrial septal defect in Ebstein's anomaly. The tricuspid valve is exposed through an oblique atriotomy. The septal and posterior leaflets are displaced downward, and the atrialized portion of the ventricle is shown. The atrioventricular node is indicated adjacent to the commissure between the displaced septal leaflet and the anterior leaflet. In order to avoid injury to the conduction system, the sutures for valve replacement are brought well posterior to the coronary sinus and membranous septum. The suture line then again follows the actual tricuspid valve ring (annulus fibrosis). The atrial septal defect is closed with a patch. APM, anterior papillary muscle; AV node, atrioventricular node; BB, branching bundle; CS, coronary sinus; PA, pulmonary artery; PB, penetrating bundle; RBB, right bundle branch; SA, sinoatrial. (Reproduced with permission from Bharati S, Lev M, Kirklin JW. Cardiac surgery and the conduction system. New York: John Wiley, 1983.)

Tricuspid Valve Repair

Although we generally recommend valve replacement when there is important tricuspid incompetence, Danielson and colleagues at the Mayo Clinic have reported good results using techniques of annuloplasty in which the anterior leaflet is allowed to function as a monocusp valve (Fig. 2). Particularly in children and infants with important tricuspid incompetence who require operation, a tricuspid valve annuloplasty, when possible, appears preferable to valve replacement. A large anterior leaflet is necessary for a successful annuloplasty. Occasionally, tricuspid valve stenosis is also present in Ebstein's anomaly. Tricuspid valvotomy plus closure of the associated atrial septal defect may provide important relief of right atrial hypertension, but caution is advised in performing the valvotomy because important tricuspid incompetence may result.

Closure of Atrial Septal Defect

Most commonly, the interatrial communication is a patent foramen ovale, though other types of atrial septal defect may exist. In general, a patch technique is recommended for closure of the atrial defect, since the tissue of the fossa ovalis is frequently very thin. Small suture leaks from direct closure may result in important right-to-left shunting and systemic desaturation. A patch of pericardium or knitted Dacron velour is used. When atrial septal defect closure is an isolated repair, cold cardioplegia is employed, and care is taken to avoid emptying the left atrium of blood. All of the air must be carefully evacuated from the left atrium before securing the suture line, followed by the usual deairing prior to discontinuation of bypass.

Plication of Atrialized Ventricle

Prior to commencing cardiopulmonary bypass, the atrialized portion of the ventricle is examined. When the atrialized portion is thin-walled with paradoxical movement during systole, plication is advised. It is generally accomplished from within the heart, using interrupted or continuous suture technique and taking care to avoid damage to the right coronary artery. In most cases, however, plication is unnecessary.

Excision of Right Atrial Wall

When the right atrium is particularly large, a portion of the wall may be excised by an elliptical excision on each side of the oblique atriotomy. On the lower side of the incision, care must be taken to stay clear of the sinoatrial node. We believe that right atrial excision is rarely necessary, and the large residual right atrium does not appear to adversely affect the late hemodynamics.

Division of Accessory Bypass Tracts

When an accessory Kent bundle is identified by preoperative electrophysiologic studies, it is nearly always a right-sided pathway, usually right free wall and less commonly posterior septal in position. Prior to or during cardiopulmonary bypass, an intraoperative electrophysiologic study is performed to confirm the preoperative findings. When the right atrium is opened, the precise location of the annulus fibrosis (tricuspid annulus) must be identified. An incision is made through the atrial endocardium 1 to 2 mm to the atrial side of the annulus fibrosis (not at the hinge point of the displaced leaflet). The incision is carried directly to the annulus fibrosis and then downward

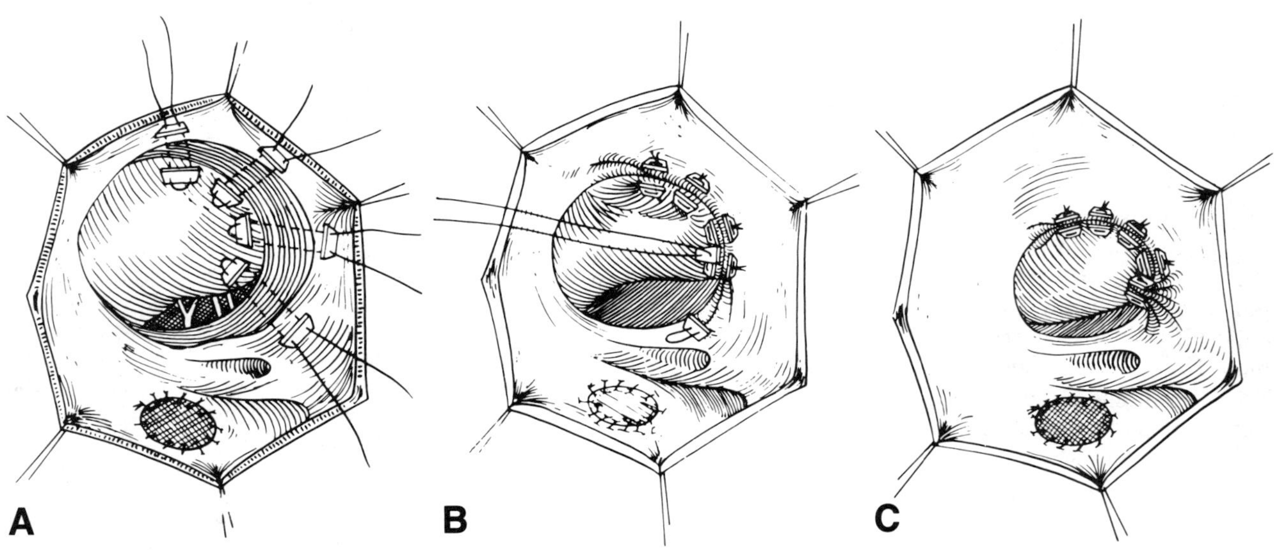

Figure 2 Annuloplasty repair of tricuspid valve in Ebstein's anomaly. *A*, The atrialized portion of the ventricle is plicated with interrupted pledgeted mattress sutures (shown from the surgeon's viewpoint, with the patient's head to the left). Care is taken to avoid the area of the conduction system. The atrial septal defect has been closed with a patch. *B*, An annuloplasty suture is placed to narrow the tricuspid annulus and includes the entire posterior leaflet. The coronary sinus marks the posterior and leftward extent of the annuloplasty, avoiding the area of the conduction system. *C*, The completed repair allows the large anterior leaflet to function as a monocusp valve. (Reproduced with permission from Danielson GK, Fuster V. Surgical repair of Ebstein's anomaly. Ann Thorac Surg 1982; 196:499–504.)

onto the underlying ventricular myocardium. In the area of atrialized ventricle the wall is extremely thin, and care must be taken to avoid "button-holing." Once the proper plane is established, the dissection of the fat and other contents of the atrioventricular groove should be carried 1 to 2 cm down onto the underlying ventricular myocardium, since the Kent bundle may lie in a subepicardial position. The dissection should be carried a distance of 2 to 3 cm along the annulus fibrosis on either side of the presumed location of the Kent bundle. Upon completing the dissection, the atrial endocardium is reapproximated with a continuous Prolene suture. In the posterior septal location, the dissection is similar to that for patients without Ebstein's anomaly.

Relief of Right Ventricular Outflow Tract Obstruction

When present, right ventricular outflow tract obstruction is relieved as for other forms of congenital heart disease. In the severely symptomatic neonate with associated valvar pulmonary stenosis, pulmonary valvotomy may significantly reduce associated tricuspid incompetence without the need for valve replacement.

Fontan Procedure

Rarely in Ebstein's anomaly, the tricuspid valve may be imperforate or the right ventricle severely hypoplastic. In such circumstances, a modified Fontan procedure may be advisable.

RESULTS OF SURGERY

With the exception of neonates and patients with advanced Class IV congestive heart failure (for which the mortality is high), hospital mortality for tricuspid valve repair or replacement and closure of the associated atrial septal defect is currently less than about 15 percent. When closure of the defect is an isolated procedure, the risk should approach that of repair of isolated secundum atrial septal defect. Repair of major associated lesions generally increases the risk, although division of accessory Kent bundles has not increased the operative mortality.

The reported long-term results with mechanical or heterograft prosthetic valves have generally been good, although such patients are subject to the same complications suffered by other patients undergoing tricuspid valve replacement. Most surviving patients are in New York Heart Association Class I or II. The operation is not curative, however, since there is a 10 to 15 percent incidence of premature late death, and up to 20 percent of patients suffer troublesome ventricular or supraventricular (not WPW) arrhythmias.

SUGGESTED READING

Barnard CN, Schrire V. Surgical correction of Ebstein's malformation with prosthetic tricuspid valve. Surgery 54:302–308.

Danielson GK, Fuster V. Surgical repair of Ebstein's anomaly. Ann Surg 1982; 196:499–504.

Hardy KL, May IA, Webster CA, Kimball KG. Ebstein's anomaly: a functional concept and successful definitive repair. J Thorac Cardiovasc Surg 1964; 48:927–940.

Sealy WC, Gallagher JJ, Pritchett ELC, Wallace AG. Surgical treatment of tachyarrhythmias in patients with both an Ebstein anomaly and a Kent bundle. J Thorac Cardiovasc Surg 1978; 75:847–853.

Westaby S, Karp RB, Kirklin JW, Waldo AL, Blackstone EH. Surgical treatment of Ebstein's malformation. Ann Thorac Surg 1982; 34:388–395.

CONGENITAL AORTIC STENOSIS

GEORGE A. TRUSLER, M.D., B.Sc.(Med), M.S., F.R.C.S.(C), F.A.C.S.
WILLIAM G. WILLIAMS, M.D., F.R.C.S.(C)

In order of frequency stenosis of the left ventricular outflow tract may be valvular, subvalvular, or supravalvular.

VALVULAR AORTIC STENOSIS

Aortic valve stenosis may occur at any age, but in infants it is usually more acute. Treatment is essentially palliative, for the valve is nearly always fundamentally abnormal, and eventually further surgery is necessary.

Indications for Surgery

We consider a left ventricular-aortic gradient of 50 mm Hg an indication for surgery. Lesser gradients are accepted if associated with other more pressing indications such as symptoms of syncope, angina, heart failure, a left ventricular strain pattern on the ECG, or an abnormal exercise test result.

Techniques of Management

Children beyond the first few months of life are managed by open aortic valvotomy with standard cardiopulmonary bypass; usually the operation is elective unless stenosis is severe. Operation is done via a sternotomy, utilizing aortic cannulation close to the innominate artery, single-cannula venous drainage in young children and two-stage venous drainage in older children, and left ventricular venting via the superior pulmonary vein. We initiate cardiopulmonary bypass at 20° C, and after the heart is cold, cross-clamp the aorta, induce cold-blood cardioplegia, and bring the systemic perfusion temperature up to normal for the remainder of the operation. Cardiac cooling is maintained by an appropriate-size plastic cooling jacket placed around the ventricles.

The aortic root is opened with an oblique incision into the noncoronary aortic sinus. The supravalvular and subvalvular areas are examined for stenosis and, if necessary, surgically treated. The valve anotomy is assessed to determine the extent to which the commissures can be opened without creating incompetence, and the orifice is measured with Hegar dilators. Very occasionally the valve is well formed with some fusion of all three commissures; opening each commissure with a small scalpel produces a fairly normal valve. The incision in the commissure should not enter the aortic wall, but should stop about 0.5 to 1 mm short. Usually the valve leaflets are thickened and abnormal, with fusion of only two commissures; in approximately 50 percent, both commissures can be opened to some extent without producing incompetence. In the other 50 percent the valve is functionally bicuspid in that one commissure is so rudimentary and nonsupporting that it cannot be opened. Truly bicuspid aortic valve stenosis in infants and children is uncommon. Rarely there is an unicuspid valve with only one commissure. Myxomatous nodules on the free edge of the valve are shaved flush with the leaflet surface with a scalpel. Again the valve orifice is measured to assess the increase in valve lumen and its potential adequacy.

The aorta is closed with a running suture and the left side of the heart allowed to fill with blood. A small "tack" or needle hole in the anterior aortic wall allows escape of any residual air. The left vent is replaced with a thin cannula in the left atrium to monitor left atrial pressure postoperatively.

Occasionally there is hypoplasia of the valve requiring aortoventriculoplasty and valve replacement. This is discussed in a separate chapter. In children a valvotomy will often produce temporary benefit, delaying the need for aortoventriculoplasty.

Early Infancy

Young infants with aortic stenosis in the first month of life often have cardiac failure and need urgent medical management with digitalis, diuretics, and sometimes respiratory assistance. Prostaglandin E_1, by increasing ductal flow, is valuable for very ill infants with metabolic acidosis, particularly to facilitate transportation for surgery. Echocardiography is now the key to diagnosis, and the infant may be too sick for cardiac catheterization. Other malformations are frequently present in association, especially endocardial fibroelastosis, mitral valve abnormalities, and left ventricular hypoplasia.

While aortic valvotomy with cardiopulmonary bypass is the standard therapy, other techniques can be used: cardiopulmonary bypass with deep hypothermia and circulatory arrest, or inflow caval occlusion with moderate hypothermia, or closed valvotomy.

Closed valvotomy has gained some favor recently. Through the seventh left interspace anteriorly a large mattress suture is placed at the apex of the left ventricle. Successively larger Hegar dilators, starting at 3 mm, are inserted briefly into the aortic valve orifice, dilating the valve until the calulated size of the aortic valve ring is attained; usually 6 to 7 mm is the largest safe size. Postmortem examinations of several infants have revealed that the valve split along its commissures. Locating the valve orifice with the tip of the dilators is aided by palpation of the aortic root and is indicated by abrupt reduction in arterial pressure. A balloon catheter can be used intraoperatively instead of a Hegar dilator, but is more difficult to position accurately.

We prefer closed valvotomy for neonates and infants when the aortic valve ring is less than 8 mm in diameter as determined by echocardiography. Since the aortic valve can be opened quickly without bypass, an infant in whom the size of the aortic valve ring and left ventricle is borderline is more likely to survive. In infants with a valve ring measuring 8 mm or more we prefer open valvotomy with cardiopulmonary bypass so that the largest possible opening can be attained.

Recently aortic valvotomy by transarterial balloon dilation in the cardiac catheterization laboratory has met with some success in both infants and older children and will likely be used more frequently in the future. This is described further in a separate chapter entitled *Percutaneous Intervention in Congenital Heart Disease.*

Results of Surgery

Our operative mortality varied by age: more than 1 year, 1 percent; between 1 month and 1 year, 15 percent; and less than 1 month, 50 percent. The size of the valve ring is a major risk factor in infants, for a small ring reduces cardiac output. No infant in our series survived in whom the valve orifice was less than 5.5 to 6.0 mm postoperatively. An infant with a ring less that 5.5 mm should be considered for a Norwood procedure or some other form of left-sided bypass. When a larger orifice is attained, most infants survive unless they have some other cardiac malformation.

Late Results

Moderate to severe aortic valve incompetence occurs in about 10 percent of cases, infective endocarditis in 4 percent and late death in about 6 percent. Of the late deaths, half were related to subsequent operations, and the other deaths were sudden, accidental, or related to endocarditis.

One-half of our series of infants who had aortic valvotomy between 1956 to 1975 have had subsequent aortic valve surgery—some repeat valvotomy and the rest aortic valve replacement. Of 148 children over 1 year of age who had valvotomy between 1956 and 1975, 40 (27 percent) have required further aortic valve surgery, mainly valve replacement. Many have required aortic root enlargement. The interval between the original operation and subsequent operation varies widely, but averages 7 to 9 years. Repeat operation is likely to be needed earlier after valvotomy in an infant than in an older child and much sooner after closed valvotomy.

SUPRAVALVULAR AORTIC STENOSIS

Supravalvular stenosis usually occurs as an hourglass narrowing of the aorta at or just beyond the free margin of the valve leaflets. The aortic intima is thickened, creating a prominent ridge that juts into the lumen. The valve leaflets are thickened, particularly at the free margins, and the combination of ridge and thickened leaflet may create a narrow opening into the sinus of Valsalva and sometimes narrow the coronary artery ostia. In one-fourth to one-third of cases the lesion is more diffuse, involving the ascending aorta and sometimes the aortic arch and its branches. Supravalvular aortic stenosis may occur in an isolated form (in approximately half the cases), a familial form, or as part of Williams' syndrome in association with peripheral pulmonary artery stenoses, elfin facies, and mental retardation.

Indications for Surgery

Indications for surgery are similar to those for aortic valve stenosis.

Technique of Management

The general management of the operation is identical to valvular stenosis employing cardiopulmonary bypass. Obstruction must be eliminated at all levels, including the opening into each aortic sinus and the coronary ostia. The primary problem in the supravalvular ridge can be relieved by an incision into the noncoronary sinus, enlarging the area with a suitable patch, roughly diamond or teardrop shaped. Although synthetic materials may be used, pericardium is effective and results in less suture line bleeding.

For severe stenosis an inverted Y-shaped patch may be used, with one limb in the noncoronary sinus and the second in the right sinus. The mobilized right commissure must be anchored securely at an appropriate level for valve competence. Rarely the left coronary sinus may be severely involved and need patching. Any heaped-up intima narrowing either coronary artery orifice or in the region of the valve commissures should be excised.

The distal end of the patch is extended beyond the obstruction, which may involve the whole ascending aorta and uncommonly the aortic arch. For more extensive lesions, femoral artery cannulation is necessary and occasionally total circulatory arrest.

Results of Surgery

Favorable results can be expected if repair is adequate and done early before myocardial damage occurs. Both early and late mortality are low, but the risk is greater with the more extensive forms of obstruction.

SUBVALVULAR AORTIC STENOSIS

Fibromuscular subaortic stenosis occurs as a diaphragm of smooth whitish yellow fibrous tissue encircling the outflow tract immediately below the valve, most prominent anteriorly over the interventricular septum, and often with a fibrous ridge across the mitral valve leaflet. The membrane often fuses superiorly with the base of the right coronary cusp of the aortic valve near its annulus; aortic valve incompetence is frequent. Occasionally the anterior portion of the diaphragm on the endocardial surface of the septum extends 1 or 2 cm inferiorly into the ventricle. Muscular hypertrophy of the left ventricle, and especially the septum underlying the membrane, is variable, related to the severity and duration of obstruction.

This lesion is acquired in certain types of congenital heart disease; it may be found incidentally with a ventricular septal defect, expecially in the presence of double-chambered right ventricle or coarctation.

Indications for Surgery

As in valvular stenosis, we consider a gradient of 50 mm Hg a general guide to indication for surgery. However, since the natural history of the lesion includes damage to the aortic valve, operative intervention is justified at the time of diagnosis, even in the absence of a pressure gradient, to prevent aortic valve dysfunction. When present in a child undergoing surgery for other cardiac lesions, the subvalvular stenosis is treated despite absence of the gradient.

Technique of Management

Exposure of the heart and cardiopulmonary bypass technique are identical to that used for aortic valvotomy.

The ascending aorta is opened obliquely, and the incision extended inferiorly into the noncoronary sinus. The aortic leaflets are carefully inspected, retracted, and protected throughout the operation. The diaphragm is visualized through the aortic orifice, and the thickness of the underlying septum is confirmed by palpation between the endocardial and epicardial surfaces.

A 5-0 figure-of-eight silk suture on a small needle is passed through the prominent anterior portion of the diaphragm for retraction. The diaphragm is then detached anteriorly immediately beneath the right coronary cusp, care being taken not to injure the cusp, by visualizing it from, both its ventricular and aortic sinus aspect. This initial incision is made parallel to and 1 or 2 mm under the surface of the left ventricular endocardium. Sharp dissection is used to detach the membrane from the intraventricular septum toward the patient's right. As the dissection approaches the membranous septum, the endocardium is preserved to protect the underlying conduction tissue. Where the diaphragm septum meets the membranous septum, the dissection then proceeds to the patient's left. Here the resection extends deeply into the muscle under the commissure between the right and left coronary cusps. A triangular wedge of muscle is excised. Finally the resection continues posteriorly onto the mitral leaflet, care being taken not to perforate the anterior cusp.

With the resection completed, the remaining septum is palpated to confirm appropriate residual thickness, and the mitral and aortic leaflets are inspected to exclude operative trauma.

In children with a ventricular septal defect the membrane can be visualized through the ventricular septal defect from a right atriotomy exposure after induction of cardioplegia. The diaphragm is usually small and incomplete, and the underlying left ventricular hypertrophy has not developed. Consequently, removing the tissue that lies anteriorly and laterally on the left side of the outflow tract is usually adequate.

Results of Surgery

Operative risk is low (less than 1 percent) and complications few. Arrhythmias, including complete atrioventricular block are rare. The left ventricle usually performs normally or is hypercontractile, so that postoperative cardiac output is almost always ideal.

Late problems are related to progression of aortic valve dysfunction. Mild aortic insufficiency present prior to operation may be cured by removal of the subaortic diaphragm; however, it often persists and may progress.

Subaortic obstruction recurs in approximately 10 percent of children at 10 years after operation. This is likely due to persistence of a small amount of obstruction and is therefore avoidable.

HYPERTROPHIC OBSTRUCTIVE CARDIOMYOPATHY

A primary muscle disorder characterized by ventricular hypertrophy without an identifiable cause, hypertrophic obstructive cardiomyopathy is usually, though not always, associated with microscopic myocardial fiber disarray. Any portion of the ventricles may be involved, although the ventricular septum is the most common site (90 percent).

Hypertrophic cardiomyopathy may be either nonobstructive (one-third of cases, involving primarily diastolic function) or obstructive (two-thirds). In the obstructive form, the mitral valve apparatus (usually the anterior leaflet) and thickened ventricular septum oppose each other in systole and impede mid to late systolic ejection. Less commonly, the obstruction may be entirely muscular, occurring either at the midventricular level where the papillary muscles insert or rarely at the apex.

The obstruction may occur at rest with each systole; it may be intermittent, appearing and disappearing for no apparent reason (labile); or it may appear because of specific provocation (latent) (Table 1). Obstruction is increased by any factor that decreases afterload or increases contractility.

Symptoms do not usually develop until late childhood or adulthood and are frequently precipitated and aggravated by atrial fibrillation. Sudden death is not uncommon. Death from congestive heart failure occurs most frequently in infants under 1 year of age or in the geriatric age group. About one-third of cases are familial.

Indication for Surgery

Symptomatic patients with resting obstruction (gradient > 50 mm Hg) who do not respond favorably to a trial of medication (disopyramide) or who are intolerant of medication should be treated surgically. Patients with symptoms from latent obstruction who do not tolerate medication (beta-adrenergic blocking drugs) are also good candidates for surgical intervention.

Technique of Management

Exposure and cannulation are similar to aortic valvotomy.

Following inspection and retraction of the aortic valve leaflets, the left ventricular outflow tract is inspected. The protruding thickened septum prevents visualization of the mitral chordae and papillary muscles. The septum is palpated between the surgeon's thumb in the left ventricular outflow tract and index finger on the outside of the heart. This allows the surgeon to determine the approximate thickness of the septum and to estimate the length of obstructive hypertrophy toward the apex.

A large block of septal muscle is then excised from the outflow tract. The initial incision is started immediately below the center of the right coronary cusp and is extended into the ventricle toward the apex until the entire thickened portion of the septum is incised. This incision is usually between 20 and 40 mm long and 10 to 20 mm deep. A second parallel incision is then made on the patient's left side, posterior to the commissure between the right and left aortic cusps and just anterior to the mitral valve. This incision is at the junction of the septum with the posterior left ventricular wall. The incision is extended into the ventricle toward the apex, passing just to the right of the anterolateral papillary muscle, and ending at the inferior border of the thickened ventricular septum.

The upper ends of these two incisions are joined by a carefully placed incision 2 to 3 mm below and parallel to the aortic annulus of the lateral half of the right coronary cusp and the anterior half of the left cusp.

These three incisions are then deepened as necessary to thin the remaining septum to an estimated 5 to 8 mm on palpation. The entire block of muscle is excised by continuing the dissection towards the apex until the apical limit of the hypertrophied section is reached. The average dimensions of myocardium removed are 25 mm wide, 15 to 20 mm deep, and 35 to 45 mm long. The mitral and aortic valves are inspected for damage and the aortotomy repaired.

Mitral insufficiency occurs in 80 percent of patients with obstructive hypertrophic cardiomyopathy as a result of the systolic anterior motion of the mitral leaflet. Preoperative investigation should elucidate whether this mechanism is present; it can be abolished by maneuvers that decrease the pressure gradient. Rarely the mitral in-

TABLE 1 Hypertrophic Cardiomyopathy

Classification	Frequency	Definition	Treatment
I Nonobstructive	⅓	Diastolic dysfunction	Calcium antagonists
II Obstructive			
1. Resting	⅓ +	Pressure gradient at rest Some diastolic dysfunction	Disopyramide/surgery
2. Labile	Rare	Intermittent pressure gradient	
3. Latent	⅓ −	Pressure gradient provocation No diastolic dysfunction	β-Blockers/surgery

sufficiency may be independent of outflow tract obstruction. In these cases, mitral valve replacement should be considered as primary surgical treatment to reduce the left ventricular outflow tract obstruction.

The usual supportive drugs used in postoperative care, such as inotropes and vasodilators, are contraindicated in patients with muscular subaortic stenosis. Adequate volume loading with colloid (blood) is the major and usually the only supportive treatment required postoperatively.

Results of Surgery

The operative risk is less than 2 percent. Postoperative atrial dysrhythmias are frequent, but are generally tolerated better than preoperatively.

Late mortality has been 1 percent per year. Successful surgery decreases or abolishes virtually all of the characteristic abnormalities of the obstruction with dramatic relief of symptoms, although troublesome arrhythmias may persist and require ongoing treatment. However, these patients continue to have the underlying hypertrophic cardiomyopathy and may develop diastolic dysfunction many years later.

DIFFUSE HYPOPLASIA OF THE LEFT VENTRICULAR OUTFLOW TRACT (TUNNEL OBSTRUCTION)

The entire outflow tract in this uncommon condition is small with a long narrow tunnel-like channel from the trabecular portion of the left ventricle to the aortic valve. In infants this type of obstruction merges with the hypoplastic left-heart syndrome and results in death during the newborn period. In children it results in severe obstruction with left ventricular hypertrophy and strain, myocardial ischemia, and death. Attempts to enlarge the outflow tract by myectomy are seldom successful and associated with a high operative risk. Survival to adulthood is unlikely. Operative management alternatives include aortoventriculoplasty and apicoaortic valved conduits, which are considered in other chapters.

SUGGESTED READING

Kean JF, Bernard WF, Nadas AS. Aortic stenosis surgery in infancy. Circulation 1975; 42:1138–1143.

Sandor GGS, Olley PM, Trusler GA, et al. Long-term follow up of patients after valvotomy for congenital valvular aortic stenosis in children. A clinical and acturial follow up. J Thorac Cardiovasc Surg 1980; 80:171–176.

Trinkle JK, Norton JB, Richardson JD, Grover FL, Noonan JA. Closed aortic valvotomy and simultaneous correction of associated anomalies in infants. J Thorac Cardiovasc Surg 1975; 69:758–762.

Wigle ED, Sasson Z, Henderson MA, et al. Hypertrophic cardiomyopathy. The importance of the site and the extent of hypertrophy. A review. Prog Cardiovasc Dis 1985; 28:1–83.

Wright GB, Keane JF, Nadas AS, Bernhard WF, Castaneda AR. Fixed subaortic stenosis in the young: medical and surgical course in 83 patients. Am J Cardiol 1983; 52:830–835.

PULMONARY VALVAR AND INFUNDIBULAR STENOSIS

WILLIS H. WILLIAMS, M.D.

Pulmonary valvar stenosis with intact ventricular septum, with or without associated right ventricular infundibular stenosis, accounts for 10 percent of congenital cardiac malformations. The stenotic pulmonary "valve" is often only a thickened membranous dome with a tiny central pinhole or eccentric orifice. At the opposite extreme, the valve may have normal tricuspid architecture with minimal commissural fusion. The dysplastic pulmonary valve with hypoplastic annulus, a markedly thickened and immobile two- or three-leaflet valve, tethering of the pulmonary artery wall at the level of commissural attachments, fibrous bands within the sinuses, and marked right ventricular hypertrophy are characteristic of Noonan's syndrome and common in tetralogy of Fallot. The right ventricle may be hypoplastic (15 percent), concentrically hypertrophic with a reduced cavity volume, or dilated and associated with tricuspid regurgitation in the later stages of the pathologic process. Infundibular stenosis may be a secondary hypertrophic response to valvar stenosis, or isolated and discrete, caused by hypertrophic parietal and septal extensions of the crista supraventricularis or, in 10 to 20 percent of patients, caused by abnormal muscle bands lying lower within the body of the right ventricle.

The pulmonary arteries, right ventricle, and tricuspid valve may be small in the neonate with pulmonary stenosis, probably as a result of diminished intrauterine pulmonary blood flow. Growth can be anticipated after relief of stenosis in all but the most severe cases of right ventricular hypoplasia. Poststenotic dilatation usually is present in the main and proximal left pulmonary arteries in older children and adults. The right atrium is hypertrophic, and an atrial septal defect or patent foramen ovale is present in 75 percent of patients, a right-to-left shunt at atrial level causing severe hypoxemia in neonates. Severe cases have intracavitary fibromuscular obstruction, tricuspid regurgitation, coronary arterial sinusoids, and myocardial ischemia.

Evaluation includes a chest roentgenogram, an electrocardiogram, a two-dimensional echocardiogram, cardiac catheterization, and cineangiography.

Pulmonary stenosis is classified as "mild, moderate, or severe," based upon the ratio of the peak right ventricular systolic pressure to the peak left ventricular (or aortic) pressure. Ratios less than 0.5 are considered "mild"; ratios between 0.5 and 0.9 are considered "moderate"; and ratios greater than 0.9 are classified as "severe."

Critically ill neonates require ventilatory support, monitoring, aggressive correction of acidosis and congestive heart failure, prostaglandin E_1 infusion, and urgent operation. Symptomatic infants over 1 month of age, all infants having severe pulmonary stenosis, symptomatic older children and young adults, and those having moderate or severe stenosis should undergo surgical correction. Progression of obstruction and emergence of symptoms are likely in moderate and severe stenosis but unlikely when stenosis is mild.

Percutaneous transluminal balloon angioplasty is an alternative to operation, particularly for those patients who have right ventricular hypoplasia or congestive heart failure, in which operative risk is increased.

Operation is performed through a median sternotomy. When infundibular resection is anticipated, anterior pericardium is excised and soaked in gluteraldehyde to increase strength. Arterial perfusion is through the ascending aorta, and venous drainage is provided through superior and inferior caval cannulas placed through the right atrium. A slitted plastic needle is sutured into the ascending aorta proximal to the perfusion cannula for administration of cardioplegic solution and continuous aspiration of possible air.

For simple pulmonary commissurotomy, I prefer normothermia without cardioplegia or aortic occlusion and with a continually beating heart while the patient is supported on total cardiopulmonary bypass. Continuous suction is applied to the plastic needle in the ascending aorta, using a cardiotomy aspirator to recover air bubbles that might enter the left side of the heart through an interatrial communication. Alternatively, moderate systemic hypothermia (28 to 32° C) with aortic occlusion and hypothermic cardioplegia provides a bloodless and motionless operative field. The left side of the heart need not be vented in most cases, but if associated anomalies justify left heart decompression, a flexible plastic catheter can be placed across the atrial septum or through the left atrial wall near the right pulmonary veins.

Traction sutures are placed to facilitate exposure. A transverse incision is made in the pulmonary artery approximately 1 cm distal to the annulus. Additional traction sutures are placed in the edges of the pulmonary arteriotomy. If the pulmonary artery or the pulmonary annulus is small, suggesting the need for an outflow tract patch, a longitudinal incision is made in the pulmonary artery. A bicuspid valve, or one that is thick and dysplastic or dome-like without architecturally defined cusps, is excised (valvectomy). If the valve is tricuspid and the leaflets are mobile, an incision is made in each fused commissure, and the commissural attachments to the pulmonary arterial wall are incised 1 to 2 mm along the annulus to enhance leaflet mobility. The pulmonary arteriotomy is repaired using continuous 5-0 polypropylene suture.

Infundibular stenosis is approached through a transverse right ventriculotomy placed directly over the palpable hypertrophic muscle, which is then excised with the septal and parietal extensions of the crista supraventricularis. Accurate excision is facilitated by passing a right-angled clamp around the muscular bands. Mild associated valvar commissural fusion is incised from below through the ventriculotomy. Anomalous muscle bundles or moderator bands causing obstruction within the body of the right ventricle are excised by incision near their attachments to the septum and free wall. Caution is required to distinguish anomalous muscle bands from papillary muscles. The right ventriculotomy is closed in two layers with continuous polypropylene suture.

When a small pulmonary annulus requiring the placement of a transannular gusset is suspected preoperatively or from intraoperative inspection, a longitudinal arteriotomy and ventriculotomy are done. After valvectomy, commissurotomy, and muscular excision are complete, Hegar's dilators are passed through the pulmonary valve annulus, and a decision is made regarding the need for a transannular patch based upon comparison of the patient's measured annular size to anticipated normal size for a patient of the same body surface area. If the patient's annulus is significantly smaller than normal, a transannular pericardial or preclotted woven Dacron patch is placed. A patent foramen ovale or atrial septal defect is closed through an atriotomy.

After weaning the patient from cardiopulmonary bypass, right and left ventricular pressures are determined and compared. A right ventricular-to-left ventricular peak systolic pressure ratio exceeding 0.65 suggests the need for further excision or placement of a transannular patch, but this decision is best made based on preoperative hemodynamic assessment combined with intraoperative measurement of annular size. When the right ventricular to left ventricular systolic pressure ratio exceeds 0.4, but is less than 0.65, a pressure monitoring catheter is placed through the right ventricular free wall into the pulmonary artery for measurement of a transannular "pullback" pressure 24 hours later. In most cases, the right ventricular pressure will be lower, indicating no need for further operative intervention.

Neonates with critical pulmonary stenosis and intact ventricular septum require individualized surgical management, depending upon the size of the right ventricle and pulmonary arteries, patency of the ductus arteriosus, size of the interatrial communication, magnitude of tricuspid regurgitation, and degree of systemic hypoxemia and acidosis. Usually a pulmonary valvectomy is performed through a pulmonary arteriotomy during 60 to 90 seconds of caval inflow occlusion with normothermic circulatory arrest. The patient is weaned slowly off of prostaglandin over the next several days. A systemic arterial to pulmonary artery shunt—usually a Blalock-Taussig shunt or modification thereof—is performed if hypoxemia (Po_2 below 30 mm Hg) persists or recurs after discontinuation of prostaglandin. Recent results of valvectomy, transannular patch, and débridement of the right ventricle while the infant is supported on cardiopulmonary bypass have been encouraging. The foramen ovale is not closed if the right ventricle is small, and a subsequent shunt may be required if hypoxemia persists.

Almost all infants, children, and young adults survive operation unless severe right ventricular hypoplasia or chronic congestive heart failure is present, and long-term prognosis for virtually asymptomatic survival, usually without reoperation, is excellent. Results following urgent valvotomy or valvectomy with or without a systemic arterial to pulmonary arterial shunt in the neonate with critical pulmonary stenosis have improved with perioperative prostaglandin infusion, but are still disappointing. Mortality approaching 50 percent has been reported for this subset, multiple operations are required, and management remains controversial and individualized. Goals include relief of right ventricular hypertension, provision for adequate pulmonary blood flow, and stimulation of growth of the tricuspid valve, right ventricle, and pulmonary arteries.

SUGGESTED READING

Brock RC. Pulmonary valvulotomy for the relief of congenital pulmonary stenosis. Br Med J 1948; 1:1121.

Coles JG, Freedom RM, Olley PM, Coceani F, Williams WG, Trusler GA. Surgical management of critical pulmonary stenosis in the neonate. Ann Thorac Surg 1984; 38:458–465.

Danilowicz D, Hoffman JIE, Rudolph AM. Serial studies of pulmonary stenosis in infancy and childhood. Br Heart J 1975; 37:808–818.

Griffith BP, Hardesty RL, Siewers RD, Lerberg DB, Ferson PF, Bahnson HT. Pulmonary valvulotomy alone for pulmonary stensosis: Results in children with and without muscular infundibular hypertrophy. J Thorac Cardiovasc Surg 1982; 83:577–583.

Mistrot J, Neal W, Lyons G, Moller J, Lucas R, Castaneda A, Varco R, Nicoloff D. Pulmonary valvulotomy under inflow stasis for isolated pulmonary stenosis. Ann Thorac Surg 1976; 21:30–37.

Polansky DB, Clark EB, Doty DB. Pulmonary stenosis in infants and young children. Ann Thorac Surg 1985; 39:159–164.

CONGENITAL MITRAL STENOSIS AND ATRESIA

JAMES W. KILMAN, M.D.

Congenital mitral stenosis and/or atresia is a rare congenital lesion and is almost always associated with other defects of the heart, such as persistent patent ductus arteriosus, aortic stenosis, ascending aortic hypoplasia, coarctation of the aorta, aortic cusp anomalies, and, rarely, ventricular septal defects. Left-sided heart syndromes seem to include many of these anomalies and are incompatible with continued survival of the neonate unless they are palliated or corrected.

EMBRYOLOGY

Congenital mitral stenosis or atresia is the result of failure of normal embryologic formation of the left-sided atrioventricular valve. It was demonstrated early that this defect is a form of persistent atrioventricular canal. The associated defects of the bulbus cordis occur at about the same time that this defect is formed from the endocardial cushions. Anatomic classification has recently been clarified by the work of Anderson, Becker, Edwards, and Van Praagh, and the group of left-sided heart syndromes is now more easily understood. The incidence of congenital mitral stenosis is very low (about 1.5 percent of all congenital heart patients presenting with symptoms), and therefore no surgeon or surgical clinic has a vast experience with the treatment of this defect.

PATHOLOGY

The mitral valve may be imperforate or only slightly fenestrated and is incompatible with life unless an atrial septal defect is present as well as a systemic-pulmonary shunt of some kind, either natural or iatrogenic. This lesion is very rare but may accompany the more complicated hypoplastic left-sided heart syndromes. Patients may have hypoplasia or atresia of the cardiac complex from the left atrial inlets to the distal aorta, and other parts of the left side of the heart may be included in or excluded from this complex.

The obstruction of congenital mitral stenosis may occur at one of the following levels or may be a combination of one or more of these levels. Type I obstruction is at the leaflet level. This is most often a long, funnel-shaped valve with narrow or absent commissures most likely accompanied by other congenital lesions such as coarctation or the left-sided heart syndromes. This is the most common type. Type II is the so-called "parachute-mitral valve" in which there is usually only one papillary muscle and the obstruction is at the chordae tendineae level. The mitral leaflets may be clefted as in a canal defect and may converge on one or two adjacent papillary muscles. Mitral valve obstruction may occur when the cleft is closed surgically at the time of repair of a complete or partial canal defect. Type III obstruction can occur at the papillary muscle level with a large, normal-looking valve and short or absent chordae tendineae and large hypertrophic papillary muscles actually obstructing almost at the annulus level. Muscular obstruction may result from the anomaly known as "mitral valve arcade." This is the result of a muscular band that crosses beneath the leaflets in which the chordae insert. Later in life, this may result in mitral insufficiency. Diagnosis can be made by careful examination of the angiograms, and "fingerprinting" of this abnormal muscle can be seen on the ventricular angiogram. The anatomy of the obstruction is quite important as to the indications for surgery.

CLINICAL DIAGNOSIS

In patients with congenital mitral obstruction it is important to study the cardiovascular system from the venae cavae to the descending aorta. During the last decade, 2-D echocardiography with Doppler studies has improved the noninvasive diagnosis of obstructive lesions of the mitral valve in the newborn infant. Total anomalous venous return and cor triatriatum may be ruled out with these studies. Contrast echocardiography, digital vascular imaging, nuclear magnetic resonance techniques, and isotope scans may provide a clearer definition of the problem, but definitive diagnosis today is made by careful cardiac catheterization and cineangiographic techniques. The typical angiographic finding of congenital mitral stenosis is delayed emptying of an enlarged left atrium. This finding alone in a sick, failing infant requires surgical exploration. Stenosis of pulmonary veins results in a small left atrium. The most difficult diagnosis to rule out is supravalvular ring, but noninvasive studies may be helpful. Children with other lesions, such as coarctation of the aorta or aortic hypoplasia, present with early symptoms because of their pulmonary and left-sided heart obstructions. At times, it is necessary to correct the most distal obstruction prior to the evaluation of the mitral involvement. Left atrial myxoma may mimic the clinical findings of congenital mitral stenosis, but this tumor is very rare in infants. Endocardial fibroelastosis may occur secondary to obstructive lesions within the heart, but it usually does not cause obstruction to the mitral valve. Primary endocardial fibroelastosis usually causes mitral insufficiency and can be differentiated by angiographic studies.

SURGICAL MANAGEMENT OF CONGENITAL MITRAL STENOSIS

The ideal approach to the treatment of these patients with congenital mitral valvular obstruction would be to relieve their symptoms with medical therapy and allow them to grow sufficiently so that the mitral valve can be worked on directly, but in most cases this is not feasible, and surgical procedures must be devised to relieve the pulmonary venous outflow obstruction. The surgical approach to congenital mitral obstruction depends on the age of the child, the presence of other associated congenital defects, and most importantly, the anatomic type of congenital mitral stenosis. The associated lesions can be relieved prior to the procedure on the mitral valve or they can be corrected at the same time as the mitral procedure. The age and condition of the patient are important factors in making this decision. Ideally in infants without failure to thrive the surgery should still be done prior to 1 year of age to protect the lungs from developing pulmonary hypertension.

The surgical procedure for Type I obstruction usually involves only the mitral leaflet, which is obstructed because of its long, narrow cone shape. Commissures, if present, may give some guidance as to where a commissurotomy should be done. Simple cuts are made in the leaflets under direct vision to allow inflow of blood. Testing of the degree of insufficiency produced can be evaluated by saline inserted with a left ventricular catheter to test the competency of the cut valve. Some insufficiency is always produced. The survival rates for surgery for congenital mitral stenosis are for patients with the best Type I obstruction and have been reported from 50 to 85 percent, depending on the experience of the surgical team.

The Type II valve is obstructed at the chordae tendineae level. The surgical procedure needed is usually a valve replacement, but attempts should be made to separate the chordae tendineae to allow the inflow of blood into the left ventricle. This can be done by the removal of obstructing chordae or by carrying an incision deep into the common papillary muscle to open a passage into the ventricle. Direct pressure measurements made with a left atrial catheter following plastic procedures on the valve or structures allow evaluation prior to decision making concerning a valve replacement. The valves in the Type II obstruction are frequently cleft as in a canal defect, and one must be cautious concerning any repair of the cleft because more obstruction can be produced by its repair. Surgical results are difficult to evaluate owing to the rare incidence of these anomalies, but reports have been published of good results with plastic procedures on this type of obstruction. However, more commonly Type II stenosis requires valve replacement.

Type III obstruction is at the papillary muscle level and most likely requires a valve replacement. Plastic procedures with muscle resection have been reported, but only with rare success. Valve replacement in small infants is limited by the annulus of the mitral valve. There is no good mitral annular enlarging procedure available at this time. Some increase in valve size can be made by backing the valve into the enlarged atrium and attaching the valve to atrial wall tissue. One must carefully size the valve and not attempt to place too large a valve in a position where it will not function or where it might obstruct the left ventricular outflow tract. Leaving a small defect in the inter-atrial septum may permit survival in these difficult patients. The size of this defect can be varied, with a pursestring suture placed around the defect and brought out through the groove between the right and left atria. It can be adjusted while the patient is coming off cardiopulmonary bypass and while left atrial and systemic blood pressures are being recorded.

Tissue valves should be avoided in children because of rapid valve tissue degeneration by early calcification. The lowprofile valve with a large central orifice should be the valve of choice in these patients with mitral obstruction and small left ventricular cavities; my preference is the St. Jude Medical valve. Anticoagulation is required. Mortality figures for valve replacement in infants and children with congenital mitral obstruction are difficult to obtain because of the small numbers of patients reported. Results have been published with mortality rates as low as 7.5 percent to as high as 33 percent.

MITRAL ATRESIA

This lesion can be defined as a lack of exit from the left atrium to the ventricle, and it requires an atrial opening for survival. A direct surgical approach is often impossible in these patients, but a palliative procedure such as atrial septostomy, either by medical or surgical means, may be required in infancy to allow the survival of those with an intact aortic outflow. If the patient has aortic as well as mitral atresia, the outlook is extremely grave. The main problem to be relieved by a surgical procedure is pulmonary venous hypertension. A palliative procedure such as an atrial septostomy by a Blalock-Hanlon procedure or a septostomy by inflow occlusion may relieve the obstruction. Following this, pulmonary blood flow may still be too great and may require banding of the pulmonary artery. A systemic-to-pulmonary shunt may be required if the pulmonary flow is not adequate after atrial septostomy. If these patients survive to middle childhood, a Fontan-like procedure to produce univentricular bypass of the right side of the heart may allow correction of the basic obstructive defect.

SUGGESTED READING

Carpentier A, Branchini B, Cour JC, et al. Congenital malformation of the mitral valve in children: pathology and surgical treatment. J Thorac Cardiovasc Surg 1976; 72:854–856.
Davachi F, Moller JH, Edwards JE. Diseases of the mitral valve in infancy: an anatomic analysis of 55 cases. Circulation 1971; 43:565–579.
Grenadier E, Sahn DJ, Valdes-Cruz LM, et al. 2D Echo Doppler study of congenital disorders of the mitral valve. Am Heart J 1984; 107:319–325.
Khalil KG, Shapiro I, Kilman JW. Congenital mitral stenosis. J Thorac Cardiovasc Surg 1975; 70:40–45.
Laks H, Hellenbrand WE, Kleinman C, Talner N. Left atrial-left ventricular conduit for relief of congenital mitral stenosis in infancy. J Thorac Cardiovasc Surg 1980; 80:782–787.

OPTIONS IN THE TREATMENT OF AORTIC AND SUBAORTIC STENOSIS IN CHILDREN: ROLE OF AORTOVENTRICULOPLASTY

DAVID R. CLARKE, M.D.

Congenital valvular aortic stenosis commonly requires surgical treatment in childhood to preserve ventricular function and prevent sudden death. Aortic valvulotomy can be accomplished by a number of methods and is effective in long-term palliation of about two-thirds of these patients. In a significant number of patients, however, aortic valve replacement is required: (1) when significant aortic regurgitation is present either before or after valvulotomy; plastic procedures are not ordinarily effective, (2) when the presence of a hypoplastic annulus or a severely dysplastic valve precludes adequate relief of stenosis by valvulotomy, and (3) when a previously placed, small artificial valve has failed.

In instances of discrete subaortic obstruction, direct resection of the fibrous membrane combined with septal myectomy is effective in about 75 percent of cases. If, however, a fibromuscular tunnel is present or subaortic obstruction recurs following direct resection, the simple approach can achieve long-term success in only 10 to 15 percent of patients. In these patients, if the aortic valve is normal, patch augmentation of the outflow septum combined with resection is useful, but since progressive aortic valve regurgitation is common with subvalvular aortic stenosis, this situation is rare. We have seen only one case in the past 8 years.

When aortic valve replacement is required during childhood, the pathologic condition is rarely simple; in a series of over 90 aortic valve operations over an 8-year period, 36 percent of children required valve replacement, and two-thirds of these required a major enlarging reconstruction of the left ventricular outflow tract. Placement of a small prosthetic device in the aortic annulus of a child is not effective therapy over the long term. Smaller prostheses tend to be obstructive even initially and, therefore, do not relieve the stenosis adequately; furthermore, fibrosis around a prosthetic device does not allow annular growth to keep pace with the growth of the child. It is wiser, if at all possible, to insert a valve that will accommodate adult flow without significant gradient at the time of initial valve replacement. This approach avoids multiple reoperative insults and repetitive episodes of damaging pressure overload on the left ventricle.

In the late 1970s, Konno and Rastan simultaneously developed the concept of aortoventriculoplasty with aortic valve replacement for treatment of complex left ventricular outflow tract obstruction. This allowed the implementation of rational therapy for aortic valve replacement of adequate size in children for the first time. Since 1978, 18 pediatric patients, 14 male and 4 female, have undergone aortoventriculoplasty at our institution. Ages ranged from 5 months to 17 years. Diagnoses included aortic stenosis and insufficiency in 10, annular hypoplasia in four, subaortic stenosis in three, and bacterial endocarditis with abscess in one. Fifteen patients had undergone aortic valve surgery previously, including four who had had pericardial valve prostheses implanted 2 to 5 years earlier.

TECHNIQUE

Aortoventriculoplasty usually is performed using cardiopulmonary bypass, moderate hypothermia (20 to 25° C), and sanguineous potassium cardioplegia for myocardial protection. In smaller infants, profound hypothermia (15° C) with circulatory arrest may be employed.

When bypass has been established and cooling accomplished, the aorta is cross-clamped and cardioplegia is infused into the coronary sinus or into the coronary ostia directly after a transverse aortotomy. If valve repair is not possible, the valve is excised, and the annulus diameter is determined. When this diameter is within 2 to 4 mm of the implantation diameter of the preferred adult size (at least 19 mm), the right section of the aortotomy can be extended downward through the noncoronary sinus and a posterior enlargement performed, as described by Manouguian. If the annulus size is very small or if the subvalvular area is stenotic, an aortoventriculoplasty is carried out.

The left part of the transverse aortotomy is extended proximally to the aortic annulus several millimeters to the left of the right coronary orifice. The right ventricular outflow tract is opened obliquely beneath the pulmonary valve, from the point at which the aortotomy meets the annulus toward the left anterior descending coronary artery. With the infundibular septum well visualized from both sides, it is relatively easy to extend the aortotomy proximally into the septum to open the left ventricular outflow tract widely (Fig. 1A). The septal incision is well anterior to the membranous septum so that conduction tissue is avoided. A double-layered, elliptical shaped Dacron patch then is fashioned so that ample annular enlargement can be accomplished. A valve sizer with the diameter of the valve to be implanted is helpful in determining the width of the patch. Initial annulus diameter can be doubled comfortably with this technique.

The patch then is sutured to the right side of the septal incision using running monofilament suture up to the level of the aortic annulus. Five or six interrupted horizontal mattress sutures with Teflon pledgets then are used to secure this suture line. A St. Jude valve, chosen because of its low-profile bileaflet design, durable all-pyrolite construction, and relative resistance to thrombi is sutured in place. The valve first is sutured into the native annulus using interrupted horizontal mattress sutures placed in standard fashion. These sutures are tied down so that the appropriate level of attachment of valve to patch can be determined. Valve suturing is completed by passing pledgeted horizontal mattress sutures through the double patch into the sewing ring and tying them individually (Fig. 1B).

When the valve is secured, the leaves of the patch are separated, and the posterior leaf is trimmed to fit the enlarged aortotomy. The aortic closure then is completed using the same running suture that was used to secure the patch to the septal incision. The aortic clamp now may be removed, taking great care to evacuate air from the aortic root and left cardiac chambers. An apical or atrioventricular vent is helpful at this juncture.

The anterior leaf of the Dacron patch is sutured into the resultant defect in the right ventricular outflow tract. Ample patch material must be used to avoid obstruction to right-sided outflow (Fig. 1C). Running monofilament suture technique is used, and the patient is rewarmed and the heart kept beating during this portion of the procedure. Atrial and ventricular pacing wires are placed. Pericardial and mediastinal drains are positioned, and when full rewarming is achieved, the patient is weaned from bypass in routine fashion.

Postoperative management after aortoventriculoplasty is very similar to that used following standard aortic valve replacement. Low cardiac output is rare, and systolic hypertension, frequently requiring afterload reduction therapy, is common. Warfarin and an antiplatelet agent are started when chest drains and intracardiac lines are removed. Patients usually are ready for discharge by the seventh postoperative day.

RESULTS

Among 18 patients, there have been three perioperative deaths (17 percent). The first death occurred following an emergency aortoventriculoplasty when unsuspected severe subaortic stenosis was detected after a period of cardiopulmonary bypass and ischemic arrest. If the aortoventriculoplasty had been planned and performed as the initial procedure, the child might have survived. The second death occurred in a 4-year-old child with an aortic annular abscess. Possibly a longer course of preoperative antibiotics or a different patching technique might have prevented the fatal aortic patch dehiscence. The third fatality was in a child with severe left ventricular dysfunction secondary to prolonged left ventricular pressure overload.

There were three patients with residual ventricular septal defects early in the series. Two required reoperation and one still has an insignificant shunt. Serious permanent arrhythmias were not encountered. One patient developed transient complete heart block but converted to sinus rhythm with complete right bundle-branch block. A total of four patients developed complete right bundle-branch block, one with accompanying left axis deviation.

No thromboembolic episodes have occurred. All mechanical valve patients received anticoagulation therapy with warfarin, and there have been no serious hemorrhagic complications. Three patients were treated with warfarin alone and 11 with warfarin plus aspirin, sulfinpyrazone, or dipyridamole. One patient who was begun on warfarin with sulfinpyrazone developed hematuria, which resolved with the discontinuation of the sulfinpyrazone. Prothrombin times were maintained at between 18 and 21 seconds.

Thirteen of the 15 survivors of the procedure remain asymptomatic 1 to 6 years later. Two late deaths occurred in patients at 1 and 3 years after surgery, respectively. One resulted from fungal endocarditis of the prosthesis and the other from severe calcific stenosis of the only tissue valve in the group.

DISCUSSION

Because the two late deaths in the aortoventriculoplasty experience were related to complications of the prosthetic device and because cryopreserved allograft aortic valve conduits are now easily available, we recently revised our approach. In the last five patients encountered

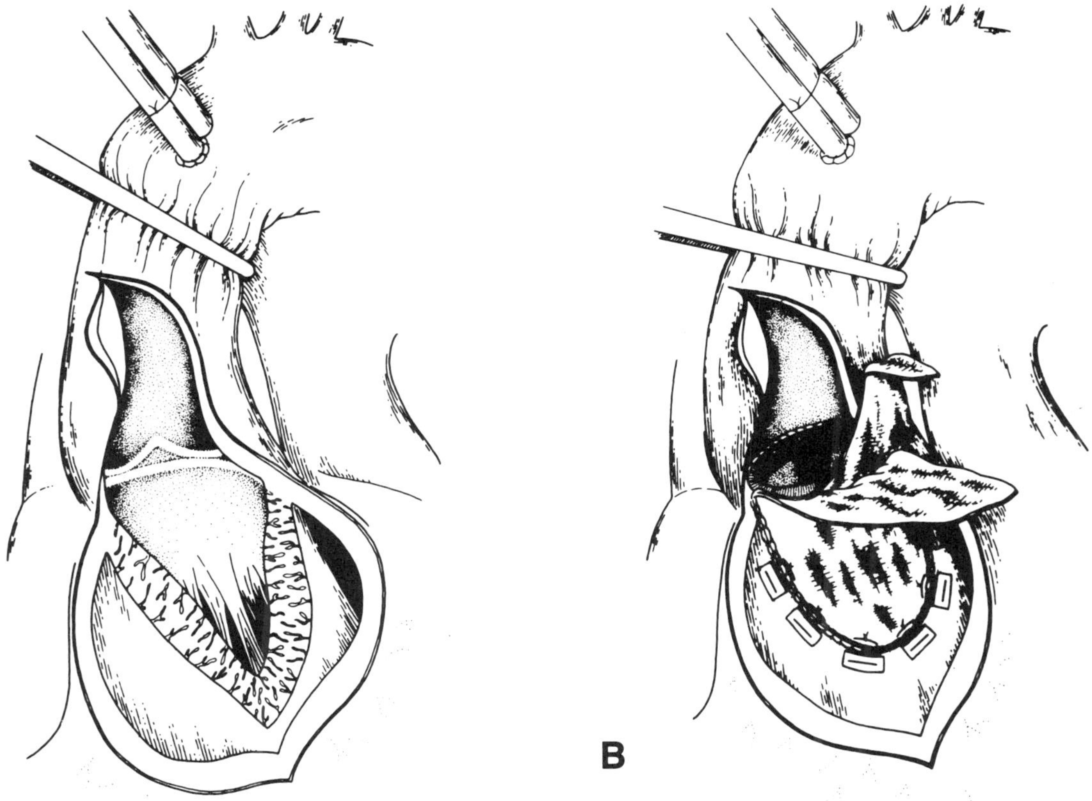

A B

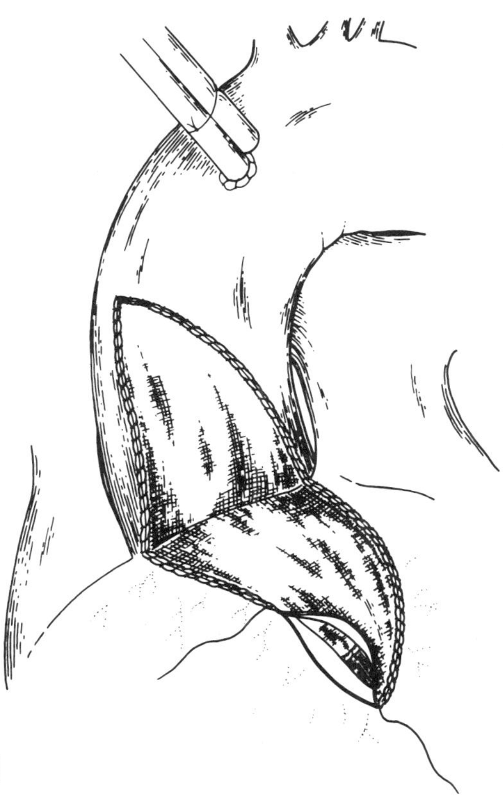

C

Figure 1 *A*, Incisions in aorta, right ventricle, and ventricular septum are made and the aortic valve excised. *B*, The bileafed Dacron patch is sutured securely to the interventricular septum and the aortic valve prosthesis is placed. *C*, The aortotomy patch is complete and, after removal of the cross-clamp, the right ventriculotomy is closed with the anterior left of patch material. (From Clarke DR. Extended aortic root replacement for treatment of left ventricular outflow tract obstruction. J Cardiac Surg 1987; (Suppl) 122.)

with complex left ventricular outflow obstruction, extended aortic root replacement (EARR) was performed. EARR combines the concept of aortoventriculoplasty with allograft aortic root replacement and coronary artery reimplantation. The valved aortic allograft is used in place of an aortic valve prosthesis, and the attached anterior mitral leaflet augments the interventricular septum to relieve the subvalvular obstruction.

The operation is performed using the same bypass technique and cardiac incisions as are used for aortoventriculoplasty. When this is accomplished, the ascending aorta is transected and the left and right coronary ostia are excised with buttons of aortic wall after minimal mobilization of the proximal portion of the coronary arteries. The aortic valve leaflets then are excised (Fig. 2A).

An antibiotic-sterilized, cryopreserved aortic allograft is selected with an internal diameter large enough to accommodate an adult cardiac output (>16 mm). The

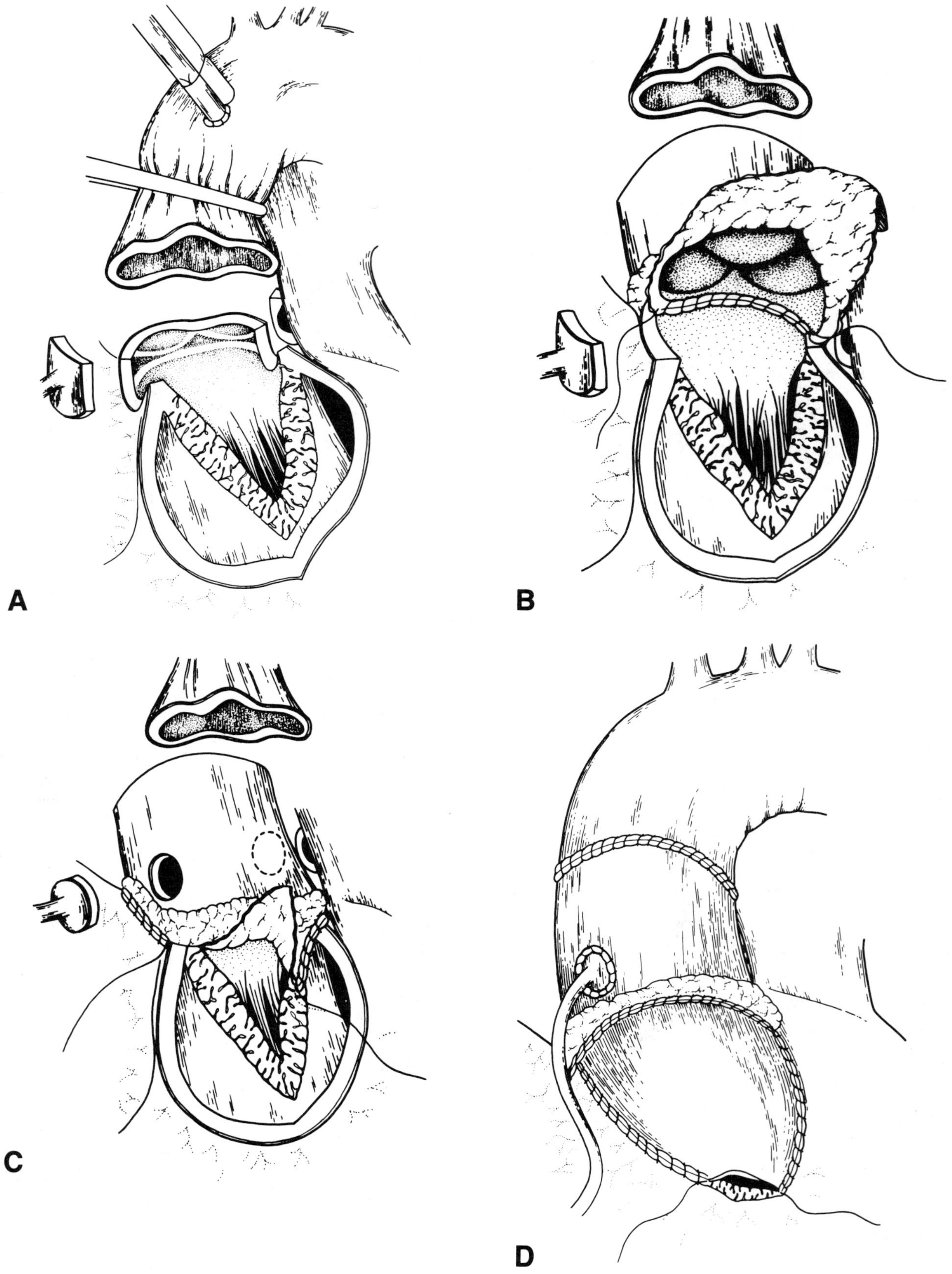

Figure 2 *A,* Cardiac incisions are similar to those for aortoventriculoplasty, but, additionally, the aorta is transected and coronary ostia are excised with buttons of aortic wall. *B,* The proximal allograft to annulus anastomosis is begun posteriorly. *C,* The donor mitral leaflet is used to widen the subvalvular area. *D,* Buttons containing coronary ostia are implanted, the distal allograft to aorta anastomosis is completed, and another piece of allograft tissue is used to patch the right ventriculotomy. (From Clarke DR. Extended aortic root replacement for treatment of left ventricular outflow tract obstruction. J Cardiac Surg 1987; (Suppl) 125, 126.)

proximal anastomosis of the allograft is begun posteriorly with running monofilament suture (Fig. 2B). The anterior mitral leaflet attached to the allograft is trimmed and sewn into the right ventricular side of the V-shaped defect in the interventricular septum, maintaining its width (Fig. 2C). The septal suture line is reinforced with Teflon pledgeted sutures. A 5-mm aortic punch is used to create sites in the aortic allograft for the coronary anastomosis. The coronary buttons then are implanted with running fine monofilament suture. The distal allograft anastomosis is accomplished using monofilament suture. The defect in the right ventricular outflow tract is patched using a triangular-shaped piece of allograft aorta, with its base along the anterior annulus of the allograft valve (Fig. 2D). The patient then is rewarmed and weaned from bypass.

All five patients had excellent hemodynamic results and easily were weaned from bypass. Transient complete heart block occurred in two cases, postpericardiotomy syndrome in one, and mediastinitis in one. None of these patients required early reoperation, but one underwent coronary bypass 6 months postoperatively after progression of his type II hyperlipidemia.

At the most recent follow-up (1 month to 1 year), all five patients are asymptomatic and not on cardiac medications or anticoagulants. Echocardiograms have revealed normal aortic valve function and wide-open left ventricular outflow tracts in all patients.

SUGGESTED READING

Cain T, Campbell D, Paton B, Clarke D. Operation for discrete subvalvular aortic stenosis. J Thorac Cardiovasc Surg 1984; 87:366-370.

Konno S, Imai Y, Iida Y, Nakajima M, Tatsuno K. A new method for prosthetic valve replacement in congenital aortic stenosis associated with hypoplasia of the aortic valve ring. J Thorac Cardiovasc Surg 1975; 70:909-917.

Manouguian S, Seybold-Epting W. Patch enlargement of the aortic valve ring by extending the aortic incision into the anterior mitral leaflet. J Thorac Cardiovasc Surg 1979; 78:402-412.

McKowen RL, Campbell DN, Woelfel GF, Wiggins JW, Clarke DR. Extended aortic root replacement with aortic allografts. J Thorac Cardiovasc Surg 1987; 93:366-377.

Rastan H, Koncz J. Aortoventriculoplasty: a new technique for the treatment of left ventricular outflow tract obstruction. J Thorac Cardiovasc Surg 1976; 71:920-927.

Schaffer MS, Campbell DN, Clarke DR, Wiggins JW, Wolfe RR. Aortoventriculoplasty in children. J Thorac Cardiovasc Surg 1986; 92:391-395.

ANOMALOUS PULMONARY VENOUS CONNECTION

CHRISTOPHER LINCOLN, F.R.C.S.

The anatomic entity of anomalous pulmonary venous connection can be conveniently divided into the partial type, in which some but not all of the pulmonary veins are directly connected to the left atrium, and the total type, in which none of the pulmonary veins are correctly connected to the left atrium. It is unfortunate that these two entities are considered together, since most of the clinical and surgical considerations are widely different. This chapter describes my personal experience in surgical correction of 83 patients with total anomalous pulmonary venous connection and 28 patients with a partial form during the years 1973 to 1986.

TOTAL ANOMALOUS PULMONARY VENOUS CONNECTION

Patient Material

Of the 83 patients under consideration, thirty-two had supracardiac drainage, most to the left vertical vein, and in one of these patients the connection was directly to the right superior vena cava. Infradiaphragmatic drainage was present in 16, and the connection was to the coronary sinus in 27 and directly to the right atrium or mixed in the remaining 8. For convenience of description and analysis, each patient is allocated to one of four groups: group 1: supracardiac; group 2: infracardiac; group 3: coronary sinus; and group 4: mixed/direct right atrium. Specifically excluded are patients with atrial isomerism and any who did not exhibit concordant atrioventricular and ventriculoarterial connections. In contrast to other groups, patients in group 2, infradiaphragmatic total anomalous pulmonary venous drainage, were smaller and tended to be more critically ill at the time of admission. The median age at operation was 14 days (range 1 to 42 days) and the median weight 3.0 kg (range 1 to 4 kg). The median body surface area was 0.2 sq m (range 0.1 to 0.2 sq m). The delay and days in hospital prior to admission were short; being a median of 1 day (range 0 to 13 days). The median pH on admission was 7.30 (range 7.20 to 7.50) (Table 1).

Risk Factors

Analysis in regard to survival within the 30-day hospital period was applied to the following "supposed" risk factors: sex of patient, year of operation in the series, age at operation in days, height and weight (each expressed as percentiles), body surface area, the number of days in the hospital prior to operation, and the pH on admission. Also included are the pulmonary artery systolic pressure and pulmonary vascular resistance in those patients who

TABLE 1 Clinical and Catheterization Data

	Group 1 Supracardiac (N = 32)	*Group 2 Infracardiac (N = 16)*	*Group 3 Coronary Sinus (N = 27)*	*Group 4 Mixed (N = 8)*
Age at operation in days	80.0 (1–180)	14.0 (1–42)	71.0 (3–240)	90.0 (2–120)
Weight in kg	4.00 (3–13)	3.00 (1–4)	4.00 (2–22)	4.00 (3–7)
Body surface area	0.26 (0.2–0.4)	0.20 (0.1–0.2)	0.25 (0.1–0.4)	0.25 (0.2–0.3)
Days in hospital prior to operation	2.00 (0–11)	1.00 (0–13)	3.00 (0–22)	5.00 (0–21)
pH on admission	7.35 (7.0–7.4)	7.30 (7.2–7.5)	7.35 (7.0–7.5)	7.39 (7.3–7.4)
PA systolic pressure	60.0 (18–130)	70.0 (41–100)	45.0 (24–114)	46.0 (20–76)
PVR	4.80 (1.0–9.0)	10.0 (2–20)	3.00 (3–20)	2.70 (1–3)
QP:QS	1.90 (0.8–7.4)	1.40 (0.6–1.9)	2.90 (1.8–4.0)	4.00 (1.0–11)
Hospital survival	30	11	24	6

All the above indices are median, with the range in parenthesis. PA = Pulmonary artery (mm Hg); PVR = Pulmonary vascular resistance units m^2.

had undergone cardiac catheterization. Account is also taken of the method of diagnosis, i.e., cardiac catheterization, cross-sectional echocardiography alone; and clinical evaluation. Finally an analysis is included of the type of perfusion used for the surgical repair, the occurrence of pulmonary hypertensive crises, the anatomy of the defect, the presence of cyanosis and heart failure, the need for preoperative ventilation, and the presence of preoperative renal failure.

Preoperative Management

Many of the patients, in particular those with the infracardiac type of total anomalous pulmonary venous connection, are critically ill when seen soon after birth. The clinical situation should be optimized, in particular, the correction of any acid-base imbalance. It is important preoperatively to maintain the patency of the arterial duct by the intravenous infusion of prostaglandin. When necessary, the patient is artificially ventilated by intermittent positive pressure. Nothing is gained from further delay; since the clinical situation can only be improved by surgically correcting the anatomic abnormality, it is my practice for the patient to undergo surgical correction at the next available operating session within the following 24 hours.

Special Investigation

Conventional cardiac catheterization and angiography can be used to establish the diagnosis and to clarify the type of anomalous venous return. More recently, 24 of the last 28 patients were diagnosed by cross-sectional echocardiography alone. Measurements are made of the pulmonary artery systolic pressure, the pulmonary vascular resistance, and the pulmonary-to-systemic flow ratio and pulmonary vascular resistance when cardiac catheterization is performed.

Operative Technique

Two methods of extracorporeal perfusion can be employed for the surgery. The first, used in only 15 patients in this series, is conventional cardiopulmonary bypass with moderate hypothermia at 28° C. The second is surface cooling followed by limited perfusion and profound hypothermia and circulatory arrest, usually reserved for those patients less than 8 kg in weight. In all patients, the heart is exposed through a conventional vertical median sternotomy incision. If it is present, a patent ductus arteriosus must be closed prior to institution of cardiopulmonary bypass. Conventional cardiopulmonary bypass is established by means of ascending aortic cannulation and two right-angled vena caval cannulas. Having established bypass, hypothermia is produced to 28° C, the aorta is cross-clamped, and the repair proceeds. Myocardial preservation is accomplished with cardioplegia and intrapericardial topical ice.

When profound hypothermic circulatory arrest technique is used, the patient is cooled by surface ice to 25° C, following which the heart is exposed through a median sternotomy. Cardiopulmonary bypass is established by means of an ascending aortic cannula and a single right atrial cannula. Core cooling of the heart and body to 15° C is then achieved, and the aorta is cross-clamped. The circulation is stopped, and blood is drained from the circulation.

Surgical Repair

Supracardiac Total Anomalous Pulmonary Venous Connection

After the aorta is cross-clamped and the heart is flaccid, it is gently retracted anteriorly and to the right, thereby exposing the back of the left atrium and the confluence of the pulmonary veins, which can be seen through the thin pericardium. The confluence is then dissected free of surrounding connective tissue and fully mobilized. An incision is made in the back wall of the left atrium commencing in the region of the left atrial appendage. A wide and open anastomosis is performed using fine monofilament suture, the anastomosis being as large as possible (Fig. 1A and B).

Infradiaphragmatic Total Anomalous Pulmonary Venous Connection

In this defect the heart is retracted anteriorly and to the right as previously described, and the confluence of the pulmonary veins is exposed in the retropericardial position. In this anomaly, there is a descending vein that emerges through the hemidiaphragm. After mobilization, it is transected at the level of the hemidiaphragm, and both cut ends are oversewn with a running suture. This allows the confluence to move freely in a cephalad direction. An incision is made in the long axis of the confluence and then in the posterior wall of the left atrium, following which the anastomosis is constructed (Fig. 2A and B).

Total Anomalous Pulmonary Venous Connection to the Coronary Sinus

The approach to this repair is via the right atrium through an incision that runs parallel to the right atrioventricular groove, sparing the crista terminalis. The superior wall of the coronary sinus is cut back, thereby allowing

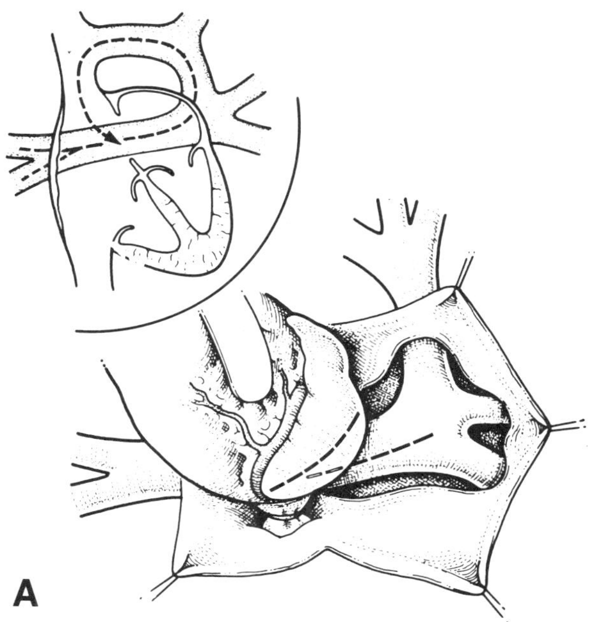

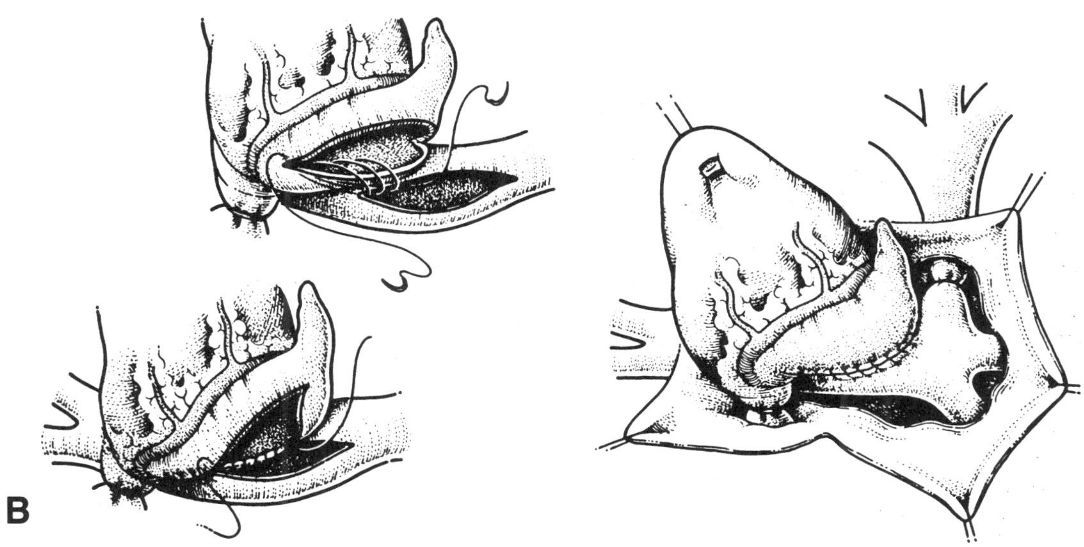

Figure 1 Incisions into the pulmonary venous confluence and left atrium (*A*) and technique of anastomosis (*B*) for supracardiac total anomalous pulmonary venous connection.

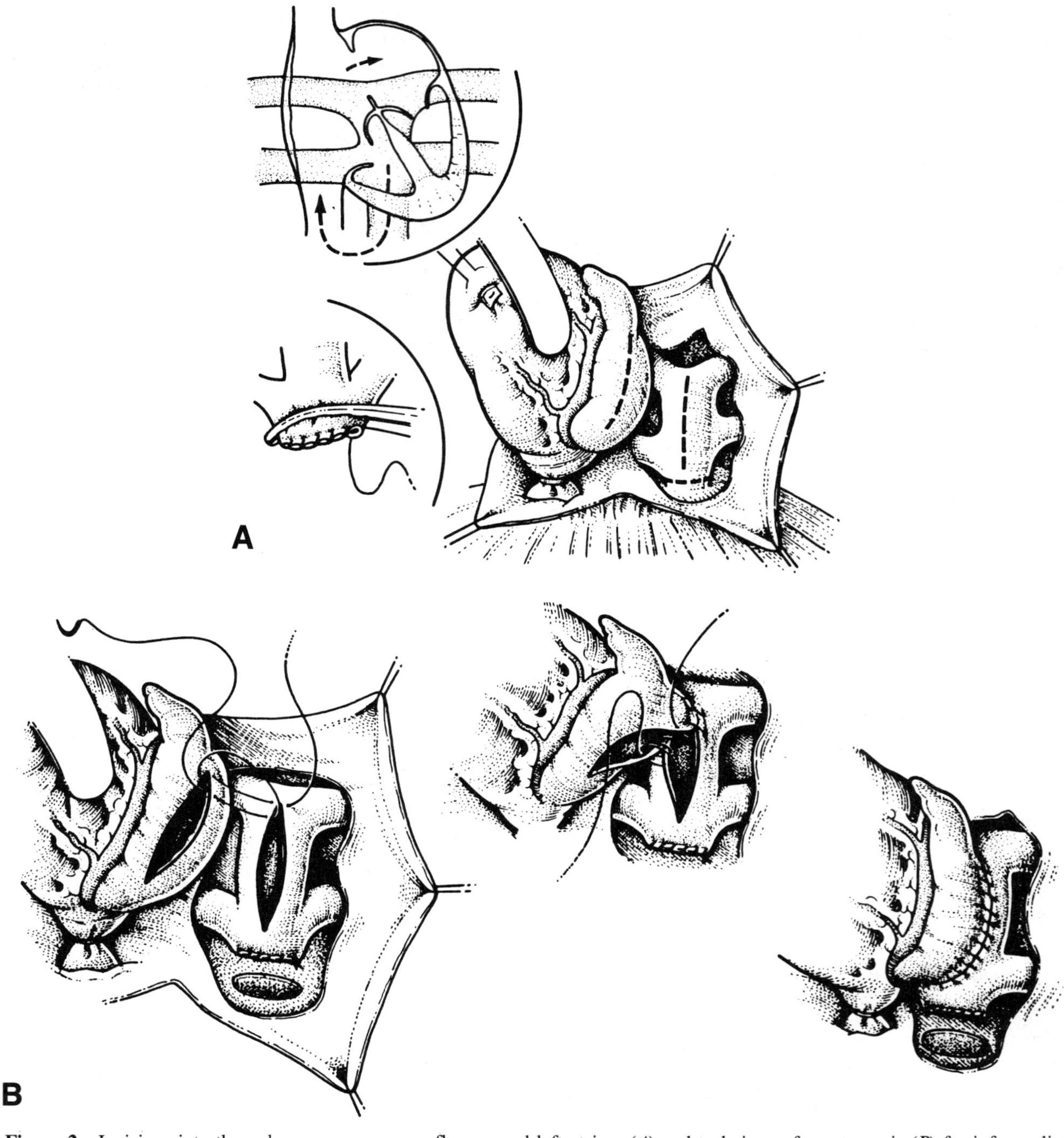

Figure 2 Incisions into the pulmonary venous confluence and left atrium (*A*) and technique of anastomosis (*B*) for infracardiac total anomalous pulmonary venous connection.

free communication with the left atrium. A full patch of Dacron cloth is then placed to roof in this new confluence, thereby directing all pulmonary venous return to the left atrium. The inferior suture line is close to the area of the atrioventricular node. Care must be taken when placing sutures here (Fig. 3).

Mixed Total Anomalous Pulmonary Venous Drainage

In this situation, a combination of any of the above techniques is used.

Other Surgical Considerations

Ligation of Left Superior Vena Cava

Obviously, to complete the repair, a persistent left superior vena cava should be ligated at the end of the operation. It is preferable to delay closure of this channel until this time. After discontinuing cardiopulmonary bypass and with a stable circulation, the left superior vena caval snare is temporarily pulled up and the systemic and pulmonary arterial pressures are monitored. Occasionally, there may be an acute elevation of the pulmonary artery pressure and

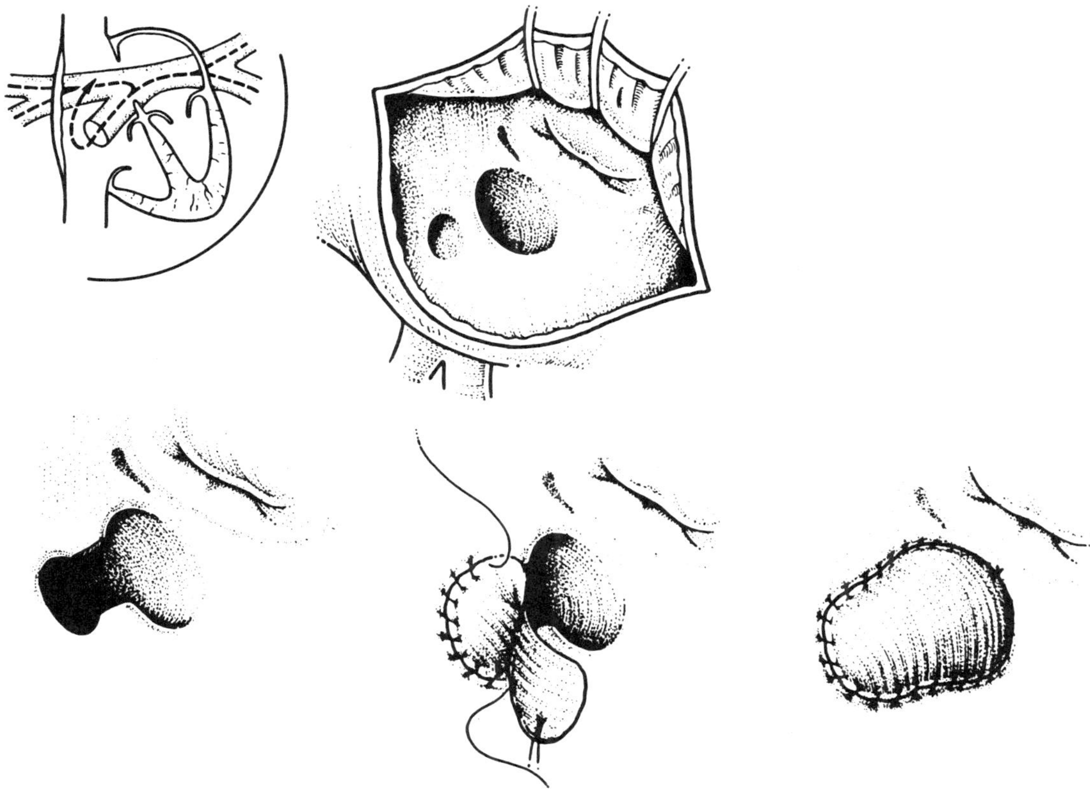

Figure 3 Total anomalous pulmonary venous connection to the coronary sinus. The superior wall of the coronary sinus is cut back as shown, and a Dacron cloth patch is then placed over this new confluence, thus directing pulmonary venous return, via the coronary sinus, into the left atrium.

a fall in the systemic arterial pressure, indicating an inadequate anastomotic size. In this circumstance, the left superior vena cava is either left unsnared or an attempt is made to widen the anastomosis.

Closure of the Atrial Septal Defect or Patent Foramen Ovale

Frequently an atrial septal defect or patent foramen ovale is present. Closure of this defect by direct suture can decrease the size of the left atrium. If according to inspection it seems likely that this will occur, a full patch is placed, thereby enlarging the left atrial cavity but at the same time closing the interatrial communication.

Other Surgical Techniques

In this experience, the trans right atrial–left atrial approach (Shumacker) can be used in particular to correct groups 1 and 2 anatomies. This incision is potentially damaging to atrial structures.

Excellent exposure of the confluence of the pulmonary veins and the posterior wall of the left atrium can be achieved through the transverse sinus by retracting the aorta to the left and the superior vena cava to the right. This approach has been successfully performed in two patients but requires further evaluation.

Postoperative Management

Since these patients are frequently in acute or chronic congestive heart failure with third space fluid, during the first 48 hours following surgery, each patient receives only 500 ml of fluid per square meter. No attempt is made to extubate the patient immediately following surgery. An indwelling pulmonary arterial monitoring line is placed at surgery in all patients in whom it is suspected or proved that pulmonary arterial pressure and pulmonary vascular resistance are elevated. Pulmonary hypertensive crises have been recognized and treated in 10 of our patients. Seven had supracardiac and three had coronary sinus forms of total anomalous pulmonary venous drainage. These crises are manifested by a sudden major clinical deterioration associated with a rise in the pulmonary artery pressure to systemic levels with concomitant evidence of a fall in cardiac output, which is not precipitated by hypercapnia or hypoxia. In eight patients an infusion of tolazoline hydrochloride initially as a bolus of 1 to 2 mg per kilogram followed by continuous intravenous infusion at 1 to 2 mg per kilogram per hour resulted in a major improvement in the clinical status associated with a fall in the pulmonary pressure and a reduction in the ratio of pulmonary artery to systemic artery pressure. Nevertheless, three out of 10 patients treated for this complication eventually died.

Reoperation

Reoperation can be necessary and was carried out in seven patients. In group 1 (supracardiac), three patients required closure of a residual atrial septal defect, and one underwent obliteration of a persistent left superior vena cava. Two patients in group 3 (coronary sinus), required reoperation. There was a persistent atrial septal defect in one, and a second patient underwent redirection of the inferior vena caval inflow into the right atrium, this having been inadvertently baffled into the left atrium at the original operation. One patient in group 4 required closure of an atrial septal defect. It is noteworthy that in four of the patients with a residual atrial septal defect, a trans-right atrial–left atrial approach had been used together with enlargement of the atrial septum.

Results

There has been a steady improvement in results of the correction of this anomaly. In this experience, 12 (14 percent) of the 83 patients died within 30 days of surgery. There were two deaths in group 1, five in group 2, three in group 3, and two in group 4. The causes of death were refractory low cardiac output in six, recurrent pulmonary hypertension crises in three, and supraventricular arrhythmias, acute renal failure, and cardiac failure each in one of three remaining patients. Six patients died more than 30 days after surgery. In two of these there was pulmonary venous obstruction at the site of the anastomosis between the pulmonary venous confluence and the morphologic left atrium. Death in the first patient was 2.5 months after the operation but was 6.5 years later in the second. The cause of death in the remaining four was not known (Table 2).

Actuarial analysis of long-term survival showed that the probability of survival, based on all 83 patients entering the study, was 75 percent at 84 months. Similar figures were obtained for group 1 and groups 3 and 4. However, the probability of survival of the 13 patients in group 2, those with infradiaphragmatic anomalous pulmonary venous connection, was 60 percent at 72 months (Table 3).

The following factors showed a significant difference with regard to survival within the 30-day hospital period. Risk of hospital death was greater in the group with infracardiac total anomalous pulmonary venous connection (group 2) ($p < 0.009$). The presence of postoperative pulmonary hypertensive crises was significant ($p < 0.025$). The first 3 years of the study (1973-1975) showed a higher risk of death than the remaining years, the break being 1975-76 ($p < 0.01$), and it was shown that females were more at risk than males ($p < 0.0025$). The presence of heart failure preoperatively was a risk factor influencing survival ($p < 0.025$). The only factor that improved the chance of survival was when the method of diagnosis was cross-sectional echocardiography associated with clinical and other radiologic examinations ($p < 0.05$).

Discussion

From 1973 to 1975, 13 patients in this series were treated with a hospital mortality of 46 percent (Table 4). Since that time, 70 patients have been treated with a mortality of 8.5 percent, giving a current overall mortality over a 13 year period of 14 percent. This in part may reflect the "era effect" on the unit and its personnel, but there must be other factors influencing the change.

The risk of surgical death was greatly increased in patients with the infracardiac type of total anomalous pulmonary venous drainage. This largely reflects the aforementioned risk factors, since the surgical technique to repair the defect is not dissimilar to that for the repair of other forms of total anomalous pulmonary venous drainage.

The recognition of postoperative pulmonary hypertensive crises by us in 1978 demonstrated that these patients are at risk from such crises and that they can be effectively treated by specific pharmacologic agents.

There can be severe leftward displacement of the interventricular septum when pulmonary hypertension is present, which encroaches on the left ventricular cavity. This reversed Bernheim's effect may corroborate the work of Laver and co-workers, who demonstrated this dynamic septal movement in patients with acute or chronic right

TABLE 2 Age at Operation with Hospital Mortality

	All Patients (N = 83)	*Group 1 Supracardiac (N = 32)*	*Group 2 Infracardiac (N = 16)*	*Group 3 Coronary Sinus (N = 27)*	*Group 4 Mixed (N = 8)*
Age at Operation:					
1–7 days	10 (1)	2 (0)	5 (1)	3 (0)	
8–14 days	12 (3)	6 (0)	6 (3)		
15–21 days	9 (0)		4 (0)	3 (0)	2 (0)
22–28 days	5 (2)	3 (1)		1 (1)	1 (0)
1–2 m	7 (1)	3 (0)	1 (1)	3 (0)	
2–3 m	10 (2)	3 (0)		6 (1)	1 (1)
3–4 m	12 (2)	6 (0)		4 (1)	2 (1)
4–5 m	5 (0)	2 (0)		1 (0)	2 (0)
5–6 m	6 (0)	4 (0)		2 (0)	
6–>12 m	7 (1)	3 (1)		4 (0)	

Number in parenthesis denotes number of hospital deaths.

TABLE 3 Total Anomalous Pulmonary Venous Connection; 30-Day Hospital Mortality

	No. Patients	*N*†	*%*	*75% Confidence Limits*
Supracardiac	32	2	6	2–16
Infradiaphragmatic	16	5	31	18–47
Coronary Sinus	27	3	11	4–21
Mixed	8	2	25	8–49
All Patients	83	12	14	10–19

† Death

ventricular volume overload. This septal displacement decreases the volume of the left ventricle, thereby impeding left ventricular filling and causing left ventricular "end diastolic tamponade." This may be one of the mechanisms leading to low cardiac output in the early postoperative period in these patients. In our analysis of risk factors, investigation by cross-sectional echocardiography alone was the sole significant factor in improving the chance of survival. By avoiding cardiac catheterization, surgical mortality is significantly reduced. It is our current practice, therefore, always to use cross-sectional echocardiography as the final arbiter in the diagnosis of total anomalous pulmonary venous connection.

PARTIAL ANOMALOUS PULMONARY VENOUS CONNECTION

Patient Material

Twenty-two patients were treated for the usual form (sinus venosus) of anomalous pulmonary venous connection. In this anomaly the right pulmonary veins drain into the lower part of the superior vena cava, communicating indirectly with the left atrium through an atrial septal defect. In four patients, all the right pulmonary veins drained into the right atrium in the presence of an intact atrial septum. Two patients had the right pulmonary veins draining into the upper part of the inferior vena cava, the Scimitar syndrome. Anomalous drainage of the left pulmonary veins was not seen in this series. The mean age of patients at the time of operation was 8 years.

Risk Factors

These patients are frequently asymptomatic at the time of surgical correction and the risk factors are few except in the elderly, in whom pulmonary hypertension may have developed. However, in the current era, it is most unusual to see older patients.

TABLE 4 Total Anomalous Pulmonary Venous Connection

Year	*No. Patients*	*Death*	
1973–1975	13	6	(46.1%)
1975–1986	70	6	(8.5%)
1973–1986	83	12	(14.0%)

Special Investigations

The diagnosis of these defects can be made by noninvasive methods, such as cross-sectional echocardiography. It is unusual for patients other than those over 40 to require cardiac catheterization.

Operative Techniques

Conventional cardiopulmonary bypass with the use of right-angled vena caval cannulas facilitates the repair. The superior vena cava is cannulated directly above the level of the azygos vein, and the inferior vena cava is cannulated at its junction with the right atrium.

Surgical Repair

Right Pulmonary Veins to Superior Vena Cava (Sinus Venosus Defect)

Following cross-clamping of the aorta and instillation of cardioplegia, an incision is made parallel and anterior to the interatrial groove, extending from the mid-right atrium cephalad up onto the lower part of the superior vena cava. This gives excellent exposure of the anomaly. A disadvantage of this incision is the possibility of damaging the artery to the sinoatrial node, which is known occasionally to encircle this junctional area. If the atrial septal defect is limiting, it is enlarged and then a full patch of Dacron cloth is placed to reroute the pulmonary veins into the left atrium (Fig. 4).

Right Pulmonary Veins to Right Atrium

In this repair, the incision begins as for the above defect but does not extend up onto the junctional area of the superior vena cava with the right atrium. When the atrial septum is intact, a vertical incision is made in the right lateral part of the atrial septum and a large section of the septum is excised up to the limbus. The right pulmonary veins are then redirected into the left atrium by a full patch of Dacron cloth roofing in this confluence (Fig. 5).

Right Pulmonary Veins to Inferior Vena Cava

In this anomaly, the right pulmonary veins drain into the inferior vena cava at its most terminal portion. Since exposure to this can be limited by the presence of the inferior vena caval cannula, the repair is facilitated by utilizing hypothermia to 20° C and low flow or even circulatory arrest when the inferior vena caval cannula can be removed. A tunnel-shaped patch is placed to reroute the pulmonary veins cephalad into the right atrium and thence into the left atrium through the atrial septal defect. Since the inferior vena caval channel is capacious in this area, the risk of causing obstruction is minimal (Fig. 6).

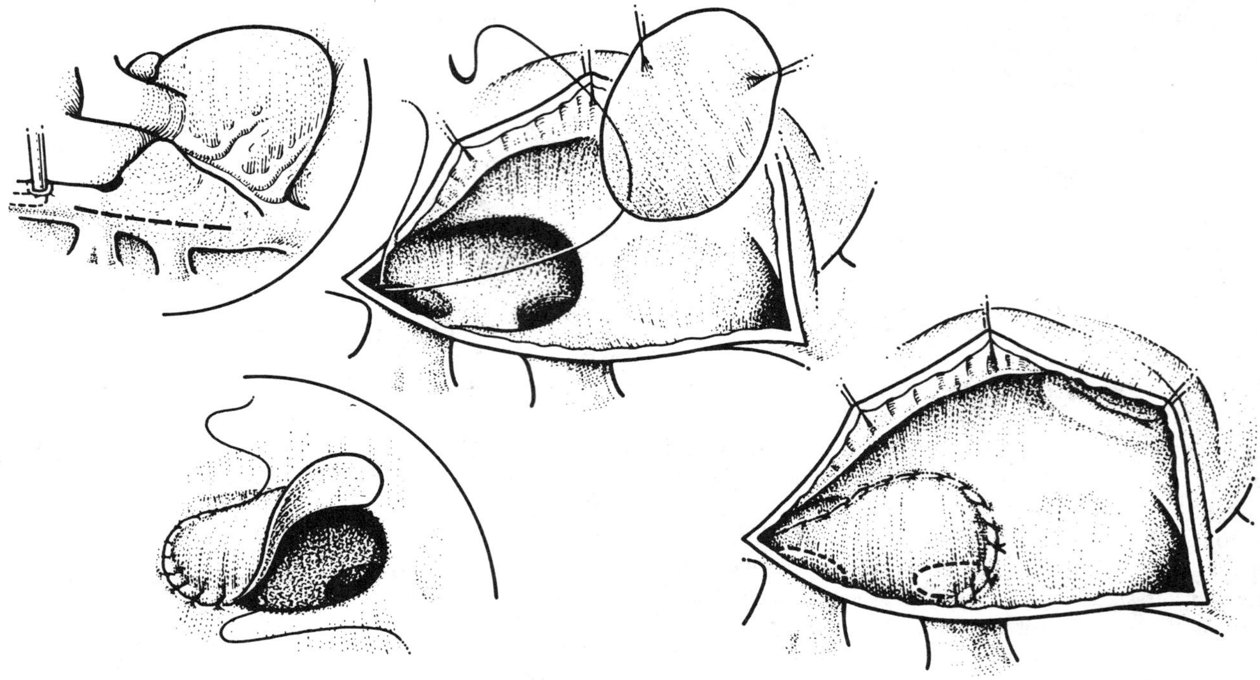

Figure 4 Sinus venosus defect with partial anomalous venous connection of the right pulmonary veins into the superior vena cava. An incision is made into the atrium, as shown. The atrial septal defect is then patched to reroute the pulmonary veins to the left atrium.

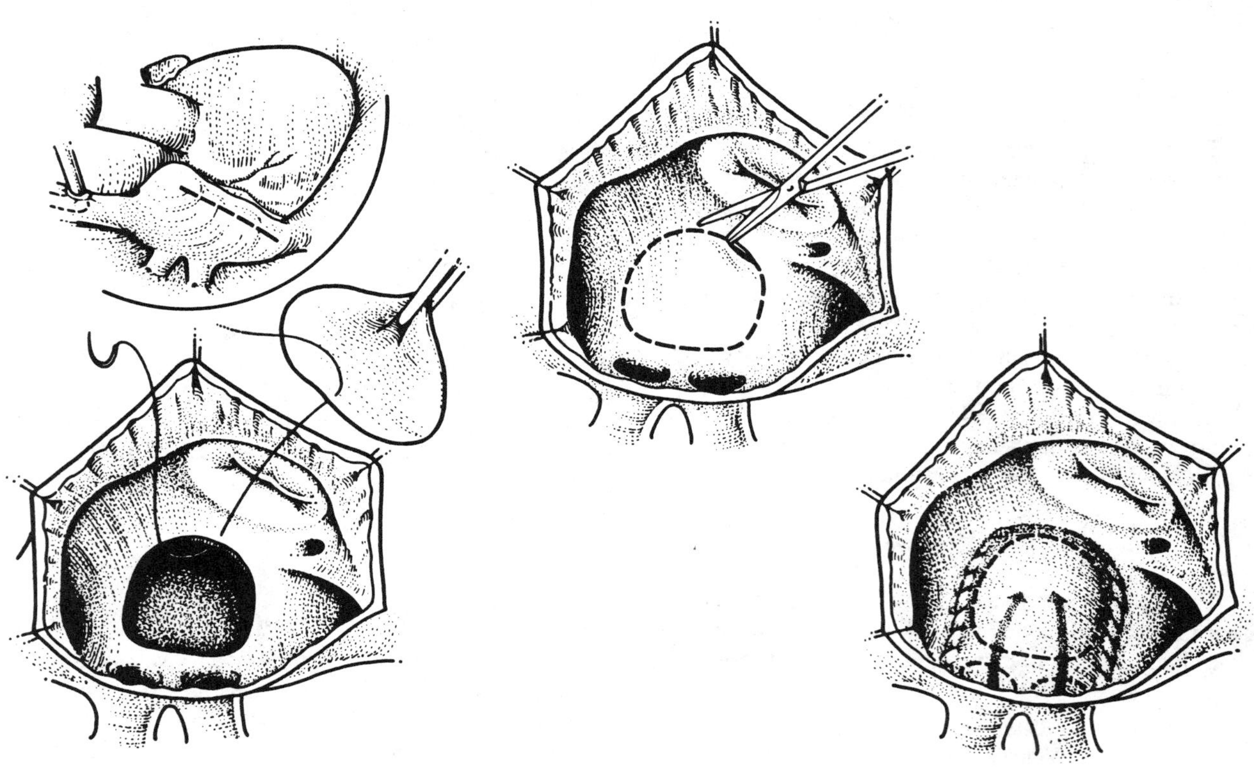

Figure 5 Partial anomalous pulmonary venous drainage with the right pulmonary veins draining into the right atrium. The right atrium is incised as shown. A portion of the interatrial septum is excised up to the limbus of the atrial septum. The right pulmonary veins are then redirected into the left atrium with a Dacron patch.

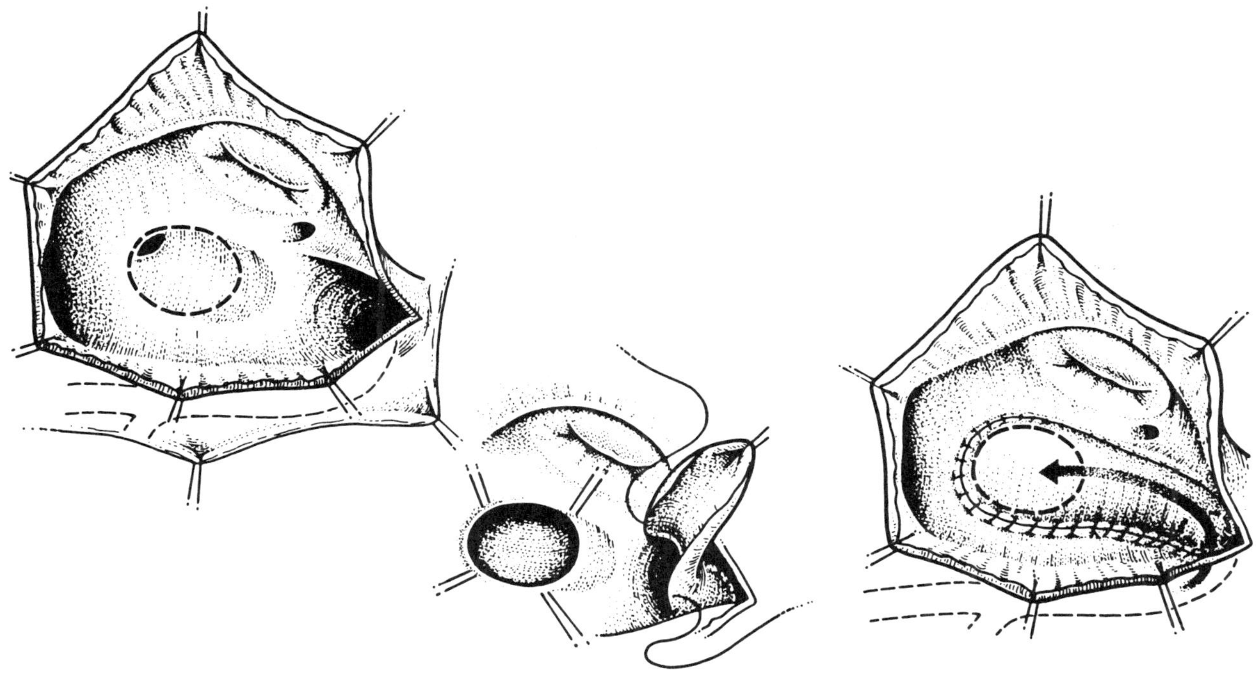

Figure 6 Partial anomalous pulmonary venous drainage with right pulmonary veins draining into the inferior vena cava. A tunnel-shaped patch is placed to reroute the right pulmonary veins cephalad, via the right atrium and thence into the left atrium.

Postoperative Management

The management of these patients is unremarkable. Anticoagulation therapy for 3 months is recommended for patients over the age of 20 years to minimize the theoretical risk of systemic emboli.

Results

In the current era, the 30-day hospital mortality for this defect is low, less than 1 percent and in this series it was 0.

SUGGESTED READING

Bove KE, Geiser CA, Meyr RA. The left ventricle in anomalous pulmonary venous return. Arch Pathol 1975; 99:522-528.

Jones ODH, Shore DF, Rigby ML, Leijala M, Scallan M, Shinebourne EA, Lincoln JCR. The use of tolazoline hypochloride as a pulmonary vaso-dilator in potentially fatal pulmonary vaso-constrictive episodes following cardiac surgery in children. Part 2C. Circulation 1981; 64:134-139.

Lincoln JCR, Rigby ML, Mercanti C, Al-Fogih M, Joseph MC, Miller GA, Shinebourne EA. Surgical risk factors in total anomalous pulmonary venous connection. Am J Cardiol 1988; 61:608–611.

Newfeld EA, Wilson A, Paul MH, Reisch JF. Pulmonary vascular disease in total anomalous pulmonary venous drainage. Circulation 1980; 61:103-109.

Yee ES, Turley K, Wen-Ren Hsieh, Ebert PA. Infant total anomalous pulmonary venous connection: factors influencing timing of presentation and operative outcome. Circulation 1987; 76:83–87.

CARDIAC TRANSPLANTATION IN CHILDREN

DOUGLAS M. BEHRENDT, M.D.
G. MICHAEL DEEB, M.D.

Heart transplantation for adults with end-stage heart disease has become an accepted therapeutic modality, but by July, 1986, only 186 cardiac transplants in children 19 years of age or less had been reported to the International Cardiac Registry. However, because there are many diseases and congenital anomalies affecting the hearts of children for which no effective conventional therapy is available and because children have such a long potential life expectancy, the possibility of achieving a definitive "cure" by means of transplantation has great appeal. Thus, these operations are being performed with increasing frequency.

INDICATIONS

Cardiac transplantation in children, as in adults, is reserved for patients judged to have less than a year to live.

There may be ventricular dysfunction from viral or nonspecific cardiomyopathy or from damage sustained during previous cardiac surgery, or the child may have a condition for which no good surgical options are available, such as severe Ebstein's anomaly, hypoplastic right or left ventricle, or uncorrectable valvular lesions.

Many patients with congenital heart disease develop pulmonary vascular obstructive disease as a result either of long-standing left-to-right shunts or of severe left atrial hypertension. Orthotopic heart transplantation is then contraindicated, because the newly transplanted normal right ventricle may fail when faced with an abruptly increased afterload. Normally, pulmonary vascular resistance should not exceed 4 Wood units, although some patients with resistances of 4 to 8 Wood units may be considered for cardiac transplantation if there is evidence that the resistance will fall with medical therapy. Our experience in children suggests that these guidelines may be exceeded, because the elevated pulmonary vascular resistance encountered in young children often falls if the patient survives operation. Evidence for potential reversibility is obtained at cardiac catheterization by administration of pulmonary vasodilators such as 100 percent oxygen, amrinone, or dobutamine. We performed a successful cardiac transplantation on one 13-year-old girl with cardiomyopathy whose preoperative pulmonary vascular resistance was 13 Wood units, falling to 8 Wood units with 100 percent oxygen and dobutamine. She survived the operation and has had a progressive fall in pulmonary vascular resistance postoperatively. Patients with severe, irreversible pulmonary hypertension may be considered for combined heart-lung transplantation procedures.

Most experience with pediatric transplantation has been with teenagers who respond very well to this form of therapy. Only 30 patients younger than 12 years old have undergone heart transplants, and only seven of these have been infants. Most recently, Bailey has reported two successful short-term survivals of three newborns who underwent cardiac transplantation for hypoplastic left heart syndrome. Although many children with uncorrectable forms of heart disease die in the first few years of life, inability to obtain appropriate donors, concerns about performing endomyocardial biopsies in small patients, and potential drug side effects have restrained progress in pediatric transplantation. We have been able to perform biopsies in children as young as 7 months of age, but we suspect that this will prove difficult in younger patients. Until better noninvasive methods of detecting rejection become available, managing the immunosuppression of infants is likely to remain a problem.

Contraindications to heart transplantation in children are basically the same as those that apply to adults: active infection, irreversible pulmonary hypertension, the presence of other diseases that might limit survival, and socioeconomic or emotional instability in either the child or the family. Since the young child cannot speak for him- or herself, the transplant team must evaluate the family's ability to adhere to the necessary rigorous follow-up care. The impact upon the rest of the family of the inevitable media attention, medical demands, and potential ultimate death of the child must all be carefully evaluated.

TECHNIQUE

The technique of heart transplantation in children is basically the same as that in adults. Procurement of the donor heart is often carried out in conjunction with surgical teams obtaining other organs. A heart is sought from a donor who is within 20 percent of body weight of the recipient. The organ is removed by dividing the inferior and superior venae cavae, pulmonary veins, and great vessels. Myocardial protection is achieved by infusing cardioplegic solution at 4 ° C and by packing the heart in sterile, cold, physiologic solution within an ice chest. Experience has shown that ischemic periods of up to 4 hours are safe utilizing these simple preservation methods.

The recipient is prepared as for any open heart procedure with appropriate monitoring lines and cannulas for cardiopulmonary bypass. The diseased heart is excised at the atrioventricular junction, leaving generous cuffs of right and left atria, ascending aorta, and main pulmonary artery. The donor heart is prepared by incisions between the four pulmonary veins to create a single left atrial cuff and by an incision from the inferior vena caval orifice to the base of the right atrial appendage to create a large right atrial cuff. The superior vena cava is ligated. The heart is then sutured to the recipient bed by anastomosing the appropriate atrial cuffs together with a continuous suture and then by anastomosing the pulmonary artery and ascending aorta. During this time, donor heart hypothermia is maintained by administration of another 5 ml per kilogram of cardioplegic solution as well as by external cardiac cooling. After the suture lines have been completed, the aortic clamp is removed and the heart is defibrillated if necessary. The acutely denervated heart must be supported with catecholamines; therefore, isoproterenol or dopamine or both are initiated prior to termination of cardiopulmonary bypass.

Some modifications have been required when the recipient has congenital heart disease with malpositioning of the great arteries. In essence, both donor pulmonary artery and aorta must be cut unusually long, with both branches of the pulmonary artery included so that these vessels can be appropriately tailored to connect with the recipient's great arteries. The recipient's right and left atria must be normally situated so that the atrial cuff may be anastomosed to the donor heart.

Donors in the pediatric age group are difficult to locate, especially newborns. This scarcity of appropriate human hearts has led to great interest in xenografting hearts from other species, and there have been some promising laboratory results. However, an early clinical attempt by Hardy with a chimpanzee heart and a recent attempt by Bailey with a baboon heart have failed.

POSTOPERATIVE CARE

Postoperatively the patient is managed according to the routines for any patient undergoing open heart surgery. In addition, one must initially administer isoproterenol or dopamine or both to support both contractility and heart rate, because the heart is acutely denervated. Atrial pacing is often used for several days. It is imperative that the patient be extubated and have catheters removed as soon as possible to reduce the likelihood of infection.

Patients with increased pulmonary vascular resistance require more prolonged monitoring. In this instance we administer a high FIO_2 along with those drugs that were shown preoperatively to reduce the resistance. The pulmonary artery pressure is monitored through an indwelling catheter as these drugs are tapered. A slightly larger than usual heart is used, and the ischemic time is kept as short as possible to minimize postoperative myocardial depression. In one such patient, the right ventricle failed, and we utilized extracorporeal membrane oxygenation for 3 days to support the patient until right ventricular function improved sufficiently to sustain cardiac output.

Patients have endomyocardial biopsies performed on a weekly basis starting 7 days following operation. They are discharged from the hospital after they are hemodynamically stable and the absence of rejection is documented by biopsy. Subsequent outpatient biopsies are then performed weekly until it is certain that no rejection is occurring. The frequency of biopsies is then reduced. Biopsies in small children are best carried out through the femoral vein utilizing a small bioptome (Cordis), whereas in teenagers they are done through the internal jugular route. Three or four pieces are obtained, and the degree of rejection is graded according to standard techniques. Interestingly, we have been able to do this on an outpatient basis in children as young as 7 months of age with only light sedation.

It is of interest that the newborns reported by Bailey have not undergone routine biopsy because of the difficulty of access. Rejection has been diagnosed by changes in clinical signs and laboratory data and then treated successfully with oral steroid pulses.

IMMUNOSUPPRESSION

We have utilized cyclosporine and steroids in the past according to a protocol similar to that for adults. Preoperatively, 17 mg per kilogram of cyclosporine are given orally. Initially, after operation 5 mg per kilogram are given through a nasogastric tube or orally twice a day and then adjusted to give cyclosporine blood levels of between 200 and 400 mg per liter (high pressure liquid chromatography assay). We have found that young children need far higher doses than adults to maintain cyclosporine at blood levels within the therapeutic range. For example, our 7-month-old patient required 28 mg per kilogram per day, roughly four times the adult dose. It must be remembered that cyclosporine causes a high incidence of seizures in children and that many drugs affect the cyclosporine blood level.

Methylprednisolone (Solu-Medrol) is initially given in a dose of 15 mg per kilogram at the termination of bypass, and three doses of 5 mg per kilogram are administered during the first 36 postoperative hours. The patient is then started on prednisone, 2 mg per kilogram per day, which is gradually tapered to 0.3 mg per kilogram per day by discharge.

This regimen has recently been modified by lowering the initial preoperative cyclosporine dose to 5 mg per kilogram by mouth and giving antithymic globulin (ATGAM)* 10 mg per kilogram per day intravenously for 7 days postoperatively, at which time the cyclosporine level should have stabilized in the therapeutic range.

Rejection episodes have been treated with intravenous or oral steroid pulses, and if these are unsuccessful, with ATGAM (17 mg per kilogram) for 14 days.

This immunosuppressive regimen has many unpleasant side effects, among which are hirsutism, osteoporosis, hypertension, renal failure, and a cushingoid appearance. Thus, at 3 to 6 months following operation we now lower the steroid and cyclosporine doses while adding azathioprine (Imuran). Whether this will reduce side effects without increasing the incidence of rejection or infection remains to be seen.

RESULTS

The early mortality from heart transplantation has been steadily improving among children as it has among adults. Graft rejection is the major factor affecting survival. The same complications can be expected to occur: infection, rejection, hypertension, and cyclosporine nephropathy. We have found that children are able to live with their siblings and engage in normal childhood activities without becoming infected unusually often. Accelerated atherosclerosis of the coronary arteries is a problem in children just as it is in adults, and several have required retransplantation for this. One of our patients, who was 2 years old, died suddenly of this condition 18 months postoperatively. She had been treated for numerous rejection episodes, suggesting that the damage to her coronary arteries was a manifestation of chronic rejection.

There has been great concern that children with heart transplants might not grow normally because of the immunosuppressive drugs, but laboratory experience with cardiac transplantation in young animals and clinical experience with renal and other transplants in infants suggest that growth and development are relatively normal. The short follow-up evidence we have obtained in our group of children supports this.

In his newborns with cardiac transplants, Bailey has avoided using steroids altogether because of concern about their possible effects on growth. Thus, his patients have been maintained on azathioprine and cyclosporine alone, with prednisone used only to reverse suspected rejection.

It had initially been hoped that neonates might have a sufficiently immature immune system that rejection would not occur. Unfortunately, Bailey's experiences have not borne this out.

Despite reservations expressed by some about the ethics of transplantation in children, the quality of life experienced postoperatively has been excellent. Most are returned to normal lives, and none of our patients has found the medications or biopsies to be troublesome. Con-

* Equine Antithymocytic Globulin, Upjohn.

sequently, we believe that transplantation will find an increasingly expanded role in treating children with otherwise untreatable heart disease.

SUGGESTED READING

Behrendt DM, Crowley D, Uzark K. Potential for reversibility of pulmonary vascular obstructive disease in children following cardiac transplantation. Am J Cardiol 1986; 58:1124–1126.

Bailey L, Li ZJ, Roost H, Jolley W. Host maturation after orthotopic cardiac transplantation during neonatal life. Heart Transplant 1984; 3:265–267.

Bailey LL, Nehlsen-Cannarella SL, Doroshaw RW, et al. Cardiac allotransplantation in newborns as therapy for hypoplastic left heart syndrome. N Engl J Med 1986; 315:949–951.

Fricker FJ, Griffith BP, Hardesty RL, et al. Experience with heart transplantation in children. Pediatrics 1987; 79:138–146.

Pennington DG, Sarafian J, Swarty M. Heart transplantation in children. J Heart Transplant 1985; 4:441–445.

Reitz BA, Jamieson SW, Gaudiani VA, et al. Method for cardiac transplantation in corrected transposition. J Cardiovasc Surg 1982; 23:293–296.

CARDIAC PACING IN CHILDREN

RICHARD B. SHEPARD, M.D.
MARK E. SAND, M.D.
EDWARD V. COLVIN, M.D.

The principal goal for cardiac pacing in children is to maintain life for an additional 60 years or more. Subgoals are to help their lives be as normal as possible and to avoid crippling complications not only now but years in the future. These goals mean that one must always consider the very long-term as well as the short-term effects of one's technical choices and procedures. The old adage "perfect is the enemy of good" may be altered to say that at times, "perfect now is the enemy of good later." The clinical questions are (1) is pacing necessary or desirable in terms of the various risk balances that apply, (2) what operative approach should be used, and (3) what modes of pacing and forms of hardware should be chosen now so that present goals are met and necessary flexibility for the future is preserved?

Small subjects destined for large growth spurts have been at risk for wound erosion, high pacing thresholds, electrode distraction, wire fracture, hardware trauma, and infection associated with the rigors of childhood. Our techniques are intended to minimize these problems.

INDICATIONS FOR CARDIAC PACING IN CHILDREN

Symptomatic bradycardia not safely or adequately treatable by medical methods is the usual indication for pacemaker implantation. Symptoms may be Stokes-Adams attacks, congestive heart failure, or dizzy spells related to exercise and bradycardia. The bradycardia or asystole may be a result of complete heart block or of sinus node dysfunction. Intermittent or constant complete heart block associated with other congenital heart disease is an indication for pacemaker implantation when the potential for a rhythm-associated death is high, whether or not symptoms are currently present. We implant pacing systems for complete wide QRS atrioventricular block that persists after repair of congenital heart abnormalities, even if the patient is asymptomatic in the hospital setting. Pacemakers may be necessary in children who have the bradycardia-tachycardia syndrome, in some instances to make antitachycardia drug use safer by setting a heart rate floor with the pacemaker, and in a few others also as active, atrial antitachycardia devices.

Usually there is no therapeutic alternative to pacemaker implantation other than continued temporary medical treatment or temporary pacing or both. We have seen postsurgical heart block in children resolve as long as 13 days after operation and have seen severe, symptomatic sinus bradycardia resolve after treatment of anorexia nervosa.

TYPES OF SURGICAL APPROACHES AVAILABLE

For children who are not undergoing a cardiopulmonary bypass operation, we have in the past nearly always utilized a left thoracotomy approach for implanting single-chamber pacemakers and a sternotomy incision for dual-chamber pacers. Now, we discuss with the parents the short- and long-term risks and imponderables of transthoracic and transvenous approaches in general and in the child's particular situation, and in larger children we use the transvenous approach. We have not used the subxiphoid approach.

Transvenous systems are implanted through a subclavian vein using an introducer, a large guidewire, and a series of dilators. In large children, the cephalic vein can be used. The pulse generator is placed posterior to the pectoralis major muscle or in the abdominal wall (see below).

Questions not yet answered regarding transvenous leads in children in the long-term statistical sense are (1) effect of growth spurts on electrode contact and function and on mediastinal anatomy, (2) whether or not the leads can be advanced or removed without opening the chest years later, and (3) whether or not transvenous screw-in electrodes compared with transvenous tined electrodes will be easier to remove years later.

The decision to utilize transthoracic atrioventricular pacing after repair of complex congenital heart disease may result in the growing child over the years having to have multiple intravascular leads or manipulation procedures, with attendant risks. We speculate that one long-term result may be occlusion of subclavian or innominate veins, with loss of these access routes for use in adulthood and old age. On the other hand, implanting epicardial electrodes initially in some circumstances may be more likely to result in early death or in multiple reoperations for high threshold problems, or in use of high output pulse generators.

TECHNIQUES OF MANAGEMENT

Whether one chooses the transthoracic or transvenous approach should depend on (1) size (our smallest child for transvenous pacing weighed 12 kg); (2) whether equally skilled persons accustomed to working with children are available for either approach; (3) the consequences of superior vena caval occlusion (e.g., does the child have an inferior vena cava draining not into the right atrium but into the superior vena cava); (4) whether the right atrioventricular valve is closed, or prosthetic, or a right-to-left shunt is present; (5) whether a transthoracic approach carries more present risk because of congestive heart failure or multiple past transthoracic operations or more future risk because of additional transthoracic congenital heart procedures needed later (epicardial leads make dissection more difficult in future operations); (6) how much caution should be exercised in balancing present thoracotomy risk against the as yet uncertain transvenous lead risks secondary to growth in very small and preadolescent children; (7) other things being equal, whether the balance should go toward transthoracic implantation of the leads because the chest will be open already. If one estimates that on the average a transvenous pacing lead will fail after 15 years of use, one might judge that a child will need at least four lead replacements during his lifetime or more if dual-chamber pacing is used. From the longterm point of view, for this child's anatomy and status, which approach should be used initially and which later?

Dual-chamber pacing is technically possible in patients of all sizes. In small children, we reserve it for those who we believe will be markedly better when atrioventricular synchronization is present. Pulse generators that increase single-chamber pacing rate with activity can be used as a partial substitute.

We usually do not implant permanent electrodes during cardiopulmonary bypass operations because of time constraints and hemostasis considerations, or because the block may be related to edema and be temporary. When we do, the patient has an anatomy problem such as a closed tricuspid valve, or has atrioventricular block, which in very high probability is not temporary (e.g., patients with septation of a single ventricle, multiple ventricular septal defects, or repair of lesions with discordant atrioventricular connection). When permanent leads are put in during a cardiopulmonary bypass operation, the pulse generator is implanted later, near the end of the intensive care unit period. We pace with temporary wires and 2 to 7 days later if complete heart block persists go ahead with pulse generator implantation. When we do go ahead, and epicardial leads have not been previously put in, we may then implant a transvenous system, if long- and short-term risk balance judgment so directs.

Long-term follow-up of serial pacing thresholds has shown an association between electrodes implanted near the end of cardiopulmonary bypass operations and subsequent high threshold syndrome occurrence. We believe this is in part related to use of the Bovie (standard electrocautery device) after the electrode has been implanted and in part to electrode motion and design. The Bovie induces radiofrequency current flow in the pacer lead and, we believe, more than the normal amount of late scar (a microburn) at the electrode site. One can hold a fluorescent lamp tube against the insulated, Bovie probe wire, without electrical contact, and the lamp will light when the Bovie is on. We do not use the Bovie after the pacing electrode is in contact with myocardium, whether or not the lead has been connected to the pulse generator. The bipolar Bovie is only slightly less likely to cause a problem than is the unipolar.

HARDWARE CONSIDERATIONS

Our choices of pulse generators are influenced by these facts:

1. Pacing threshold rises for about 10 days, and then becomes stable in most patients. In some children, threshold continues to rise for 6 to 9 months after implantation and may rise still more after late additional congenital heart procedures.
2. High thresholds are probably more apt to occur in children after cardiopulmonary bypass operations, when pacemaker implantation subtleties may not be fully appreciated in light of the overall situation.
3. Important up and down changes in pacing threshold occur, superimposed on chronic threshold levels. They can be tracked and measured over the telephone when a pulse generator with the pacing voltage threshold Vario test capability has been used. For example, 44 months following Fontan's operation and pacemaker implantation for univentricular heart one child developed a marked rise in pacing threshold with varicella, which later decreased; she might have died if the threshold increase had not been detected and output increased.

We have used the Medtronic 6917A screw in electrodes (-35T in smaller patients and -53T in larger patients) on the ventricles. Chronic thresholds are usually between 1.5 and 3 V, but there have been important exceptions. The Medtronic model 5951 stick-on electrode has usually shown 2- to 3-V chronic thresholds. This electrode has also been employed for atrial pacing; some surgeons have considered its fishhook configuration dangerous in thin-walled, pediatric atria. Medtronic model 5815 spring-coil electrodes have been used with the coil spring carefully bent flat against the baseplate for atrial sensing (excellent), and in some instances for atrial pacing (with low voltage but with relatively high current chronic pacing thresholds). We have also used a porous platinum suture-on electrode from Cordis (model 325–452) when the myocardial surface was bare and not scarred. In 1988, this has become our electrode-of-choice. The incidence of very high threshold occurrences has been higher in all direct myocardial electrodes than in transvenous electrodes but is confounded with cardiopulmonary bypass and Bovie use with the direct operation. Among the transvenous electrodes now available we have been most pleased with the handling characteristics and electrical performance of the Cordis model 327 and 328 series because of the low chronic threshold (0.7 to 1.3 V), the very small diameter, and the ease of maneuvering. We have used a few transvenous screw-in electrodes (Medtronic 6957 and Intermedics 479-01) without problem.

For VVI pacing, the Siemens-Elema 668/688/748 pulse generator series has been our preferred device because of its ability to measure and transmit the pacing voltage threshold (the Vario test)—as contrasted with the much less quantitative "threshold margin test" of other pulse generators—over the telephone. It also has 2.5-, 5-, and 10-V output capability. The Medtronic Activitrax single-chamber pulse generator does not have high output or Vario test capability but is very useful when pacing rate increase with exercise is certain to be the more important factor. The Pacesetter 242-6 and 251-6 pulse generators are extremely small and are useful in very small children. No pulse generator that will automatically adjust its output to just suprathreshold level is available in the United States in 1988.

For dual-chamber pacing we now use the Pacesetter models 283 and 277 and the Intermedics models 283-01 and 271-03. These have extensive multiprogrammable and low and high output capabilities and both small and large programmers. Dual-chamber pulse generators with Vario capability are desirable and are in the testing stage.

TECHNIQUE OF OPERATION

Prophylactic antibiotics are begun prior to the procedure and continued for 48 hours. General anesthesia is necessary except in some older children who are undergoing pulse generator changes. All electrical measuring equipment is assembled, and proper function is confirmed before proceeding. A median sternotomy incision is employed only if it involves reopening a very recent wound or when dual-chamber pacing is elected. Generally we have employed a limited left anterior thoracotomy for lead placement and a separate abdominal incision for the pulse generator. In our experience this has provided excellent exposure, optimum placement of the pulse generator just anterior to the posterior sheath of the rectus muscle in the midabdomen, and very little morbidity. We have made only sparing use of midline incisions for both lead and pulse generator placement. Wound edges are covered with antibiotic damp E-tapes to reduce pacemaker hardware contamination by skin organisms. The pulse generator pouch is made. A pouch posterior to the rectus muscle protects the pulse generator, is cosmetically superior in thin patients, and lowers the risk of wound breakdown in very small subjects. This position does enhance the likelihood of rectus muscle stimulation if bipolar pacing is not employed, and it makes reoperation somewhat more involved. A tunnel between the two wounds is formed. Hemostasis is achieved before electrode placement. The electrode should be kept lint- and powder-free, and stable once it is in the myocardium. Suturing of the electrode pad should assure mechanical stability and produce no ischemia at the electrode. We make large curves in the lead leading away from the electrode to allow for growth, and when possible we stabilize the curves with pericardial fat. Usually we implant one or two spare electrodes for future use. Threshold and electrogram measurements are conducted in a standardized manner. Acute thresholds less than 0.9 V (stimulus duration 0.5 msec) are acceptable. Atrial thresholds tend to be somewhat higher (1.0 to 1.5 V). Ventricular electrograms should usually exceed 6 to 8 mV peak-to-peak amplitude and atrial electrograms should exceed 1.5 to 2 mV for proper sensing, measured between the electrode and the pulse generator pouch. Also, if testing with 5 or 10 V stimuli produces phrenic nerve or direct diaphragm stimulation, the electrode position is unsatisfactory. Electrode placement directly posterior to the sternum should be avoided because electrode baseplate adherence to the sternum has been associated with shearing of the electrode at the myocardium. If present, retrograde conduction is detected and measured by pacing the ventricles while recording the surface ECG and the atrial electrogram (dual-chamber pacemaker loop tachycardia generally can be prevented or managed by pulse generator reprogramming). The leads are tunneled medially or brought over the lowest portion of the costochondral junction in curves to avoid late fracture. The pulse generator is then chosen. It is tested against manufacturer's specifications. The pin ends of the leads are cleansed to remove blood and salt and to minimize shunt current flow and they are mated with the pulse generator, which is then bathed in antibiotic solution and secured in the pouch. Redundant lead is placed posterior to the pulse generator. Unipolar pulse generators are placed in the pouches with the uninsulated side facing away from muscle. The wounds are closed in layers, with particular attention to skin edge blood supply.

Patients are monitored until discharge, and threshold measurements are obtained serially either by transtelephonic Vario test or office visit during the acute phase rise. Families are instructed on the importance of continuing pacemaker and threshold checks, on the need for precautions against infection (following the same American Heart Association guidelines as for prosthetic valves), and on staying away from illegal CB booster amplifiers. Some very active young children are fitted with protective pulse generator shields to prevent direct trauma.

Last, for children at high risk for high thresholds after cardiopulmonary bypass procedures, we now pace at 7 to 10 V at the time of hospital discharge. About 6 months later, the pulse generator is reprogrammed according to the threshold as measured then.

RESULTS

As of April 1, 1987, we had implanted 304 pacing leads in 119 patients less than 20 years old. One hundred and two of these had cardiopulmonary bypass operations for congenital heart disease. Most of these patients had two to four leads implanted during the bypass procedure, some shortly thereafter. Nine screw-in and one stick-on leads were taken out of use because of high thresholds. The mean out-use time was 45 months, the range 7 to 119 months, and the median 37 months. Among the other leads, two broke, one was replaced because of infection, and two were taken out of service because of diaphragm stimulation. Twenty-six children we follow have both a Variothreshold measuring pulse generator and screw-in leads. For these screw-in leads in place more than 1 month, the median threshold is 2.5 V and the mean 3.1 V as determined by the Vario measurements made during telephone checks (mean 7.9 observations per patient). For adults, the similarly measured mean chronic threshold for screw-in leads has been 2.7 V, with a mean of 10.4 observations per patient. A 1985 UAB review of thresholds in 40 children operated on by four surgeons showed ($p < 0.01$) that high threshold occurrence varied by surgeon. Whether the high threshold rate differences were related to lead implantation technique or to case selection was not determined.

The 5-year actuarial survival for 74 children under 10 years of age (all but 10 with complex congenital heart disease), most of whose pacemakers were implanted about the time of cardiopulmonary bypass, has been 75 percent ± 5.4 percent at 33 months and at 5 years (Fig. 1). These data are for the period 1964 to June 1987. For patients (n=48) whose ages at the time of repair and pacemaker implantation were 10 through 19 years, the actuarial survival at 24 months and at 5 years has been 82 percent ± 5.9 percent (Fig. 2). In this institution the 5-year survival rate in paced children under 10 was better before 1980 (see Fig. 1). This may be related in part to the earlier phases of the present shift toward doing more complex repair operations at a younger age.

Since 1973 (i.e., after lithium cells came into use), pulse generator use time in children before replacement

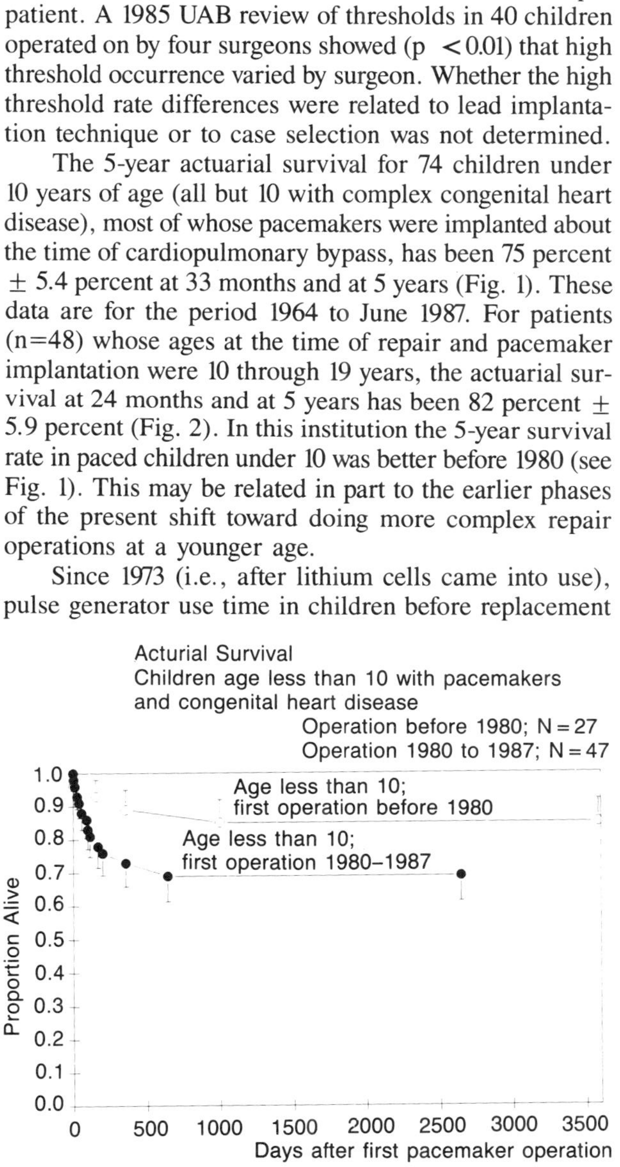

Figure 1 Actuarial survival in children under 10 years of age with pacemakers and congenital heart disease. Operation before 1980, N=27; operation 1980 to 1987, N=47.

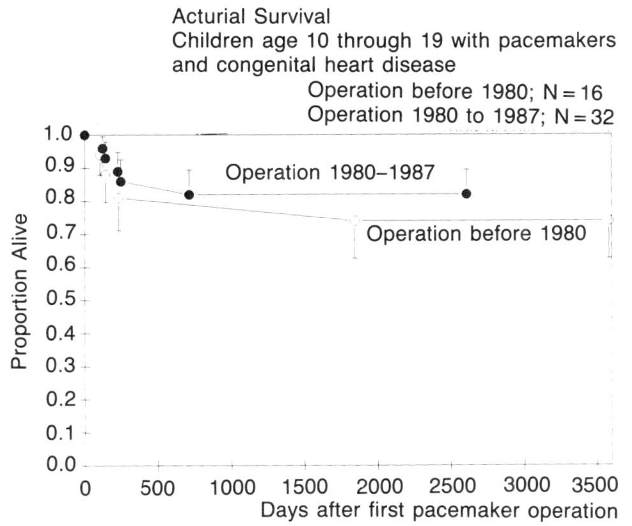

Figure 2 Actuarial survival in children age 10 through 19 with pacemakers and congenital heart disease. Operation before 1980, N=16; operation 1980 to 1987, N=32.

for cell depletion has been from 2 years to 10 years. Pulse generator life expectancy depends on the lead impedance, the pulse generator voltage setting, the pulse rate, the percentage of time pacing, whether two chambers or one are being paced, and on other factors lumped together as statistical chance. In our "worst-case" experiences, when a pulse generator is set at 10 V output and paces at a rate of 90 or 100 all the time into a screw-in lead with 400 ohms impedance, the safe use time is about 2.5 years. For other situations, the pulse generator life expectancy has been 3 to 8 years. For pulse generators removed from children at battery end of life since 1980, the mean use time was 46.6 months and the median time 45.0 months (n=12). For seven pulse generators removed for reasons other than battery replacement, the mean time has been 9.9 months and the median 10.0 months. For 55 pulse generators pacing children currently followed by us, the mean time in use is now 43.1 months, the median 37.7 months, and the maximum still in use time is 123.1 months.

SUGGESTED READING

Gillette PC, Wampler DG, Shannon C, Ott D. Use of cardiac pacing after the Mustard operation for transposition of the great arteries. J Am Coll Cardiol 1986; 7:138–141.

Mugica J, Ripart A. Twelve years' experience with cardiac pacing leads: clinical conclusions for 8,004 cases. Clin Prog Pacing Electro 1984; 2:513–532.

Shepard RB. The use of pacemakers in children. In: Stark J, deLeval M, eds. Surgery for congenital heart disease. London: Grune & Stratton, 1983:111.

INDEX

Note: Page numbers followed by t indicate tables; those followed by f indicate figures.

C

D

F

I

J

K

L

Q

R

S

U

V